PATHOLOGY

A Dynamic Introduction
to Medicine and Surgery

PATHOLOGY

A Dynamic Introduction to Medicine and Surgery

Second Edition

THOMAS MARTIN PEERY, M.D.
Professor and Chairman, Department of Pathology
FRANK NELSON MILLER, JR., M.D.
Professor of Pathology
The George Washington University School of Medicine,
Washington, D.C.

Little, Brown and Company
Boston

Library of Congress catalog card No. 71-146338

Second Edition

Third Printing

ISBN 0-316-69749 (C)
ISBN 0-316-69748 (P)

Printed in the United States of America

PREFACE TO THE SECOND EDITION

PATHOLOGY, well-learned, is a two-way bridge between the basic medical sciences and clinical practice. In one direction, the medical student moving toward his clinical clerkship finds in pathology his first real contact with disease processes and actual cases. In the other direction, the graduate physician seeking to use in his practice the new discoveries of biochemistry, physiology, microbiology, immunology, and genetics finds in clinical pathology the natural access to these sciences.

Three basic aspects of pathology deserve special attention and are emphasized throughout this volume. First, the causes of disease are of particular importance, because knowledge of cause brings hope of prevention and prospect of cure.

Second, a disease is a continuously changing current, not a simple ebb-and-flow tide. No two patients afflicted with the same disease show precisely the same signs, nor is any single patient clinically the same on two succeeding days. The student must learn the sequence in which the clinical alterations tend to appear, the duration of their effects, and the factors which tend to modify their development. With this knowledge he can recognize a disease whether he sees the patient early or late in its course, can foretell its outcome to some degree, and can judge the effects of therapy.

Third, the gross and microscopic alterations that occur in the organs in disease are of great importance. For the student, a knowledge of these changes, viewed in the light of anatomy, biochemistry, and physiology, provides an understanding of the essential nature of a disease and of its complications or sequelae. For the clinician, a knowledge of these changes provides a reasonable explanation of the symptoms and physical signs of the disease, as observed in the living patient. For the pathologist, these tissue changes serve to define the disease and permit its recognition.

Of these three basic aspects of pathology, the most difficult to get across to the student is the concept of continual change; pictures of lesions tend to give the contrary impression. Since this fourth dimension of disease – time – is fundamental and cannot be shown in still pictures, the authors have settled upon a textbook rather than a picture book to present their ideas of pathology.

This book is planned primarily for medical students; for them it should be supplemented with gross and microscopic materials from actual cases and with clinical case histories. The presentation begins with a consideration of the basic concepts of disease, using terms with which the student is familiar from his study of anatomy, biochemistry, physiology, and microbiology. From this beginning the vocabulary and factual data are gradually expanded. Clinical manifestations are correlated with pathologic changes to increase the significance of each. In order to encourage an orderly process of learning, the subject matter of each chapter is organized under sectional topics, and these in turn are developed further under marginal headings. Key words and phrases are printed in italics for emphasis. References have been provided at the ends of chapters so that the student will be encouraged to undertake supplemental reading.

In the decade since the publication of the first edition of this book momentous progress has been achieved in many fields of medicine. The advances in knowledge concerning chromosomal abnormalities, enzyme deficiencies, immunology, tissue transplantation, drug reactions, and viruses have been explosive. The authors have sought to cover these changes, as well as others which have become apparent during the past ten years, in this new edition in a concise, thorough, and, hopefully, exciting manner.

For the second-year medical student, the study of pathology is usually an exciting experience. His earlier courses have dealt with theories and generalities, the significance of which is often obscure. In pathology the teaching comes down to cases. This fact undoubtedly accounts for the sudden awakening of interest that the medical student feels during his course in pathology. He has come to medical school to learn to be a doctor; in pathology he sees for the first time a vision of his goal.

The authors hope that this textbook will help the medical student to see that vision and to attain that goal.

T. M. P.
F. N. M., Jr.

Washington, D.C.

CONTENTS

PATHOLOGY

A Dynamic Introduction
to Medicine and Surgery

1 INTRODUCTION TO PATHOLOGY; CELL DEGENERATION AND NECROSIS

CONCEPTS OF DISEASE

1. Basic Definitions

Disease is any disturbance of the structure or function of the body or its constituent parts, an imbalance between the individual and his environment: a lack of perfect health. *Pathogenesis* means the sequence of events in the development of a disease from its earliest beginnings, including the factors which influence its development. The usual course of a disease from beginning to end, without treatment, is known as the *natural history* of that disease. *Lesions* are the structural alterations in the tissues, recognizable by gross and microscopic examination, which occur with many diseases. Lesions often serve to distinguish one disease from another, as fingerprints identify criminals. These structural alterations, and the functional disturbances which accompany them, result in the *clinical manifestations* of disease: symptoms and physical signs. *Symptoms are subjective* complaints of the patient, as pain in the chest, nausea, or weakness, usually not subject to confirmation by the physician. *Physical signs are objective* findings, such as heart murmur, swelling of the feet, or jaundice, sometimes noted by the patient himself and confirmed by the physician, more commonly first detected by the physician at the time of his examination. In their early stages many diseases have no clinical manifestations, and can be detected only – if at all – by laboratory examination of blood or other body fluids, or by x-ray examination of the lungs or bones. By a careful analysis and interpretation of all the facts in a given case the experienced physician is usually able to reach a *diagnosis,* i.e., a determination of the nature of the disease process and of the organ(s) and tissue(s) affected. A correct and complete diagnosis is essential; otherwise treatment, whether medical or surgical, is haphazard, usually ineffective, and sometimes dangerous. *Prognosis,* the prediction of outcome, is contingent upon accurate diagnosis, and is based upon knowledge of the natural history of a disease and its response to treatment.

Disease: its course and effects

Pathology is the study of disease. More specifically, it is the study of the pathogenesis of disease, and of the structural and functional alterations which result from disease, including the natural history of these changes. In its broadest sense pathology covers the whole realm of biology and has such major subdivisions as human pathology, veterinary pathology, and plant pathology. (Note that pathology is a science, a field of study. Do not make the error of saying,

Pathology

(Warning!)

"There is no evidence of pathology in the lungs." Pathology does not mean abnormality.)

Basic science and clinical specialty

Pathology is unique among the basic sciences of modern medicine in that it is also a clinical specialty. As a basic scientist the pathologist studies the causes and mechanisms of disease and the characteristics of tissue alterations at autopsy, and teaches these essential biologic concepts to his students. As a clinical specialist the pathologist is an important member of the medical care team, bringing the knowledge and techniques of the basic sciences to aid other physicians in the diagnosis and treatment of their patients. Thus the clinical pathologist directs the laboratories – including the chemical, bacteriologic, and histologic laboratories – in which the body fluids and tissues of living patients are examined in order to recognize and identify evidence of disease.

Divisions of human pathology: anatomic pathology

Anatomic pathology is the study of structure (morphology) of cells, organs, and tissues in disease. Its methods include direct (gross) examination of organs, supplemented by microscopic study of tissues stained by various methods to bring out the histochemical changes of disease. Anatomic pathology includes cytology, surgical pathology, and necropsy (autopsy) pathology. *Cytology is the study of cells;* its usual application is the examination of smears prepared from body secretions, especially those of the cervix uteri, bronchi, breast, and prostate, as a screening test for cancer in patients having no clinical evidence of the disease. *Surgical pathology is the study of organs or tissues removed surgically;* if the tissue is removed primarily for the purpose of the examination, the removal and examination together are known as *biopsy. Necropsy pathology is the study of organs and tissues removed from the body post mortem,* to confirm or correct the diagnosis, evaluate the results of treatment, and extend the knowledge of disease. The autopsy is thus the final yardstick, the quality control system of medical practice.

clinical pathology

Clinical pathology has two slightly different meanings, as the term is used. It usually means the application of all types of laboratory techniques to the study of individual living patients; as such, it includes cytology and surgical pathology as well as clinical chemistry, clinical microbiology, hematology, immunohematology (blood bank), and serology. In a more restricted sense, clinical pathology is often used in contrast to anatomic pathology, thus excluding cytology and surgical pathology from the list above.

2. *Normal and Abnormal, Health and Disease*

Individuality

Each of us is different, in some degree, from every other person. Height, weight, coloration of skin and hair, pattern of hair growth on scalp and elsewhere, color of iris, size and shape of forehead, nose, mouth, teeth, and, of course, fingerprints – these and many other characteristics define our individuality. In addition to these obvious differences between individuals, there are also functional, cellular, and biochemical differences. Some of these, such as the blood groups, are well known; others, such as differences in cellular enzyme pattern, are just beginning to be understood.

Normal and abnormal

With such wide variations it is obviously impossible to give a sharp definition to *normal* and *abnormal.* For most parameters of individual variation we usually think in terms of *average* instead of normal. Even this requires further definition. Thus the average height of United States college freshmen has increased significantly in recent generations, and the average height of one ethnic group may be quite different from that of another. Normal thus becomes, for most individual characteristics, a *range of values clustered closely about the average; values outside this range are considered abnormal.* For example, the normal range for fasting blood sugar, measured as true glucose, is 60 to 100 mg. per 100 ml. of blood. We must recognize, however, that this range is only a guide. Someone with a fasting blood glucose of 100 mg. per 100 ml. is not necessarily free of diabetes, nor is one with 101 mg. necessarily diabetic.

Health and disease

Definitions of health and disease are similarly elusive. We have defined disease as any disturbance of the structure or function of the body or any of its constituent parts, or, negatively, as a lack of perfect health. But since disease is sometimes well advanced before abnormality of structure or function is detectable, i.e., before there are symptoms or signs of disease, the concept of absolute health is purely theoretical, subject to the limitations of the examining methods used. On the other hand, disease is sometimes recognized as being present although there may be no disturbance of structure or function in the ordinary sense. Disease of this type may be spoken of as *subclinical disease,* meaning disease recognized by x-ray or laboratory examinations, but not manifest by subjective complaints of the patient and not demonstrable on physical examination by the physician. In contrast, disease which is manifest by complaints or demonstrable on physical examination is sometimes referred to as *clinical disease.*

Health is harmony

Health is a state of harmony between the organism and its environment; in the case of man and other complex forms of life, it also signifies an internal harmony among the individual's own cells, fluids, organs, and tissues. Since the internal and external conditions are constantly changing, and these changes threaten to disrupt the state of harmony, *the organism must be able to adapt to change if it is to remain healthy.* When conditions change beyond the limits of adaptation, a disturbance of normal structure or function results, which we recognize as a state of disease. If harmony subsequently comes about, either spontaneously or as a result of treatment, the state of health is restored. If the imbalance persists, and if the parts affected are not essential for the survival of the whole organism, the disease state may persist indefinitely; under these circumstances, the disease state is said to have become chronic. If the imbalance is severe, or if it disrupts the vital functions of the organism, the individual dies.

Adaptability depends upon stage of development

The capability of the organism to adapt to change depends upon many factors. One is the *stage of development* of the organism at the time the imbalance occurs. An influence that would be overpowering at one stage may be harmless at another. *Prior to conception,* the genetic material in the sex cells in the gonads of each parent is halved in preparation for the union of the chromosomes of sperm and ovum. A harmful influence at this stage, affecting only a single sex cell, may modify the number of chromosomes in the daughter cells, producing gross abnormalities in the resulting individual, if indeed it is able to survive at all. A similar influence acting upon a mature somatic cell may destroy that cell but have no significant effect upon the organism as a whole. *In the embryo* the multipotential cells divide and differentiate into various cell strains under the control of the embryonic organizer. Infection of the mother at this stage by the virus of German measles may affect the embryo and cause defective development of the heart, resulting in serious congenital heart disease, although the virus may have no significant effect upon the tissues of the mother. *In infancy and childhood,* organs and tissues continue to grow under the influence of the pituitary growth hormone and other factors; defective production of this hormone by the pituitary in childhood may result in dwarfing. *In older persons* various cells of the body have accumulated damage as a result of wear and tear and perhaps of mutation [1]; some of these cells may break away from the restraint of specific cell inhibitors and give rise to uncontrolled growth, i.e., cancer.

Adaptability depends upon level of organization

The capability of the organism to adapt to change is also dependent upon whether the imbalance occurs at the cellular level, or at a higher level of organization and function. *At the cellular level* each healthy cell absorbs from the intercellular fluids those substances which it requires; its lysosomal enzymes break down the large molecules to provide usable fuel for the mitochondrial engines. When cell injury occurs, these enzymes may cause lysis of the cell's own nuclear chromatin and cytoplasmic organelles, resulting in cell death. This lytic cellular process is perfectly normal and necessary at certain stages of development of multicellular organisms – for example, it accounts for the disappearance of certain embryonic organs [2]. This process is also commonplace in the adult in epidermis, intestinal epithelium, and blood cells, where new cells are continually formed to take the place of lysed ones. The organism adapts readily to this level of disease without any evidence of disturbance in the whole organism. *At the level of individual organs and parts of the body,* needs are normally supplied by the circulation of blood and lymph, and specific organ functions such as respiration, digestion, and elimination are carried out under the regulation of hormones and the autonomic nervous system. Blockage of the blood flow locally, as by a thrombus in the popliteal artery, may result in death of the cells of the skin and connective tissues of the foot, and a concomitant impairment of function of the whole part, i.e., the leg. *At the level of the body as a whole* there is, in health, a *subconscious coordination* of the activities of all component parts through the autonomic nervous system, and a *conscious, purposeful adaptation* in response to internal and external stimuli such as hunger, thirst, fatigue, discomfort, ambition, and fear. Disease at this level may be due to aging, or to such circumstances as atomic radiation, anoxia, or starvation, and may result in widespread cell death throughout the organism or in destruction of the higher centers of control.

Disease is failure of adaptation

Disease is thus seen as a failure of adaptation of the organism to change, resulting in biochemical, functional, or structural alterations in the organism. Manifestations of disease, i.e., symptoms and physical signs, are usually a result of these functional or structural changes.

3. Causes of Disease

Etiology

Etiology is the study of causes. It is not a synonym for cause, although the word is often used erroneously in this way. Every disease has more than one cause, just as every automobile accident and every war does. It is important to know causes: without knowledge of cause, prevention is, of course, difficult. The *immediate* or *inciting cause* is the trigger factor which initiates the disease, as *Diplococcus pneumoniae* in the case of pneumonia, or the blow on the head in the case of skull fracture. The immediate cause is not known (or there may be no immediate cause) for many of the chronic diseases which are the great killers, such as cancer, coronary thrombosis, and diabetes mellitus. *Precipitating causes* are those conditioning factors which permit the immediate cause to act, as wetting and chilling of the body in the case of pneumonia, or the automobile accident which resulted in the blow on the head. *Predisposing causes* are those general circumstances which pave the way for the immediate cause to act, as acute alcoholism in some cases of pneumonia and automobile accidents; other predisposing causes may be malnutrition, chronic disease, genetic defects, inability to manufacture protective antibodies, or old age.

It should be noted that the mere presence of an inciting agent does not prove that the disease commonly associated with that agent is also present. Thus *D. pneumoniae* may be present in the sputum without the patient having pneumonia, and every blow on the head is not associated with skull fracture.

4. Types of Disease

In the unicellular organism, disease usually results from such easily understood disturbances as starvation, poisoning, physical injury, or freezing. In a multicellular organism such as man, these same harmful influences cause disease, but the process is much more complex because of the dependence of one cell upon another, and because of the role of the intercellular fluids and supporting tissues.

Inherited or *familial* diseases, such as hemophilia, are due to faults which are inherent in the chromosomes of one or both parents and are transmitted to the offspring.

Congenital diseases are those present at birth. Some are inherited; some are developmental defects of unknown cause; others, like congenital syphilis, are infections acquired in utero.

Toxic diseases are due to various poisons, such as snake venom or methanol, which cause cell degeneration or cell death. The outcome depends upon the reversibility of the process, and the importance of the injured cells to the body as a whole.

Infectious diseases are due to invasion of the body by living pathogenic agents, usually bacteria (tuberculosis, diphtheria) or viruses (poliomyelitis), but sometimes fungi (thrush), protozoa (amebiasis), or helminths (ascariasis). Many infectious diseases are also *contagious,* i.e., capable of being spread from one person to another.

Traumatic diseases, such as fractures, sprains, and wounds, are due to direct physical injury. Closely allied are diseases due to physical agents, such as heat, cold, electricity, and irradiation.

Degenerative diseases, while undoubtedly having more specific chemical causes than we realize, are generally considered to be the result of aging or wear and tear. Included are some of the most common diseases of the elderly, such as stroke, arteriosclerosis, and osteoarthritis.

Allergic diseases result from unusual sensitivity to some exciting agent (antigen) such as drugs (penicillin reaction) or pollens (hay fever). People who are allergic or hypersensitive react in a violent or unusual manner to substances which produce little or no reaction in others.

Auto-immune diseases are somewhat similar to allergic diseases, but in this group the patient becomes sensitized to some product of his own cells or tissues. Rheumatic fever and one type of thyroid disease are thought to belong to this poorly understood group.

Neoplastic diseases (cancers of various organs, as breast or bone) are those in which certain cells become "outlaw" cells, multiplying rapidly and invading and destroying surrounding tissues and cells, and often spreading to distant organs.

Nutritional diseases usually result from a dietary intake deficient in total amount (starvation) or in some essential ingredient (vitamin C deficiency is scurvy), or from an excessive food intake (obesity). Occasionally a nutritional disease may be a result of an abnormality of the digestive tract, leading to malabsorption.

Metabolic diseases are those in which certain physiologic processes become deranged. Included are most of the dysfunctions of the endocrine system (diabetes mellitus, hyperthyroidism).

Molecular diseases are metabolic diseases in which the molecular products of cellular activity are abnormal in composition. Included are certain hereditary diseases such as phenylketonuria and sickle cell anemia.

Psychosomatic diseases have their beginnings in the emotions and are mediated largely through the autonomic nervous system. Thus duodenal ulcer in some people seems to be a result of malfunction of the autonomic nervous system due to fear or frustration, accompanied by an oversecretion of acid gastric juice.

A *factitious* disease is one produced artificially. Thus convulsions may be due to hypoglycemia produced when an emotionally disturbed patient surreptitiously gives himself an overdose of insulin.

An *iatrogenic* disease is one arising from the actions or words of the doctor. Drugs used in the treatment of disease may themselves produce disease. Bad effects of surgery, skin cancer following x-ray therapy, or "cardiac neurosis" following careless or misunderstood statements by the physician, are examples.

Many diseases overlap several of these categories, and many patients have more than one category of disease at a time. For many other diseases, including some of the most common, such as hypertension and rheumatoid arthritis, the true nature of the disease is uncertain or even completely unknown.

5. *Incidence of Disease*

Morbidity

Certain diseases are encountered infrequently or not at all in death statistics but nevertheless cause a great deal of sickness, absence from work, and economic loss, i.e., *morbidity.* On the basis of interviews conducted by the National Health Survey [3], it has been estimated that the civilian, noninstitutional population of the United States experiences more than 3 billion man-days per year of restricted activity due to illness or injury, equivalent to 16 days for each man, woman, and child. Included are more than a billion man-days of confinement to bed, plus 385 million days lost from work, and 200 million days lost from school. Acute illness accounts for more than half of this total record of disability, corresponding to more than 380 million separate illnesses. More than 200 million of these acute illnesses are respiratory infections, including the common cold; 55 million are nonrespiratory infections, including childhood diseases; about the same number are injuries from accidents; and 20 million are digestive illnesses. While acute illnesses account for more than half the days lost from work or school as reported in this study, chronic diseases have an even greater social significance. Chronic diseases more commonly affect family breadwinners rather than children, and the economic dislocation is great in affected families. Chronic diseases, especially neurologic and mental diseases, arthritis, and cancer, account for far more patient days in hospital than do the acute diseases. The number of patients affected is large and the duration of the confinement per patient is generally long.

Mortality [4]

The *crude death rate* or *mortality rate,* defined as the ratio of total deaths in a given year to the total population in that year, remained relatively constant in the United States over the decade 1955 to 1964, after having fallen gradually in earlier years. There are about 1,800,000 deaths each year giving a death rate of 940 per 100,000 estimated population. The *infant mortality rate,* often used as a measure of the quality and availability of medical care, has also fallen more slowly in the last decade; now there are 100,000 infant deaths (under 1 year), a rate of 24.8 per 1000 live births. The *expectation of life at birth* is 66.9 years for males and 73.7 years for females, these being approximately the same values that applied for several previous years. In each category these rates reflect the fact that no great new life-saving medical discoveries were applied during that decade. Previous improvements had been due to the better control of infectious diseases as a result of improved sanitary methods and the use of antibiotics, and improved surgical and obstetrical results related to asepsis, anesthesia, and blood transfusions. But the *great killers of today* – heart disease, cancer, and stroke – have yielded hardly at all to the research efforts of recent years. Certain discoveries give promise of greatly reducing mortality from these diseases, however; it is highly probable that the elimination of cigarette smoking and the reduction of the fat content of the diet could greatly reduce these hazards to life and health.

Major causes of death [4]

Most of the major *causes of death are age-related,* and hence the death rates, and the causes of death, show striking variations in relation to age. The death rate during the first 28 days after birth is many times higher than for any other equal period of life; this is a result of the hazards peculiar to intra-uterine existence and to birth, plus the effects of lethal congenital malformations. The decade 5 to 14 has the lowest mortality rate of any 10-year age period, and accidents account for almost half the deaths in this decade. *Deaths from accidents* reach their peak in the decade 15 to 24 years, and are largely motor vehicle accidents. *Diseases of the heart and blood vessels,* generally considered to be degenerative diseases resulting from the aging of tissues, together account for almost exactly half the total deaths in the United States and take an increasing toll with each decade of life. Heart disease in particular has a rapidly rising slope; the death rate from heart disease increases by a factor of nearly four for each decade from 5 to 14 through 55 to 64, thereafter rising more slowly.

Population control

It should be noted that disease and death are universal biologic processes. They provide a built-in population control specific for each species. If all major human diseases were eradicated and everyone lived to be as old as the biblical Methuselah, some artificial and perhaps less friendly means of population control would probably have to be invented. Think of the crowding, the unemployables, the food shortages – and the strain on the Social Security system!

6. *Manifestations of Disease*

A disease becomes clinically manifest when it causes structural or functional changes which can be recognized as abnormal, i.e., when it produces symptoms or signs. Many chronic internal diseases, such as arteriosclerosis and cirrhosis of the liver, are far advanced when they first become manifest. A few of the more important disease manifestations (symptoms and signs) are listed in Table 1-1, together with certain mechanisms by which they may be produced, and some of the diseases with which they may be associated.

TABLE 1-1. Some Important Disease Manifestations and Some of Their Associated Mechanisms and Diseases

Manifestation	Mechanism	Diseases
Cyanosis	Anoxia	Drowning Morphine poisoning Heart disease
Swelling, pain	Inflammation	Sunburn Bacterial infection Hay fever
Jaundice	Blockage of common bile duct	Stone in common bile duct Cancer of duodenal papilla Stricture of bile duct
Headache	Increased intracranial pressure	Hemorrhage Brain tumor Meningitis
Vomiting	Intestinal obstruction	Strangulated hernia Cancer of colon Peritoneal adhesions

Differential diagnosis

The diagnostician must differentiate between the various diseases which may cause the symptoms and signs manifest in his patient, so that his treatment will be properly directed. He does this by carefully tracing the course of events in the *history of the present illness;* by considering factors in the *past history, family history, occupation, environment, habits,* and *diet;* by noting all abnormalities on the *physical examination;* by obtaining the necessary *clinical pathology tests, radiographic examinations,* and *special studies* such as electrocardiogram or consultation. These together constitute the clinician's resources for differential diagnosis.

THE SIMPLEST FORMS OF DISEASE

1. Introduction: Cell Structure and Function

Concepts of cell structure and cell function have been greatly modified in recent years as a result of research studies in electron microscopy [5] and cell chemistry. While some of these new concepts are still conjectural, many are well established. It is necessary to review these advances in order to understand the nature and significance of cell injury.

Cell differences

Of course, there is really no such thing as a typical cell, as Brachet [6] and others have pointed out, any more than there is a typical human being or a typical atom. Each cell strain – as cartilage or squamous epithelium – is different from all other cell strains, even at a very early stage of its development, and each strain has its specific morphologic and biochemical characteristics. Cells of the same strain differ from each other according to age, nutritional status, stage of functional cycle, and environmental influences. Most cells, nevertheless, have certain characteristics in common.

Cell structures: cell membrane

The *cell membrane* is a wall, retaining the cell contents and isolating the cell from its environment; at the same time it is an actively functioning structure, capable of selectively passing one ion while retaining another of similar size and electric charge. The cell membrane also permits larger particles and molecules to enter the cell by wrapping a bit of membrane about the particle and ingesting it *(pinocytosis)*.

cytoplasmic "organelles"

The *cell cytoplasm* is not a simple gel, as we used to think, but a highly organized, complicated chemical factory. Everywhere it is interlaced by a spongelike system of internal membranes and canaliculi – the *endoplasmic reticulum* – which provides a mazelike communication between the external membrane of the cell and the nuclear membrane, permitting certain substances to enter or leave the cytoplasm and perhaps even the nucleus itself. These internal membranes are lined with granules *(ribosomes)* which are thought to synthesize enzymes and perhaps other cell proteins. The *Golgi apparatus* is apparently continuous with the endoplasmic reticulum, and is thought to provide pockets for the storage of synthesized protein. Energy for the cell factory is provided by the *mitochondria* (sing., mitochondrion), which are cucumber-shaped structures having a well-defined internal organization. The mitochondria extract energy from the chemical bonds of cell nutrients by the process of oxidation, and make this energy available in the phosphate bonds of adenosine triphosphate, for various cellular functions.

Lysosomes [7, 8] are specialized cytoplasmic structures or "bags" containing enzymes capable of breaking down the large molecules of most forms of living matter; the smaller molecules can then be oxidized by the mitochondrial enzymes. Although lysosomes cannot always be identified from other cytoplasmic granules in electron micrographs, they can be spotted by cytochemical methods that identify the hydrolytic enzymes and other substances they contain – nucleases, phosphatases, cathepsins, glycosides, and others. The lysosomal membrane isolates these enzymes from the rest of the cell cytoplasm. Polymorphonuclear leukocytes and macrophages are especially rich in lysosomes – the granules of the neutrophilic granulocyte are lysosomes – thus endowing these cells with special functions such as phagocytosis of bacteria and autolysis of cellular debris. Lysosomes are thought to participate in many vital functions, including penetration of ovum by sperm, resorption of outmoded embryonic organs, osteoclastic destruction of bone, and the continuing lysis and renewal of other cytoplasmic structures. (The cytoplasmic structures called lysosomes must not be confused with the lytic enzyme known as lysozyme which may be contained within the lysosome.)

Centrosomes are tiny structures that apparently function only to provide the poles of the mitotic spindle; between times of cell mitosis, these "cell muscles" apparently rest.

nucleus

The cell nucleus is enveloped in a double-layered *nuclear membrane,* the outer layer of which apparently has holes which communicate with the cytoplasm and permit movement of molecules in either direction. The nucleus contains all the cell *chromatin,* or *genetic material.* Deoxyribonucleic acid *(DNA)* is localized in the nuclear chromatin; between times of cell division it "presides" over the synthesis of ribonucleic acid *(RNA)* in both nucleus and cytoplasm. The RNA, in turn, arranges the various amino acids in proper relationship for the synthesis of the specific types of protein required by the particular cell. In anticipation of cell division, the chromatin filament breaks up into *chromosomes,* always the same number for all cell strains of a given species (except that the sex cells, in anticipation of conception, contain half as many chromosomes as the other cell strains of a given species). When cell division occurs, each chromosome is divided between the two daughter cells. The DNA of the nuclear chromatin brings the genetic information to both daughter cells, so that, at an appropriate time, the postmitotic cells will have the same special characteristics and capabilities as the parent cell with regard to morphology, protein synthesis, and cellular function. The *nucleolus* is a closely packed area within the nucleus consisting of granules of RNA, without a well-defined nucleolar membrane. The nucleoli apparently are centers for protein synthesis. The *nuclear sap* is the protein-rich material bathing the chromatin filaments and the nucleoli, and contained within the nuclear membrane.

Cell reproduction

Some cell strains (skin epithelium, bone marrow, intestinal epithelium) continue to reproduce throughout the life of the organism; others (cardiac muscle, neurones) do not divide once the organism has attained its full growth. Still other cell strains (fibrous connective tissue, bone, liver cells) tend to remain static but may be stimulated to reproduce under certain circumstances. All living cells, however, are in a *perpetual state of internal change,* using externally derived nutrient materials to rebuild elements of internal structure. Except for the germ cells, all cells of each tissue strain develop along one of two mutually exclusive pathways, the intermitotic or the postmitotic. Under ordinary circumstances the *intermitotic cells never mature and never die;* they are destined only to divide. *Postmitotic cells,* on the other hand, *never reproduce;* they mature, carrying out the specific function which characterizes the cell strain, age, and, in some instances, die.

Regulation of cell division

Obviously some strain-specific mechanism is required to control cell division. Apparently this is accomplished by *a chemical feedback of type-specific inhibitors of cell division,* released into the circulation [9]. Thus, as an organ or tissue gains mass, its cells increase their output of inhibiting substance until eventually growth of the organ or tissue is suppressed. Removal of a part of the cell mass reduces the quantity of circulating inhibitors and permits renewed cell division until cell mass is restored. Thus, after surgical removal of a portion of the liver, there is renewed division of the hepatic and Kupffer cells and of the cells of the bile ducts, until equilibrium is again reached. The wild, uninhibited cell growth which we call cancer is undoubtedly due to some defect in this mechanism of control.

2. *Cell Injury*

Causes and effects

This fine, well-ordered balance of structure and function, within the cell and between cells, can be disturbed by a variety of influences. Anoxia, dehydration, excess heat or cold, starvation, chemical poisoning, physical trauma, bacterial agents – any of these may cause cell injury. If the injury is mild and brief and the cell is otherwise healthy, the sick cell will adapt and survive. If the injury is severe or prolonged, or if the cell was already defective in some way, the sick cell will die. Thus, even at the cellular level, disease is an imbalance between the individual and its environment, a failure of homeostasis. At first the *reaction* to injury is apt to be *biochemical,* a modification of substrate; later it is *functional,* perhaps due to reduction in output of a normal cellular product or alteration of a metabolic pathway. *Structural* alterations in nucleus and cytoplasm usually follow.

Variability of response

Cells having different functions may be affected differently by injurious agents. Thus liver cells may be seriously affected by carbon tetrachloride as a result of accidental poisoning, but the intestinal epithelium, exposed to much higher concentrations of the agent, may be relatively unaffected. Intermitotic cells usually show nuclear alterations and cessation of mitosis as their earliest evidence of injury, while postmitotic cells react first by failing to carry out such usual functions as synthesis of enzymes and transport of water across cell membranes.

General nature of reaction

The effects of *cytotoxic agents* have been studied most extensively in the case of liver cells, but identical changes have been observed in other cell strains, both in vivo and in vitro. Carbon tetrachloride, phosphorus, dimethylnitrosamine, thioacetamide, ethionine, and beryllium are some of the substances that have been used experimentally. Similar results have been observed after simple cell anoxia. It seems likely that the first effect upon cells is an interaction between the specific toxic molecules (in the case of cytotoxic agents) and some specific cellular component, resulting in a *"biochemical lesion"* specific for the particular toxic agent and the particular cell type; however, this has not been proved. Following this initial and specific injury there is *impairment of some cell function,* such as protein synthesis or perhaps the mechanism for transport of molecules across cell membranes. These functional changes are probably not specific for the different toxic agents. Similarly, the *structural changes* that can be observed are identical, no matter what has caused the cellular injury [10].

Spectrum of structural alterations, cell injury to cell death: postmitotic cells

With the light microscope, the earliest evident morphologic change seen in postmitotic cells after a low dose of a cytotoxic agent is an *overall enlargement of the cell* and an *increased granularity of the cytoplasm.* Electron microscopy at this stage reveals [11] *alterations in the endoplasmic reticulum and ribosomes,* thought to signify impairment of protein synthesis, and *swelling of the mitochondria* from increased water content. Somewhat later (16 to 24 hours after minimal injury), *lipid droplets accumulate in the endoplastic reticulum.* Apparently this lipid is predominantly triglyceride; its accumulation is thought to be a result of the inability of the injured cell to manufacture the protein moiety of lipoprotein at a rate equivalent to the normal cellular intake of triglyceride, hence the latter accumulates [12]. Still later, some of the *mitochondria may disintegrate* and *be engulfed by the lysosomes,* forming *dense abnormal cytoplasmic inclusions.* Along with and following these cytoplasmic changes, *nuclear changes* may become evident. The earliest nuclear change is a shriveling and condensation of nuclear chromatin, a process known as *pyknosis.* Later there is fragmentation *(karyorrhexis)* and disappearance *(karyolysis)* of the nucleus as a whole, apparently a result of the release of hydrolases from the lysosomes into the cytoplasm, whence they can attack the nuclear membrane. Finally the cell membrane ruptures, the liquid content of the cell becomes mixed with the intercellular fluid, and the particulate matter of the cell membranes is engulfed by circulating phagocytes and lysed by their lysosomal enzymes.

intermitotic cells

The changes outlined are seen characteristically in postmitotic cells. In intermitotic cells, as exemplified by certain experimental cell strains derived from malignant neoplasms, the first change noted following injury is in the nucleus [13]; DNA is lost and mitosis abruptly ceases. Thereafter the cell is apparently unable to carry out its normal activities, such as synthesis of enzymes, production of energy, repair of structural deficiencies, and maintenance of ionic environment, and as a consequence changes occur in the cytoplasm. Potassium is lost from the cell, and sodium and water are taken up, resulting in swelling of the cell as a whole. Finally the cell bursts and the fragments of cell structure shrivel up and coagulate.

When is a cell dead?

It is customary to speak of these changes as being reversible up to a certain point, and irreversible, i.e., leading inevitably to cell death, if they continue beyond that point. It would probably be more accurate to refer to these changes simply as nonlethal or lethal, since it is very likely that injured cells do not fully recover but carry the effects of prior injury throughout their life span: the *aging of cells is probably the result of the accumulation of nonlethal cell injuries.* Polymorphonuclear leukocytes, after they have matured and entered the circulation, show many of the changes noted above, particularly loss of mitochondria and endoplasmic reticulum and the appearance of cytoplasmic dense bodies. Mitochondrial swelling and even disruption do not necessarily mean that cell death is inevitable. Cells may also recover after a certain amount of lipid has accumulated in the cytoplasm. After extensive disruption of cytoplasmic organelles has occurred, and especially after changes have come about in the nuclear chromatin, it is generally held that cell death is inevitable, although certain cellular functions may persist for some time, perhaps carried on at a different pace. As Brachet [6] has pointed out, "Life in the case of the cell and its constituents, is more a quantitative than an all-or-none concept." Even after the removal of the nucleus, unicellular organisms may continue certain activities that are generally thought to signify life: cilia may continue to beat, specific enzymes may still be synthesized and limited cytoplasmic regeneration may still occur. This might have been anticipated, since it is well known that, under favorable circumstances in multicellular organisms, the cells of certain relatively inert tissues may remain "alive" for many days after heartbeat and respiration have ceased. This fact is the basis for the numerous tissue banks – cornea, cartilage, bone, blood cells – and for the recent success of whole-organ transplants, in which tissue or organs from the bodies of suitable, recently dead individuals are used to replace tissues or organs damaged by disease or injury. Human erythrocytes are known to carry out vital functions for some 120 days after disappearance of their nuclei.

Effects of cell death

Even in those instances where cell death occurs, the effect on the body as a whole may be negligible. In the case of tissues capable of regeneration, dead cells may be replaced by new cells; in the case of other cells, they may be lost from the organ mass without impairment of organ function. It is likely that the reduction in size of organs that occurs with old age is the result of the elimination of dead cells in this way.

3. *Cloudy Swelling*

Gross changes

When the cells of an organ are affected *diffusely* by an adverse circumstance, as by bacterial toxins in the case of bacterial infections or by inadequate oxygen supply in the case of severe anemia, the affected organs are increased in size and weight by perhaps one-third, and the tissues lose their normal glistening translucency and resemble parboiled meat. *Cloudy swelling* is the name ordinarily used to designate these changes; synonyms are *parenchymatous degeneration, albuminous degeneration, hydropic degeneration,* and *vacuolar degeneration.*

Micro-scopic picture

Chiefly affected are certain *highly specialized cells:* the epithelial cells of the convoluted tubules of the kidney, the cells of the hepatic cords, the leukocytes of the circulating blood, myocardial fibrils. Affected cells are swollen due to water imbibition, and fine granules and vacuoles can be noted in the cytoplasm with the ordinary light microscope. Nuclei are usually not affected. (These changes are, of course, the same as those described in the preceding section as occurring in single cells as a result of minimal injury.)

Functional effects

Functional manifestations of these cell alterations are usually *minimal;* the transient mild proteinuria and hypotension common during febrile illnesses may reflect these changes as they occur in the kidney tubules and myocardial cells, respectively. If the patient recovers from the underlying condition, the toxic changes in the parenchymatous cells usually disappear and their functional expression also disappears. The end result to the patient depends upon the seriousness of the primary underlying infection or other cause, and its response to treatment.

4. *Fatty Change*

Use of terms

Fatty change or *fatty metamorphosis,* also known as *fatty degeneration* and *fatty infiltration,* must be distinguished from the normal deposition of neutral fat that occurs in obese persons in subcutaneous connective tissues, omentum, mesentery, breasts, and buttocks. In these latter instances, *normal fat cells* in great excess are noted in these sites. This is *fatty deposition,* a different matter from fatty metamorphosis in which fat vacuoles appear in the cytoplasm of functional cells of parenchymatous organs, especially the liver cords, renal convoluted tubules, and myocardial cells.

Types of fatty liver

There are still grounds for confusion, however, since fat vacuoles, at least in liver cells, may occur under *either physiologic or pathologic conditions,* and there may be little microscopic difference between the two. The so-called *physiologic type* of fatty liver may occur *after a fatty meal,* or, as noted by Rees [14], as a result of unusual requirements, such as in *starvation.* In the latter, fat is mobilized from the fat depots and deposited in the liver cells; the amount of fat is relatively small, liver function is not affected, and the proportion of the several fatty components in the cell is not altered. The *pathologic type* of fatty liver may occur as a result of *poisoning* by hepatotoxic agents such as chloroform or phosphorus, from *nutritional causes* such as protein or choline deficiency, *following severe infections* such as diphtheria, in *prolonged anemia,* and in *toxemia of pregnancy.* In the pathologic type of fatty liver, huge amounts of fat may be present in the liver, liver function may be greatly impaired, and the composition of the fat is abnormal. It appears that *the basic defect in the pathologic type of fatty liver is a reduction in the capability of the liver cells to synthesize the protein moiety of the lipoprotein;* as a consequence, the lipid moiety accumulates in the liver cells, there is a failure to deliver lipoprotein to the circulation, and plasma lipoprotein falls.

Causes of fatty change

With certain exceptions as noted above in the case of the liver, *fatty metamorphosis is a pathologic process, usually resulting from prolonged cell injury.* Not all parenchymatous organs are equally affected in a given case, probably because the causative circumstance "poisons" the enzyme system of certain cell strains but does not affect the different enzyme systems of other strains. Thus phosphorus poisoning, choline deficiency, and toxemia of pregnancy cause fatty change in the liver; diphtheria toxins and anoxia from severe prolonged anemia usually cause fatty degeneration of the myocardium; and an unknown metabolic disturbance associated with diabetes mellitus often causes fatty degeneration of the epithelium of the convoluted tubules of the kidney.

Gross appearance: liver

When the *liver* is affected by severe fatty change, as in a patient with severe and prolonged alcoholism whose diet is inadequate and unbalanced, the organ is often palpably *enlarged,* and at autopsy may weigh 2500 to 5000 gm. instead of the normal weight of about 1800 gm. The *edges are rounded* as a result of the enlargement, and the *cut surface is yellow and greasy.* Some degree of fibrous scarring (cirrhosis) is also commonly noted in such cases. Usually the degree of dysfunction is relatively mild, but occasionally there may be total hepatic failure, with jaundice, coma, increased serum ammonia level, and portal hypertension.

kidney

Fatty metamorphosis of the *kidney* is rarely so advanced that it produces any functional effect, such as proteinuria or uremia. Both kidneys are somewhat *enlarged* and *pale,* but their gross appearance is not particularly characteristic.

heart

Fatty change in the *heart* results in a rather characteristic gross alteration. The heart is *soft* and *flabby* but ordinarily not increased in weight. The changes affect chiefly those muscle fibers which lie just beneath the endocardium of either the right or left ventricle. The condition can be recognized grossly by a *speckled yellow appearance,* or sometimes by *alternate bars of yellow and brown in the papillary muscles* as seen from the endocardial surface ("thrush breast" or "tabby cat" appearance). No distinctive functional effect is recognized from the myocardial changes.

Microscopic picture

Microscopically *droplets of lipid material are deposited in the cytoplasm of affected cells:* liver cells, heart muscle cells, epithelial cells of the kidney tubules. Most of the lipid is in the form of triglyceride. Earliest stages show it finely dispersed in the cytoplasm, apparently within the lumen of the endoplasmic reticulum. In more advanced cases, especially in the liver, these tiny droplets may coalesce to form large collections of lipid (giant liposome) which may displace the cell nucleus. In *routine paraffin sections,* from which fat is removed by the usual processing solvents, these small or large droplets are seen as empty spaces or vacuoles. When the nucleus is displaced by fat, the empty space appears to compress the nucleus and gives the cell a signet-ring appearance. In severe cases these vacuoles will obscure the normal structure and make the liver difficult to identify. In *frozen sections* the fat can be demonstrated positively with fat-soluble dyes such as Sudan III or Scarlach R. Using other histologic techniques, fat can be demonstrated by virtue of its molecular union with osmic acid or Nile blue sulfate.

Other disorders of lipids

Other conditions affecting body lipids, but different from fatty metamorphosis of parenchymatous organs, are: (1) the *lipoid storage diseases,* genetically transmitted enzymatic defects in which various lipoid substances are deposited in the *reticuloendothelial cells;* (2) *Wallerian degeneration,* an alteration in the lipid-containing *myelin sheath* of injured nerve fibers; (3) *fat necrosis,* a change in *adipose tissues* as a result of trauma or action of lipase; (4) *lipoid deposits* (cholesterol and cholesterol esters), commonly noted in the *subintimal layer of arteries* in atherosclerosis of later life; (5) *intestinal lipodystrophy,* in which fat is deposited in the *intestinal mucosa* as a result of a defect in fat absorption or transport; (6) unusual conditions in which fats or oils reach the pulmonary alveoli, presumably by inhalation, to give *lipoid pneumonia,* or are deposited in cells lining the sinuses of spleen or lymph nodes *(lipoid granuloma).*

5. Necrosis

Definition

Necrosis means the death of a group of cells as a result of injurious influences, while the cells are still in contact with the living body. This definition attempts to distinguish necrosis from *somatic death,* i.e., death of the body as a whole, and from *necrobiosis,* the more or less normal process by which, in certain tissues, individual cells die and are replaced by new cells.

Causes

Any harmful influence capable of causing injury of single cells, as described earlier, may, by acting longer or with greater intensity, cause the death of a group of cells, i.e., necrosis. Usual causes include *anoxia* (as by blockage of arterial supply), *physical agents* (trauma, heat, cold, radiant energy), *chemical agents* (solvents, acids, hygroscopic substances), and *biologic agents* (pathogenic bacteria, viruses, fungi, protozoa).

Types:

When a group of cells becomes necrotic, certain gross differences between the living and dead tissues can be noted with the naked eye. These vary with the tissue affected and to some extent with the nature of the insult causing cell death; the variations are usually considered different types of necrosis.

coagulation necrosis

Coagulation necrosis occurs characteristically in the *lung, kidney,* and *spleen,* as a result of the sudden, complete blockage of a branch of the arterial tree. As a consequence there is anoxia of that part of the affected organ, the affected cells of the organ die, cytoplasmic and intercellular fluids coagulate, and fibrin forms in the interstices between the dead cells. The area affected becomes firm and rubbery. Microscopically, faint outlines of tissue structure can often be recognized in the area of necrosis; dead cells show nuclear alterations as previously described; a zone of cellular reaction separates normal and necrotic tissues (see Infarction in Chapter 2).

liquefaction necrosis

Liquefaction necrosis occurs characteristically in the *brain* or *spinal cord* as a result of the sudden, complete blockage of an arterial branch; although the precise cause of the liquefaction or lysis of tissue is not known, it is presumably due to some characteristic inherent in the chemistry of the central nervous system. Liquefaction necrosis also occurs in *abscesses* in any organ or tissue, as a result of the invasion of the tissues by pyogenic bacteria and the consequent outpouring of leukocytes. From these leukocytes, lytic enzymes are released into the tissues, the mass of dead cells is liquefied, and a cavity filled with fluid and phagocytic cells develops.

caseation necrosis

Caseation necrosis occurs characteristically as a result of infection by *Mycobacterium tuberculosis,* no matter what tissue is affected. The lipid content of the capsule of the organism apparently accounts for the peculiar change. The affected tissues are somewhat coagulated and converted to yellow, cheesy, crumbly material. Microscopically the underlying tissue is often unrecognizable, and is replaced by granular eosinophilic material, often with a fine sprinkling of basophilic calcium granules.

fibrinoid necrosis

Fibrinoid necrosis, sometimes called fibrinoid degeneration, occurs characteristically in the *walls of small arteries* and in *fibrous connective tissues* generally, sometimes as a result of local interaction between antigen and antibody (autoimmune disease). The fibrillar structure which normally gives a layered pattern to the tissue is lost focally and replaced by a granular smudgy material which stains intensely with eosin. The new material, probably a modified tissue protein, gives histochemical reactions similar to those seen with fibrin in ordinary thrombi.

fat necrosis

Fat necrosis occurs in *adipose tissue* and may be a result of trauma, bacterial invasion, or chemical injury. As a result of enzyme action, there is hydrolysis of fat, and white chalky deposits of calcium soaps are formed in the tissues. In the omentum and mesentery, fat necrosis usually means chemical injury due to the escape of pancreatic lipase into the peritoneal cavity as a result of pancreatic disease. Microscopically the fat no longer appears as vacuoles but as globular masses of homogeneous material surrounded by inflamed tissue.

Dystrophic calcification

In areas of fat necrosis, and in other sites of old tissue degeneration and injury, *calcium* is often deposited. This type of calcium deposition is called dystrophic calcification to distinguish it from the normal calcification that occurs in bone and from calcium deposits that occur in normal tissues as a consequence of hypercalcemia (metastatic calcification). Dystrophic calcification, like the normal calcification of bone, is usually associated with *local increase in phosphatase enzymes.* Calcium is evident grossly by its *gritty* character, sandlike when in granular form or eggshell-like when deposited in layered structures like the aorta. Microscopically the deposits are usually granular or amorphous, and basophilic. Chemically the calcium is present in the form of *carbonates* and *phosphates,* much like that in normal bone. *Cholesterol* is often present in conjunction with calcium.

Gangrene

Gangrene is a complex and variable form of necrosis which is described in Chapter 2.

End results

Final resolution of necrotic tissue and restoration of the part are a result of the action of enzymes, phagocytic cells, and other factors, plus regeneration and repair (see Chapter 3).

6. *Aging of Cells and Tissues; Hyaline Degeneration and Related Disorders*

Nature of aging

Aging of cells, and of the body as a whole, is presumably a result of the *accumulation of injuries* from all causes occurring over the lifetime of the individual. Cells that have been damaged sublethally often retain in their cytoplasm fragments of damaged organelles, secretory products, and incompletely metabolized substances which can be recognized by electron microscopy. While the mechanisms of cell aging are poorly understood, it is generally believed [1, 15] that *aging results from decreased enzyme activity, accumulation of pigments derived from lipids, damage to DNA strands,* and *free-radical reactions* resulting in *crosslinking in macromolecules* such as collagen.

Effects of aging

Whatever the mechanisms of cellular damage, the effect at the level of organs and whole body is a general reduction in functional reserve related to stress, such as breathing capacity, cardiac output, formation of urine, neuromuscular responses, and integration of skills. This impaired function is associated with a decrease in the size and number of cells of parenchymatous organs, such as liver and brain, and frequently also a decrease in the number of functional units, such as nephrons.

Aging in connective tissues

The effects of aging are particularly evident in the *connective tissues.* Both the amount and the character of connective tissues undergo changes with age. Collagen about joints becomes tougher and less plastic; elastic tissues of the dermis, lens of the eye, and blood vessels become stretched and lose their ability to recoil. These changes are easily recognized by both the patient and the physician. While the physical changes are not fully understood, they are thought to be chiefly a *result of chemical modification of the extracellular mucopolysaccharides of the connective tissues,* particularly *collagen.* Sinex [15] suggests that aging may also affect *elastin,* another extracellular protein; this alteration may be a result of "thermal denaturation" from "a lifetime of incubation at 38°C." These changes may also be accounted for, at least in part, by *arteriocapillary fibrosis* in aging tissues. That aging may be accelerated by the accumulation of unusual tissue injury is likely but unproved.

Hyaline degeneration:

One of the most common and important types of connective tissue alteration, often associated with aging, is *hyaline degeneration.* The noun *hyalin* is applied to a number of poorly understood protein or mucopolysaccharide substances which may be deposited in the tissues. All these substances have certain physical and chemical characteristics in common: grossly they cause affected tissues to become *stiff, resilient, translucent,* and *gristly,* and microscopically they are *stained by acid dyes* such as eosin.

connective tissue hyalin

Hyalin is formed in inert connective tissue such as *old scars,* in *blood vessel walls,* in *serous membranes* such as pleura and peritoneum, and in the *capsules of organs* such as the spleen. Hyalin also forms in *old blood clots* and *thrombi,* probably as a result of the aging of fibrin. Undoubtedly the *most common and important site* for deposition of hyalin is in the *inner layers* of arteries, especially large arteries such as the aorta. Its presence here is a characteristic early change in that important disease of the arteries of the elderly known as *atherosclerosis* (see Chapter 18). In this condition hyalin is grossly evident as glistening, resilient *plaques in the intima,* often containing lipid and calcific deposits. When these localized areas of intimal thickening occur in small arteries, they may reduce the lumen and thus impair blood flow to an organ or part. Microscopically these intimal hyaline plaques consist of deposits of homogeneous eosinophilic material in which cholesterol crystals and calcium granules are often evident. Hyalin is also seen in the *muscular layer of small arterioles* in patients with increased blood pressure (hypertension).

cellular hyalin

While hyaline degeneration as a grossly evident tissue change is largely confined to connective tissues, as noted above, tiny bodies usually described as *hyaline droplets* may also be seen microscopically in the cytoplasm of various cells. Such droplets – glistening, homogeneous, and eosinophilic – are commonly seen in the epithelial cells lining the convoluted tubules of the *kidney* in patients having advanced renal disease. In patients with various types of hepatic disease, similar droplets (Mallory bodies) may be seen in the *liver* cells. *Plasmocytes,* when they accumulate in large numbers, often show similar cytoplasmic droplets, known in this case as Russell bodies. In each of these instances, the hyaline material is thought to be a *residue of old cellular injury,* such as cloudy swelling. It is doubtful if cellular hyalin has much in common with connective tissue hyalin except in staining reaction.

related conditions

Related conditions in which hyaline material having a similar microscopic appearance is deposited in the tissues include: (1) *amyloidosis,* an important disease (see Chapter 4) in which hyaline material of specific chemical composition and clinical significance is found in various tissues; (2) *fibrinoid necrosis,* an alteration in blood vessel walls and connective tissues described in an earlier section; (3) *Zenker's degeneration of muscle,* a condition which occurs in typhoid and other fevers, characterized by swelling of the fibers and loss of cross striations of certain voluntary muscles, especially those of the rectus abdominis; (4) *hyaline casts* in the tubules of the kidney, found also in the urine, representing plasma protein leaked through the glomerular filter and inspissated in the renal tubules; (5) *corpora amylacea,* small bodies of unknown significance seen in the lumen of prostatic glands, in the central nervous system, and in the stroma of certain papillary tumors. *Viral inclusions* may also appear as hyaline droplets when seen in the cytoplasm of affected cells.

Mucinous degeneration:

Mucinous degeneration, also known as mucoid or myxomatous degeneration, is somewhat akin to hyaline degeneration. *Mucin (mucus),* the natural substance after which this process is named, is a clear, viscid, sticky fluid, like raw egg white, normally secreted on mucosal surfaces by the *mucous glands.* (Note that the noun is spelled mucus; the adjective, mucous.) Mucin is formed in excess when mucous membranes are inflamed (catarrhal inflammation). It is normally present in the connective tissues of the *fetus* and in the umbilical cord (Wharton's jelly), but it is not normally present in the connective tissues of the adult. In tissue sections, mucus usually stains faintly with the basic dyes and can be positively identified by its reddish color with carmine (mucicarmine).

epithelial mucin

Epithelial mucin may collect in glandular organs when their ducts are obstructed, as by stone, forming mucus-containing *cysts.* It may also accumulate in an organ that is the seat of an abnormal growth arising from mucin-secreting cells. These cells, no longer connected with a duct or surface, may be ballooned by the mucin in their cytoplasm so that the nucleus is displaced, giving another type of signet-ring cell. Later these cells may rupture and small mucous cysts may be formed in the areas where the cell infiltration occurred. Most *mucous cysts,* formed as above, continue to enlarge and are finally removed surgically. Occasionally a cystic structure in the abdomen may rupture, spilling living mucus-secreting epithelial cells into the peritoneal cavity, where they grow as on tissue culture producing great masses of mucin. This condition, known as *pseudomyxoma peritonei,* may cause peritoneal adhesions and intestinal obstruction.

connective tissue mucin

Strictly speaking, epithelial mucin is not formed by degeneration but by cell secretion; the formation of connective tissue mucin is more truly a degenerative process related to aging. Mucin may form, presumably as a result of alteration in collagen, in fibrous connective tissue neoplasms of the extremities in the elderly. If the mucin is abundant, such tumors *(myxomas* or *fibromyxomas)* may be soft, translucent, and sticky on the cut surface. *Myxedema* is the subcutaneous accumulation of mucoid (mucin-like) material in cases of thyroid hypofunction.

SOMATIC DEATH

Definition

When heart action and respirations cease permanently, the whole organism is said to be dead; this is *somatic death,* as contrasted with cell death. What with the cardiac pacemaker and supported respiration, it is not always easy to determine when death has occurred, but the following *signs of death* are usually observed and help to establish the time of death:

Signs of death

1. *Cessation of vital functions.* When respirations and heart action are no longer detectable by any means, and cannot be restored by appropriate stimula-

tion, the individual is usually pronounced dead. Sometimes the electrocardiogram or electroencephalogram may be required to make the determination.

2. *Rigor mortis.* This is a tight muscular contraction due to chemical changes in skeletal muscle, which causes a stiffening of the entire body. The process begins within minutes after death in the muscular soldier killed during the violent action and heat of battle, but may be delayed many hours in the chronically ill, emaciated, anemic cancer patient with subnormal body temperature. The rigidity begins in the face and neck and extends in a few hours to the trunk and then to the extremities; it disappears 2 to 5 days later in the same order.

3. *Livor mortis.* This is a bluish purple discoloration of the skin over the dependent portions of the body, due to diffusion of blood and pigment through vessel walls. Since the location of the staining is determined by the position of the body in the first few hours after death, the medical examiner takes special notice of it in determining the circumstances of death.

4. *Algor mortis.* This is the cooling of the body post mortem, and is purely a physical matter determined by the body temperature at the time of death, the nature of the clothing, and the temperature of the environment.

5. *Clotting of blood* within the vessels and chambers of the heart. This occurs within hours after death, somewhat more rapidly in those who were vigorous and healthy than in those wasted by disease. Several days after death the clot liquefies.

6. *Postmortem changes in the viscera.* These result from the action of lytic enzymes of the cells, plus bacterial invasion. The stomach, pancreas, intestine, and gallbladder are the first organs to undergo lysis because of their own digestive enzymes. Eventually all tissues will undergo such changes. At the cellular level, postmortem changes are manifest by loss of cell detail, particularly loss of differential staining between nucleus and cytoplasm as nucleic acids diffuse through the nuclear membrane.

7. Other changes occur post mortem, depending upon the circumstances. *Softening of the eyeballs* and *drying of the cornea* occur regularly. *Putrefaction* occurs from invasion of tissues by gas-forming organisms, usually from the intestinal tract, and causes a greenish black discoloration of the peritoneal membranes and eventually of the abdominal wall.

REFERENCES

1. Comfort, A. The prevention of ageing in cells. *Lancet* 1:1325, 1966.
2. Saunders, J. W., Jr. Death in embryonic systems. *Science* 154:604, 1966.
3. Linder, F. E. The health of the American people. *Sci. Amer.* 214:21, 1966.
4. Derived from: Final mortality statistics, 1964. *Monthly Vital Statistics Report,* vol. 14, no. 10, Suppl. U.S. Dept. of Health, Education, and Welfare, Jan. 14, 1966.
5. Fawcett, D. W. *The cell: Its Organelles and Inclusions.* Philadelphia: Saunders, 1966. (A fascinating book, with clearly worded text and sharp, well-chosen electron micrographs mapping the sites of cell function.)
6. Brachet, J. The living cell. *Sci. Amer.* 205:50, 1961. (A classic study of the

internal structure of the cell, as revealed by electron microscopy and cytochemistry.)

7. de Duve, C. The lysosome. *Sci. Amer.* 208:64, 1963. (An excellent, easily followed discussion of this important organelle by the scientist who first described it.)
8. de Reuck, A. V. S., and Cameron, M. P. (Eds.). *Lysosomes.* A Ciba Foundation Symposium. Boston: Little, Brown, 1963. (A thorough presentation of the subject from many points of view, in which controversial facets are explored.)
9. Weiss, P. The cell in development. *Lab. Invest.* 8:413, 1959. (The lead paper of a group "Chemical Organization of Cells, Normal and Abnormal"; all are valuable.)
10. Magee, P. N. Toxic liver necrosis. *Lab. Invest.* 15:111, 1966. (One of a series of excellent papers from a symposium "Biochemical Pathology." The entire series, which has been published as a unit in *Laboratory Investigation,* is recommended for the serious student of cellular pathology.)
11. Ashworth, C. T., Werner, D. J., Glass, M. D., and Arnold, N. J. Spectrum of fine structural changes in hepatocellular injury due to thioacetamide. *Amer. J. Path.* 47:917, 1965. (A significant article, well illustrated and logically presented.)
12. Lombardi, B. Considerations on the pathogenesis of fatty liver. *Lab. Invest.* 15:1, 1966.
13. King, D. W., Paulson, S. R., Puckett, N. L., and Krebs, A. T. Cell death. IV. The effect of injury on the entrance of vital dye in Ehrlich tumor cells. *Amer. J. Path.* 35:1067, 1959. (The last in a series of four papers reporting a classic study, brilliantly conceived and concisely presented, of biochemical and morphologic changes following cell injury.)
14. Rees, K. R. The biochemical lesions in the development of a fatty liver. In Wartman, W. B. (Ed.), *Yearbook of Pathology and Clinical Pathology.* Chicago: Yearbook Medical Publishers, 1962–63.
15. Sinex, F. M. Biochemistry of aging. *Science* 134:1402, 1961. (A thoughtful summary of a very complex subject.)

2 CIRCULATORY DISTURBANCES

DISTURBANCES IN THE DISTRIBUTION OF BLOOD

The distribution of blood within the vascular tree, which normally is marvelously controlled so as to supply oxygen and nutritional needs to cells in all parts of the body, may under pathologic conditions be disturbed in three ways: a local increase (hyperemia) or generalized increase (plethora) in the amount of blood, or a local decrease in or absence of blood (ischemia).

1. Hyperemia

Hyperemia (congestion) is the presence of an abnormally increased amount of blood within the finer vessels of a tissue.

ACTIVE HYPEREMIA

Active hyperemia is a dynamic congestion due to an increased flow of arterial blood to a part, e.g., flushing of the face and acute inflammations. It results from the dilatation of arterioles produced by nervous or noxious stimuli. There is increased oxidation, which leads to increased activity and temperature in the part involved.

PASSIVE CONGESTION: Causes

Passive congestion results from obstruction or hindrance to the outflow of venous blood from a part. It may be general (as in cardiac failure) or local. The *causes* of passive congestion include defective cardiac action (congestive heart failure); pressure of a mass (tumor, enlarged lymph nodes) or scar tissue on a vein; pregnancy (by pressure on pelvic veins); venous thrombosis (formation of a clot within a vessel during life); twisting of the intestinal mesentery or a cyst pedicle with venous compression; and compression of a vein by a tight bandage, tourniquet, or ligature. Passive hyperemia causes decreased circulation, leading to decreased metabolism and functional activity. The capillary blood pressure is increased and the oxygen supply decreased, causing increased capillary permeability, escape of plasma protein, and edema.

Pathologic changes

The *lungs* are heavy and dark red. Most of the increased weight is due to pink, frothy edema fluid which exudes from the cut surface. The changes are most marked in the dependent portions of the lungs. *Microscopically* the pulmonary veins and capillaries are dilated and engorged with blood. The alveolar walls are thickened, and acidophilic proteinaceous fluid fills the alveolar spaces. Erythrocytes and brown blood pigment-laden macrophages *(heart-failure cells)* are found within the alveoli. These cells, mixed with mucus and desquamated mucosal cells, are present in the bronchioles and bronchi in chronic congestion. The *liver* is enlarged and purplish red early, with a tense capsule. On the cut surface it is dark red in acute congestion and a mottled yellow and brown *(nutmeg liver)* after long-standing congestion *(chronic passive congestion). Microscopically* the hyperemia is mainly centrolobular, the central veins and sinusoids being dilated and engorged. There may be necrosis of a varying number of centrolobular hepatic parenchymal cells. Granular, brown lipofuscin pigment is present within the cytoplasm of hepatic cells [1]. The peripheral zones of the lobules are pale and may be fatty. Fibrosis occurs centrally and peripherally in severe congestion of prolonged duration *(cardiac cirrhosis of the liver).* The *spleen* is enlarged and tense. *Microscopically* the sinusoids of the red pulp are dilated and engorged with erythrocytes. The *kidneys* are enlarged and dark red. *Microscopically* the glomerular and peritubular capillaries are congested. The tubular epithelium shows varying degrees of degeneration, such as cloudy swelling and fatty changes.

Brown induration

Brown induration is produced by very long-standing congestion. The firm consistency of the involved organs results from fibrosis due to prolonged hypoxia and the deposition of blood pigments, mainly hemosiderin. This condition is seen in the lungs, liver, and spleen especially. The term *brown induration* is no longer widely used.

2. *Plethora*

Plethora is an overfullness of the vascular tree due to a marked increase in the blood volume. It may affect the entire body or only a part.

Primary plethora

Primary plethora is an increase in both the cells and the fluid of the blood. It is seen in polycythemia vera, in which there is an abnormally high number of red cells (6 to 12 million per cubic millimeter).

Hydremic plethora

Hydremic plethora (water intoxication) is an increase of fluid only. It is usually temporary because the homeostatic mechanisms of the body react quickly to excrete or transfer the excess fluid out of the bloodstream. It occurs in the rapid administration of large amounts of parenteral fluids. A serious sudden increase in intravascular fluid may result. Water intoxication is probably due as much or more to the dilution of the body salts as to the excess of fluid. *Pathologic changes* are inconstant and minor. In patients with diseases of the myocardium a sudden increase in blood volume may cause acute cardiac failure with severe edema of the lungs.

Local plethora

Localized plethora occurs rarely in the abdomen when, after it has been greatly distended by a tumor, ascites, or pregnancy, the cause of the distention is suddenly removed. The great veins may dilate and withhold large amounts of blood from the circulation. If cardiac disease is present, death from acute heart failure may occur within a few minutes.

3. *Ischemia*

Ischemia is a local decrease in the volume of blood, or an absence of blood, due to cutting off of the arterial supply to a part. Obstruction of the arterial blood supply may be sudden or gradual.

Ischemia due to sudden obstruction

Sudden obstruction of the arterial blood supply is caused by thrombosis, embolism (the impaction of foreign material in the bloodstream), a ligature, or traumatic spasm. The *result* of sudden obstruction depends on the collateral circulation: if it is adequate, there is little or no change in the tissues supplied by the blocked artery; if it is inadequate, infarction (death of tissue due to the loss of its blood supply) results.

Ischemia due to gradual obstruction

Gradual obstruction is usually due to arteriosclerosis, but may also be caused by spasm (as in the fingers in Raynaud's disease and ergot poisoning) or external pressure (as in bed sores). It may lead to *ischemic necrosis,* in which the tissues are replaced by fibrosis.

DISTURBANCES IN THE DISTRIBUTION OF BODY FLUIDS

NORMAL DISTRIBUTION OF BODY FLUIDS:

The adult human male is about 60 percent water by weight, and his total body water averages 42 liters. About two-thirds of this water is intracellular. Of the extracellular water 25 percent is in the plasma volume (about 3.5 liters) and 75 percent is interstitial fluid (15 percent of the body weight). The *volume of body water* is normally carefully regulated by the interplay of a number of physiologic mechanisms. Water intake is a function of thirst, while water in excess of body needs is mainly excreted as urine and sweat. Urinary excretion of water is controlled by vasopressin, an antidiuretic hormone (ADH), and, indirectly, by aldosterone, the sodium-conserving hormone produced by the adrenal cortex. *Arginine vasopressin* is formed by neurosecretory hypothalamic cells and stored in dilated nerve endings in the neurohypophysis. It acts directly on the distal convoluted renal tubular epithelium so that these cells reabsorb a hypotonic solution. There is also a fluid homeostatic mechanism sensitive to variations in the extracellular fluid volume and possibly mediated through stretch receptors in the atrial myocardium. At the capillary level, where a constant interchange of intravascular and extravascular fluid takes place, the *normal fluid balance* is maintained by the interrelationship of four factors: the capillary blood pressure, the osmotic pressure of the plasma proteins, the extravascular tissue pressure, and the extravascular osmotic pressure. The *hydrostatic pressure of the blood* in the capillary tends to push fluid out of the vessel, while the *plasma osmotic pressure* tends to hold fluid within it. The serum proteins and, to a much lesser extent, lipids produce the osmotic pressure by their molecular concentration. Because of its smaller molecules and higher concentration, the serum albumin is responsible for about 90 percent of the osmotic pressure within the capillary.

Role of the endothelium

Essential to normal fluid balance at the capillary level is the *integrity of the endothelium.* It acts as a membrane through which water, electrolytes, and organic solutes pass freely, but it normally allows only small amounts of albumin to pass through. The diffusion of lipid-soluble substances (oxygen and carbon dioxide) occurs throughout the capillary surface, but lipid-insoluble ones, such as water, sodium chloride, urea, and glucose, are filtered through an area constituting less than 0.2 percent of the capillary surface, probably the intercellular spaces.

1. Edema

Edema is a dynamic pathologic process characterized by the accumulation of an abnormal amount of fluid in the cells, intercellular spaces, and/or cavities of the body due to conditions which upset the mechanism of fluid balance or which interfere with normal lymph flow.

CAUSES

The *basic causes* of edema are obstruction to lymph flow (lymphedema), abnormal permeability of capillary endothelium, increased capillary blood pressure, decreased plasma colloidal osmotic pressure, decreased extravascular tissue pressure, and excessive sodium ion retention. The causes of edema are complex, however, and edema probably can never be ascribed to an abnormality in only one of these processes.

LYMPHEDEMA:

Lymphedema is an increase of tissue fluid resulting from obstruction of the lymph flow from an area. Occasionally large collections of lymph accumulate in the pleural or peritoneal cavities, the latter being called *chylous ascites. Lymphatic blockage* may be due to malignant neoplastic cells within lymph channels or nodes, parasites (especially filaria, which cause elephantiasis) within lymph channels, chronic inflammation (by causing scar tissue to form about lymph channels), or removal of a lymph node group by surgery. The edema is localized to the tissues normally drained by the obstructed lymph channels.

Congenital edema

Congenital edema (Milroy's disease, hereditary trophedema) is a chronic, usually bilateral, mild edema which may appear shortly after birth or later. It is inherited as a simple autosomal dominant of variable penetrance and affects the lower limbs. The edema is apparently due to a congenital lymphatic defect, with an overgrowth and dilatation of lymph vessels (congenital lymphangiectasis). The subcutaneous fat may be partly replaced by lymphatic vessels.

Lymphedema praecox

Lymphedema praecox is a form of idiopathic lymphedema [2] which usually has its onset between the ages of 10 and 14 years. It is much more common in females than males and almost always involves the lower extremities. In about half the cases both legs are affected. The *cause* is unknown. *Grossly* the skin of the involved extremity is roughened and slightly hyperpigmented. The skin and subcutaneous tissue are markedly thickened. *Microscopically* there are fibroblastic proliferation and increased collagen deposits in the dermis and subcutaneous tissue. The subcutaneous fat is abundant. The *superficial lymphatic vessels* are not dilated nor increased in number. They are often surrounded by a cuff of lymphocytes and plasmocytes. The *deep lymphatics* are moderately dilated, and there are perilymphatic lymphocytic and plasmocytic infiltrates. *Complications* include single or recurrent episodes of lymphangitis or cellulitis and rarely the development of lymphangiosarcoma (a malignant neoplasm arising from lymphatic endothelium) in very prolonged cases. Lymphangiosarcoma in chronic lymphedema of a lower extremity is known as Kettle's syndrome.

EDEMA DUE TO INCREASED ENDOTHELIAL PERMEABILITY:

Edema due to increased endothelial permeability is very frequent. It is caused by a wide variety of endothelial poisons and hypoxia. Increased endothelial permeability occurs in severe infections, due to bacterial toxins; metabolic intoxications such as eclampsia and diabetic acidosis; hypersensitivity reactions, such as hay fever and anaphylactic shock; abdominal catastrophes, such as visceral perforations; anoxia, especially when due to carbon monoxide; poisoning with various drugs, such as the barbiturates; severe injuries; and burns. Edema due to increased endothelial permeability is seen especially in the soft viscera of the chest and abdomen and is usually accompanied by serous effusions.

Inflammatory edema

Inflammatory edema is localized and results from increased endothelial permeability. Examples are wheals, insect bites, stings, burns, infections, and irritations from drugs or chemicals. Vesicles or bullae may result, because the fluid pressure produces separation of the epidermis from the dermis. In the *mechanism of inflammatory edema,* cell injury releases a cytoplasmic substance which causes dilatation and increased permeability of the adjacent capillaries. The process is summed up as the *triple response* of Lewis: arteriolar dilatation, due to axon reflex stimulation (the *flare*); capillary and venular hyperemia, due to the chemical action of histamine liberated by the injured tissue (the *red reaction*); and edema, due to exudation of plasma into the tissues (the *wheal*). Inflammatory edema fluid has a high plasma protein content, including fibrinogen, if the endothelial permeability is greatly increased. The protein molecules may pass out of the capillaries through the endothelial cells or through the intercellular spaces. Leukocytes are also present in the edema fluid. Electron microscopic studies show that these cells, as well as particulate matter, leave capillaries and venules through gaps which develop between endothelial cells [3].

Angioneurotic edema

Angioneurotic edema (Quincke's edema) is an intermittent and rapidly developing local swelling of the skin, lips, respiratory mucosa, stomach and intestines, urogenital tract, and occasionally the brain. In the *sporadic type* the swelling results from a hypersensitivity (allergic) reaction. In the uncommon *hereditary type,* which is transmitted as a simple autosomal dominant, the cause is presumably neurogenic. In either type the escape of fluid from the capillaries is due to increased endothelial permeability. *Gastrointestinal edema* may cause abdominal pain which leads to exploratory surgery. At laparotomy marked focal and circumferential edema of the gastrointestinal mucosa and intraperitoneal collection of serous fluid are found. Acute laryngeal edema is a fairly common cause of sudden death in cases of angioneurotic edema.

EDEMA DUE TO INCREASED CAPILLARY PRESSURE:

Edema due to increased capillary blood pressure results from an abnormally high venous pressure which causes an increased capillary hydrostatic pressure. If this more than counterbalances the colloidal osmotic pressure, fluid accumulates in the tissues.

Postural edema

Postural edema due to an elevated capillary blood pressure may develop from standing too long in one position. It occurs usually in the subcutaneous tissues of the feet and ankles and is transient.

Venous obstruction

Mechanical venous obstruction leads to increased local venous pressure, which in turn elevates the capillary pressure. The obstruction is due to venous thrombosis, pressure from a tumor or other mass, or pregnancy. Increased capillary permeability becomes a factor in these edemas because of the hypoxia produced by the stasis of blood.

EDEMA DUE TO DECREASED PLASMA PROTEINS

Edema due to a decrease in plasma proteins usually occurs when the plasma protein level falls below 4 gm. per 100 ml. or the plasma albumin level is below 3 gm. per 100 ml., because the colloidal osmotic pressure is not sufficient to counteract the hydrostatic pressure of the blood; this tends to drive fluid into the tissue spaces. Examples are *nutritional (famine) edema,* in which the plasma proteins may be greatly decreased by prolonged malnutrition, and the rare *hypoproteinemic edema,* due to a congenital defect in protein formation [4]. In nutritional edema, decreased extravascular tissue pressure due to the loss of fat and cardiac failure due to thiamine deficiency are contributory factors in the development of edema. Hypoproteinemic edema may appear in children or adults. The only sign is a moderate edema. An absence of or decrease in gamma globulin has been demonstrated in some of these patients.

EDEMA DUE TO DECREASED EXTERNAL PRESSURE

Edema due to decreased external pressure is uncommon and occurs in aviators at high altitudes, workers in low pressure chambers, and the application of a vacuum cup to the skin.

PATHOLOGIC CHANGES IN EDEMA

All tissues may be involved by edema except the hair, nails, and bone. Soft tissues such as the lungs, mucous membranes, glandular structures, and areolar connective tissues are especially affected. Slight subcutaneous edema is seen first in the soft parts, such as the eyelids and external genitalia. *Edematous tissue* is translucent, pale (unless congestion is also present), and swollen. It is doughy in consistency and may pit. Such tissue appears gelatinous when cut, and fluid oozes from it. The fluid may be clear, yellowish, or pink. *Microscopically* the collagenous fibers are swollen by the absorbed fluid. Coagulated protein in the intercellular spaces is faintly acidophilic and may be homogeneous or granular.

PATHOLOGIC PHYSIOLOGY

Edema is secondary to other conditions, and usually the primary condition is more important than the edema. Large accumulations of fluid may embarrass function; e.g., pericardial and pleural effusions may compress the heart or lungs. Edema contributes to infection, since albuminous fluid is a good medium for bacterial growth. Patients with pulmonary edema often develop hypostatic bronchopneumonia.

SPECIAL FORMS OF EDEMA

Certain forms of edema are of particular interest clinically, because of the high frequency of their occurrence and/or the importance of the edema as a manifestation of the underlying disease process. These are the edemas resulting from cardiac failure, hepatic cirrhosis, and various renal disorders, and edema of the lungs, whatever the cause.

Edema due to cardiac failure:

Edema due to cardiac failure is one of the most common and most important forms. *Cardiac failure (congestive heart failure, cardiac decompensation)* may be acute or chronic and left-sided or right-sided, or both ventricles may fail together. *Left ventricular failure* is caused by systemic hypertension (high blood pressure), coronary artery disease, aortic valvular stenosis (narrowing) or insufficiency, mitral valvular insufficiency, and certain congenital defects. *Right ventricular failure* may be due to pulmonary hypertension, mitral valvular stenosis, pulmonary valvular stenosis or insufficiency, and certain congenital defects. *Failure of both ventricles* occurs in diseases involving inflammation of the myocardium, such as rheumatic fever, and in coronary artery disease.

mechanism

The mechanism of cardiac failure is still unsettled. The classic *backward failure* theory states that when the heart becomes unable to eject in systole the amount of blood entering it in diastole, the blood becomes dammed back in the atria and veins; consequently the venous and capillary hydrostatic pressures rise. The edema results from this increase in capillary pressure.

The *"forward failure"* theory considers the formation of edema as due to the retention of sodium (and thus water) and to increased capillary permeability from tissue hypoxia caused by inadequate circulation. An inadequate cardiac output leads to tissue hypoxia, which produces the increased capillary endothelial permeability. Increased discharge of adrenal cortical aldosterone and posterior pituitary antidiuretic hormone (ADH) results in sodium and water retention by the kidneys. This is aggravated by the decreased renal blood flow caused by the deficient cardiac output, so that glomerulotubular imbalance leads to further retention of sodium and water. According to this theory the increased venous pressure of cardiac failure results from an increased plasma volume and occurs after edema has appeared, as is often observed clinically.

pathologic changes

In *acute left ventricular failure* the edema fluid collects rapidly in the lungs. In *chronic left ventricular failure* the edema fluid appears first in the dependent portions of the body, such as the ankles, legs, scrotum, and sacral regions. The edema pits under pressure. In *right ventricular failure* the venae cavae and the liver become engorged early. Later, fluid collects in the peritoneal cavity (ascites) and peripherally. *Autopsy findings in congestive heart failure* [5] include: increased organ weights throughout the body due to congestion and edema; pericardial effusion in about 15 percent of the cases; pleural effusion larger than 200 ml. in over 50 percent; ascites in 15 percent; esophageal and gastrointestinal venous dilatation and capillary engorgement; erythroid bone marrow hyperplasia in 50 percent, probably as a result of the prolonged hypoxia; and pulmonary infarction in 20 percent.

Edema in hepatic cirrhosis

Edema in portal cirrhosis (fibrosis) *of the liver* is due in part to increased capillary pressure in the portal system and to a decrease in the plasma osmotic pressure. The former is due to portal hypertension, and the latter to failure of the liver to produce adequate plasma protein. Another factor in the development of this type of edema is water retention due to failure of the damaged liver to detoxify aldosterone and possibly antidiuretic hormone, and to lymphatic "weeping" from the liver. The edema is mainly in the form of ascites. Portal cirrhosis is discussed on page 528.

Nephritic edema

Nephritic edema occurs in acute glomerulonephritis and eclampsia (a toxic condition occurring during late pregnancy). The edema has been attributed to an increased endothelial permeability (caused by severe arteriolar constriction which leads to endothelial hypoxia), retention of sodium, and the loss of albumin in the urine (which causes a decreased plasma osmotic pressure). Cardiac failure, due to the sudden development of hypertension and the increased blood volume resulting from fluid retention caused by oliguria (decreased urine volume), is a factor in the production of nephritic edema. The edema characteristically begins in the soft eyelids, does not pit, and may become generalized.

Nephrotic edema

Nephrotic edema occurs in subacute glomerulonephritis and other renal disorders which are characterized by massive proteinuria (loss of protein, mainly albumin, in the urine). The albumin-globulin ratio (A/G) in the blood is reversed, and systemic edema results. Another factor in this edema is the retention of sodium by the kidneys and in the tissues, elevating the tissue "osmotic" pressure and thus drawing water there.

Edema of the lungs:

Edema of the lungs is characterized by the transudation of plasma into the alveoli and by its extension by air currents into the bronchial tree. It is caused by left ventricular failure, increased resistance to the outflow of blood through the pulmonary veins (such as occurs in mitral stenosis), obstruction of the lymphatic outflow of the lungs (rarely), inflammation of the lungs (such as occurs in pneumonia), noxious gases, and sudden hypervolemia (excessive blood volume) produced by intravenous fluids in patients with decreased left ventricular reserve. In sudden hypervolemia the systemic return to the right side of the heart is overloaded, and the right ventricular output exceeds the pulmonary venous runoff. *Factors involved* in pulmonary edema include: the hydrostatic pressure in pulmonary capillaries (normally 10 mm. of mercury); the osmotic pressure of plasma proteins (normally 25 to 30 mm. of mercury); the permeability of the pulmonary capillary endothelium (increased permeability is caused by hypoxia and noxious agents); the intrathoracic pressure (−5 to −10 mm. of mercury); the lymphatic runoff of the lungs; and neurogenic factors (pulmonary edema occurs in brain and spinal cord injuries, cerebral hemorrhage, and other types of brain damage and is thought to be due to neural impulses which mediate increased capillary permeability).

clinical features

Clinically congestion and edema of the lungs causes dyspnea (difficulty in breathing), cyanosis (blueness of the skin and mucosa due to decreased oxygenation of hemoglobin), orthopnea (difficulty in breathing while lying down), and cough, sometimes with expectoration of blood-tinged sputum. Bubbling rales are heard, especially at the base of the lungs. Bronchopneumonia is a common complication.

pathologic changes

Pathologic changes in pulmonary edema are those discussed under passive congestion of the lungs on page 21, except in the rare cases of edema of the lungs due to lymphatic obstruction. In such cases congestion is absent.

DISTRIBUTION OF EDEMA FLUID

Edema may be localized or general. In those types produced by venous or lymphatic obstruction, *edema fluid* collects only in the parts normally drained by the blocked vein or lymph channels; e.g., during pregnancy the lower extremities are commonly swollen because of compression of the iliac veins by the enlarged uterus. Even those types of edema which may become generalized usually appear first in particular local areas. In the edema of cardiac failure, swelling of the feet and ankles is typically the first clinical sign. Patients with cardiac failure remain ambulatory until the decompensation is severe, and the edema fluid appears in the dependent parts first. As more fluid collects, the rest of the lower extremities and the sacral region become edematous. Patients with renal failure due to nephritis, on the other hand, are so ill that they are bedridden early; in this case the edema fluid is apparent first in the softest tissues, the eyelids and scrotum.

DEFINITIONS RELATING TO EDEMA

Some terms relating to edema are defined below.

Anasarca. Edema of the body as a whole.

Ascites (hydroperitoneum). A collection of edema fluid in the peritoneal cavity.

Dropsy. Abnormal accumulation of serous fluid in the tissues or body cavities. The term is often used synonymously with edema.

Exudate. Edema fluid with a specific gravity above 1.015 and a protein level above 3 mg. per 100 ml. It occurs in acute inflammations as a result of increased capillary endothelial permeability.

Pericardial effusion (hydropericardium). An excessive collection of fluid in the pericardial sac.

Pleural effusion (hydrothorax). A collection of fluid in one or both pleural spaces.

Spongiosis. Intercellular edema in the epidermis.

Transudate. Edema fluid with a specific gravity below 1.015 and a protein content below 3 mg. per 100 ml. (usually below 1 percent). It results from increased capillary hydrostatic pressure with normal endothelial permeability.

Vesicle (blister). A focal elevation of the epidermis (1) due to a collection of fluid beneath it and separating it from the underlying dermis, or (2) due to marked intracellular edema in the epidermis (ballooning degeneration). A *bulla* (bleb) is similar to but larger than vesicle (1), measuring over 5 mm. in diameter.

2. Dehydration

Dehydration is characterized by a marked decrease in the total fluids of the body. It may result from a primary loss of water or of salt.

Dehydration from water loss

Dehydration from loss of water occurs when there is an excessive loss through the skin (as in fever or a high environmental temperature) or through the kidneys (as in diabetes insipidus), or when there is a decreased intake of water. The salt concentration in the body fluids increases, producing a shift of fluid from intracellular to extracellular compartments. Severe intracellular dehydration results.

Dehydration from salt loss

Dehydration from loss of salt occurs in adrenal cortical insufficiency, diabetic ketosis, and diarrhea or vomiting.

In dehydration the tissues are excessively dry, and the subcutaneous fat is relatively opaque.

HEMORRHAGE AND SHOCK

HEMORRHAGE:

Hemorrhage is the escape of blood from a vessel incident to a mechanical defect in the vascular or cardiac wall. Such a defect may result from trauma, excessive blood pressure, or disease of the vessel wall.

Causes

The *causes* include injury, infection, or ulceration of a blood vessel wall; atherosclerosis, in which the arterial wall becomes brittle; rupture of an aneurysm (a bulge in a vessel wall); purpuras (bleeding diseases in which small hemorrhages occur in the skin and mucosa); leukemia, because of the suppression of platelet formation; avitaminosis K, because of the deficiency of prothrombin formation; scurvy (avitaminosis C), because of fragility of the vessel walls; certain poisons and bacterial toxins; and anoxia.

Systemic effects

When even a large amount of blood is lost over a long period of time, as in chronically bleeding hemorrhoids, the body is able to compensate fairly well by increasing the activity of the bone marrow (compensatory hyperplasia) to replace the shed erythrocytes. Eventually the blood loss will outstrip the body's remarkable ability to replace, and anemia ensues.

When a large amount of blood is lost suddenly, a decrease in both blood pressure and blood volume flow develops. The body reacts quickly to counteract the loss. Reduced blood pressure or flow stimulates the carotid sinus reflex. This produces increased cardiac action and selective vasoconstriction. Release of epinephrine from the adrenal medulla leads to peripheral arteriolar constriction, increased cardiac output, and an augmented coagulability of the blood by increasing its viscosity. Norepinephrine exerts a powerful pressor effect by causing vasoconstriction in peripheral vessels. If the blood pressure cannot be maintained, the decreased capillary blood pressure results in the movement of fluid from the tissues into the blood vessels. Thus the blood volume is partly restored by hemodilution. Eventually the erythrocyte loss produces tissue hypoxia which leads to increased capillary endothelial permeability and capillary dilatation. The outcome of this is *secondary shock* (discussed on page 31). While there is some individual variability, the sudden loss of 30 percent or more of the blood volume is usually fatal. Following nonshock-producing *venous bleeding of 10 to 20 percent of the blood volume* [6], there is a movement of water and albumin from the tissues into the circulation. The *plasma volume refill rate* is about 100 ml. per hour in the first 2 hours, drops to 50 ml. per hour at between 6 and 10 hours, then decreases steadily until the refill is complete after 30 to 40 hours. By that time the plasma volume refill almost exactly equals the total volume of shed plasma and erythrocytes. Increased *erythrocyte synthesis* in the bone marrow begins almost immediately. A transient hypoalbuminemia sometimes develops, but within 4 to 6 hours the plasma albumin level begins to increase rapidly. This albumin is derived from the shift of preformed protein from the extravascular tissues into the bloodstream and probably from increased albumin synthesis in the liver. *Endocrine changes* following such bleedings include increased aldosterone, renin, erythropoietin, epinephrine, norepinephrine, and antidiuretic hormone secretion. These changes achieve sodium and water conservation (aldosterone and ADH), pressor effects to maintain the blood pressure (renin and the epinephrines), and stimulation of red cell synthesis (erythropoietin). Within about 6 weeks the lost erythrocytes are completely replaced, and the blood is restored to normal.

Local effects

Hemorrhage into the gastrointestinal tract or abdominal cavity has the same effect as external hemorrhage. *Pleural or pericardial hemorrhage* may compress the lungs or heart (cardiac tamponade). *Cerebral hemorrhage* infiltrates the adjacent soft brain substance and destroys it.

Pathologic changes

Severe or fatal hemorrhage causes ischemia of all organs. The mucosa, skin, and organs are pale. The organ weights are decreased, and the tissues are dry. *Internal, nonfatal hemorrhage* produces a mild inflammatory response. *Local extravasations of blood* cause a foreign body reaction. Blood pigments appear, with fibrosis. *Large hematomata* are encapsulated, and *small hemorrhages* may be resorbed without a trace.

Definitions relating to hemorrhage

Some terms relating to hemorrhage are defined below.

Ecchymosis. A blotchy, purplish hemorrhage (greater than 1 cm. in diameter) into the subcutaneous tissue due to leakage from a capillary or venule.

Epistaxis. A hemorrhage from the nose.

Hematemesis. The presence of a significant amount of blood in the vomitus.

Hematocele. The escape of blood into a cavity, especially into the tunica vaginalis testis. A hematocele may also be pelvic (into the cul-de-sac of Douglas), pudendal (into a labium), or vaginal.

Hematoma. A localized mass of blood, usually clotted, within a tissue.

Hematometra. An accumulation of blood in the uterine cavity.

Hematomyelia. A hemorrhage into the spinal cord.

Hematosalpinx. A hemorrhage into the lumen of a uterine tube.

Hematuria. The presence of blood in the urine.

Hemopericardium (hematopericardium). A hemorrhage into the pericardial sac.

Hemoperitoneum (hematoperitoneum). A hemorrhage into the peritoneal cavity.

Hemoptysis. The presence of blood in the sputum.

Hemostasis. The stopping of blood flow from the vascular tree.

Hemothorax. A collection of blood in a pleural cavity.

Melena. The presence of dark, digested blood in the feces.

Menorrhagia. Excessive endometrial bleeding during a menstrual period.

Metrorrhagia. Irregular endometrial bleeding between menstrual periods.

Petechia. A tiny hemorrhage (less than 1 mm. in diameter) due to leakage from a capillary or venule.

SHOCK:

Shock is a profound and emergent circulatory disturbance characterized by a disparity between the effective blood volume and the volume capacity of the vascular system.

Primary shock

Primary shock (vasovagal state) is a transient neurovascular collapse indistinguishable from syncope (fainting). Nociceptive impulses originated by an emotional disturbance, pain, or nonsensory nerve impulses arising in traumatized tissue initiate the neurovascular reaction. *Clinically* there are a short period of unconsciousness and a slight blood pressure drop, often with bradycardia. Not all authorities recognize this as a true form of shock, but in some cases, where hemorrhage has occurred or injury has been severe, the reaction may be profound and merge with secondary shock.

Secondary shock:

Secondary shock may be hypovolemic or normovolemic, depending on whether the total blood volume is decreased or normal. *Hypovolemic shock* occurs when about one-third of the normal blood volume is suddenly lost. This loss may be in the form of whole blood, as in hemorrhage; plasma, as in burns, acute pancreatitis, acute peritonitis, and extensive soft tissue injury; or water and electrolytes, as in severe vomiting or diarrhea. *Normovolemic shock* may result from acute myocardial failure *(cardiogenic shock);* acute adrenal insufficiency (Waterhouse-Friderichsen syndrome) due to meningococcemia; anaphylactic and other severe hypersensitivity reactions; body injury, including surgical trauma, with little blood loss; intoxication due to a drug or poison; and overwhelming septicemia (the presence of bacteria in the bloodstream with accompanying clinical manifestations). *Shock occurs in about 25 percent of patients with a gram-negative septicemia,* and such shock carries a high mortality rate. These septicemias are most often due to *Escherichia coli,* but the fatality rate is highest in *Proteus* species septicemia. *Irreversible shock* is the lethal end stage of cases of severe shock which become intractable to treatment.

underlying causes

Except for shock secondary to the loss of a large volume of blood by hemorrhage, the *underlying causes* of the circulatory disparity in shock are uncertain. The onset of shock has been attributed to an increased permeability of the capillary endothelium, to a generalized capillary atony and dilatation due to vasodepressor material (VDM), and/or to severe plasma loss. The last factor certainly is a potent one in shock following a burn. The cause of the shock in gram-negative septicemia is endotoxin released from the bacterial cell walls on lysis *(endotoxic shock)* [7]. In experimental animals irreversible shock and death within 24 hours are produced by injection of a lethal dose of endotoxin. The endotoxin apparently alters the reactivity of small blood vessels to epinephrine by the release of serotonin (5-hydroxytryptamine) and/or histamine. After a prolonged and intense constriction of arterioles and venules, vasodilatation and venous pooling of blood occur. Decreased venous return to the heart and a consequent decreased cardiac output result. The development of *irreversible shock* has been attributed to acute myocardial failure resulting from myocardial ischemia caused by sharply decreased coronary arterial flow [8], to endotoxins released from gram-negative intestinal bacteria [9], and to widespread coagulation of blood within capillaries due to endothelial damage [10]. Experimental studies indicate that intravascular clotting in endotoxic and hemorrhagic shock is related to the secretion of large amounts of catecholamines during the period of shock [11].

clinical features

Clinically the patient in a state of shock is apprehensive, cold, clammy, pale, and ashen gray. Respirations are rapid and shallow, and there is a tachycardia (fast pulse rate). The blood pressure is typically less than 90/60 mm. of mercury. *Chemical changes* include an elevated blood sugar with a terminal fall to hypoglycemic levels, presumably due to a depletion of liver and muscle glycogen; increased blood ammonia late in shock; and decreased blood pH and CO_2 levels due to the development of metabolic acidosis. Unless it is treated promptly and vigorously, shock may become irreversible and produce death within a few hours.

pathologic changes

Dilatation and engorgement of the capillaries and venules in the thoracic and abdominal viscera occur. *Petechiae* appear on the serous and mucosal surfaces, and *serous effusions* into the body cavities are common. *Pulmonary congestion and edema* are among the most constant changes in shock. The lungs may attain two to three times their normal weight. Pneumonia is common if the state of shock is prolonged. In the *heart,* fatty degeneration of the myocardial fibers appears after 18 hours in about half the fatal cases, due to the hypoxia. Fatty metamorphosis and centrolobular necrosis occur in the *liver* due to hypoxia. In the early phase of shock the cortex of the *adrenal glands* is slightly enlarged and bright yellow due to an increase of cortical lipids. Later the lipids are depleted, and the cortex is thinner than normal, the cortical cells being shrunken and focally necrotic. Their cytoplasm is eosinophilic and granular and lacks the normal vacuolated or foamy appearance. The changes in the *kidneys* vary somewhat according to the initiating cause of the shock. In general, on gross examination the kidneys appear normal or slightly enlarged in size. On section the cortex is pale reddish brown and swollen; the medulla is dark reddish brown. Microscopically the tubular epithelium shows all degrees of degeneration from cloudy swelling to necrosis, and hemoglobin casts may be present in the tubular lumina. This *hypoxic nephrosis* is typical of shock following a crushing muscle injury (crush syndrome), but it also appears in other cases of severe shock. Many of the renal changes are due to hypoxia which is apparently produced by shunting of the blood from the cortex to the medulla. The *gastric and small intestinal walls* are congested and edematous, and petechiae appear in their mucosa.

Homologous-blood syndrome

A situation analogous to shock occurs in the *homologous-blood syndrome during extracorporeal circulation* established for open heart surgery in which the blood is shunted through a pump-oxygenator. A decreased circulating blood volume (hypovolemia) is noted in the patient during or following such surgery despite the careful replacement of all measured blood loss. The hypovolemia is due to the sequestration of the administered blood, apparently in the lungs [12].

DISTURBANCES OF COAGULATION

COAGULATION:

Coagulation (clotting) *of the blood* is a protective physiologic mechanism to prevent excessive loss of blood from injuries or other causes of hemorrhage. The mechanism is extremely complex; the known factors involved in coagulation include [13]:

Coagulation factors

Factor	Name	Factor	Name
Factor I	Fibrinogen	Factor VIII	Antihemophilic globulin (AHG) (thromboplastinogen, antihemophilic factor A)
Factor II	Prothrombin		
Factor III	Thromboplastin	Factor IX	Plasma thromboplastin component (PTC) (Christmas factor, antihemophilic factor B)
Factor IV	Calcium		
Factor V	Proaccelerin (plasma Ac-globulin, labile factor)	Factor X	Stuart factor (Prower factor)
		Factor XI	Plasma thromboplastin antecedent (PTA) (antihemophilic factor C)
Factor VII	Proconvertin (serum prothrombin conversion accelerator [SPCA], stable factor)	Factor XII	Hageman factor (glass factor)
		Factor XIII	Fibrin-stabilizing factor (FSF) (fibrinase, Laki-Lorand factor)

Coagulation mechanism:

Coagulation is thought to occur in three stages: (1) the elaboration of plasma thromboplastin, (2) the elaboration of thrombin, and (3) the formation of fibrin. *Thromboplastin elaboration* requires a platelet factor (a phospholipid derived from the plasma membranes of aggregated platelets), antihemophilic globulin, plasma thromboplastin component, plasma thromboplastin antecedent, and the Stuart (X) and Hageman (XII) factors. *Thrombin elaboration* requires prothrombin, thromboplastin, calcium ions, accelerator factors (V and VII), and the Stuart factor. *Fibrin formation* is mediated from fibrinogen by thrombin and calcium. A *waterfall sequence* has been proposed [14], in which as one protein clotting factor is activated it acts as an enzyme to tumble the activation of the next factor. In this mechanism the *intrinsic clotting system* is accomplished in cascade-like steps beginning in vitro with the conversion of Hageman factor to its activated form. Then, in order, plasma thromboplastin antecedent, plasma thromboplastin component, antihemophilic globulin, Stuart factor, proaccelerin, prothrombin, and fibrinogen are converted to their activated forms. The last two are changed to thrombin and fibrin, respectively. In the *extrinsic system,* which requires the participation of substances outside the blood, tissue thromboplastin and proconvertin activate Stuart factor, initiating the waterfall sequence at that level and bypassing the earlier steps.

initiation of clotting [15]

platelet thrombus [17]

When a blood vessel wall is damaged or disrupted, platelets aggregate at the site of injury. Through breaks in the endothelial lining, the platelets come in contact with subendothelial collagen [16]. They swell up and degranulate, releasing adenosine diphosphate (ADP) and serotonin. In the presence of fibrinogen the ADP causes rapid thrombocytic aggregation to form a *platelet thrombus.* The serotonin enhances the contraction which occurs in injured blood vessels. In small vessels, such as venules and capillaries, the formation of a platelet thrombus and the vascular constriction are sufficient to produce *hemostasis.* This explains the normal bleeding time in nonthrombocytopenic coagulation disorders, since only tiny vessels are punctured in performing this test.

coagulation

The *coagulation mechanism* is triggered by release of tissue thromboplastin into the injured blood vessel through the break in its endothelial surface. Activation of Stuart factor X initiates the *extrinsic system.* Exposed subendothelial collagen fibers act as an electronegative, wettable surface on which Hageman factor XII is transformed to its active form to begin the cascade of the *intrinsic system.* By both systems thrombin is evolved and a definitive fibrin clot develops. Thrombin also stimulates further platelet aggregation, the clumps becoming enmeshed in fibrin strands within the coagulum of blood.

1. Hemorrhagic Diseases

Hemorrhagic diatheses due to a deficiency or lack of every known coagulation factor, except calcium and the Hageman factor, have been described. Hypocalcemia does not result in bleeding because a plasma level of only 2.5 mg. of calcium per 100 ml. is needed for coagulation, and a level below 5 mg. is incompatible with life. *Hageman factor (factor XII) deficiency* is rare and surprisingly causes little or no evidence of a bleeding tendency even though the coagulation time is greatly prolonged. The Hageman factor is evidently necessary for clotting to occur at a normal rate in vitro, but *its absence does not interfere with coagulation in vivo in any detectable manner.* The Hageman factor is involved in the very earliest stages of the clotting process, and patients with deficiencies show impaired thromboplastin generation and prothrombin consumption.

LABORATORY TESTS:

An extensive battery of *laboratory tests* is used in the differential diagnosis of hemorrhagic diseases.

Coagulation time

The Lee-White *coagulation or clotting time* is determined by placing venous blood in two or three test tubes. The first tube is tilted every 30 seconds until clotting occurs, and the definitive end point is determined by timing clot formation in the second or third tube. The coagulation time is normally 8 to 15 minutes. It is *prolonged* in hemophilia, Christmas disease, plasma thromboplastin antecedent deficiency, Hageman factor deficiency, proaccelerin deficiency, and hypofibrinogenemia, and it is infinite in afibrinogenemia. The clotting time is *normal* in thrombocytopenia, because only small numbers of platelets are needed to initiate thromboplastin generation. The test is more sensitive when siliconized or Lusteroid tubes are used, the normal time with this technique being 25 to 40 minutes.

Bleeding time

The *bleeding time* is determined by needle puncture of the fingertip or ear lobe (normal bleeding time, 1 to 3 minutes) or by a tiny forearm incision with elevated venous pressure (normal bleeding time, 1 to 7 minutes), the time being measured until bleeding stops from the small wound. The bleeding time is *prolonged* in thrombocytopenia, thrombocythemia, and thrombocytopathic purpura, as well as pseudohemophilia. The prolongation is due to failure of formation of a platelet clot or to a vascular defect.

Capillary fragility test

The Rumpel-Leede *capillary fragility or tourniquet test* is performed by inflating a pressure cuff above the elbow to about 100 mm. of mercury for about 5 minutes. In a positive test, numerous petechiae appear on the flexor surface of the forearm. The test is usually *positive* in thrombocytopenia.

Prothrombin time

The *prothrombin time* is determined by adding tissue thromboplastin to recalcified oxalated plasma. The normal time for clotting to occur is 11 to 15 seconds. *Prolonged* prothrombin times are found in hypoprothrombinemia; proaccelerin, proconvertin, and Stuart factor deficiencies; hypofibrinogenemia (the time is infinite in afibrinogenemia); and bishydroxycoumarin therapy.

Clot retraction time

Clot retraction time is determined by periodic observation of clotted venous blood in a test tube. Retraction should begin at 1 hour and be complete within 24 hours. *Clot retraction is dependent on platelets,* so that impaired retraction occurs in thrombocytopenia and thrombocytopathic purpura.

Platelet count

A *platelet count* can be done by (1) the indirect method of Dameshek in which thrombocytes are counted relative to the number of erythrocytes in diluted blood (normal 400,000 to 800,000 per cubic millimeter), or (2) a direct method on a counting chamber using cresyl blue or phase microscopy (normal 150,000 to 300,000 per cubic millimeter). A decrease of platelets below 100,000 per cubic millimeter occurs in the thrombocytopenias.

Other differential tests include the *prothrombin consumption time,* the *partial thromboplastin time,* and the *thromboplastin generation test.*

THROMBOCYTOPENIC PURPURA:

Thrombocytopenic purpura is characterized by a deficiency or absence of platelets and may be primary or secondary. *Thrombocytopenia may be due to a decreased production of platelets, decreased life span of platelets* (normal survival time is 8 to 10 days), *dilution of platelets by the transfusion of platelet-poor blood, or unknown causes. Decreased production of platelets* results from: a decrease in or absence of megakaryocytes in the bone marrow, as in depression due to exposure to ionizing radiation or to toxic drugs and chemicals; infiltration of the marrow by abnormal cells as in leukemia, multiple myeloma, and metastatic carcinoma; or bone marrow depression during certain infections. A *decreased platelet life span* may be due to: the development of *antiplatelet antibodies,* as in primary thrombocytopenic purpura, thrombotic thrombocytopenic purpura, systemic lupus erythematosus, some hemolytic anemias, and sensitivity to certain drugs; and sequestration or excessive destruction or use of platelets, as in congestive splenomegaly and intravascular coagulation (e.g., amniotic fluid embolism). *Thrombocytopenia due to platelet dilution* occurs in multiple blood transfusions with stored blood. *Bleeding manifestations in thrombocytopenia* develop when the platelet count falls below 100,000 per cubic millimeter and are usually marked when levels are below 60,000.

Primary thrombocytopenic purpura: cause

Primary thrombocytopenic purpura (purpura hemorrhagica, Werlhof's disease) [18] is now thought to be *an auto-immune disease. Antiplatelet antibodies are found in about 60 percent* of the cases, and as many as 85 percent may be due to an immune mechanism. Transient thrombocytopenia has been found in the infants born of mothers with this disease, indicating the transplacental transference of a humoral substance into the fetal circulation. The spleen plays a causative role in this disease by destroying platelets coated by auto-antibodies and by producing these antibodies. Splenectomy leads to remission or cure in most cases.

clinical features

Clinically primary thrombocytopenic purpura is more common in women than in men by 3:1 and usually appears between the ages of 12 and 45. In numerous cases the disease has become manifest during pregnancy, and purpura has occurred cyclically during menstruation. There is purpura, and the *platelet count* is commonly reduced to below 50,000 per cubic millimeter. The bleeding time is prolonged, and the coagulation time is normal unless the platelets are reduced to an extremely low level. Clot retraction does not occur. There is increased capillary fragility, as shown by the Rumpel-Leede tourniquet test. *Platelet survival time* is strikingly reduced.

pathologic changes

Small hemorrhages occur in the skin, brain, and respiratory, gastrointestinal, and genitourinary mucosa. The *spleen* may be enlarged to 200 to 400 gm. Its germinal centers are large and active, and the sinusoids are nearly empty but may contain *"hyaline" megakaryocytes.* These lack cytoplasmic granules and show deficient platelet budding. Similar megakaryocytes are found in the *hepatic sinusoids.* In the *bone marrow* the number of megakaryocytes is usually increased, but many of them are immature forms.

Thrombotic thrombocytopenic purpura

Thrombotic thrombocytopenic purpura (Moschcowitz syndrome) is a rare and paradoxical entity characterized by purpura, a reduction in platelets, hemolytic anemia (an anemia in which there is destruction of erythrocytes), and the blocking of small arteries and arterioles by fibrin thrombi. The disease has an acute onset and is characterized by fever, petechiae, ecchymoses, and neurologic disturbances such as weakness, headaches, speech defects, paralysis, convulsions, confusion, hallucinations, and coma. Women are affected more frequently than men, and the *disease is usually rapidly fatal.* The *cause* is unknown but *appears to be a type of hypersensitivity reaction* which is sometimes due to drugs such as sulfonamides or penicillin. The thrombocytopenia is frequently explained by the utilization of large numbers of platelets in the many small thrombi; however, by the fluorescent antibody technique these thrombi have been shown to consist of fibrin and they give a negative reaction with antiplatelet antibodies. *Pathologically* multiple fibrin thrombi are found in small arteries, arterioles, and capillaries with surrounding hemorrhages. Changes are most severe in the kidneys, adrenals, liver, myocardium, and brain.

Hemolytic-uremic syndrome

Apparently related to but distinct from thrombotic thrombocytopenic purpura is the idiopathic *hemolytic-uremic syndrome* [19]. Most cases occur in children under 2 years of age. Usually following the sudden onset of vomiting and/or diarrhea, the child develops skin, gastrointestinal, or urinary bleeding, moderate hypertension, and severe pallor. A Coombs test (see page 283) negative hemolytic anemia is found, and most patients develop thrombocytopenia. Proteinuria and hematuria are present. *Bone marrow aspirations* disclose erythroid hyperplasia. *Renal biopsies* early reveal focal glomerular necrosis, fibrin microthrombi in some glomerular capillaries, and numerous erythrocyte and hemoglobin casts within tubules. In fatal cases (the mortality rate is about 25 percent) the *kidneys* show patchy to almost complete bilateral cortical necrosis.

Secondary thrombocytopenic purpura

Secondary thrombocytopenic purpura is caused by a very large number of therapeutic agents. *Drugs which produce thrombocytopenia by direct depression of the production of platelets in the bone marrow* include: cancer chemotherapeutic agents such as nitrogen mustard, cyclophosphamide, folic acid antagonists, 6-mercaptopurine, 5-fluorouracil, and urethane; antibiotics such as streptomycin and chloramphenicol; sulfonamides such as sulfamethoxypyridazine; arsphenamine and other organic arsenicals; barbiturates; anticonvulsants such as methyl phenyl ethyl hydantoin (Mesantoin) and phenylacetylurea; tranquilizers such as meprobamate; and methimazole. *Drugs which produce thrombocytopenia by decreasing the life span of platelets* through the development of an immune mechanism include: quinine and quinidine, the diuretics chlorothiazide and hydrochlorothiazide, sulfonamides such as acetazolamide, the hypoglycemic drug chlorpropamide, and the antihistaminics diphenhydramine and chlorpheniramine.

Thrombocytopenic purpura also occurs in the leukemias, metastatic carcinoma in bone marrow, aplastic anemia, benzene poisoning, radiation therapy, or chronic infection. In all of these, platelet formation is interfered with by direct invasion of the bone marrow or by marrow hypoplasia caused by the action of toxins.

THROMBOCYTHEMIA

Bleeding manifestations occur not only with thrombocytopenia but also with *thrombocythemia,* in which the number of platelets is above 600,000 per cubic millimeter, and in the *thrombocytopathies,* in which the platelets are present in normal numbers but are functionally defective. *Thrombocythemia* [20] may occur as a primary disease, but is more often a feature of polycythemia vera, in which the erythrocytes are abnormally increased in number, in chronic myelogenous leukemia, and following splenectomy (operative removal of the spleen). *About 75 percent of patients with thrombocythemia develop hemorrhagic manifestations* such as epistaxes and gingival and gastrointestinal bleeding. Cutaneous petechiae and ecchymoses are rare. Patients with thrombocythemia also have a tendency to thrombosis which is possibly related to the increased viscosity of the blood. In thrombocythemia the bleeding time is greatly prolonged, while the clotting time and other tests are normal.

THROMBOCYTOPATHIC PURPURA

Thrombocytopathic purpura may manifest itself by impaired clot retraction or impaired blood clotting. Both types are rare. The platelets often appear abnormal on blood smears, and bizarre or giant forms are common. They frequently do not form the clusters usually seen in normal blood smears. In both forms the bleeding time is prolonged. Thrombocytopathic purpura with impaired blood clotting is familial, and fatal bleeding is relatively common.

HEMOPHILIA:

Hemophilia is inherited as a recessive sex-linked characteristic, occurs almost always in males, and is *due to a congenital deficiency of antihemophilic globulin.* It occurs about five times as frequently as Christmas disease. In hemophilia the coagulation time is prolonged and the bleeding time normal. Clot retraction is prompt, once coagulation occurs.

Pathologic changes

There is *excessive* and sometimes fatal *bleeding from minor wounds as well as spontaneous hemorrhages* in the gums, gastrointestinal tract, and joints *(hemarthroses).* Hemarthroses occur in about half the cases – the knees, ankles, and elbows being most frequently involved. Hyperplasia of the synovial lining may lead to the formation of a vascular pannus. Erosion and thinning of the joint cartilage and small cyst formation in the cartilage and adjacent bone sometimes occur, and these changes may lead to limitation of motion and deformity of the affected joint.

VASCULAR HEMOPHILIA

Vascular hemophilia (pseudohemophilia, von Willebrand's disease) is a hereditary bleeding disease *transmitted as an autosomal dominant.* It is probably the most common widespread bleeding disorder, but because its manifestations are very mild and its diagnostic features ill defined, most cases are never identified [21]. The bleeding time is prolonged, and the tourniquet test is mildly positive. The coagulation time is normal. The antihemophilic globulin level is usually low, and platelet adhesiveness is decreased. The *bleeding is capillary in type* and usually begins in childhood. There are easy bruising, repeated epistaxes, bleeding from the gums and other mucous membranes, excessive bleeding from small wounds, and menorrhagia.

PTC DEFICIENCY

Plasma thromboplastin component deficiency (Christmas disease) is a hemophilioid state due to the absence of the Christmas factor of the thromboplastin generating system. It is rare, occurs almost always in males, and has a sex-linked recessive transmission. Distinction from hemophilia is made by the thromboplastin generation test. *Excessive bleeding* occurs from wounds such as tooth extractions.

PTA DEFICIENCY

Plasma thromboplastin antecedent (factor XI) deficiency is rare and is apparently transmitted as an autosomal dominant. Bleeding is usually mild and follows tooth extractions and surgery.

PROACCELERIN DEFICIENCY

Proaccelerin (factor V, labile factor) deficiency may be hereditary *(parahemophilia)* or acquired due to hepatic disease. Hereditary factor V deficiency is uncommon and may be associated with hemophilia [22]. *Bleeding is mainly capillary in type* and includes spontaneous mucous membrane hemorrhages, epistaxes, and menorrhagia. Prolonged bleeding following tooth extractions and other surgical procedures and easy bruising are common. The prothrombin time is markedly prolonged, and the coagulation time is increased. Bleeding begins when the concentration of factor V is reduced to 30 percent of normal, and in severe deficiencies little or no proaccelerin is detectable in the plasma.

PROCONVERTIN DEFICIENCY

Proconvertin (factor VII) deficiency is transmitted as a highly penetrant, incomplete autosomal recessive. It occurs in both sexes. Bleeding is usually mild.

HYPOPROTHROMBINEMIA

Hypoprothrombinemia is due to vitamin K deficiency, bishydroxycoumarin administration, or severe liver disease. Spontaneous *hemorrhages* occur in the skin, the gastrointestinal and genitourinary mucosa, and the brain in the newborn infant.

STUART FACTOR DEFICIENCY

Stuart factor (factor X) deficiency is rare and is inherited as an autosomal recessive. The clinical manifestations are mild in heterozygous patients. However, in homozygotes with a marked deficiency of factor X, there is severe bleeding in the form of epistaxes, hematomas following mild trauma, and hemarthroses.

AFIBRINOGENEMIA

Afibrinogenemia is an absence or a deficiency of fibrinogen *(factor I).* Normally there is 0.2 to 0.4 gm. of fibrinogen per 100 ml. of plasma. In afibrinogenemia the blood is completely incoagulable. The erythrocyte sedimentation rate is very slow. The disease is rare, has no sex predilection, and is usually congenital. The *congenital type* is probably transmitted by a recessive gene. The *acquired (secondary) type* appears in cases of severe liver disease and of carcinoma (epithelial cancer) with widespread bone marrow replacement.

Pathologic changes

In infants uncontrollable bleeding may occur from the umbilicus. Later, excessive bleeding may appear following minor trauma or the eruption of teeth. *In acquired cases* severe bleeding has sometimes followed surgery or delivery.

FIBRIN-STABILIZING FACTOR DEFICIENCY

Fibrin-stabilizing factor (factor XIII) deficiency [23] is rare; it is transmitted as an autosomal recessive. In its activated form factor XIII acts as a transpeptidase, so that firm peptide bonds are formed between fibrin molecules. When FSF is deficient, fibrin clot formation is defective. Bleeding is severe, almost always beginning as massive bleeding from the umbilical stump.

CONSUMPTION COAGULOPATHIES

The *consumption coagulopathies* [24] are a group of disorders characterized by bleeding resulting from the using up of coagulation factors by excessive intravascular clotting. They develop in a variety of situations. In the human equivalent of the *Sanarelli-Shwartzman phenomenon,* which occurs in septicemia due to gram-negative bacteria, widespread intracapillary fibrin thrombosis is triggered by activation of Hageman factor and the release of thromboplastin. The latter also initiates disseminated intravascular clotting in premature placental separation; *amniotic fluid embolism* (see page 44); injection of *certain snake venoms,* such as that of the viper; and in the *hemolytic-uremic syndrome.* In the consumption coagulopathies various hemorrhagic phenomena occur. The platelet count and the blood levels of proaccelerin, antihemophilic globulin, prothrombin, and fibrinogen are low.

2. *Thrombolysis*

Thrombolysis [25] is the dissolution of a fibrin clot and takes place by the action of fibrinolytic enzymes. *Plasminogen (profibrinolysin)* is a proenzyme which in the presence of certain activators is converted to *plasmin (fibrinolysin),* an active proteolytic enzyme capable of lysing fibrin clots and certain plasma proteins. Three different plasmins (alpha, beta, and gamma) have been postulated. *Plasminogen activators include streptokinase,* a protein derived from beta-hemolytic streptococci; *staphylokinase,* from filtrates of staphylococcal cultures; *urokinase,* normally present in urine; tissue activators in the microsomes of the cells of the uterus, prostate, and other organs; *a blood activator;* and pharmacologic agents such as nicotinic acid and thrombin-E (esterase-thrombin). Only the fibrin of recent thrombi and emboli are susceptible to lysis. Coagula older than 72 hours cannot be dissolved. Fibrinolytic system inhibitors are present in the plasma as antiplasmins and activator inhibitors. The streptokinase inhibitor is an antibody. Platelets are carriers of antiplasmin, and the increased fibrinolytic activity in cases of thrombocytopenic bleeding may be related to a deficiency of platelet antiplasmin or to the release from degenerating platelets of a plasminogen activator [26].

3. *Thrombosis*

Thrombosis is the formation of a coagulum of blood (thrombus) within the lumen of a vessel or the heart during life. Thrombi consist of platelets, fibrin, erythrocytes, and leukocytes, the relative proportion of each depending on the rate of thrombus formation and the surrounding conditions. A *white thrombus* consisting of platelets enmeshed in fibrin forms when the rates of blood flow and thrombosis are slow. A *red thrombus* contains much fibrin and many red corpuscles. *Lines of Zahn* are pale and consist of agglutinated platelets in a fibrin meshwork. They alternate with masses of erythrocytes, leukocytes, and fibrin to give the thrombus a corrugated appearance.

Mechanism

Thrombosis is initiated by the adherence of platelets to the vessel wall. A mass of agglutinated and fused platelets builds up *(conglutination thrombus).* When this mass becomes sufficiently large to alter the blood flow past it, a fibrin coagulum containing erythrocytes and leukocytes forms on its surface *(coagulation thrombus).* In this way the laminated thrombus with its alternating pale and dark zones is constructed. The *propagation* of a thrombus is its extension along a vessel, usually a vein, by continued laying down of the constituents of the thrombus. Propagation usually occurs in the direction of blood flow, but may extend in the opposite direction if the vessel is occluded.

Causes:

The *basic causes* of thrombosis are injury, inflammation, or degeneration of a blood vessel wall; slowing, stasis, or eddying of the blood flow; and increased coagulability of the blood.

blood vessel injury, inflammation, or degeneration

Blood vessel injury may be due to mechanical trauma, such as fractures and bullet or knife wounds; ligation or clamping during surgery; strenuous muscular exercise; burns (toxins may also be involved); and cold (stasis may also be involved). *Blood vessel inflammation* occurs in thrombophlebitis, in which clotting occurs within veins, especially in those of the lower extremities; thromboangiitis obliterans, an inflammation of the arteries and veins, particularly of the extremities; periarteritis nodosa, a hypersensitivity reaction in medium-sized arteries in various organs; and in foci of acute inflammation (see Chapter 3). *Septic thrombosis* occurs when an infectious process invades the vessel and extends into the thrombus. Infected thrombi tend to soften, liquefy, and disintegrate. Septic thrombosis of the pelvic and iliac vessels is common in puerperal sepsis. Infections of the face, nose, or orbit may lead to septic cavernous sinus thrombosis. Septic thrombosis of the portal vein (pylephlebitis) may follow appendicitis or other abdominal infections. *Blood vessel degeneration* develops in the arteries, veins, or heart. Arterial degeneration occurs as *atherosclerosis,* with hyalin and lipid deposits and calcification in the intima. Thrombi frequently form on atherosclerotic plaques at the zone of initial degeneration. Such thrombi seldom become large, because of the swiftness of the blood flow in arteries. Atheromatous plaques in large vessels may be produced by the organization of thrombi. In veins *phlebosclerosis* occurs, with hyaline thickening of the intima; thrombosis may occur on the roughened endothelium. In the heart, principally in the left ventricle, mural thrombosis frequently occurs on the endocardium overlying a myocardial infarct.

stasis or eddying of blood

Slowing or eddying of the blood in an auricular appendage, such as in auricular fibrillation, often leads to thrombosis. Such a thrombus as well as a mural one may become pedunculated and act as a *ball-valve thrombus.* Thrombosis may also occur in an aneurysmal sac due to eddying within the bulged-out portion of the vessel. Varicose (dilated and tortuous) veins, especially in the pampiniform plexus (varicocele) or in the perirectal veins (hemorrhoids), are common sites of thrombosis due to slowing or stasis of the blood flow within them. Postoperatively thrombosis often occurs in vessels that have been ligated, because of stasis and damage to the vessel wall. More commonly postoperative thrombosis is due to inactivity, occurring most frequently in the calf and thigh veins. Thrombosis occurring without precedent alteration in a vein wall is *phlebothrombosis* and is usually due to slowing or stasis of the blood within the vein. Pressure of a space-occupying mass or of a fetus on veins produces slowing of the venous flow distally, and thrombosis sometimes follows. The general circulatory slowing in congestive heart failure, together with the inactivity of the cardiac patient, is accompanied by a tendency to venous thrombosis.

increased coagulability

Increased coagulability of the blood is caused by the discharge of epinephrine after fright, wounds, burns, or hemorrhages, due to an increase in blood viscosity; by certain snake venoms such as that of Russell's viper; and by foreign sera. A migratory phlebothrombosis complicates some cases of abdominal (especially pancreatic) cancer, due to increased coagulability of the blood. In pancreatic cancer this is probably due to the thromboplastin-like activity of released trypsin.

Pathologic changes

Occlusion of a vein produces stasis in the area drained, causing acute passive hyperemia or even necrosis of the involved tissues. Thrombosis of a mesenteric vein often causes gangrene of the intestine, and thrombosed varicose veins in the thigh may lead to ulceration *(varicose ulcer). Occlusion of an artery* causes ischemia of the tissue supplied. Unless collateral circulation is present and adequate, infarction will follow. If the thrombus becomes detached and free in the circulation, it is known as an *embolus.* Some thrombi are removed by lysis. If a thrombus remains attached and the organism survives, it becomes organized from the lining of the vessel [27]. Capillaries bud into the thrombotic mass, fibroblasts proliferate, and gradually the thrombus is replaced. New vascular channels develop through it *(recanalization)* or the mass becomes fibrous. A phlebolith results if this scar becomes calcified in a vein.

Agonal clots

Agonal clots occur in the heart usually just before death. They show a mixture of the elements of antemortem thrombi and postmortem clots and are loosely adherent to the endocardium. In persons dying gradually, adherent agonal thrombi may form along the valve cusps in the heart and resemble vegetations *(terminal endocardiosis,* nonbacterial endocarditis). This condition occurs most often in patients with types of cancer in which the malignant cells secrete mucin [28]. Usually the thrombi are of no clinical significance. However, they occasionally form days or weeks before death, and portions may break off to become arterial emboli.

Postmortem clots

After death, blood in the heart and great vessels usually clots. If coagulation is prompt and rapid, the clots are dark red and homogeneous *(currant-jelly clots).* If clotting is slow, plasma and red cells separate, producing a clot with a deep red lower layer and pale yellow upper portion *(chicken-fat clot). Postmortem clots* are moist, tough, homogeneous (as compared to the laminated antemortem thrombus), and easily removed from the vessels (as contrasted with the often firmly adherent thrombus). No lines of Zahn are present in the postmortem clot.

EMBOLISM, INFARCTION, AND GANGRENE

EMBOLISM:

Embolism is the lodging of an embolus in a blood vessel at a point beyond which it cannot pass. An *embolus* is a foreign substance such as a thrombus or fragments of a thrombus, tissue cells, clumps of bacteria, parasites, globules of fat, or bubbles or gas carried in the bloodstream. Fragments of or entire thrombi are the most common type of emboli. Movement or manipulation of the thrombosed part may produce detachment of the thrombus, and thus embolism. *Venous emboli* originate in the peripheral veins and almost always lodge in a pulmonary artery, producing infarction of a lung, or sudden death in cases of massive embolism. Venous emboli are more common than arterial emboli, so that embolism in the pulmonary circulation is more frequent than in the peripheral circulation.

Pulmonary embolism

Pulmonary embolism is a fairly common sequela of congestive heart failure, surgery, and obstetric delivery. It occurs in about 1 percent of hospital patients and causes 5 percent of postoperative deaths and 1 maternal fatality in about every 50,000 deliveries. Pulmonary embolism causes about 30,000 deaths annually in the United States and is found in about 10 percent of adult autopsies. However, the clinical diagnosis is made in only 20 to 50 percent of the cases in which it is discovered at autopsy. In over 90 percent of the cases pulmonary emboli arise in veins of the lower extremities, especially the deep calf veins; less often the pelvic veins are the foci of origin. Small or large thrombi break off from a site of phlebothrombosis and are carried in the venous bloodstream up the inferior vena cava and through the right side of the heart into the pulmonary arterial circulation, where they impact. Embolism is more common in the right pulmonary artery and its branches than in the left. When a *large embolus* is suddenly jammed into the main pulmonary artery or is impacted astride the bifurcation to block both great pulmonary trunks *(saddle embolus),* the pulmonary circulation is completely obstructed and an enormous strain is immediately placed on the right ventricle. There is a rapid rise in the pulmonary arterial pressure proximal to the block, and the right ventricle and atrium become dilated (acute cor pulmonale). *Death* usually ensues within a few minutes due to the profound shock resulting from the failure of venous return to the left side of the heart. A *shower of small emboli* which lodge in numerous pulmonary arterial branches may produce similar results. In this case the pulmonary hypertension appears to be due to arterial spasm caused by a reflex mediated through efferent fibers of the vagus nerve [29].

In healthy young individuals who survive the initial insult of pulmonary embolism, ischemic necrosis generally does not occur in the lung unless the embolus is large. Infarction is prevented by the continuous oxygen exchange in the lung and the terminal anastomoses between the pulmonary and bronchial arteries. However, in individuals with any significant deficiency in pulmonary or cardiac function, *infarction of the lung* will occur following pulmonary embolism if the patient survives for several hours. In nonfatal cases of pulmonary embolism the greater part of the impacted thrombotic material is often completely lysed; the undissolved portion becomes organized into a small fibrous intimal plaque. Some pulmonary arterial atheromatous plaques consisting of hyalinized fibrous tissue with cholesterol deposits arise by the organization of emboli. Occasionally the end result of the organization of a pulmonary thromboembolus is the formation of an intra-arterial fibrous cord, band, or web [30]. Such structures are found most commonly in primary, secondary, and tertiary pulmonary arterial branches and rarely in the main pulmonary arteries. The cords and bands are typically covered by endothelium and are attached to the arterial wall at both ends.

Arterial embolism

Arterial emboli originate from the left side of the heart (auricular appendage, ventricular mural thrombus, or vegetative thrombus on the mitral or aortic valve), an aneurysmal sac, an atheromatous plaque on a large arterial trunk, or, rarely, the pulmonary veins. The effects of arterial emboli depend on the size and nature of the embolus, the organ involved, and the state of collateral circulation. If collateral circulation is absent or deficient, an embolus of any size will produce infarction in the heart, brain, spleen, intestine, kidney, or an extremity.

Paradoxical embolism

Paradoxical embolism results when a venous embolus enters the arterial circulation through a patent foramen ovale or other septal defect.

Septic embolism

Septic (mycotic) embolism is the lodgment of infected foreign material in a blood vessel. Masses of bacteria, usually within a septic embolus, are carried in the bloodstream. Septic infarcts or abscesses (localized collections of pus) are produced where the emboli lodge. In some cases necrosis of the artery in which the infected embolus lodges leads to thinning and outpouching of the wall *(mycotic aneurysm).*

Fat embolism: causes

Neutral fats from injured tissue or the bone marrow, or injected fats and oils, may act as *fat emboli,* obstructing capillaries in the lungs, brain, and elsewhere. *Most cases follow fractures* or other trauma to fat. Fat embolism also occurs in cases of fatty liver in acute and chronic alcoholism, carbon tetrachloride poisoning and diabetes mellitus, and in decompression sickness.

pathogenesis [31]

Fat embolism occurs when lipid globules 10 to 15 microns in diameter are present in the circulating blood. *Exogenous embolism* occurs when oily liquids are accidentally introduced into the blood and lymph streams during diagnostic or therapeutic procedures. Most fat embolism is *endogenous* in type. Because the *classic mechanical theory* of the entrance of free fat into the blood or lymph stream secondary to tearing of small vessels in fractured bones or areas of trauma to fat does not explain all features of fat embolism, it has been proposed that the fat emboli arise intravascularly rather than from extravascular adipose tissue. It has been postulated that *fat emboli may arise from the loss of stability within the emulsion of chylomicrons of fat* normally measuring 1 to 7μ in diameter *in the venous blood* with a resulting coalescence of fat to form larger globules. This would explain the development of fat embolism in cases without trauma, which occur in influenzal pneumonia and fatty liver associated with diabetes mellitus, acute and chronic alcoholism, and poisons such as carbon tetrachloride.

embolic phase

Fat embolism has been divided into four phases. In the *embolic phase* large globules of fat reach the pulmonary circulation, occluding arterioles and capillaries. If a large number of small vessels are blocked, the pulmonary arterial pressure rises, and acute right heart failure may occur. The patient shows dyspnea, tachypnea, tachycardia, and cyanosis. Peripheral vascular collapse due to a decreased left ventricular output and shock ensue. Death may occur within a short time as a result of the massive pulmonary capillary embolism. Some of the fat globules in the pulmonary circulation will pass through the capillaries in the *ameboid phase.* These globules enter the arterial circulation through the left heart and are carried to the coronary, cerebral, and renal arteries mainly. The *enzymatic phase* develops on the second or third day. A rise in serum lipase breaks down the only slightly toxic neutral fat to highly irritating free fatty acids. Unsaturated fatty acids disrupt the capillary endothelium, producing intra-alveolar hemorrhages and an acute inflammatory reaction in the lungs and petechiae in the brain and skin. Small hemorrhages are especially common in the axillae and over the chest wall. In the lungs a *chemical pneumonitis* with fever, chest pain, cough, dyspnea, and tachypnea develops. The x-ray picture of the

ameboid phase

enzymatic phase

lungs resembles a snowstorm. *Cerebral fat embolism* produces confusion, restlessness, excitement, convulsions, and/or coma. Free fat may be found in the urine when emboli reach the kidneys. There is a progressive drop in the hemoglobin level throughout the clinical course of fat embolism. The fourth phase is characterized by *death or recovery.* If the patient survives, marked improvement – presumably due to the unsludging of the pulmonary capillaries by enzymatic breakdown of fat – occurs after about a week.

fourth phase

pathologic changes

In fatal cases of fat embolism the *lungs* are heavy due to marked congestion. *Microscopically* in frozen sections fat particles can be distinguished in capillaries by special stains such as Sudan IV. When the *brain* is involved, there are petechiae in the meninges and throughout the brain. Fat globules can be identified in the capillaries. Areas of softening are seen microscopically. No pathologic changes occur in the kidneys, although fat may often be seen in the glomeruli.

Bone marrow embolism

Bone marrow embolism in the pulmonary arterial circulation occurs most commonly in fractures, but has been reported in cases of "medullary fracture" from bony "concussion" during surgical manipulation and closed chest cardiac massage [32]; sternal marrow puncture [33]; sickle cell anemia and hemoglobin-C disease secondary to small infarcts of the bone marrow; and convulsive states such as eclampsia, tetanus, and electroshock therapy. Such embolism is uncommon and is rarely massive enough to be the primary cause of death. In this type of embolism masses of bone marrow containing hematopoietic elements and fat cells are found in small pulmonary arteries.

Calcium embolism

Calcium embolism occurs occasionally in the cerebral and other arteries. It is due to the dislodging of calcified material from a valve during cardiac surgery or to *atheromatous embolism.* The latter is due to the spontaneous breaking off of an atheromatous plaque, usually from the intima of the aorta. A foreign body reaction is produced about the artery in which it lodges, due to the cholesterol in the plaque. Either type of calcium embolism may produce infarction in the tissue supplied by the occluded artery.

Neoplastic cell embolism

Neoplastic cell embolism is a means of spread in cancer. Malignant cells in a neoplasm (an uncontrolled new growth of tissue) invade lymphatic vessels or venules. They are carried in the lymph or blood and lodge in the sinusoids of a lymph node or the capillaries of an organ, often the lung or liver. Metastases (malignant growths at a distance from the primary neoplasm) may develop where the cells impact. In some cases a large *neoplastic cell thrombus* may fill a vein such as the renal or portal vein or inferior vena cava. Neoplastic cell embolism is discussed in detail on page 336.

Amniotic fluid embolism

Amniotic fluid embolism [34] is rare. It characteristically occurs during a difficult labor, amniotic fluid entering the maternal circulation through a tear in the fetal membranes, with dissection of fluid between the membranes and uterine wall to enter the venous sinuses. Emboli consisting of squamous cells, vernix caseosa, mucin, and meconium impact in the small pulmonary arterioles and capillaries of the mother. *Clinically,* when amniotic fluid reaches the pulmonary circulation in significant amounts, there are chilliness, hyperpnea, and cyanosis. Shock and acute pulmonary edema follow. Convulsions due to cerebral anoxia are common. Death usually occurs within 2 to 3 hours. It is probable that, besides the mechanical obstruction of pulmonary circulation by the amniotic fluid contents, *reflex vasospasm* occurs in nonoccluded arterioles due to an anaphylactoid reaction. Mechanical and spastic obstruction of the pulmonary circulation produces a sudden drop in blood flow to the left heart, and peripheral vascular collapse develops rapidly because of the reduced left ventricular output. The *consumption coagulopathy* which has been reported in a number of cases of amniotic fluid embolism may be due to increased plasma fibrinolytic activity, as well as to the depletion of fibrinogen in intravascular clotting initiated by increased thromboplastic activity. The release of a heparin-like substance in amniotic fluid may also be a factor in the coagulation disorder by blocking the conversion of prothrombin to thrombin.

Air embolism

Air embolism results when air is drawn or forced into the circulation as into the jugular vein during neck surgery, uterine veins during a criminal abortion, and during pneumothorax. The air tends to lodge in the right ventricle, mixing with blood and producing a frothy mass which obstructs blood flow. At autopsy in suspected cases the great vessels should be tied and the heart opened under water to determine whether bubbles of air are present.

Aeroembolism

Aeroembolism refers to the presence of tiny bubbles of gas, especially nitrogen, in the bloodstream. The nitrogen is released by sudden lowering of the air pressure such as may occur in the raising of divers *(bends),* the decompressing of workers in tunnels *(caisson disease),* or the rapid ascent of fliers to high altitudes. The gas comes out of solution in the blood and lodges in the capillaries of the heart, lungs, muscles, and bones, producing severe pain. Infarcts of bone may occur.

Miscellaneous forms of embolism

Other forms of embolism include the impaction in the pulmonary circulation of a segment of skin after a venipuncture [35]; fragments of brain tissue, following severe head injury [36]; liver tissue or bile after hepatic trauma [37]; bile thrombi from the liver in cases of biliary obstruction [38]; polyethylene catheters used for venous infusions; cotton fibers and green soap introduced into uterine venous sinuses during criminal abortions [39]; silicone antifoam from pump oxygenators used in open-heart surgery (with entrance of emboli into the arterial circulation to produce small cerebral infarcts and reduced renal function) [40]; barium sulfate used as a contrast medium for radiologic studies [41]; and gastric contents following rupture of the stomach [42].

INFARCTION:

Infarction is the production of an infarct, a local focus of necrosis resulting from vascular obstruction. When an artery is occluded suddenly, cell death occurs in the tissues supplied by it. The vessels and capillaries deprived of blood later dilate and fill with blood from surrounding anastomoses. A fresh infarct is therefore dark and congested. The capillary walls break down, and hemorrhage occurs into the affected tissue. In soft organs, such as the lungs and intestines, *hemorrhagic infarcts* occur. In a firm organ, such as the kidney, swelling of parenchymal cells presses the blood out of small vessels so that a *pale (anemic) infarct* occurs. This area is surrounded by a hemorrhagic zone.

Pathologic changes

Infarcts correspond roughly in size and shape to the distribution of the occluded artery. They are usually pyramidal or conical in shape, with the base toward the periphery of the organ. *Fresh infarcts* are swollen, congested or pale, and have sharply defined, hyperemic margins. *Microscopically* the hyperemic zone is infiltrated with polymorphonuclear leukocytes. The infarct is hemorrhagic or shows ghostly outlines of tissue in a stage of coagulation necrosis.

Infarction of the lung:

Infarction of the lung results from occlusion of a branch of the pulmonary artery from either thrombosis or embolism. However, a large embolus occluding the main pulmonary artery or lodged in the right or left pulmonary artery usually causes almost immediate death without infarction.

clinical features

Clinically pulmonary infarction is characterized by a sudden, sharp chest pain which later localizes over the infarct and is worsened by deep inspiration, a pleural friction rub due to fibrin, hemoptysis, fever, tachycardia, and dyspnea. Pleural effusion sometimes develops, and with large infarcts in cases of congestive failure there may be a slight jaundice. *A significant rise in the serum lactic dehydrogenase (LDH) activity* has been found in cases of pulmonary embolism and infarction. Increased serum LDH and bilirubin concentrations in patients with a normal serum glutamic oxalacetic transaminase (SGOT) level are valuable aids in differentiating pulmonary infarction from acute myocardial infarction and pneumonia [43]. The elevated bilirubin results from the breakdown of hemoglobin pigments in the hemorrhagic infarct. After about 24 hours the infarct appears on an x-ray film of the chest as a wedge-shaped subpleural area of increased density.

pathologic changes

The *pulmonary infarct* is dark red and pyramidal with its base at the pleura. Early it is moist, blood oozing from the cut surface. By the second day it is dry and firm. Organization begins at the margins, and after several weeks the infarct is replaced by a pigmented scar. The thrombus or embolus which caused the infarct becomes recanalized and eventually is converted into fibrous bands within the artery.

Infarction of the myocardium

Infarction of the myocardium results from coronary artery occlusion, usually by thrombosis. Blockage of a large artery often causes sudden death without producing a myocardial infarct. This important condition is discussed in detail on page 428.

Infarction of the kidney:

Infarcts of the kidneys are caused by emboli arising in the left auricular appendage, a mural thrombus in the left ventricle, a vegetation on a mitral or aortic valve in endocarditis, or an aortic aneurysmal sac. *Clinically* there is a sudden onset of costovertebral angle pain and tenderness. Showers of erythrocytes appear grossly or microscopically in the urine.

pathologic changes

The infarct is pale with a surrounding zone of hyperemia infiltrated with polymorphonuclear leukocytes. Because of the capsular vessels, a thin zone of tissue beneath the capsule is often spared. Old infarcts appear as dense contracted scars.

Infarction of the spleen:

Infarcts of the spleen may be either pale or hemorrhagic, the large ones tending to be pale. Emboli entering the splenic artery arise from the same sources as those causing renal infarcts. Infarcts are common in cases of leukemia and polycythemia vera due to splenic artery thrombosis resulting from increased blood viscosity.

clinical features

Clinically the only sign of splenic infarction is a sudden sharp pain in the left upper quadrant of the abdomen, typically in a patient with evidence of a bacterial endocarditis, a recent myocardial infarct (with mural thrombosis), auricular fibrillation, or an aortic aneurysm.

Infarction of the intestines:

Infarction of the small or large intestine may result from embolism or thrombosis in a mesenteric artery or vein, or from compression of a vein by pressure or twisting. About 90 percent of the occlusions occur in the superior mesenteric artery or vein and its tributaries. In most of these cases the occlusion is in the superior mesenteric artery. Thrombotic and even embolic obstruction of mesenteric arterial branches can occur without producing intestinal infarction [44]. On the other hand, extensive intestinal infarction can occur without mesenteric vascular occlusion in cases of aortic valvular insufficiency, presumably on the basis of decreased mesenteric circulation resulting from lowered aortic blood pressure [45]. Focal infarction of the small intestine and colon has been observed as a terminal event in patients in shock who have received extensive vasopressor therapy, such as levarterenol, due to an arteriolar constriction. *Ischemic changes in the intestine* are common in prolonged shock because of the stagnant hypoxia which results from a markedly decreased mesenteric arterial flow. Large amounts of 5-hydroxytryptamine (5-HT) are released from the ischemic bowel, and bacteria enter the devitalized intestinal wall. The entrance of 5-HT and bacteria into the bloodstream is an important factor in the production of the systemic effects of shock [46].

clinical features

Clinically mesenteric vascular occlusion is more common in men than in women by about 3:1 and is most frequent in the 40 to 60 age group. Embolism is most common in patients with auricular fibrillation. Arterial thrombosis is usually associated with atherosclerosis, especially in diabetic patients. Venous thrombosis is most often a sequela of upper abdominal surgery. When intestinal infarction occurs, there is an acute onset of severe abdominal pain with nausea, vomiting, and sometimes bloody diarrhea. Profound shock ensues and bowel sounds are decreased in intensity or absent.

pathologic changes

Early the *infarcted segment of intestine,* commonly the entire jejunum, ileum, and ascending colon, is extremely congested and edematous. Later the infarct becomes gangrenous, being dark green to reddish black. The intestinal wall is markedly hemorrhagic, and its structure is destroyed. There is hemorrhage into the lumen. Within a day the serosa becomes dull and covered with a fibrinous or fibrinopurulent exudate due to bacterial invasion of the wall.

Extremity arterial occlusion

Occlusion of an artery to an extremity, usually a lower extremity, is due to arterial embolism, thrombosis, or sclerosis; it results in dry gangrene unless the collateral circulation is sufficient, as it frequently is in the upper extremities.

Cerebral infarction

Infarction of the brain is due to thrombosis or embolism in a cerebral or cerebellar artery. The affected portion of the brain becomes soft and creamy, undergoing liquefactive necrosis. Cerebral infarction is discussed in detail on page 696.

Septic infarction

Septic infarction results from embolism of an infected thrombus. Such thrombi often fragment and produce multiple emboli and infarcts. Valvular vegetations in acute bacterial endocarditis are the most common source of septic emboli, the infarcts developing most frequently in the spleen and kidneys.

GANGRENE:

Gangrene is a massive necrosis of tissue with superadded putrefaction, due to the action of saprophytic bacteria. The blackening of gangrenous areas is due to the action of the saprophytic organisms on blood, black ferrous sulfide being produced by the breakdown of hemoglobin.

Dry gangrene:

Dry gangrene results from occlusion of a large artery. It is most common in the extremities. The occlusion may be due to embolism, thrombosis, arteriosclerosis *(senile gangrene)*, diabetes mellitus associated with arteriosclerosis *(diabetic gangrene)*, thromboangiitis obliterans, or spasm (as in small arteries of the hand in Raynaud's disease and chronic ergot poisoning). Strong caustic acids produce dry gangrene by direct contact.

pathologic changes

Dry gangrene develops slowly because of the difficulty of bacterial growth in ischemic tissue. The affected part becomes black and mummified. At the level of separation of gangrenous and viable tissue there is a zone of inflammatory granulation tissue. In the gangrenous tissue there is a complete loss of all structure.

Moist gangrene:

Moist (wet) gangrene usually occurs in internal organs (lungs, intestines, uterus). It develops rapidly and is often due to blockage of first the venous and later the arterial supply to a part by twisting or strangulation, as in a hernia. In moist tissues such as the intestines this type of gangrene follows arterial or venous occlusion, as in mesenteric embolism or thrombosis. Strong caustic alkalis may produce liquefaction and moist gangrene by direct contact.

pathologic changes

The gangrenous tissue is reddish or purplish black and foul-smelling. It is partly liquefied, and gas may be produced. No definite line of demarcation between gangrenous and viable tissue develops, as in dry gangrene. Moist gangrene may be superimposed on inflammation due to thrombosis of small vessels, as in *gangrenous appendicitis.*

Gas gangrene is discussed with the Acute Bacterial Infections on page 93.

REFERENCES

1. Roberts, W. C. Hepatic-cell pigment in congestive heart failure. *Arch. Path.* (Chicago) 82:566, 1966.
2. Schirger, A., Harrison, E. G., Jr., and Janes, J. M. Idiopathic lymphedema. *J.A.M.A.* 182:14, 1962.
3. Movat, H. Z., and Fernando, N. V. P. Acute inflammation. The earliest fine structural changes at the blood-tissue barrier. *Lab. Invest.* 12:895, 1963.
4. Schick, B., and Greenbaum, J. W. Edema with hypoproteinemia due to a congenital defect in protein formation. *J. Pediat.* 27:241, 1945.
5. Paul, O., Vawter, G. F., Schweitzer, A. W., and Hass, G. M. Pathological changes in congestive heart failure. *A.M.A. Arch. Path.* 64:363, 1957.
6. Moore, F. D. The effects of hemorrhage on body constitution. *New Eng. J. Med.* 273:567, 1965.
7. Shubin, H., and Weil, M. H. Bacterial shock. *J.A.M.A.* 185:850, 1963.
8. Bing, R. J., and Ramos, H. The role of the heart in shock. *J.A.M.A.* 181:871, 1962.
9. Rosen, F. S. The endotoxins of Gram-negative bacteria and host resistance. *New Eng. J. Med.* 264:919, 1961.
10. Berdjis, C. C., and Vick, J. A. Endotoxin and traumatic shock. Role of the capillaries and small blood vessels. *J.A.M.A.* 204:191, 1968.
11. Whitaker, A. N., McKay, D. G., and Csavossy, I. Studies of catecholamine shock. I. Disseminated intravascular coagulation. *Amer. J. Path.* 56:153, 1969.
12. Litwak, R. S., Slonim, R., Wisoff, G., and Gadboys, H. L. Homologous-blood syndrome during extracorporeal circulation in man. II. Phenomena of sequestration and desequestration. *New Eng. J. Med.* 268:1377, 1963.

13. Gaston, L. W. The blood-clotting factors. *New Eng. J. Med.* 270:236, 290, 1964.
14. Davie, E. W., and Ratnoff, O. D. Waterfall sequence for intrinsic blood clotting. *Science* 145:1310, 1964.
15. Deykin, D. Thrombogenesis. *New Eng. J. Med.* 276:622, 1967.
16. Ashford, T. P., and Freiman, D. G. The role of the endothelium in the initial phase of thrombosis. *Amer. J. Path.* 50:257, 1967.
17. Marcus, A. J. Platelet function. *New Eng. J. Med.* 280:1213, 1969. (The first of 3 parts of a résumé of the roles of platelets in hemostasis and coagulation. The others are 280:1278 and 280:1330.)
18. Baldini, M. Idiopathic thrombocytopenic purpura. *New Eng. J. Med.* 274:1245, 1301, 1966.
19. Lieberman, E., Heuser, E., Donnell, G. N., Landing, B. H., and Hammond, G. D. Hemolytic-uremic syndrome. *New Eng. J. Med.* 275:227, 1966.
20. Hall, W. J., III. Hemorrhagic thrombocythemia. *J.A.M.A.* 192:912, 1965.
21. Quick, A. J. Hereditary bleeding diseases. *J.A.M.A.* 178:941, 1961.
22. Friedman, I. A., Quick, A. J., Higgins, F., Hussey, C. V., and Hickey, M. E. Hereditary labile factor (factor V) deficiency. *J.A.M.A.* 175:370, 1961.
23. Zahir, M. Congenital deficiency of fibrin-stabilizing factor. *J.A.M.A.* 207:751, 1969.
24. Rodriguez-Erdmann, F. Bleeding due to increased intravascular blood coagulation. *New Eng. J. Med.* 273:1370, 1965.
25. Brinkhous, K. M., and Roberts, H. R. Thrombolysis and thrombolytic agents. *J.A.M.A.* 175:284, 1961.
26. Reid, W. O., Somylo, A. V., Somylo, A. P., and Custer, R. P. Role of the platelet in fibrinolysis. *Amer. J. Clin. Path.* 37:561, 1962.
27. Scott, G. B. D., and Gracey, L. R. H. Analysis of the factors concerned in the organization of occlusive thrombi. *Arch. Path.* (Chicago) 87:643, 1969.
28. Rohner, R. F., Priar, J. T., and Sipple, J. H. Mucinous malignancies, venous thrombosis and terminal endocarditis with emboli. *Cancer* 19:1805, 1966.
29. Jaques, W. E., and Hyman, A. L. Experimental pulmonary embolism in dogs. *A.M.A. Arch. Path.* 64:487, 1957.
30. Korn, D., Gore, I., Blenke, A., and Collins, D. P. Pulmonary arterial bands and webs: An unrecognized manifestation of organized pulmonary emboli. *Amer. J. Path.* 40:129, 1962.
31. Ellis, H. A., and Watson, A. J. Studies on the genesis of traumatic fat embolism in man. *Amer. J. Path.* 53:245, 1968.
32. Yanoff, M. Incidence of bone-marrow embolism due to closed-chest cardiac massage. *New Eng. J. Med.* 269:837, 1963.
33. Yoell, J. H. Bone marrow embolism to lung following sternal puncture. *A.M.A. Arch. Path.* 67:373, 1959.
34. Liban, E., and Raz, S. A clinicopathologic study of fourteen cases of amniotic fluid embolism. *Amer. J. Clin. Path.* 51:477, 1969.
35. Nosanchuk, J. S., and Littler, E. R. Skin embolus to lung. *Arch. Path.* (Chicago) 87:542, 1969.
36. Tackett, L. R. Brain tissue pulmonary emboli. *Arch. Path.* (Chicago) 78:292, 1964.
37. Doyle, W. F., and Gray, J. M. Bile embolization following hepatic trauma. *Arch. Path.* (Chicago) 85:559, 1968.
38. Mehta, H., and Rubenstone, A. I. Pulmonary bile thrombo-emboli. *Amer. J. Clin. Path.* 47:490, 1967.
39. Adelson, L. Recent progress in forensic pathology. *J. Forensic Sci.* 4:250, 1959.

40. Lindberg, D. A. B., Lucas, F. V., Sheagren, J., and Malm, J. R. Silicone embolization during clinical and experimental heart surgery employing a bubble oxygenator. *Amer. J. Path.* 39:129, 1961.
41. Truemner, K. M., White, S., and Vanlandingham, H. Fatal embolization of pulmonary capillaries. *J.A.M.A.* 173:1089, 1960.
42. Graham, J. W., and Breitenecker, R. Embolization of gastric contents associated with rupture of the stomach. *Arch. Path.* (Chicago) 84:659, 1967.
43. Wacker, W. E. C., Rosenthal, M., Snodgrass, P. J., and Amador, E. A triad for the diagnosis of pulmonary embolism and infarction. *J.A.M.A.* 178:8, 1961.
44. Reiner, L., Rodriguez, F. L., Jimenez, F. A., and Platt, R. Injection studies on mesenteric arterial circulation. III. Occlusions without intestinal infarction. *A.M.A. Arch. Path.* 73:461, 1962.
45. Hoffman, F. G., Zimmerman, S. L., and Cardwell, E. S., Jr. Massive intestinal infarction without vascular occlusion associated with aortic insufficiency. *New Eng. J. Med.* 263:436, 1960.
46. Zweifach, B. W. Tissue mediators in the genesis of experimental shock. *J.A.M.A.* 181:866, 1962.

GENERAL REFERENCES

French, J. E., MacFarlane, R. G., and Roberts, K. B. In Florey, H. (Ed.), *General Pathology* (4th ed.). Philadelphia: Saunders, 1970, pp. 273–336, 370–393. (Excellent critical presentation of the pathology of coagulative disorders, hermorrhage, shock, and edema.)

Walter, J. B., and Israel, M. S. *General Pathology*. Boston: Little, Brown, 1963, pp. 588–607, 614–696. (A thoughtful exposition of the pathology of thrombosis, embolism, infarction, hemorrhage, and edema.)

3 LOCAL AND SYSTEMIC REACTIONS TO INJURY

INJURIOUS AGENTS: THE IMMEDIATE CAUSES OF DISEASE

Nature of injurious agents

Most injurious agents can be divided into three large categories: physical agents, chemical agents, and living agents. *Physical agents* include excesses of heat, light, radiant energy, electricity, cold, and trauma. *Chemical agents* include poisons of exogenous origin, such as acids and alkalis, and poisons of endogenous origin – such as uric acid in gout, and calcium in certain bone diseases. *Living agents* include pathogenic bacteria, fungi, rickettsiae, viruses, protozoa, and animal parasites.

Variations in response

A given agent is sometimes harmless or beneficial under one circumstance, whereas under another it may be injurious and even fatal. For example, many useful drugs are poisonous when the therapeutic dose is exceeded; vitamin D, an essential substance for the formation of growing bones, may be definitely toxic when taken in excessively large doses. Furthermore, there are individual differences in the reaction to injurious substances. Thus some people, because of a specific sensitivity, react violently to the poison in *Rhus toxicodendron* (poison ivy); others react little or not at all.

Defenses against injurious substances

The human body is well equipped to protect itself against injurious substances. The skin and mucous membranes form effective barriers against most minor injuries. Neuromuscular reflexes also serve to protect us. Thus the hand is jerked back quickly from a hot object. One coughs to expel an inhaled particle, and vomiting is commonly a means to eliminate a swallowed poison. These defenses serve primarily to *prevent* injury. In addition, the body has a generally effective mechanism of reaction to minimize tissue damage resulting from injurious agents (see below).

INFLAMMATION: LOCAL REACTION TO INJURY

1. *Nature of the Inflammatory Response*

Definition

The local reaction of the tissues to an injurious agent is known as inflammation. Note that inflammation is a *vital, changing process,* part of a continuum that begins with tissue injury and ends with healing and restoration of structure and function. It must be understood as a motion picture, not a "still."

Usually beneficial

We ordinarily think of the inflammatory response as *beneficial,* serving to localize, destroy, neutralize, dilute, or remove the injurious agent and the injured cells, in preparation for the process of healing. There appears to be a specific and direct relationship between the severity of the inflammatory reaction and the speed of the subsequent repair. It should be noted, however, that *occasionally the inflammatory process itself is harmful;* this is particularly true in sensitized or allergic individuals overreacting to an irritant and injuring their own tissues in so doing.

Terminology

Every organ and part of the body is subject to inflammation. An inflammatory process in a specific organ is ordinarily identified by *attaching the suffix -itis to the proper form for the organ or part;* thus we speak of *tonsillitis, appendicitis, endocarditis,* and *encephalitis.* Other word forms are also used to imply inflammation. Thus *pneumonia* has much the same meaning as *pneumonitis,* and *pleurisy* as *pleuritis.* Note that *inflammation is not synonymous with infection.* The former signifies the reaction of the tissues to injury, whether chemical, thermal, bacterial, or any other; the latter signifies invasion of the body by living pathogenic microorganisms.

Acute and chronic inflammation

When the injurious agent is particularly irritating, the reaction is quick and violent, and the inflammation is said to be acute. Illnesses characterized by *acute inflammation* generally last hours or days, constitutional symptoms such as fever are prominent, and the patient can usually recall exactly the time and manner of onset. Illnesses characterized by *chronic inflammation* are usually less severe and more protracted: the process may last weeks or months, constitutional symptoms are usually minimal, and the patient often cannot recall the precise time or manner of onset. Pain and swelling are usually less conspicuous in chronic inflammation than in acute, and the proliferative features of repair are more evident. In most instances chemical and biologic *factors inherent in the injurious agents* account for the differences in the reaction of the host, i.e., whether it is an acute or a chronic inflammatory response. In some instances the differences are due to *factors inherent in the host;* thus a first exposure to a particular agent may be characterized by a mild or chronic reaction, while subsequent contacts result in an acute response because of prior sensitization.

Activation of the inflammatory reaction

The casual observer thinks of the injurious agent as activating the inflammatory response by penetrating the tissues of the body and stirring them up to reaction. Note, however, that some physical agents, such as heat or ultraviolet light, may incite a violent inflammatory response without any particulate substance penetrating the body. This shows that the inflammatory response may be activated by *some substance derived from injured body cells* as well as by the injurious agent itself. Boyden [1] suggests that inflammation results from an *antigen-antibody reaction at the site of the tissue injury.* He has shown that adult animals, but not newborn ones, normally have antibodies against their own cells, probably as a result of prior cell injury. He postulates that injured cells release antigen which is bound locally by antibodies to form complexes to which the tissues react by the inflammatory response. Certainly the humoral and cellular events following cell injury are quite similar to those which occur in an immunized animal following injection of the corresponding antigen.

Methods of study

The inflammatory reaction consists of a series of events which can be observed by studying injured living tissues microscopically. The phenomenon does not occur in the dead body when it is subjected to the same injury. In Cohnheim's classic experiment, published in 1873, the web of a frog's tongue was stretched across the opening in the microscope stage and a chemical irritant was applied to the transparent membrane. The modern method is to use a transparent chamber inserted in the skin of a rabbit's ear, as described by Florey [2]. In this chamber the full development and evolution of the process can be studied, from initial injury to wound healing.

Sequence of events

As seen under the microscope, the following events occur when the tissues are inoculated with a *small quantity of living culture of virulent bacteria.* Those cells coming into contact with the highest concentration of bacterial toxins die, while those less severely injured undergo *cloudy swelling.* Next a series of *vascular changes* takes place [3], beginning with a transient constriction of blood vessels, presumably due to a stimulation of nerve endings. Soon thereafter the *arterioles* dilate, causing a speeding of blood flow. Next the *venules,* and finally the *capillaries,* dilate, resulting in hyperemia, with stagnation of the circulation. As the vessels dilate and the flow of blood slows, the *vessel walls become more permeable:* leukocytes and plasma move out of vessels into the connective tissues, forming the *inflammatory exudate* which separates the fixed tissue elements. This stage of inflammation, in which the tissue spaces are filled with plasma and leukocytes but massive necrosis has not occurred, is often referred to as *cellulitis.* Subsequent developments *depend chiefly upon the amount of tissue destroyed.* If tissue destruction is minimal, the dead cells are removed, hyperemia subsides, and the tissues return almost to normal, leaving no scar. If there is extensive destruction of tissue, great numbers of leukocytes come into the area and release their lytic enzymes; the central portion of the affected tissues liquefies, forming an *abscess,* or, if at a surface, an *ulcer.* Under these circumstances the defect is filled in by the multiplication and migration of tissue cells in the slower process known as *granulation tissue formation;* the scar is larger and may interfere with the normal function of the part. Or if bacterial multiplication gets ahead of the host's response, the *infection may spread to adjacent parts,* and the process may end with the death of the host due to *systemic effects of the toxemia.*

2. Biochemical and Physiologic Aspects of Inflammation

Chemical activation

Let us now consider in detail the functional changes which underlie the alterations that have been described. From the lysosomes of dead or injured cells an *activator* (Hageman factor) is released which reacts with an *inactive precursor substance* (kallikreinogen) in blood, releasing into the tissue spaces *certain enzymes* (kallikrein, others) which in turn react with *plasma globulin* to release the active substances known as *kinins* (kallidin, bradykinin). Many of the subsequent events in the inflammatory response are a result of the physiologic effects of the kinins [4, 5]. (Many of the compounds given here have other names, as well as the German ones taken from early reports.)

Kinins: mediators of the inflammatory response

The *kinins* are a group of peptides, formed locally in the tissues where needed. Under normal conditions, they serve to regulate the activity of secretory glands by inciting local vasodilatation, and hence have been called *local hormones.* Kinins have been identified in the venom of certain wasps and poisonous snakes. Under abnormal conditions, as following tissue injury, kinins *serve to incite the inflammatory response:* vascular dilatation, increased vascular permeability, and emigration of leukocytes. There is evidence also that kinins stimulate the *increased formation of leukocytes in the bone marrow.* This release of kinins in the tissues in inflammation has been compared [5] to the deposition of fibrin in wounds: both are standby physiologic systems set in motion by abnormal local conditions; both systems are based upon the activation of precursor substances normally present in blood. Even more remarkable, the two systems apparently are triggered by the same activating substance, the so-called *Hageman factor.*

bradykinin

Bradykinin is the member of the kinin family which has been studied in most detail. It is a nine-amino-acid peptide which, when injected locally, causes severe pain and tissue changes which closely simulate those occurring naturally in acute inflammation. When injected intravenously, it causes a fall in the blood pressure and constriction of the bronchioles. Certain *anti-inflammatory agents* such as salicylates and phenylbutazone *antagonize some of its actions. Steroids* interfere with the release of kinins from their plasma precursors; it may be that this is the mechanism of the known anti-inflammatory effect of cortisol [6]. It seems likely that leukotaxine, a vessel-dilating and leukocyte-attracting substance identified in inflammatory exudates by Menkin [7] in the '30s, was in fact a crude mixture of kinins [4]. The action of bradykinin is in many ways similar to that of histamine, a substance which was thought earlier to mediate the inflammatory response.

Vascular response

The vascular phenomena of inflammation apparently occur as the result of the action of two mechanisms, as noted by Majno [3]. Often, as in burns, there is *direct injury to the vessel walls* by the injurious agent, causing local increase in permeability and perhaps hemorrhage; this type of injury is long-lasting, and affects all types of vessels. More regularly, the increased vascular permeability comes about indirectly as a result of the action of paralytic agents, i.e., the kinins; this effect is short-lived unless kinin release continues. Increased vascular permeability resulting from kinins occurs chiefly in the venules and is apparently based upon acquired characteristics. Majno [3] noted that it did not occur in the newborn rat; Boyden [1] reported the same lack of response in newborn rabbits, and suggested auto-immunity as its basis.

Migration of leukocytes

Even without evident direct injury of the vessel walls, leukocytes escape from the bloodstream into the affected tissues. First the cells move out of the axial stream and adhere to the vascular lining; this shift is spoken of as *margination* or *pavementing* of leukocytes. As the muscle coat of the venule relaxes further, the *endothelial cells lining the vessel are pulled apart,* exposing the underlying basement membrane to the leukocytes. These cells then emigrate into the perivascular connective tissues, passing through the normal pores in the basement membrane by *ameboid motion.*

Chemotaxis

Cells are attracted to the area of tissue injury by a positive force known as *chemotaxis,* which may derive either from bacteria, or, presumably through the action of kinins, from injured host cells. Particulate matter such as carbon and quartz have no chemotactic effect [8]. Ward and his co-workers [9] showed that bacteria-free filtrates of a wide variety of gram-positive and gram-negative bacteria were actively chemotactic, but filtrates of *M. tuberculosis* were not. Bessis [10], using laser microbeam and time lapse cinematography in human blood, was able to demonstrate migration of leukocytes toward a single dead cell. Certain bacteria seem to attract specific types of leukocytes. Thus *Staphylococcus aureus attracts polymorphonuclear leukocytes* and *Salmonella typhi attracts monocytes.* (Negative chemotaxis, in which leukocytes are repelled, has also been described.) As the leukocytes move into the area of tissue injury, they provide an additional source of kinins. Plasma always seeps out of the vessels along with the leukocytes. This exudation of leukocytes and plasma separates the fixed tissues of the affected part and leads to swelling: *inflammatory edema.* Plasma brings with it its various ingredients such as the plasma proteins, including, in some instances, *specific antibodies* capable of acting against the infectious agent or neutralizing its toxins.

Role of leukocytes

That the leukocytes have an especial role in inflammation was suggested by Metchnikoff in 1891. It is the *polymorphonuclear (PMN) leukocyte* in particular that *is important in acute inflammation.* These remarkable cells constitute a mobile force, a ready reserve of shock troops, for battling infections in any part of the body. The polymorphonuclear cells ("polys") are *formed in the bone marrow,* and, when passed into the bloodstream as postmitotic cells, they have an average prospective life span of about 7 hours [11]. The PMNs are armed with great numbers of *lysosomes,* represented by the neutrophilic granules in the cytoplasm. These granules contain several potent lytic enzymes which make it possible for these cells to *destroy many types of bacteria* and to *liquefy the cell fragments* resulting from tissue injury. Polys derive their energy largely from *glycolysis.* When actively engaged in phagocytosis, they show a great increase in consumption of glucose and oxygen, and a marked depletion of their own glycogen stores. Along with these changes there occurs a *large accumulation of lactic acid,* both in the cytoplasm of the cells and in the intercellular spaces. This local increase in acidity tends to inactivate the enzyme *kininase* [4], whose function normally is to inhibit kinins; hence the *acidity enhances the inflammatory response.*

Phagocytosis: general features

The polymorphonuclear leukocyte and the macrophage have special significance in the inflammatory exudate because of their capability as *phagocytes.* Phagocytosis is the process by which tiny particles – bacteria, cell fragments, foreign matter – are taken into the living cell. Phagocytes provide an effective form of antibacterial defense, provided the cells can trap the bacterial invaders [11]. Tissues having a generous blood supply and a structure that promotes cellular "infighting" are better defended by leukocytes than are avascular surface tissues; thus lung is more favorable for phagocytic action than is peritoneum or cornea. On the other hand, bacteria having a well-developed capsule are able to resist the lytic action of enzymes concerned in phagocytosis. Phagocytosis is accelerated by the presence in the plasma of anticapsular antibodies, opsonins, and complement, as may result from *prior exposure of the host to the specific bacterial agent.*

clinical importance

The special role of leukocytes is emphasized by the peculiar *susceptibility to infection* of those individuals whose *leukocytes are reduced in number* or *impaired in quality.* Patients with marked leukopenia are very *susceptible to infections.* Patients receiving cancer chemotherapy may show a leukocyte count of 1000 or less per cubic millimeter, as a result of the cytotoxic effect of the drug upon leukocyte precursors in the bone marrow. Such patients often develop *"opportunistic" infections* – bacterial, fungal, or viral – to which they succumb. In such cases the inflammatory exudate may contain fewer leukocytes than is usual with the organism in question, making microscopic diagnosis difficult. Perhaps even more remarkable are the instances in which leukocytes are present in normal numbers but are somehow impaired in quality. Since leukocyte dysfunctions are usually due to inborn, often hereditary, disorders, the effects are usually manifest in infancy or early childhood as an unusual susceptibility to infection. Ward and Schlegel [12] have listed three different *types of leukocytic dysfunctions.* In the first of these – the associated clinical syndrome is called *chronic granulomatous disease* – the defect usually occurs in males and is generally believed to be linked to the X chromosome [13], although exceptions occur [14]. In this type, the *bactericidal process within the phagocyte is defective,* and the defect can be measured with the nitroblue tetrazolium test [13]. In a second type of leukocytic dysfunction there is apparently a *deficiency of a humoral phagocytosis-promoting factor,* tentatively identified as the fifth component of human complement. In a third type the *normal chemotactic response of the leukocytes is prevented by an inhibitor substance* present in the patient's serum. In each of these types of disorder – there may be others – the leukocytes are ineffective in combatting bacterial infections and the affected individual usually dies in infancy or early childhood after a series of severe infections.

details of action

The activity that occurs within the living cell during phagocytosis has been referred to as *intracellular inflammation* by Rogers [11]. The process can be observed directly with the phase-contrast microscope. When bacteria are encountered under suitable circumstances, polys and macrophages – the two major cell types participating in phagocytosis – throw out pseudopods to surround the bacteria. As the pseudopods merge to engulf a bacterium, a bit of cell membrane is pinched off so that a vacuole, lined with cell membrane and containing the bacterium, is formed in the cell cytoplasm. (This process is presumably identical with *pinocytosis,* the mechanism by which the cell normally engulfs food particles.) Cytoplasmic granules (lysosomes) then merge with the pinocytic vesicles and release their lytic enzymes to digest the bacterium [15]. Presumably the lysosomal enzymes are aided by *phagocytin,* another antibacterial substance that has been identified in the cytoplasmic granules of the leukocyte [11]. Soluble products of the lytic process are passed into the cytoplasm and then through the cell wall; insoluble particles may either be extruded from the cell within the lysosomal bag or retained harmlessly as a residual body. Thus, under favorable circumstances, the cell recovers. If circumstances are not favorable, the *bacteria may multiply* within the lysosome and bacterial toxins may damage the lysosomal membrane which then ruptures, liberating the lytic enzymes into the cell cytoplasm. The *cell* itself may thus be liquefied, the cell membrane may rupture, and contained organisms may be spilled into the tissue spaces where they may attack, and be attacked by, other cells. A third possibility also exists. Under certain circumstances *bacteria may survive within the cell* in a sort of symbiotic balance; in such infections – brucellosis is an example – the bacteria seem to have a biologic advantage which leads to *persistence of infection* within the cells.

Role of fibrin

Meanwhile *other changes* have occurred in the area of injury. The blood in the small vessels, already stagnant from vasodilatation, has become more viscous; *thrombosis of small vessels* commonly occurs. Strands of *fibrin* also form in tissue interstices as the result of the interaction of the coagulation-promoting factors present in the exudate. The fibrin web tends to block the movement of tissue fluids, thereby *localizing the bacterial agent* in the case of staphylococcal infections; in streptococcal infections fibrinolytic enzymes are active in the exudate and there is less tendency for the infection to remain localized. Although not much is known about the balance between fibrin formation and fibrin lysis in wound healing, the relationship may well be a critical one in determining spread of infection or wound healing.

End results

The outcome in acute inflammation is dependent upon a number of forces, including the *nature, virulence,* and *dose* of the *phlogogenic* (inflammation-causing) *substance.* Perhaps equally important are the general state of *nutrition and health* of the host, the *specific immunity* of the host against the infectious agent, the *site of tissue injury,* and the *effectiveness of the therapeutic agents* employed. The end result may be any of the following:

1. *Complete healing* without loss of tissue (e.g., sunburn). Leukocytic enzymes liquefy dead cells, dissolved material is resorbed, fixed tissue cells regenerate, and the hyperemia subsides. The part is totally restored, anatomically and functionally, and there is no scar.

2. *Abscess formation or ulceration* followed by healing (e.g., moderately virulent staphylococcal infection of the skin). Bacteria multiply within a localized area walled off by a fibrin barrier, the *pyogenic membrane;* fixed tissue cells of the host are destroyed en masse by bacterial toxins; leukocytes are attracted in large numbers; and *leukocytic enzymes liquefy fibrin and dead tissue cells* (liquefaction necrosis). If the area of injury is deep in the tissues, a *cavity* is formed, filled with *pus;* this *abscess* must be drained surgically before healing can occur. If the area of injury involves the skin or a mucosal surface, an *ulcer* is formed. In either event *healing is slow* and imperfect, and is followed by *scar* formation.

3. *Gradual modification of the reaction* (e.g., tuberculosis). The infectious agent and the host may reach a status of coexistence, *scarring* and repair going on slowly over a long period in the face of continuing infection. Sometimes, following extensive damage to tissues, there is severe *impairment of the circulation* to the part as a result of scarring and venous thrombosis. Under these circumstances *healing may be incomplete* in spite of the fact that the bacterial infection may be under control. In such cases a *chronic ulcer* or a *fistulous tract* may persist, necessitating surgical excision and grafting before complete healing can take place.

4. *Spread of the infection* (e.g., extremely virulent *Clostridium welchii* infections). Fibrinolytic and histolytic enzymes (spreading factors) of certain bacteria may destroy the usual barriers to infection, and bacteria may be disseminated via blood or lymph to other organs, where new foci of inflammation develop.

5. *Death of the host.* This may result from spread of infection to vital organs as above, from constitutional inability to form protective antibodies (agammaglobulinemia) or to manufacture leukocytes (agranulocytosis), from the systemic effect of bacterial toxins, or from general debility and exhaustion of the host.

3. The Inflammatory Exudate

Exudate vs. transudate

The fluid formed in the area of tissue injury as a result of the active migration of blood cells and plasma is known as an *exudate.* It differs physically, chemically, and microscopically from a *transudate,* which is the fluid formed passively by leakage from obstructed hemic or lymphatic vessels. Thus peritoneal fluid due to tuberculous peritonitis (an exudate) can be differentiated in the laboratory from that due to heart failure (a transudate). A *transudate is sterile, contains few cells,* and has a *specific gravity less than 1.015* and a *protein content less than 3.0 gm. per 100 ml.* An *exudate usually contains bacteria,* has a *high cell count, high specific gravity,* and *high protein content.*

Amount of exudate

The amount of the inflammatory exudate depends in large part upon the portion of the body affected. In inflammations of serous sacs (pleura, pericardium, peritoneum, meninges, and synovia), fluid may collect in large quantities. In such tissues as cornea, bone, and cartilage, little exudate can form. In soft tissues and organs of the body, such as the thigh, breast, or liver, a small amount of exudate may accumulate in tissue spaces, leading to an increased firmness of the tissues, the so-called inflammatory edema; if the exudate is abundant, tissue necrosis occurs and there is a softening of the area as an abscess cavity forms, filled with liquid exudate (pus). If the area of inflammation is on the skin and exposed to the air, it "weeps" exudate for a while; gradually the exudate dries, forming a scab or crust.

Types of exudate

The character of the exudate is determined by the nature and severity of the inflammatory reaction and the stage of its development. Appearance of the exudate is best studied in those cases in which the fluid can be carefully withdrawn from a body cavity or abscess via needle or trocar. In mild inflammation, such as viral meningitis, the fluid is usually clear or faintly yellow and is relatively poor in cells and protein; a watery fluid of this type is spoken of as a *serous exudate,* and the process may be called *serous inflammation.* When protein is more abundant, as in tuberculous pleuritis, the fluid is more yellowish and opalescent and either contains fibrin or tends to form fibrin on standing; it is spoken of as *fibrinous.* The exudate in staphylococcic and other pyogenic infections is thick, often yellow, gray, or green, and contains large numbers of cells, particularly polymorphonuclear leukocytes; it is said to be *purulent* or *suppurative.* In some exudates, particularly those associated with trauma, the fluid has a red color from the large number of erythrocytes it contains *(sanguineous* or *hemorrhagic).* When a mucous membrane, such as the nasal or bronchial mucosa, is inflamed, there is an increased secretion of mucus along with the other elements. This results in a thick, ropy, whitish exudate *(mucous* or *catarrhal* inflammation). In a given case the character of the exudate may change; thus with the common cold the exudate may be serous for a few hours, later catarrhal, and finally after a few days frankly purulent.

Inflammatory cells:

All exudates contain cells derived from the blood. When leukocytes are found outside the blood vessels, they signify inflammation and are often spoken of as *inflammatory cells.*

poly

The neutrophilic *polymorphonuclear leukocyte* is the characteristic cell in inflammations due to pyogenic cocci and is sometimes loosely termed the pus cell. These cells, also known as *microphages,* are actively phagocytic and provide the important proteolytic enzymes that aid in liquefaction of dead tissue. These cells are formed only in hemopoietic foci and have a life of 3 to 5 days, of which normally the last 7 hours are spent in the bloodstream.

macrophage

The *macrophage* is also phagocytic. In the circulating blood this cell is usually called a *monocyte;* in the tissues, a *histiocyte.* Somewhat larger than the poly, the macrophage has a pale, usually oval nucleus and abundant cytoplasm. The Kupffer cells of the liver and the reticulum cells of the sinusoids of spleen and lymph nodes are closely related cells and are also capable of phagocytosis. Macrophages are seen in the *later phases of acute inflammation,* and also in *chronic infections* such as *syphilis* and *tuberculosis.* Monocytes live several months, and subsequent generations may arise by direct division of cells in an area of inflammation. *Epithelioid cells,* found in great numbers in tuberculous lesions, are stringy, elongated cells generally believed to be derived from monocytes [16].

eosinophil

Eosinophils are frequently seen in the tissues in *subacute* and *chronic inflammation,* and especially in allergic inflammation (e.g., bronchial asthma, parasitic infestations). The exact role of eosinophils is not known but they are thought to carry in their granules the mechanism for the release of fibrinolysin [17].

Lymphocytes are important elements of the exudate in instances of *chronic inflammation* and in the *healing* stage of acute inflammation. Lymphocytes are believed to interact with antigen to *initiate antibody responses.* Their roles in rejection of homografts and in tissue invasion by neoplastic cells are under intense investigation [18]. Lymphocytes are formed in the lymph nodes, spleen, and Peyer's patches, and circulate in both lymphatic- and bloodstreams. Their life span is said to be a year or more.

lymphocytes

Plasma cells are probably lymphocytes that have been modified as a result of their *involvement in antibody formation.* They occur in chronic inflammation, particularly syphilis, and may be seen in the tissues in the stage of healing after acute inflammation.

plasma cells

Multinucleated giant cells, formed by the fusion of histiocytes [19], appear in response to foreign particles in areas of inflammation. They engulf such things as hair, vegetable matter, and suture material in a contaminated wound.

giant cells

Erythrocytes are present in the inflammatory exudate only by accident; apparently they serve no useful purpose in the inflammatory reaction. The *fluid of the exudate is derived from blood plasma* and carries plasma proteins, glucose, fibrinogen, electrolytes, and antibodies in solution. Other substances are inconstantly present in the exudate, depending upon circumstances: foreign material such as dirt, bacteria, vegetable matter, and glass; chemical agents used in therapy; fibrin, dead tissue cells, and the like.

other elements

4. *Gross Features of Inflammation*

Much time and space has been devoted to the microscopic features of inflammation. The gross features are equally important, because they provide the visible evidence that leads the physician to recognize the nature of the process. These "cardinal signs" of inflammation have been known for centuries, long before their microscopic basis was understood. *Calor* (heat) and *rubor* (redness) are manifestations of the active hyperemia in the affected part. *Tumor* (swelling) is due chiefly to the accumulation of the inflammatory exudate but also to hyperemia. *Dolor* (pain) and *functio laesa* (disturbed function) are due to a combination of factors, including the stimulation of sensory nerve endings as the exudate stretches the tissues, and the direct effect of kinins.

Cardinal signs

5. *Special Features of Inflammation in Different Tissues*

While the general features of inflammation are remarkably similar, no matter what the phlogogenic agent may be or which tissues are affected, there are certain important differences in the response of different tissues to various injurious agents.

In the skin, *mild inflammation,* perhaps resulting from a slight burn, is evidenced by transient swelling, redness, pain, and itching; healing occurs in a few days without scar. *Severe inflammation,* usually due to pyogenic cocci and often associated with trauma, is manifest by severe pain, marked swelling, often extensive liquefaction necrosis, with abscess formation or ulceration. These may heal slowly, by granulation tissue. In other cases the infection may spread along fascial

Skin

planes, and inflammatory edema may make the tissues almost wooden in their tenseness and rigidity; this is spoken of as *phlegmon* or *phlegmonous inflammation.* Infection may also spread along lymphatic channels, giving reddish streaks in the skin *(lymphangitis)* extending from the primary lesion toward the regional lymph nodes, where signs of acute inflammation may also appear *(lymphadenitis).* Thus in severely infected wounds or burns there may be bacteremia as well as toxemia, great loss of fluids from the exuding surface, dehydration, electrolyte imbalance, and death.

Mucous membranes

In the mucous membranes of the nasal passages, pharynx, larynx, and bronchi, *mild inflammation* (common cold) is usually manifest by edema of the membranes, resulting in some degree of obstruction of the air passages (stuffiness), plus excess mucus secretion leading to nasal discharge, cough, and expectoration. This mucinous exudate is sometimes called *catarrh,* and the process may be spoken of as *catarrhal inflammation.* More *severe inflammation,* as with diphtheria, may lead to superficial ulceration of the mucosa and formation of a fibrinous *membrane* which may block the air passages and cause death from suffocation. In the mucous membranes of the digestive tract, mild inflammation, as with food allergy, usually causes edema of the intestinal wall, excess mucus production, increased peristaltic activity, and *diarrhea.* Severe inflammation, as with *Salmonella typhosa,* may lead to *extensive ulceration of the mucosa,* even affecting the full thickness of the intestinal wall, thus resulting in perforation of the bowel, peritonitis, and death. In other cases, ulceration may involve the submucosal blood vessels and may lead to massive, even fatal, *hemorrhage into the intestinal tract.*

Heart and blood vessels

In the vascular system (heart, arteries, veins), *mild inflammation,* as due to trauma or low-grade infection, is usually followed by formation of fibrin on the vascular lining (thrombus), leading to interference with the circulation. If the inflammation is in an artery, the result may be ischemia of the part; in a vein, edema may develop; in a heart valve, perhaps a murmur may be heard. Fibrinolysis may lead to recovery, with gradual, more or less complete restoration of circulation and disappearance of symptoms. *Severe inflammation* of the vascular system, usually due to *trauma plus pyogenic infection,* causes fibrin formation along with destruction of the vascular structure, resulting in *rupture.* If an artery or vein is affected, rupture may lead to hemorrhage, or if a heart valve is involved, rupture may lead to valve leakage, heart failure, and death. In other cases, *fragmentation of an infected thrombus* may occur as a result of action of bacterial and leukocytic enzymes, leading to septic *embolism.*

Serous sacs

In the pleura, pericardium, peritoneum, meninges, or joints, even *mild inflammation,* as due to a virus, may lead to accumulation of fibrin on the surface *(fibrinous inflammation),* or to formation of a thin watery exudate in the sac, usually spoken of as a *serous effusion* or *serous inflammation.* While this is usually not critical, sometimes the amount of fluid is so massive that it results in *compression of vital structures* and death. *Severe inflammation* of these sacs, usually due to pyogenic cocci such as *Diplococcus pneumoniae,* may cause massive accumulation of pus in the cavity, or *empyema,* with extreme *toxemia* as well as pressure effects. With antibiotics and surgery, most such patients now survive, but extensive *adhesions* between opposing serous surfaces often persist after the acute inflammation subsides, and this may lead to deformity and eventual disability.

Viscera and soft tissues

In *internal organs* such as kidney, liver, or lung, or in the *soft tissues* of the extremities or the breast, *mild inflammation* is usually manifest by swelling and discomfort due to exudation into the tissues, followed by evidence of dysfunction of the specific organ affected – hematuria, jaundice, cough, or localized pain. If there is minimal tissue destruction, the inflammatory lesions may heal without scar, or may *persist as a chronic process,* with fibrosis and gradual failure of the affected organ. *Severe inflammation* of these viscera or parts, often due to pyogenic cocci or *Mycobacterium tuberculosis,* often leads to liquefaction necrosis and cavity formation, with sepsis, in addition to signs of organ dysfunction. If the individual recovers from such infections, perhaps as a result of surgery and/or antibiotics, there is often extensive scarring and deformity, and perhaps also chronic draining sinuses.

Bone

Mild injuries of bone, usually traumatic, normally heal readily if the bone fragments are in good position and no soft tissue is interposed between the ends of bone. Severe inflammation, usually a result of pyogenic cocci, sometimes bloodborne from a distant infection and sometimes due to compound fracture, often brings complications. As exudate accumulates in the unyielding bony canals, it compresses blood vessels, leading to thrombosis. This causes foci of bone necrosis which cannot be liquefied by cell enzymes. As a result, fragments of dead bone (sequestra) remain, and inflammation continues until the bone fragments are removed surgically. Draining sinuses often extend from the area of bone inflammation to the skin surface.

6. Chronic Inflammation

Proliferative changes

In certain instances the injurious agent acts over a longer period of time but is less damaging than in the examples of acute inflammation just cited. In such cases, tissue destruction, hyperemia, and exudation may be minimal or nonexistent, *lymphocytes and macrophages may outnumber polymorphonuclear leukocytes* in the exudate, and *proliferative tissue changes may be dominant.* Thus the continuous friction of a jagged tooth against the lip, or of a gallstone in the gallbladder, may stimulate both fibrous and epithelial cells to divide. In the case of the jagged tooth, a localized, slightly tender, firm wartlike growth comprising surface epithelium may develop on the mucous membrane of the lip, and the underlying fibrous tissue may be infiltrated with lymphocytes. In the case of the gallbladder, lymphocytes and macrophages will infiltrate the walls, the lining epithelium will develop areas of overgrowth, and the thin muscle layer will become thickened by fibrous scar tissue which will contract to reduce the size of the gallbladder by about half. The patient will experience discomfort after fatty meals, when the gallbladder is stimulated to empty itself.

Granulomatous inflammation

A special form of chronic inflammation is seen in response to tissue invasion by *Mycobacterium tuberculosis.* Macrophages and giant cells accumulate about the organisms, and fibrous tissue forms about these small focal lesions or *tubercles.* This combination of macrophages and fibrosis is known as *granulomatous inflammation.* These lesions may heal by scarring and become calcified, or they may undergo a distinctive form of necrosis known as *caseation,* whose characteristic cheesy yellow appearance is due to the waxy material from the capsule of the organisms. Similar focal collections of macrophages may be seen in *certain other diseases* (fungus infections, syphilis, sarcoid, brucellosis); these focal lesions are often spoken of as *tuberculoid granulomas.* The chemical element beryllium, when inhaled into the lung or deposited in a wound, may also incite a similar granulomatous inflammation.

Foreign body reaction

Another form of chronic inflammation is seen as a reaction to foreign material in the tissues. Usually the material in question is organic matter such as vegetable fibers or hair, but a similar reaction occurs with the use of chromic or other types of suture material. Macrophages are attracted to the area, and a number of them – perhaps a dozen or even as many as 50 – will merge their cytoplasm while their nuclei remain distinct, resulting in a *multinucleated giant cell.* These cells will engulf the foreign matter. Lymphocytes and fibrous tissue formation are always seen in conjunction with the giant cells.

The really distinctive feature of chronic inflammation is the remarkable tendency for the proliferative changes of healing to be active at the same time that the mild inflammatory response is going on.

WOUND HEALING

Relation to inflammation

When the inflammatory response has been fully effective, the irritant and all cell debris have been removed from the wound and vascular channels have been established for supply and drainage; then wound healing is ready to begin. *Inflammation and healing should be looked upon as two parts of a single vital function, the physiologic response to tissue injury,* the objective of which is *restoration of normal structure and function.*

Cell regeneration

Perfect restoration of function is dependent upon the replacement of lost cells by like cells *(regeneration),* and the orderly arrangement of these new cells in relation to preexisting cells so that intercellular functions are restored. This is not possible in all human tissues, although in lower animals such as the earthworm, near-perfect regeneration occurs, even the restoration of a large part of the whole body. In the human infant, regeneration is more complete than in the adult, in whom certain cells are incapable of reproducing their kind; loss of these cells results in replacement by other cell types. *Repair,* i.e., filling in of a wound or tissue defect, may restore lost tissue mass, but this is not the same as regeneration. In the discussion of cell types (Chapter 1) it was noted that certain cell strains – epidermis, intestinal epithelium, endothelium, and hematopoietic tissues – continue to undergo cell division throughout life, whereas others – neurons, skeletal tissue, and cardiac muscle – do not. This difference in reproductive capability is apparently due to the presence or absence of intermitotic cells in adult tissues: tissues which have them are able to regenerate after injury; tissues which lack them cannot [20, 21]. Intermediate between these two extremes are liver cells, cells of other solid epithelial viscera, and connective tissues in general. Tissues composed of these cells normally contain few intermitotic cells, but when tissue is lost, surviving cells are capable of rapid increase in the rate of cell division [21]. This knowledge makes it possible to understand the differences in the quality of regeneration or repair after injury in the different tissues.

Basic concepts

All wounds heal in roughly the same way: *new cells are formed from preexisting cells* and *fill in the area of tissue loss,* receiving support and nourishment from connective tissue and blood vessels as they grow. Small wounds heal quickly, large wounds slowly. A clean, dry surgical wound heals rapidly and readily by *primary union (first intention).* By contrast, the gaping perineal wound after resection of a rectal cancer must fill in by a process known as *granulation* before the skin epithelium can cover it over; healing is then said to have occurred by *secondary union (second intention).*

Healing of surgical wounds

In a *clean surgical wound* of the abdominal wall, cut blood vessels are ligated so that the wound remains relatively dry, the various layers of tissue – peritoneum, muscle, fascia, skin – are sutured together neatly one at a time so that no gaps remain and there is relatively little bacterial infection or foreign matter in the wound. Since the zone in which the cells have been injured by the surgeon's knife is narrow, the *inflammatory response is minimal;* it is, nevertheless, important. Capillaries and venules dilate to provide abundant nutrition to the tissues, and leukocytes are attracted into the wound where their digestive enzymes can remove fragments of dead cells. In such a wound, fibrin forms a *delicate web* between the two edges, but has no tensile strength: for the first few days sutures are required to hold the wound together. Intermitotic *fibrocytes* from the several layers (peritoneum, muscle sheath, subcutaneous tissues) respond to the injury by undergoing cell division, growing on the fibrin scaffold to bridge the gap, and *laying down collagen fibers* to *bind the edges of the wound together.* Epidermis of the skin surface is similarly stimulated to grow; intermitotic *epidermal cells undergo accelerated cell division,* project themselves on the surface of the wound, and intermingle with their fellows on the opposite side to seal the gap. Union is generally complete enough by the seventh day for sutures to be removed. This type of wound healing is commonly known as healing by *primary union, or by first intention.*

Healing of large wounds: inflammation

In larger wounds, with significant tissue loss, the picture is different. A gunshot wound of an extremity may leave a *tissue defect* at the skin surface which is several centimeters in diameter and in depth, so that suturing cannot be done. *Bacteria* inevitably contaminate such a wound, and the *tissue injury* resulting from the combination of trauma and infection may be severe. After the surgeon has effected *debridement* (removal of foreign matter and dead tissue from the wound), blood and exudate accumulate and dry to form a *crust* or *scab.* Beneath this crust, an *active inflammatory reaction* develops: capillaries and venules in the base of the wound dilate, leukocytes and plasma exude into the tissues, and fibrin forms on the surface. Viable intermitotic cells in the wound are stimulated to undergo mitosis. Thus *fibrocytes* and *capillary endothelial cells divide* and *project themselves into the wound* beneath the crust as the fibrin is reduced in amount by the action of fibrinolytic enzymes.

granulation

By the second or third day, endothelial cells can be seen growing as *buds* from preexisting capillaries. These capillary buds connect with other buds to form a looping strand, and the strand is hollowed out so that a *new capillary loop is formed,* bringing increased blood into the base of the wound. *Fibrocytes grow along with the capillaries into the wound,* extending their cytoplasmic processes along the fibrin scaffold beneath the crust. If the crust should be removed at this time, it would be noted that the *wound has a granular appearance* and bleeds easily. The delicate *granulations* at the base of the wound correspond to the capillary loops and their fibrocytic covering. This network of fibrin, endothelial cells, and fibrocytes is continuously remodeled until the missing tissue beneath the crust is replaced. By this time the *epidermal cells at the edge of the wound* have begun to show mitoses and to project themselves over the capillary loops and bed of fibrocytes until they cover the surface of the wound. Commonly the crust drops off spontaneously at about this time, and a thin, fragile, milky-white layer of epidermis can be seen covering the wound. This type of wound healing, in which *granulation tissue* (capillary loops and fibrocytes, with accompanying inflammatory cells) is interposed, is known as *healing by secondary union, or by second intention.* It is necessarily much slower than healing by primary union. Note that highly specialized fixed tissue elements normally present in such a tissue (striated muscle, sweat glands, hair follicles, and nerve fibers) do not regenerate as the wound is healing. As a result, large scars are hairless and they do not perspire.

Scar formation

Once a large wound has been filled in by granulation tissue and covered over by epithelium, it must *undergo revision* before a stable, healthy state is reached. Because of the persistent hyperemia and interstitial exudate, the *surface of the wound is elevated slightly* above surrounding tissues. As inflammation subsides, the thin, fragile capillaries shrink back to normal size, excess loops are obliterated, and the plump young fibroblasts mature to thin adult fibrocytes as *collagen is laid down* in the scar.

Collagen

Collagen is the chief constituent of scar tissue, just as it is the major constituent of skin, tendon, and bone. The collagen molecule is made up of three polypeptide chains, each containing approximately 1000 amino acids [22] in which glycine, proline, and hydroxyproline seem to be critically spaced. Collagen apparently owes its physical properties to the fact that the polypeptide chains are coiled about each other to make a *twisted fiber.* That the fiber structure is a result of its molecular form is shown by the fact that, after dissolving completely in acid, it can be exactly reconstituted when the acid is neutralized. Collagen is apparently synthesized by the fibroblast and extruded into the extracellular space where it polymerizes to form the fibrils. These fibrils then arrange themselves at right angles to each other to form an orderly sheet. As collagen ages, the bond between fibrils continues to grow stronger. Thus the healed wound continues to gain tensile strength.

Favorable factors

The following systemic factors *promote wound healing:* (1) youth (wound healing is a slower process in the elderly person), (2) warmth, (3) ultraviolet light, and (4) good nutrition, particularly adequate reserves of protein. Feeding of zinc sulfate apparently accelerates wound healing in both man and animals [23].

Unfavorable factors

The following systemic factors *delay or prevent wound healing,* probably by interfering with protein synthesis: (1) vitamin C deficiency, (2) protein starvation, (3) prolonged therapy with steroids (apparently by suppressing the vascular phase of inflammation), and (4) ionizing radiation. Local factors which inhibit wound healing include presence of foreign matter, poor blood supply, and persistence of infection.

Continuum of wound healing

Note that *acute inflammation and wound healing comprise a continuum.* Hyperemia and cell exudation are necessary first steps in healing. They make it possible for dead cells to be removed and for processes of tissue reconstruction to come into play.

SYSTEMIC REACTIONS TO INJURY

Noxious substances, most of them unidentified, may be absorbed from the area of local tissue injury and produce systemic manifestations. With mild irritants there may be no systemic reaction.

Fever

Fever occurs in varying degree in most instances of acute inflammation, and in many cases in which the local tissue reaction is subacute or chronic. Fever is believed to be due to *systemic absorption* of the products of local cell destruction; pyrogens – substances capable of causing fever – can be demonstrated by injecting intravenously into rabbits the protein fractions of the inflammatory exudate.

Leukocytosis is a feature of most pyogenic infections; it is probably due to circulation of the *chemotactic substances* liberated in the area of tissue injury. The bone marrow is stimulated to form leukocytes in excess of usual requirements, and spills them, both mature and immature, into the bloodstream as a sort of ready reserve for the local combat with the irritant.

Leukocytosis

Anorexia, lassitude, and generalized *aching* are commonly noted but have not been adequately explained. They may be related in some way to the metabolic disturbances that are known to occur in association with serious infections; these include negative nitrogen balance, proteinuria, disturbed utilization of carbohydrates and vitamins, and a tendency to ketosis. The cause of these metabolic derangements is not known for certain, but it may be that they are manifestations of degeneration of parenchymatous organs such as the liver and kidneys.

Other symptoms and signs

REFERENCES

1. Boyden, S. Autoimmunity and inflammation. *Nature* (London) 201:200, 1964.
2. Florey, H. W. *General Pathology* (4th ed.). Philadelphia: Saunders, 1970.
3. Majno, G. Mechanisms of abnormal vascular permeability in acute inflammation. In Thomas, L., Uhr, J. W., and Grant, L. (Eds.), *Injury, Inflammation and Immunity.* Baltimore: Williams & Wilkins, 1964. (This small volume, the proceedings of an international symposium presented in 1962, brings together much valuable information.)
4. Lewis, G. P. The role of peptides in the first stages of inflammation. In Thomas, L., Uhr, J. W., and Grant, L. (Eds.), *Injury, Inflammation and Immunity.* Baltimore: Williams & Wilkins, 1964.
5. Collier, H. O. J. Kinins. *Sci. Amer.* 207:111, 1962. (A clear exposition of the nature and mode of action of an important group of chemicals in the inflammatory response.)
6. Cline, M. J., and Melmon, K. L. Plasma kinins and cortisol: A possible explanation of the anti-inflammatory action of cortisol. *Science* 153:1135, 1966.
7. Menkin, V. Biology of inflammation. *Science* 123:527, 1956. (A summary of a lifetime of research in inflammation.)
8. Gordon, G. B., and King, D. W. Phagocytosis. *Amer. J. Path.* 37:279, 1960.
9. Ward, P. A., Lepow, I. H., and Newman, L. J. Bacterial factors chemotactic for polymorphonuclear leukocytes. *Amer. J. Path.* 52:725, 1968.
10. Bessis, M. C. Use of partial cell irradiation by laser microbeam as a microsurgical tool. *Israel J. Med. Sci.* 1:1284, 1965.
11. Rogers, D. E. Intracellular inflammation: dynamic and metabolic changes in polymorphonuclear leukocytes participating in phagocytosis. In Thomas, L., Uhr, J. W., and Grant, L. (Eds.), *Injury, Inflammation and Immunity.* Baltimore: Williams & Wilkins, 1964.
12. Ward, P. A., and Schlegel, R. J. Impaired leucotactic responsiveness in a child with recurrent infections. *Lancet* 2:344, 1969.
13. Baehner, R. L., and Nathan, D. G. Quantitative nitroblue tetrazolium test in chronic granulomatous disease. *New Eng. J. Med.* 278:971, 1968.
14. Quie, P. G., Kaplan, E. L., Page, A. R., Gruskay, F. L., and Malawista, S. E. Defective polymorphonuclear-leukocyte function and chronic granulomatous disease in two female children. *New Eng. J. Med.* 278:976, 1968.
15. De Duve, C. Lysosomes and cell injury. In Thomas, L., Uhr, J. W., and Grant, L. (Eds.), *Injury, Inflammation and Immunity.* Baltimore: Williams &

Wilkins, 1964. (The role of lysosomes in cell injury and inflammation has recently received much attention. This excellent paper, by the scientist who first described the lysosome, deserves careful reading.)

16. Epstein, W. L., and Krasnobrod, H. The origin of epithelioid cells in experimental granulomas in man. *Lab. Invest.* 18:190, 1968.
17. Riddle, J. M., and Barnhart, M. I. The eosinophile as a source of profibrinolysin in acute inflammation. *Blood* 25:776, 1965.
18. Gowans, J. L. Immunobiology of the small lymphocyte. *Hosp. Practice* 3:34, 1968. (A fascinating report on the activity of the lymphocyte in graft rejection and other immunologic responses.)
19. Silverman, L., and Shorter, R. G. Histogenesis of the multinucleated giant cell. *Lab. Invest.* 12:985, 1963.
20. Edwards, J. L., and Klein, R. E. Cell renewal in adult mouse tissues. *Amer. J. Path.* 38:437, 1961. (A meticulous study, in which tritium-labelled thymidine was used to mark cells synthesizing DNA.)
21. Post, J., and Hoffman, J. Cell renewal patterns. *New Eng. J. Med.* 279:248, 1968.
22. Gross, J. Collagen. *Sci. Amer.* 204:121, 1961. (The author describes the physical arrangement of the collagen molecule and relates its properties to this arrangement.)
23. Pories, W. J., Henzel, J. H., Rob, C. G., and Strain, W. H. Acceleration of wound healing in man with zinc sulphate given by mouth. *Lancet* 1:121, 1967.

4 HYPERSENSITIVITY STATES; COLLAGEN VASCULAR DISEASES

HYPERSENSITIVITY STATES

1. Basic Concepts

ANTIGEN

An *antigen* is a substance that stimulates the formation of antibodies within the host and reacts with them specifically. Any of the following may serve as antigens at various times and in various individuals: bacteria and their products, many foods, certain drugs, and a variety of biologic materials containing protein (such as kidney extracts, horse serum, plant pollen, molds, dog hair, etc.). A *complete antigen* is one which, when administered to a sensitive animal, stimulates the formation of antibodies, which react with it. A *haptene* is a partial antigen and is capable of stimulating antibody formation only when combined with protein.

ANTIBODY:

An *antibody* is a substance that usually appears in the bloodstream or body fluids in consequence of the introduction of an antigen, and reacts specifically with that antigen. Antibodies are protein substances present in the gamma globulin fraction of the serum proteins or body fluids. *Bivalent antibody* has two reactive sites for an antigen. *Precipitin antibodies* are bivalent and play a role in immediate hypersensitivity reactions. With the proper proportion of such antibodies and antigen, a precipitate is formed. A *univalent antibody* has only one reactive site; this type is present in most allergies. *Cellular antibody* is bound and expresses itself only when the cell to which it is bound reacts with an antigen; this occurs in tuberculin-type (delayed) hypersensitivity. Reagins and blocking antibodies are univalent. *Reagins* do not form precipitates with antigens and do not fix complement. *Blocking antibodies* react with antigen interstitially, thus preventing its contact with reagin bound to the cells of an organ.

Formation of antibodies [1, 2]

The mechanism of *antibody formation* is incompletely understood, but it is generally believed that antibodies are produced by cells of the reticuloendothelial system. Antigen is probably processed by macrophages. The altered antigenic material stimulates antibody formation by plasmocytes. These cells have developed from thymus-independent lymphocytes (immunoblasts). The latter also give rise to small lymphocytes which carry an immunologic memory. This enables them to react to further exposure to the same antigen.

Tests for antibodies

Often it is possible to demonstrate the presence of a *specific antibody* in a patient's serum by mixing the serum with a suspension of the specific antigen.

This is the basis for the agglutination, precipitation, flocculation, complement fixation, and other tests that are used for the *serologic diagnosis* of certain infectious diseases. Some antibodies can be demonstrated by means of a *skin test* when serologic methods are not effective.

Beneficial antibodies

Antibodies are responsible, in large part, for whatever *acquired immunity* we may have, and as such are ordinarily beneficial. In the host, antibody is believed to unite, directly or indirectly, with its specific antigen if the antigen is present. When the antigen is a free chemical substance such as a bacterial toxin, the new substance formed by union with the antitoxin is ordinarily harmless. When the antigen is part of a bacterial cell, the antibody attaches itself to the cell, sometimes destroying it, in other instances immobilizing it so as to prevent its spread, and sometimes rendering it more susceptible to phagocytosis.

Gamma globulins

Most of the plasma *antibodies are contained in the gamma globulin fraction* of the blood proteins. Studies of this fraction have yielded much information about antibodies. By means of radioactive labels, the catabolic *half-life* (time required for 50 percent of the molecules to be destroyed or degraded) of the antibodies has been estimated at about 20 days [3]. The gamma globulins of the newborn infant approximate those of the mother, both in kind and in grams per 100 ml., because the *infant's antibodies are derived from the mother* by transfer across the placenta. As a result of normal catabolism, the infant's gamma globulins decrease progressively until about the fourth to the 12th week after birth, when the synthesis of antibodies by the baby begins to catch up with antibody destruction. Thereafter the baby's gamma globulins rise slowly, reaching the normal adult level at from 6 months to 7 years of age, depending on many factors.

AGAMMAGLOBULINEMIA [4]

Much has been learned about the significance of antibodies by a study of patients with *agammaglobulinemia.* For one reason or another they are *unable to manufacture antibodies.* They develop delayed (tuberculin-type) hypersensitivity, but it is short-lived. These patients show extreme *susceptibility to infection,* both acute and chronic. In a number of patients with this syndrome a wide mediastinal shadow has been noted on x-ray, due to an *enlarged thymus.* Lymphoid tissue generally is diminished; the liver and spleen are often palpable. Plasmocytes are absent in lymph nodes challenged with antigen. Laboratory studies reveal almost complete absence of gamma globulins, including the naturally occurring hemagglutinins. Neutropenia and lymphocytopenia are commonly noted. In some instances the disease is hereditary, occurring as a sex-linked recessive evident chiefly in males.

HYPERGAMMAGLOBULINEMIA [5]

The opposite state, *hypergammaglobulinemia,* is not evidence of unusual immunity to infection nor is it in itself a disease, but it is a feature of a number of different conditions. *Chronic granulomatous diseases* (tuberculosis, leprosy, lymphogranuloma venereum, kala-azar), *liver diseases* (cirrhosis, toxic or viral hepatitis), *malnutrition, hypersensitivity states, collagen diseases, multiple myeloma, Waldenström's macroglobulinemia,* and *sarcoidosis* account for most instances in which the plasma gamma globulin level is elevated. Rarely the increase may be due to unusually large molecular forms of globulins, the *macroglobulins,* or to globulins which become insoluble at cold temperatures, the *cryoglobulins;* both these rare findings are associated with *blood dyscrasias.*

Although hypergammaglobulinemia often is found in association with hypersensitivity states, *high levels of plasma gamma globulin do not account directly for the occurrence of hypersensitivity.* Hypersensitivity states and collagen diseases may occur even in patients with congenital agammaglobulinemia, being apparently related to antibodies within the leukocytes rather than in the plasma. Hypersensitivity states may be related to antibodies contained within blood cells or tissue cells as well as to antibodies in the blood plasma.

BLOOD GLOBULINS AND HYPERSENSITIVITY STATES

In some circumstances it appears that antibodies may be harmful. They may cause a *too-violent reaction* when the host encounters the antigen on subsequent occasions (hypersensitivity reaction), and this may result in death or serious illness. Under other circumstances the new substance formed by the union of antigen and antibody (the antigen-antibody complex) may itself be harmful even though the original substances separately were not.

HARMFUL ANTIBODIES

Hypersensitivity, or *allergy,* is a phenomenon whereby an immunologic response is the cause of reactions damaging to body cells. Antigens producing such harmful effects may be called *allergens.* Allergens may be bacterial or nonbacterial, or even simple chemical substances. The nature of a hypersensitivity reaction depends on many factors, including the nature of the allergen, the method of contact (skin, nose, gastrointestinal tract), the frequency and recentness of prior contacts, and the ability of the host to form antibodies.

HYPERSENSITIVITY

2. *Anaphylaxis*

Anaphylaxis is a type of hypersensitivity reaction that is usually a result of an initial *parenteral sensitization* followed some time later by a *second injection* of the sensitizing antigen. An interval of 8 to 28 days after the sensitizing injection is necessary for the development of hypersensitivity, but once it has developed, it may persist indefinitely. A naturally occurring reaction of this type is sometimes observed following insect stings. Anaphylactic reactions also occur in persons sensitive to certain drugs, especially penicillin.

PRINCIPLES

In order to avoid an anaphylactic reaction, the physician customarily *tests for sensitivity* before giving a therapeutic injection of a substance that may cause trouble. A minute quantity of the substance is injected *intradermally;* if the individual is sensitive, a wheal develops at the site of injection. In such a case, if it is essential that the treatment be given, either some other form of the substance may be used (e.g., a product derived from sheep serum instead of horse serum), or the patient may be desensitized by serial injections of the substance given in small doses.

PREVENTION

Anaphylaxis occurs in two forms: a systemic form usually known as *anaphylactic shock,* and a local form known as the *Arthus phenomenon.* The systemic form usually occurs when the sensitized individual receives his second or later injection of the antigen by the intravenous, intramuscular, or subcutaneous route, whereas the local form occurs when the injected antigen remains locally, as at the site of an intracutaneous injection.

FORMS:

Anaphylactic shock varies in different species. In guinea pigs it is manifested by constriction of the bronchi, severe respiratory distress, and death in about 10 minutes. Electron microscopy reveals extensive antigen-antibody precipitation

ANAPHYLACTIC SHOCK

and thrombosis in pulmonary capillaries [6]. Antigen-antibody complexes are found within the cytoplasm of eosinophils. The *Schultz-Dale reaction* is the violent contraction in vitro of smooth muscle from a sensitized guinea pig when specific antigen is applied. In dogs a large fall in blood pressure, pooling of the blood in the liver, and death in 1 to 2 hours occur. Features common to anaphylactic shock in all species are *contraction of smooth muscle* and *capillary endothelial damage,* often followed by *death.* The blood becomes less coagulable due to an increase in the amount of heparin and a decrease in the number of platelets. Leukopenia is commonly noted. The functional manifestations of anaphylactic shock are apparently due to toxic products similar to histamine liberated in the blood by the liver; these products can be demonstrated in perfusion experiments and can be neutralized by certain antihistamines.

Arthus phenomenon

The *Arthus phenomenon* ("local anaphylaxis") is a violent *local inflammatory reaction* occurring at the site of intracutaneous injection, or occasionally after topical application, of an antigen in a sensitized individual. There is marked damage to endothelial cells and blood vessel walls with hemorrhage, thrombosis, *necrosis,* and *slough.* Antigen localizes on the vessel walls, and an antigen-antibody reaction occurs there [7]. A heavy neutrophilic infiltrate accumulates. The neutrophils phagocytize antigen-antibody complex. Later, thrombosis occurs within the vessels.

PASSIVE TRANSFER

Both anaphylaxis and the Arthus reaction can be transferred passively by injecting serum from a sensitized animal into a normal animal. If the second animal is then injected with the antigen to which the first animal was sensitive, it will develop an anaphylactic reaction. This may sometimes have clinical importance if a patient receives a transfusion of blood from a sensitized individual.

3. Serum Sickness

Serum sickness is unusual in that it *often occurs without prior sensitization.* A large dose of antigen (e.g., 100 ml. or more of horse serum) is generally necessary to cause the reaction. There is usually a *latent period* of 6 to 12 days after the injection of the inciting antigen before the reaction occurs; presumably this time is required for the body to manufacture antibodies. The latent period is shortened if the patient has been previously sensitized to the antigen *(accelerated serum sickness).* Symptoms (urticaria, joint swellings, and edema) then appear, all a result of increased capillary permeability. Certain drugs such as the sulfonamides and penicillin may produce a delayed *"drug sickness,"* which is comparable in all respects to serum sickness.

Inherent dangers

When serum or drug sickness reaction occurs, the patient should be warned that *subsequent use* of the agent, or even of different but chemically related agents, *may be dangerous.* The hypersensitive state is often due to a *substance incidentally present along with the therapeutic agent.* Thus a person who develops serum sickness following the injection of tetanus antitoxin which has been prepared by injecting a horse with tetanus toxin is usually not sensitive to the tetanus antitoxin per se but to other protein substances present in horse serum. Such a person might have a dangerous anaphylactic shock following the subsequent injection of any horse-serum product, such as diphtheria antitoxin, but no reaction whatever to a second injection of tetanus antitoxin prepared in the goat.

4. Atopy

Atopy is a form of hypersensitivity that is usually determined by hereditary influence. Apparently it is the general predisposition to become sensitive that is inherited rather than a sensitivity to a particular allergen. In this group of diseases are sensitivities to *foods* (strawberries, crustaceans), *airborne particles* (ragweed and other pollens, house dust, dog hair), and *drugs* (aspirin, barbiturates). The reaction usually occurs promptly after contact with the allergen. The *Prausnitz-Küstner reaction* demonstrates the occurrence of an antigen-antibody reaction in atopy. When the serum of a sensitive person is injected intradermally into a nonsensitive one, subsequent injection of antigen causes a local wheal.

Hereditary influences

Prausnitz-Küstner reaction

The *nature of the reaction* is often determined by the manner of contact. Thus airborne particles like pollens usually cause nasal discharge and weeping eyes (hay fever), or bronchial spasm and exudation (asthma); foods usually cause digestive upsets. Sometimes the relationship of the allergen to the *"shock tissue,"* i.e., the organ manifesting symptoms, is so indefinite that the nature of the reaction is not recognized. Thus a common symptom of allergy to crabmeat is violent itching of the skin. When this occurs after eating a meal that includes a salad in which crabmeat is not recognized by taste, it may take a bit of medical detective work to establish a relationship. If sensitization is suspected, the specific substance to which the individual is sensitive can usually be determined by *skin tests.* Eosinophils are often numerous in the mucous secretions of the nose in a case of hay fever, and sometimes are increased in the circulating blood as well.

"Shock tissue"

5. Contact Dermatitis

Repeated or continuous contact of the skin with chemical substances may cause sensitization resulting in a *weeping or crusting skin disorder.* Synthetic fiber underclothing, plastic watch bands, cosmetics, and occupational materials (inks, cleansers, darkroom chemicals) are frequent offenders. Ordinarily the skin lesion *corresponds directly to the area of contact.* The skin lesion is customarily delayed some time after exposure; features of chronicity are usually present when the patient is first seen.

6. Delayed (Tuberculin-Type) Hypersensitivity

The clinical manifestations of many infectious diseases include symptoms of allergy. Because it takes time for antibodies to develop, allergic manifestations are more often noted during the course of *chronic infections* such as tuberculosis, fungus diseases, and diseases due to animal parasites than in the acute bacterial diseases. The sensitization may be due to some chemical constituent of the presence of the infecting organism. Circulating antibodies are not found in this delayed type of hypersensitivity. Allergy in these diseases is often evident as an *unduly violent reaction* to the infecting agent. This type of hypersensitivity can be demonstrated by a *skin test;* the classic example is the tuberculin test (see page 127).

7. Transfusion Reactions

Bloods from different individuals contain various combinations of antigens and antibodies that permit their classification into *blood groups.* Within a single

Blood groups

blood group, all the individuals show the same antigens *(agglutinogens)* on their erythrocytes and the same antibodies *(agglutinins)* in their serum, and their bloods mix without clumping, i.e., their bloods are *compatible.* When the blood of an individual of one blood group is mixed with the blood of an individual of another group, the agglutinins in the serum of the one blood cause the clumping of the erythrocytes in the other blood, i.e., their bloods are *incompatible.*

ABO INCOMPATIBILITY

Some antibodies against erythrocytes that cause incompatibility between two bloods are naturally occurring, i.e., they are present without there having been any known prior sensitization; these are the agglutinins anti-A and anti-B. If blood from a person whose erythrocytes possess the agglutinogen A is injected intravenously into a person whose serum contains agglutinin anti-A, the donor's cells are agglutinated in vivo by the recipient's antibodies. The result is a serious if not fatal *transfusion reaction,* usually accompanied by *intravascular hemolysis, icterus,* and *anuria.*

Rh INCOMPATIBILITY

In other instances the antibodies against erythrocytes are not naturally occurring and appear only following sensitization. This sensitization may come about by the *transfusion of blood* possessing the agglutinogens C, D, or E (Rh', Rh_0, or Rh'', respectively) into a person whose red cells do not have these substances, or in the case of a female, by a *pregnancy* in which the erythrocytes of the fetus possess these agglutinogens but the mother's erythrocytes do not. Ordinarily no reaction occurs with the sensitizing transfusion or pregnancy, but if blood containing these agglutinogens is given following such sensitization, a serious transfusion reaction may occur, identical in all respects to that following an incompatibility in the ABO system.

FETAL REACTIONS

The fetus is also apt to be a victim of blood incompatibilities, especially those of the CDE (Rh) system. Antibodies from the mother can pass freely *through the placental barrier* into the fetal circulation, causing the equivalent of a transfusion reaction in the fetus in utero. This condition, *erythroblastosis fetalis,* is considered in more detail on page 368.

8. Auto-immunization

AUTO-IMMUNIZATION [8]

Auto-immunity is the development of hypersensitivity to an endogenous antigen from the body's own cells. It ordinarily does not develop because of immunotolerance to the body's own proteins. Autosensitization may come about by an alteration in the antibody-producing cells, by a change in a cell protein, or possibly by the coincident presence of a reactive site on a body protein that is identical with one on an exogenous antigen to which the body is sensitive.

AUTO-IMMUNE DISORDERS

Diseases in which the development of auto-immunity plays a pathogenetic role include idiopathic thrombocytopenic purpura (page 36), disseminated lupus erythematosus (page 78), auto-immune hemolytic anemia (page 289), pernicious anemia (page 291), myasthenia gravis (page 695), lymphocytic thyroiditis (page 727), and sympathetic ophthalmia (page 801).

TISSUE AND ORGAN TRANSPLANTATION [9]

1. General Considerations

TYPES

An *autograft* (autologous graft) is one in which the recipient's own tissue is transferred from one part of his body to another. Such transfers may be in the form of a *free graft,* in which the tissue is completely separated initially from its original location, or a *pedicle or flap graft,* in which the tissue is left partly attached to its original site until a new blood supply develops at the graft site. Autografts are usually successful as long as circulation is established within 3 or 4 days. An *allograft (homograft,* allogeneic or homologous graft) is the transfer of a tissue or organ from one member of a species to another. An *isograft* (syngeneic or isogeneic graft) is a within-strain allograft, i.e., a transfer between members of closely inbred strains or between identical twins. Genetically it is an autograft. A *heterograft* (xenograft, xenogeneic or heterologous graft) is a transfer between members of different species.

An *orthotopic graft* is one in which a tissue or organ is transplanted to an anatomically similar location, i.e., skin to skin gap. A *heterotopic graft* is one in which the transplantation is to an abnormal anatomic environment, such as the use of a segment of vein as an arterial graft.

An *allovital graft* is one which is expected to carry on complete function at the new site. On the other hand, an *allostatic graft* is intended to serve only a mechanical function in its new site and need not remain viable.

REJECTION:

Rejection typically occurs in allografts, due to antibody formation against the graft. The exact nature of this immune reaction is not clear. Circulating serum antibodies against homologous cells have been demonstrated in some cases [10]. Host cells (lymphocytes and plasmocytes) apparently must be present within the allograft for its destruction to occur, and such cells carry antibodies.

Patients with agammaglobulinemia – who are unable to produce antibodies – tolerate skin and other allografts like autografts. No rejection occurs in identical twins, who are genetically identical. Skin exchanges from mothers to their infants may last up to 28 months, and an infant's skin also survives on its mother for a long period. Transfers from mothers to boys show female sex chromatin in the graft for months. The epidermis is normal but hairs and sweat and sebaceous glands are absent, and the dermis is densely infiltrated by lymphocytes. All skin grafts between fathers and children are rejected, although they may last grossly for about 3 weeks.

Tolerance to an allograft may be relative or complete. Fully tolerated grafts are like autografts. Grafts which survive for at least 30 days are considered to show relative tolerance. In a skin graft, relative tolerance is characterized by fibrous tissue growth, with contraction and eczematous (vesicular) changes in the epidermis. Patients with severe burns tolerate allografts longer than those without burns, but eventually such grafts are rejected.

Modification

The allograft rejection reaction can be modified by agents which depress the recipient's immunologic reaction [11]. These include adrenocortical steroids (cortisone and cortisol), whole body x-radiation, and immunosuppressive drugs such as azathioprine (1-methyl-4-nitro-5-imidoazolyl thiopurine), azaserine, and actinomycin-D.

SUCCESSFUL GRAFTS

In successful transplantations, blood vessels in the grafted tissue or organ tend to survive. If circulation is not established within 3 to 4 days, cells in the graft will die if the tissue is vascular. Anastomoses between graft and host blood vessels are not necessarily end to end, but this is the earliest pattern. Vessels in the graft which are occluded by thrombi become recanalized within 7 to 8 days. Replacement of dead cells in a graft is often by mitosis of other graft cells. In grafts of cartilage, cancellous bone, fascia, and tendon, the parenchymal cells tend to survive, and the matrix structure is retained. In free skin autografts, epidermal cells persist, as do dermal fibroblasts. Specialized sensory endings, hair follicles, and melanocytes also tend to survive in autografts.

2. Skin Allografts

SKIN ALLOGRAFTS

Except when the graft is from an identical twin, or from mother to infant, or when the recipient has agammaglobulinemia, in *skin allografts* the first to fifth postoperative days are characterized by marked engorgement of the dermal vessels and an extensive accumulation of neutrophils at the host-graft junction, with a slight neutrophilic infiltration of the allograft. Beginning on about the fifth day lymphocytes and plasmocytes infiltrate the graft, and rejection begins typically on the seventh to ninth day. Grossly the previously pink homograft becomes swollen and cherry red and then cyanotic. Microscopically during this rejection period the mononuclear cell infiltrate becomes intense, and both the graft blood vessels and newly ingrown capillaries disappear. By about 2 weeks postoperatively the graft dries and becomes covered by a brownish eschar (scab) consisting of desiccated epidermis and blood elements. The graft is typically sloughed within about 3 weeks.

3. Corneal Allografts

CORNEAL ALLOGRAFTS

Corneal allografts are possible because the cornea is avascular and thus is less subject to the immune graft-rejection reaction. Corneas from eyes refrigerated for several days can be used for transplantation. The corneal epithelium is not essential for graft transparency. Only the collagenous stromal lamellae and the endothelium are essential for a successful graft. If the lamellar structure is preserved, host macrophages can penetrate it and become keratoblasts. Two types of partial or total corneal transplantation are performed, the *lamellar keratoplasty,* in which one-half to two-thirds of the corneal thickness is used, and the *penetrating keratoplasty,* in which the entire thickness is employed.

An *allograft reaction* is much less common in lamellar than in penetrating grafts. The formation of cholesterol crystals at the zone of contact is the most common cause of delayed opacification in lamellar grafts. Allograft clouding within the first 3 weeks postoperatively is due to: poor donor material from which the endothelium has peeled off, faulty apposition of the edges, infection, or traumatic displacement of the graft. Delayed opacification is due to an allograft reaction and typically occurs at about 6 months. The cornea becomes edematous because of endothelial sloughing, and a fibrous membrane grows over the back of the graft. The longer after grafting this reaction occurs, the better is the chance for a successful graft. Delayed clouding may also be due to keratinization of corneal and conjunctival epithelium overlying the graft surface or to retention of infectious agents, such as the virus of herpes simplex, in residual host cornea.

4. Kidney Transplants

KIDNEY TRANSPLANTS:

Kidney allografts in humans have been carried out with success by transplantation of a kidney from one identical twin to the other and by immunosuppression of the recipient's immune response by whole body x-radiation, adrenocortical steroids, and/or appropriate drugs when the donor kidney is from a person other than an identical twin. In renal transplants the donor kidney is implanted in an iliac fossa and anastomoses are established between the renal artery and an artery such as the hypogastric, the renal vein and one such as the external iliac, and the ureter and the host ureter. Kidney transplants are used in patients with chronic renal disease with intractable uremia (renal failure). Evidence of normal renal function and the absence of urinary tract infection in the donor are essential, and major and minor blood group, leuko-agglutinin, and platelet agglutinin compatibilities are desirable.

Rejection [12]:

Clinical signs of *incipient renal allograft rejection* include fever, decreased urine output, increased proteinuria, the presence of cellular or granular casts in the urine, and an elevation in the blood urea nitrogen level. *Rejection* may occur almost immediately after implantation of a kidney, or weeks, months, or even years later.

hyperacute rejection

Hyperacute (immediate) rejection appears within minutes after restoration of circulation in the transplanted kidney, which becomes cyanotic due to diffuse capillary thrombosis. Neutrophils are found along the endothelial surfaces of capillaries and venules. The intravascular coagulation is confined to the kidney and is not part of a generalized Shwartzman reaction (see page 88) with a consumption coagulopathy [13]. Hyperacute rejection is caused by preexisting circulating antibodies to antigens in the graft, such as blood group A or B agglutinogens or leukocyte antigens (HL-A).

early acute rejection

Early acute rejection occurs within the first 2 weeks after transplantation. The kidney is enlarged to up to two to three times its normal size due to diffuse interstitial edema. There is a moderate to heavy interstitial infiltrate consisting of small lymphocytes, immunoblasts, plasmocytes, and macrophages. The immunoblasts are large lymphoid cells in which the cytoplasm stains red with methyl green pyronine because of a high ribonucleic acid content.

late acute rejection

Late acute rejection develops during the third or fourth post-transplantation weeks. The kidney is swollen and there are subcapsular petechiae. A moderate interstitial mononuclear cell infiltrate is present. Necrosis of arteriolar walls is found, and there are subendothelial deposits of immunoglobulins G (IgG) and M (IgM) and β_1C globulin, as shown by immunofluorescent studies.

late rejection

In *late (chronic) rejection* the kidney is shrunken and firm. The glomeruli [14] are enlarged and show diffuse and focal basement membrane thickening, and increased amounts of basement membrane-like material are found in the mesangium. Subendothelial accumulations of amorphous material are present. The epithelial foot processes are fused focally. Immunofluorescent studies have demonstrated the presence of IgG, IgM, complement, and fibrinogen in the subendothelial deposits [15]. Those accumulations are assumed to represent the reaction of circulating antibodies and antigen located on the basement membranes. An obliterative endarteritis is also found in kidneys rejected after 2 months.

In renal transplants, rejection may involve the inserted segment of ureter [16]. After 3 weeks ureteral arterial lumina are obliterated by endothelial cellular proliferation and intimal infiltration by lymphocytes and lipid-laden macrophages.

Complications: recurrence of glomerulonephritis

Glomerulonephritis (see page 572) has developed in transplanted kidneys in a number of cases. Subepithelial humps have been found on glomerular basement membranes by electron microscopy in such instances. Immunofluorescence has revealed the presence of IgG, IgM, and complement along the epithelial side of the basement membranes.

transplantation of neoplasm

In rare cases a *malignant neoplasm* has been inadvertently transplanted to the recipient in a kidney [17]. Widespread metastases have developed in some, but immunologic rejection of a transplanted tumor has occurred [18].

complications due to immunosuppressive agents: infections

Infections are common in patients who have received a renal transplant and have been administered immunosuppressive drugs [19]. The infections are related to the suppression of the body's immune and inflammatory responses to infectious organisms and the depression of granulopoiesis in the bone marrow by these agents. Such infections are commonly due to staphylococci (see page 90), gram-negative bacteria, especially *Pseudomonas* species (see page 101), fungi (see Chapter 8), and *Pneumocystis carinii* (see page 185). The lungs are frequently involved in post-transplantation infections [20].

hepatic injury pancreatitis

Mild changes have been observed in the liver in renal transplant patients on adrenal corticosteroids and azathioprine [21]. Iron deposition in hepatocytes, loss of glycogen in parenchymal cells, and slight cholestasis are found. In a few cases *acute hemorrhagic pancreatitis* (page 547) has developed, presumably related to the use of steroids [22].

5. *Liver Transplants*

LIVER TRANSPLANTS

Orthotopic *liver transplantation,* in which the patient's organ is removed and replaced with a donor liver, has proved more successful than heterotopic transplantation, in which an accessory liver is implanted in an abnormal location. When early rejection occurs, the transplanted liver shows a periportal infiltrate of lymphocytes and plasmocytes [23]. In livers that have survived several weeks, fibrous fingers link the central vein regions together. Inspissated bile is found in intrahepatic bile channels. In some early transplants large abscesses developed in the right lobe of the liver because of kinking of the right branch of the hepatic artery.

6. *Lung Transplants*

LUNG TRANSPLANTS

The *lung* is not especially difficult to transplant technically. However, postoperative infection is a major problem and has caused the deaths of most patients who have received a pulmonary transplant.

7. *Heart Transplants*

HEART TRANSPLANTS

The *heart transplant* is vulnerable to rejection. Early clinical signs of trouble are fatigue, tachycardia, and a diastolic gallop rhythm. The electrocardiogram shows diminished voltage, right axis deviation, and heart block. Later fever, dyspnea, and indications of mainly right-sided heart failure appear. In *early rejection* [24] the heart is dusky red and edematous. Microscopically the myocardium shows widespread focal hydropic vacuolization of myocytes, necrosis, and infiltration of lymphocytes and plasmocytes. Small coronary arteries reveal intimal thickening due to cellular proliferation. In *chronic rejection* [25] the coronary arteries show fibrous intimal thickening, with infiltration by lymphocytes, plasmocytes, and lipid-vacuolated macrophages. The myocardium has foci of necrosis and is infiltrated with lymphocytes, plasmocytes, and macrophages. Small hemorrhages are also present.

8. Bone Marrow Transplants

BONE MARROW TRANSPLANTS

Bone marrow allografts have been employed in patients with acute leukemia after total body radiation. Rejection in marrow grafts differs from that with other tissues in that the transplanted cells react against the host. This graft rejection of the host is called *secondary disease.* In rodents it results in *runt disease* [25a]. When a newborn animal is given a graft containing lymphocytes (lymph nodes or spleen) from a homozygous parent, the graft cells produce antibodies against antigens in the host inherited from the other parent. Thus the transplant launches an immunologic attack on the host. The animal's growth is blighted, and it dies in a few months.

COLLAGEN VASCULAR DISEASES

1. Chronic Allergy

Allergens and chronic diseases

There is some evidence, chiefly experimental, that certain chronic diseases may be a result of a persistent or recurring interaction between antigens and antibodies. Certain *foods, drugs, bacterial products,* and *bacterial variants* (L organisms) are among the substances which have been suggested as the antigens. These diseases are tentatively grouped together as the collagen vascular diseases, because the connective tissues and the blood vessels are principally affected.

2. Collagen Vascular Diseases Generally

No other group of diseases is the subject of so much study and controversy at the present time as are the collagen vascular diseases. There is a pronounced tendency to assign any disease of unknown cause or uncertain pathogenesis to this group. Clinically the diagnosis of collagen vascular disease always seems to be considered if a case is obscure and uncertain.

Drugs

It appears that many of the diseases in this category are of *relatively recent origin.* Whenever a new disease appears we must suspect that it might be due to some *new therapeutic agent* or some *new factor in the environment.* It seems that this suspicion has been confirmed, for at least one of the diseases in this group, disseminated lupus erythematosus, or a disease practically indistinguishable from it, has been reported to have followed the therapeutic use of the drugs, *hydralazine and procainamide* in a number of cases. The relationship of drug therapy to lupus erythematosus is discussed further on page 78.

Group features

Certain features are common to the so-called collagen vascular diseases: (1) *young adults* are chiefly affected; (2) many patients give a *history of allergy,* or there has been evidence of the development of allergy during a recent illness; (3) clinical features include *recurrent fever, arthralgia, skin lesions,* and *splenomegaly;* (4) laboratory studies often reveal *hyperglobulinemia* and *biologically false positive serologic tests for syphilis;* (5) *temporary improvement* may occur following administration of *hormones of the adrenal cortex;* and (6) pathologic changes consist chiefly of *"fibrinoid degeneration"* of the connective tissues and blood vessels of affected organs, and a variable *cell exudate in relation to the blood vessels* [26].

3. Polyarteritis Nodosa (Necrotizing Angiitis, Panarteritis, Periarteritis Nodosa, Allergic Vasculitis)

POLY-ARTERITIS NODOSA: Although certain clinical and pathologic differences have been described [27] among the various members of this group of diseases, there is no obvious reason to separate them. In many instances the *vascular disease appears to have developed following an allergic reaction* to serum, sulfonamides, penicillin, or iodides, or during the course of an allergic disorder such as bronchial asthma or Löffler's syndrome, but in a number of cases no such relationship is evident.

Clinical features

Clinically most cases are manifest by fever, weakness, hypertension, tachycardia, and evidence of functional disturbance of several body systems. Gastrointestinal symptoms (abdominal pain, nausea, diarrhea) are among the most common manifestations; neurologic symptoms (convulsions, blindness, paralyses, paresthesias), respiratory symptoms (dyspnea, cough, wheezing), skin lesions, joint inflammation, and renal symptoms (proteinuria, hypertension, uremia) are commonly noted, and correspond to the localization of the vascular lesions.

Pathologic changes

The tissue changes are of varying severity and distribution. Multiple *small and medium-sized arteries* are usually affected; arterioles, venules, and capillaries (including the glomerular tufts) may also be involved. In acute cases there is *smudgy necrosis* of the walls of the vessels, obliterating evidence of the normal muscular layers, and *eosinophils* and other inflammatory cells are found throughout all portions of the vessel walls including the adventitia. *Thrombosis* and related areas of infarction are commonly seen. In more chronic cases, and especially in instances of temporal arteritis, there is often a *foreign body reaction* in the vessel walls in relation to fragments of broken elastica; this reaction may merge with one in which *sclerotic changes* predominate. Sometimes there are grossly visible *nodules* along the course of the medium-sized vessels, and sometimes multiple *aneurysms* are noted. The renal lesions are generally believed to be responsible for the hypertension that commonly occurs.

4. Disseminated Lupus Erythematosus

LUPUS ERYTHEMATOSUS: Causes

Disseminated lupus erythematosus is an autosensitivity disease which occurs most commonly in women between 18 and 35 years of age. Antinuclear, antinucleolar [28], antilysosome, antithyroglobulin, antierythrocyte, antithrombin, and Wassermann antibodies have been identified in cases of lupus erythematosus [29]. Significantly increased titers of myxovirus antibodies have been found in patients with lupus, and persistent viral infection may be a pathogenetic factor in this disease [30]. Lupus erythematosus has developed in a number of patients receiving hydralazine hydrochloride over a prolonged period for hypertension [31]. An almost identical disorder has occurred in several patients using procainamide hydrochloride [31a]. Symptoms of lupus are often first evident following *exposure to sunlight,* and many patients give a history of unusual sensitivity to sun. In most patients with lupus erythematosus, however, there is no apparent cause.

Clinical manifestations

Clinically any of the following may be noted at one time or another during the illness: *joint pain and swelling* (80 percent of the cases); *reddened skin lesions*

(50 percent) particularly of the face and in response to sunlight; *proteinuria* or other evidence of renal disease (60 percent); *cardiac involvement* (50 percent); *lymph node enlargement; fever;* and blood changes – *anemia, thrombocytopenia, leukopenia, and hyperglobulinemia.* When the erythematous "butterfly" rash is present over the nose, the prognosis is grave.

Pathologic changes [32]

Pathologic changes are often meager in proportion to the clinical symptoms. The following lesions are classic but are often lacking even in fatal cases of presumed disseminated lupus. The *kidneys* may be large and pale on gross examination; microscopically *eosinophilic deposits* may be seen *in the basement membrane of the glomerular tuft* ("wire loop" lesions). The *heart* often shows no changes grossly; however, in some cases small *sterile fibrinous masses* are seen *along the line of closure of the valve cusps* and on the endocardium of the left atrium (nonbacterial endocarditis of Libman and Sachs). Microscopically *hematoxylin bodies* [33] may be seen beneath the atrial endocardium; these bodies give a positive Feulgen reaction and are thereby shown to contain *nucleic acid derivatives.* The *spleen* is usually enlarged. Microscopically, concentric *rings of fibrous tissue* may be noted *about the small blood vessels. Skin* changes include *fibrinoid changes* in the collagen just beneath the epidermis and vacuoles in the basal layer of epithelium. Inflammatory cells are noted about small vessels in the dermis. *Small blood vessels* generally may show eosinophilic deposits in their walls. Electron microscopy reveals deposits, which probably represent antigen-antibody complex, at the epidermodermal junction and subendothelially in small blood vessels [34].

L.E. cells

An important laboratory finding is the *L.E. cell phenomenon,* due to antinuclear antibodies in the plasma. When the patient's plasma is added to his own or another's blood cells, basophilic masses appear and are engulfed by polymorphonuclear cells. These masses are Feulgen-positive and are probably identical with the hematoxylin bodies sometimes seen on postmortem examination in other organs. The leukocyte with its phagocytosed basophilic material is known as the L.E. cell; search for these cells is an important diagnostic test for the disease. The severity of the disease generally parallels the degree of positiveness of the L.E. cell test.

5. *Scleroderma*

SCLERODERMA

This rare disease in which the *skin* becomes *thickened* and *stiff* occurs in two forms: (1) *circumscribed scleroderma (morphea),* in which the lesions are localized, usually about the joints of the fingers, and which may go on to the diffuse form or may clear completely; and (2) *diffuse scleroderma,* a slowly fatal disease which may involve, in addition to the skin, the *mucous membranes, fascial layers,* and *serous membranes.* Microscopically there are a peculiar fibrillar change and *sclerosis of the dermis* which results in *atrophy of the epidermis* and a gradual *disappearance of the dermal appendages.* Vascular lesions are variable. Terminally many cases show severe *pulmonary symptoms;* thickening of the alveolar walls of the lungs is sometimes seen, apparently a result of extension of the process to these organs. Death is usually a result of an intercurrent infection.

6. *Dermatomyositis*

DERMATOMYOSITIS

Dermatomyositis is a rare and poorly defined disorder, often developing after an upper respiratory infection, and characterized by *muscle tenderness* and *weakness* and by *variable skin lesions.* Microscopically there are vascular and perivascular inflammation of the dermis and voluntary muscles, and later *muscle atrophy.* Involvement of the heart or other viscera is rare. Malignant neoplasms (cancers) are present in about 5 percent of cases of dermatomyositis. The latter disease in such cases may be due to the development of hypersensitivity to cellular products of the malignant tumor [35].

7. Amyloidosis

AMYLOIDOSIS [36]: Chemistry

Amyloidosis is the accumulation of amyloid in various body tissues. *Amyloid* is an abnormal, complex protein substance containing alpha and gamma globulin and glycoprotein. By electron microscopy amyloid appears as fibrils consisting of filaments measuring about 75 angstroms in diameter [37]. Occasional stellate formations (amyloid stars) are found.

Artificial amyloid

Experimentally amyloid deposits can be produced in mice by the continuous feeding of casein; discontinuance of casein results in the disappearance of the deposits. Horses receiving injections of diphtheria toxin (for antitoxin production) for a number of years develop amyloid deposits in their organs.

Types:

In man amyloidosis occurs in three forms: (1) *primary* atypical amyloidosis, (2) *secondary* (systemic) amyloidosis, and (3) *amyloid tumors.* Secondary amyloidosis is the most common form.

primary amyloidosis

Primary amyloidosis is a rare disease having no demonstrable cause. In a few instances it has developed in patients with *multiple myeloma.* The amyloid deposits occur in the *tongue, skin, heart* [38], *gastrointestinal tract,* and occasionally in and about the *large joints,* more or less diffusely and without any demonstrable relationship to blood vessels. The liver, spleen, kidneys, and adrenal glands – the organs characteristically affected in secondary amyloidosis – are ordinarily not affected in the primary form. The deposits may or may not give the usual histochemical staining reactions described hereafter; when these reactions are negative, it may be impossible to differentiate the disease from scleroderma.

secondary amyloidosis

Secondary amyloidosis is usually the late result of a *long-continued destructive process involving bones, joints,* or *lungs.* It is generally believed that, as these tissues are destroyed, the ground substance liberates chondroitin sulfuric acid, which then serves as an antigen to call forth an antibody. The amyloid deposits are believed to be this antigen-antibody complex, localized in the reticuloendothelial system. Since most patients dying with amyloidosis are already seriously ill with their underlying disease (such as pulmonary tuberculosis or chronic osteomyelitis), it is common for amyloidosis to be undiagnosed prior to autopsy.

One or all of the following organs are characteristically affected: liver, spleen, kidneys, and adrenal glands. The *liver* is often palpably enlarged and is firm and waxy; microscopically the deposits are found between the liver cords and the endothelium lining the sinusoids. Ordinarily there is no functional effect, such as jaundice or ascites, from the liver disease. The *spleen* is often palpably enlarged and is firm. In some cases the amyloid is seen on the cut surface of the spleen as rounded translucent masses replacing the lymphoid follicles (sago spleen); in other cases the deposits are more diffuse, filling in the walls of the sinuses of the red pulp and giving a streaked appearance (bacon spleen). The *kidneys are the organs most likely to show the functional effects of amyloid deposits:* massive *proteinuria* and severe *hypoproteinemia* are common, but hypertension and uremia are rare. The kidneys are usually firm but their size is often not affected, and the deposits are ordinarily not visible grossly without specific stains. Microscopically the deposits are noted in the glomeruli between the endothelial and epithelial layers of the capillary tuft; in advanced cases they may also be evident in the walls of the small vessels in the renal medulla. The *adrenal glands* are often affected. The deposits occur in the walls of the sinusoids and may compress the cells of the cortex. Usually no functional effects are evident, but occasionally there may be signs of chronic adrenal insufficiency (Addison's disease).

amyloid tumors

Amyloid tumors occur in those locations where solitary plasma cell tumors are sometimes found: the *nasopharynx* and *larynx*. They are not true neoplasms. There is a suspicion that amyloid tumors are really plasma cell tumors in which retrogressive changes have occurred.

Staining reactions of amyloid

In tissues stained with hematoxylin and eosin, amyloid appears as a *glistening eosinophilic substance* without granules or fibers, i.e., it is a form of *"hyalin."* It cannot be certainly differentiated from other hyaline substances except by special staining methods.

For the *gross confirmation* of amyloid at the autopsy table, it is usually satisfactory simply to treat organ slices with an *aqueous iodine solution,* such as Lugol's solution. By this method amyloid is stained mahogany brown. When this color is characteristically located, as in punctate dots in the renal cortex, amyloid is almost certainly present. As a second step, *dilute sulfuric acid* may be added; this produces a bluish black discoloration similar to that occurring when starch is treated with iodine and acid (hence the name *amyloid,* or starchlike). This second color change is not constant in deposits staining as amyloid by other methods.

For the demonstration of amyloid in *microscopic sections, methyl violet* or *gentian violet* is usually recommended; these stain amyloid a rose red. A somewhat less reliable agent for staining amyloid in tissue sections is *Congo red.* As this dye is nontoxic and has a specific affinity for amyloid, it may be used for *in vivo tests.* Following intravenous administration of the dye, 60 percent or more of the injected dose is removed from the blood within an hour if amyloid deposits are present. This method should be avoided for cosmetic reasons if it is suspected that amyloid is present in the skin.

REFERENCES

1. Roitt, I. M., Greaves, M. F., Torrigiani, G., Brostoff, J., and Playfair, J. H. L. The cellular basis of immunological responses. *Lancet* 2:367, 1969.
2. Schlossman, S. F. The immune response. *New Eng. J. Med.* 277:1355, 1967.
3. Gitlin, D., Gross, P. A. M., and Janeway, C. A. The gamma globulins and their clinical significance. *New Eng. J. Med.* 260:21, 72, 121, 170, 1959.
4. Rosen, F. S., and Janeway, C. A. The gamma globulins. III. The antibody deficiency syndromes. *New Eng. J. Med.* 275:709, 1966.
5. Alper, C. A., Rosen, F. A., and Janeway, C. A. The gamma globulins. II. Hyperglobulinemia. *New Eng. J. Med.* 275:591, 652, 1966.

6. Sabesin, S. M. Electron microscopy of hypersensitivity reactions. Intravascular antigen-antibody precipitation in acute anaphylactic shock. *Amer. J. Path.* 44:889, 1964.
7. Sabesin, S. M., and Banfield, W. G. Electron microscopy of hypersensitivity reactions. The Arthus phenomenon. *Amer. J. Path.* 42:551, 1963.
8. Witebsky, E. The clinical pathology of auto-immunization. *Amer. J. Clin. Path.* 49:301, 1968.
9. Russell, P. S., and Monaco, A. P. *The Biology of Tissue Transplantation.* Boston: Little, Brown, 1965.
10. Jeannet, M., Pinn, V. W., Flax, M. H., Winn, H. J., and Russell, P. S. Humoral antibodies in renal allotransplantation in man. *New Eng. J. Med.* 282:111, 1970.
11. Murray, J. E., Merrill, J. P., Harrison, J. H., Wilson, R. E., and Dammin, G. J. Prolonged survival of human-kidney homografts by immunosuppressive drug therapy. *New Eng. J. Med.* 268:1315, 1963.
12. Russell, P. S., and Winn, H. J. Transplantation. *New Eng. J. Med.* 282:896, 1970.
13. Colman, R. W., Braun, W. E., Busch, G. J., Dammin, G. J., and Merrill, J. P. Coagulation studies in the hyperacute and other forms of renal-allograft reaction. *New Eng. J. Med.* 281:685, 1969.
14. Porter, K. A., Dossetor, J. B., Marchioro, T. L., Peart, W. S., Rendall, J. M., Starzl, T. E., and Terasaki, P. I. Human renal transplants. I. Glomerular changes. *Lab. Invest.* 16:153, 1967.
15. Porter, K. A., Andres, G. A., Calder, M. W., Dossetor, J. B., Hsu, K. C., Rendall, J. M., Seegal, B. C., and Starzl, T. E. Human renal transplants. II. Immunofluorescent and immunoferritin studies. *Lab. Invest.* 18:159, 1968.
16. Haber, M. H., and Putong, P. B. Ureteral vascular rejection in human renal transplants. *J.A.M.A.* 192:417, 1965.
17. Martin, D. C., Rubini, M., and Rosen, V. J. Cadaveric renal homotransplantation with inadvertent transplantation of carcinoma. *J.A.M.A.* 192:752, 1965.
18. Wilson, R. E., Hager, E. B., Hampers, C. L., Corson, J. M., Merrill, J. P., and Murray, J. E. Immunologic rejection of human cancer transplanted with a renal allograft. *New Eng. J. Med.* 278:479, 1968.
19. Rifkind, D., Marchioro, T. L., Waddell, W. R., and Starzl, T. E. Infectious diseases associated with renal homotransplantation. *J.A.M.A.* 189:397, 1964.
20. Rifkind, D., Starzl, T. E., Marchioro, T. L., Waddell, W. R., Rowlands, D. T., Jr., and Hill, R. B., Jr. Transplantation pneumonia. *J.A.M.A.* 189:808, 1964.
21. Hill, R. B., Jr., Porter, K. A., and Massion, C. G. Hepatic reaction to renal transplants modified by immunosuppressive therapy. *Arch. Path.* (Chicago) 81:71, 1966.
22. Tilney, N. L., Collins, J. J., Jr., and Wilson, R. E. Hemorrhagic pancreatitis. A fatal complication of renal transplantation. *New Eng. J. Med.* 274:1051, 1966.
23. Russell, P. S., and Winn, H. J. Transplantation. *New Eng. J. Med.* 282:896, 1970.
24. Stinson, E. B., Dong, E., Jr., Bieber, C. P., Schroeder, J. S., and Shumway, N. E. Cardiac transplantation in man. I. Early rejection. *J.A.M.A.* 207:2233, 1969.

25. Nora, J. J., Cooley, D. A., Fernbach, D. J., Rochelle, D. G., Milam, J. D., Montgomery, J. R., Leachman, R. D., Butler, W. T., Rossen, R. D., Bloodwell, R. D., Hallman, G. L., and Trentin, J. J. Rejection of the transplanted human heart. *New Eng. J. Med.* 280:1079, 1969.
25a. Hildemann, W. H., Gallagher, R. E., and Walford, R. L. Pathologic changes in lymphoid tissues in early transplantation (runt) disease in mice. *Amer. J. Path.* 45:481, 1964.
26. Strukov, A. General morphology of collagen diseases. *Arch. Path.* (Chicago) 78:409, 1964.
27. Zeek, P. M. Periarteritis nodosa: A critical review. *Amer. J. Clin. Path.* 22:777, 1952.
28. Ritchie, R. F. Antinucleolar antibodies. *New Eng. J. Med.* 282:1174, 1970.
29. Vaughan, J. H., Barnett, E. V., and Leddy, J. P. Autosensitivity diseases. Immunologic and pathogenetic concepts in lupus erythematosus, rheumatoid arthritis and hemolytic anemia. *New Eng. J. Med.* 275:1426, 1966.
30. Phillips, P. E., and Christian, C. L. Myxovirus antibody increases in human connective tissue disease. *Science* 168:982, 1970.
31. Perry, H. M., Jr., and Schroeder, H. A. Syndrome simulating collagen disease caused by hydralazine (Apresoline). *J.A.M.A.* 154:670, 1954.
31a. Kaplan, J. M., Wachtel, H. L., Czarnecki, S. W., and Sampson, J. J. Lupus-like illness precipitated by procainamide hydrochloride. *J.A.M.A.* 192:444, 1965.
32. Teilum, G., and Poulsen, H. E. Disseminated lupus erythematosus. Histopathology, morphogenesis, and relation to allergy. *A.M.A. Arch. Path.* 64:414, 1957.
33. Worthington, J. W., Baggenstoss, A. H., and Hargraves, M. M. Significance of hematoxylin bodies in the necropsy diagnosis of systemic lupus erythematosus. *Amer. J. Path.* 25:955, 1959.
34. Grishman, E., and Churg, J. Ultrastructure of dermal lesions in systemic lupus erythematosus. *Lab. Invest.* 22:189, 1970.
35. Grace, J. T., Jr., and Dao, T. L. Dermatomyositis in cancer. A possible etiological mechanism. *Cancer* 12:648, 1959.
36. Cohen, A. S. Amyloidosis. *New Eng. J. Med.* 277:522, 574, 628, 1967.
37. Gueft, B., and Ghidoni, J. J. The site of formation and ultrastructure of amyloid. *Amer. J. Path.* 43:837, 1963.
38. Mulligan, R. M. Amyloidosis of the heart. *A.M.A. Arch. Path.* 65:615, 1958.

GENERAL REFERENCES

Gowans, J. L. The immunology of tissue transplantation. In Florey, H. W. (Ed.), *General Pathology* (4th ed.). Philadelphia: Saunders, 1970.

Porter, K. A. Tissue transplantation. In Harrison, C. V. (Ed.), *Recent Advances in Pathology* (8th ed.). Boston: Little, Brown, 1966.

5 ACUTE BACTERIAL DISEASES

INFECTIOUS DISEASES IN GENERAL

Diseases caused by living agents are known as the infectious diseases and the communicable diseases, because the etiologic agents can be passed from man to man or from lower animal to man. Before 1900, infectious diseases were perhaps the major cause of human death and were certainly the principal factor in deaths during childhood and early adult life. Through the truly magnificent achievements in microbiology, preventive medicine, and therapeutics within the past century, most of the infectious diseases, including the dreadful scourges such as bubonic plague and cholera, have been brought under control and some have been almost eradicated.

The spectrum of living organisms which produce disease in man includes bacteria, fungi, rickettsiae, viruses, protozoa, helminths, insects, and arachnids.

1. Infection

INFECTION:

Infection is the invasion of tissue by pathogenic microorganisms or animal parasites and the local and general reactions that follow. Infectious lesions are inflammatory in nature, and the general principles of inflammation (see Chapter 3) apply to them. The *modes of infection* include surface contact (skin or mucous membranes) and the inhalation or ingestion of organisms.

Factors determining outcome of infection

The *factors determining the result of infection* include the following:

1. *Number of organisms.* The greater the number of organisms, the greater is the chance for the development of infection and the more severe is the resultant infection. Small numbers of bacteria are quickly killed, except for *Mycobacterium tuberculosis.*

2. *Kind of organisms.* Many organisms cause a specific disease entity, and the immunity of the host varies from agent to agent.

3. *Virulence of the organisms.* Virulence is a measure of the ability of a living agent to overcome the body defenses and cause disease, as well as of its invasiveness and toxicity. The greater the virulence, the more severe is the resultant infection.

4. *Type of tissue involved.* Many organisms have a definite predilection for particular tissues and cannot gain a foothold elsewhere.

5. *Tissue defenses.* These are discussed as the mechanical, cellular, and vascular responses in inflammation on pages 52–56.

6. *Humoral defenses.* In both normal and immune sera there are numerous *antibodies* which are of great importance in localizing living agents, especially bacteria, and rendering them ineffective. The antibodies may be specific (i.e., affect only one type of living agent in the immune animal) or nonspecific. They include *agglutinins,* which coat the surfaces of bacteria and promote the adherence of one organism to another to form clumps in the immune individual; *precipitins,* which cause the precipitation of specific bacteria in gel-like masses; *lysins,* which dissolve bacteria; *ablastins,* which inhibit the reproduction of bacteria; *antitoxins,* which neutralize the exotoxins produced by specific agents, usually bacteria; *opsonins,* specific or nonspecific substances that so affect the surfaces of bacteria as to render them more easily phagocytized; and *properdin,* a euglobulin which appears to be important in natural immunity and which is destroyed by radiation.

7. *General state of health of the host,* especially as to protein balance. Antibodies derive from the gamma globulin, and good protein reserves are essential for the repair of injury.

The resultant vector of these factors determines whether infection will occur and, if so, the degree of its severity. When infection occurs, there is a local inflammatory reaction at the site of entry. The *organisms may spread* from the site of entry through the tissues, via the bloodstream or lymphatics, and over body surfaces.

Special features of infection

Special features of infection as compared to other types of inflammation include: (1) the ability of living organisms to proliferate within the body, so that prolonged and dynamic stimulation of an inflammatory reaction is possible; (2) the ability of living agents to spread because of their reproductive capacity, motility, and secretion of a spreading factor (hyaluronidase); (3) the elaboration by living organisms of a variety of agents and substances which modify the host body's inflammatory response; and (4) the formation of specific antibodies which may alter the usual inflammatory response and produce a superimposed inflammatory response of their own (antigen-antibody reaction).

Clinical features of infectious diseases:

While living agents produce a wide variety of specific disease entities, certain general features are common to most. There is usually an *incubation period* of days or weeks between the time of exposure to the organism and the onset of clinical disease. During this period the agent is gaining a foothold and proliferating in the body of the host. In many diseases there is a short *prodromal period* in which early nonspecific manifestations of a disease, usually those of an upper respiratory infection (fever, malaise, nasal congestion, sore throat, and headache), appear. The *onset* of an infectious disease is usually sudden, although in chronic infections such as tuberculosis it is often insidious.

signs and symptoms

General signs and symptoms of acute infectious diseases include fever, chills, sweating, malaise, muscle aches, headache, weakness or prostration, tachycardia (rapid heart rate), and leukocytosis (elevated white blood cell count). These systemic manifestations are due to circulating toxins and/or a bacteremia, protozoemia, or viremia (the presence of these organisms in the bloodstream). There are important exceptions to these rules; e.g., in typhoid fever there is a relative bradycardia (slow heart rate), and in most viral, protozoan, and helminthic infections there is no leukocytosis. *Most acute bacterial infections cause a shift to the left in the leukocytes* with the appearance of many young forms of the polymorphonuclear leukocytic series in the peripheral blood. However, in pertussis there is a marked increase in lymphocytes (lymphocytosis). In helminthic infections there is often an increase in the number of eosinophils (eosinophilia). In many bacterial, rickettsial, and viral infections there is a *skin rash (exanthem);* the rash may involve the mucous membranes *(enanthem).* The rash is often characteristic of the disease. Many infectious diseases have special features, such as the lower motor neuron type of paralysis in poliomyelitis or the yellowish gray pharyngeal membrane of diphtheria, which enable the physician to make a clinical diagnosis.

identification of organisms

Infectious diseases often mimic each other as well as some noninfectious disorders. Therefore it is essential, whenever feasible, *to identify the causative organism* by smear or culture in order to establish a definite diagnosis. Material for such identification should be obtained before the administration of antibiotics, because these make the isolation of bacteria difficult or impossible.

course

The height of an infectious disease is known as the *fastigium.* If the patient survives, an acute infectious disease may either run out its course gradually (by *lysis*), or clear suddenly (by *crisis*). The return of the elevated temperature to normal is *defervescence.* There then follows a short or prolonged period of *convalescence,* during which the body regains its full vigor. The convalescence may be punctuated by a *recurrence* (return of a disease). A number of bacterial, protozoan, and helminthic infections are chronic and have a slowly progressive course unless treated.

ACUTE BACTERIAL INFECTIONS

BACTERIA:

Bacteria are microscopic, unicellular plants which are devoid of chlorophyll and grow independently of sunlight. They are classified among the fungi as Schizomycetes. Reproduction is asexual by binary fission. Morphologically the bacteria may be spherical (cocci), cylindrical (bacilli), rigidly curved (vibrios, spirilla), or spiral (spirochetes). Of the 1600 known species of bacteria most are harmless – and many are actually beneficial – to man. However, a number of species are pathogenic, i.e., capable of producing disease. Bacteria cause disease by invading and proliferating in the tissues of the host and by elaborating a variety of toxic (poisonous) substances.

Exotoxins

Toxins that are excreted from the living bacterial body are called *exotoxins.* Most of these are enzymes or enzyme-like. Some exotoxins are incredibly poisonous to the animal body; e.g., the A toxin of *Clostridium botulinum* has an LD_{50} (median lethal dose) in mice of 4.5×10^{-9} mg. Many organisms release powerful trypsin-like proteolytic enzymes which cause tissue necrosis. Other exotoxins include leukocidins, which kill leukocytes; fibrinolysins (fibrinokinases), which dissolve fibrin clots; and hemolysins, which dissolve erythrocytes.

Endotoxins:

Endotoxins (somatic or O antigens, bacterial pyrogen, Shwartzman material) [1] are partly or completely a constituent of the bacterial cell wall which is released by lysis of the bacteria. They are most commonly present *in the cell walls of gram-negative bacteria* showing smooth colonial growth. Small amounts have been isolated from gram-positive bacteria and from colonially rough gram-negative organisms. No correlation has been found between the virulence of gram-negative bacteria and their endotoxin content. Chemically endotoxins are large protein-lipopolysaccharide-carbohydrate complexes. The *toxic fraction* of the endotoxin molecule appears to be the lipid A component extracted by acid hydrolysis. When administered in sufficient amount, endotoxin is lethal through the production of *irreversible shock.* Nonlethal doses of endotoxin produce *tolerance,* a state of refractoriness to the effects of further increased doses of endotoxin. *Tolerance is nonspecific,* animals which have been made refractory by one endotoxin exhibiting tolerance to all. Therefore, tolerance is not due to the formation of antibody against antigenic endotoxin.

role in fever

The *pyrogenicity of endotoxin* is demonstrated by the febrile response following intravenous administration of very minute amounts. A *latent period* of 15 to 30 minutes, during which a definite leukopenia develops, precedes the fever spike. The *fever* subsides after about an hour, coincident with a rapid rise in the leukocyte count which persists for 4 to 6 hours. When substantial doses of endotoxin have been injected, a *second temperature rise* occurs shortly after the subsidence of the first peak and lasts for 4 to 6 hours. Since all endotoxin has been cleared from the circulation by this time, the second peak appears to be due to the release of *endogenous pyrogen* from injured leukocytes. Animals which have been rendered tolerant to endotoxin are refractory to the secondary rise in temperature.

role in shock

Irreversible shock, and death within 24 hours, are produced by the injection of a lethal dose of endotoxin. After 1 to 2 hours the animal becomes weak and lethargic and develops marked hypothermia or hyperpyrexia. Terminally the animal has convulsions. At autopsy gastrointestinal hemorrhages are the only morphologic evidence of the shock. It is possible that endotoxin causes an altered reactivity of small blood vessels to epinephrine by the release of serotonin and/or histamine. There is evidence that endotoxin from gram-negative bacteria in the intestine is the final underlying factor in the production of irreversible shock. In the shock state the reticuloendothelial cells are damaged to a degree sufficient to lose their capacity to inactivate endotoxin.

Shwartzman phenomenon

The *Shwartzman phenomenon of focal dermal hemorrhagic necrosis* is produced by a preparatory intradermal endotoxin injection followed in 18 to 24 hours by the intravenous administration of endotoxin. This *provoking dose* produces necrosis in the prepared skin site where neutrophils have been collecting about blood vessels in the interim. The intravenous administration of both the preparatory and provoking doses produces the generalized Shwartzman reaction characterized by bilateral cortical necrosis of the kidneys. Cortisone or reticuloendothelial blockage by thorium dioxide prepares the body for a generalized Shwartzman reaction to a single dose of endotoxin. The provoking dose of endotoxin appears to be thromboplastic; the generalized reaction in experimental animals and probably in humans is triggered by intravascular coagulation of blood, especially in the glomerular capillaries [2]. Renal cortical necrosis in endotoxin-induced generalized Shwartzman reaction can be prevented by the use of anticoagulants.

role in pregnancy

Endotoxin produces *decidual injury* by causing the stasis of blood flow, thrombus formation, and hemorrhage. It is possible that *premature birth and increased perinatal mortality* may be caused by decidual damage produced by circulating endotoxins from genitourinary infections due to gram-negative bacteria. Pregnant animals are highly sensitive to the effects of endotoxins.

host defense reaction

Host defense mechanisms against endotoxin begin with the surface adsorption or possibly ingestion of circulating endotoxin by leukocytes. The material is also rapidly cleared from the circulation by reticuloendothelial cells. *Specific antibody formation is not protective against endotoxin,* and in fact endotoxin combined with specific antibody is sometimes more toxic than the endotoxin alone. *Endotoxin also produces protective effects.* A single dose stimulates the *phagocytic activity of neutrophils and macrophages.* The injection of endotoxin also increases the opsonic activity against gram-negative bacteria and causes a rise in serum properdin levels. The *granulopectic* (granule fixing) *activity of the reticuloendothelial cells* is enhanced by small endotoxin doses. Animals made tolerant to endotoxin have an *increased resistance to the development of traumatic shock and the effects of gamma radiation and x-radiation.* The protein component of endotoxin causes an accelerated and increased, but not prolonged, *stimulation of antibody production.*

Bacteremia

Bacteremia is the simple presence of bacteria in the bloodstream without clinical manifestations. It probably occurs in all deep wounds and tooth extractions, and it provides a means whereby infections spread to distant foci.

Toxemia

Toxemia is a clinical state produced by the sum total of the effects of bacterial toxins. It is *not* dependent on the presence of organisms in the blood. Clinical manifestations of toxemia are malaise, fatigue, general aching, and spasm or paralysis of muscles. Examples of pure toxemia are tetanus and botulism. However, toxemia plays a role in the clinical picture of most infectious diseases.

Septicemia:

Septicemia is a clinical state in which, in addition to bacteremia, there are chills, fever, and petechial hemorrhages. It represents the failure of the body defenses to localize an infection. Organisms may enter the blood by direct extension and entrance into a vessel, by thrombosis in an area of inflammation with subsequent infection of the thrombus and release of mycotic emboli, by infection of lymphatics with subsequent entrance into the venous system, and by direct injection. *Common causes of septicemia* include beta-hemolytic streptococci, coagulase-positive staphylococci, *Escherichia coli* and other gram-negative coliform bacteria, and *Pseudomonas aeruginosa.*

pathologic changes

Degenerative changes in septicemia include cloudy swelling of the myocardium, liver, and kidneys, fatty metamorphosis of the liver, waxy (Zenker's) degeneration of skeletal muscle (especially in typhoid fever), focal necrosis in the liver, spleen, and lymph nodes (typhoid fever), hemolysis with icterus, multiple petechiae due to capillary damage, extensive adrenal hemorrhage (meningococcemia), and thrombi in the capillaries in many organs. The *host defense reaction,* manifested clinically by fever, tachycardia, and leukocytosis, includes reticuloendothelial hyperplasia in the spleen, lymph nodes, liver, and bone marrow. In *acute septic splenitis* the spleen is enlarged and mushy. *Microscopically* the germinal centers are hyperplastic, large, and poorly defined. The reticular elements are hyperplastic, and the sinusoids are engorged with erythrocytes and polymorphonuclear leukocytes. In overwhelming infections the lymph follicles may be depleted. The *local effects of bacteria* are foci of acute inflammation, sometimes with abscess formation, or a chronic granulomatous reaction. *Fulminating septicemia* may cause death in a few hours with few pathologic findings.

Pyemia

Pyemia is a condition in which pyogenic (pus-producing) organisms, especially *Staphylococcus aureus,* are carried in the bloodstream and initiate multiple focal abscesses.

Sapremia

Sapremia is the presence in the bloodstream of toxic metabolites resulting from the growth of saprophytic organisms in necrotic tissue.

1. Staphylococcal Infections

Staphylococci: toxins

Staphylococci are gram-positive cocci which grow in grapelike clusters. The *toxins* they produce are: a *leukocidin* which damages neutrophils; *dermonecrotoxin* which produces skin necrosis; *lethal toxin; enterotoxin;* and five *hemolysins.* Their *enzymes* include: free and bound *coagulase,* which produces clotting of plasma; *staphylokinase,* a fibrinolysin; *hyaluronidase; phosphatase; protease; lipase; desoxyribonuclease;* and *penicillinase,* which inactivates penicillin and is thus responsible for resistance to this antibiotic, being found only in penicillin-resistant strains. Coagulase-positive and mannitol-fermenting staphylococci are classified as *Staphylococcus aureus,* regardless of whether they produce golden yellow pigment. Coagulase-negative and nonmannitol-fermenting organisms are classified as *Staphylococcus epidermidis (S. albus).* The *ability to produce coagulase* is the criterion of pathogenicity in staphylococci. *Coagulase-positive strains are* more resistant to phagocytosis than coagulase-negative strains. Staphylococci can also survive within neutrophils. The appearance of a satellite zone of multiple discrete foci of clearing of blood agar at some distance from a staphylococcal colony *(staphylococcal satellite proteolysis, Mueller phenomenon)* is peculiar to coagulase-positive staphylococci. *Antibiotic resistance* may also be due to the induction of degraded G or L forms of staphylococci by antibiotics. A *capsule* has been visualized on staphylococci, and it has been shown that a specific, probably polysaccharide surface antigen is responsible for resistance to phagocytosis [3].

antibiotic-resistant strains

Due largely to the development of *antibiotic-resistant strains,* serious staphylococcal infections have become common in recent years. *Hospital infections* have become a major problem in medical and especially surgical cases. *Staphylococcus aureus* of bacteriophage type 80/81 and more recently of type 54 have been the principal causes of such hospital infections [4]. Factors involved in hospital staphylococcal infections include: (1) the *susceptible patient,* (2) a *"person with a lesion"* or a persistent, intermittent, or occasional *carrier* among hospital personnel or other patients, and (3) *articles in the hospital environment* such as clothes, mattresses, bed linen, soap, and personal effects [5]. *Postoperative wound infections* are largely due to aerial contamination within the operating room or endogenous infection in a carrier-patient. *Nursery infections* of newborn infants result from mothers who are carriers or have staphylococcal infections, nursery personnel, fomites, and other infants carrying staphylococci, especially the "cloud-babies" who expel vast numbers of staphylococci from their nasal passages on coughing or sneezing.

increased susceptibility

Increased susceptibility to staphylococcal infection is present in patients with eczema and other dermatitides; hepatic disease; diabetes mellitus; malignant neoplasms; agammaglobulinemia; agranulocytosis, in which leukocyte count is markedly depressed; influenza and other viral infections; trauma; operative wounds; burns; urinary catheterization; intravenous injections; and steroid and/or antibiotic therapy [6]. Antibiotic therapy predisposes to staphylococcal infection by the elimination of normal or pathogenic bacterial flora.

Pathologic changes

Lesions due to staphylococci include furuncles, carbuncles, abscesses, impetigo contagiosa (a skin infection usually occurring in infants), acne vulgaris (a chronic infection about the hair follicles and sebaceous glands of the face, especially in adolescents), tonsillitis, sinusitis, otitis media (middle ear infection), bronchopneumonia (a patchy pulmonary infection, often with abscess formation), acute bacterial endocarditis, gastroenteritis, antibiotic enteritis (an acute intestinal inflammation following the use of oral antibiotics), osteomyelitis (infection of bone), septicemia, and pyemia. The *pathologic changes* are those of acute inflammation. Infections are usually localized, and abscesses are common.

Furuncle

A *furuncle (boil)* is an abscess of a hair follicle or sebaceous gland. It is common on the buttocks and on the back of the neck. *Microscopically* it has a necrotic, often liquefied center with polymorphonuclear leukocytes, a marked fibroblastic proliferation, and fibrin. Furuncles are common in diabetics.

Carbuncle

A *carbuncle* is a focal suppurative lesion resulting from lateral extension through the subcutaneous fibroadipose tissue of an infectious process such as a boil, or from the coalescence of infections of several adjacent hair follicles. Fat necrosis results, as well as numerous sinuses which extend to the surface of the skin. It occurs most commonly on the back of the neck.

Gastroenteritis

Staphylococcal gastroenteritis is a common type of food poisoning due to strains which contain a heat-stable *enterotoxin.* Cream pastries, potato or chicken salad, and meat preparations are commonly contaminated. The incubation period is 3 to 6 hours. There is marked hyperemia and edema of the gastric and intestinal mucosa.

Botryomycosis

Botryomycosis (bacterial pseudomycosis) [7] is a chronic, somewhat granulomatous lesion caused by staphylococci, including *S. aureus,* as well as *Escherichia coli, Pseudomonas* and *Proteus* species, and streptococci. Skin lesions are usually on the hand or foot and resemble mycetoma. Visceral involvement includes abscesses of the lungs, liver, and kidneys. Grapelike fungoid granules are found in the suppurative foci. Eosinophilic knobby or smooth shells ("clubs"), representing a hypersensitivity reaction, form about the causative organisms.

2. Streptococcal Infections

Streptococci:

Streptococci are gram-positive organisms occurring in chains. On blood agar they may show alpha hemolysis – a greenish discoloration due to formation of methemoglobin and partial hemolysis of surrounding erythrocytes – *(Streptococcus viridans);* beta hemolysis – complete hemolysis – *(Streptococcus hemolyticus);* or gamma hemolysis – no hemolysis. Streptococci have been classified antigenically into Lancefield groups A through O (except I and J). *Most of the streptococci pathogenic for man are in group A. Group B beta-hemolytic streptococci,* which are commonly pathogenic for cattle, occasionally produce human infection [8]. Such infections tend to originate in the genitourinary tract and are typically suppurative. The *enterococci,* including *Streptococcus faecalis, in group D* are sometimes isolated as infective agents, especially in the intestines, appendix, and genitourinary system.

toxins

Pathogenic strains of streptococci contain streptolysins S and O, which are hemolytic; spreading factor (hyaluronidase), which degrades mucopolysaccharides; erythrogenic toxin (scarlatinal or Dick toxin); fibrinolysin (streptokinase); streptodornase, which depolymerizes desoxyribonucleoproteins; and a leukocidin (which may be streptolysin O).

Pathologic changes

Lesions due to streptococci include wound infections, impetigo, scarlet fever, erysipelas, cellulitis, tonsillitis, pharyngitis, sinusitis, otitis media, bronchopneumonia, bacterial endocarditis, meningitis, appendicitis, puerperal sepsis, and septicemia. Glomerulonephritis and rheumatic fever (noninfectious inflammations of the kidneys and of the heart and joints, respectively) are evidently caused by hypersensitivity reactions to streptococci. The *pathologic changes* are characterized by pyogenicity (pus formation) and invasiveness. The lesions are less often localized than those due to staphylococci. However, streptococcal infections tend to be more localized in children than in adults.

Scarlet fever:

Scarlet fever (scarlatina) is an acute infectious and communicable disease due to strains of streptococci containing erythrogenic toxin. Most cases occur from January to May. About 350,000 cases of scarlet fever and septic sore throat are reported yearly in the United States. The incubation period is 2 to 5 days.

clinical features

Clinical manifestations are chills, fever, sore throat, lymphadenopathy, a generalized punctate rash, strawberry tongue (reddened papillae on a gray-coated background), and proteinuria. When the skin of a patient with scarlet fever is injected with convalescent serum, the bright red rash will disappear locally in 6 to 12 hours *(Schultz-Charlton blanching phenomenon)*.

pathologic changes

Microscopically the vessels in the *skin* are dilated, due to vasoparalysis caused by the erythrogenic toxin. The epidermis is infiltrated with polymorphonuclear leukocytes. *Lymph nodes* show hyperplasia with enlargement of the germinal centers and dilation of the sinusoids. In the kidneys there may be an *acute nonsuppurative interstitial nephritis,* with an infiltration of lymphocytes and other mononuclear cells into the fibrous interstitium.

complications

Complications include otitis media, meningitis, bronchopneumonia, septicemia, and glomerulonephritis.

Septic sore throat:

Septic sore throat ("strep throat") is a nasopharyngitis, characterized *clinically* by chills, fever, malaise, muscle aching, a painful throat, a swollen, red, velvety pharynx, and tonsillar crypts filled with pus.

pathologic changes

Acute inflammation, with redness and swelling, occurs in both the nasopharyngeal mucosa and the tonsils.

complications

Complications include peritonsillar abscess (quinsy), Ludwig's angina (phlegmon of the floor of the mouth), and retropharyngeal abscess due to suppuration of cervical lymph nodes with extension along fascial planes.

Erysipelas

Erysipelas (St. Anthony's fire) is an acute inflammation of the lymphatics of the skin produced by beta-hemolytic streptococci. Bacteria enter by large or small breaks in the skin and spread outward from the site of inoculation, producing a bright red, indurated area with a sharp margin. At the periphery of the apparent lesion, and even beyond it, the lymphatics are filled with streptococci. Erysipelas is seen most frequently on the scalp and face. There may be a systemic reaction due to *toxemia.*

3. Clostridial Infections

TETANUS (lockjaw): Cause

The cause of *tetanus (lockjaw)* is *Clostridium tetani,* an anaerobic, gram-positive, spore-forming rod. It is found in soil and in the feces of horses, cattle, and human beings. The organism is saprophytic, does not invade tissue, and produces a powerful *neurotoxin.* The organisms remain localized at their point of entry; however, the toxin reaches the anterior horn motor cells via the axis cylinders (or possibly the endoneural and perineural lymphatics or the bloodstream). The toxin violently stimulates the motor cells of the spinal cord and cranial nerve nuclei.

Clinical features

Clinically the incubation period varies from 3 to over 30 days. In general, the shorter the period, the more severe is the case. Tetanus follows a puncture wound, deep laceration, or infection of the umbilical cord *(tetanus neonatorum).* Wounds which are especially likely to be contaminated with the spores of tetanus bacilli are war wounds, umbilical cord stumps, injuries from blank cartridges and fireworks, smallpox vaccinations, and wounds closed with contaminated catgut sutures. Trismus, risus sardonicus, opisthotonos, and tonic convulsions occur. Roughly 500 cases are reported annually in the United States, with a mortality rate of about 50 percent.

Pathologic changes

No specific changes are found in the spinal motor neurons despite the profound toxic effects upon them.

GAS GANGRENE: Causes

Gas gangrene is produced by several gas-forming *clostridia,* principally *C. perfringens (C. welchii),* which is present in 80 percent of the cases; *C. septicum (Vibrion septique); C. novyi (C. oedematiens);* and *C. sporogenes.* All cause infections by contaminating wounds in which the organisms grow anaerobically. They are all saccharolytic and thrive in tissues abundant in carbohydrates, such as muscle and liver. *Clostridium perfringens* elaborates α (alpha) toxin (lecithinase), δ (delta) toxin, and θ (theta) toxin, which are hemolytic; β (beta) toxin (Z factor), which is lethal and produces skin necrosis; the lethal γ (gamma) and η (eta) toxins; ϵ (epsilon) toxin, which is dermonecrotic; and the lethal κ (kappa) toxin, a collagenase, which causes necrosis. This organism is found widely in soil, the intestinal contents of humans and animals, bile, and the vagina. In recent years an increasing number of infections due to *Clostridium perfringens* have been reported. *Clostridial septicemia* has occurred following gallbladder and biliary tract surgery [9]; necrotic enteritis secondary to leukemia, intestinal perforation or surgery, or tuberculous intestinal ulcers; and intestinal ulceration in shock, uremia, or adrenocorticosteroid and antimetabolite therapy for leukemia [10]. *Hemorrhagic intestinal necrosis due to Clostridium perfringens* has been called darmbrand ("fire in the bowel"). *Gas gangrene* has developed following intramuscular and other parenteral injection of therapeutic agents [11]. *Clostridium perfringens* contaminates about 15 percent of skin wounds (25 percent of war wounds), and *gas gangrene is especially liable to develop in traumatized necrotic, ischemic, walled-off, and contaminated soft tissue* [12].

Pathologic changes

The affected *muscle* is dull red at first, then becomes dark green to black. Bubbles of foul-smelling gas and pink or raspberry-colored fluid can be pressed along the muscle. The muscle fibers are separated from their sheaths by the sanguineous fluid. The bacteria are found in the interstitial tissue. In *gas bacillus septicemia* or in *postmortem infection* the liver, brain, and other organs become crepitant and are filled with bubbles due to gas formation. Profound *intravascular hemolysis* may be produced by the hemolytic toxins of *C. perfringens.* In one of the authors' cases the serum hemoglobin level suddenly rose to over 1300 mg. per cubic millimeter. The aorta and kidneys had a brilliant scarlet color due to the massive release of hemoglobin from lysed erythrocytes.

BOTULISM: Cause

Botulism is a toxemia caused by the ingested exotoxins of *Clostridium botulinum* [13], a large, motile, subterminally sporulated, anaerobic, gram-positive rod. The exotoxins can be subdivided into types A, B, C, D, and E on the basis of immunologic differences. Those of types A and B, which produce most of the cases in humans, are usually proteolytic; those of types C, D, and E are saccharolytic. All are resistant to proteolytic digestion. They enter the body by being ingested in improperly canned, smoked, or pickled foods, such as vegetables, tuna fish [14], ham, or sausage (the disease's name is derived from the Latin word *botulus,* a sausage). The number of cases reported annually in the United States averages about 20, with a mortality rate of about 70 percent.

Clinical features

The exotoxins of C. botulinum interfere with acetylcholine release at myoneural junctions, especially in muscles supplied by the cranial nerves. *Clinical manifestations* usually appear in less than 24 hours after ingestion of the contaminated food. They include nausea, vomiting, constipation, headache, difficulty in swallowing due to pharyngeal muscle paralyses, diplopia (double vision), and breathing difficulties due to paralysis of respiratory muscles. Death is caused by respiratory failure and may occur from 1 to 7 days after the onset of symptoms.

Pathologic changes

The *lesions are nonspecific* and consist largely of congestion, hemorrhages, and thrombosis of small blood vessels, especially in the *brain.* No morphologic changes are found in the cranial or peripheral nerves, motor end-plates, or muscles [15]. *Bronchopneumonia* sometimes develops, due to the aspiration of regurgitated food or liquids. The *liver* may show fatty metamorphosis.

4. Diphtheria

DIPHTHERIA: Cause

Diphtheria is caused by *Corynebacterium diphtheriae* (Klebs-Loeffler bacillus), a slender, aerobic, gram-positive rod with segmented appearance and polar club-shaped swellings. Three strains are known: gravis, intermedius, and mitis. The organism produces a powerful *exotoxin. Transmission* is usually by droplet infection from human carriers; about 1 percent of the population harbors virulent organisms. The *incidence* is highest between the ages of 1 and 5. Most cases occur from October to December; about 1000 cases and 75 deaths are reported yearly in the United States.

Schick test

The *Schick test* is performed by the intradermal injection of a minute amount of diphtheria toxin. In the *nonimmune individual* the toxin produces a local erythema (reddening of the skin), followed by necrosis and desquamation; this reaction is called positive. In the *immune individual* antitoxin neutralizes the toxin and the characteristic reaction does not occur; this result is called negative.

Reh's test introduces diphtheria toxin by punctate scarification of the skin. Its results are parallel to those of the Schick test in both nonimmune and immune individuals.

Clinical features

The *incubation period* is 1 to 7 days. The *clinical manifestations* are malaise, headache, sore throat, and cervical lymphadenopathy. A yellow-gray membrane is present over the nasal and pharyngeal mucosa, tonsils, larynx, and tracheal mucosa. *Complications* include peripheral nerve paralyses, cardiac failure (myocarditis is present in about 70 percent of fatal cases), and bronchopneumonia.

Pathologic changes

Local changes are due to the presence of *C. diphtheriae* with the focal elaboration of exotoxin. There is a *membranous exudate* consisting of polymorphonuclear leukocytes, bacteria, and desquamated epithelial cells enmeshed in a dense fibrinous network. The underlying mucosa is necrotic. The submucosa is hyperemic and edematous. There is little tendency for the organisms to invade. The characteristic membrane is usually found over the mucosa of the nose, mouth, pharynx, larynx, trachea, and bronchi, but it may occur on the skin and mucosa of the esophagus, stomach, conjunctiva, or vagina. *Systemic changes* are produced by the powerful exotoxin. The lymph nodes, especially those draining the area of infection, show hyperplasia and focal necrosis. The spleen is slightly hyperplastic. The heart [16] is slightly pale and swollen, and *microscopically* there is interstitial edema and hyalinization. Fine lipid granules may appear in the myocardial fibers. In some cases there is an interstitial myocarditis with an infiltrate of lymphocytes and macrophages. The liver and kidneys show cloudy swelling. Peripheral nerves may show myelin degeneration and swelling of the axis cylinders.

Cutaneous diphtheria

Primary cutaneous diphtheria [17] results from infection of the skin by *Corynebacterium diphtheriae* at the site of an abrasion or other injury of the skin. It is rare in the United States, where most cases are due to the mitis strain, and occurs almost entirely in warm and humid or tropical climates. The *lesion begins as a pustule* which develops into an *anesthetic ulcer covered by a gray or brown membrane* which later hardens to a *leathery, adherent eschar* (scab) *or* into an *eczematoid dermatitis* (a weeping, scaly skin inflammation). The ulcer is punched out and oval or round, and exudes seropurulent fluid when the eschar is removed. It heals with a depressed scar. *Diphtheritic myocarditis* occurs in 5 percent and *polyneuritis* in 35 percent of cases of cutaneous diphtheria, due to the absorption of exotoxin.

5. Pertussis (Whooping Cough)

PERTUSSIS: Cause

Bordetella pertussis (Hemophilus pertussis), a short, gram-negative, nonmotile, encapsulated (in its smooth form) rod which releases an endotoxin on disintegration, causes *pertussis.*

Clinical features

Clinically 90 percent of the cases occur in children under 5 years. The incubation period is 7 to 14 days. After a coldlike *catarrhal stage* of about a week, there is a prolonged (2 to 4 weeks) *paroxysmal stage* characterized by short violent coughs with whoops. During the *convalescent stage,* paroxysms are less frequent and less severe, but the typical cough may return following an upper respiratory infection months after the apparent end of the disease. Leukocytosis averaging 30,000 white blood cells per cubic millimeter with over 70 percent lymphocytes is characteristic. Incidence is highest between January and August, and about 40,000 cases with 250 deaths are reported each year in the United States.

Pathologic changes

In the bronchioles, bronchi, trachea, and larynx, the mucosa is red, swollen, and covered by a mucous exudate. *Microscopically* bacteria are enmeshed in the cilia, and there are lymphocytes, plasmocytes, and macrophages in the mucosa and submucosa, which is edematous and hyperemic. There may be a superficial necrosis of the mucosa. The presence of polymorphonuclear leukocytes indicates a secondary bronchopneumonia.

Complications

Complications include bronchopneumonia, cerebral hemorrhage, emphysema, bronchiectasis, umbilical hernia, and rectal prolapse. All but the first of these are due to the enormous intrathoracic and intra-abdominal pressures attained during episodes of whooping.

6. *Hemophilus Influenzae Infections*

Hemophilus influenzae

Hemophilus influenzae is a short, gram-negative rod occurring singly, in pairs, or in short chains. Some strains are encapsulated. *Transmission* is by airborne droplets and possibly by fomites. Most infections occur in infants and children under the age of 3 years. The organism may cause acute nasopharyngitis, paranasal sinusitis, otitis media, epiglottitis, and tracheitis; acute septic meningitis; subacute bacterial endocarditis; suppurative arthritis; and occasionally septicemia. In *Hemophilus influenzae* infections there is an *acute pyogenic reaction* with a heavy neutrophilic infiltration.

7. *Pasteurella Infections*

TULAREMIA: Cause

The cause of *tularemia* (rabbit fever) is *Pasteurella tularensis,* a gram-negative, pleomorphic bacillus, which occurs as coccal and bacillary forms. Rabbits and ground squirrels are reservoirs of infection. *Transmission* is by handling infected animals (the organism passes through unbroken skin), laboratory infections, insect bites (wood or rabbit ticks and deer flies), and occasionally by ingesting poorly cooked infected meat or drinking contaminated water. About 600 cases occur annually in the United States.

Clinical features

The incubation period is 3 to 5 days. The symptoms are headache, chills, fever, aching, and prostration. At the infection site there is a red papule, followed by a punched-out ulcer. Within 36 to 48 hours of the onset the regional lymph nodes become swollen and painful. Four clinical types are recognized: ulceroglandular, oculoglandular (infection via the conjunctiva), glandular, and typhoidal.

Pathologic changes

The *acute lesions* in the lymph nodes are focal necrosis and suppuration. The *chronic lesions* resemble those of fungus infections. In the liver, spleen, lungs, and lymph nodes, hard nodules, 2 to 3 mm. in diameter, appear. Larger granulomatous nodules show central necrosis. *Microscopically* the nodules have a fibrous wall about collections of mononuclear cells and occasional giant cells. There may be central caseation, the caseous material often containing polymorphonuclear leukocytes.

PLAGUE: Cause

Plague is caused by *Pasteurella pestis,* a gram-negative, nonmotile, encapsulated coccobacillus transmitted by the bite of a rat flea, especially *Xenopsylla cheopis,* or by droplet infection. *Sylvatic plague* is due to infection from nondomestic rodents (other than the rat) and is found in western United States.

Clinical features

Clinically bubonic plague (black death) is a severe acute infection with an abrupt onset of high fever, chills, and headache, with later delirium. The site of the flea bite may show a pustule, and the regional lymph nodes are enlarged. Foci of hemorrhagic necrosis may appear in the skin. Before antibiotic therapy up to 75 percent of the cases were fatal. In *pneumonic plague,* which is transmitted by droplet infection, there are dyspnea and a cough productive of large amounts of bloody sputum. Circulatory failure in plague is probably due to a direct toxic effect on the myocardium [18].

Pathologic changes

Bubonic plague is characterized by markedly soft, matted, plum-colored lymph nodes *(buboes)* measuring up to 4 to 5 cm. in diameter; these nodes show marked *hemorrhagic necrosis. Septicemic plague* may or may not develop buboes; since it is almost always rapidly fatal, the tissue changes are not marked. In *pneumonic plague* death is rapid, so that there is little inflammatory response in the lungs; necrosis of alveolar walls and hemorrhages are found. In all forms of *plague* there is *marked endotoxic damage to the walls of small blood vessels,* resulting in petechiae or ecchymoses in the skin and mucous membranes and hemorrhage into viscera and serous cavities.

PASTEURELLA MULTOCIDA INFECTIONS [19]

Pasteurella multocida is a small, nonmotile, gram-negative rod which is pathogenic in a number of animals. Most human infections follow bites, especially those inflicted by dogs and cats. Local cellulitis or abscess formation, with lymphangitis and regional lymphadenitis, develops. Occasionally osteomyelitis due to perforation of the periosteum, septicemia, or meningitis occurs. In cases in which organisms are inhaled or in which there is pulmonary localization during a septicemia, lung abscess with pulmonary cavitation may be found.

8. Salmonella Infections

TYPHOID FEVER: Cause

The *cause of typhoid fever* is *Salmonella typhi (Salmonella typhosa),* a gram-negative, plump, flagellated, motile rod with O (somatic), H (flagellar), and Vi antigens.

Transmission

Transmission occurs directly or indirectly from active or convalescent patients or carriers. The five Fs of spread are: food, fingers, flies, fomites, and feces. Urine is also a major factor in spread. The organisms enter the body through the mouth and are carried to the small intestine, where they reach the mesenteric lymph nodes, whence they enter the liver and, through the thoracic duct, the bloodstream.

Clinical features

Clinically the *incubation period* is 10 to 14 days. Typhoid fever is protean and difficult to diagnose early. In the septicemic stage the symptoms include headaches, malaise, fever and chills, and prostration. Splenomegaly and bradycardia are found. Leukopenia (2000 to 5000 white blood cells per cubic millimeter) is characteristic, with a marked neutropenia and eosinopenia due to depression of bone marrow function. Blood cultures are positive in 80 to 90 percent of the cases during the first week. Rose spots appear in the second week on the abdomen; they persist only a few days. Intestinal hemorrhage and other signs of organ damage also appear in the second week. Debility and wasting are marked. Transient local paralyses may occur, and mental signs are common. During the second and third weeks urine and stool cultures are positive in 80 percent of the cases. The *Widal agglutination test* is positive in 20 percent of the cases in the first week, 50 percent in the second week, and 70 to 90 percent in the third week. Convalescence is prolonged, and relapses appear in 5 to 10 percent of the cases. *Death* may result from the septicemia or from one of the complications. Before chloramphenicol and chlortetracycline therapy, the mortality was 10 to 20 percent. Less than 1000 cases with about 25 deaths are now reported annually in the United States.

Pathologic changes:

The *predominant cell* of reaction is the *macrophage,* and there is a distinct paucity of polymorphonuclear leukocytes in the lesions. In the *septicemic stage,* reticuloendothelial hyperplasia is pronounced in the lymph nodes (especially in the Peyer's patches and solitary lymph follicles of the ileum and cecum and the mesenteric nodes), the Kupffer cells of the liver, the spleen, and the bone marrow. Skeletal muscles may undergo Zenker's waxy degeneration, especially the intercostals, diaphragm, and rectus abdominis. Occasionally the rectus abdominis muscle ruptures, with hemorrhage. *Rose spots* are due to bacterial emboli in the skin, with local hyperemia and small foci of macrophages in the dermis.

stage of local injury

In the *stage of local injury* the ileum ulcerates over the button-like protrusions of the enlarged Peyer's patches. The ulcers are long, oval, and parallel to the longitudinal axis of the intestine. Smaller punctate ulcers overlying lymph follicles are found in the cecum. The margins are elevated, and the ulcers extend to the submucosa or muscularis. *Microscopically* there is an abundance of macrophages *(Mallory cells)* in the floor and edges of the ulcer. These cells are actively phagocytic and contain erythrocytes, lymphocytes, and other cellular debris in their cytoplasm. Lymphocytes and plasma cells are also present in the ulcer. Healing occurs by granulation tissue and re-epithelialization; scarring is minimal. The Peyer's patches and mesenteric lymph nodes show foci of necrosis up to several millimeters in diameter. The sinusoids are filled with macrophages. The spleen may weigh 800 to 900 gm. A tense capsule covers a mushy, cherry-red pulp. Foci of necrosis are found about clusters of macrophages. The liver is enlarged and swollen, with a tense capsule and rounded edges. Microscopically cloudy swelling is marked. There are microscopic, haphazardly distributed *typhoid nodules* consisting of aggregates of macrophages with necrosis of a few surrounding hepatic cells (focal necrosis).

cholecystitis

The *gallbladder* is always infected, the organisms thriving in the bile. Most of the bacilli in the feces originate in the bile. Lesions are slight in the gallbladder, but development of a chronic cholecystitis after recovery from the acute illness leads to the *carrier state,* organisms being passed in the feces for years. The kidneys and ureters may be involved during the bacteremia, but few lesions develop. Organisms are passed in the urine. The bone marrow shows reticuloendothelial hyperplasia and focal necrosis about macrophage aggregates.

Complications

Complications include: (1) massive *intestinal hemorrhage* (in 5 to 10 percent of the cases); (2) *perforation of an ulcer,* usually in the terminal ileum in the second or third week, resulting in generalized peritonitis; (3) *rupture of a mesenteric lymph node,* producing an *S. typhosa* peritonitis; (4) *thrombophlebitis of the femoral or saphenous veins* (in 5 to 10 percent); and (5) *meningitis, endocarditis, nephritis,* or *osteomyelitis,* which may result from the bacteremia. The osteomyelitis may be chronic and suppurative and is most common in the tibiae, sternum, ribs, and vertebrae. Periosteitis also occurs.

Paratyphoid fever

Paratyphoid fever is caused by *Salmonella paratyphi A (S. paratyphi), S. paratyphi B (S. schottmuelleri),* and *S. paratyphi C (S. hirschfeldii).* All are motile, flagellated, gram-negative rods. *Clinically and pathologically* paratyphoid fever is similar to typhoid fever, except that the course and the lesions are less severe.

OTHER SALMONELLA INFECTIONS [20]: Gastroenteritis

Salmonella gastroenteritis (food poisoning) is the clinical form in about 70 percent of cases of salmonella infections. *Salmonella typhimurium* is the most common cause in the United States; other causative organisms are *S. enteritidis* and *S. choleraesuis.* All are gram-negative, flagellated rods which liberate endotoxins. Most human infections are acquired by eating food contaminated with rodent feces or eggs from infected hens. Salmonella gastroenteritis has a short incubation period (as little as 12 hours) and an acute onset of nausea, vomiting, foul-smelling diarrhea, and fever. Recovery is usually rapid, and the mortality rate is about 0.5 percent. The gastrointestinal mucosa, especially that of the ileum, is inflamed and edematous. *Postgastrectomy salmonella gastroenteritis is* probably due to the failure of the normal destruction of such organisms by gastric acid and enzymes following removal of most of the stomach. *Salmonella appendicitis* is uncommon and is probably secondary to inflammation in the ileocecal region. *Acute salmonella infections following abdominal surgery* may be due to spillage of organisms from the gallbladder, intestinal tract, or an intra-abdominal abscess, or to the removal of competitive bacterial flora in the intestine by preoperative or postoperative antibiotic therapy. *Salmonella bacteremia is common in patients with liver disease,* such as viral hepatitis and cirrhosis, presumably due to the loss of the normal filtering action by which such organisms are destroyed in the liver. In *salmonella septicemia,* most often due to *S. choleraesuis,* localization may occur in numerous sites. *Osteomyelitis* develops most commonly in long bones, especially the humerus and femur, and in vertebrae. Multiple foci of involvement are common. *Mycotic aneurysm* of the aorta or other major arteries occurs occasionally. *Salmonella meningitis* develops most often in premature and other young infants. *The incidence of salmonella infections is increased in patients given antibiotic therapy,* by which the normal flora of the oropharynx or intestine is eliminated, allowing pathogenic salmonella organisms to thrive, *and in patients on cortisone therapy,* due to decreased resistance to bacterial infection.

Septicemia

9. Bacillary Dysentery

BACILLARY DYSENTERY: Causes

Bacillary dysentery is produced by *Shigella dysenteriae,* a gram-negative, nonmotile, short rod which produces a powerful neurotropic exotoxin. Other causative bacilli are the closely related *Shigella paradysenteriae (S. flexneri), S. boydii, S. ambigua (S. schmitzii),* and *S. sonnei,* which produce no exotoxin. All produce endotoxins. *Transmission* is mainly by eating contaminated foods.

Clinical features

Clinically this disease is common in both temperate and tropical zones, especially in conditions of crowding and poor sanitation, as in field armies. The dysentery is a diarrhea with mucus, pus, and blood *(bloody flux)* in the stools, and marked straining and tenesmus. A peripheral neuritis is common due to the exotoxins of *S. dysenteriae.* The disease may become chronic. The *mortality* before sulfonamide and antibiotic therapy averaged 5 percent, being as high as 50 percent in epidemics. Roughly 13,000 cases with a mortality rate of 0.1 percent now occur each year in the United States.

Pathologic changes [21]

The organisms remain localized in the colon and terminal ileum in most cases. An acute inflammation in the mucosa is soon followed by small patches of *ulceration,* which often coalesce to form large ulcers. The intervening mucosa often becomes heaped up, and even papillomatous. The ulcers are clean-cut and seldom penetrate the muscularis mucosa, although they occasionally perforate the intestinal wall. The surface is covered by fibrin, polymorphonuclear leukocytes, and necrotic material *(membranous exudate).* The intestinal wall is edematous and infiltrated with polymorphonuclear leukocytes; many *shigella* organisms are found in the wall. *Healing* occurs by granulation tissue and re-epithelialization, with little scarring except where the ulcers are deep. Mucous glands containing bacilli may become embedded in the wall, leading to the production of mucous cysts which may later rupture and produce reinfection. Focal necrosis occurs in the liver. Degenerative and minute hemorrhagic lesions resembling those of acute poliomyelitis occur in the brain stem and anterior horns of the spinal cord, due to the neurotropic exotoxin of *S. dysenteriae.*

Complications

Complications include: (1) *perforation of an ulcer* to produce generalized peritonitis (uncommon); (2) *stenosis of the terminal ileum or colon* due to scarring in healing of a deep ulcer; (3) *chronic ulcerative colitis* from development of chronic infection; (4) *bacterial endocarditis, arthritis,* or *nephritis* resulting from an occasional bacteremia; (5) *prolapse of the rectum;* and (6) *inflammation of the anus or perianal region.*

10. Cholera

CHOLERA: Cause

Cholera is caused by *Vibrio cholerae (V. comma),* a short, gently curved and twisted, motile, gram-negative rod which liberates a powerful endotoxin. *Transmission* is by drinking polluted water.

Clinical features

Cholera is a serious problem in Asia and some tropical countries. *Clinical signs* are explosive diarrhea, collapse, dehydration, delirium, and coma. In the algid phase the body temperature may fall precipitously. The feces are thin and watery *(rice-water stools).* Death may occur in a few hours.

Pathologic changes

The infection is localized in the intestines, the changes in other organs being due to toxemia. The small and large intestines are greatly distended with a watery fluid like thin barley soup. The mucosa throughout is deep red due to severe congestion. Hemorrhages are common, but ulceration does not occur. The covering epithelium is desquamated throughout the intestine. *Biopsies during the acute illness* in cholera show that the intestinal epithelium is intact, so that the sloughing noted at autopsy is agonal or postmortem [22]. The basement membrane becomes ill defined, and there is marked hyperemia of the lamina propria with edema and a mononuclear inflammatory infiltrate. In surviving patients no sequelae are found in the intestinal wall. The *rice water* is a transudate from the capillaries of the lamina propria. The albumin and sodium levels in the fluid are lower than those in plasma. The potassium level is higher in the rice water. Endotoxin probably acts on the capillaries of the lamina propria to produce the fluid loss and electrolyte imbalance. At *autopsy* the body is markedly dehydrated, and the blood is dark and viscous. Rigor mortis is extreme, the arms and legs being "stiff as iron rods."

11. Coliform Bacterial Infections

COLIFORM BACTERIAL INFECTIONS

Coliform organisms are part of the normal bacterial flora of the intestines. Within recent years *these usually mildly pathogenic organisms have become important because of the extensive use of antibiotics in combatting gram-positive bacterial infections.* The major coliform organisms are *Escherichia coli,* which is a small, gram-negative rod with peritrichous flagella, and *Aerobacter (Klebsiella) aerogenes,* a nonmotile, encapsulated, gram-negative rod. Disease results from auto-infection by endogenous organisms, personal contact, and the ingestion of fecally contaminated food and water. *Coliform organisms may cause* an acute appendicitis or gastroenteritis; peritonitis, following intestinal surgery or perforation of a viscus; cystitis and ascending pyelonephritis; cholecystitis; bronchopneumonia; meningitis; and skin wound infection. Abscess formation is common at the infection site. The abscesses are filled with neutrophils, macrophages, and lymphocytes. *Septicemia* with peripheral vascular collapse secondary to endotoxic shock may occur. In bronchopneumonia due to *E. coli* [23] the lungs are heavy, and empyema is common. Typically there are foci of consolidation with abscess formation in the lower lobes. The alveoli are filled with proteinaceous fluid, erythrocytes, macrophages, and some neutrophils.

12. Klebsiella Infections

KLEBSIELLA PNEUMONIAE INFECTIONS: Friedländer's pneumonia

Klebsiella pneumoniae (Friedländer's bacillus) is a heavily encapsulated, short, thick, gram-negative rod with K (capsular) antigen and O and R (somatic) antigens. Culturally it is very similar to *Aerobacter (Klebsiella) aerogenes.* It produces about 1 percent of cases of pneumonitis. *Friedländer's pneumonia* occurs most frequently in men over the age of 40, especially those with debilitating disease, malnutrition, and alcoholism. It is usually lobar in distribution, the affected lobe or lung being voluminous. Foci of consolidation are uniformly gray, and the cut surface is sticky because of mucin secretion. The tissue is friable. *Microscopically* the exudate is predominantly mononuclear, and many bacilli are found. The most common site of *Klebsiella pneumoniae* infection is the gastrointestinal tract, but the organism also may cause a sinusitis, mastoiditis, meningitis, cystitis, appendicitis, salpingitis, and osteomyelitis, as well as the pneumonitis described above.

RHINOSCLEROMA

Rhinoscleroma [24] is caused by *Klebsiella rhinoscleromatis.* The disease is endemic in the Mediterranean region. *Clinically* there are nodular, often ulcerated, masses in the nose, with a foul discharge. In the nodules there is a plasmocytic and lymphocytic infiltration. Hyaline *Russell-Fuchs bodies* are found in degenerating plasmocytes. In the deeper portions typical foamy macrophages *(Mikulicz cells)* are present.

13. Proteus Infections

PROTEUS INFECTIONS

Infections by Proteus species, especially *Proteus vulgaris* and *P. mirabilis,* are becoming increasingly common in this era of extensive antibiotic therapy. These are straight, gram-negative rods occurring singly and in pairs, and having peritrichous flagella. Auto-infection by fecal contamination of the fingers, personal contact, and bath water are means of transmission of these bacteria. *They may produce* an acute gastroenteritis, peritonitis, cystitis and ascending pyelonephritis, bronchopneumonia, meningitis, and otitis media. There is an *acute pyogenic reaction,* sometimes with abscess formation. Double or multiple infections with *Proteus* species or infections in combination with *E. coli* and *Staphylococcus* are common. *Proteus septicemia* occasionally occurs.

14. Pseudomonas Infections

PSEUDOMONAS INFECTIONS:

Pseudomonas aeruginosa (Bacillus pyocyaneus) is a small, slender, gram-negative rod with polar flagella. It is frequently part of the normal flora of the skin and intestines. The organism is usually of low pathogenicity and is a secondary invader in wounds and other inflammations. However, in debilitated individuals, infants, and the aged, it may produce severe and resistant infections [25]. *Antibiotic-resistant strains* of *Pseudomonas aeruginosa* are common, and these may produce severe infections, including septicemia, in patients on prolonged antibiotic therapy.

Pathologic changes

The *general lesions* in *Pseudomonas* infections are tissue necrosis, abscess formation, massive infiltration of polymorphonuclear leukocytes, and acute suppurative arteritis. The *pus* produced is *typically bluish green. Pseudomonas aeruginosa may cause* otitis media, bronchopneumonia, purulent conjunctivitis, and acute serpiginous keratitis (a destructive inflammation of the cornea), acute gastroenteritis, bacterial endocarditis, septic meningitis, and septicemia. *Pseudomonas septicemia* is not uncommon in children with leukemia. In cases treated with steroids and/or antimetabolites, an *acute vasculitis* characterized by a smudgelike necrosis of vessel walls caused by bacterial invasion occurs. Reddish black infarct-like foci are common in tissue surrounding such vessels.

Melioidosis

Melioidosis [26] is caused by *Pseudomonas pseudomallei (Malleomyces pseudomallei)*, a motile, small, gram-negative rod, resembling *Actinobacillus mallei*. The disease occurs mainly in Burma, Thailand, Vietnam, the Malay peninsula, and Ceylon. Man is infected by eating food contaminated with the excreta of diseased rats. Clinically and pathologically melioidosis is similar to the acute form of glanders, pyemic abscesses being widespread. The abscesses are filled with macrophages and neutrophils, with some large cells containing multiple or multilobate nuclei. The mortality rate is high in untreated cases.

15. Glanders and Farcy

GLANDERS: Cause

Actinobacillus mallei (Malleomyces mallei), a pleomorphic gram-negative rod, causes glanders, a disease of horses and mules. *Transmission* to human beings occurs in stables and laboratories. The organisms probably enter through skin abrasions and by inhalation. When the peritoneal cavity of a male guinea pig is inoculated, the organism produces acute inflammation in the tunica vaginalis testis *(Straus test)*.

Pathologic changes

Glanders is an acute, almost always fatal disease. It is a pyemia, with numerous abscesses in many viscera. *Farcy* is chronic and affects the skin and lymphatics. *Farcy buds* are granulomatous nodules in the subcutaneous tissues along lymphatics. The granuloma may contain a few giant cells but does not caseate. The overlying skin may ulcerate and discharge a thick, sticky, sanguineo-purulent material.

16. Brucellosis

BRUCELLOSIS: Cause

Three species of *Brucella* produce *brucellosis* (undulant or Malta fever) in man: *B. abortus* (cattle), *B. melitensis* (goat), and *B. suis* (swine). *Brucella* are small, nonmotile, coccobacillary organisms which are encapsulated in their smooth form.

Transmission

Transmission to man is by ingestion of milk and dairy products from infected animals, by handling infected meat, and by exposure to laboratory cultures.

Clinical features

Clinically diagnosis is often difficult because of the vagueness or protean nature of the manifestations. The onset is insidious with fever (sometimes undulating), weakness, excessive sweating, and muscle and joint pains. Splenomegaly and lymphadenopathy are common. The disease lasts for months. About 1000 cases are diagnosed yearly in the United States; the mortality is low.

Pathologic changes

The lesions are essentially those of a *granuloma with reticuloendothelial hyperplasia*. In the spleen, lymph nodes, liver, and bone marrow there are small granulomatous foci with lymphocytes, epithelioid cells, and giant cells. *Fatal cases* show hyperplasia of Peyer's patches, with ulceration and hemorrhage in the ileum. *Brucellar endocarditis* is found in about 80 percent of the established cases, almost always males, and in 95 percent of those cases due to *B. abortus* [27]. The endocardial lesions are especially common on the aortic valve (about 85 percent of the cases), the mitral valve being involved in 45 percent. Previously normal valves are apparently directly invaded by the organisms. Nodular hyaline and calcific vegetations form on the affected valvular cusps. The commissures are destroyed, and microabscesses are found within the cusps. Myocardial abscesses occasionally occur, and paravascular granulomatous lesions resembling Aschoff bodies are sometimes found. Because of the close resemblance of brucellar endocarditic lesions to those of calcific aortic stenosis, it has been suggested that the latter may be produced by brucellar infection. *Less common lesions* are abscesses in the liver, kidneys, lymph nodes, and bone marrow; bronchopneumonia, meningoencephalitis, myelitis, neuritis, and subarachnoid hemorrhage due to a ruptured mycotic aneurysm [28]; salpingo-oophoritis; orchitis; and osteomyelitis.

17. Anthrax

ANTHRAX: Cause

Bacillus anthracis, a large, gram-positive, spore-forming rod, is the cause of *anthrax* [29], a disease of sheep and cattle from which human beings are sometimes infected. *Transmission* to man is by inhalation of spores (woolsorter's disease), by handling infected animals (farmers, veterinarians, and butchers), and by the use of a shaving brush with infected bristles.

Clinical features

Clinically the usual form of anthrax in man is the *malignant pustule* on the face or neck. This begins as a papule, then progresses to an ulcerated pustule. Pulmonary and intestinal types occur also.

Pathologic changes

The *typical lesion* is an acute *hemorrhagic inflammation.* The *malignant pustule* passes through papular and vesicular phases, ending in a fibrinous "scab" which undergoes central necrosis to develop a black *ulcer.* The *intestinal type* of anthrax produces malignant pustules in the intestinal mucosa or a phlegmonous gastritis. *Inhalation anthrax* [30] occurs among sheep shearers, workers in animal hair processing mills, and tannery workers. It is due to the breathing in of spores which reach the alveoli. The spores are carried by macrophages to the hilar and mediastinal lymph nodes. Here the spores germinate and the bacteria multiply, causing a hemorrhagic necrosis in the nodes and paranodal tissue and frequently a mediastinitis with massive edema, hemorrhage, and focal suppuration. Organisms enter the bloodstream, producing *a septicemia* and being disseminated widely. Blood-borne organisms localize to produce meningitis, gastrointestinal ulceration, and a hemorrhagic necrosis in the lungs. Thus *anthrax pneumonia* is a result of septicemia. *Death* is probably due to shock resulting from hemorrhage and fluid loss caused by a toxin of *B. anthracis.*

18. Erysipeloid

ERYSIPELOID: Cause

Erysipelothrix insidiosa (rhusiopathiae), a slender, slightly curved, nonmotile, nonsporulating, gram-positive rod occurring in long chains, causes *erysipeloid.* The great majority of human infections are acquired from contact with swine or pork products, especially in abattoir workers. Other common sources of infection are the handling and cleaning of fish or shellfish and the bite of a crab.

Pathologic changes

Typically purplish red elevated lesions with a paler, less swollen central focus appear on the hand. *Microscopically* intense hyperemia, edema, and hemorrhage into the dermis are found. The basal cells of the epidermis are vacuolated. Lymphocytic infiltration is found, and there is no suppuration.

19. Bartonellosis

BARTONELLOSIS: Cause

Bartonellosis (Carrion's disease) is caused by *Bartonella bacilliformis,* a small motile, aerobic, ricksettia-like gram-negative bacillus which is *transmitted by* the *sand flies, Phlebotomus verrucarum* and *noguchi.* The disease is found on the western slopes of the Andes, and there are two forms, Oroya fever and verruca peruviana.

Oroya fever:

Oroya fever is characterized by an acute course and profound anemia, the mortality averaging 30 percent. The anemia is due to a hemolytic effect of the bacteria and to hemorrhages. An irregular, intermittent fever, bone and joint pains, and headache occur.

pathologic changes

The skin, mucous membranes, and viscera are pale. Lymph nodes are enlarged and soft, the reticuloendothelial cells being swollen, hyperplastic, and filled with *Bartonella* organisms. The liver shows focal and central necrosis, the spleen is enlarged, and the bone marrow is intensely hyperplastic. The Kupffer cells and reticuloendothelial cells of the spleen and bone marrow are stuffed with microorganisms.

Verruca peruviana: pathologic changes

Verruca peruviana is chronic, with an anemia and a nodular eruption. On the skin, especially on the extensor surfaces of the extremities, are small, bright red, sessile or pedunculated nodules up to 1 cm. in diameter. Similar nodules are found on the mucous membranes. *Microscopically* there is proliferation of the capillary endothelium in the dermis or submucosa. Many organisms are found in the endothelial cells. Small foci of necrosis or hemorrhage are common.

20. Mimeae Infections

MIMEAE INFECTIONS

Mimeae are short, nonmotile, gram-negative rods or diplococci with a remarkable ability to mimic infections due to *Neisseria* species. This group of organisms includes *Mima polymorpha, Herellea vaginicola,* and *Colloides anoxydana.* Among the infections caused by these often penicillin-resistant organisms are *acute and chronic meningitis* [31], acute bacterial endocarditis [32], urinary tract infection, dermatitis, *urethritis (gonorrhea-like syndrome)* [33], and *fulminating septicemia.* In acute infections the involved tissues are infiltrated with neutrophils. Prolonged infections, especially chronic meningitis, with a lymphocytic infiltration are common. The mimiae causing urethritis are transmitted during coitus. Other mimiae infections are probably airborne.

21. Mycoplasma Infections

MYCOPLASMA INFECTIONS [34]

Mycoplasma species (pleuropneumonia-like organisms, PPLO) which are capable of infecting human beings are *Mycoplasma hominis* types 1 and 2, and *M. fermentans,* found in the male and female genital tracts; *M. salivarum,* found in the mouth and throat; and *M. pneumoniae* (Eaton agent), the cause of primary atypical pneumonia (see page 459). The pneumonitis is contracted by inhalation of the organism. Mycoplasma are extremely pleomorphic, appearing as small or large rods, coccoid bodies, spirals, filaments, or granules. Some are small enough to be filtrable. Thick films of cultures are gram-negative. On solid media these organisms grow as masses of protoplasts resembling L bacterial forms. *Infections* produced by *Mycoplasma* include an acute mucopurulent urethritis, which is probably transmitted by sexual intercourse; Reiter's disease (urethritis, conjunctivitis, and arthritis); prostatitis; cervicitis; and possibly rheumatoid arthritis.

22. Borrelia Infections

FUSOSPIROCHETOSIS: Cause

Fusospirochetosis is due to the association of two or more saprophytic organisms which act synergistically to cause disease under anaerobic conditions in previously injured or poorly nourished tissue. One is *Borrelia vincentii,* a gram-negative, anaerobic organism with three to eight shallow wavy spirals. The other is a *Fusobacterium,* such as *F. fusiforme (F. plauti-vincenti), F. polymorphum, or F. nucleatum.* These are anaerobic, gram-negative (with frequent gram-positive granules), short or long, slender rods occurring singly, in pairs, or in short chains. *Auto-infection from organisms present in the mouth* occurs in patients with nutritional deficiencies, trauma, or debilitating disease. The mouth lesions include an ulcerative gingivostomatitis *(trench mouth),* necrotizing ulcerative stomatitis *(Vincent's angina),* gangrenous stomatitis (noma, cancrum oris), and pyorrhea. In the lung these organisms are commonly found in areas of gangrenous necrosis. The fusospirochetes produce *an acute necrotizing inflammation* with a fibrinous mucosal membrane in the mouth, and neutrophilic infiltration.

RELAPSING FEVER: Cause

Relapsing fever is caused by *Borrelia recurrentis, B. duttonii,* and *B. novyi,* which are transmitted in most of the world by scratching the bite of the body louse and in the United States and South Africa by the bite of ticks of the *Ornithodorus* genus. These microorganisms are cylindrical, gram-negative spirochetes with irregular wavy spirals.

Clinical features

Clinically after an incubation period of 5 to 10 days there is a sudden onset of high fever, chills, headache, muscle aches, nausea, vomiting, petechiae, and sometimes jaundice. After 2 to 7 days the temperature drops rapidly to normal. About a week later another febrile episode occurs, again with a sharp temperature drop at the end. There are typically four to five febrile attacks. In roughly 10 percent of the cases there is a false positive serologic test for syphilis. The mortality is about 5 percent.

Pathologic changes [35]

The spleen is moderately enlarged (300 to 500 gm.) and firm, with conspicuous malpighian bodies. Microscopically hemorrhages into the pulp and reticulum cell hyperplasia are seen. Focal necroses occur in the liver. Hemorrhages are common in the central nervous system. Death is usually due to a secondary bronchopneumonia.

23. Leptospira Infections

LEPTOSPIROSIS: Cause

Leptospirosis (Weil's disease) is caused by *Leptospira icterohaemorrhagiae,* a motile spirochete with fine, tightly wound spirals about an axial filament. Human beings acquire the disease by contact with water contaminated by the feces and urine of rats. The organisms may enter the body through the conjunctival or respiratory mucosa. *Pretibial (Fort Bragg) fever* is due to the autumnalis AB serotype of *Leptospira icterohaemorrhagiae.*

Clinical features

Clinically there is an abrupt onset with fever, chills, muscle aches and tenderness, nausea and vomiting, headache, nuchal rigidity (due to meningeal irritation), and jaundice (in over 70 percent of the cases). Petechiae and ecchymoses may appear in the skin and conjunctivae; the latter are markedly injected. After a week oliguria (decrease in urine volume) or anuria (absence of urine output) may develop. Surviving patients undergo a prolonged convalescence.

Pathologic changes [36]

The liver is slightly enlarged and bile-stained. Microscopically proliferation and necrosis of parenchymal cells, cloudy swelling, and fatty changes are found. There is a slight infiltration of polymorphonuclear leukocytes. The kidneys are large and yellow. The tubular epithelium shows cloudy swelling, necrosis, and deposits of bile pigment. The skeletal muscles show vacuolation, hyalinization, and swelling of the fibers. Hemorrhages due to capillary damage are common in the viscera, mucosa, and skin.

OTHER LEPTOSPIRAL INFECTIONS

Canicola fever is similar to Weil's disease and is caused by *Leptospira canicola.* Infection in man is due to contact with infected dogs. *Swineherd's disease* is caused by *Leptospira pomona,* and *swamp fever* by *Leptospira grippotyphosa.*

24. Rat-Bite Fever

SPIRILLUM RAT-BITE FEVER

Rat-bite fever, as the name implies, is transmitted by the bite of a rat or a mouse. One form *(sodoku)* is caused by *Spirillum minus,* a short, thick, flagellated, gram-negative organism with two or three thick, regular, spiral windings. *Clinically* after an incubation period of about 2 weeks the patient suddenly develops fever, headache, malaise, nausea and vomiting, joint and muscle pains, and in severe infections stupor or delirium. The *rat-bite site* becomes firm and may ulcerate like a chancre. A *reddish blue maculopapular skin rash* appears. The serologic test for syphilis is positive in about 50 percent of cases. The fever persists for up to a week and may reappear several times after apparent remissions. *Pathologically* at the bite site the epidermis is ulcerated, and there is an intense lymphocytic dermal infiltrate. In the occasional fatal cases fatty metamorphosis is found in the liver, the renal tubular epithelium shows degenerative changes varying from cloudy swelling to necrosis, and there is myocardial fibrillar cloudy swelling. The *general inflammatory reaction* is hyperemia and edema with little cellular response.

STREPTOBACILLUS RAT-BITE FEVER

Rat-bite fever is also caused by *Streptobacillus moniliformis,* a gram-negative, pleomorphic rod in chains. Infection with this organism may also occur by the ingestion of food, milk, or water contaminated with rodent excreta *(Haverhill fever).* The incubation period is about a week. The initial rat bite heals during this period and is not reactivated. In both rat-bite and Haverhill fever there is a sudden onset of chills and fever, severe headache, vomiting, malaise, and generalized weakness. A *red or reddish blue maculopapular skin rash* is often present. Painful swelling of several joints is common. The duration varies from 2 to many weeks. About 10 percent of the cases are fatal. *Pathologically* hepatocytic cloudy swelling or fatty metamorphosis, ulceration of the cardiac valvular endocardium, infarcts of the spleen and kidney resulting from embolism, and increased synovial fluid within joint cavities are found. Secondary bronchopneumonia occurs frequently. Streptobacilli may be identified by culture or animal inoculation using blood or joint fluid.

Information on many bacterial infections is summarized in Table 5-1.

Disease	Cause	Characteristics of organism	Mode of transmission	Principal organs or sites involved	Type of cellular reaction	Principal cell(s) in reaction	Special features
Staphylococcal infections	*Staphylococcus aureus*	Gram + cocci in clusters; antibiotic-resistant strains are common; virulent strains are coagulase +	Airborne droplet infection from infected cases or carriers; direct contact; fomites; auto-infection; food contaminated with enterotoxin	Skin (furuncle [boil], carbuncle, impetigo contagiosa, abscesses, botryomycosis) Lungs (bronchopneumonia with abscess formation) Heart (acute bacterial endocarditis, abscesses in pyemia) Gastrointestinal tract (gastroenteritis due to strains with heat-stable enterotoxin, antibiotic enterocolitis) Bone (acute osteomyelitis) Brain (abscess, meningitis)	Acute pyogenic reaction with abscess formation	Neutrophil	*S. epidermidis* causes mild infections of skin such as furuncles, impetigo, and acne vulgaris Septicemia and pyemia are commonly due to *S. aureus* Hospital infections are common, especially due to bacteriophage types 80/81 and 54 of *S. aureus*. Patients with burns, hepatic disease, diabetes mellitus, renal failure, cancer, and skin disorders have increased susceptibility
Streptococcal infections	Streptococci	Gram + cocci in chains; virulent strains are hemolytic; most human infections are due to organisms in Lancefield Group A; some are caused by β-hemolytic	Airborne droplet infection; direct contact; fomites	Skin (scarlet fever, erysipelas, impetigo, cellulitis) Upper respiratory tract (scarlet fever, pharyngitis, tonsillitis, sinusitis, otitis media) Lungs (bronchopneumonia)	Acute pyogenic reaction	Neutrophil	Scarlet fever is caused by strains with vasoparalytic erythrogenic (Dick) toxin Septicemia is common with β-hemolytic Group A streptococci

Table 5-1 continued on pages 108–121

TABLE 5-1. Bacterial Infections (Continued)

Disease	Cause	Characteristics of organism	Mode of transmission	Principal organs or sites involved	Type of cellular reaction	Principal cell(s) in reaction	Special features
Streptococcal infections (Cont.)		Group B or by Group D *(S. faecalis)* organisms		Heart (acute bacterial endocarditis [β-hemolytic strains], subacute bacterial endocarditis [α-hemolytic *S. viridans*]) Gastrointestinal tract (appendicitis) Uterus (puerperal sepsis) CNS (meningitis)			Rheumatic fever and glomerulonephritis are due to hypersensitivity to streptococci
Pneumococcal infections (page 456)*	*Diplococcus pneumoniae*	Gram +, encapsulated coccus often occurring in pairs; produces α-hemolysis; capsule undergoes swelling (quellung) with type-specific antibody	Airborne droplet infection	Lung (lobar pneumonia, bronchopneumonia) Heart (acute bacterial endocarditis, pericarditis) Ear (acute otitis media, mastoiditis) CNS (meningitis)	Acute pyogenic reaction with fibrin	Neutrophil	Lobar pneumonia classically passes through phases of red and gray hepatization and resolution, with occasional organization of the exudate by intra-alveolar fibrosis
Meningococcal infections (page 674)*	*Neisseria meningitidis*	Gram – cocci occurring singly or in pairs; found intra- and extracellularly in exudate	Airborne droplet infection	CNS (meningitis, sometimes epidemic) Upper respiratory tract (nasopharyngitis) Heart (acute bacterial endocarditis, or pericarditis rarely)	Acute pyogenic reaction	Neutrophil	Meningococcemia may result in Waterhouse-Friderichsen syndrome with massive adrenal hemorrhages, purpura, and shock

*Page references are given for bacterial infections which are not discussed in Chapters 5 and 6

Gonorrhea (page 606)*	*Neisseria gonorrhoeae*	Gram – cocci occurring singly or in pairs; often found intracellularly in exudate	Sexual contact; fomites (in girls)	Urethra, periurethral and vulvovaginal glands, vagina and cervix. Genital complications include prostatitis, epididymitis, urethral stricture, salpingitis, tubo-ovarian abscess, and pelvic peritonitis (in women). Hematogenous complications include septic arthritis, keratoderma blennorrhagica, acute bacterial endocarditis (sometimes right-sided), and pyemia	Acute pyogenic reaction	Neutrophil [illegible]	[illegible] (ophthalmia neonatorum) is due to intranatal infection
Tetanus	*Clostridium tetani*	Gram +, anaerobic, terminal spore-forming rods; saprophytic, elaborate powerful neurotoxin	Organisms introduced by puncture or gunshot wounds or deep lacerations	Skin (organisms remain localized in wound) Spinal cord and cranial nerve nuclei (motor neurons stimulated by neurotoxin)	None	None	Toxemia
Gas gangrene	Gas-forming *Clostridia*, esp. *Cl. perfringens (welchii)* and *novyi*	Gram +, anaerobic, spore-forming, saccharolytic, hemolytic, and sometimes proteolytic rods	Organisms introduced in wounds with tissue devitalization or during intestinal or gallbladder surgery	Skeletal muscle Liver and other viscera (in gas bacillus septicemia)	Massive necrosis with little inflammatory reaction	Few neutrophils	—

TABLE 5-1. Bacterial Infections (Continued)

Disease	Cause	Characteristics of organism	Mode of transmission	Principal organs or sites involved	Type of cellular reaction	Principal cell(s) in reaction	Special features
Botulism	*Clostridium botulinum*	Gram +, anaerobic, subterminal, spore-forming rods; elaborate highly poisonous exotoxins	Exotoxins ingested in improperly smoked or canned foods	Myoneural junction (toxins interfere with acetylcholine release, especially in muscles innervated by cranial nerves)	Hyperemia, petechiae, and ecchymoses; and thrombosis in small vessels	None	Toxemia Types A, B, and E of *Cl. botulinum* produce human disease
Diphtheria	*Corynebacterium diphtheriae*	Gram + rod with club-shaped terminal swellings; elaborates powerful exotoxin; gravis, intermedius, and mitis strains	Airborne droplet infection from infected individuals and carriers	Bacteria (nasal, pharyngeal, laryngeal, tracheal, and bronchial mucosa; occasionally skin, esophagus, or vagina) Exotoxin (myocardium, peripheral nerves)	Bacteria incite acute membranous inflammation with fibrin	Neutrophil	Combination of local infection + toxemia. Death is due to respiratory obstruction, secondary bronchopneumonia, or myocarditis
Pertussis (whooping cough)	*Bordetella (Hemophilus) pertussis*	Short, gram −, encapsulated, nonmotile rod	Airborne droplet infection	Bronchiolar, bronchial, and tracheal mucosa Lungs (secondary bacterial or *B. pertussis* bronchopneumonia or interstitial pneumonia)	Acute catarrhal inflammation	Lymphocyte	Bacteria are enmeshed in cilia Lymphocytic leukocytosis is characteristic
Influenza bacillus infections	*Hemophilus influenzae*	Short, gram − rod occurring singly and in pairs or short chains; some strains	Airborne droplet infection and possibly fomites	Nasopharynx and paranasal sinuses Middle ear Larynx and trachea Leptomeninges	Acute pyogenic reaction	Neutrophil	Most infections occur in infants and children under 3 years of age

		almost all severe infections caused by type B		terial endocarditis) Joints (suppurative arthritis)			septicemia
Pinkeye (acute conjunctivitis) (page 796)*	*Hemophilus aegyptius* (Koch-Weeks bacillus)	Short, gram – rod morphologically almost identical with *H. influenzae*	Personal contact and fomites	Bulbar and palpebral conjunctiva	Acute catarrhal inflammation (Gonococci cause purulent conjunctivitis)	Neutrophil	Bacterial conjunctivitis is also caused by *Moraxella lacunata*, pneumococci, streptococci, and staphylococci
Chancroid (page 608)*	*Hemophilus ducreyi*	Short, gram – rod in pairs and chains	Sexual contact	Prepuce and glans penis, vulva, inguinal lymph nodes	Acute pyogenic reaction with ulceration and abscesses	Neutrophil	Genital lesion passes from vesicle to pustule to deep ragged ulcer
Tularemia (rabbit fever)	*Pasteurella tularensis*	Small, gram – bacillus with coccoid and rod forms; obligate aerobe	Handling infected rabbits or squirrels or eating their poorly cooked meat; bite of deer fly or dog or rabbit tick	Skin (papule → pustule → ulcer at inoculation site) Conjunctiva Lymph nodes draining inoculation site Lungs (necrotizing pneumonitis) Liver and spleen	Acute necrotizing reaction in initial lesions and lungs Granuloma formation with central suppuration in lymph nodes, liver, and spleen	Neutrophil Epithelioid cell	Ulceroglandular, oculoglandular, glandular, and typhoidal forms
Plague	*Pasteurella pestis*	Small, nonmotile, encapsulated, gram – rod	Bite of rat flea; airborne droplet infection	Lymph nodes (bubonic plague) Lungs (pneumonic plague)	Acute necrotizing and hemorrhagic inflammation	Neutrophil	Septicemic plague is highly fatal terminal phase

TABLE 5-1. Bacterial Infections (Continued)

Disease	Cause	Characteristics of organism	Mode of transmission	Principal organs or sites involved	Type of cellular reaction	Principal cell(s) in reaction	Special features
Typhoid fever	*Salmonella typhosa (S. typhi)*	Plump, flagellated, gram – rod with O (somatic), H (flagellar), and Vi antigens	Contaminated water, milk, or food	Ileum (ulcers over hyperplastic Peyer's patches) Mesenteric lymph nodes, liver, spleen, bone marrow (focal necrosis) Gallbladder Lungs (bronchitis and pneumonitis)	Acute granulomatous reaction with ulceration or focal necrosis	Macrophage	Cholecystitis is responsible for carrier state Septicemia occasionally leads to meningitis, endocarditis, pyelonephritis, or osteomyelitis
Paratyphoid fever	*Salmonella paratyphi A (S. paratyphi), B (S. schottmuelleri), C (S. hirschfeldii)*	—	—	—	—	—	Similar to but less severe than typhoid fever
Salmonella gastroenteritis (food poisoning)	*Salmonella typhimurium, S. enteritidis, S. choleraesuis*	Gram –, flagellated rods; liberate endotoxins (somatic antigens)	Contaminated water, milk, other dairy products, fish, and eggs	Gastrointestinal tract, especially ileum	Mucosal hyperemia and edema	Little cellular response	Septicemia is not uncommon in *S. choleraesuis* infections
Bacillary dysentery	*Shigella* species: *S. dysenteriae, S. paradysenteriae, S. ambigua, S. sonnei*	Short, gram –, nonmotile rods; all produce endotoxins; *S. dysenteriae* elaborates powerful neurotropic exotoxin	Eating contaminated food or water	Colon (membranous ulcerative colitis) Brain stem and spinal cord (motor neuron degeneration due to exotoxin)	Acute membranous inflammation	Neutrophil	Occasional bacteremia with endocarditis, pyelonephritis, or arthritis Chronic ulcerative colitis sometimes

Cholera	*Vibrio cholerae*	Short, gently curved, gram – rod; elaborates powerful endotoxin	Drinking contaminated water	Small intestine and colon	Mucosal hyperemia and edema; lymphoid hyperplasia	Little cellular response	Profound dehydration due to vomiting and diarrhea (rice-water feces)
Coliform bacterial infections	*Escherichia coli, Klebsiella (Aerobacter) aerogenes*	Small, gram – rods; *E. coli* has peritrichous flagella; frequently in normal intestinal flora	Auto-infection, personal contact, food, water, fomites	Gastrointestinal tract (acute appendicitis, gastroenteritis) Peritoneum (following surgery or perforated viscus) Urinary bladder and kidneys (ascending pyelonephritis Gallbladder and bile ducts Lungs (bronchopneumonia) Leptomeninges Skin (wound infections)	Acute pyogenic reaction	Macrophage Neutrophil	Septicemia with shock due to peripheral vascular collapse may occur
Klebsiella pneumoniae infections	*Klebsiella pneumoniae*	Short, heavily encapsulated, gram – rod with O and R (somatic) and K (capsular) antigens; culturally very similar to *Aerobacter aerogenes*	Inhalation; auto-infection	Lungs (lobar pneumonia) Gastrointestinal tract (appendicitis) Peritoneum Urinary bladder and kidneys Paranasal sinuses Leptomeninges	Acute mononuclear reaction in lung	Macrophage	Bronchiolar and alveolar exudate is sticky due to mucin and contains little fibrin Neutrophils predominate in some cases
Rhinoscleroma	*Klebsiella rhinoscleromatis*	Encapsulated, gram – rod	Inhalation	Nasal, buccal, pharyngeal, and laryngeal mucosa	Granuloma formation	Lymphocyte	Russell-Fuchs bodies from degenerated plasmocytes and Mikulicz cells (foamy macrophages) are common in granulomata

TABLE 5-1. Bacterial Infections (Continued)

Disease	Cause	Characteristics of organism	Mode of transmission	Principal organs or sites involved	Type of cellular reaction	Principal cell(s) in reaction	Special features
Proteus infections	*Proteus* species, especially *P. vulgaris* and *P. mirabilis*	Straight, gram – rods, occurring singly and in pairs; peritrichous flagella	Auto-infection, personal contact, bath water	Gastrointestinal tract (gastroenteritis) Peritoneum Urinary bladder and kidneys (ascending pyelonephritis) Lungs (bronchopneumonia) Leptomeninges, middle ear	Acute pyogenic reaction, sometimes with abscess formation	Neutrophil	Double or multiple infections with *Proteus* species or infections in combination with *E. coli* or *Staphylococcus* are common Septicemia may occur
Pseudomonas infections	*Pseudomonas aeruginosa (Bacillus pyocyaneus)*	Small, slender, gram – rod with polar flagella; frequently part of normal flora of skin and intestine	Auto-infection, personal contact, fomites	Skin (surgical or other wound infection) Peritoneum (following surgery or perforated viscus) Upper respiratory tract, middle ear, and mastoid cells Lungs (necrotizing bronchopneumonia) Heart (acute bacterial endocarditis) Gastrointestinal tract (gastroenteritis) Leptomeninges Urinary bladder and kidneys Eye (purulent conjunctivitis and acute serpiginous	Acute pyogenic reaction with typical bluish green pus in abscesses	Neutrophil	Antibiotic-resistant strains are common. Usually of low pathogenicity, but may produce severe infections in debilitated individuals and infants, especially those on prolonged antibiotic therapy

	(Actinobacillus, Malleomyces) pseudomallei	gram – rod with polar flagella	food contaminated with infected rat excreta	abscesses in lungs and other organs	genic reaction with small abscesses	phage Neutrophil	of glanders Chronic form also occurs
Glanders and farcy	*Actinobacillus mallei*	Nonmotile, gram – rod	From horses and mules through skin wounds or inhalation	Skin (papule → pustule → ulcer) Lymph nodes Lungs (bronchopneumonia with abscesses)	Acute pyogenic reaction with abscess formation	Neutrophil	Pyemia is frequent in acute form Farcy is chronic form with epithelioid cell granulomata in skin and lymphatics (farcy buds)
Brucellosis (Malta fever)	*Brucella abortus, B. melitensis, B. suis*	Small, nonmotile, encapsulated, gram – coccobacillus	Milk from infected cows or goats, meat from infected animals, laboratory cultures	Ileum (ulcers) Liver, spleen, lymph nodes, and bone marrow Heart (vegetative endocarditis)	Granuloma formation; marked reticuloendothelial response	Epithelioid cell	Endocarditis may result in calcific aortic stenosis Pneumonitis, meningitis, pyelonephritis, and osteomyelitis may occur
Anthrax	*Bacillus anthracis*	Large, gram +, nonmotile, spore-forming rod	Inhalation of spores, using infected shaving brushes, handling infected sheep or cattle	Skin (papule → vesicle → malignant pustule → black ulcer) Lungs (bronchopneumonia) Gastrointestinal tract	Acute hemorrhagic inflammation	Neutrophil	—
Erysipeloid	*Erysipelothrix (rhusiopathiae) insidiosa*	Slender, slightly curved, nonmotile, gram + rod in long chains	Contact with infected pork, fish or shellfish, crab bite	Skin of hand (purplish red papule)	Acute mononuclear reaction	Lymphocyte	Occasional hematogenous dissemination

TABLE 5-1. Bacterial Infections (Continued)

Disease	Cause	Characteristics of organism	Mode of transmission	Principal organs or sites involved	Type of cellular reaction	Principal cell(s) in reaction	Special features
Listeria infections (page 676)*	*Listeria monocytogenes*	Short, gram +, motile (flagellated) rod; produces β hemolysis	Probably airborne droplets; intrauterine infections	Leptomeninges (purulent meningitis)	Acute pyogenic reaction	Neutrophil	Usually causes infections in infants and young children Hematogenously disseminated miliary granulomatosis occasionally occurs in newborn
Bartonellosis (Carrion's disease)	*Bartonella bacilliformis*	Small, motile, aerobic, gram – bacillus	Bite of sand fly, *Phlebotomus noguchi* and *verrucarum*	Lymph nodes, spleen, liver, and bone marrow in acute form (Oroya fever) Skin and mucous membranes in chronic form (verruca peruviana)	Reticuloendothelial hyperplasia	Endothelial cell	Organisms are rickettsia-like and proliferate in capillary endothelial cells
Granuloma inguinale (page 609)*	*Donovania (Calymmatobacterium) granulomatis* (Donovan body)	Gram –, encapsulated, leishmanioid body with polar or bipolar chromatin condensation	Probably sexual contact	External genitalia (papules → pustules → ulcers on penis, vulva, perineum, inner thighs)	Granulation tissue response in ulcer base	Macrophage	Organisms are found in intracytoplasmic cysts in macrophages (granuloma cells)
Mimeae infections	*Mima polymorpha, Herellea vaginicola, Colloides anoxydana*	Short, gram –, nonmotile rods or diplococci which mimic *Neisseria*	Sexual contact ("gonorrhea"); airborne droplets	Urethra (penicillin-resistant gonorrhea) Leptomeninges Heart (subacute bacterial endocarditis)	Acute pyogenic reaction	Neutrophil	Prolonged infections, especially chronic meningitis, with lymphocytic infiltration are common

Mycoplasma (pleuropneumonia-like organism, PPLO) infections	*Mycoplasma pneumoniae* (Eaton agent); *M. hominis; M. fermentans; M. salivarum*	Extremely pleomorphic rods, coccoid bodies, spirals, filaments, or granules; thick films gram –; grow on solid media as protoplasts like L bacterial forms; small forms are filtrable	Airborne droplets, personal contact, sexual intercourse	Lungs (interstitial pneumonitis) Pharyngeal and tracheobronchial mucosa Urethra Conjunctiva Joints	Pleomorphic intra-alveolar and septal infiltrates in lungs; mucopurulent urethritis	Histio[illegible]phic in lungs; neutrophils in urethra and conjunctiva	*M. pneumoniae* [illegible] commonest cause of primary atypical pneumonia when cold agglutinins are +. *Mycoplasma* cause Reiter's disease (urethritis, conjunctivitis, and arthritis), prostatitis, cervicitis, and possibly rheumatoid arthritis
Fusospirochetosis	*Borrelia vincentii* plus *Fusobacterium fusiforme (F. plautivincent), F. polymorphum,* or *F. nucleatum*	*Borrelia:* gram – organism with 3–8 shallow wavy spirals *Fusobacterium:* gram – (with frequent gram + granules), short or long, slender rods occurring singly, in pairs, or in short chains; anaerobic	Auto-infection in persons with nutritional deficiencies, trauma, or debilitating diseases	Mouth (ulcerative gingivostomatitis [trench mouth]); necrotizing ulcerative stomatitis (Vincent's angina); gangrenous stomatitis (noma, cancrum oris), pyorrhea Lung (gangrene)	Acute necrotizing inflammation (with fibrinous membrane in mouth)	Neutrophil	Organisms are saprophytes which act synergistically to cause disease under anaerobic conditions in previously injured or poorly nourished tissue
Relapsing fever	*Borrelia recurrentis, B. duttonii, B. noyvi*	Gram –, cylindrical spirochetes with irregular, large, wavy spirals	Scratching of body louse bite, bite of ticks of *Ornithodorus genus*	Spleen Liver	Reticular hyperplasia; hemorrhages	Reticulum cell	Recurrent episodes of high fever lasting 2–7 days with remissions of about a week. Death often due to secondary bronchopneumonia
Leptospirosis (Weil's disease)	*Leptospira icterohaemorrhagiae;* occasionally *L. canicola*	Spirochete with fine, tightly wound spirals about an axial filament	Water contaminated with infected rat urine or	Liver (fatty metamorphosis, necrosis, bile stasis) Kidneys (tubular epithelial degeneration,	Acute inflammation; capillary hemorrhages in	Neutrophil (with lymphocyte in meningitis)	Pretibial (Fort Bragg) fever is due to autumnalis AB serotype of *L. icterohaemorrhagiae*

(Continued on next page)

TABLE 5-1. Bacterial Infections (Continued)

Disease	Cause	Characteristics of organism	Mode of transmission	Principal organs or sites involved	Type of cellular reaction	Principal cell(s) in reaction	Special features
Leptospirosis (Cont.)			feces (dog excreta for *L. canicola*); organisms enter skin, conjunctivae, and respiratory or intestinal mucosa	bile pigment casts) Skeletal muscles Leptomeninges	skin, mucosa, and viscera		Swineherd's disease is caused by *Leptospira pomona* and swamp fever by *L. grippotyphosa*
Rat-bite fever	*Spirillum minus*	Short, thick, flagellated, gram – organisms with 2–3 thick, regular spiral windings	Rat or mouse bite	Skin (reddish blue maculopapular rash) Liver (fatty metamorphosis) Kidneys (tubular degeneration) Joints (polyarthritis)	Hyperemia and edema	Little cellular response	Also caused by *Streptobacillus moniliformis,* a gram –, pleomorphic rod in chains Haverhill fever (erythema arthriticum epidemicum), also caused by the *Streptobacillus,* is transmitted by contaminated milk, food, or water
Tuberculosis	*Mycobacterium tuberculosis*	Acid-fast, gram +, unencapsulated, obligatively aerobic rod; human, bovine, and avian strains; BCG (bacille Calmette	Airborne droplet infection, occasionally milk from infected cows	Lungs (primary lesion in periphery of lower lobe and hilar lymph nodes; reinfection lesion begins in apex; primary [Ghon] lesion)	Granuloma formation with caseation necrosis in primary infection lesions, and	Epithelioid cell	Primary complex is Ghon lesion + caseous hilar nodes Scrofula is tuberculous cervical lymphadenitis Cold abscess is a

Guerin) strain is used in tuberculin-negative individuals as vaccine; acid-fastness and epithelioid and Langhans giant cell reactions are due to lipid fraction in organisms; protein fraction is responsible for hypersensitivity response in progressive 1st-infection tuberculosis (after 2–3 weeks) and in 2nd-infection tuberculosis	usually calcifies; reinfection lesion may calcify, may spread peripherally as fibrocaseous tuberculosis, may cavitate, or may spread endobronchially to infect same or opposite lung; sometimes as tuberculous pneumonia; either primary or reinfection lesions may spread hematogenously to cause miliary tuberculosis) Lymph nodes (caseating granulomata in primary infections) Ileum and cecum (ulcers girdling lumen; due to swallowing infected sputum or milk) Peritoneum (from salpingitis or mesenteric lymphadenitis or hematogenous spread) Pleura and pericardium (by direct extension) Adrenals, kidneys, uterine tubes, prostate, epididymes; joints, bones, and leptomeninges (by hematogenous spread) Skin (through wound or hematogenously)	liquefaction in reinfection	liquefied bone or joint lesion Psoas abscess is a cold abscess extending within psoas sheath from thoracic vertebral osteomyelitis to groin Pott's disease is tuberculous spondylitis Miliary tuberculosis is the presence of numerous small (millet seed-sized) tubercles in the lungs, meninges, liver, spleen, etc. due to hematogenous spread

TABLE 5-1. Bacterial Infections (Continued)

Disease	Cause	Characteristics of organism	Mode of transmission	Principal organs or sites involved	Type of cellular reaction	Principal cell(s) in reaction	Special features
Leprosy (Hansen's disease)	*Mycobacterium leprae*	Acid-fast, gram +, slightly curved, beaded rod; incites reagin formation, causing biologically false positive test for syphilis in 2/3 of cases	Personal contact	Skin (lepromatous or nodular leprosy) Peripheral nerves (tuberculoid leprosy)	Granuloma formation	Macrophage (leproma cell) Epithelioid cell (tuberculoid granuloma)	Many organisms are found in foamy lepra cells Organisms are difficult to find in tuberculoid leprosy Miliary lepromas are found in liver and spleen
Syphilis (lues, pox, bad blood)	*Treponema pallidum*	Thin, delicate spirochete with tightly and evenly twisted spirals; reagin is a readily diffusible antibody-like substance in serum and cerebrospinal fluid which makes possible the flocculation and complement fixation tests for syphilis; immobilizing antibody is the basis of the TPI *(Treponema pallidum* immobilization) test	Sexual contact, transplacental infection of fetus (congenital syphilis)	Primary stage (glans penis, vulva, vagina, cervix, occasionally lip or nipple – chancre) Secondary stage (skin – macular, papular, and pustular syphilids; mucous membranes – mucous patches, condyloma latum; lymph nodes – hyperplasia) Tertiary stage (ascendint aorta – saccular aneurysm; CNS – meningovascular syphilis, tabes dorsalis, general paresis, gummata; liver, testes, etc.	Chronic interstitial inflammation and proliferative endarteritis with perivascular plasmocytic and lymphocytic cuffing; gummatous necrosis in tertiary stage	Plasmocyte	In congenital syphilis no primary lesion develops. Fetus may die in utero, infant may be born with manifestations of syphilis, or these may appear after birth (syphilis tarda). Osteitis, epiphysitis, and periosteitis interfere with bone development (saber shins, saddle nose); notched, narrow-edged incisors (Hutchinson's teeth), interstitial keratitis, and nerve deafness make up Hutchinson's triad Pneumonia alba is a fine pulmonary fibrosis in

Yaws, pinta, and bejel	*Treponema pallidum* (organism producing yaws is called *T. pertenue;* that of pinta, *T. carateum)*	As listed under syphilis	with infectious skin lesion		syphilis are positive

REFERENCES

1. Rosen, F. S. The endotoxins of Gram-negative bacteria and host resistance. *New Eng. J. Med.* 264:919, 980, 1961.
2. Rapaport, S. I., Tatter, D., Coeur-Barron, N., and Hjort, P. F. *Pseudomonas* septicemia with intravascular clotting leading to the generalized Shwartzman reaction. *New Eng. J. Med.* 271:80, 1964.
3. Morse, S. I. Isolation and properties of surface antigen of *Staphylococcus aureus*. *J. Exp. Med.* 115:295, 1962.
4. Cohen, L. S., Fekety, F. R., and Cluff, L. E. Studies of the epidemiology of staphylococcal infection. IV. The changing ecology of hospital staphylococci. *New Eng. J. Med.* 266:367, 1962.
5. Nahmias, A. J., and Eickhoff, T. C. Staphylococcal infections in hospitals. *New Eng. J. Med.* 265:74, 120, 177, 1961.
6. Keene, W. R., Minchew, B. H., and Cluff, L. E. Studies in the epidemiology of staphylococcal infection. III. Clinical factors in susceptibility to staphylococcal disease. *New Eng. J. Med.* 265:1128, 1961.
7. Winslow, D. J. Botryomycosis. *Amer. J. Path.* 35:153, 1959.
8. Mannik, M., Baringer, J. R., and Stokes, J. Infections due to Group B beta-hemolytic streptococci. *New Eng. J. Med.* 266:910, 1962.
9. Pyrtek, L. J., and Bartus, S. H. *Clostridium welchii* infection complicating biliary-tract surgery. *New Eng. J. Med.* 266:689, 1962.
10. Jarkowski, T. L., and Wolf, P. L. Unusual gas bacillus infections including necrotic enteritis. *J.A.M.A.* 181:845, 1962.
11. Berggren, R. B., Batterton, T. D., McArdle, G., and Erb, W. H. Clostridial myositis after parenteral injections. *J.A.M.A.* 188:1044, 1964.
12. Roberts, J. M., and Bassett, F. H. Gas gangrene: Recent cases. *J.A.M.A.* 177:148, 1961.
13. Lamanna, C. The most poisonous poison. *Science* 130:763, 1959.
14. Eadie, G. A., Molner, J. G., Solomon, R. J., and Aach, R. D. Type E botulism. *J.A.M.A.* 187:496, 1964.
15. Tyler, H. R. Pathology of the neuromuscular apparatus in botulism. *Arch. Path.* (Chicago) 76:55, 1963.
16. Gore, I. Myocardial changes in fatal diphtheria. *Amer. J. Med. Sci.* 215:257, 1948.
17. Funt, T. Primary cutaneous diphtheria. *J.A.M.A.* 176:273, 1961.
18. Mengis, C. L. Plague. *New Eng. J. Med.* 267:543, 1962.
19. Holloway, W. J., Scott, E. G., and Adams, Y. B. *Pasteurella multocida* infection in man. *Amer. J. Clin. Path.* 51:705, 1969.
20. Black, P. H., Kunz, L. J., and Swartz, M. N. Salmonellosis – a review of some unusual aspects. *New Eng. J. Med.* 262:811, 864, 1960.
21. Macumber, H. H. Acute bacillary dysentery. *Arch. Intern. Med.* 69:624, 1942.
22. Fresh, J. W., Versage, P. M., and Reyes, V. Intestinal morphology in human and experimental cholera. *Arch. Path.* (Chicago) 77:529, 1964.
23. Tillotson, J. R., and Lerner, A. M. Characteristics of pneumonias caused by *Escherichia coli*. *New Eng. J. Med.* 277:115, 1967.
24. Fisher, E. R., and Dimling, C. Rhinoscleroma. *Arch. Path.* (Chicago) 78:501, 1964.
25. Hubbard, J. D., King, H., and Beamer, P. R. The pathogenicity of *Pseudomonas aeruginosa (Bacillus pyocyaneus)*. *Amer. J. Clin. Path.* 28:243, 1957.
26. Greenawald, K. A., Nash, G., and Foley, F. D. Acute systemic melioidosis. *Amer. J. Clin. Path.* 52:188, 1969.

27. Peery, T. M., and Belter, L. F. Brucellosis and heart disease. II. Fatal brucellosis: A review of the literature and report of new cases. *Amer. J. Path.* 36:673, 1960.
28. Fincham, R. W., Sahs, A. L., and Joynt, R. J. Protean manifestations of nervous system brucellosis. *J.A.M.A.* 184:269, 1963.
29. Gold, H. Anthrax. *A.M.A. Arch. Intern. Med.* 96:387, 1955.
30. Albrink, W. S., Brooks, S. M., Biron, R. E., and Kopel, M. Human inhalation anthrax. *Amer. J. Path.* 36:457, 1960.
31. Sprecace, G. A., and Dunkelberg, W. E., Jr. *Mima polymorpha* – causative agent in acute and chronic meningitis. *J.A.M.A.* 177:706, 1961.
32. Hirsch, S. R., and Koch, M. L. *Herellea (Bacterium anitratum)* endocarditis. *J.A.M.A.* 187:148, 1964.
33. Svihus, R. H., Lucero, E. M., Mikolajczyk, R. J., and Carter, E. E. Gonorrhea-like syndrome caused by penicillin-resistant mimeae. *J.A.M.A.* 177:121, 1961.
34. Chanock, R. M. Mycoplasma infections of man. *New Eng. J. Med.* 273:1199, 1257, 1965.
35. Anderson, T. R., and Zimmerman, L. E. Relapsing fever in Korea. *Amer. J. Path.* 31:1083, 1955.
36. Arean, V. M. The pathologic anatomy and pathogenesis of fatal human leptospirosis (Weil's disease). *Amer. J. Path.* 40:393, 1962.

GENERAL REFERENCES

Burrows, W. *Textbook of Microbiology* (19th ed.). Philadelphia: Saunders, 1968.

Gladstone, G. P., and van Heyningen, W. E. In Florey, H. (Ed.), *General Pathology* (4th ed.). Philadelphia: Saunders, 1970, pp. 823–897. (An excellent critical study of the pathogenicity and virulence of microorganisms.)

Walter, J. B., and Israel, M. S. *General Pathology.* Boston: Little Brown, 1963, pp. 74–83, 108–126, 265–302. (A concise, practical discussion of infection in general and some specific infections.)

6 TUBERCULOSIS AND THE TUBERCULOID GRANULOMAS; SYPHILIS AND OTHER TREPONEMATOSES

GRANULOMATOUS DISEASES

CHRONIC BACTERIAL INFECTIONS

Most bacterial agents, as noted in the preceding chapter, cause an acute inflammatory reaction in the tissues. A few characteristically incite a granulomatous reaction. In most instances the resulting granulomatous diseases are chronic, lasting months or years. Proliferation of *fibroblasts* and new *capillaries* is the outstanding pathologic feature; *monocytes, lymphocytes,* and frequently *giant cells* characterize the cellular exudate, although other cells are also present.

SPECIFIC AND NONSPECIFIC GRANULOMAS

When the disease is incited by a specific infectious agent, as is the case with tuberculosis or syphilis, the granulomatous response is often referred to as a *specific granuloma,* or a *specific infectious granuloma.* These terms recognize that there are also *nonspecific granulomas,* often of noninfectious origin. It is often impossible to identify the cause of a granulomatous tissue reaction by means of routine stains, because the tissue reactions in these different diseases may be indistinguishable, and the causative agent may be unstained and invisible. In order to make the differentiation, it is frequently necessary to apply specific staining methods to identify the etiologic agent. Thus the carbolfuchsin method is used to identify the acid-fast *Mycobacterium tuberculosis,* the Levaditi method to demonstrate the presence of the *Treponema pallidum,* and the periodic acid-Schiff method or the Gomori silver stain to demonstrate and identify fungi in tissues.

The two most important specific infectious granulomata in the United States at the present time are *tuberculosis* and *syphilis.* Most of the *fungus diseases* are also members of this group; they have increased in importance in recent years. Certain *viral* and *protozoan diseases* are also properly included among the specific infectious granulomata.

TUBERCULOSIS AND THE TUBERCULOID GRANULOMAS

1. Tuberculosis

The causative agent

Tuberculosis is a specific infectious granulomatous disease due to *Mycobacterium tuberculosis,* commonly known as the tubercle bacillus. Two strains of this species are recognized. The *human strain is the chief cause of tuberculosis of all organ systems at all ages in man;* it may also infect monkeys, house pets, and domestic animals. The *bovine strain* may also cause human tuberculosis, especially of the tonsils, cervical lymph nodes, and gastrointestinal tract in children, but it is much less important now than previously due to the control of tuberculosis in cattle. A related organism, *M. avium,* causes tuberculosis in birds but is apparently unimportant in human disease; it has been suspected from time to time as the cause of Hodgkin's disease, sarcoidosis, and other chronic infections. Other acid-fast organisms of this genus cause a disease resembling tuberculosis in snakes, frogs, and turtles, but are apparently not pathogenic to man. *M. muris* (the vole bacillus) is capable of producing local disease and of inciting an immune reaction in man, but it is not known to cause spontaneous human disease.

Chemical constituents The protein and lipid fractions of *M. tuberculosis* have been held responsible for certain characteristics of the disease in man [1]. The *protein fraction* is responsible for the local and systemic reactions of the tuberculous individual *to reinfection.* The *lipid fraction* accounts for the acid-fast property of the organism and the development of epithelioid and giant cells in the tissues. In spite of these statements, it should be noted that there is no conclusive evidence that the *M. tuberculosis* or any of its fractions or products on culture media are ordinarily toxic to normal, nontuberculous individuals. Mononuclear cells grow, migrate normally on tissue culture, and survive even when they contain great numbers of bacilli.

Prevalence: in man Tuberculosis is widespread throughout all parts of the world. It is said that about 5 million people die each year of tuberculosis [2]. The death rate from this disease in the United States is about 3.5 per 100,000 population per year [3]; in 1900 the death rate was nearly 200. Much higher rates, about 150 per 100,000 per year, occur in Asia, and parts of South America. Although death rates from tuberculosis have declined remarkably in recent years, partly as a result of effective antibiotic agents, the number of new cases of tuberculosis discovered each year remains high.

in animals Tuberculosis is an important problem in captive wild animals, although it is rarely a problem in wild animals in their native habitats. In autopsies on zoo animals, we have found evidence of active lesions containing acid-fast bacilli in snakes, turtles, birds, monkeys, bison, capybara, and almost every variety of creature. In several instances the organisms in these animals have been identified as the human strain of the tubercle bacillus. Domesticated animals such as cattle, pigs, cats, dogs, and fowls are especially susceptible to human infection; they may in turn reinfect man.

Natural resistance and susceptibility Human tuberculosis has been studied at all ages, in a great variety of population groups, and for a number of years. From these studies it has been learned that there is both a *natural resistance* and a *natural susceptibility* to infection. The American Negro, American Indian, and Eskimo are all very susceptible. This was thought at one time to be due to recent exposure of these peoples to the disease, or to diet, inadequate housing, and the like. It has, however, been shown that either resistance or susceptibility to tuberculosis can be developed by *inbreeding* [1]. This suggests that differences between the frequency of tuberculosis in the various racial strains may be due to a variety of causes. *Sex* apparently has little influence on natural resistance to tuberculosis; females are slightly more susceptible than males in adolescence and young adulthood, but this is not universally the case. Susceptibility to tuberculosis is much influenced by *age. In infants it is a highly fatal disease,* gradually becoming less so at about 5 years. Death from tuberculosis is rare between the ages of 5 and 15. Thereafter the death rate gradually rises, reaching its maximum at the end of the scale (75 years). These age differences in the death rate from tuberculosis are probably due more to the *degree and frequency of exposure* rather than to true susceptibility. These same factors are probably responsible in large part for the high mortality and morbidity rates in *city slums,* where infected individuals come in close contact with the uninfected. *Occupation* may also provide unusual opportunities for exposure to the tubercle bacillus. Thus physicians, nurses, medical students, hospital employees, bacteriologists, and research workers in the field of tuberculosis have a higher than average incidence of infection.

Acquired resistance; hypersensitivity

Infection by *M. tuberculosis* results in both *acquired resistance* and *hypersensitivity.* Although produced by the same stimulus and occurring together, acquired resistance and hypersensitivity are apparently not the same phenomenon. Acquired *resistance to tuberculosis is partial* and seems to be largely a phenomenon of the *mononuclear macrophage:* in the immune animal macrophages assemble more quickly and in larger numbers about injected bacilli and are more effective in destroying or localizing those bacilli than is the case in the nonimmune animal [2]. There is no known means of measuring resistance. Resistance is apparently *not dependent upon circulating antibodies.* The blood serum of immunized animals is not protective. Hypersensitivity to tuberculosis can be induced only by the injection of the whole bacterial cell. However, once induced, it can be demonstrated or measured by skin tests using either filtrates of cultures of *M. tuberculosis* (tuberculin or "old tuberculin" – O.T.) or purified protein derivatives (P.P.D.) of *M. tuberculosis. The tuberculin test indicates prior infection by the tubercle bacillus or lack of it;* a positive test does not mean active infection, except perhaps in very young children or when it is known that the test was negative shortly before. Hypersensitivity accounts for the acute inflammatory reaction, tissue destruction, and liquefaction which characterize the local reaction to reinfection by the tubercle bacillus. Hypersensitivity also accounts for the constitutional symptoms, such as fever, that are commonly noted in reinfection tuberculosis. These local and systemic reactions do not occur in first-infection tuberculosis unless the dosage is massive.

Koch phenomenon

The *Koch phenomenon* provides the experimental evidence for the significance of *hypersensitivity in tuberculosis.* If a tuberculous guinea pig is reinoculated with tubercle bacilli 4 to 6 weeks after the first infection, a *violent inflammatory reaction* develops at the site of the second injection and results in swelling and ulceration of the skin, but there is *no spread of the bacilli to regional lymph nodes.*

BCG vaccine

BCG vaccine has been developed to take advantage of the benefits of acquired resistance to tuberculosis and to reduce the risk from tuberculous infection. The value of this vaccine has been the subject of much controversy. A special committee appointed by the Surgeon General of the United States Public Health Service to evaluate the evidence concerning BCG vaccine [4] noted that, although affording some protection to uninfected persons, the vaccine cannot be used in persons already reacting to tuberculoprotein and therefore it does not help the group needing protection. Furthermore, the *use of the vaccine renders the tuberculin test valueless.* The committee recommended that its use be limited to those individuals who react negatively to the tuberculin test and who have a definite risk of infection by virtue of their occupation. Included in this group are many physicians, nurses, and medical students.

Exogenous and endogenous infection

Without doubt the most important source of human infection is direct contact with persons having open tuberculous lung lesions, i.e., tuberculous cavities communicating with bronchi; these cavities contain great numbers of living organisms. This type of exposure gives rise to *exogenous infection.* Of secondary importance is *endogenous infection,* meaning reinfection of an individual as a result of the breakdown of his own old tuberculous lesions. Of minimal importance at the present time is the swallowing of living tubercle bacilli in the milk from cows with tuberculosis of the udders.

Avenues of infection

The chief portal of entry of the organism is the *respiratory tract.* Bacilli may thus be inhaled directly by droplet infection or indirectly in contaminated dust. *Pulmonary tuberculosis* is the result of entry of organisms by this avenue. Today the *alimentary tract* is rarely a portal of entry, but occasionally, if very large numbers of viable bacilli are swallowed, this route may lead to tuberculous lesions of the tonsils or intestines. Rarely cuts or scratches of the hands may serve as the portal of entry for bacilli; only those persons working with heavily infected material have any risk from this route. Rarer still is the possibility of infection of the fetus via the placental circulation from a mother with disseminated infection.

Pathogenesis

The *character, distribution,* and *extent* of the lesions of human tuberculosis are determined largely by the following factors: (1) *avenue of infection,* (2) *dosage of bacilli,* (3) *degree of natural immunity,* and (4) presence or absence of *acquired resistance and hypersensitivity.* With the human strain of the organism, virulence is generally of a high order and is rarely an important variable. Since the course of events in first-infection tuberculosis is often radically different from that in reinfection tuberculosis, in which sensitization plays a major role, the development of the lesions in these two conditions is presented in some detail.

First-infection tuberculosis

First-infection tuberculosis, formerly known as childhood tuberculosis, is the usual form of tuberculosis in children. The parenchymal lung lesion (Ghon lesion) is usually in the lower lobe of one lung; a cavity rarely develops. The parenchymal lung lesion plus the lesions in the regional lymph nodes are known as the *primary complex.* A patient whose tuberculin test is positive usually has a primary lung lesion, although it may not be demonstrable by x-ray. There are usually *no symptoms in first-infection tuberculosis;* toxic symptoms appear only after sensitization to tuberculoprotein has developed. In first-infection tuberculosis the size of the lesion and the end result are probably determined largely by the size of the infecting dose. Children usually either recover from tuberculosis or die from it; chronic disease is uncommon. Miliary tuberculosis and tuberculous meningitis are important manifestations of tuberculosis during the first few years of life. Tuberculosis of cervical lymph nodes and tonsils may occur. Older children have a very low mortality from tuberculosis.

Reinfection tuberculosis

Reinfection tuberculosis (adult tuberculosis) is the usual form of tuberculosis in adults. It features parenchymal lung lesions with no lymph node lesions. Cavities are common, usually in the apices of the upper lobes of the lungs. Symptoms are numerous. Tuberculosis of specific organs, and especially pulmonary tuberculosis, is considered in more detail in subsequent chapters.

COMPARISON OF FIRST-INFECTION AND REINFECTION TUBERCULOSIS OF THE LUNGS

First-infection tuberculosis	*Reinfection tuberculosis*
1. Small numbers of polymorphonuclear cells are attracted by the bacilli but are destroyed.	1. Same as in first-infection tuberculosis.
2. Macrophages gather slowly and engulf the bacilli, which continue to multiply. Macrophage becomes stringy and poorly outlined – the epithelioid cell. These cells fuse to form Langhans' giant cells, each containing 10 to 100 nuclei.	2. Hyperemia occurs, and macrophages and polymorphonuclear cells gather rapidly. Bacterial multiplication is inhibited and the infection may die out. Epithelioid cells and giant cells are formed, as in first infection.
3. Center of the lesion becomes granular, structureless, and eosinophilic – *caseation necrosis.* New epithelioid cells and giant cells form at periphery. Lymphocytes and fibroblasts surround the lesion. Slowly the tubercle is formed – a *proliferative lesion.* Sensitization to tuberculoprotein usually has developed by this time.	3. Lytic enzymes from assembled cells and thrombosis of small vessels cause *liquefaction necrosis.* There is little walling off of the lesion. Rapidly the tubercle is formed – *an exudative lesion.* (Dosage of bacilli and degree of sensitization are the chief factors determining the outcome.)
4. Newly formed bacteria are carried by macrophages to the periphery. The caseous center enlarges, sometimes to several centimeters. Daughter tubercles form about the larger lesion. Lesions are usually subpleural, in a *lower lobe. There is no cavitation.*	4. As bacilli multiply and are carried to the periphery of the tubercle, the liquefied area enlarges until it ruptures into a bronchus, producing a *cavity.* The organisms now multiply rapidly, because they are aerobic. Lesions, often bilateral, are usually in *apices of upper lobes.*
5. Macrophages carry bacilli *via lymphatics* to *regional lymph nodes,* causing identical lesions. Rarely bacilli may extend to the thoracic duct, leading to *miliary tuberculosis.* If caseous lesions in a lung or lymph node break down at a later date, permitting spread of bacilli *(endogenous reinfection),* consequent lesions show the features of sensitization, including cavity formation.	5. Spread of the infection is chiefly *along natural passages by aspiration of infected material* from a cavity *into the lower portions of both lungs,* destroying more and more lung tissue. There is *no tendency to involvement of the regional nodes.* Miliary tuberculosis may occur but is less common than in first-infection tuberculosis.
6. In most cases the lesions in the lung and lymph nodes heal without symptoms or treatment. Fibroblasts wall off the lesions, hyaline changes ensue, calcium is deposited, and the bacilli tend to die out.	6. With modern therapy the bacilli may be destroyed, but scarring may lead to distortion of the bronchi, mediastinum, and spine. The remaining cavities are susceptible to recurring pyogenic infection. Calcification seldom occurs.

Manner of spread

In progressive tuberculosis, tubercle bacilli may be disseminated within the host in any of the following ways: (1) *by direct extension,* involving contiguous tissues; (2) *by natural passages,* such as along the bronchial tree from an upper lobe cavity to a lower lobe on the same or opposite side (this is the usual manner of spread in reinfection tuberculosis); (3) *by lymphatic channels* to regional lymph nodes (this method is practically restricted to first-infection tuberculosis); (4) *by hematogenous spread,* resulting in miliary tuberculosis; or (5) *by implantation* in a body cavity (thus tuberculous peritonitis often complicates tuberculous salpingitis, and tuberculous pericarditis may develop from a tuberculous mediastinal node).

Special forms of tuberculosis

Certain special forms of tuberculosis require brief consideration. *Miliary tuberculosis* is the usually fatal consequence of tuberculous bacteremia, either via the thoracic duct and the superior vena cava in first-infection tuberculosis, or more rarely by dissemination of bacilli from an eroded vein in reinfection tuberculosis. Small (1 to 2 mm.) caseous lesions appear in the lungs (where they may sometimes be recognized by x-ray), liver, spleen, meninges, kidneys, and in almost any other organ. *Intestinal tuberculosis* may be primary, as a result of drinking infectious milk, or it may be secondary to the swallowing of infectious material from cavities in the lungs. *Urogenital tuberculosis* (kidneys, uterine tubes, epididymis) may arise as a result of transient hematogenous dissemination at the time of first infection, the miliary lesions becoming activated months or years after healing of the primary focus. *Bone and joint tuberculosis* (spine and hips chiefly) may occur following the first infection and be activated later, as above. *Tuberculous meningitis* is most often encountered in infancy. It is often a terminal feature of miliary tuberculosis. Examination of the spinal fluid may reveal the causative organism. *Skin tuberculosis,* commonly called *lupus vulgaris,* sometimes is a result of infection of skin cuts or scratches, but may also be a manifestation of systemic infection. *Cervical lymph node tuberculosis* (scrofula) is usually a result of tuberculosis of the tonsils, which may be either of respiratory or alimentary origin. *Cold abscesses* of bones, joints, or lymph node masses signify liquefied tuberculous lesions similar to pyogenic abscesses but lacking the clinical features of acute inflammation (hence "cold"). The liquefied material burrows along fascial planes in the direction of least resistance. Such a lesion beginning in a thoracic vertebra may extend along the sheath of the psoas muscles to a point in the groin – a *psoas abscess.* If it ruptures through the skin, a *tuberculous sinus* forms, which may persist for months or years.

2. *Tuberculoid Granulomas*

Tuberculous-like lesions

There are a number of chronic granulomatous diseases in which the tissue changes resemble tuberculosis, but in which tubercle bacilli cannot be identified. These are commonly grouped together as the tuberculoid granulomas. These lesions serve to emphasize that the histologic pattern in tuberculosis is not absolutely diagnostic in most instances. For a positive diagnosis of tuberculosis, acid-fast organisms must be demonstrated in tissue sections, or, better still, *M. tuberculosis* must be identified by culture and virulence studies in animals.

Various causes

Tuberculoid granulomas may be encountered as a feature of the reaction of the tissues to specific living agents: (1) certain *fungi,* such as *Coccidioides, Cryptococcus,* and *Actinomyces;* (2) certain *helminths,* particularly *Schistosoma,* in which the ova are distributed in the tissues; (3) certain *bacteria,* especially *Treponema, Brucella,* and *Pasteurella;* and (4) certain chlamydiae, including the causative agents of cat-scratch fever and lymphopathia (lymphogranuloma) venereum. Tuberculoid granulomas are seen in certain diseases of unknown cause, but are possibly related to *antigen-antibody reaction;* the subcutaneous nodules of rheumatoid arthritis are an example. Similar tuberculoid lesions may be seen in tissues in which relatively *insoluble endogenous products* have been deposited, including keratin, hair, and cholesterol, as from the rupture of a dermoid or pilonidal cyst. *Exogenous matter* may also incite such lesions: (1) beryllium, used in the manufacture of fluorescent lights, (2) talc, (3) suture material, (4) fragments of an insect body remaining in the skin after an insect bite, (5) aspirated mineral or vegetable oils, and (6) aspirated vegetable or other organic fibers. Tuberculoid granulomas are encountered chiefly in the skin, lungs, and lymph nodes. The most important disease exhibiting tuberculoid granulomas is *sarcoidosis.*

3. *Sarcoidosis* (Boeck's Sarcoid; Besnier-Boeck-Schaumann Disease; Benign Lymphogranulomatosis)

Definition

Boeck's sarcoid is a *chronic granulomatous disease* of unknown cause. It resembles tuberculosis in many respects and is characterized pathologically by *noncaseating tuberculoid granulomas,* chemically by an *increase in plasma globulin,* and clinically by a *benign protracted course,* often without symptoms.

Etiology

The cause of Boeck's sarcoid is unknown. For many years it was thought to be an atypical form of tuberculosis, but acid-fast bacilli cannot be demonstrated in the affected organs. Virus studies have resulted in negative findings. Boeck's sarcoid may be a reaction to *pine pollen* [5]. This idea is based chiefly upon the geographic distribution of the disease, but also upon a peculiar chemical and immunologic kinship between pine pollen and the tubercle bacillus. Most patients with Boeck's sarcoid are young adults, ages 20 to 39 years. Sexes are equally affected. Negroes have a high incidence of the disease in the United States, but this probably is a result of the geographic distribution of the disease in the southeastern United States rather than a true racial susceptibility. Boeck's sarcoid is quite common in the Scandinavian countries.

Pathologic changes

Early lesions are about the *size of miliary tubercles.* They are composed of great numbers of *epithelioid cells,* with a ring of lymphocytes in some instances, and often with giant cells resembling Langhans' cells. The giant cells sometimes contain *crystalline material,* or *asteroid bodies,* or *laminated iron-containing structures.* These inclusion bodies are found in about 40 percent of the cases, but may also be noted in other conditions.

Organs affected

Sarcoid nodules may occur in almost any organ or tissue of the body. Clinical manifestations are usually due to involvement of the skin, lungs, lymph nodes, or eyes. In fatal cases the lesions are often widespread. The percentage figures given below show the frequency of involvement of the different organs in fatal cases, as reported by Longcope and Freiman [6]. The lungs (86 percent) show minute scattered parenchymal lesions resembling miliary tuberculosis on x-ray; the hilar lymph nodes were involved concurrently in most cases. The lymph nodes (86 percent) are often enlarged, firm, and painless, and on gross examination are rubbery. While any nodes may be affected, the cervical, axillary, and mediastinal nodes are most commonly involved. The liver (65 percent) commonly shows lesions in fatal cases, but clinical evidence of liver involvement is rare in mild cases. The spleen (63 percent) is often palpable in generalized sarcoidosis. Heart (20 percent) involvement is rarely noted in mild cases; confluent granulomas may affect the myocardium diffusely, resulting in heart block and occasionally in sudden death. Eye involvement is an important clinical manifestation of the disease; iritis is the usual manifestation and may lead to blindness. The parotid gland is sometimes involved concurrently with the eye (uveoparotid fever); in these cases the cranial nerves are sometimes affected, particularly the facial and auditory nerves. The skin is often involved in mild cases, but curiously may remain unaffected in fatal cases; the lesions are usually distinctly nodular and well defined (lupus pernio). Bones, especially the phalanges, sometimes show decalcified areas on x-ray, but clinical symptoms of bone involvement are unusual.

Blood chemistry

Certain blood chemical findings occur with sufficient frequency in Boeck's sarcoid to be of value in clinical diagnosis. The *serum proteins* are usually elevated, primarily because of an increase in the globulin fraction. The blood *calcium* is elevated at one time or another in about half the cases; this is apparently due to increased absorption of dietary calcium. In some instances hypercalciuria reaches such proportions that renal stones and metastatic calcification result, suggesting hyperparathyroidism.

Anergy to tuberculin

Patients with sarcoid give a *negative tuberculin reaction* in about 70 percent of the cases. This *anergy* to tuberculoprotein, thought at first to signify some relationship between sarcoid and tuberculosis, may be due to the immunologic kinship of pine pollen and tuberculin.

4. *Leprosy* (Hansen's Disease)

Leprosy is an infectious disease of long incubation (usually about 5 years, rarely as long as 30 years). It is caused by *Mycobacterium leprae,* which invokes a chronic granulomatous reaction, chiefly of the skin and nerves.

Distribution

Leprosy is widely distributed in *Asia, Equatorial Africa,* and the *islands of the Pacific.* There are over 5 million lepers in the world, of whom about 2000 are in the United States.

Pathologic changes

The most characteristic lesion, the *leproma,* is a superficial nodule of the corium and is composed of stringy, foamy macrophages – the lepra cells – often packed with great numbers of acid-fast bacilli. These nodules appear in crops, accompanied by irregular fever *(leprous fever),* and are most common on the forehead, brows, cheeks, ears, and alae nasae, giving rise to the "leonine facies." This form of the disease, known as *lepromatous* (nodular) leprosy, is by far the most common type in the United States [7]. The *neural* (tuberculoid) form of leprosy is usually manifest by areas of analgesia or anesthesia, leading in some instances to loss of fingers or toes and to severe deformity. Skin macules and other skin lesions may accompany this type of leprosy. The nerve changes are due to *granulomatous lesions in the peripheral nerves* and their sheaths. It may be difficult to demonstrate organisms in this form of leprosy. Occasionally there is a mixture of the features of lepromatous and neural leprosy in a single case. Scrapings taken from the nasopharynx, even in cases showing no evident disease of this portion of the body, may reveal the organisms. This means that lesions of the nasopharynx are very common in leprosy although they may not be clinically evident. In later stages of the disease, marked deformity of the nose may occur. In fatal cases there is dissemination of the organisms to the liver and spleen, where foci of lepra cells *(miliary lepromas)* are formed.

Causes of death

While leprosy is rarely a direct cause of death, there is much disability (blindness, contractures, ulcers, renal insufficiency). *Secondary amyloidosis* is common and accounts for the high incidence of renal insufficiency (38 percent of the fatal cases) [7]. Serologic *tests for syphilis are positive* in about 68 percent of the cases of leprosy; this is generally considered to be a biologically false positive reaction.

SYPHILIS AND OTHER TREPONEMATOSES

1. Syphilis

Definition

Syphilis is a specific infectious disease due to *Treponema pallidum,* manifest clinically by *genital, dermal, mucosal,* and *visceral lesions* and pathologically by a *chronic granulomatous inflammation.*

Treponema pallidum

Treponema pallidum is a spiral organism whose loops are tightly and evenly twisted. It cannot be seen in tissues stained by ordinary methods, but after silver impregnation (Levaditi's method) it is seen as a black, well-outlined organism. In moist hanging-drop specimens prepared from syphilitic sores and viewed by dark-field illumination, the spirochete is seen to be actively motile and twisting. The organism is easily killed by heat, cold, or drying. It is destroyed in vivo by most modern antibiotic agents.

Serologic tests for syphilis (STS)

Infection by this agent incites the production of antibodies. *The demonstration of these antibodies in blood serum is the standard means by which the diagnosis of syphilis is made;* the absence of these antibodies is almost certain evidence that syphilis is not present. Syphilitic antibodies occur in the serum in several forms. Some arrest the motility of suspensions of living treponemas; these serve as the basis for the *Treponema pallidum* immobilization (TPI) test, generally believed to be the most *specific* of the various serologic tests for syphilis, i.e., giving fewest false positive results in nonsyphilitic patients. Other antibodies in syphilitic patients have been noted empirically to cause the flocculation of nonspirochetal antigenic substances present in beef heart (such as in the Kahn, Kline, Eagle, Mazzini, or Venereal Disease Research Laboratory [VDRL] flocculation tests), and to bind these substances in the presence of complement (Wassermann, Kolmer, and other complement fixation tests). These empirical tests, such as the VDRL flocculation test, probably are more *sensitive* than the TPI test, i.e., give fewer false negative results in syphilitic patients, but are generally thought to be less specific. (The usefulness of a particular serologic test for syphilis is determined by both its *specificity* and its *sensitivity.*)

Reagin

The substance in the serum of syphilitic patients which causes flocculation of the nonspirochetal antigenic substances used in these tests is known as reagin. Reagin is a *readily diffusible* substance. It can be demonstrated *in the spinal fluid* of many patients with syphilis. It is also present *in the blood of a newborn child whose mother's blood contains reagin,* whether or not the child has syphilis. Reagin in the serum of syphilitic patients seems identical with the substance which is present in the serum of certain nonsyphilitic patients with leprosy, malaria, collagen vascular diseases, or infectious mononucleosis and which accounts for the frequent *biologically false positive* reactions in these diseases. The reagin antibody differs from the antibody responsible for the positive TPI test; the latter antibody apparently occurs only in syphilitic patients.

Prevalence

The incidence of syphilis has been greatly reduced by public health measures, by public education, and by the incidental use of antibiotics for other infectious diseases. In 1939 there were in the United States 11.8 deaths due to syphilis per 100,000 population; this had fallen to 2.3 per 100,000 in 1956 [8]. The number of reported cases of primary and secondary syphilis in the United States was about 20,000 in 1969. As the incidence of syphilis has been reduced, the importance of *the biologically false positive serologic test for syphilis has become greatly increased;* Moore and Mohr [9] estimated that nearly half the positive standard serologic tests for syphilis discovered in routine blood testing are due not to syphilis but to false positive tests. Syphilis is more common in males than in females, in Negroes than in whites, in low income groups than in the well-to-do, and in city dwellers than in a rural population.

Mode of infection

The *only known source of infection in syphilis is another infected human being;* animals are apparently not susceptible, and insect transmission is unproved. Since the organisms die rapidly on exposure to air, *direct contact* with syphilitic lesions is necessary for transmission of the disease. In about 95 percent of the cases this contact is *venereal,* by direct inoculation of the genitalia with living organisms from an open lesion on the genitals of a sexual partner. Rarely, as a result of unusual sexual practices, the *Treponema* may be transmitted from the genitals to the lips, buccal mucosa, tonsils, or anal region. Occasionally an individual with a syphilitic ulcer of the mouth may infect another by kissing. Very rarely syphilis may be acquired as a wound infection. The fetus in utero may be infected from a syphilitic placenta, which in turn is infected from a syphilitic mother. Theoretically syphilis in a blood donor can be transmitted to a recipient, but this is extremely rare in modern transfusion practice; the usual refrigeration of blood before use will cause the organisms to die out; in addition, serologic tests for syphilis are used to screen out all bloods giving a positive reaction.

Inoculation

The spirochetes penetrate the mucosa at the site of contact; no wound of entry is necessary. They *spread rapidly throughout the body* even before the local lesion appears. *Treponemal bacteremia* may persist for many months and is commonly present during both the primary and the secondary stages of the disease, but rarely persists into the tertiary stage.

Primary stage

The *chancre* is the lesion characteristic of the primary stage of syphilis, and appears 2 to 6 weeks after infection. It occurs at the site of inoculation; it is usually seen *on the genitals* but may appear on the lips or buccal mucosa. In the female this stage often goes unrecognized because the lesion is hidden from self-examination in the vagina or on the cervix. There is no chancre in congenital syphilis or in syphilis acquired by transfusion. The chancre is a firm, round, relatively *painless, button-like lesion;* it usually is single and generally is 0.5 to 2.0 cm. in diameter. Initially *papular,* it later becomes *ulcerated.* The chancre can be distinguished from other ulcerative genital lesions by demonstrating the characteristic spirochetes on *dark-field examination* of tissue fluid expressed from the lesion. In routine sections there is dilatation of the capillaries, and the perivascular spaces are packed with an infiltrate composed chiefly of *lymphocytes, plasma cells,* and *mononuclear phagocytes.* The chancre usually persists for 3 to 8 weeks and heals with little scarring. *Regional lymph nodes may be enlarged* during the primary stage of syphilis but they show no distinctive microscopic features. Serologic tests for syphilis usually become positive shortly after the appearance of the chancre. Immunity against new syphilitic infection also develops at about this time and persists for the duration of the disease.

Antibiotic therapy brings about a rapid cure of the chancre and prevents the appearance of secondary and tertiary lesions. Even without therapy the infection is said to die out in about 25 percent of syphilitic patients. With cure or spontaneous recovery, the serologic tests for syphilis become negative. After a time immunity against syphilis may also be lost; the patient may then contract a new chancre after a new exposure.

Secondary stage

The characteristic lesions of the secondary stage affect chiefly the *skin* and *mucous membranes.* The interval between the disappearance of the chancre and the appearance of the skin lesions is usually 2 to 6 months, but is extremely variable; occasionally the chancre and the skin lesions occur together. The skin lesions may resemble many other skin diseases. Characteristically they are *macular* (nonelevated, and pink to coppery brown), or *papular* (elevated, reddish brown, peaked nodule), or *pustular* (papule with a small collection of pus at the top). These lesions are usually most evident over the back, chest, and upper arms, and are usually rather symmetric in distribution. *Alopecia* (patchy hair loss) is a common feature of this stage, but alopecia is more often due to causes other than syphilis. The most characteristic lesions of the mucous membranes in this stage are the *mucous patches.* These are superficial ulcers noted in the buccal mucosa and pharynx, commonly causing a *chronic sore throat.* The mucosal lesions and, to a somewhat lesser degree, the skin lesions contain numerous treponemas and may serve to spread the infection to others. Another mucocutaneous lesion of the secondary stage of syphilis is the *condyloma latum,* a flat nodular lesion which occurs most often in the moist areas such as those about the anus or genitals. Microscopic examination of the skin and mucosal lesions shows numerous blood and lymphatic channels surrounded by a cellular infiltrate composed chiefly of plasma cells and lymphocytes; the microscopic picture is not absolutely diagnostic. *Generalized lymph node enlargement* is commonly observed during the secondary stage of syphilis.

Tertiary stage

After a variable interval, which may occasionally be as short as 6 months after the primary infection but is more often a matter of some years, the lesions characteristic of the tertiary stage appear. There are two general types of tertiary lesions: (1) the *gumma,* and (2) a *diffuse inflammatory fibrosis.* Both show an *inflammatory reaction in the walls of small blood vessels* and more especially *in the adventitial spaces.* This involvement of small blood vessels leads to ischemia, fibrosis, and impaired function of affected organs. It is probably the basic cause of the gumma, which is a *rubbery, well-defined, infarct-like lesion,* usually several centimeters in diameter, occurring especially in the liver but occasionally in the testes, breast, bones, tongue, or central nervous system. Microscopically it is necrotic; there are some features of coagulation necrosis and others of caseation necrosis. Usually the outline of organ architecture can still be recognized in the necrotic zone. At the periphery of the gumma there is fibrous tissue proliferation, perivascular plasma cell and lymphocytic infiltration, and occasionally a few giant cells. In the other type of reaction of the tertiary stage, the *inflammatory fibrosis,* there is replacement of specialized cells by *fibrous connective tissue, lymphocytes,* and *plasma cells,* resulting in impairment of function. The aorta and central nervous system are the sites chiefly affected, but the liver, skin, eyes, testes, and nearly every other organ or tissue may sometimes be involved. Detailed consideration of these manifestations of syphilis is given later under the organ systems.

Congenital syphilis:

Congenital *syphilis* has been greatly reduced in prevalence by two public health measures: (1) premarital tests for syphilis, and (2) testing for syphilis on the first prenatal visit of the pregnant woman. (Treatment of the pregnant mother begun in the first trimester of pregnancy is almost certain to prevent syphilis in the infant.)

intra-uterine infection

Syphilis in the infant is a result of syphilis in the mother. The treponema is transmitted to the placenta and thence to the fetus. If pregnancy occurs during the primary or secondary stage of syphilis, and if the infection is untreated, the spirochetemia is usually so heavy that it causes the *death of the fetus in utero* and the result is a prematurely born dead child (stillbirth). A subsequent pregnancy in the same mother may result in a living child born at term but with clinical *evidence of congenital syphilis.* Pregnancies still later in the course of maternal syphilis (when bacteremia is less likely and less severe) may result in the birth of syphilitic children without evidence of the disease at birth, or the child may be completely free of the disease.

clinical and pathologic manifestations

Congenital syphilis differs from syphilis acquired in later life in several regards. *There is no chancre.* The syphilitic infection *interferes with bone growth* and results in stunting and frequently in bone deformities. Among the most characteristic syphilitic deformities are those of the nasal septum resulting in the *saddle-back nose,* and the anterior bowing of the tibiae which gives them an unduly sharp anterior edge known as *saber shin.* In early infancy the lesions of the *bone epiphyses* may be recognized on x-ray or at autopsy; there is an irregular and broadened line of junction between the epiphysis and the diaphysis. Often the spleen and liver are enlarged at birth. (However, it is probable that some of the cases considered by earlier workers to be congenital syphilis, and manifested by early neonatal death with jaundice and splenomegaly, were in fact cases of erythroblastosis fetalis.) As in syphilis of adults, the treponema produces a *diffuse fibrosis of many organs,* but the liver shows the most evident damage in most cases and the treponemas are probably most numerous in preparations of this organ. If the infant survives the neonatal period, manifestations of syphilis may appear later, particularly those due to the following: (1) *skeletal deformity,* (2) *defective dentition* (Hutchinson's teeth), (3) *interstitial keratitis,* (4) *nerve deafness,* or (5) *central nervous system disease.* Findings (2), (3), and (4) are sometimes known as *Hutchinson's triad*, and when present together are strong presumptive evidence of congenital syphilis. Cardiovascular syphilis is rarely encountered in congenital syphilis. *Pneumonia alba* is a form of *chronic pneumonia* seen in stillborn and newborn infants dying from congenital syphilis. *Syphilitic nephritis* sometimes occurs and causes generalized edema.

serologic tests

The infant's blood at birth will give the same results with serologic tests for syphilis as does the mother's; *after 8 weeks* a positive test on the infant's blood usually means congenital syphilis.

2. Other Treponematoses

YAWS

Yaws (frambesia, pian) is a tropical form of treponematosis which is apparently nonvenereal, and which is chiefly manifest by *skin lesions.* The causative agent *(Treponema pertenue)* is indistinguishable from *T. pallidum;* it induces the same type of reaction in animals, and *serologic tests for syphilis are positive.* The disease is often spread from an infected mother to her nursing infant: contact with infectious skin lesions seems to be the important source of spread. The disease is prevalent in Equatorial Africa, Malay Peninsula, Haiti, certain Pacific islands, etc. Yaws has the same late complications in the cardiovascular and nervous systems as does syphilis.

PINTA

Pinta is a disease of the American tropics (Mexico and Colombia particularly) and is caused by an organism known as *Treponema carateum,* which is morphologically identical with *T. pallidum.* Its manifestations are largely cutaneous, consisting of itching granulomatous lesions often associated with depigmentation. Serologic tests for syphilis are usually positive.

BEJEL

Bejel is a nonvenereal treponematosis occurring in Syria and Iraq. It is said that the disease often affects infants and children and involves entire communities. Serologic tests for syphilis are positive.

Relationship to syphilis

It is likely that the causative agents in these diseases are essentially identical with *T. pallidum,* and that the clinical manifestations and modes of spread differ from those in syphilis because of differences in climate, dress, and habits. It may be, too, that intercurrent skin infections (bacterial and fungus) modify the development and course of the skin lesions. The character of the late visceral manifestations – so far as they are known – and the positive serologic tests for syphilis in each of these diseases indicate the essential oneness of all these treponematoses.

Information on tuberculosis, leprosy, and syphilis is summarized in Table 5-1.

REFERENCES

1. Rich, A. R. *The Pathogenesis of Tuberculosis.* Springfield, Ill.: Thomas, 1944. (A monumental source of information on the chemistry and particularly the immunology of the tubercle bacillus.)
2. Florey, H. W. *General Pathology* (4th ed.). Philadelphia: Saunders, 1970, Chapter 42. (An excellent presentation of experimental and other data on tuberculosis.)
3. *Vital Statistics of the United States.* Mortality, vol. 2, part A, pp. 1–53. Washington, D.C.: U.S. Government Printing Office, 1966.
4. Report of the Advisory Committee on BCG to the Surgeon General of the Public Health Service. In *Tuberculosis Abstracts* 31:No. 1, 1958.
5. Cummings, M. M., and Hudgins, P. C. Chemical constituents of pine pollen and their possible relationship to sarcoidosis. *Amer. J. Med. Sci.* 236:311, 1958.
6. Longcope, W. T., and Freiman, D. G. A study of sarcoidosis. *Quart. J. Med.* 31:1, 1952.
7. Powell, C. S., and Swan, L. L. Leprosy: Pathologic changes observed in fifty consecutive necropsies. *Amer. J. Path.* 31:1131, 1955.
8. Brown, W. J., Sellers, T. F., and Thomas, E. W. Challenge to the private physician in the epidemiology of syphilis. *J.A.M.A.* 171:389, 1959.
9. Moore, J. E., and Mohr, C. F. Incidence and etiologic background of chronic biologic false positive reactions in serologic tests for syphilis. *Ann. Intern. Med.* 37:1156, 1952.

7 RICKETTSIAL, CHLAMYDIAL, AND VIRAL DISEASES

RICKETTSIAL INFECTIONS

RICKETTSIAE:

Rickettsiae are gram-negative, bacterium-like, obligate intracellular parasites. They are very small (0.3 to 0.5μ) and are seen best with the Giemsa stain. Together with the chlamydiae and viruses, the rickettsiae form the class *Microtatobiotes,* the smallest living organisms. The known rickettsial diseases of man fall into five main groups: typhus, spotted fever, tsutsugamushi, Q fever, and trench fever. Insects and arachnids are the direct vectors of all rickettsial diseases. Most are transmitted by the Acarina order of arachnids (ticks, mites). Infection with a rickettsial disease usually confers lifelong immunity. Several rickettsiae cross agglutinate with various strains of *Proteus vulgaris (Weil-Felix reaction)* (see Table 7-1). Probably the rickettsiae and the *Proteus* organisms contain a common antigenic substance.

General pathologic changes

The *gross changes* are not distinctive and consist mainly of petechiae or ecchymoses. The *typical microscopic change* in rickettsial infections is a mononuclear cell inflammatory reaction (lymphocytes, plasmocytes, and macrophages) about small blood vessels. The rickettsiae enter the bloodstream and are carried to the capillary bed throughout the body. They enter and proliferate in the endothelial cells lining arterioles and capillaries in many parts of the body. Electron microscopic studies have shown that the proliferating rickettsiae appear to cause lysis of the cytoplasmic organelles [1]. Eventually the affected cells become rickettsiae-filled sacs which rupture to release the organisms. *Rickettsia prowazekii* (and probably the other rickettsiae) produces unstable toxins on disintegration and a soluble capsular antigen. The latter indicates that some manifestations of these diseases may be allergic.

1. Epidemic and Endemic Typhus

EPIDEMIC TYPHUS: Cause

Rickettsia prowazekii is the cause of *typhus. Transmission* is by the body louse *(Pediculus humanus corporis).* The organisms are passed in the louse feces during biting and enter the puncture wound of the bite.

Clinical features

Clinically epidemic typhus fever has been one of the great scourges, especially in times of war or famine. The incubation period is 10 to 14 days, and the onset is usually abrupt with high fever, severe headache, muscle aches, constipation, and occasional shaking chills. Usually on the fifth day a maculopapular rash

TABLE 7-1. Weil-Felix Reaction of Rickettsiae – Cross Agglutination with *Proteus* Strains

Disease	Organism	Agglutination with *Proteus* strain		
		OX-19	OX-2	OX-K
Epidemic typhus	*Rickettsia prowazekii*	4+	1+	0
Endemic typhus	*Rickettsia typhi*	4+	1+	0
Tsutsugamushi	*Rickettsia tsutsugamushi*	0	0	4+
Q fever	*Coxiella burnetii*	0	0	0
Spotted fever	*Rickettsia rickettsii*	2+	2+	0

appears on the trunk and spreads to the extremities, sparing the face, palms, and soles except in very severe cases. The average mortality in epidemics is about 20 percent. Death may be due to cerebral or myocardial involvement, toxemia, or bacterial bronchopneumonia. *Brill's disease* is a mild type of louse-borne typhus which occurs in Europe and the eastern United States. Some cases are a recrudescence of previous typhus.

Pathologic changes

Grossly there is a maculopapular rash on the skin, especially on the trunk. The heart is dilated, and the myocardium is pale and yellow. In most fatal cases there are foci of bronchopneumonia. The brain is slightly edematous and congested. The *typical microscopic lesion* is a nodular inflammation associated with the small blood vessels. The capillary endothelium is swollen and filled with rickettsiae. About the involved vessels there are lymphocytes, plasmocytes, macrophages, and a few polymorphonuclear leukocytes. There is rarely necrosis of the vessel walls. The heart shows a diffuse myocarditis with focal necrosis of the myofibrils. The skeletal muscles have focal lesions about the vessels and may show Zenker's degeneration. Throughout the brain, more in the gray than in the white matter, there are typical *typhus nodules,* usually about capillaries. These consist of swollen endothelium and peripheral collections of microglia, macrophages, and lymphocytes. Elsewhere in the brain there is a perivascular lymphocytic infiltrate.

ENDEMIC TYPHUS

Endemic typhus (murine typhus, tabardillo of Mexico, shop typhus of Malaya) is a relatively mild form of typhus transmitted by the rat flea, *Xenopsylla cheopis,* or the rat louse, *Polyplax spinulosus.* It is caused by *Rickettsia typhi (R. muricola, R. mooseri)* and occurs more frequently in men than in women by 2:1. The rickettsia of endemic typhus differs antigenically and in virulence from that of epidemic typhus. The *pathologic changes* are similar to those of epidemic typhus, but less severe.

2. *Spotted Fever*

SPOTTED FEVER: Cause

The causative organism of *spotted fever* is *Rickettsia rickettsii (Dermacentroxenus rickettsi) (R. conorii,* for fièvre boutonneuse). In explants of infected spleens the rickettsiae grow within the nuclei, a pathognomonic characteristic of spotted fever rickettsiae. The organisms are injected into the skin during the bite of the wood tick, *Dermacentor andersoni,* in the Rocky Mountain region *(Rocky Mountain spotted fever),* and by the dog tick, *Dermacentor variablis,* in the central and eastern United States *(Eastern spotted fever).*

Clinical features

Clinically spotted fever resembles epidemic typhus. However, the rash in spotted fever usually appears on the third day, beginning on the extremities and face and later extending to the trunk. The palms, soles, and scalp are involved. The rash is more hemorrhagic than that of typhus, with numerous petechiae and ecchymoses, because of the greater extent of vascular necrosis in spotted fever. The incubation period varies from 2 to 14 days. In treated cases the mortality is about 5 percent. In the United States about 200 cases are reported annually, most of them occurring from May to September. *São Paulo typhus* of Brazil and the *fièvre boutonneuse* of the Mediterranean region are varieties of spotted fever.

Pathologic changes

The *gross and microscopic changes* are similar to those in epidemic typhus, except that necrosis of small vessel walls and thrombosis are much more common. The lesions occur in the skin and viscera. The rickettsiae are found in the endothelial and smooth muscle cells of arterioles and venules. In the brain there are proliferation of glial tissue to form nodules, sometimes around small blood vessels; perivascular infiltration of lymphocytes, with endothelial swelling; and necrosis and thrombosis of arterioles, with miliary infarcts of the brain.

3. Tsutsugamushi (Scrub Typhus)

TSUTSUGAMUSHI: Cause

Rickettsia tsutsugamushi is the cause of *tsutsugamushi.* Agglutination with OX-K becomes positive in the second week of the disease. *Transmission* is by the bite of the larvae of mites of the *Trombicula* genus, especially *T. akamushi.*

Pathologic changes

At the site of the bite there is a small *eschar* (a crusted ulcer) 0.5 to 1 cm. in diameter, with necrosis and little cell reaction. The regional nodes are enlarged and show foci of necrosis, with hyperplasia of lymphocytes and reticulum cells. The heart is dilated and flabby; microscopically the myocardium is edematous and infiltrated by mononuclear cells *(interstitial myocarditis).* Scattered arteriolar and capillary lesions typical of rickettsial disease are found. Glial nodules are present in the brain. Bronchopneumonia appears terminally.

4. Rickettsial Pox

RICKETTSIAL POX: Cause

Rickettsia (Dermacentroxenus) akari causes *rickettsial pox.* Except for occasional low titers, the Weil-Felix test is negative. *Transmission* is by the bite of the rodent mite, *Allodermanyssus sanguineus.*

Pathologic changes

The *initial lesion* is a round, red macule which grows to 5 to 15 mm. and becomes centrally vesiculated. The *vesicle* is intra-epidermal. There is a dermal infiltration of lymphocytes and a few polymorphonuclear leukocytes. Later a black *eschar* forms. In the lesions of the *rash* there are dilatation of vessels and heavy perivascular infiltration by lymphocytes in the dermis. Some capillaries are thrombosed.

5. Trench Fever

TRENCH FEVER: Cause

Trench fever is due to *Rickettsia quintana. Transmission* is by the feces of the body louse. The organisms exist extracellularly in the louse.

Clinical features

Clinically the disease has occurred mainly in field troops during World Wars I and II. Trench fever is an acute febrile disease with chills, headache, myalgia, and a red macular rash. It is not fatal.

Pathologic changes

The skin rash shows nonspecific perivascular lymphocytic infiltration and endothelial hyperplasia. The internal changes are unknown.

6. Q Fever (Nine-Mile Fever of Montana)

Q FEVER: Cause

Coxiella (Rickettsia) burnetii (Rickettsia diaporica) causes Q (for query) *fever. The Weil-Felix test is negative. Transmission* is uncertain, but it appears to be by ticks and contaminated dust. The disease is harbored by the bandicoot, a small marsupial, in Australia. Sheep and cattle are the reservoir in the United States.

Pathologic changes

The principal lesion is in the lungs, where there is an *interstitial pneumonitis,* with large amounts of fibrin and infiltration of the edematous alveolar septa by lymphocytes, plasmocytes, and macrophages. The alveolar epithelium is swollen and may become cuboidal. Intra-alveolar hemorrhages are common. About 15 percent of the cases develop a hepatitis with focal degeneration of hepatocytes early and the formation of small granulomata with multinucleated giant cells later in the course [2]. Occasionally there may be a meningitis, encephalitis, pericarditis, pancreatitis or orchitis in cases of Q fever.

Information on rickettsial infections is summarized in Table 7-2, page 144.

CHLAMYDIAL INFECTIONS

CHLA-MYDIA

Chlamydia make up the Chlamydiaceae, a family of tiny (0.1 to 0.4μ in diameter) spherical organisms which were formerly classified among the viruses. Now they are considered to be more closely related to rickettsiae. Chlamydiae contain both deoxyribonucleic acid (DNA) and ribonucleic acid (RNA). They are filtrable through unglazed porcelain. These obligate intracellular parasites may appear in infected cells as inclusion bodies. Diseases attributed to chlamydiae are trachoma, psittacosis, lymphogranuloma venereum (discussed on page 609), and cat-scratch fever.

1. Trachoma

TRA-CHOMA: Cause

Trachoma is caused by *Chlamydia trachomatis (Chlamydozoon trachomatis),* which measures 150 to 390 mμ. *Transmission* is by close personal contact. *Inclusion blennorrhea* and *swimming-pool conjunctivitis* are produced by the closely related *Chlamydia oculogenitalis;* the lesions in these conditions are much less severe than those in trachoma, and healing is spontaneous.

Clinical features

Clinically trachoma is common in Egypt and the Near East, and there are endemic areas in the United States. It is the most common cause of blindness. Trachoma begins as tiny white or red dots on the palpebral conjunctiva and upper cornea. In the second phase the dots enlarge into follicles, and the cornea becomes vascularized and superficially eroded. The upper lids are heavy and partially ptosed ("melancholic eyes"). In the cicatricial phase the tarsal conjunctiva becomes pale and blotchy and shows crisscross white lines. The last phase is characterized by corneal dryness, ulcerations, and opacities sometimes resulting in blindness. Lid distortions (entropion, symblepharon) result from scarring.

Pathologic changes

The first changes are those of an *acute conjunctivitis.* In about 7 to 10 days numerous small red or yellow *follicles* form on the intensely hyperemic mucosa.

In the *hypertrophic stage* these follicles enlarge and involve almost the entire palpebral and retrotarsal conjunctiva. From the upper limbus a *vascularized white membrane* grows down as a pannus over the cornea. In the *cicatricial stage* gray or white scars appear in the conjunctiva. *Microscopically* in the early stages there are congestion, edema, and focal collections of lymphocytes and plasma cells (the *follicles*) in the conjunctiva. Small basophilic intracytoplasmic inclusion bodies are found in the conjunctival epithelial cells *(Halbertstädter-Prowazek Körperchen, H.P.K.).*

2. Psittacosis

PSITTACOSIS: Cause

Psittacosis (parrot fever) is caused by *Miyagawanella psittaci,* which measures 275 mμ in diameter. It is classified in the Chlamydiaceae family. Man is infected by contact with parrots or their excreta.

Clinical features

Clinically the incubation period is 1 to 2 weeks. There is a sudden onset of chills and fever, headache, sore throat, and a persistent, only slightly productive cough. Delirium or stupor may develop. The disease lasts about 2 weeks and has a mortality rate of about 20 percent.

Pathologic changes

There is a nodular, discrete *pneumonitis,* the lungs being voluminous, dark purplish red, and irregularly firm. During the first few days the alveoli are filled with erythrocytes, polymorphonuclear leukocytes, and fibrin. Later the infiltrate becomes mononuclear in character. In the cuboidal alveolar epithelial cells, intracytoplasmic inclusion (Leventhal-Cole-Lillie, L.C.L.) bodies may be seen. The liver and spleen are enlarged and show tiny foci of necrosis. The meninges and brain may be edematous and hyperemic.

ORNITHOSIS

Ornithosis is caused by a chlamydia identical with or similar to that of psittacosis, *M. ornithosis.* The organism is found in pigeons, turkeys, and other birds, and may be transmitted from them to man.

3. Cat-Scratch Fever

CAT-SCRATCH FEVER: Cause

The *cause* of *cat-scratch fever* [3] is probably a chlamydia of the psittacosis-lymphogranuloma family. *Transmission* is by a cat scratch, inhalation of cat's urine, or the prick of a thorn, beef bone, or splinter contaminated by feline saliva or urine. The *incubation period* is usually 7 to 14 days, but it may vary from 4 to 60 days.

Clinical features

Clinically a raised erythematous nodule surmounted by a vesicle, pustule, or eschar appears at the site of the scratch or prick a few days after inoculation. The regional lymph nodes become swollen (up to the size of a tangerine), tender, and warm, 4 to 30 days after inoculation. They remain enlarged for a week to a few months. Suppuration and sinus tract formation may occur. A macular or vesicular rash may appear on the skin. Some cases of Parinaud's conjunctivitis with preauricular lymphadenopathy are due to cat-scratch fever. Occasionally thrombocytopenic purpura or encephalitis with headache, convulsions, and transient limb weakness occurs in cases of cat-scratch disease.

Pathologic changes

The lesions resemble those of tularemia. Grossly the lymph nodes are enlarged (1 to 8 cm.), gray, and soft. Satellite nodes are common. *Microscopically* mild cases show only lymphoid hyperplasia. In more severe cases there is nodular

TABLE 7-2. Rickettsial Infections

Disease	Cause	Characteristics of organism	Mode of transmission	Principal organs or sites involved	Type of tissue reaction	Principal cell(s) in reaction	Special features
Rickettsial diseases in general	(Rickettsiae are small, gram –, bacteria-like, obligate intracellular parasites classed with chlamydiae and filtrable viruses as Microtatobiotes)		Insects and arachnids, especially Acarina order of arachnids (ticks, mites)	Cytoplasm of capillary and arteriolar endothelial cells; organisms proliferate and cause rupture of cells	Acute mononuclear reaction, petechiae and thrombosis due to capillary endothelial damage	Lymphocyte, plasmocyte, macrophage	Specific complement fixation tests are more useful for diagnosis than Weil-Felix reaction
Epidemic typhus	*Rickettsia prowazekii*	Weil-Felix: OX-19 4+ OX-2 1+ OX-K 0	Feces of body louse *(Pediculus humanus corporis)*	Skin (maculopapular rash, petechiae) Brain (typhus nodules – swollen endothelium, microglial cells, macrophages, and lymphocytes) Heart (myocarditis) Skeletal muscle (Zenker's degeneration)	Same as for general rickettsial diseases	Same as for general rickettsial diseases	Epidemic typhus occurs mainly in Europe Brill's disease is mild louse-borne typhus of Europe and eastern U.S.
Endemic typhus (murine typhus)	*Rickettsia typhi (R. mooseri, R. muricola)*	Same as for epidemic typhus	Feces of rat flea or rat louse	Same as for epidemic typhus but less severe	Same as for general rickettsial diseases	Same as for general rickettsial diseases	–
Spotted fever Fièvre boutonneuse	*Rickettsia rickettsii* *R. conorii*	Weil-Felix: OX-19 2+ OX-2 2+ OX-K 0 Grow intranuclearly in explants of infected spleens	Bite of wood tick or dog tick	Skin (maculopapular rash, hemorrhages) Brain (perivascular mononuclear cuffing, arteriolar thrombosis, miliary infarcts)	Same as for general rickettsial diseases (endothelial damage is more severe than in typhus)	Same as for general rickettsial diseases	–

Tsutsugamushi (scrub typhus)	*Rickettsia tsutsugamushi*	Weil-Felix: OX-19 0 OX-2 0 OX-K 4+	Bite of larva of *Trombicula* mites, especially *T. akamushi*	Skin (crusted ulcer at bite) Heart (interstitial myocarditis) Brain (typhus-like nodules)	Same as for general rickettsial diseases	Same as for general rickettsial diseases	Mainly in Asia
Rickettsial pox	*Rickettsia (Dermacentroxenus) akari*	Weil-Felix: all 0	Bite of rodent mite	Skin (red macule → vesicle → eschar at bite; maculopapular rash)	Same as for general rickettsial diseases	Same as for general rickettsial diseases	Mainly in New York City
Trench fever	*Rickettsia quintana (R. wolhynica)*	—	Feces of body louse	Skin (macular rash)	Same as for general rickettsial diseases	Same as for general rickettsial diseases	Mainly in Europe
Q (for query) fever (nine-mile fever)	*Coxiella (Rickettsia) burnetii (R. diaporica)*	Weil-Felix: all 0	Probably by ticks and contaminated dust	Lungs (atypical interstitial pneumonia with mononuclear infiltrate) Liver (hepatitis in 15%)	Same as for general rickettsial diseases, with relatively little endothelial damage	Same as for general rickettsial diseases	In Australia, U.S., Mediterranean region

lymphoid hyperplasia with central necrosis. Polymorphonuclear leukocytes fill the necrotic centers. There may be a palisading of epithelioid cells about the necrotic foci, and a few giant cells may appear. In some cases there is an increase in reticulum fibers. The skin lesions show infiltration of the dermis by lymphocytes and plasma cells.

Information on chlamydial infections is summarized in Table 7-3.

VIRAL INFECTIONS

VIRUSES: *Viruses* are a heterogeneous group of disease-producing agents which are smaller than the finest particle resolvable by the compound microscope. They are obligate intracellular parasites. In general viruses are more labile than bacteria, and thus transmission of a virus from one person to another requires intimate contact or an intermediate host. In size viruses vary from 10 to 300 mμ in diameter. Most will pass through unglazed porcelain filters *(filtrable viruses).* The ultimate nature of viruses is incompletely understood. That they are living agents has been disputed, but they unquestionably reproduce and at least some evidently have an incomplete respiratory mechanism. Chemically they consist of a protein coat, which makes up roughly 75 to 90 percent of the virion (complete infectious particle), 5 to 25 percent nucleoprotein, and small lipid and carbohydrate fractions. The nucleoprotein in a true virus may be either ribonucleic acid (RNA) or deoxyribonucleic acid (DNA), but not both. Many viruses have a definite specificity for proliferation in one or a few cell types; e.g., the poliomyelitis virus has a special affinity for the anterior horn motor neurons of the spinal cord. Other viruses are less finicky and survive in a variety of cells. It is not certain whether the inflammatory reactions which occur in virus diseases are due to toxins or antigens present in or on the viruses, or to the breakdown products of body cells killed by viruses. Cell death may be produced either by inability of the cell to compete with the proliferating virus for nutrient metabolites or by toxic waste products of the virus.

Inclusion bodies: Histologic study of tissues in many viral diseases reveals small or large, usually acidophilic *inclusion bodies* which may be cytoplasmic or nuclear. About the nuclear inclusions there is a clear halo, and the basophilic chromatin is marginated at the nuclear membrane. The inclusion bodies appear to vary from virus to virus. In most cases they represent aggregations of virus particles. An *elementary body* is a single mature virus particle.

Humoral immunity: *One attack of many viral diseases confers lifetime immunity.* This has been explained by some on the basis of the persistence of the virus in the animal organism. *Naked or free viral nucleic acids are infectious,* although less efficiently so than intact viruses. It is possible that the continued presence of infectious viral nucleic acids sustains a very low level of infection which explains the permanent immunity [4]. Neutralizing antibodies appear in the serum within a few days to a week of the onset of viral diseases. This serum will then protect another animal from a lethal dose of the virus. There is also a cellular immunity independent of circulating antibodies. However, in certain viral diseases immunity is transient or nonexistent, e.g., the common cold.

Pathogenesis of cellular infection: From observations on bacteriophages (viruses which parasitize bacteria) it is thought that viral invasion of a cell begins with intimate *attachment* of the virus

Disease	Characteristics of organism	Inclusion body	Mode of transmission	Principal organs or sites involved	Types of tissue reaction	Special features
Trachoma	*Chlamydia trachomatis*, measures 150–390 mμ	Halberstädter-Prowazek body (C)*	Close personal contact	Conjunctiva (acute conjunctivitis → hypertrophic stage [lymphoid follicles in palpebral conjunctiva] → cicatrization of lids and corneal pannus)	Marked lymph follicle proliferation	Inclusion blenorrhea and swimming-pool conjunctivitis are caused by the closely related *C. oculogenitalis*
Psittacosis	*Miyagawanella psittaci*, about 275 mμ; IP† 7–14 days; divides by binary fission	Leventhal-Cole-Little (L.C.L.) body (C)*	Contact with parrots or their excreta	Lung (nodular pneumonitis)	Neutrophilic (early) and mononuclear (later) intra-alveolar infiltrate	Ornithosis is due to an identical or similar body and is transmitted from pigeons, turkeys, and other birds to man.
Lymphogranuloma (lymphopathia) venereum‡	Classified in *Miyagawanella* genus of Chlamydiaceae; measures 150 mμ; IP† 3–21 days	—	Sexual contact	Prepuce (ulcerated vesicle) Vulva ulcerated vesicle) Inguinal lymph nodes (buboes) Rectum (stricture)	Hydropic epidermal degeneration; lymph node hyperplasia with coalescent foci of necrosis (stellate abscesses)	Rectal stricture in females is due to proctitis caused by lymphatic drainage; in males, to homosexual activity Frei test is tuberculin-like reaction indicating present or past infection
Cat-scratch fever	Organism probably of psittacosis-lymphopathia venereum family; IP† usually 7–14 days (varies from 4–60 days)	—	Cat scratch, inhalation of cat's urine, contaminated thorn prick	Skin (erythematous vesicle, pustule, or eschar at inoculation site) Regional lymph nodes (vary from hyperplasia to epithelioid granulomata with central suppuration)	—	Lesions resemble those of tularemia Some cases of Parinaud's conjunctivitis with preauricular lymph node enlargement are due to cat-scratch chlamydia Thrombocytopenic purpura occurs rarely

*C, intracytoplasmic.
†IP, incubation period.
‡See Page 609.

to the surface receptor area of the cell membrane. Naked viral nucleic acid enters the cell during the *penetration phase,* leaving the protein envelope to be carried away in the circulation. The intracellular nucleic acid becomes inapparent during the *eclipse phase.* During this phase the cellular metabolism is redirected to synthesize specific viral nucleic acid and protein. The viral material becomes recognizable during the *phases of maturation and proliferation,* in which for many viruses elementary and inclusion bodies are formed within the cell nucleus or cytoplasm. When a virus enters a cell, the latter produces a protein *interferon* [5] which renders it resistant to infection by other viruses. On the other hand, viruses are capable of coding the formation of protein *stimulons* which are antagonistic to interferons and which enhance viral activity within cells [6].

interferon

stimulon

General pathologic changes:

The changes due to viruses are quite varied, but there are certain general features. In the *skin,* marked *hydropic degeneration of the epidermal cells* (especially in the basal layer), known as ballooning or reticular degeneration, is common in the dermotropic diseases. While many viruses produce *necrosis* of the cells they parasitize – e.g., the poliomyelitis virus causes degeneration of the anterior horn cells – other viruses induce *proliferation* – e.g., the common verruca (wart). This ability to cause marked proliferation of epithelial cells and the production of both benign and malignant (cancerous) neoplasms in animals indicate that viruses or viral mutants may play a role in the development of human neoplasms. Both RNA viruses and DNA viruses are capable of producing tumors in animals and neoplastic transformation in tissue culture cells [7]. At least some oncogenic (tumor-producing) viruses cause a disturbance in the regulation of DNA formation in infected cells [8]. An increase in host cell DNA synthesis results. There is evidence that all or part of the viral genome persists in malignant cells [9]. Virus-like particles have been demonstrated in lymph node and bone marrow material from patients with acute leukemia [10] and Burkitt's tumor, a lymphatic neoplasm occurring mainly in East African children [11].

relationship of viruses to neoplasia

cellular reaction

There is often a transient infiltration of polymorphonuclear leukocytes in the early stages of viral diseases, but *mononuclear cells, especially lymphocytes, are the major components of the cellular infiltrate.* Often the lymphocytes are arranged about small blood vessels *(perivascular infiltration),* especially in the central nervous system. The later return of polymorphonuclear leukocytes usually is due to secondary bacterial invasion of the lesions.

1. Dermotropic Viral Diseases

VACCINIA: Cause

Vaccinia (cowpox) is caused by *Poxvirus officinale (P. bovis),* which contains double-stranded deoxyribonucleic acid (DNA), is spherical or brick-shaped, and measures about 230 mμ in diameter. The virus produces a cross immunization with that of smallpox. It is introduced into the skin of the arm or leg during vaccination and is also transmissible to man by the handling of infected cows.

Clinical features

Clinically at the vaccination site any one of four reactions may occur: (1) vaccinia (primary reaction), (2) vaccinoid (accelerated reaction), (3) reaction of immunity (immediate reaction), or (4) negative reaction. The first three result in a depressed, depigmented scar on healing. Occasionally *generalized vaccinia* develops, especially in patients with chronic eczema. Rarely a demyelinating encephalomyelitis follows vaccination.

Pathologic changes

Grossly the lesion at the *vaccination site* is successively a *macule* (a well-defined flat area of altered skin coloration), a *papule* (a raised, circumscribed area of skin discoloration), a *vesicle* (a blister), and a *pustule* (a vesicle containing pus). *Early microscopic changes* are ballooning degeneration of the epidermis, formation of inclusion bodies, and development of an intra-epidermal vesicle. The inclusion bodies *(Guarnieri bodies)* are intracytoplasmic and acidophilic and probably represent aggregates of minute elementary bodies *(Paschen corpuscles).* Guarnieri bodies are ovoid and measure up to 10μ. The dermis is edematous, congested, and infiltrated by lymphocytes and plasmocytes. In the pustule there are necrosis of the epidermis and infiltration by polymorphonuclear leukocytes. Occasionally a regional *lymphadenitis* follows vaccination. The enlarged lymph node shows diffuse and follicular lymphocytic hyperplasia, an increased number of reticular lymphocytes, and variable numbers of eosinophils, plasmocytes, and mast cells [12]. The pattern may simulate that of a malignant lymphoma.

VARIOLA: Cause

Variola (smallpox) is produced by *Poxvirus variolae,* a spherical or brick-shaped virus measuring about 200 mμ in diameter and containing DNA. *Transmission* of the causative virus is by direct contact through the desquamated crusts and through respiratory secretions (air-borne droplet infection). Intrauterine infections occur transplacentally.

Clinical features

Clinically the incubation period is usually 8 to 12 days. There is a sudden onset of severe headache, back and muscle aches, high fever, convulsions and vomiting in children, prostration, delirium, and sometimes coma. The characteristic rash is described below. Mortality varies from 1 to 20 percent of the cases, and death is usually due to bacterial bronchopneumonia. *Alastrim* is a mild form of smallpox (variola minor).

Pathologic changes

The *initial lesion* is a small area of redness of the face. Within 24 hours the eruption spreads to all parts of the body. The lesions are, successively: red macules, papules, vesicles, and pustules. The pustules appear by the sixth to seventh day, and drying begins on the tenth day. In *hemorrhagic smallpox* numerous hemorrhages appear in the dermis about the skin lesions. Vesicles and pustules may occur on the buccal mucosa and pharynx. The heart, liver, and kidneys may show cloudy swelling, petechiae, focal necroses, or fatty changes. *Bronchopneumonia* is common. *Guarnieri bodies* are found in the cytoplasm of epidermal cells or in areas of ballooning degeneration. They are not as abundant as in vaccinia. *Microscopic changes* in the skin are like those of vaccinia.

Variolation

Variolation is an old procedure of inoculating well persons with unmodified smallpox virus during mild epidemics to protect them against the disease in severe epidemics.

VARICELLA: Cause

The virus of *varicella (chickenpox)* is brick-shaped, measures 210 to 250 mμ, and contains double-stranded DNA. *Transmission* of the virus is by direct contact from child to child. Cases have been reported of contraction of varicella from adults with *herpes zoster,* which is caused by the same virus.

Clinical features

Clinically varicella is typically a mild exanthem of childhood. The incubation period is 14 to 21 days. There is a prodromal period with sore throat, slight fever, headache, and malaise for 1 to 2 days. The characteristic rash then appears and is the most prominent feature. The uncomplicated disease is mild. However, several fatal cases have occurred in patients on cortisone or other steroid therapy and in pregnant women. Almost all cases of varicella pneumonitis occur in adults, especially men.

Pathologic changes

The initial lesion is a small macule, which disappears on pressure. In a few hours the *macules* become *papules,* and later vesicles. Some lesions go on to pustulation. At any time the lesions are pleomorphic, in contrast to variola in which they are all the same. The rash appears first on the face and back, then spreads to the rest of the body. Eosinophilic *intranuclear inclusion bodies* (Lipschütz or Tyzzer bodies) are found in epithelial cells at the bases of the vesicles. The latter are intra-epidermal, and scarring does not occur except from scratching or secondary infection. *Varicella pneumonitis* usually involves the lungs patchily, but these may be coalescent foci of consolidation. The involved areas show proliferation and desquamation of alveolar septal cells, within which intranuclear inclusion bodies are found. There is an interstitial infiltration by lymphocytes, macrophages, and a few neutrophils.

RUBELLA: Cause

Rubella (German measles) is caused by a virus which passes through a 320 mμ but not a 260 mμ gradocol filter. Electron microscopy reveals that the virus particles are variable. They are threadlike and show helical filaments characteristic of paramyxoviruses. *Transmission* is by direct contact, droplet infection, and transplacentally.

Clinical features

The *incubation period* is 14 to 21 days. *Clinically* rubella is a mild childhood exanthem, the rash being maculopapular and purplish red. There are slight fever, malaise, posterior cervical lymphadenopathy, and leukopenia. Numerous *congenital anomalies* are related to the incidence of rubella in women during the first trimester of pregnancy. Rubella virus has been isolated from defective newborns. The most common anomalies are those of the heart, deaf-mutism, microcephaly, and lenticular cataracts. Rubella accounts for about 1 percent of all congenital cardiac defects, including patent ductus arteriosus, septal defects, tetralogy of Fallot, Eisenmenger's complex, pulmonary or aortic stenosis, and coarctation of the aorta. Occasional cases show neonatal hepatitis [13] or thrombocytopenic purpura. The fetal changes are due to an intra-uterine viremia with cell invasion and destruction by rubella virus, which interferes with embryonic cell metabolism [14]. Increased numbers of chromosomal breaks are produced by rubella virus in embryonic tissue cultures and in vivo [15], indicating that the virus induces teratogenesis by altering genetic material.

Pathologic changes

The *pathologic changes* in rubella are little known. There is a lymphocytic dermal infiltrate in the skin macules and papules. The posterior cervical lymph nodes show lymphoid and reticular hyperplasia. *Rubella arthritis* is a common complication in young adults, especially women. Finger joints, wrists, knees, ankles, and toes are often involved. The synovial inflammation clears after about 2 weeks. Rarely a sometimes fatal *encephalitis* complicates rubella in children [16]. The brain is edematous, and there is a sparse perivascular lymphocytic infiltrate.

RUBEOLA: Cause

Rubeola (*measles,* morbilli) is caused by a filtrable myxovirus which is spherical and measures 90 to 100 mμ in diameter. It is antigenically related to the virus of canine distemper. *Transmission* of the virus is by direct contact and droplet infection from secretion of the nose, mouth, and eyes.

Clinical features

Clinically this exanthem is an almost inevitable childhood disease. About 400,000 cases with 400 deaths are reported annually in the United States. Epidemics occur every 2 to 3 years in large cities in late winter. The *incubation period* is usually 10 to 12 days. There is a period of invasion lasting 2 to 3 days with fever, malaise, lacrimation, photophobia, conjunctival injection, and signs of an upper respiratory infection. The earliest characteristic sign is the Koplik spot. The period of eruption usually begins about 14 days after exposure, and the maculopapular rash lasts 4 to 7 days. It begins on the forehead and neck and gradually involves the entire body. A slight, brown, branlike scale is left on desquamation. Deaths are rare (less than 0.2 percent of reported cases) and are due to complications.

Pathologic changes:

The *Koplik spot* is a small, grayish yellow focus with a red halo on the buccal mucosa opposite the first molar. Microscopically there is an infiltration of polymorphonuclear leukocytes, with capillary dilatation and small hemorrhages. In the *skin lesions* the dermis is edematous and infiltrated by lymphocytes and macrophages. Small hemorrhages may occur. The formation of multinucleated giant cells is the most specific change in rubeola. Reticuloendothelial *(Warthin-Finkeldey) giant cells,* with up to 100 closely packed nuclei, are found in the tonsils, lymph nodes, spleen, and lymphatic tissue of the intestines and appendix. Their appearance may precede the exanthem. *Epithelial giant cells* have been found in the tracheobronchial mucosa and in nasal and bronchial secretions. These may contain eosinophilic cytoplasmic or nuclear inclusions. Similar cells may be found in the urine of children with measles or who have received measles vaccine. Hecht's *giant cell pneumonia* [17] is a rare lesion produced by the rubeola virus. It occurs in infants, children, and young adults. There is an *interstitial pneumonitis* characterized by the presence of large multinucleated giant cells which appear to be formed by the proliferation and fusion of cells lining the alveolar ducts and bronchioles. Large eosinophilic cytoplasmic and nuclear inclusion bodies are found in these cells. The thickened alveolar septa are infiltrated with lymphocytes and plasmocytes. Hyaline membranes may line alveolar walls. *Grossly* the lungs are heavy and hypocrepitant. A rare complication of rubeola is *myocarditis,* which is characterized by interstitial edema and infiltration with lymphocytes and Anitschkow myocytes and by minute foci of myocardial necrosis [18]. *Encephalitis,* with perivascular lymphocytic infiltration and neuron degeneration, is an unusual complication occurring in about 0.5 percent of the cases. Many changes in measles, such as otitis media and bronchopneumonia, are caused by secondary bacterial infection.

giant cell pneumonia

ROSEOLA INFANTUM

Roseola infantum (exanthema subitum, sixth disease) is a mild macular exanthem which occurs in infants and children below the age of 3 years. It is presumably due to a virus, but the agent has not been isolated. Binucleate epithelial cells have been found in the urine of patients with roseola infantum [19].

HERPES SIMPLEX: Cause

Herpes simplex (fever blister, cold sore) is usually caused by *Herpesvirus hominis,* which is spherical or doughnut-shaped, contains double-stranded DNA, and measures about 180 mμ in diameter. Type 1 causes oral lesions, and type 2 produces genital herpes. Occasional cases are due to herpes virus B *(Herpesvirus simiae)* following monkey bites. *Transmission* of the type 1 human virus is by intimate contact, such as kissing, but most cases occur from virus carried normally in the skin or nervous tissue, usually appearing in association with some other disease in which there is a rise in body temperature. Type 2 virus is probably transmitted during coitus. Disseminated herpes in the newborn is acquired transplacentally, in the birth canal from vulvovaginal herpetic lesions, or postnatally.

Clinical features

Herpes lesions occur most frequently on the lips and external genitalia. They also appear on the face, buccal mucosa, vagina, cervix uteri, and conjunctiva.

Disseminated herpes simplex of the newborn usually occurs in prematures and is characterized by vesicles of the skin and mucous membranes, hepatomegaly, lymphadenopathy, signs of pneumonitis, thrombocytopenia, and anemia.

Pathologic changes

The *herpetic vesicle* is formed by ballooning and reticular degeneration of the epidermal cells. Typical eosinophilic intranuclear inclusions *(type A Lipschütz bodies)* are found in epidermal cells. In the dermis there is a heavy infiltration of polymorphonuclear leukocytes, with edema and congestion. *Herpetic encephalitis,* a rare complication, is discussed on page 684, and *herpetic keratitis,* on page 798. In *disseminated herpes simplex of the newborn* [20], besides the skin and mucosal vesicles, there are a bilateral pneumonitis with foci of necrosis at the margins of which alveoli are filled with fibrin, neutrophils, and cellular debris; central and midzonal necrosis in the liver; cortical necrosis in the adrenal glands [21]; and encephalitis. Intranuclear inclusion bodies are found in the skin and visceral lesions.

Relationship to neoplasia

A number of herpes viruses have been implicated in the induction of malignant neoplasms in humans and lower animals [22]. The Epstein-Barr (EB) virus isolated from cell cultures of Burkitt's tumor is herpes virus-like. *Type 2 herpes virus* has been implicated as an etiologic agent in *cervical carcinoma.* There is a significantly increased incidence of cervical dysplasia and in situ and invasive carcinoma in women with genital herpes [23]. Antibodies to type 2 virus are found much more frequently in patients with cervical cancer than in controls [24].

VERRUCA VULGARIS: Cause

The virus which causes *verruca vulgaris (wart)* belongs to the papova group. It measures 45 to 55 mμ in diameter and contains DNA. *Transmission* of the wart is by direct contact and auto-inoculation. *Clinically* the wart is asymptomatic. Several types are recognized: verruca plana juvenalis (flat wart), verruca plantaris (plantar wart), verruca filiformis (pedunculated wart), and condyloma acuminatum (venereal wart).

Pathologic changes

In the involved *epidermis* there are hyperkeratosis (thickening of the stratum corneum), acanthosis (hyperplastic thickening of the rete Malpighi), and elongation and widening of the rete pegs. There is edema of the underlying dermis with infiltration by lymphocytes. Satellite warts about the original lesion are common. Eosinophilic cytoplasmic and nuclear inclusion bodies are found in the epidermal cells of the prickle layer in some warts. By electron microscopy virus-like particles are found in both the cytoplasm and nuclei of such cells [25].

MOLLUSCUM CONTAGIOSUM: Cause

Molluscum contagiosum is caused by a poxvirus which is closely related to that of variola. It is rectangular to ovoid, contains DNA, and measures 220 by 300 mμ. *Transmission* is by personal contact and auto-inoculation.

Clinical features

Clinically one or more waxy elevations appear on the skin, especially in children. Dry, cheesy material may be squeezed from them. The lesions usually disappear spontaneously after several months.

Pathologic changes

The well-developed lesion is a small firm *papule* up to 2 mm. in diameter, with a minute orifice at its apex through which a pearly white core may be seen. The epidermis is hyperplastic, and there are large, eosinophilic hyaline masses in the midepidermis *(molluscum bodies),* with the epidermal cells compressed about them. These bodies represent fused, dried elementary bodies. Within the surrounding intact cells there are similar eosinophilic intracytoplasmic inclusion bodies (Henderson-Patterson bodies).

ORF

Orf (ecthyma contagiosum) [26] is a disease of sheep and goats which is uncommonly transmitted to men who handle infected animals. Its cause is a poxvirus which contains DNA. In man there is typically a single lesion on a hand or finger. It passes through maculopapular, target, nodular, regenerative, and papillomatous phases before healing without a scar. *Microscopically* the epidermal cells are vacuolated and contain eosinophilic intracytoplasmic and intranuclear inclusions. The dermis is heavily infiltrated with lymphocytes, plasmocytes, and macrophages. A few patients have fever and epitrochlear lymphadenopathy.

FOOT AND MOUTH DISEASE

Foot and mouth disease, a viral disease of cloven-hoofed animals, infects man rarely by means of contact or by ingestion of contaminated food. Intra-epidermal vesicles appear on the skin of the soles, palms, and fingers, and on the buccal mucosa. There is a polymorphonuclear leukocytic infiltration. Intranuclear inclusions are found.

2. Conjunctivotropic Viral Disease

EPIDEMIC KERATO-CONJUNCTIVITIS:

The *causes* of *epidemic keratoconjunctivitis* (EKC) are adenoviruses, chiefly serotype 8. *Transmission* is by personal contact.

Clinical features

Clinically there is a sudden onset of burning and injection beginning in the palpebral conjunctiva and spreading in 12 to 36 hours to the bulbar conjunctiva. The lids may be swollen. Visual impairment may follow corneal involvement.

Pathologic changes

The *conjunctival submucosa* is congested and edematous and infiltrated with mononuclear cells. Focal infiltration with resultant opacities of the cornea may occur.

3. Viscerotropic Viral Diseases

MUMPS: Cause

Mumps (epidemic parotitis) is caused by a paramyxovirus which contains ribonucleic acid (RNA). It is variable in size and shape, averaging about 200 mμ in largest diameter. *Transmission* of the virus is by droplet infection and direct contact. The virus probably reaches the parotid glands via the excretory ducts, but there is also a definite viremia. Intra-uterine infection by mumps virus has been implicated in the development of primary endocardial fibroelastosis [27].

Clinical features

Clinically most cases of mumps occur in children, but adult infections are not rare and may be severe. The incubation period is about 3 weeks, and the first symptom is usually pain below the ear. Soon parotid enlargement is noted, along with fever, malaise, and headache. In about 70 percent of the cases there is bilateral parotid involvement, and in about 10 percent other salivary glands are involved. Rarely mumps may occur without parotid enlargement. The disease lasts approximately a week, but recurrences are seen in about 10 percent of the cases. Mumps meningoencephalitis develops in up to 20 percent of the cases in epidemics and is characterized by high fever, headache, neck stiffness, and delirium. Permanent deafness may result.

Pathologic changes

Mumps is a *systemic disease* with localization in the parotid glands, testes or ovaries, pancreas, and meninges. The *parotid glands* are enlarged and pink, the edematous interstitial tissue being infiltrated by mononuclear cells. The changes are most pronounced about the ducts – some of the duct epithelium is swollen or necrotic. Similar changes are found in the *testes.* The orchitis is usually unilateral and patchy and is rarely followed by sterility. Acute hemorrhagic necrosis of the pancreas occurs rarely. In *acute meningoencephalitis* the meninges are infiltrated by lymphocytes, up to 200 per cubic millimeter appearing in the cerebrospinal fluid. The brain is edematous and shows perivascular lymphocytic cuffing.

CYTOMEGALIC INCLUSION DISEASE:

The causative virus of *cytomegalic inclusion disease* is transmitted transplacentally to the fetus in utero; probably by airborne droplets; and possibly via blood transfusions. It is classified in the herpes virus group and contains double-stranded DNA. *Clinically* in infants the disease occurs in a localized, asymptomatic form involving the salivary glands and in a disseminated form characterized by jaundice, pneumonitis, signs of brain involvement such as cerebral palsy, anemia, thrombocytopenia, and petechiae of the skin and mucous membranes. Cytomegalovirus antibodies are often present in infants with microcephaly [28]. In adults cytomegalovirus is most often associated with a pneumonitis in patients with debilitating diseases, such as leukemia, lymphomas, or refractory anemia.

Pathologic changes

In stillborn fetuses, infants, and young children whose deaths were due to various causes such as mucoviscidosis and lipid nephrosis, *intracytoplasmic and intranuclear inclusions* have been found in the salivary glands and other organs. The cytoplasmic inclusions are small and basophilic, and the nuclear bodies are large reddish violet masses surrounded by clear halos. The most common sites of involvement in disseminated disease are the brain, lungs, liver, gastrointestinal tract, pancreas, kidneys, and adrenal glands. Many newborn infants are smaller than normal for their gestational age, indicating fetal growth retardation by the virus [29]. In infants and children, viral inclusions are found mainly in epithelial cells, while in adults they are predominantly in endothelial cells and macrophages [30]. In the lungs the viral inclusion bodies are frequently associated with infection by *Pneumocystis carinii.* The pneumonitis is characterized by an interstitial plasmocytic infiltrate. In the brain there are foci of necrosis with calcification.

COMMON COLD: Cause

Common cold (acute coryza), one of the most common of all human ailments, is caused by numerous respiratory viruses such as rhinoviruses, para-influenza viruses, respiratory syncytial (RS) virus, and JH (ECHO-28) virus. *Rhinoviruses* are very small (15 to 30 mμ), RNA-containing picornaviruses of which about 75 serotypes are known. They are the most common cause of colds in adults. *Transmission* of the causative virus is by droplet infection and personal contact. There are predisposing factors such as exposure to wet or cold. The incubation period is 2 to 5 days.

Clinical features

Clinically there is a sudden onset of slight fever, malaise, and muscle aches. The nasal discharge is serous at first, and later becomes mucopurulent. Secondary bacterial infections of the nose and throat are common. The usual duration of the infection is 3 to 10 days.

Pathologic changes

The *nasal mucosa* is red, edematous, and velvety. Early a thin, serous fluid is present in the nasal cavity. Later this becomes mucopurulent. Edema of the mucosa produces obstruction of the nasal passages. *Microscopically* the submucosa is edematous and infiltrated with polymorphonuclear leukocytes and some lymphocytes. The blood vessels are dilated and congested. Involvement of the mucosa of the paranasal sinuses and pharynx is common.

RESPIRATORY SYNCYTIAL VIRUS INFECTIONS

Respiratory syncytial (RS) *virus* (chimpanzee coryza agent [CCA]) is thought to cause up to 20 percent of serious lower respiratory illness in infants and young children. It is a myxovirus, contains RNA, and produces a typical syncytium in HeLa cell cultures after 5 or 6 days. *Transmission* is by airborne droplets and personal contact. This virus causes the common cold syndrome and a *necrotizing bronchiolitis,* in which there are bronchial and bronchiolar epithelium with syncytium formation and a submucosal mononuclear cell infiltrate. Cytoplasmic inclusion bodies are found in the epithelial cells.

ADENOVIRUS INFECTIONS:

There are over 30 serotypes of *adenovirus.* They average about 75 mμ in diameter, contain double-stranded DNA, and are transmitted by airborne droplets and personal contact. Intranuclear eosinophilic inclusions are found in HeLa cells infected by serotypes 1, 2, 5, and 6. A number of strains of adenovirus (3, 7, 12, 14, 16, 18, 31) have produced *malignant neoplasia in animals.* In general adenoviruses produce catarrhal inflammation of the respiratory and ocular mucosa, lymphocytic submucosal infiltration, and lymphoid hyperplasia in the regional nodes. *Pharyngoconjunctival fever* (PCF) is most commonly caused by serotypes 1, 3, 4, 5, and 7. Other syndromes induced by adenoviruses include *acute febrile pharyngitis* (types 1 and 2); *acute respiratory disease* (ARD) (types 3, 4, 7, and 14); *viral pneumonitis* (cold agglutinins are not developed as in primary atypical pneumonia); *acute follicular conjunctivitis* (types 3 and 4); and *epidemic keratoconjunctivitis* (EKC) (type 8). Sources of summer epidemics of pharyngoconjunctival fever are almost always traced to swimming pools.

Clinical features

Clinically PCF may occur at any age but appears predominantly in children. The incubation period is 5 to 6 days. The symptoms are fever, sore throat, and conjunctival burning and injection.

Pathologic changes

In pharyngoconjunctival fever the *pharyngitis* and *conjunctivitis* are follicular and nonpurulent. The cell infiltrate is mainly lymphocytic. The cervical nodes show lymphoid hyperplasia.

INFLUENZA: Causes

Influenza (la grippe) is caused by influenza viruses A, B, and, uncommonly, C. They are spherical to ovoid myxoviruses which measure about 100 mμ and contain RNA. "Asian flu" is caused by a variant of type A (A_2). Secondary bacterial invasion is very common in cases of influenza, and it is difficult to separate lesions due to the virus from those due to the secondary invaders. *Transmission* is by droplet infection and personal contact. The *incubation period* is 2 days.

Clinical features

Clinically influenza is characterized by headache, prostration, muscle aches, dyspnea, cough, and cyanosis. In "intestinal flu" nausea, vomiting, and/or diarrhea are present.

Pathologic changes

The pharynx is red and velvety. The tracheobronchial mucosa is dark red, swollen, and velvety, and there may be small mucosal ulcerations. Serofibrinous fluid is present in the pleural cavity, and a fibrinous exudate is found on the pleural surfaces. The affected portions of the lungs are collapsed, dark purple, and leathery. The surrounding areas are voluminous due to compensatory emphysema (alveolar overdistention). The bronchioles are filled with a yellow, thick fluid. *Microscopically* the bronchiolar walls are edematous and infiltrated with polymorphonuclear leukocytes and fibrin. Many alveoli are collapsed; others contain a small amount of exudate with polymorphonuclear leukocytes and lymphocytes. The typical lesion is a thin, eosinophilic, adherent *hyaline membrane* lining the walls of the alveolar spaces. The membrane appears to be formed by the inspissation of albuminous edema fluid. In up to 50 percent of the cases, especially in men, there is a squamous metaplasia of the tracheal and bronchial mucosa. The tracheobronchial lymph nodes are swollen, edematous, and hyperplastic. *Complications* include empyema, otitis media, meningitis, and pyemia, and are due to secondary bacterial infection.

PARA-INFLUENZA VIRUS INFECTIONS

There are four types of *para-influenza virus.* They are myxoviruses and contain RNA. Type 2, the *croup-associated* (CA) *virus* causes an acute laryngotracheobronchitis. The others usually produce a mild upper respiratory infection with pharyngitis. Types 1 and 3 sometimes cause a pneumonitis.

COXSACKIE VIRUS INFECTIONS:

Coxsackie viruses, of which there are about 32 serotypes in groups A and B, are classified with the ECHO viruses and polioviruses as *enteroviruses* [31], because they are found in the intestinal tract. Because of their small size the enteroviruses and adenoviruses are grouped together as *picornaviruses.* The Coxsackie viruses measure about 20 mμ and contain RNA. They are transmitted by direct contact with nasal secretions or infected feces. These viruses are highly infectious, especially in infants and children, and cause a variety of disease states.

Clinical features

Clinically the *group A* viruses produce an *aseptic meningitis,* with fever, headache, neck stiffness, up to 500 lymphocytes per cubic millimeter in the spinal fluid, and in some cases muscle weakness or flaccid paralysis *(poliomyelitis-like disease); herpangina,* with fever, sore throat, and painful, rosily areolated, 1 to 2 mm. grayish white papules or vesicles on the anterior pillars, soft palate, uvula, tongue, or tonsils; *acute respiratory disease* (types A21 and A24); and *maculopapular and vesicular exanthemata* (types A9 and A16). The vesicular form may involve the hands, feet, and mouth. The *group B* viruses cause *aseptic meningitis; epidemic pleurodynia* (Bornholm disease, devil's grip), in which there is a sometimes excruciating chest (less often abdominal) pain with exquisite focal muscle tenderness; *myocarditis* in infants, with circulatory collapse, sudden hepatomegaly, and cyanosis; *pericarditis;* and *hepatitis* (type B5). Paralytic poliomyelitis has been caused by types A7, A9, B3, B4, and B5.

Pathologic changes

The *pathologic changes* in fatal cases include an interstitial *pneumonitis* with a mononuclear cell infiltrate; *hepatitis* with central hepatocytic necrosis; *myocarditis* with necrosis of myocardial fibers and an interstitial mononuclear cell infiltrate; and *meningoencephalomyelitis* with hyperemia, edema, and lymphocytic cuffing in the central nervous system and meninges [32].

ECHO VIRUS INFECTIONS:

About 28 antigenic types of *ECHO* (enteric cytopathogenic human orphan) *viruses* have been recognized. Except for type 10, they measure approximately 18 mμ. ECHO 10 and antigenically related viruses, which measure about 72 mμ have been reclassified as *reoviruses* because they are distinctly larger than the enteroviruses and have an affinity for the respiratory as well as the intestinal system. ECHO viruses are classified as *enteroviruses* and *picornaviruses.* In tissue cultures the cytopathologic changes produced by the enteroviruses are remarkably similar. They include the development of large nuclear eosinophilic masses, with later nuclear pyknosis and cell degeneration [33].

Clinical features

Clinically the viruses produce an *aseptic meningitis* (ECHO types 2, 3, 4, 5, 6, 7, 9, 14, 16, 18, and 21) with rare paralyses; a *maculopapular rash* on the skin (exanthem) and mucosa of the mouth (enanthem) (especially types 4, 9, and 16) with pharyngitis (sore throat) and fever (concurrent rash and meningitis – meningitis-rash syndrome – have occurred with type 9 infections); and an *enteritis* with nausea, vomiting, abdominal pain, and sometimes diarrhea. Diarrhea is usually due to types 4, 8, 18, and 20 and is most common in infants and young children.

In children and adults the diarrhea may occur as a steatorrhea with bulky, foul-smelling stools. In infants it is usually in the form of *epidemic diarrhea of the newborn infant,* the intestinal contents being watery and greenish yellow, with large amounts of mucus. Isolated cases of mild *paralytic poliomyelitis* have been attributed to types 2, 4, 6, 9, 11, and 16.

Pathologic changes

In *diarrhea of the newborn infant* the intestinal mucosa is edematous and shows petechiae. There may be small ulcers. The lesions in the other syndromes are little known.

VIRAL HEPATITIS: Causes

Infectious hepatitis is produced by an unidentified hepatitis virus A. *Serum hepatitis* (homologous serum jaundice) is caused by hepatitis virus B, which measures about 26 mμ in diameter. Australia antigen (AU) (hepatitis-associated antigen) (HAA) is present during the incubation period and the acute phase of serum hepatitis [33a]. The two hepatitis viruses are distinct immunologically. Infectious hepatitis virus is transmitted by ingestion of fecally contaminated food and occasionally by blood transfusion or injection. Serum hepatitis virus is transmitted by plasma and blood transfusions, vaccines containing human serum, injections with contaminated needles, and tattoo needles. A few cases of serum hepatitis are apparently transmitted by fecal contamination. Hepatitis is also caused by a number of other organisms, including herpes simplex and Coxsackie viruses and cytomegalovirus.

Clinical features

Clinically the *incubation period of infectious hepatitis* varies from 15 to 40 days, while *that of serum hepatitis* is 60 to 160 days. The *clinical* course of these conditions is varied, most cases showing jaundice, fever, nausea and vomiting, right upper quadrant pain and tenderness, and hemorrhages. Their *mortality* is 0.2 to 0.4 percent. About 5 percent of the cases develop postnecrotic cirrhosis.

Pathologic changes [34]:

The *gross and microscopic appearance of the liver* in these conditions depends on the severity of the disease. In *nonfatal cases* biopsies show early degeneration of the parenchymal cells. The orderly columnar pattern of the lobules is lost. In the central zone the changes are most marked, with necrosis and loss of cells. The associated inflammatory reaction may be perilobular or intralobular; it is mainly a lymphocytic reaction with some neutrophils and eosinophils. Electron microscopy reveals dilatation of the endoplasmic reticulum and fingerprint-like arrays of glycogen granules within hepatocytes [35]. Degenerative changes in the form of hyalinization of hepatic cells similar to the Councilman bodies of yellow fever may occur in hepatitis. By electron microscopy these eosinophilic bodies consist of condensed ground cytoplasm with a few organelles [36]. Ribosomal particles are almost completely absent.

Councilman-like bodies

fulminating cases

In *fulminating cases* [37] with early death the liver is usually moderately reduced in size, very soft, dark reddish brown, and has a wrinkled capsule. The cut surface is mottled without any pattern, congested, and purplish red. *Microscopically* there is massive destruction of liver cells, but the supporting reticulum is preserved. The remaining sinusoids are congested and dilated. Bile ductules may show proliferative changes. The inflammatory response – mainly macrophages, lymphocytes, and plasma cells, with fewer neutrophils and eosinophils – is most marked at the periphery of the lobule.

subacute hepatitis

In patients who survive for several weeks or a few months *subacute hepatitis* [38] sometimes develops. The liver is markedly reduced in size and weight and is deformed. The surface shows several projecting coarse nodules. The cut surface is variegated, with dark red areas of parenchymal destruction and nodular pale or greenish areas of regenerative hyperplasia. *Microscopically* foci of both parenchymal cell necrosis with inflammation and the formation of large new parenchymal cells are found. The hyperplastic hepatic cells are usually arranged in an atypical fashion with little lobular architecture. Intralobular cholestasis and bile ductule proliferation may be marked.

The severity of the *jaundice* in viral hepatitis does not necessarily correlate with the hepatic damage, the jaundice being due mainly to obstruction of bile canaliculi by bile plugs. *Extrahepatic* changes include ascites, pleural effusion, and peripheral edema. *Hemorrhages* may occur in various tissues due to a disturbance of prothrombin formation. The kidneys may show changes in the convoluted tubular epithelium varying from fatty metamorphosis to bile nephrosis. In the brain in about 15 percent of the cases there is a nonspecific degeneration of ganglion cells, and slight lymphocytic collections may be seen about small blood vessels and in the meninges.

YELLOW FEVER:

Yellow fever is caused by an arbovirus measuring about 22 mμ in diameter and containing RNA. *Transmission* of the virus is by the bite of female *Aedes aegypti* mosquitoes. In Brazil there is a jungle yellow fever which is transmitted by other mosquitoes (*Haemogogous* and *Aedes* species).

Clinical features

Clinically the incubation period is 3 to 6 days. The onset is sudden, with fever, headache, muscle aches, and prostration. After 2 to 3 days there is a characteristic fall in temperature followed by a secondary rise. Jaundice appears, and there may be petechiae in the skin. The pulse, which is rapid initially, falls progressively, and sometimes is less than 50 beats per minute. Vomiting of altered blood (coffee-ground material) is a prominent feature ("black vomit"). Albuminuria and the passage of dark urine are often noted, and there is a leukopenia. The disease lasts 7 to 8 days, and the mortality rate is about 5 percent. Death may be due to uremia (renal failure), hepatic failure, toxemia, or bronchopneumonia.

Pathologic changes

The liver is normal in size and reddish or yellowish gray in color; on section the parenchyma bulges from beneath the capsule and shows occasional petechiae. On cut surface the lobular architecture is partially obscured. The characteristic microscopic change is necrosis, affecting the midzonal region of each hepatic lobule. Within the cytoplasm there are foci of hyaline necrosis, known as *Councilman bodies.* In some cases there are characteristic multiple, small, acidophilic, *intranuclear inclusion bodies* (Torres bodies). The spleen is normal in size, soft, and dark red. Microscopically depletion of the lymphoid tissue and slight hyperplasia of the endothelial cells about the follicles are noted. The heart is pale and may show fatty degeneration. In the brain there are small foci of perivascular hemorrhage and occasional perivascular lymphocytic infiltrations. The kidneys are slightly enlarged and pale. Microscopically all grades of cloudy swelling, fatty degeneration, and necrosis of the epithelium of the proximal convoluted tubules are seen. In the mucosa of the gastrointestinal tract, throughout many of the viscera, and in the skin there are petechiae and ecchymoses. The lumen of the gastrointestinal tract is partially filled with dark blood. The lymph nodes are enlarged and may show small foci of necrosis. The degree of icterus varies.

EPIDEMIC HEMORRHAGIC FEVER:

Epidemic hemorrhagic fever is caused by a filtrable virus which has been found in gamasid mites. It is likely that contact with infected rodent excreta transmits the disease to humans.

Clinical features

Clinically the disease has long been endemic in Manchuria and Siberia and it was a serious problem among field troops during the Korean War. There are hemorrhagic manifestations such as petechiae in the skin, hematuria, and hematemesis. Headache, blurred vision, fever, nausea, and vomiting are common. The white cell count varies from 20,000 to 93,000 per cubic millimeter with a shift to the left. The course may be fulminating, with death in 2 to 8 days.

Pathologic changes [39]

Hemorrhages are found in most of the organs, but especially in the renal pelvis, renal medulla, right atrium (subendocardially), and submucosa of the gastrointestinal tract. There is a peculiar type of necrosis (probably due to small infarcts) in the renal medulla, anterior pituitary body, adrenal cortex, and islets of Langerhans. A mononuclear cell infiltrate is found in the myocardium, pancreas, spleen, and liver. Despite the widespread capillary hemorrhages, there is no evidence of capillary damage.

Related diseases [40]

Related diseases include *South American hemorrhagic fever,* which is due to the Junin virus [41] in Argentina and the Machupo virus in Bolivia [42]; *Crimean* and *Central Asia hemorrhagic fevers,* the viruses of which are probably transmitted by *Hyalomma* ticks; *Kyasanur forest disease* (KFD) of southern India, which is an epizootic viral infection of monkeys and is thought to be transmitted to man by a tick, possibly *Haemaphysalis spinigera;* and *Thailand hemorrhagic fever,* which is an acute viral infection of children characterized by fever, petechiae, gastrointestinal hemorrhage, and shock.

4. *Miscellaneous Viral Diseases*

There are numerous virus diseases about whose pathologic changes little is known because the diseases are rare or their clinical courses are nonfatal.

COLORADO TICK FEVER

Colorado tick fever is caused by a virus measuring about 25 mμ and transmitted by the wood tick, *Dermacentor andersoni.* The incubation period is about 5 days. The virus is present in the blood of patients. The pathologic changes are little known in man. In rodents and rabbits the virus produces degeneration and cerebellar Purkinje cells and ischemic necrosis in the hippocampus and pons [43].

DENGUE

Dengue (breakbone fever) is caused by a dumbbell- or rod-shaped arbovirus measuring 17 to 25 mμ in greatest diameter. It is transmitted by the bite of the *Aedes aegypti* mosquito. After an incubation period of 5 to 8 days the patient develops prostrating bone and muscle pains, a maculopapular skin rash, and severe leukopenia. The skin lesions show hemorrhages and perivascular mononuclear cell infiltrates.

PHLEBOTOMUS

Phlebotomus (pappataci, sandfly) *fever* is due to an arbovirus measuring about 50 mμ. It is transmitted by the bite of the female sandfly, *Phlebotomus papatasii.* The incubation period is 3 to 4 days. Clinically it is typified by myalgia, fever, and leukopenia.

RIFT VALLEY FEVER

Rift Valley fever occurs in herders in this East African valley, is mainly a disease of cattle and sheep (enzootic hepatitis), and is probably transmitted by mosquitoes. In Rift Valley fever foci of necrosis and intranuclear acidophilic inclusions are found in the liver.

ALEUTIAN MINK DISEASE

Aleutian mink disease is a viral disease of mink which has rarely infected their raisers and handlers [44]. Clinically there are episodes of fever, lymphocytosis with monocytoid and plasmacytoid lymphocytes in the peripheral blood, and hepatosplenomegaly. In the liver there are granular foci about 1 mm. in diameter. Microscopically these consist almost entirely of plasmocytes. There are also plasmocytic infiltrates in the spleen, lymph nodes, bone marrow, and kidneys. Glomerular lesions in mink resemble those of lupus erythematosus and appear to be due to an immune reaction [45].

OTHER VIRAL DISEASES

Infectious mononucleosis is treated on page 391. The *neurotropic viral diseases* (rabies, poliomyelitis, lymphocytic choriomeningitis, encephalitis, and herpes zoster) are discussed in Chapter 26.

Information on viral infections is summarized in Table 7-4.

Disease	Characteristics of virus*	Inclusion body†	Mode of transmission	Principal organs or sites involved	Type of tissue reaction‡	Special features
Vaccinia (cowpox)	*Poxvirus officinale* or *bovis;* about 230 mμ, spherical or brick-shaped; cross immunity with variola virus; contains double-stranded DNA; IP 6–12 days	Guarnieri body (C) made up of Paschen corpuscles	Inoculation for smallpox vaccination; handling infected cows	Skin at inoculation site (macule → papule → vesicle → pustule)	A (hydropic degeneration of epidermal cells)	Generalized vaccinia occurs occasionally; rarely demyelinizing encephalomyelitis develops; regional lymphadenitis simulating a malignant lymphoma may occur
Variola (smallpox)	*Poxvirus variolae;* about 200 mμ, spherical or brick-shaped; contains DNA; IP 8–12 days	Same as vaccinia	Direct contact; airborne droplets; fomites; transplacentally	Skin and buccal mucosa (eruption of macules → papules → vesicles → pustules; hemorrhages into lesions in hemorrhagic smallpox) Lungs (bacterial bronchopneumonia)	A (same as vaccinia)	Alastrim is mild form (variola minor)
Varicella (chickenpox)	210–250 mμ, brick-shaped; also causes herpes zoster; contains DNA; double-stranded; IP 14–21 days	Tyzzer body (N)	Direct contact; airborne droplets	Skin (exanthem of macules → papules → vesicles → some pustules; no scarring) Lungs (patchy viral pneumonitis in adults)	A (same as vaccinia)	Infection is severe (and may be fatal) in patients on steroids and during pregnancy
Rubella (German measles)	Passes 320 mμ but not 260 mμ gradocol filter; morphologically a paramyxovirus; contains RNA; IP 14–21 days	—	Direct contact; airborne droplets; transplacentally	Skin (mild maculopapular exanthem) Posterior cervical nodes (hyperplasia) Joints (arthritis common in young adults)	Dermal lymphocytic infiltrate	Congenital anomalies (cardiac defects, deaf-mutism, cataracts, microcephaly) are common with infection during 1st trimester of pregnancy

See footnotes on page 169.

TABLE 7-4. Viral Infections (Continued)

Disease	Characteristics of virus*	Inclusion body†	Mode of transmission	Principal organs or sites involved	Type of tissue reaction‡	Special features
Rubeola (measles)	90–100 mμ; spherical; a paramyxovirus; contains RNA; antigenically related to canine distemper virus; IP 10–12 days	—	Direct contact; airborne droplets	Skin (maculopapular rash) Buccal mucosa (Koplik spot) Lungs and middle ear (secondary bacterial infection)	Warthin-Finkeldey (reticuloendothelial) giant cells found in tonsils, lymph nodes, spleen, appendix	Epithelial giant cells in respiratory secretions. Virus occasionally causes Hecht's giant cell pneumonia Encephalitis occurs rarely
Roseola infantum (6th disease)	Not known; IP about 14 days	—	—	Skin (macular exanthem)	—	Occurs only in children < 3 years
Herpes simplex (fever blister)	About 180 mμ; spherical, somewhat doughnut-shaped; contains double-stranded DNA; IP ?; type 1 causes oral lesions; type 2 produces genital herpes; herpes virus B (of monkeys) occasionally infects man	Type A Lipschütz body (N)	Type 1: direct contact (kissing); type 2: sexual contact; fetus infected transplacentally or during passage through birth canal	Lip, skin, buccal mucosa, conjunctiva, cornea (dendritic ulcer), external genitalia (vesicle)	A (hydropic degeneration of epidermal cells)	Most cases are due to recrudescence of virus already present in skin or mucosa. Disseminated herpes may produce encephalitis, hepatitis, and/or hepatoadrenal necrosis; occurs mainly in newborn
Verruca vulgaris (wart)	45–55 mμ in diameter; contains DNA	—	Direct contact; autoinocula-tion	Skin, external genitalia	B (proliferation of epidermal cells)	—

Molluscum contagiosum	220 x 300 mμ; rectangular to ovoid shape; a poxvirus; contains DNA; IP 14+ days	Molluscum body (C)	Direct contact; autoinoculation	Skin	B (same as verruca vulgaris)	—
Foot and mouth disease	—	(N)	Contact with infected cattle, sheep, or pigs	Skin of fingers, palms, or soles (intraepidermal vesicles)	A (neutrophils)	—
Epidemic keratoconjunctivitis	Adenoviruses, chiefly serotype 8; about 75 mμ	—	Personal contact	Conjunctiva and cornea	Submucosal lymphocytic infiltrate	—
Mumps (epidemic parotitis)	About 200 mμ, variable in size and shape; a paramyxovirus; contains RNA; IP about 21 days	—	Direct contact; airborne droplets; fomites	Salivary glands, especially parotid; pancreas, testis, ovary CNS (mild meningoencephalitis)	Interstitial mononuclear infiltrate	Bilateral parotid involvement in 70%
Cytomegalic inclusion disease	Classified in herpes virus family; contains double-stranded DNA; 2 immunologic types	(N) large, acido- or amphophilic (C) small, basophilic	Transplacentally, probably by airborne droplets	Salivary glands, liver, renal tubular epithelium, pancreas, adrenals in young Lungs (interstitial pneumonitis) in adults and infants	Epithelial cell swelling with inclusion bodies	Found in stillborn fetuses and in infants and children dead from various causes such as mucoviscidosis or lipid nephrosis *Pneumocystis carinii* often associated in pneumonia
Acute coryza (common cold)	Numerous respiratory viruses such as rhinoviruses, parainfluenza viruses, RS (CCA) and JH (ECHO-28) viruses; IP 2–5 days		Airborne droplets; personal contact	Nasal and pharyngeal mucosa	Edema and congestion, catarrhal inflammation	—

See footnotes on page 169.

TABLE 7-4. Viral Infections (Continued)

Disease	Characteristics of virus*	Inclusion body†	Mode of transmission	Principal organs or sites involved	Type of tissue reaction‡	Special features
Respiratory syncytial (RS) virus infections	A paramyxovirus; also called chimpanzee coryza agent (CCA); causes typical syncytium in HeLa cell cultures after 5–6 days	(C)	Airborne droplets; personal contact	Nasal mucosa Bronchi and bronchioles (necrotizing bronchiolitis, bronchial epithelial proliferation with syncytium formation)	Submucosal mononuclear cell infiltrate	May cause up to 20% of serious lower respiratory illness in infants and young children
Adenovirus infections	> 30 sterotypes; contain double-stranded DNA; measure 60–90 mμ. Several types have produced neoplasms in experimental animals	–	Airborne droplets; personal contact	Nasal and pharyngeal mucosa Conjunctiva and cornea Lungs (interstitial pneumonitis) Lymph nodes (hyperplasia, mesenteric, lymphadenitis in infants)	Submucosal lymphocytic infiltrate, catarrhal inflammation	Pharyngoconjunctival fever (PCF) – serotypes 1, 3, 4, 5, 7 Acute febrile pharyngitis – 1, 2, 3, 5 Acute respiratory disease (ARD) – 3, 4, 7, 14 Acute follicular conjunctivitis – 3, 4 Epidemic keratoconjunctivitis (EKC) – 8
Influenza (la grippe)	Viruses A, B, and C; about 100 mμ, spherical to ovoid; myxovirus; contain RNA; IP 2 days	–	Airborne droplets; personal contact	Pharyngeal and tracheobronchial mucosa Lung (interstitial pneumonitis)	Congestion and edema; hyaline alveolar membranes; squamous metaplasia, interstitial lymphocytic infiltrate in lungs, with neutrophils in fulminant cases and secondary bac-	Occasional cases have associated myocarditis and/or pericarditis

Primary atypical pneumonia	Influenza, parainfluenza, and psittacosis viruses, adenoviruses, and *C. burnetii* are causes	—	Airborne droplets; personal contact	Lung (patchy interstitial pneumonitis)	Pleomorphic intra-alveolar and septal infiltrate	When cold agglutinins are +, cause in 90% of cases is *Mycoplasma pneumoniae*, a pleuropneumonia-like organism
Rhinovirus infections	About 75 serotypes; measure 15–30 mμ; classified as picornaviruses; contain RNA	—	Airborne droplets; personal contact	Nasal and pharyngeal mucosa	Congestion and edema; catarrhal inflammation	—
Coxsackie virus infections	Groups A and B with about 32 serotypes; about 20 mμ; classified in picornaviruses; contain single-stranded RNA	—	Direct contact with secretions or infected feces	*Group A* viruses cause aseptic meningitis (poliomyelitis-like disease) with a lymphocytic meningeal infiltrate; herpangina; acute respiratory disease (types A21 and A24); and maculopapular and vesicular exanthemata (types A9 and A16) *Group B* viruses cause aseptic meningitis; epidemic pleurodynia (Bornholm disease, devil's grip); myocarditis; pericarditis; and hepatitis (type B5). Paralytic poliomyelitis has been caused by types A7, A9, B3, B4, and B5		
ECHO virus infections	About 28 serotypes; classified as picornaviruses; about 18 mμ, except for serotype 10 now classified with reoviruses (respiratory enteric orphan viruses); contain single-stranded RNA	—	Same as Coxsackie viruses	Aseptic meningitis (types 2, 3, 4, 5, 6, 7, 9, 14, 16, 18, 21) Meningitis-rash syndrome (9) Maculopapular rash (4, 9, 16) Enteritis (epidemic diarrhea of newborn) (4, 8, 18, 20)	—	Isolated cases of paralytic poliomyelitis (2, 4, 6, 9, 11, 16) and pleurodynia (8) have been reported
Viral hepatitis	Infectious hepatitis; unidentified virus A; IP 15–40 days	—	Infectious: ingestion of fecally	Liver (mild to fulminating necrosis) Kidneys (tubular	A (Hepatocellular necrosis with lymphocytic and	Rarely pancytopenia has developed in viral hepatitis Occasional cases of serum

See footnotes on page 169.

TABLE 7-4. Viral Infections (Continued)

Disease	Characteristics of virus*	Inclusion body†	Mode of transmission	Principal organs or sites involved	Type of tissue reaction‡	Special features
Viral hepatitis (Cont.)	Serum hepatitis (homologous serum jaundice) virus B; about 26 mμ in diameter; Australia antigen (AU) present during incubation period and acute phase; IP 60–160 days		contaminated food; occasionally by transfusion or injection Serum: plasma and blood transfusions; vaccines containing human serum; infections with contaminated needles	epithelial degeneration [bile nephrosis]) CNS (meningoencephalitis) with perivascular lymphocytic cuffing in 15% of cases	some neutrophilic infiltrate)	hepatitis are apparently transmitted by fecal contamination
Yellow fever	About 22 mμ; an arbovirus; contains RNA; IP about 4 days	(N)	Bite of *Aedes aegypti* mosquito	Liver (midzonal necrosis) Gastrointestinal tract (hemorrhages)	A (Councilman bodies are foci of hyaline necrosis in hepatocytes)	Small nuclear inclusion bodies are sometimes present in hepatocytes
Epidemic hemorrhagic fever	Virus	—	Mite and tick bites	Skin, renal pelvis, gastrointestinal tract, right atrium Myocardium, liver, spleen Adrenal cortex, anterior pituitary	Hemorrhages Mononuclear cell infiltrates Small infarcts	No evidence of capillary damage is found Endemic in Manchuria, Korea, and Siberia South American hemorrhagic fever is caused by Junin and Machupo viruses
Colorado tick fever	About 25 mμ; an arbovirus; IP 5 days	(C)	Bite of wood tick *(D. andersoni)*	Little known in man	A (Degeneration of Purkinje cells; ischemic necrosis)	Virus is present in blood stream Lesions in experimental animals resemble those

Dengue (breakbone fever)	17–25 mμ, dumb-bell- or rod-shaped; an arbovirus; IP usually 5–8 days	—	Bite of *Aedes aegypti* mosquito	Skin (maculopapular rash)	Hemorrhages, perivascular mononuclear cell infiltrate	Severe bone and muscle pains and leukopenia
Phlebotomus (sandfly, pappataci) fever	About 50 mμ; an arbovirus; IP 3–4 days	—	Bite of female sandfly, *Phlebotomus papatasii*	Little known	—	Myalgia, fever, and leukopenia
Rift Valley fever	—	(N)	Probably mosquitoes	Liver	A (hepatocellular necrosis)	Disease of cattle and sheep in East Africa; occasional infections in herders
Lymphocytic choriomeningitis[§]	About 50 mμ; IP 7–21 days	—	Probably inhalation	Leptomeninges and choroid plexus	Lymphocytic infiltration	—
Type A encephalitis (von Economo's disease)[§]	Virus not identified	—	—	Midbrain, substantia nigra, diencephalon, basal ganglia, pons, and medulla	A (neuronal degeneration; perivascular cuffing by lymphocytes)	Postencephalitic parkinsonism is due to substantia nigral lesions
St. Louis encephalitis[§]	20–30 mμ; an arbovirus; IP 4–21 days	—	Mosquito bite	Cerebral cortex, basal ganglia, and brain stem	A (same as type A encephalitis)	—
Japanese B encephalitis[§]	About 18 mμ; similar to St. Louis virus; an arbovirus; IP about 8–15 days	—	Probably mosquito bite	Cerebrum, basal ganglia, midbrain (especially substantia nigra and red nuclei), cerebellum, and spinal cord	A (neuronal degeneration; perivascular cuffing)	—
Russian spring and summer encephalitis[§]	15–25 mμ; an arbovirus; IP 7–21 days	—	Bite of forest tick	Similar to Japanese B encephalitis	A (same as Japanese encephalitis)	—

See footnotes on page 169.

TABLE 7-4. Viral Infections (Continued)

Disease	Characteristics of virus*	Inclusion body†	Mode of transmission	Principal organs or sites involved	Type of tissue reaction‡	Special features
Equine encephalomyelitis§	30–50 mμ, spherical; an arbovirus; IP usually 5–10 days	–	Probably mosquito bite	Cerebrum, basal ganglia, pons, medulla, spinal cord	A (neuronal degeneration; acute arteritis; perivascular neutrophilic cuffing)	Eastern form more severe clinically and pathologically than Western type
Poliomyelitis (infantile paralysis)§	*Poliovirus* is a small (8–12 mμ) picornavirus; serologic types 1 (Brunhilde), 2 (Lansing), and 3 (Leon); IP 7–14 days (4–10 days for abortive cases); contain RNA	–	Ingestion of fecally contaminated water and food; possibly airborne droplets	Spinal cord (anterior horns) especially in lumbar segment Brain stem (bulbar poliomyelitis) Skeletal muscles (atrophy) Liver (focal necrosis) Heart (myocarditis in some fatal cases)	A (necrosis and neuronophagia of motor neurons; perivascular lymphocytic cuffing)	In spinal form virus reaches intestine, multiplies in epithelial cells, and reaches anterior horns via nerve fibers or hematogenously In bulbar form virus penetrates oropharyngeal mucosa, especially in tonsillar region, and reaches cranial nerve motor nuclei along nerve fibers or hematogenously
Rabies (hydrophobia)§	About 125 mμ; bullet-shaped; contains RNA; IP 15–150+ days	Negri body (C)	Bite of infected dog, cat, fox, wolf, bat, etc.	Hippocampus major, medulla, Purkinje cells of cerebellum	Perivascular lymphocytic cuffing	Street virus, isolated from naturally infected animals, forms Negri bodies Fixed virus is attenuated by passage through experimental animals
Herpes zoster (shingles)§	210–250 mμ, brick-shaped; identical with varicella virus; IP 7–14 days	Lipschütz body (N)	Probably direct contact and airborne droplets	Posterior spinal ganglia, peripheral nerve and corresponding skin segment	Crusted vesicles on skin; edema of nerves and ganglia	Generalized herpes zoster occurs occasionally in cases of leukemia or lymphoma

Infectious mononucleosis (see page 391)	Probably the EB virus, a herpes-type virus	—	Kissing; airborne droplets	Lymph nodes, spleen, liver, blood	Lymphoid hyperplasia	Abnormal lymphocytes with strongly basophilic, foamy cytoplasm make up 50–90% of peripheral blood leukocytes Heterophile antibodies are present in over 50% of cases
Aleutian mink disease	Virus of minks which rarely infects raisers and handlers	—	Contact with contaminated mink	Liver, spleen, lymph nodes, bone marrow and kidneys	Plasmocytic infiltrates	Monocytoid and plasma cytoid lymphocytes found in peripheral blood. Glomerular lesions resemble those of lupus erythematosus

*IP, incubation period.

†C, intracytoplasmic; N, intranuclear.

‡A, necrosis of parasitized cells – hydropic (ballooning) degeneration of epidermal cells or mucosal epithelium, anterior horn neuronophagia, etc.; B, proliferation of parasitized cells (epidermal cells in verruca vulgaris), especially when intermitotic cells are infected.

§Page references are given for viral infections not treated in Chapter 7. See Chapter 26 for a discussion of these diseases.

REFERENCES

1. Wissig, S. L., Caro, L. G., Jackson, R., and Smadel, J. E. Electron microscopic observations on intracellular rickettsiae. *Amer. J. Path.* 32:1117, 1956.
2. Gallaher, W. H. Q fever. *J.A.M.A.* 177:187, 1961.
3. Carithers, H. A., Carithers, C. M., and Edwards, R. O., Jr. Cat-scratch disease. *J.A.M.A.* 207:312, 1969.
4. Herriott, R. M. Infectious nucleic acids, a new dimension in virology. *Science* 134:256, 1961.
5. Ho, M. Interferons. *New Eng. J. Med.* 266:1258, 1313, 1367, 1962.
6. Chany, C., and Brailovsky, C. Stimulating interaction between viruses (stimulons). *Proc. Nat. Acad. Sci. U.S.A.* 57:87, 1967.
7. Dulbecco, R. Cell transformation by viruses. *Science* 166:962, 1969.
8. Black, P. H. Recent advances in the study of oncogenic viruses. *New Eng. J. Med.* 275:377, 1966.
9. Goodheart, C. R. Molecular virology and cancer. *J.A.M.A.* 194:48, 1965.
10. Murphy, W. H., Ertel, I. J., and Zarafonetis, C. J. D. Virus studies of human leukemia. *Cancer* 18:1329, 1965.
11. Bell, T. M. Viruses associated with Burkitt's tumor. *Progr. Med. Virol.* 9:1, 1967.
12. Hartsock, R. J. Postvaccinial lymphadenitis. *Cancer* 21:632, 1968.
13. Strauss, L., and Bernstein, J. Neonatal hepatitis in congenital rubella. *Arch. Path.* (Chicago) 86:317, 1968.
14. Gray, J. E. Rubella in pregnancy. *Brit. Med. J.* 1:1388, 1960.
15. Nusbacher, J., Hirschhorn, K., and Cooper, L. Z. Chromosomal abnormalities in congenital rubella. *New Eng. J. Med.* 276:1409, 1967.
16. Sherman, F. E., Michaels, R. H., and Kenny, F. M. Acute encephalopathy (encephalitis) complicating rubella. *J.A.M.A.* 192:675, 1965.
17. Koffler, D. Giant cell pneumonia. *Arch. Path.* (Chicago) 78:267, 1964.
18. Cohen, N. A. Myocarditis in prodromal measles. *Amer. J. Clin. Path.* 40:50, 1963.
19. Gittes, R. F. Observation of nucleogeminy in urinary-sediment cells in the roseola-infantum syndrome. *New Eng. J. Med.* 269:446, 1963.
20. Wheeler, C. E., Jr., and Huffines, W. D. Primary disseminated herpes simplex of the newborn. *J.A.M.A.* 191:455, 1965.
21. Patrizi, G., Middelkamp, J. N., and Reed, C. A. Fine structure of herpes simplex virus hepatoadrenal necrosis in the newborn. *Amer. J. Clin. Path.* 49:325, 1968.
22. Goodheart, C. R. Herpesviruses and cancer. *J.A.M.A.* 211:91, 1970.
23. Naib, Z. M., Nahmias, A. J., Josey, W. E., and Kramer, J. H. Genital herpetic infection: Association with cervical dysplasia and carcinoma. *Cancer* 23:940, 1969.
24. Rawls, W. E., Tompkins, W. A. F., Figueroa, M. E., and Melnick, J. L. Herpesvirus type 2: Association with carcinoma of the cervix. *Science* 161:1255, 1968.
25. Chapman, G. B., Drusin, L. M., and Todd, J. E. Fine structure of the human wart. *Amer. J. Path.* 42:619, 1963.
26. Leavell, U. W., Jr., MacNamara, M. J., Muelling, R., Talbert, W. M., Rucker, R. C., and Dalton, A. J. Orf. *J.A.M.A.* 204:657, 1968.
27. Gerne, J. W. S., Jr., Noren, G. R., and Adams, P., Jr. Proposed embryopathic relation between mumps virus and primary endocardial fibroelastosis. *New Eng. J. Med.* 275:339, 1966.

28. Hanshaw, J. B. Cytomegalovirus complement-fixing antibody in microcephaly. *New Eng. J. Med.* 275:476, 1966.
29. Naeye, R. L. Cytomegalic inclusion disease. *Amer. J. Clin. Path.* 47:738, 1967.
30. Wong, T., and Warner, N. E. Cytomegalic inclusion disease in adults. *Arch. Path.* (Chicago) 74:403, 1962.
31. Ashkenazi, A., and Melnick, J. L. Enteroviruses – a review of their properties and associated diseases. *Amer. J. Clin. Path.* 38:209, 1962.
32. Fechner, R. E., Smith, M. G., and Middelkamp, J. N. Coxsackie B virus infection of the newborn. *Amer. J. Path.* 43:493, 1963.
33. Shaver, D. N., Barron, A. L., and Karzon, D. T. Cytopathology of human enteric viruses in tissue culture. *Amer. J. Path.* 34:943, 1958.
33a. London, W. T., Sutnick, A. I., and Blumberg, B. S. Australia antigen and acute viral hepatitis. *Ann. Intern. Med.* 70:55, 1969.
34. Lucké, B. The pathology of fatal epidemic hepatitis. *Amer. J. Path.* 20:471, 1944.
35. Wills, E. J. Acute infective hepatitis. *Arch. Path.* (Chicago) 86:184, 1968.
36. Biava, C., and Mukhlova-Montiel, M. Electron microscopic observations on Councilman-like acidophilic bodies and other forms of acidophilic changes in human liver cells. *Amer. J. Path.* 46:775, 1965.
37. Lucké, B., and Mallory, T. B. The fulminant form of epidemic hepatitis. *Amer. J. Path.* 22:867, 1946.
38. Tisdale, W. A. Subacute hepatitis. *New Eng. J. Med.* 268:85, 138, 1963.
39. Steer, A. Pathology of hemorrhagic fever. *Amer. J. Path.* 31:201, 1955.
40. Kremers, M. Y. Arthropod-borne viral hemorrhagic fevers. *Bull. Int. Acad. Path.* 6:57, 1965.
41. Rapp, F., and Buckley, S. M. Studies with the etiologic agent of Argentinian epidemic hemorrhagic fever (Junin virus). *Amer. J. Path.* 40:63, 1962.
42. Child, P. L., MacKenzie, R. B., Valverde, L. R., and Johnson, K. M. Bolivian hemorrhagic fever. *Arch. Path.* (Chicago) 83:434, 1967.
43. Miller, J. K., Tompkins, V. N., and Sieracki, J. C. Pathology of Colorado tick fever in experimental animals. *Arch. Path.* (Chicago) 72:149, 1961.
44. Chapman, I., and Jimenez, F. A. Aleutian-mink disease in man. *New Eng. J. Med.* 269:1171, 1963.
45. Henson, J. B., Gorham, J. R., Padgett, G. A., and Davis, W. C. Pathogenesis of the glomerular lesions in Aleutian disease of mink. *Arch. Path.* (Chicago) 87:21, 1969.

GENERAL REFERENCES

Fenwick, M. L., and Watkins, J. F. Viruses and viral infection. In Florey, H. W. (Ed.), *General Pathology* (4th ed.). Philadelphia: Saunders, 1970, pp. 898–931. (An excellent, concise discussion of the general nature of viruses and the mechanism of viral infections.)

Horsfall, F. L., Jr., and Tamm, I. (Eds.). *Viral and Rickettsial Infections of Man* (4th ed.). Philadelphia: Lippincott, 1965. (An authoritative review of the biologic, morphologic, and clinical aspects of these infections.)

8 FUNGUS, PROTOZOAN, HELMINTHIC, AND ARTHROPODAL DISEASES

FUNGUS INFECTIONS

A *fungus* is a thallophytic plant which is destitute of chlorophyll and which usually reproduces through asexual spores. The classes of true fungi *(Eumycetes)* are: (1) *phycomycetes* (genus *Mucor*), characterized by nonseptate hyphae and the presence of zygospores; (2) *ascomycetes,* which are almost entirely nonpathogenic and are characterized by septate hyphae and ascospore production; (3) *basidiomycetes* (rusts, smuts, mushrooms), which are nonpathogenic and have clublike hyphae bearing spores; and (4) *deuteromycetes (fungi imperfecti)* (genera *Blastomyces, Cryptococcus, Coccidiodes, Histoplasma, Candida, Sporotrichum, Penicillium, Aspergillus, Trichophyton,* and *Epidermophyton*), which have septate hyphae and freeborn spores or conidia and in which no sexual cycle is known. Another class, *pseudomycetes* (genera *Actinomyces, Nocardia, Streptothrix,* and *Erysipelothrix*), has forms with thin, branching hyphae; the genera are variously grouped as higher bacteria or fungi. FUNGI:

Yeasts are oval or spherical unicellular fungi, ordinarily without hyphae, which usually reproduce by gemmation (budding). True yeasts rarely cause disease in man. Pathogenic yeastlike fungi include *Blastomyces* species, *Candida albicans, Cryptococcus neoformans, Coccidioides immitis,* and *Histoplasma capsulatum.* Yeasts

Some terms relating to fungi are defined below.

Hypha. Threadlike filament formed by many fungi. The *thallus* is the main hypha. Definitions

Mycelium. Network or matted mass of branching hyphae.

Spore. Primitive, usually unicellular reproductive body produced by many fungi.

Arthrospore. Asexual spore formed of hypha segments and released by disarticulation.

Ascospore. Sexual spore enclosed, usually in groups of 4 or 8, in a sac *(ascus).*

Blastospore. Asexual spore produced by budding *(gemmation).*

Chlamydospore. Large asexual intercalary or terminal spore with a tough, frequently double-contoured wall, undergoing encystment.

Conidium. Asexual spore formed from the vegetative portion of a fungus by the development of a dividing partition *(abstriction),* budding, or septate division.

Conidiophore. Hypha bearing conidia by abstriction.

Endospore. Spore formed within an outer envelope.

Oöspore. Spore resulting from union of a male *(antheridium)* and female *(oosporangium)* spore.

Zygospore. Spore resulting from union of two similar sexual cells *(gametes).*

Coenocyte. Fungus composed of a number of protoplasts united in a single large cell.

Systemic infections:

Systemic fungus infections are not common in the United States, but are increasing in frequency, especially as *opportunistic fungus infections* [1] in persons with diabetes mellitus, avitaminosis, malnutrition, leukemia, Hodgkin's disease, aplastic anemia, and burns. Widespread systemic fungus infections, especially candidiasis, have occurred in persons undergoing prolonged antibiotic therapy, presumably because of suppression of the bacterial flora ordinarily checking fungus growth, and/or adrenocorticosteroid therapy, because of suppression of the inflammatory response [2]. Experimentally the administration of cortisone with antibiotics or alone renders animals highly susceptible to fatal pulmonary infection by inhalation of *Aspergillus flavus* spores [3]. In patients with leukemia the neutropenia which may be a manifestation of the disease or the result of antileukemic therapy is the most important factor in the development of fungus infections [4]. The frequent use of antibiotics and steroids in such patients is also a predisposing factor. Less commonly, deep mycoses occur in other types of malignant neoplasm due to the suppression of granulocytopoiesis by cancer chemotherapeutic agents and of the inflammatory response by the use of adrenocorticosteroid therapy.

clinical features

Many fungus infections closely resemble tuberculosis clinically and histologically. *Pulmonary mycoses* are characterized *clinically* by fever, malaise, weakness, night sweats, weight loss, cough, and bloody and/or purulent sputum. *Meningitic mycoses* produce headache, nuchal rigidity, dizziness, and cerebrospinal fluid changes (increased pressure and protein, 50 to 500 lymphocytes per cubic millimeter of fluid, decreased sugar and chloride levels). Since systemic fungus infections are not distinctive clinically, *diagnosis* depends on smear, tissue section, or culture. The causative organism is often easily identified in the lesions. The best techniques are the periodic acid-Schiff (PAS), Gomori silver methenamine, and Gridley stains.

pathologic changes

The *lesions* in deep fungus infections are granulomatous, frequently with accompanying suppuration. Much of the tissue necrosis is due to the development of hypersensitivity to the proteins of the fungi.

Superficial infections

Superficial fungus infections such as ringworm, athlete's foot, and thrush are very common in the United States and elsewhere. Unless they become secondarily infected, the lesions are usually not important except for the itching they produce.

1. Systemic Fungus Infections

ACTINOMYCOSIS: Cause

The *cause of actinomycosis* is *Actinomyces israeli* (*A. bovis,* ray fungus), an anaerobic pseudomycete with gram-positive hyphae and gram-negative, club-shaped peripheral bodies.

Incidence

Actinomycosis is a common mycosis in man, especially in farmers. It is more common in horses, cattle, and pigs than in humans.

Transmission

Infections of the jaw (lumpy jaw) arise through breaks in the buccal mucosa from chewing grain or through the root of a carious tooth. Primary lesions of the *intestines* are due to ingestion of fungi, and of the *lungs,* to inhalation.

Pathologic changes

The *most common lesion* (50 percent of the cases) occurs in the *lower jaw* and *neck* (cervicofacial actinomycosis). A firm mass develops, breaks down, and becomes riddled with abscesses, multiple sinuses opening onto the skin. There is destruction of fibrous tissue, muscle, and bone. The lesions extend by direct contiguity. Similar changes occur in the cecum, appendix, and rectum, with numerous sinuses forming. Multiple abscesses develop in the lungs, which may become involved by transdiaphragmatic spread of abdominal actinomycosis. The central nervous system, kidneys, or legs (mycetoma) may be involved. Liver abscesses may occur via the portal vein or by direct extension. *Microscopically the lesions are granulomatous* (fibrosis, lymphocytes, epithelioid cells, and multinucleated giant cells) *and suppurative* (clusters of polymorphonuclear leukocytes), and contain tiny yellow sulfur granules called *Drusen.* These granules show a central felted mass of mycelial filaments, with peripheral club-shaped bodies.

NOCARDIOSIS

Nocardiosis is an uncommon fungus infection caused by the aerobic, gram-positive, and sometimes acid-fast *Nocardia asteroides.* It occasionally occurs in apparently healthy individuals, but most cases develop in patients with debilitating diseases [5]. Those with malignant neoplasms, such as Hodgkin's disease, leukemia, and carcinoma of the breast or colon, are especially susceptible. The infection is usually primary in the *lungs* due to inhalation of the fungi. Hematogenous dissemination leads to involvement of the heart, spleen, kidneys, and brain. The *lesions* are abscesses, sometimes with a surrounding granulomatous reaction. *Nocardia* species are occasionally the causative organism in mycetoma.

MYCETOMA: Causes

Mycetoma (maduromycosis) is caused by a variety of fungi including *Madurella mycetomi, M. grisea, Phialophora jeanselmei, Allescheria boydii, Cephalosporium* species, *Nocardia* species, *Streptomyces* species, and *Actinomyces bovis.* The *distribution* is usually tropical, especially in people customarily going barefoot. The fungi enter the skin via wounds caused by thorns or fish bones.

Pathologic changes

There is subcutaneous swelling of the foot (Madura foot) or occasionally the hand, and numerous sinuses appear on the skin. The deeper tissues and even bones of the foot may become extensively involved. *Grains* 1 to 2 mm. in diameter are discharged through the sinus tracts. These may be yellow, red, brown, or black. *Microscopically* they consist of masses of hyphae or branching filaments of the causative fungus, surrounded by an irregular, homogeneous, eosinophilic coating [6]. This probably represents an antigen-antibody reaction.

NORTH AMERICAN BLASTOMYCOSIS: Cause

Blastomyces dermatiditis, a yeastlike, double-contoured fungus, 5 to 15μ in diameter, which buds in tissue, produces *North American blastomycosis* (Gilchrist's disease). It occurs mainly in the United States and rarely in Canada and England. Men are infected more often than women.

Transmission

The primary cutaneous form is due to inoculation; the pulmonary type (which usually leads to generalized blastomycosis), to inhalation.

Pathologic changes

Cutaneous blastomycosis [7] begins as a papule, which breaks down after weeks or months to produce single or multiple elevated red ulcers; the organisms are in small abscesses in the raised edges of the ulcers (and/or within giant cells). The marked hyperplasia of the surrounding epidermis and the lengthening of the rete pegs may cause diagnostic confusion with epidermoid carcinoma. *Generalized blastomycosis* (usually fatal) is characterized by pyemia, with abscesses in the lungs, bones, subcutaneous tissues, and elsewhere. Caseous nodules with many giant cells may surround the suppurative zone.

SOUTH AMERICAN BLASTOMYCOSIS

South American blastomycosis (paracoccidioidal granuloma) is caused by *B. brasiliensis* and is similar to North American blastomycosis, except that lesions in lymph nodes and mucous membranes are prominent.

CRYPTOCOCCOSIS (TORULOSIS): Cause

Cryptococcus neoformans (Torula histolytica, Debaryomyces hominis), a yeastlike fungus, 5 to 10μ in diameter, which buds and has a thick mucinous capsule, causes *cryptococcosis.* Some strains are saprophytic or of low pathogenicity, and infections with such strains may be endogenous. Its *distribution* is worldwide and the reported incidence of cryptococcosis is increasing. Cryptococcosis occurs more frequently in patients with Hodgkin's disease, lymphosarcoma, leukemia, or multiple myeloma than in healthy persons or in patients with other malignant diseases. *Transmission* is by inhalation in most cases.

Pathologic changes [8]

Primary lesions are often in the *lungs,* where they are mucinous or fibrotic, or in the *skin,* where one or more abscesses may form. Hematogenous spread is common. The most important lesions are in the *central nervous system,* by hematogenous metastasis from the lungs, cryptococcosis being the most common type of mycotic meningitis. Many organisms are found in the spinal fluid, meninges *(torula meningitis),* and perivascular cerebral spaces. The yeast may occur in free, jelly-like masses. A chronic inflammatory reaction in the meninges, with giant cells and fibrosis, may occur, but in some cases it is surprisingly slight. Cysts 1 to 2 mm. in diameter may form in the brain. The meningoencephalitis is usually fatal within a period of months.

TORULOPSIS INFECTIONS

Infections due to *Torulopsis glabrata* [9], a yeast of the Cryptococcaceae family, are rare and usually occur in patients with leukemia, lymphoma, or a carcinoma. This organism is round or ovoid, measures 2 to 4μ in diameter, and reproduces by budding. Lesions develop in the esophagus, lungs, and kidneys in the form of microabscesses which sometimes have a surrounding granulomatous reaction.

COCCIDIOIDOMYCOSIS: Cause

The cause of *coccidioidomycosis* is *Coccidioides immitis,* a double-contoured, encapsulated fungus which reproduces by endosporulation, is 10 to 80μ in diameter, and may contain over 100 endospores. The disease occurs in the southwestern United States, especially San Joaquin Valley in California. The coccidioidin skin test is positive in about 75 percent of the Valley residents. *Transmission* is by inhalation of the fungus in dust.

Pathologic changes

Primary pulmonary coccidioidomycosis (San Joaquin Valley fever, desert rheumatism) is mild and often subclinical, lasting 1 to 2 weeks. Organisms are present in the sputum. X-rays show pneumonic consolidation in the lungs and enlargement of the mediastinal lymph nodes. Calcified nodules form in the lungs and lymph nodes. Caseous foci may occur in these sites, and organisms may be found in both caseous and calcified lesions. Subcutaneous nodules, allergic in type, occasionally appear late in the disease. *Progressive coccidioidomycosis (coccidioidal granuloma),* with about 50 percent fatality, develops in approximately 0.2 percent of the cases. Granulomatous nodules and abscesses form in the subcutaneous tissues, bones, viscera, and brain.

RHINOSPORIDIOSIS: Cause

The cause of *rhinosporidiosis* is *Rhinosporidium seeberi,* a large, endosporulating fungus. The disease is endemic in India and Ceylon; females are rarely affected.

Pathologic changes

Pinkish red, friable polypoid masses form on the *nasal mucosa* and less commonly on the conjunctiva or in the urethra. *Sporocysts,* measuring 200 to 300μ and packed with endospores, appear as white or yellow dots in these masses. Smaller sporocysts have a double-contoured wall. The submucosal cellular reaction consists of lymphocytes, plasmocytes, and foreign-body giant cells.

HISTOPLASMOSIS: Cause

Histoplasmosis is caused by *Histoplasma capsulatum,* a tiny (1 to 5μ), budding, yeastlike fungus. Its *distribution* is mainly in the United States, but is probably worldwide. *Transmission* is usually by oral ingestion or inhalation. *H. capsulatum* is commonly found in soil, starling excreta, chicken coops, pigeon lofts, caves, and silos.

Clinical features

Fever, ulcers in the mouth, larynx, and pharynx, hepatomegaly, splenomegaly, lymphadenopathy, leukopenia, anemia, and emaciation occur. Sometimes there are signs of a pulmonary mycosis; in the mild form these are influenza-like. In most cases the histoplasmin skin test is positive after a few weeks.

Pathologic changes

The entire reticuloendothelial system is invaded, organisms being most common in the *liver, spleen, lymph nodes,* and *bone marrow.* Granuloma formation with caseation or reticuloendothelial cell proliferation may occur. Chronic granulomatous lesions in the lungs are now frequently recognized as due to *Histoplasma capsulatum,* which has been demonstrated in granulomatous nodules previously considered tuberculous [10]. A healed primary complex has been demonstrated in histoplasmosis. Occasional cases of fibrous constrictive pericarditis have been caused by *H. capsulatum* [11]. Ulceration of the oral mucosa or intestine may be prominent. The central nervous system is involved in about 10 percent of the cases. Progressive disease is usually fatal in less than a year, the adrenal glands often being involved in fatal cases. Addison's disease may result from bilateral adrenal destruction. Experimentally in *primary infection* spores are engulfed by neutrophils and epithelioid cells and other macrophages. Rupture of spore walls liberates the infective yeastlike bodies, which are disseminated through the bloodstream. Severe tissue destruction occurs at the primary site. In *reinfection histoplasmosis* the process is restricted locally, and often heals within a few weeks [12].

SPOROTRICHOSIS: Cause

Sporotrichum schenckii is the cause of *sporotrichosis.* The disease is common in gardners and florists, who acquire it through a break in the skin, especially from thorn pricks.

Pathologic changes

Nodules, which may soften and ulcerate, form at the entry site *(sporotrichotic chancre)*, usually the hand, and along the lymphatics of the arm. *Microscopically* there is an abscess surrounded by a granulomatous zone and giant cells. *Asteroid bodies*, each consisting of a central chlamydospore surrounded by a stellate arrangement of eosinophilic material, are found in the skin lesions [13]. This material probably represents an antigen-antibody reaction. Generalized disease is rare, but pulmonary sporotrichosis and leptomeningitis [14] occasionally occur.

CHROMOBLASTOMYCOSIS:

The cause of *chromoblastomycosis, Hormodendrum pedrosoi (Fonsecaea pedrosoi)*, is transmitted through a skin injury, especially a thorn prick.

Pathologic changes

Warty nodules, which contain the brown septate organisms in giant cells or tiny abscesses, appear on the lower (occasionally upper) extremities. The epidermis is hyperplastic. Granulomatous nodules appear also in subcutaneous tissue.

CANDIDIASIS: Cause

Candida (Monilia) albicans, a yeastlike fungus, causes *candidiasis (moniliasis)*. Its *distribution* is worldwide, and about 15 percent of normal persons harbor the fungus. Infection is more common in diabetics than nondiabetics, and infants are frequently affected. Generalized candidiasis may occur following prolonged antibiotic therapy.

Pathologic changes

Infection, usually surface in type, is called *thrush* when on the mucous membranes of the mouth. The esophageal and vaginal mucosa are also commonly involved. Grayish white membranes (patches composing mycelia) appear, with destruction of the mucosal epithelium and often with secondary bacterial infection. Skin infections are usually superficial, paronychia being common. Involved in systemic candidiasis are the lungs, kidneys, retina, meninges, and valvular endocardium. Candidial endocarditis occurs in drug addicts and following cardiac surgery [15].

PENICILLIOSIS

Penicilliosis is rare; it is caused by *Penicillium* species such as *P. crustaceum* and *P. commune* [16]. These fungi form septate and branching hyphae and chlamydospores. Infections are primary in the lungs and occur in otherwise healthy persons or those with leukemia or chronic bronchitis. The *pulmonary lesions* may be hemorrhagic infarcts due to blocking of pulmonary arteries by mycelial masses of fungi and thrombi. Hemorrhagic infarction may occur in the brain and other organs due to hematogenous dissemination of the fungi.

ASPERGILLOSIS: Causes

The most common cause of *aspergillosis* is *Aspergillus fumigatus*, a blue-green mold. *A. nidulans, A. flavus*, and *A. niger* occasionally infect man. Nonpathogenic species are found on bread. Internal aspergillus infections usually occur in patients with a debilitating disease, especially those on prolonged antibiotic or steroid therapy, and in diabetics.

Pathologic changes

The most frequent lesion is in the external ear and auditory canal *(otomycosis)*, masses of mycelium sometimes plugging the meatus. *Ulcers* and *wounds* are common sites of infection. Rarely the lungs, paranasal sinuses, heart valves, and brain are involved, with tissue necrosis and suppuration. *Pulmonary aspergillosis* may occur as an intracavitary fungus mass *(aspergilloma)* or as a frequently bilateral bronchopneumonia [17]. Abscesses develop in the pulmonary parenchyma. These consist of a mycelium of sinuous, septate hyphae radiating from a center and branching freely. The mycelium is surrounded by degenerated neutrophils and necrotic tissue.

MUCORMYCOSIS: Cause

Mucormycosis (phycomycosis) [18] is caused by *Mucor* and *Rhizopus* species, especially *Mucor corymbifer*. These are phycomycetes with nonseptate coenocytic hyphae 4 to 20μ wide and up to 200μ long. Spores are inhaled or ingested. Infections are increasing in the United States, particularly in patients on steroids, antibiotics, or cancer chemotherapy. About 80 percent of the associated malignancies have been lymphomas [19]. About 25 percent of cases of mucormycosis occur in diabetics. A few cases have developed in patients with severe burns [20].

Pathologic changes

Vascular invasion is common, and thrombi containing hyphae may be encountered. Infection progresses rapidly in the lungs where the lesions are a combination of acute inflammation and infarction due to vascular obstruction by masses of hyphae [21]. The brain may be invaded by direct extension from the nose and paranasal sinuses or by hematogenous spread. Foci of necrosis containing polymorphonuclear leukocytes and the large hyphae of the organism occur in the cerebrum [22]. The meninges are also involved. The eyes are commonly infected in the form of a severe keratitis which may perforate the cornea.

2. Superficial Fungus Infections (Dermatomycoses)

Though other fungi (such as *Candida albicans*), and even bacteria, can produce indistinguishable infections, the true dermatophytes are *Trichophyton* (infecting hair, skin, and nails), *Microsporum* (hair and skin), and *Epidermophyton* (skin and nails). Because of hypersensitivity to the dermatophytes *(dermatophytid)*, a nonspecific id reaction, with small vesicles (blisters) and scales, may occur at a distance from the infection site.

TINEA PEDIS

In *tinea pedis (athlete's foot)* the fungi are picked up on floors of baths or gymnasiums. Lesions, which are more common in men than in women, usually begin interdigitally, spreading to the soles and toenails. Minute intra-epidermal vesicles as well as deep fissures appear. Fungi occur in the keratinized epidermis of skin and nails. Secondary streptococcal infection, with lymphangitis and inguinal lymphadenitis, is common.

TINEA CRURIS

Tinea cruris ("jock itch") occurs as itching, reddish brown patches or rings in the groin and the perianal and axillary regions.

TINEA CORPORIS

Tinea corporis (ringworm) infects the general body surface. The rings often coalesce. Papules are present at the peripheries. Ulceration may occur. The epidermis is hyperplastic and contains the fungi. There is a chronic inflammatory reaction in the superficial dermis; when this is marked, with polymorphonuclear leukocytes and giant cells, it is a localized immune reaction called a *kerion*.

TINEA CAPITIS

Tinea capitis (ringworm of the scalp) is commonly caused by *Microsporum audouini* and *M. lanosum*. The hair is brittle and lusterless; scaly reddish patches with areas of loss of hair (alopecia) occur. Organisms are found in the epidermis and hair follicles. Deep abscesses with giant cells may form. Infections of the beard are called *tinea barbae (mycosis parasitica)*.

TINEA FAVOSA

Tinea favosa infects the scalp or other skin surfaces and produces cup-shaped crusts composed of fungi and necrotic epidermal cells. The lesions have a mousy odor.

TINEA VERSICOLOR

Tinea (pityriasis) versicolor is a mild macular eruption with scaling and browning of the affected skin. It is caused by *Malassezia furfur (Microsporon furfur).* Fungi are found in the scaling epidermis as fragments of mycelia and clusters of spores.

PROTOZOAN INFECTIONS

PROTOZOA

Protozoa are unicellular animals occurring singly or in colonies. The parasitic protozoa of man are grouped in four classes: (1) *Sarcodina* (Rhizopoda) – characterized by the formation of pseudopodia; contains the pathogenic amebae, such as *Entamoeba histolytica, Dientamoeba fragilis,* and *Iodamoeba butschlii;* (2) *Infusoria* – characterized by cilia; the only pathogen is *Balantidium coli;* (3) *Mastigophora* – characterized by flagella; includes three pathogenic genera, *Trichomonas, Leishmania,* and *Trypanosoma;* nonpathogenic species include *Enteromonas hominis, Chilomastix mesnili,* and *Giardia lamblia;* and (4) *Sporozoa* – characterized by lack of definite organs for locomotion and food procurement; all members are parasitic; the genera are *Isospora, Plasmodium, Sarcocystis,* and possibly *Toxoplasma.*

1. Amebic Infections

AMEBIASIS: Cause

Amebiasis is caused by *Entamoeba histolytica,* a protozoan found in feces as trophozoites, precystic forms, and cysts. The *trophozoite,* the only form found in tissues, is 18 to 30μ in diameter and moves by pseudopodia. Its cytoplasm may contain erythrocytes and vacuoles. This distinguishes *E. histolytica* from the harmless *Entamoeba coli.* The *cyst* of *E. histolytica* is spherical with a refractile wall and measures 5 to 20μ. Its cytoplasm contains 1 to 4 nuclei.

Transmission

Usually transmission occurs by ingestion of food or water contaminated with human feces containing cysts of *E. histolytica.* Food is contaminated by flies and the soiled fingers of food handlers. Night soil is a source of infection in the Orient. Cysts are ingested and pass into the small intestine where they excyst, each releasing four amebulae. These travel to the colon and develop into trophozoites which invade the mucosa and multiply in colonies in the submucosa. The organisms secrete proteolytic enzymes, which aid in their spread through the tissues. They also enter the portal venules and lymphatics.

Clinical features

Clinically amebiasis occurs in both temperate and tropical regions, being more prevalent in the latter. It is more common in males than females, and in rural than urban areas. Many persons are carriers without clinical symptoms. Those persons with clinical amebiasis (amebic dysentery) have diarrhea with tenesmus. Blood, mucus, trophozoites, cysts, "mouse-eaten" macrophages, "pyknotic bodies" (from nuclear fragments), and Charcot-Leyden crystals are present in the feces. Liver "abscess" may be relatively silent until perforation. Lung "abscess" is rapidly fatal. About 3500 cases of amebiasis with 100 deaths occur in the United States annually.

Pathologic changes

In many cases a state of equilibrium develops between the organisms and the host, with small or minimal lesions and chronic infection (carrier state). *Amebic dysentery* is characterized by the formation of *deep, ragged ulcers with undermined edges in the colon and rectum.* Because of the undermining, amebic lesions are called *flask-shaped* or *water-bottle ulcers.* The intervening mucosa appears intact. *Microscopically* the ulcer margins and floor show little inflammatory reaction, with only a few macrophages and lymphocytes, unless secondary bacterial infection is present. Hordes of amebae are found in the submucosa.

Complications

Complications of amebic dysentery include:

1. *Liver "abscess."* This is common (in 40 percent of the autopsied cases) due to infiltration of the portal venules. In the majority of cases there are multiple abscesses, occurring in the right lobe. The abscesses are due to liquefactive necrosis of liver cells by the proteolytic enzymes of the amebae. Brown "anchovy sauce" material fills the cavity. The wall consists of necrotic liver cells infiltrated with lymphocytes and plasma cells, and there are many amebae. Liver "abscess" occurs more frequently in men than in women by 10:1.

2. *Rupture of a liver "abscess"* into the right pleural cavity, right lung, pericardial sac, stomach, lumbar region, colon, bile ducts, or duodenum (in decreasing order of frequency).

3. *Lung "abscess."* This is most common at the base of the right lung due to perforation of the diaphragm by a liver "abscess.". Multiple lung abscesses may result from embolism of amebae-containing thrombi from the hepatic veins. The process in the lung is similar to that in the liver.

4. *Brain "abscess."* This is rare, usually being associated with liver involvement. It develops by extension of a leptomeningitis which is hematogenous in origin. The brain lesion is usually single and in a cerebral hemisphere. It may be up to 10 cm. in diameter and is similar to the abscess in the liver.

5. *Amebiasis of the skin.* This usually results from cutaneous rupture of a hepatic abscess or from surgery on a patient with amebiasis. The abdominal skin drains "anchovy sauce" material.

6. *Amebic granuloma (ameboma) of the colon.* This is secondary to ulceration, a dense mass of fibrous adhesions developing in the cecum, hepatic and splenic flexures, or sigmoid colon.

DIENTAMEBIASIS: Cause

Dientamoeba fragilis, an erythrocytophagic ameba of relatively low pathogenicity, occasionally causes human infection. Only a binucleated trophozoite form about 10μ in diameter is known. *Transmission* is by the ingestion of trophozoites.

Pathologic changes

This ameba has been implicated in several cases of *acute appendicitis* and fibrosis of the appendix. They remain in the appendiceal lumen and do not invade tissues. In most cases they are found in association with other parasites such as *Chilomastix mesnili, Entamoeba coli, Giardia lamblia, Enterobius vermicularis,* or *Strongyloides stercoralis.*

2. Infusorial Infection

BALANTIDIASIS: Cause

The cause of *balantidiasis* is *Balantidium coli,* a large ciliated, infusorial parasite of pigs. The cyst is round or ovoid and measures 40 to 60μ in diameter. The trophozoite is 30 to 150μ long and 40 to 55μ wide. Man is occasionally infected by the ingestion of cysts.

Pathologic changes [23]

In some persons the organism causes only slight lesions in the colon; in others there is a *balantidial colitis* similar to that caused by *E. histolytica.* The more acute lesions tend to become gangrenous, and hemorrhage and perforation of the undermined ulcers is common. Rarely balantidia have caused acute appendicitis, and a few cases of chronic balantidial appendicitis have been reported. Liver abscess does not occur.

3. Flagellate Infections

TRICHOMONIASIS: Cause

Trichomoniasis is usually due to *Trichomonas vaginalis,* a protozoan with 3 to 5 anterior flagella. Two other trichomonads found in man, *T. hominis,* an inhabitant of the intestine, and *T. tenax,* which lives in the mouth, have not been proved to be pathogenic.

Pathologic changes

In *trichomonal vaginitis* the vaginal wall is injected and shows petechiae. The mucosa may be focally eroded. The submucosa is infiltrated with lymphocytes and a few polymorphonuclear leukocytes. In the male similar changes may occur in the urethra, prostate, and seminal vesicles, so that husband-wife infections are common. Some or perhaps most of the pathologic changes are due to secondary bacterial invaders.

CUTANEOUS LEISHMANIASIS: Cause

The cause of *cutaneous leishmaniasis* is *Leishmania tropica,* an ovoid, nonflagellated body measuring 2 by 2.5μ. *Transmission* is by the sandfly *Phlebotomus papatasii* and by direct contact. *Synonyms* are Oriental sore, tropical ulcer, Bagdad button, Aleppo boil, and Lahore sore.

Pathologic changes

The typical *papule* appears on an exposed part of the body. This enlarges and ulcerates, forming a sharply punched-out *crater* with raised, indurated edges. *Microscopically* the base consists of granulation tissue, and the dermis is infiltrated by mononuclear cells. The epidermis is hyperplastic, and the rete pegs extend down into the dermis, simulating epidermoid carcinoma.

MUCOCUTANEOUS LEISHMANIASIS:

Mucocutaneous leishmaniasis (American leishmaniasis, espundia, forest yaws) is caused by *Leishmania braziliensis. Transmission* is probably by sandflies, especially *Phlebotomus intermedius.*

Pathologic changes

The skin lesions are like those of cutaneous leishmaniasis. In about 20 percent of the cases there are also lesions of the mucous membranes of the nose, pharynx, larynx, and buccal cavity. The mucosa is red, elevated, firm, and granular. It is infiltrated by mononuclear cells, some of which contain protozoa.

KALA-AZAR: Cause

Kala-azar (visceral leishmaniasis, dumdum fever) is caused by *Leishmania donovani,* an ovoid, nonflagellated body measuring 2 to 4 by 1 to 2μ. *Transmission* is by the bite of sandflies such as *Phlebotomus argentipes* in India.

Clinical features

Clinically the disease is characterized by fever, hepatomegaly and splenomegaly, lymphadenopathy, leukopenia, anemia, and hyperglobulinemia. Death usually occurs within 2 years in untreated patients.

Pathologic changes

Kala-azar is characterized by the presence of hordes of *Leishman-Donovan bodies* in the reticuloendothelial cells. The spleen is dark red (congestion), and the malpighian corpuscles are conspicuous; the organ may weigh over 4000 gm. The liver is next most frequently affected, being enlarged (sometimes weighing over 2000 gm.) and presenting a grayish yellow parenchyma. The bone marrow is soft and red. The lymph nodes are enlarged, soft, and gray. In all organs there is a multiplication of the reticuloendothelial cells.

Complications

Complications include noma (an ulcerative, gangrenous stomatitis), pneumonia, and ulcerative colitis.

AFRICAN SLEEPING SICKNESS: Cause

African sleeping sickness is produced by two morphologically identical trypanosomes, *Trypanosoma rhodesiense,* the etiologic agent of East African sleeping sickness, and *Trypanosoma gambiense,* the cause of the mid-African type. *Transmission* is by the bite of a tsetse fly, usually *Glossina morsitans* for *T. rhodesiense* and *Glossina palpalis* for *T. gambiense.*

Clinical features

Clinically the two types are similar, but the course is more acute and epidemics much less common in the East African form. The incubation period is usually 1 to 2 weeks. The stage of lymph node invasion is characterized by episodes of fever as organisms are released, lymphadenopathy (especially in the posterior cervical triangle), hepatomegaly, and splenomegaly. In the later stage of nervous system invasion there are severe headaches with progressive mental dullness, apathy, and somnolence. Emaciation becomes extreme in chronic cases.

Pathologic changes

The lymph nodes in the early stages are enlarged, soft, and pinkish red. Many trypanosomes can be expressed from them. Later the nodes become small and firm. There is an increased amount of slightly cloudy cerebrospinal fluid. The brain is edematous, and the Virchow-Robin spaces are filled with lymphocytes, plasmocytes, and macrophages. In the meninges and brain are characteristic *morular cells,* presumably macrophages which have ingested foreign material in the form of vacuoles, each of which projects onto the surface, giving the cell a mulberry appearance.

CHAGAS' DISEASE:

The cause of *Chagas' disease* is *Trypanosoma cruzi.* In the blood these are typically thin, undulating organisms with a free flagellum and about 20μ long. The nonflagellated leishmanial form is 1.5 to 4μ long and pear-shaped. *Transmission* is by rubbing the feces of a reduviid bug (most commonly *Panstrongylus megistus*) into an abrasion or bite on the skin or a mucous membrane.

Clinical features

Clinically the incubation period is 1 to 4 weeks. Children are the most common victims. The acute form, which lasts about a month, is typified by high fever, severe edema of one or both eyelids (Romaña's sign), a myxedema-like swelling of the skin, lymphadenopathy, hepatomegaly, splenomegaly, nervousness, and tachycardia. Trypanosomes are found in the blood. In children who survive the acute form and more often in adults, a chronic form occurs. The clinical picture depends on the organ involvement – cardiac, meningoencephalitic, myxedematous, and adrenal types occur.

Pathologic changes

A *chagoma* may occur beneath the site of entry, which is commonly at the outer canthus of the eye or at an angle of the lips. The skin is edematous, and the dermis is infiltrated with neutrophils, lymphocytes, and macrophages. The lesion becomes encapsulated. Leishmania multiply in the lymph nodes and enter the blood as trypanosomes during febrile episodes. Localization is common in the heart, which is dilated and flabby, with a pale, soft myocardium. The muscle fibers are enlarged and laden with parasites in their leishmanial form. There is an intense infiltration by mononuclear cells and a few eosinophils.

4. Sporozoan Infections

MALARIA: Cause

Malaria is caused by several *species of plasmodia.* The important ones are *Plasmodium vivax* (tertian malaria), *P. malariae* (quartan malaria), and *P. falciparum* (malignant tertian or estivo-autumnal malaria). *P. knowlesi* is used in the treatment of general paresis. *Transmission* is by the bite of the *female anopheles mosquito.* A few cases result from blood transfusions or transplacental transmission. About 20 million new cases of malaria appear throughout the world each year.

Clinical features

Clinically malaria is characterized by periodic paroxysms of chills and high fever. The paroxysms coincide with the cyclic release of merozoites by rupture of infested erythrocytes. In *P. vivax* infections the attacks of chills and fever occur every 48 hours; in *P. malariae* infections, every 72 hours; and in *P. falciparum* infections, every 24 to 48 hours. During the paroxysms there are also headache, sweating, and prostration. Progressive hepatomegaly and splenomegaly develop. Patients with malaria sometimes show a false positive serologic test for syphilis.

Pathologic changes

There are four basic processes: (1) hypertrophy and hyperplasia of the reticuloendothelial cells, (2) elaboration of the characteristic malarial pigment by the parasites, (3) blockage of capillaries by parasitized red cells, and (4) secondary effects of the destruction of red cells. *Malarial pigment* is closely related to hematin.

Acute malaria

In *acute malaria* the spleen is moderately enlarged and soft. The sinusoids are distended by erythrocytes and macrophages. The erythrocytes contain parasites, and the phagocytic cells are filled with fine granules of brown or black pigment. The liver is enlarged and brown, with hyperplasia of the Kupffer cells which are filled with pigment. In the brain the cortex is slate gray throughout. The capillaries are distended and many are occluded by agglutinated parasitized red cells. The endothelial cells are filled with pigment. The bone marrow is red and fleshy, with a normoblastic type of hyperplasia.

Chronic malaria

In *chronic malaria* the *characteristic pathologic change* is the enlarged "ague cake" spleen, weighing 500 to 2000 gm. Its capsule is thick and gray, and the organ cuts with increased difficulty. There is marked fibrous proliferation. In and about the malpighian bodies are extensive pigment deposits. The liver is enlarged and microscopically shows Kupffer cell hyperplasia and pigment deposition. Gallstones are common in the thick bile because of excessive bilirubin formation in the prolonged hemolytic process. In the bone marrow there is a prominent hyperplasia of the reticuloendothelial cells and erythropoietic tissue. The brain shows atrophy and a slate gray discoloration. The patient is emaciated.

Blackwater fever

In *blackwater fever* (hemoglobinuric fever), a serious complication of malignant tertian malaria, there is a massive *intravascular hemolysis.* Part of the liberated hemoglobin is excreted in the form of red or black urine; the remainder is converted into bilirubin and excreted in the bile. *Hemoglobin casts* are found in the renal tubules, and the reticuloendothelial cells are filled with pigment.

SARCOCYSTIASIS: Cause

Sarcocystiasis is caused by *Sarcocystis lindemanni,* a sporozoan which elaborates a toxin, sarcocystin. *Transmission* is by ingestion of food or water contaminated with *Sarcocystis.* Spores are liberated in the small intestine, multiply in the intestinal mucosal cells, enter the bloodstream, and lodge in skeletal muscles and the myocardium.

Clinical features

Clinically the infection is rare and mild in man, being principally a disease of sheep, cattle, and horses.

Pathologic changes

In the *myocardium* and in the *muscles* of the larynx, tongue, and extremities, tiny white streaks are seen grossly *(Miescher's tubes).* These are cylindrical cysts within the muscle fibers and consist of outer and inner hyaline membranes; the inner one contains myriads of spherical, ovoid, or sickle-shaped spores *(Rainey's corpuscles)* measuring 4 to 16μ in diameter.

TOXOPLASMOSIS: Cause

Toxoplasmosis is caused by *Toxoplasma gondii,* an obligate intracellular parasite measuring 5 by 2.5μ. *Transmission* is by transplacental infection in the congenital form. The mode of transmission in acquired cases is unknown, but may be by droplet inhalation.

Clinical features

Clinically in the *congenital type* the fetus may be stillborn. If the fetus survives, the neonatal period is marked by convulsions, nystagmus, bilateral patches of chorioretinitis (inflammation of the choroid and retina) with macular involvement, microphthalmos (symmetric smallness of the eye), and internal hydrocephalus (enlargement of the head due to an accumulation of cerebrospinal fluid in the ventricles). Many foci of intracerebral calcification may be demonstrated by x-ray. In the *acquired type* the symptoms are fever, a maculopapular, typhus-like rash, cough, muscle and joint pains, and signs of cardiac failure. A hemagglutination test has been developed for the diagnosis of toxoplasmosis.

Pathologic changes

In the *congenital type* [24] the outstanding lesions are in the brain, the gray matter showing a variety of lesions varying from infiltration by polymorphonuclear leukocytes, lymphocytes, and plasma cells to foci of necrosis and cyst formation. *Calcification* may occur in the foci of necrosis. Small granulomatous lesions may be found in the adrenal glands, liver, spleen, myocardium, and lungs. There may be an interstitial pneumonitis. Chorioretinitis is common. The retina is edematous and the choroid is infiltrated with mononuclear cells. Organisms are found in all lesions. In the *acquired type* [25], changes in the brain are less marked, and granulomatous changes in other organs are more prominent. Chorioretinitis and uveitis are fairly common. The lymph nodes are commonly enlarged and show lymphoid and reticular hyperplasia. Organisms are found within phagocytes. Myocardial involvement is characterized by small foci of necrosis with a mononuclear cell infiltrate, and the organisms parasitize the myofibrils.

PNEUMOCYSTIASIS: Cause

The cause of *pneumocystiasis* is *Pneumocystis carinii,* a protozoan of undetermined classification, or possibly a yeast. It reproduces by binary fission and exists as "cysts" containing eight single-nucleated bodies and measuring about 5μ long. The mode of *transmission* is unknown.

Clinical features

Clinically the infection occurs mainly in infants. Adult infections are usually in patients with leukemia or a lymphoma. There is a notable frequency of coexistent pneumocystis infection and cytomegalic inclusion disease in infants and cytomegaly in the lungs of adults. The course is acute, with fever, marked tachypnea (rapid respiratory rate), dyspnea, and cyanosis. The mortality is about 35 percent.

Pathologic changes [26]

Grossly the lungs show a uniform grayish white consolidation of all lobes. *Microscopically* there is a marked infiltration of the alveolar septa with plasmocytes *(interstitial plasmocytic pneumonitis).* The alveoli are filled with edema fluid or a foamy material consisting of conglomerate parasites. Phagocytized organisms are found in the alveolar septa. Electron microscopic studies reveal that the causative organisms are spherical and contain round or crescentic inner bodies connected by membranes [27].

HELMINTHIC INFECTIONS

HELMINTHS:

The *helminths* which cause disease in man can be classified as follows:

Phylum – Nemathelminthes (roundworms)
  Class – Nematoda (elongated, cylindroid, bilaterally symmetric helminths)
    Genera – *Trichinella*, *Ascaris*, *Trichuris*, *Toxocara*, *Strongyloides*, *Wuchereria (Filaria)*, *Ancylostoma*, *Loa*, *Necator*, *Onchocerca*, *Enterobius*, *Dracunculus*

Phylum – Platyhelminthes (flatworms) (bilaterally symmetric helminths lacking a body cavity and circulatory system)
  Class – Trematoda (exclusively parasitic helminths with suckers and with a digestive system without an anal opening; excretory system terminates in ciliated solenocytes – flame cells)
    Genera – *Schistosoma*, *Paragonimus*, *Fasciolopsis*, *Fasciola*, *Heterophyes*, *Opisthorchis*, *Metagonimus*, *Clonorchis*
  Subclass – Cestoda (exclusively parasitic, hermaphroditic helminths without a digestive system and with a hooked head piece – scolex – and a tape consisting of proglottides)
    Genera – *Diphyllobothrium*, *Taenia*, *Echinococcus*, *Hymenolepis*

Incidence of infection

The *incidence of helminthic infections* depends on climatic and sanitary conditions. The important *climatic factors* are rainfall, type of soil, and temperature; wet, warm areas are especially suitable for the growth of helminths. Important *sanitary factors* are the use of human excreta for fertilizer and the careless disposal of human excreta. Many persons carry worms in their gastrointestinal tracts without ill effects, so that distinction must be made between infestation with a worm and disease caused by a worm.

Pathologic changes

Helminths produce their effects on the body by (1) *mechanical irritation* – they may partially or completely obstruct the intestine or cause cramps or diarrhea by irritating the musculature; (2) *loss of blood or lymph* – anemia may be profound due to the ingestion of blood by intestinal worms; and (3) *action of toxic substances* – this is seen with the tapeworms, especially *Diphyllobothrium latum* which produces a macrocytic anemia, most likely due to a toxic substance elaborated by the worm. The *tissue reaction* to invasive helminths is fibrosis and infiltration by lymphocytes and eosinophils.

1. Nematode (Roundworm) Infections

TRICHINOSIS: Cause

The cause of *trichinosis* (trichinelliasis) is *Trichinella spiralis,* a white, slender, cylindrical, viviparous worm. Adults measure 1.5 to 3.5 mm. by 0.02 mm. The encysted larva is about 1000 by 40μ. About 250 cases of trichinosis are reported annually in the United States.

Transmission

Man contracts trichinosis by eating uncooked or poorly cooked *pork* or *pork products* containing encysted larvae. The cyst is digested in the stomach, and the liberated larvae develop in the duodenum, where after copulation the female invades the wall and bears larvae. Most of the resulting larvae enter the blood or lymph and are carried through the lungs into the systemic circulation. Muscles poor in glycogen are more readily invaded.

Clinical features

Clinically larvae may be found in the blood or spinal fluid. A leukocytosis with an eosinophilia of 20 to 75 percent may be found during larval migration. The diagnosis is established by finding the encysted larvae in a biopsy from a deltoid or gastrocnemius muscle. Such larvae are present without producing clinical manifestations in about 5 percent of adults in the United States.

Pathologic changes

Trichinella larvae are present as white calcified nodules, 1 to 1.5 mm. in diameter, throughout the skeletal muscles. Partly or fully preserved worms, each surrounded by a focus of fibrosis with a few lymphocytes and eosinophils are also found. In *active trichinelliasis* female worms are present within the duodenal crypts or in the muscularis. The skeletal muscles are pale and swollen, with many small white or red foci. The typical *coiled larvae* are seen microscopically within the muscle fibers. The adjacent connective tissue is edematous and infiltrated by lymphocytes and eosinophils. In *severe infections* any organ or tissue may be involved, especially the heart and brain. The heart is pale, flabby, and dilated, with petechiae or ecchymoses in the pericardium, endocardium, and myocardium. Microscopically larvae are found in the myocardial fibers. The larvae are usually necrotic and do not encyst in the myocardium. The interstitial tissue is heavily infiltrated by lymphocytes, with a few eosinophils. The brain is hyperemic. Microscopically there is a diffuse lymphocytic infiltration in the leptomeninges and Virchow-Robin spaces. Necrotic and living larvae can be found in nodules of lymphocytes and glial cells within the brain.

TRICHURIASIS: Cause

Trichuriasis is due to *Trichuris trichiura,* the whipworm. Pinkish gray adults measure 30 to 50 mm. by 1.5 mm., and the anterior three-fifths is whiplike. The lemon-shaped ova measure 50 by 25μ. Ova are ingested and develop through a larval stage to the adults in the intestine. About 400,000 persons are infested in the United States.

Pathologic changes

Minimal infection causes few changes in the intestines. In *severe infection* many worms are found in the cecum, the mucosa being swollen and congested. *Microscopically* there are minute ulcerations, with infiltration by lymphocytes and eosinophils. Other changes are due to the resulting *anemia* (paleness of the viscera, with fatty changes in the heart, liver, and kidneys).

STRONGYLOIDIASIS: Cause

Strongyloidiasis is caused by *Strongyloides stercoralis,* the threadworm. The translucent parasitic adults measure 2 by 0.04 mm. (female) and 0.7 by 0.04 mm. (male). The ovum of the parasitic form is about 50 by 30μ. *Clinically* in the blood the *eosinophils* may reach 40 percent during active infection. An estimated 400,000 individuals are infested in the United States.

Transmission

Filariform (elongated) *larvae* penetrate the skin along the hair shafts, causing a local edema and hyperemia, with small hemorrhages in the dermis. Many larvae remain in the skin, with resulting fibrosis. Others enter the venules and are carried to the lungs. As they migrate from the capillaries into the alveolar spaces, hemorrhages occur into the alveoli, and there is an acute inflammatory reaction. Some larvae invade the bronchial and tracheal mucosa, establishing a parasitic existence there. Occasionally ova are found in the sputum. Other larvae are swallowed and enter the small intestine. They become adults and inhabit the duodenum and upper jejunum. Parasitic males are rarely found, so that reproduction is probably by parthenogenesis. Ova laid in the intestinal mucosa are carried downward in the fecal stream. In *hyperinfection* the *rhabditiform* (rod-shaped) *larvae* metamorphose into dwarf *filariform larvae,* invade the rectal mucosa or perianal skin, and start a new cycle. Outside the host, free-living rhabditiform larvae develop into infective filariform larvae directly or indirectly through a generation of free-living adults.

Pathologic changes

In *mild infections* there are edema and congestion of the small *intestine,* especially the duodenum. In more *severe infections* focal or confluent ulceration occurs. The mucosa of the pancreatic and common bile ducts may show similar changes. *Microscopically* the female *Strongyloides* are found in the crypts of Lieberkühn and in submucosa of the villi with their oviposited eggs. There is an infiltration by lymphocytes, polymorphonuclear leukocytes, and eosinophils. After several months each worm in the tissue is surrounded by a sheath of fibroblasts, with a few mononuclear, epithelioid, and giant cells in the surrounding tissue. Invasion below the muscularis mucosa does not occur.

ANCYLOSTOMIASIS: Cause

Four species of *hookworm* are pathogenic for man: *Ancylostoma duodenale, A. braziliense, A. ceylonicum,* and *Necator americanus. A. braziliense* does not invade the body, but migrates about through the subcutaneous tissues *(creeping eruption, cutaneous larva migrans).* Adult hookworms are grayish and fusiform and measure about 10 by 0.5 mm. They have a buccal capsule with teeth and lancets by which they attach to the intestinal mucosa. The ova measure about 60 by 40μ. Almost 2 million persons are infested with hookworms in the United States.

Transmission

Females deposit eggs in the intestine, and these are passed in the feces. The ova hatch into *rhabditiform larvae* in the ground. Developed *filariform larvae* enter the skin, especially of the feet, causing a slight inflammation in the dermis, with itching *(ground itch).* The larvae pass through the bloodstream to the lungs, causing slight hemorrhages and infiltration by lymphocytes and eosinophils as they enter the alveoli. The larvae migrate up the trachea, being swallowed to enter the jejunum.

Pathologic changes

Typically the first 50 cm. of the jejunum are involved, the mucosa showing petechiae and sometimes ulceration or gangrene, and the submucosa being edematous and infiltrated by polymorphonuclear leukocytes and eosinophils. Pieces of mucosa are clamped in the mouths of the worms. A single hookworm can ingest 0.4 to 0.8 ml. of blood daily. The mesenteric lymph nodes are hyperplastic. The bone marrow may be largely replaced by eosinophils, which accounts in part for the anemia. Due to the anemia, the heart is dilated and sometimes hypertrophic, with fatty degeneration of the myocardium. The liver and kidneys also show fatty changes but to a lesser degree. Hemosiderin may be found in the liver and spleen.

ENTEROBIASIS (OXYURIASIS): Cause

Enterobiasis is caused by *Enterobius vermicularis,* the pinworm. The cylindrical, white adults measure 2 to 5 mm. by 0.15 mm. (male) and 8 to 13 mm. by 0.4 mm. (female). Ova are 55 by 25μ and contain a folded embryo. There are about 18 million cases of pinworm infestation in the United States.

Transmission

Females migrate onto the perianal skin and discharge their eggs, which are carried to the mouth on the fingers or to another host on fomites. The swallowed eggs hatch in the duodenum, and the larvae pass down to the cecal region.

Pathologic changes

In the cecum, appendix, and adjacent colon and ileum there may be a catarrhal inflammation of the mucosa and slight lymphoid hyperplasia. Perianal and perineal inflammation is common due to the migration of gravid females and to scratching.

ASCARIASIS: Cause

Ascaris lumbricoides, the roundworm, causes *ascariasis.* The large white or reddish adult measures about 25 by 0.3 cm. (male) and 30 by 0.5 cm. (female). The serrated ovum is about 60 by 45μ and may contain a folded larva. There are roughly 3 million cases of ascariasis in the United States.

Transmission

Embryos within the ova passed in feces develop into larvae outside the body. Infective ova containing second-stage larvae are swallowed in food or water. The larvae migrate into the intestinal wall, enter the bloodstream, and pass to the liver and lungs. They cause hemorrhage and a mild inflammation in the lungs before passing up the respiratory tree and down the digestive tract into the small intestine, where they establish themselves and mature. Occasionally larvae enter the systemic circulation, to lodge in the spleen, meninges, and elsewhere.

Pathologic changes

Infestation is usually minimal, as are the pathologic changes. When the infestation is heavy, the mass of worms in the intestine may produce obstruction. Occasionally adult worms are found in the peritoneal cavity, bile ducts, or lungs, with resulting purulent inflammation and abscess formation. *Ascaris* ova may produce tuberculoid granulomata in the peritoneum and mesentery. It is possible that *pulmonary calcification* may result from infestation with *Ascaris.*

VISCERAL LARVA MIGRANS: Causes

The causes of *visceral larva migrans* are most commonly *Toxocara canis,* the dog ascarid, less often *Toxocara cati,* the cat ascarid, and occasionally *Strongyloides stercoralis* and certain filaria. The dog and cat ascarids are closely related to *Ascaris lumbricoides.* Infection occurs when the larvae of nematode worms gain access to the extra-intestinal viscera of unnatural hosts or of natural hosts under unfavorable conditions. It is of some importance, since these are helminthic infections which can be transmitted from pets to children.

Transmission

Ova containing second-stage larvae are ingested. The larvae are freed in the upper small intestine, invade the wall, enter the mesenteric venules or lymphatics, and are carried to the liver and other viscera.

Clinical features

Clinically the picture varies from mild cases with only persistent eosinophilia to severe cases with marked eosinophilia, fever, cough, hepatomegaly, hyperglobulinemia, and evidence of cardiac, renal, ocular, and/or cerebral involvement.

Pathologic changes [28]

Miliary white nodules are found mainly in the liver, but also in the lungs, heart, kidneys, brain, eyes, and skeletal muscles. *Microscopically* these are *granulomata,* each formed about a second-stage larva of *T. canis* or *T. cati.* The larva is surrounded by eosinophils and macrophages. At the periphery there are epithelioid cells with occasional giant cells.

FILARIASIS: Causes

Filariasis is infestation by *Wuchereria bancrofti* or *Wuchereria (Brugia) malayi.* The slender, creamy white adults are 40 by 0.1 mm. (male) and 80 by 0.25 mm. (viviparous female). Microfilariae (embryos) of *W. bancrofti* average 26 by 8μ. *W. bancrofti* is transmitted by *Culex, Aedes,* and *Anopheles* mosquitoes; *W. malayi,* by *Mansonia* and *Anopheles* mosquitoes.

Pathologic changes

In early stages of the disease or in patients infected only a few times, the lymph nodes show a granulomatous reaction, with eosinophilic infiltration. Chronic, massively infected cases develop *elephantiasis,* which involves the legs, scrotum, and penis in men, and the legs, external genitalia, and breasts in women (not over 5 percent of infected persons develop elephantiasis). The affected part is greatly enlarged, and its skin is thickened and hyperkeratotic. The lymphatic vessels are dilated and filled with adult filarial worms. About the worms are fibrin thrombi which completely occlude the vessels. The surrounding tissue is fibrotic and infiltrated by lymphocytes, plasma cells, and eosinophils. Filarial complement-fixation tests indicate that *tropical eosinophilia (eosinophilic lung)* may be due to hypersensitivity to filariae. There is a prolonged eosinophilia, and the lungs show scattered granulomatous foci with foreign-body giant cells and a surrounding alveolar eosinophilic and neutrophilic infiltrate [29]. The dog heartworm, *Dirofilaria immitis,* has been proposed as the causative agent of tropical eosinophilia [30].

LOAIASIS: Cause

Loaiasis is due to *Loa loa (Filaria oculi),* the eye worm. The white, tapering adults measure 32 by 0.35 mm. (male) and 60 by 0.5 mm. (viviparous female). Microfilariae are about 275 by 7.5μ. Man is infected with microfilariae by the bite of flies, *Chrysops dimidiata* and *C. silacea* in Africa.

Clinical features

Clinically adult worms migrate through the subcutaneous tissues, causing a shifting inflammatory edema (fugitive or Calabar swellings). These are painful, measure up to 5 cm. in diameter, and persist for 2 to 3 days. Huge red urticarial swellings occasionally appear. An eosinophilia of 50 to 70 percent is not uncommon. Adults may cross the bridge of the nose, or the front of the eye in the conjunctiva.

Pathologic changes

A few worms may become encapsulated and even calcified in the subcutaneous tissues.

ONCHOCERCIASIS: Cause

Onchocerca volvulus, which is endemic in Africa, Guatemala, and southern Mexico, causes *onchocerciasis* (blinding filariasis) [31]. Opalescent adults with bluntly rounded heads measure 30 by 0.15 mm. (male) and 400 by 0.35 mm. (viviparous female). Microfilariae average 25 by 7μ. *Transmission* is by the bite of black gnats of the genus *Simulium,* especially *S. damnosum,* infective larvae entering the wound. An estimated 20 million people suffer from onchocerciasis, and about 400,000 persons are blind due to it.

Pathologic changes

The adults encyst in the *subcutaneous tissues,* small firm nodules being formed most commonly about the great joints and in the temporal and occipital regions of the scalp. A fibrous capsule encloses softer cavernous tissue within which the adults and microfilariae are found. Occasionally the periorbital tissues are involved, with resulting atrophy of the optic nerve.

DRACUNCULIASIS: Cause

Dracunculiasis is caused by *Dracunculus medinensis,* the guinea worm, which is common in Egypt, India, and southern Russia. The long adult female measures about 1000 by 1.5 mm., and the rarely seen male is 20 by 0.4 mm.

Transmission

Females eject motile larvae into water. These are ingested by crustaceans of the genus *Cyclops.* Man is infested by drinking water contaminated by *Cyclops.* The larvae develop in man, invade the intestinal wall, and migrate through the tissues for 8 to 12 months, some arriving in the foot to complete the cycle.

Pathologic changes

Infestation is characterized by the appearance of a small papule, usually on the *sole of the foot.* This develops into a vesicle which ruptures, a single large worm protruding from the skin.

2. Trematode (Fluke) Infections

SCHISTOSOMIASIS: Causes

Schistosomiasis is caused by the blood flukes, *Schistosoma haematobium* (urinary schistosomiasis or bilharziasis), *Schistosoma mansoni* (Manson's intestinal schistosomiasis), and *Schistosoma japonicum* (Oriental schistosomiasis). Schistosomal adults are roughly 1 to 2 cm. by 0.01 to 0.1 cm. and have oral and ventral suckers. Cercariae have pear-shaped bodies with long tails which divide near the end. Their bodies measure about 200 by 50μ. Miracidia average 130 by 60μ. The brown ova are about 150 by 50μ and are spined (laterally in *S. mansoni,* terminally in the others). There are roughly 125 million cases of schistosomiasis in the world.

Transmission

Cercariae enter the skin of persons wading or swimming in infested water and gain entrance to venules, becoming *metacercariae.* They pass through the lungs into the general circulation. Via the portal circulation they reach the liver where they develop into adult sexual forms. These adults leave the liver through the portal vein, going against its current, and settle in the tissues of the intestine, mesentery, peritoneum, or urinary bladder, where the worms mate and the fertile females lay eggs. Ova and larvae leave the human body in the urine or feces. *Miracidia* develop and become *cercariae* in certain species of snails.

Clinical features

Clinically the three flukes evoke similar patterns, although the organ location differs. During a *developmental stage* of 1 to 2 months the symptoms are fever, cough, hemoptysis, chest pain, tender hepatomegaly, leukocytosis, and up to 50 percent eosinophilia. The *active stage* lasts up to 18 months and is usually most severe in *S. japonicum* infections. Fever, weight loss, and allergic phenomena occur in all types of schistosomiasis. Intestinal infection is characterized by attacks of diarrhea and/or dysentery with bloody, mucous stools. Vesical infection produces urinary burning and frequency, painless or painful hematuria, suprapubic pain, and seminal vesiculitis. The *chronic stage* may persist for years and shows emaciation, anemia, bloody diarrhea and/or dysentery or hematuria, signs of hepatic cirrhosis (rare in *S. haematobium* infections), splenomegaly, and occasionally evidence of pulmonary or cerebral invasion.

Pathologic changes:

At the *sites of cercarial penetration,* transitory petechiae and a papular rash develop. In the lungs during cercarial migration, petechial bronchial hemorrhages with eosinophilic and neutrophilic infiltration occur. *S. haematobium* infections are predominantly in the urinary bladder, whereas *S. mansoni* and *S. japonicum* infect the colon and liver mainly. In vesical and intestinal schistosomiasis the adult female worms lay ova within the venules of all layers of the walls. The embryos break through the venule walls and come to lie in the tissues. They cause an intense edema, congestion, and infiltration by polymorphonuclear leukocytes, eosinophils, lymphocytes, and macrophages. The area may undergo necrosis and ulcerate into the lumen. Many ova die and become surrounded by foreign-body giant cells; calcification follows. Similar lesions are found in the mesentery, peritoneum, mesenteric lymph nodes and seminal vesicles, and occasionally in the uterus and vagina. In the late stages there is extreme mucosal hyperplasia; not infrequently neoplastic proliferation occurs, forming polyps or carcinoma of the urinary bladder and colon.

schistosomal cirrhosis

Schistosomal cirrhosis of the liver (Symmer's pipe stem cirrhosis) probably represents a reinfection, ova from the bladder and intestine having reached the liver through branches of the portal vein. The fibrosis is most marked about the larger portal vein branches, rapidly diminishing with vein size. Bile duct proliferation occurs. Schistosomal pigment, which appears to be identical with malarial pigment, is found within enlarged Kupffer cells. Larvae are embedded in the connective tissue, which is infiltrated by polymorphonuclear leukocytes, eosinophils, and mononuclear cells.

embolism of ova

Embolism of ova to the lungs sometimes occurs and causes an allergic necrotizing and obliterative arteritis which leads to pulmonary hypertension and right ventricular hypertrophy (cor pulmonale). Cerebral embolism of ova is unusual and occurs mainly in *S. japonicum* infections. Tuberculoid granulomata develop about the ova.

SCHISTOSOMAL DERMATITIS: Cause

Schistosomal dermatitis is produced by penetration of the skin by the cercariae of various nonhuman schistosomes. These include members of the genera *Trichobilharzia* and *Gigantobilharzia* as well as *Schistosomatium douthitti.* The cercariae derive from snails in infested water.

Pathologic changes

There is a *papular rash* with severe itching *(swimmer's itch). Microscopically* [32] there is marked edema and an acute inflammatory reaction. The cercariae in the dermis are walled off by fibrous tissue and die. They are later phagocytized.

INTESTINAL DISTOMIASIS: Causes

Intestinal distomiasis is principally due to *Fasciolopsis buski, Heterophyes heterophyes,* and *Metagonimus yokogawai. F. buski* is pinkish white, has an elongated ovoid shape and suckers, and measures 2 to 7.5 cm. by 1 to 2 cm. The others are much smaller.

Transmission

Man is infected with *F. buski* (found chiefly in China, Formosa, and Indochina) by ingesting metacercariae on uncooked water plants, especially the water caltrop and water chestnut. Infection with *H. heterophyes* and *M. yokogawai* (found in the Far East, Egypt, and southeast Europe) is incurred by eating raw or poorly cooked fish infested with metacercariae.

Pathologic changes

The adult worm attaches to the *duodenal or jejunal mucosa,* causing hemorrhage, ulceration, and an eosinophilic infiltrate.

PULMONARY DISTOMIASIS: Cause

Paragonimus westermani causes *pulmonary distomiasis.* The reddish brown adult fluke measures about 10 by 6 mm. and is covered with spines. Ova are yellowish brown, ovoid, and thick-shelled, and measure 85 by 55μ.

Transmission

The adult worm encapsulates in a thick-walled, fluid-filled cyst in the lung. Ova escape into the bronchi and are coughed up. Some are swallowed and passed in the feces. After passage first through certain snails and then into crustaceans (freshwater crabs or crayfishes), metacercariae return to man by ingestion of the raw meat of the second intermediary host. They pass through the intestinal wall into the peritoneum, then through the diaphragm into the pleural cavity and lungs.

Pathologic changes

In the lungs there is an infiltration of polymorphonuclear leukocytes and eosinophils. The worms become encapsulated in white fibrous tissue and encyst. Typically up to 20 cysts, measuring about 1 cm. in diameter, are present, especially subpleurally. Occasionally cysts develop in the liver, spleen, mesentery, peritoneum, or brain.

HEPATIC DISTOMIASIS: Causes

The most important causes of *hepatic distomiasis* are *Fasciola hepatica (sheep liver fluke), Opisthorchis felineus (cat liver fluke),* and *Clonorchis sinensis (Chinese liver fluke). C. sinesis* is long, flabby, and gray, measuring about 15 by 4 mm. The yellowish brown ovum is 30 by 15μ and contains a miracidium. *O. felineus* is similar, and the leaf-shaped *F. hepatica* is larger.

Transmission

The eggs are excreted in human feces. They develop to cercariae in snails, then enter the muscles of fish or encyst on vegetation, in or on which they are ingested, reaching the bile ducts via the duodenum.

Pathologic changes

The adult worms are found within the intrahepatic bile ductules and, less often, the pancreatic ducts. There are hyperplasia of the biliary epithelium, fibrosis of the periductal tissues, and infiltration by lymphocytes and eosinophils.

3. *Cestode (Tapeworm) Infections*

DIPHYLLOBOTHRIASIS: Cause

Diphyllobothrium latum, the broad fish tapeworm, causes *diphyllobothriasis.* The ivory-colored adult (strobila) has a small scolex (head) with two suctorial grooves. It may become 10 meters long with over 3000 proglottides (segments). The ovum averages 60 by 50μ and is knob-shaped at one end. *D. latum* infection is common in the Scandinavian countries, Baltic states, northern Minnesota and Michigan, and central and western Canada.

Transmission

Plerocercoid larvae are ingested by man in the raw fish whence they have come from crustaceans eaten by the fish. They develop to adults in the middle ileum, ova being passed in the feces.

Pathologic changes

Usually infection is by a single worm, and intestinal lesions are slight. In about 1 percent of infections there is a pernicious-like anemia of unknown cause. Associated pathologic findings are megaloblastic hyperplasia of the bone marrow, hemosiderosis of the spleen, hypertrophy, dilation and fatty degeneration of the heart, and occasionally subacute combined degeneration of the spinal cord.

SPARGANOSIS: Cause

Sparganosis [33] is due to the unusual extra-intestinal infestation with the sparganum larva of several species of *Diphyllobothrium,* subgenus *Spirometra.*

These include *D. mansoni* and *D. ranarum* in the Orient, and *D. mansonoides* in the United States. In sparganosis the human patient is the second intermediate host of these species; the adult worms usually infest dogs or cats.

Trans-mission

Ova from the feces of dogs or cats develop in water into ciliated coracidia. Procercoid larvae infest the first intermediate host, the water flea, *Cyclops,* for *D. mansonoides.* The sparganum (plerocercoid) larvae infest the second intermediate host, usually frogs, lizards, snakes, or mice. These larvae measure up to 8 cm. long and 0.3 cm. wide, have a scolex, and are motile. Microscopically they consist of a cuticle, large subcuticular cells, and bundles of smooth muscle. Man becomes infested by drinking water in which there are fleas containing procercoid larvae; by eating or handling the meat of raw or poorly cooked frogs, snakes, or mice infected with plerocercoid larvae; or by applying the flesh of frogs or other secondary intermediate hosts to skin or mucosal wounds.

Pathologic changes

Most sparganum larvae lodge in the subcutaneous tissues, where each produces a slowly moving, fluctuant mass. Microscopically the larva lies in a cavity surrounded by a zone of fibrinoid necrosis with adjacent eosinophils and epithelioid cells. In skeletal muscle the larva evokes severe edema and results in focal coagulation necrosis. Rarely man is infested by *Sparganum proliferum,* the adult of which is unknown. This form has lateral branching processes which split off and develop into separate individuals. Thousands of larvae may lodge in the skin and all internal structures except bones. Lymphatic involvement can produce elephantiasis. Grossly these lesions are cystic and gelatinous, and microscopically they are like those of other sparganum larvae.

TAENIASIS: Causes

Taeniasis is caused by *Taenia solium (pork tapeworm),* most common in the Balkans, but found frequently in Mexico, India, northern China, and Manchuria; *Taenia saginata (beef tapeworm),* which has a worldwide distribution in beef-eating areas, especially in North Africa and the Near East; and *Hymenolepis nana,* the cause of over 90 percent of all tapeworm disease in the United States. In the southern United States 1 to 2 percent of the population is infested with *H. nana.* The scolex of *T. solium* attaches by suckers and rostellar hooklets. The worm grows to about 4 meters with roughly 1000 proglottides. *T. saginata* lacks the hooklets but is larger than *T. solium. H. nana* is small, having up to 200 proglottides and measuring about 20 by 0.7 mm.

Trans-mission

Man is infected by *T. solium* and *T. saginata* by eating pork or beef infested with cysticerci. *H. nana* ova are transmitted directly by personal contact; this infection is more common in children than in adults.

Pathologic changes

There may be a petechia or minute ulcer at the site of attachment of the scolex. Rarely a mass of worms may obstruct the intestine, or a proglottis may block the lumen of the appendix. Peritonitis may result from perforation of the intestine by a scolex.

CYSTICERCIASIS: Cause

Cysticerciasis is due to the larval form of *Taenia solium,* which was at one time given the name *Cysticercus cellulosae.* The translucent cyst measures 10 by 5 mm. and contains an invaginated scolex with suckers and hooklets.

Trans-mission

This disease is transmitted by the ingestion of the ova of *T. solium* in fecal contamination or by the forcing of mature proglottides into the stomach by reverse peristalsis. The embryos are released by the action of gastric juice.

Pathologic changes

Oncospheres (hexacanth ova) invade the intestine and enter the bloodstream. *Cysts* form in the subcutaneous tissues, brain, orbit, heart, skeletal muscles, liver, lungs, and peritoneum. Each cyst is a clear, translucent membrane with an opaque white spot at one point, representing the larva. *Microscopically* the fibrous capsule is infiltrated by eosinophils and polymorphonuclear leukocytes. After months or years the worms die, causing a marked reaction, with necrosis of the worm and the surrounding tissue, infiltration by polymorphonuclear leukocytes and eosinophils, giant cell formation, and calcification.

ECHINOCOCCIASIS: Cause

Echinococciasis is usually due to *Echinococcus granulosus,* the adult of which measures 2.5 by 9 mm. and has a scolex with four suckers and numerous rostellar hooklets. There are three proglottides. The ovum is about 35μ in diameter and contains an embryo.

Transmission

Transmission is by contamination of food or drink by ova in the feces of dogs, wolves, or cats which have eaten the flesh of infested sheep, cattle, pigs, horses, camels, or goats. It is most common in great sheep and cattle areas, such as Iceland, New Zealand, Australia, and Argentina. An embryo is hatched from each ovum in the duodenum. *Embryos* enter the intestinal lymphatics and venules, causing an infiltration of macrophages and eosinophils. Many embryos are destroyed, but the survivors develop a cyst or cysts slowly.

Pathologic changes

The *typical lesion* is the formation of a cyst or cysts in the viscera and other tissues. Of such cysts about 70 percent are in the liver, 20 percent in the lungs, and less than 5 percent each in the kidneys, bones, and brain. Typically there are five to six cysts; each may measure up to 20 cm. About the cyst wall are epithelioid and giant cells and eosinophils, surrounded by a layer of fibrous tissue. By about the fifth month the cyst is 1 cm. in diameter and the wall intrinsic to the cyst separates into two parts, an *outer opaque, non-nucleated layer* and an *inner nucleated germinal layer.* Numerous small *brood capsules* project into the cavity from the inner layer. From the inner wall of these capsules the *scolices* develop and invaginate, so that rostellar hooklets are embedded. A fertile cyst contains about 2 million scolices. Rupture of a brood capsule releases scolices into the cyst fluid as *"hydatid sand."* If the cyst ruptures at one point, the scolices are forced into surrounding tissue and daughter cysts are formed.

ALVEOLAR ECHINOCOCCIASIS

Alveolar echinococciasis (alveolar hydatid disease) [34] is caused by *Echinococcus sibiricensis* in Siberia, Alaska, and Canada, and by *E. multilocularis* in southern Germany. Voles and lemmings are the intermediate hosts of the former, and dogs and foxes are the definitive hosts of both species. Man becomes infested by ingesting the ova. Alveolar cysts are characterized by outward budding. Germinal tissue breaks through the outer laminated membrane, and daughter and granddaughter cysts continue to grow in the same organ or metastasize through the bloodstream.

ARTHROPODAL DISEASES

Insects and arachnids are of immense importance medically as vectors for numerous bacteria, rickettsiae, viruses, protozoa, and helminths. *Crustacea* are intermediate hosts for a few helminths. Besides the transmission of pathogenic organisms, insect and arachnid bites or infestations may be of clinical importance in themselves.

STINGS: Hymenoptera

Stings are inflicted by a number of insects, especially those of the Hymenoptera order. These inject venom through a stinger. Bee venom contains choline, glycerol, fatty acids, and probably tryptophan and saponin [35]. The venom of Hymenoptera causes localized erythema, and edema. All members of this group, with the exception of the honeybee, remove the stinger. The bee is disemboweled as it tugs to free itself, and the stinger, venom sac, muscles, and intestine are left behind. In persons who are hypersensitive to the venom of bees, wasps [36], hornets, or yellow jackets, an often fatal *anaphylactic reaction* occurs following a sting. In such cases at autopsy the lungs show congestion and edema, the larynx is edematous, and there is generalized congestion.

Caterpillars

Among *stinging caterpillars* the puss caterpillar, *Megalopyge opercularis,* causes the severest reaction [37]. This larval form of the flannel moth stings through hollow spines on its dorsal surface, a toxic substance being secreted by underlying glands. A few or many spines break off and may remain in the skin. A gridlike pattern of small hemorrhages and sometimes vesicles is produced at the sting site.

BITES:

Insect and tick bites may cause a microscopic picture in the skin much like that of Hodgkin's disease or other lymphomas, with infiltration of the dermis with eosinophils, lymphocytes, plasmocytes, and reticulum cells. This may persist for months. There may also be a pseudoepitheliomatous hyperplasia of the epidermis.

Arachnidism

Arachnidism [38] is the clinical syndrome which follows the bite of a spider. The *black widow spider, Latrodectus mactans,* and other *Latrodectus* species cause most of the severe spider bites in the United States. Venom from poison glands is injected through fangs called cheliceras. It is neurotoxic, principally affecting the spinal cord. Many black widows spin their webs across the seats of outdoor latrines, so their bites are frequent on the buttocks and scrotum. The venoms of *lycosid* spiders *(tarantulas)* are cytotoxic, causing localized dermal necrosis. Bites result in erythema, edema, vesiculation, and in severe cases ulceration with later eschar formation. *Necrotic arachnidism* [39] is caused by the bite of the brown recluse spider, *Loxosceles reclusus.* The pain of the bite becomes increasingly severe for several hours. A bulla forms and later ruptures. The surrounding zone of erythema becomes violaceous. A central black eschar remains for several weeks and then sloughs off, leaving a necrotic base. In severe cases there is an acute systemic reaction with fever, skin rash, joint pains, and hemoglobinuria. Death is unusual following spider bites. *Pathologic changes in fatal cases* show pulmonary congestion and edema, generalized congestion, and fatty metamorphosis of the liver.

Tick paralysis

Tick paralysis occasionally occurs in human beings due to the bite of the gravid female of the wood tick, *Dermacentor andersoni,* and less often of the dog tick, *D. variabilis.* A neurotoxin is injected from the salivary gland of the feeding tick. The paralysis is due to a failure in the liberation of acetylcholine at the neuromuscular junction, resulting from a conduction block in the somatic motor fibers [40]. An ascending flaccid paralysis may include respiratory failure. Mortality is about 10 percent.

SCABIES: Cause

Scabies is caused by *Sarcoptes scabiei,* a mite which lives in cutaneous burrows where the female lays her ova. These develop into six-legged larvae which produce lateral tunnels.

Pathologic changes

Papules appear on the skin, especially of the fingers, toes, flexor surfaces of the forearms, and the genitalia. About the burrows there is slight fibrosis, with infiltration by lymphocytes and eosinophils. Fecal pellets cause edema of the dermis and vesicles in the epidermis.

CHIGGER INFESTATION:

Six-legged mite larvae *(Eutrombicula* species in the United States), which attach to the skin from vegetation, produce *chigger infestation.* The larvae, after becoming engorged with blood, fall to the ground, become nymphs, and mature.

Pathologic changes

A macule with edema, hyperemia, and lymphocytic and eosinophilic infiltration in the dermis appears, due to the salivary secretion from the larvae.

DEMODEX FOLLICULORUM INFESTATION

Infestation of the hair follicles and sebaceous glands by the mite *Demodex folliculorum* [41] is common but seldom causes clinical manifestations. Adult mites burrow into the skin and form colonies in the accessory structures. When large numbers of mites are present, there may be an erythema with scaling of the epidermis.

PEDICULOSIS: Causes

Pediculus humanus capitis (head louse), *P. h. corporis* (body louse), and *Phthirius pubis* (crab louse), which infests the genital region, cause *pediculosis.*

Pathologic changes

Saliva from the nymphs or adults causes a papule which is roseate and elevated. There are hemorrhage, edema, and infiltration by lymphocytes. Prolonged infestation produces hyperpigmentation, mostly due to scratching.

MYIASIS

Myiasis is the invasion of the tissues by the larvae of certain flies. They may involve the skin *(creeping eruption),* eyes, nose, ear, larynx, or vulva. Swallowed eggs may develop into larvae which may attach to the gastric or intestinal mucosa.

REFERENCES

1. Utz, J. P. The spectrum of opportunistic fungus infections. *Lab. Invest.* 11:1018, 1962.
2. Frenkel, J. K. Role of corticosteroids as predisposing factors in fungal diseases. *Lab. Invest.* 11:1192, 1962.
3. Sidransky, H., and Friedman, L. The effect of cortisone and antibiotic agents on experimental pulmonary aspergillosis. *Amer. J. Path.* 35:169, 1959.
4. Baker, R. D. Leukopenia and therapy in leukemia as factors predisposing to fatal mycoses. *Amer. J. Clin. Path.* 37:358, 1962.
5. Saltzman, H. A., Chick, E. W., and Conant, N. F. Nocardiosis as a complication of other diseases. *Lab. Invest.* 11:1110, 1962.
6. Winslow, D. J., and Steen, F. G. Considerations in the histologic diagnosis of mycetoma. *Amer. J. Clin. Path.* 42:164, 1964.
7. Wilson, J. W., Cawley, E. P., Weidman, F. D., and Gilmer, W. S. Primary cutaneous North American blastomycosis. *A.M.A. Arch. Derm.* 71:39, 1955.
8. Littman, M. L., and Zimmerman, L. E. *Crytococcosis.* New York: Grune & Stratton, 1956, pp. 53–99, 116–120.
9. Grimley, P. M., Wright, L. D., Jr., and Jennings, A. E. *Torulopsis glabrata* infection in man. *Amer. J. Clin. Path.* 43:216, 1965.
10. Zimmerman, L. E. Demonstration of histoplasma and coccidioides in so-called tuberculomas of lung. *A.M.A. Arch. Intern. Med.* 94:690, 1954.

11. Klieger, H. L., and Fisher, E. R. Fibrocalcific constrictive pericarditis due to *Histoplasma capsulatum*. *New Eng. J. Med.* 267:593, 1962.
12. Farid, Z., and Barclay, W. R. Histoplasmosis: In vivo studies in the rabbit ear chamber. *A.M.A. Arch. Path.* 68:413, 1959.
13. Lurie, H. I. Histopathology of sporotrichosis. *Arch. Path.* (Chicago) 75:421, 1963.
14. Shoemaker, E. H., Bennett, H. D., Fields, W. S., Whitcomb, F. C., and Halpert, B. Leptomeningitis due to *Sporotrichum schenckii*. *A.M.A. Arch. Path.* 64:222, 1957.
15. Sanger, P. W., Taylor, F. H., Robicsek, F., Germuth, F., Senterfit, L., and McKinnon, G. *Candida* infection as a complication of heart surgery. *J.A.M.A.* 181:88, 1962.
16. Huang, S., and Harris, L. S. Acute disseminated penicilliosis. *Amer. J. Clin. Path.* 39:167, 1963.
17. Naji, A. F. Bronchopulmonary aspergillosis. *A.M.A. Arch. Path.* 68:282, 1959.
18. Straatsma, B. R., Zimmerman, L. E., and Gass, J. D. M. Phycomycosis. *Lab. Invest.* 11:963, 1962.
19. Hutter, R. V. P. Phycomycetous infection (mucormycosis) in cancer patients: A complication of therapy. *Cancer* 12:330, 1959.
20. Rabin, E. R., Lundberg, G. D., and Mitchell, E. T. Mucormycosis in severely burned patients. *New Eng. J. Med.* 264:1286, 1961.
21. Baker, R. D. Pulmonary mucormycosis. *Amer. J. Path.* 32:287, 1956.
22. Smith, M. E., Burnham, D. K., and Black, M. B. Cerebral mucormycosis. *A.M.A. Arch. Path.* 66:468, 1958.
23. Arean, V. M., and Koppisch, E. Balantidiasis. *Amer. J. Path.* 32:1089, 1956.
24. Alexander, G. M., and Callister, J. W. Toxoplasmosis of newborn. *A.M.A. Arch. Path.* 60:563, 1955.
25. Budzilovich, G. N. Acquired toxoplasmosis: A clinico-pathologic study of a case. *Amer. J. Clin. Path.* 35:66, 1961.
26. Hamperl, H. Pneumocystis infection and cytomegaly of the lungs in the newborn and adult. *Amer. J. Path.* 32:1, 1956.
27. Huneycutt, H. C., Anderson, W. R., and Hendry, W. S. *Pneumocystis carinii* pneumonia. Case studies with electron microscopy. *Amer. J. Clin. Path.* 41:411, 1964.
28. Dent, J. H., Nichols, R. L., Beaver, P. C., Carrera, G. M., and Staggers, R. J. Visceral larva migrans. *Amer. J. Path.* 32:777, 1956.
29. Danaraj, T. J. Pathologic studies in eosinophilic lung (tropical eosinophilia). *A.M.A. Arch. Path.* 67:515, 1959.
30. Donohugh, D. L. Tropical eosinophilia. An etiologic inquiry. *New Eng. J. Med.* 269:1357, 1963.
31. Steen, F. G., and Price, D. L. Onchocerciasis. *Bull. Int. Acad. Path.* 5:27, 1964.
32. Batten, P. J., Jr. The histopathology of swimmer's itch. *Amer. J. Path.* 32:363, 1956.
33. Wirth, W. A., and Farrow, C. C. Human sparganosis. *J.A.M.A.* 177:6, 1961.
34. Smith, E. M. G., and Hanson, S. Alveolar echinococcosis. *Amer. J. Clin. Path.* 35:160, 1961.
35. Shaffer, J. H. Stinging insects – a threat to life. *J.A.M.A.* 177:473, 1961.
36. McCormick, W. F. Fatal anaphylactic reactions to wasp stings. *Amer. J. Clin. Path.* 39:485, 1963.
37. McGovern, J. P., Barkin, G. D., McElhenney, T. R., and Wende, R. Megalopyge opercularis. *J.A.M.A.* 175:1155, 1961.
38. Horen, W. P. Arachnidism in the United States. *J.A.M.A.* 185:839, 1963.

39. Dillaha, C. J., Jansen, G. T., Honeycutt, W. M., and Hayden, C. R. North American loxoscelism. *J.A.M.A.* 188:33, 1964.
40. Murnaghan, M. F. Site and mechanism of tick paralysis. *Science* 131:418, 1960.
41. Breckenridge, R. L. Infestation of the skin with *Demodex folliculorum. Amer. J. Clin. Path.* 23:348, 1953.

GENERAL REFERENCES

Belding, D. L. *Textbook of Parasitology* (3d ed.). New York: Appleton-Century-Crofts, 1965. (An exhaustive discussion of the protozoan, helminthic, and arthropodal parasites.)

Brown, H. W., and Belding, D. L. *Basic Clinical Parasitology* (3d ed.). New York: Appleton-Century-Crofts, 1969. (An invaluable, concise presentation of all aspects of parasitic diseases.)

Faust, E. C., and Russell, P. F. *Clinical Parasitology* (7th ed.). Philadelphia: Lea & Febiger, 1964. (An authoritative treatment of the clinical and morphologic features of parasitic infections.)

Wilson, J. W., and Plunkett, O. A. *The Fungous Diseases of Man.* Berkeley: University of California Press, 1965. (A well-organized and abundantly illustrated treatise on mycotic infections.)

9 INJURIES DUE TO PHYSICAL AGENTS

MECHANICAL INJURIES

Mechanical injury is caused by force, that which changes or tends to change the state of rest or uniform motion of a body. The *characteristics* of a mechanical injury are determined either by the way in which the state of rest of the tissues is changed by a moving object, or by the way in which the uniform motion of the tissues is altered by a resisting object. A *wound (injury, trauma)* is the disruption of normal anatomic relationships resulting from force. The potential of a moving object to produce a wound is a function of its kinetic energy – its capacity to do work by reason of its weight and motion. The kinetic energy of a moving object equals $mv^2/2g$, where m is the weight of the object, v its velocity, and g, the acceleration due to gravity. Trauma is of tremendous importance medicolegally because of the compensation, civil, and criminal implications.

Factors determining outcome

When a moving object strikes the body, the impact tends to displace the tissues in the direction of the motion of the object. If the force and rate of the impact are sufficient to accelerate the tissues rapidly, a wound results. When a moving body strikes a stationary object, the impact tends to interrupt the forward motion of the tissues. If the rate of deceleration is rapid, a wound results. The *rate of acceleration or deceleration* is the most important factor in wound production. Other factors include:

1. *State of muscular contraction* at the time of impact. Perfectly coordinated muscular opposition is the best protection against injury, complete relaxation being next best.

2. *Plasticity (resilience) of the object or tissue struck.* The greater the plasticity, the longer the period of impact, thus lessening the potential for injury.

3. *Amount of surface area of the impact.* The greater the area against which a fixed amount of energy is dissipated, the smaller is its destructive capacity.

4. *Transmission of the energy of impact* into the deeper tissues, as through delicate tissues to strong ones such as bone, or through gases or liquids which exert pneumostatic or hydrostatic forces.

Tissue reaction

The *reaction of the tissues to injury* is that of acute inflammation, with later regeneration and repair. *Secondary effects of injury* include: (1) *hemorrhage,* which varies from slight to exsanguinating; (2) *infection,* which depends on the type and extent of the wound and the type of organisms introduced; (3) *shock,* both primary (neurogenic) and secondary; (4) *crush syndrome;* and (5) *embolism* (of fat from fractures, of air, or of detached thrombi).

1. Types of Mechanical Injury

ABRASION

Abrasion (scratch) is the superficial tearing away of epidermal cells by friction. It may or may not penetrate the epidermis. *Fingernails often produce characteristic abrasions,* especially about the neck during manual strangulation. Distinctive *abrasion patterns* are produced by grillwork and tire marks, and these have often aided in identifying automobiles in hit-and-run cases. It is sometimes impossible to distinguish antemortem and postmortem superficial abrasions. In those lesions extending into the dermis, the extravasation of erythrocytes and the presence of inflammatory cells identify antemortem abrasions.

LACERATION

Laceration (tear) is a wound resulting from excessive stretching of tissue. A laceration may be internal or external and may or may not communicate with a surface. If the crushing or stretching force is unidirectional, the wound produced is usually linear or curved. If the force is multidirectional, the wound is stellate and ragged. Laceration produced by a crushing blow typically has ragged margins; a strong oblique blow usually causes a flaplike tear. Incisions differ from lacerations in that, in the latter, tags of fibrous tissue traverse across the wound, while they are absent in incisions. *Scalp lacerations* are common in persons found lying in the street, and such wounds often provide valuable medicolegal evidence. In wounds resulting from a blow on the head from above by a moving object, the flap of torn scalp is usually raised posteriorly. When the head is struck from below by a stationary object, such as a curb edge, during a fall, the torn flap is typically raised anteriorly. *Laceration of internal organs,* such as the brain, lungs, heart, liver, and spleen, is caused by compression or displacement of the organ by a blunt force impacting against the body surfaces without penetrating it or by a force piercing the skin surface and the organ. Splenic laceration occasionally occurs during "belly-whopping" on a sled. *Air blasts* may cause lung lacerations without apparent external injury. Similarly *immersion blast* may produce intestinal lacerations.

CHOPPING WOUND

Chopping wound is one caused by a blow with the sharp splitting edge of a rather heavy weapon such as an ax, hatchet, cleaver, sword, or saber. This type of wound is usually homicidal and occurs commonly on the head, neck, shoulders, or extremities. Wounds on the upper extremities are made as the victim attempts to stave off the attack with his arms *(defense wounds).* Such defense wounds may also occur in cuttings and stabbings.

INCISION

Incision (incised wound) is a wound produced by pressure or friction against the skin by a sharp-edged object, such as a scalpel, razor, knife, or piece of glass. Incised wounds are surgical, accidental (often occupational), homicidal, or suicidal. *Occupational incisions* usually involve the hands, and most are superficial. In *homicides,* multiple incised wounds often represent purposeless mutilation of the body, the incisions having no pattern *(homicidal frenzy).* A patterned mutilation often indicates a revengeful motivation. The genitalia are sometimes amputated. *Suicidal incisions* are usually cutthroat wounds. Right-handed persons begin such wounds high up on the left side of the neck and carry the incision across and down to the lower right side of the neck. The head is held back, and the wound is above the thyroid cartilage. The jugular veins are severed, but the carotid arteries usually are not cut. Other common suicidal incisions are slashings of the wrists. *Hesitation marks* are common. Sometimes neurotic persons, in order to get attention, also make such multiple tentative incisions at the wrists or neck. These are usually quite superficial and are made in parallel lines or crossing one another. *Homicidal cutthroat wounds* are usually below the thyroid cartilage, the head being held down. There are no hesitation marks.

STAB WOUND

Stab (penetrating, puncture) wound is a deep defect with a narrow opening, produced by a sharp, slender object such as an ice pick, stiletto, scissors, hat pin, knitting needle, skewer, or sharp end of a knife. Bone splinters from fractures may cause internal penetrating wounds. The *skin opening may be inapparent,* and external bleeding is often absent or minimal. In stabbings with closed scissors, both wound edges are covered with introverted epidermis; in stabbings with one scissors blade, one edge is introverted and the other reveals torn elastic fibers [1]. *Internal injuries may be severe or fatal,* especially if a large artery is torn. Wounds of the atria, pulmonary artery, aorta, or coronary arteries hemorrhage more rapidly than those of the more muscular left ventricle. With fatal stab wounds of the heart the victims may live 5 to 15 minutes. Death is due to cardiac tamponade, or to exsanguination if the pericardium is rent open. Penetrating wounds are accidental (such as in automobile accidents), homicidal, or suicidal; most are homicidal; suicidal ones are usually into the heart. *Infection, especially tetanus,* is a common complication of such wounds.

CONTUSION

Contusion (bruise) is an injury of such force as to be transmitted through the skin and disrupt small blood vessels, causing hemorrhage, without interrupting the epidermal surface. The cause is usually a forcible impact acting over a large surface area. *Internal organs,* such as the brain, *may be contused* by the violent agitation caused by such an impact. *Patterned contusions* are often produced by the grillwork or other parts of an automobile, by fingers in manual strangulation, or by ropes or cords used in hangings or strangulation. Early the bruise is dark or bluish red due to the extravasated blood. Within a few hours the red cells break down, releasing blood pigments. With time the color of the contusion passes through blue, dark blue, brown, yellow, and yellowish green color phases, as the blood pigments form and are then removed by phagocytic cells. A *hematoma* may develop in a contusion. Such a hematoma may resolve, persist as a cyst, or calcify. *Necrosis of subcutaneous fat* may occur at the site of contusion, especially in the breast. *Muscles* contracted at the moment of impact may show extensive contusion. Similar wounds occur in the *myocardium* in blows over the left side of the chest during systole. Massive myocardial contusion has occurred during cardiac massage. *Bones* may be contused, with tearing of the "hairpin" vessels at the metaphyseo-diaphyseal junction.

FRACTURE:

Fracture is a mechanically produced disruption in the continuity of bone. It may be caused by direct crushing trauma to the bone, by a force transmitted along an extremity, or by poorly coordinated muscular action at the time of impact. A fracture is designated as *simple* when the bone is separated into only two parts. When there are three or more bone fragments, the fracture is called *comminuted.* In an *impacted fracture,* cortical bone is jammed into cancellous bone, with or without lateral displacement. If the break extends only part way through the bone, it is an *incomplete fracture.* Types of incomplete breaks include *fissure fraction,* in which a transverse or longitidinal crack develops partly through a bone; *puncture fracture,* in which a hole is produced through a bone, usually by a bullet; and *greenstick fracture,* which is caused by marked bending of bone and in which the bone is broken on the convex but not on the concave side. A *stress fracture* is due to excessive overuse of bone. It may be preceded by periosteal proliferations to strengthen the bone and occurs when this is insufficient. A break produced by slight trauma in a diseased area in a bone, as in a cyst or neoplasm, is called a *pathologic fracture.* When a piece of broken bone pierces the skin surface, the term *compound fracture* is applied. *Nonunion* is a failure of a fracture to heal. It may be due to infection with liquefaction of the clot between the bone ends; interposition of tissue, such as muscle or fascia, between the fractured parts; impairment of the blood supply due to severe damage to surrounding tissues; or deficiencies of vitamins C or D or of calcium.

Complications

Complications of fractures include:

1. *Infection.* This may lyse the clot or actually invade the bone to produce osteomyelitis. Infection is most common in compound fractures.

2. *Injury to muscles and soft tissues.* Sharp bone fragments may severely damage tissues. Perforation of the pleura by rib fractures or of the urinary bladder in hip fractures, and laceration of the meninges and brain in skull fractures are especially common and serious.

3. *Volkmann's ischemic contracture.* Rarely, some weeks or months after a fracture in the upper extremity, muscles of the forearm become replaced by fibrous tissue, with only an occasional atrophic muscle fiber. This condition is caused by an interference with the venous return without cutting off the arterial supply, due to a too tight cast or severe edema of the part.

4. *Ossification of a hematoma or a muscle.* Rarely a hematoma about a fracture becomes calcified and later ossifies. Injured muscle may undergo the same changes (myositis ossificans). *Muscle injury related to fractures* is most severe halfway between the skin and bone surface. The first phase of *myositis ossificans* is pseudosarcomatous. This has led to a misdiagnosis of fibrosarcoma or osteogenic sarcoma and unnecessary limb amputations. Later there is cellular differentiation in myositis ossificans, and finally a hollow shell of bone remains.

5. *Injury to blood vessels and nerves.* These may lead to gangrene or paralysis below the fracture.

6. *Injury to joints* (traumatic arthritis).

7. *Acute traumatic atrophy of bone.* Slight atrophy and osteoporosis occur in all bones immobilized for some time. Rarely this may be severe and widespread, even involving the surrounding bones as well *(Sudeck's atrophy).*

8. *Fat embolism.*

Skull fracture

Skull fracture may be due to a blow on the head by a solid object, crushing of the head between two solid objects, or impaction of the moving head against a stationary solid object. At the moment and site of the impact, the skull is slightly flattened. In children the skull is often resilient enough to recoil without fracture. If the distortion of bone is sufficient, it will be fractured, the lines of force from the site of impact being transmitted through the vault and base of the skull.

Occasionally a fracture is contrecoup (opposite the point of impact), especially in an orbital roof in parietal or occipital fractures. The *fracture lines* follow the paths of least resistance. These are through the vault between the reinforcing pillars; through the base within the fossae, not at the junctions of the fossae; and along the suture lines. All lines of fracture directed toward the base will converge on the body of the sphenoid bone. In *basal skull fractures* bleeding from the ear is common, and *Battle's sign* is discoloration of the skin along the course of the posterior auricular artery, beginning as an ecchymosis near the tip of the mastoid process. A *ring fracture* of the occipital bone about the foramen magnum may occur in injuries in which the base of the skull is jammed against the atlas. A *depressed fracture* occurs when a piece of bone is displaced inward and presses on or lacerates the brain. A *linear fracture* consists of a single line of fracture without bone displacement. A *composite fracture* is one in which the fracture lines branch without bone displacement. Skull fractures may also be comminuted or compound. If the fracture line passes through an accessory nasal sinus, air may enter the cranial cavity *(pneumocephalus),* and cerebrospinal fluid may escape through the nose. The *most common cause of death* from a skull fracture is laceration of the brain. Other causes are subdural hematoma, cerebral concussion, extradural hemorrhage, and meningitis.

Vertebral fracture

Fractures of the vertebrae are produced by hyperflexion, hyperextension, or vertical compression of the spine. The most common sites of fracture are the second, fifth, and sixth cervical vertebrae and the first lumbar vertebra. In about half the cases there is injury to the cord and permanent paralysis below the point of fracture. In healing, the callus may impinge on the cord or the peripheral nerves as they pass through the foramina.

DISLOCATION

SUBLUXATION

SPRAIN

Dislocation is the complete and persistent displacement of the articular surface of one of the bones of a joint from that of its fellow. *Subluxation* is a partial dislocation, in which the normal relation of the articular surfaces is disturbed although they remain partly in contact. *Sprain* is a temporary subluxation, in which the articular surfaces return to their normal positions with some damage to the ligaments, tendons, and muscles about the joint. *Sprain fracture* is a sprain in which a small piece of bone is pulled off. It is very common in the malleoli of the ankles.

NECK INJURIES:

Whiplash injury

Neck injuries [2] usually involve the cervical vertebrae, spinal cord, and muscles and ligaments of that region. Such injuries are fairly common, especially in automobile accidents. Cervical trauma may be caused by blunt force to the neck, hyperflexion or hyperextension of the neck, or the so-called whiplash mechanism. *Whiplash (necklash) injury* usually occurs in an automobile passenger when the car is struck sharply from behind. The impact accelerates the automobile momentarily, and the passenger's torso, padded against the seat, moves forward. The unprotected neck and head are thrown violently backward because of their inertia. The neck muscles react to right the head, usually overcompensating and snapping the head forward. This latter action probably causes the most severe damage in the neck. The extent of the cervical injuries depends on the degree of violence of the whiplash effect. Such *injuries include* transient muscle strain, cervical nerve root damage (radiculitis), subluxation of one or more vertebra(e) due to rupture of ligaments, compression fracture of one or more vertebra(e), especially the fifth and sixth cervical ones, and herniation of an intervertebral disk. Injury to the sympathetic chain may produce Horner's syndrome. In about 25 percent of the cases there is cerebral concussion due to the rapid deceleration of the brain. Post-traumatic psychoneuroses are also common. *Blunt-force neck injuries* produce soft tissue contusion, hematoma formation, and sometimes tracheal or laryngeal damage. Blows to the back of the neck may fracture a vertebral spinal process or even a vertebral body by causing hyperflexion of the neck.

CRUSH SYNDROME

Crush syndrome occurs when there is trauma due to the falling of heavy objects – as during a bombing – on the legs, with crushing of muscle. The changes in the body are due to the hemoglobin and myohemoglobin released from the damaged muscle and to vasoconstrictive renal ischemia. The latter leads to oliguria and aciduria, with the precipitation of pigment casts in the distal convoluted tubules and loops of Henle. The epithelium of these tubules shows cloudy swelling and necrosis *(hypoxic nephrosis)*. Brown, granular pigment casts are found in the lumina. The casts give a positive Prussian blue reaction for iron. Grossly the kidney is enlarged and swollen, the cut surface being dark red. The *injured muscle* shows necrosis, edema, and hemorrhage.

BULLET WOUNDS:

Bullet wounds [3, 4] have peculiar characteristics due to high velocity (up to over 2000 feet per second). The force of impact is projected laterally from the path of the bullet, so that trauma may occur at a distance from the path. Bone fragments may become secondary missiles. A *bullet from a rifled bore* has two sources of energy: (1) forward motion, K.E. = $mv^2/2g$, and (2) rotary motion, K.E. = $I\omega^2/2g$, where I is the rotary inertia and is equal to ½ Mr^2 where M is the weight of the bullet and r its radius. ω is the angular velocity in radians per second and equals $2Rg$, where R is the number of rotations per second and g is the acceleration due to gravity. Even with rifling, which imparts a spin to the bullet and stabilizes its flight, a bullet is likely to wobble for a few microseconds after leaving the barrel. Such wobbling partly accounts for the severe damage caused by bullets striking the body at close range.

Cavitation

A bullet traveling through the heart or other hollow viscus filled with fluid exerts an explosive force and pushes the fluid away from its track. This force may be sufficient to rupture a hollow viscus, even the heart and aorta. Even while traversing solid tissues, bullets produce a momentary explosive *cavitation* in which the wound track becomes much larger than the caliber of the bullet. *The degree of cavitation varies directly with the velocity of the bullet.* Forces transmitted radially from the path of the speeding bullet initiate the cavitation and thus cause tissue destruction at some distance around the actual missile track. High-speed camera studies of a bullet fired through gelatin blocks reveal that its track enlarges to many times its diameter within 2 to 3 milliseconds and collapses after about 4 milliseconds [5].

Entrance wound

The *hole of entrance* is characteristically smaller than that of exit except in contact wounds. It is funnel-shaped, with depressed edges, and there is marginal abrasion and bruising of the epidermis *(contact ring)*. If the entrance wound is concentric, the bullet entered perpendicularly to the skin surface. Pieces of subcutaneous tissue may extrude from the opening due to "*splashback.*" The *wound of exit* is usually irregularly lacerated, with everted edges. The bullet moves more slowly at its exit and may be tumbling.

Exit wound

Contact wound

If the gun muzzle is in contact with or very close to the skin, the rapidly expanding gases may enter the wound and explosively tear the tissues. A gram of smokeless powder (nitrocellulose and nitroglycerin) used as the propellant in cartridges forms 800 to 900 cc. of gases with a solid residue of nitrates and nitrites. Therefore, bullet wounds at contact or short range are especially destructive.

Pathologic changes

A *microscopic study of bullet wounds* [6] reveals that epidermal and dermal changes result from a combination of mechanical and thermal trauma. In *contact wounds,* thermal injury is due to muzzle flame and the hot missile. The flame of burning gases may carbonize the epidermis, with nuclear swelling and vacuolization of the basal cells. The hot bullet produces coagulation necrosis of the epidermis. The *dermal collagen* about the wound is fused and homogeneous, indicating *thermal coagulation necrosis. Powder residue* (PR) is seen as black amorphous clumps or collections of brownish yellow needles in abundance on the surface of the skin defect and in the subcutaneous tissues in contact entrance wounds. Powder residue may be found deep within the wound tract. Relatively little powder residue is found on the skin surface adjacent to the defect in *tight contact wounds,* but moderate quantities are found there in *loose contact wounds.* In *near (close-range) wounds* in which the gun muzzle is within 6 to 8 inches of the body surface, a heavy, spotted deposit of powder residue is found on the intact skin surface about the wound and may even be present in viscera deep within the wound tract. In *distant wounds,* powder residue is sparse or absent about the skin defect, the PR which is present having rubbed off the bullet surface. *Reentrance wounds* are similar to distant wounds. In *exit wounds,* powder residue is typically absent or minute in amount. The epithelial perforation is sharply demarcated from the adjacent skin surfaces. *Coagulation necrosis* is frequently found in dermal collagen, indicating hotness of the bullet partly due to heat created by friction.

Fatal bullet wounds

Among patients with *fatal gunshot wounds* about 80 percent collapse promptly, 15 percent more become prostrate following minor activity within 5 minutes, and 5 percent collapse more than 5 minutes after sustaining the injury [7]. Comparable figures for *fatal stab wounds* are prompt collapse in 25 percent, collapse within 5 minutes in 50 percent more, and collapse after 5 minutes in the remaining 25 percent. These differences are explained on the basis that bullets cause holes from which bleeding is often rapid, whereas stab wounds produce a slit. The average *internal blood loss with fatal gunshot and stab wounds* is 1200 to 1800 ml. Those collapsing promptly have a greater blood loss than those who remain active for several minutes.

SHOTGUN WOUNDS

Shotgun wounds [8] are similar to bullet wounds, except that the velocity is slower and multiple wounds are made by the metal pellets of shot after the wad has separated. Pieces of cardboard and felt from the cartridge may be carried into the wounds at ranges under 6 feet. *At very close range shotgun wounds are destructive* because of the large amounts of gas and flame emitted from the muzzle. Most fatal gunshot wounds are suicidal, and the head and chest are the most common injury sites, death being due to massive damage to the brain, lungs, or heart, or to exsanguination.

2. Motor Vehicular Injuries

Motor vehicular injuries [9] kill over 55,000 persons in the United States annually, and over a million other individuals receive significant injuries in traffic accidents. About 25 percent of the fatalities are pedestrians, the rest being occupants of automobiles involved in collisions with other vehicles or objects or in overturns. Most pedestrian deaths occur in children and persons over 50, while about 75 percent of occupant deaths are in those from 15 to 50 years of age. Almost *three times as many males as females are killed* in motor vehicular accidents, and in the 20 to 40 age range the ratio is 6:1 [10]. *Ethyl alcohol* plays an important causative role in many accidents, definite evidence of recent alcohol ingestion being found in about 55 percent of fatally injured pedestrians and in 60 percent of drivers and 35 percent of passengers killed in automobile accidents. A person whose blood alcohol is 0.10 percent is more than twice as likely to become involved in such an accident as a person whose level is 0.05 percent, and in one whose blood alcohol is above 0.15 percent the likelihood is increased 10 times. Drugs such as barbiturates and tranquilizers are becoming increasingly important factors in traffic accidents, and physicians should warn patients using such drugs of their potential dangers, especially in relation to driving.

The *types of injuries* sustained in vehicular accidents run the gamut of mechanical wounds, and only general principles and common forms of trauma can be mentioned here.

INJURIES TO PEDESTRIANS

Injuries to pedestrians are due to the *initial impact* from the automobile or other vehicle; *crushing injuries* due to the wheels, especially common in children; and *secondary impact* with the pavement, ground, or other objects after being thrown by the initial impact. *Most fatal injuries are caused by the initial impact.* The speed of the vehicle is the major factor in determining the force of impact. Typically the front bumper strikes the adult pedestrian below the knee, and *"bumper fractures"* of the tibia and fibula together are very common and often compound and comminuted. Bilateral "bumper fractures" occur fairly frequently. The pelvis, abdomen, and chest sustain injury from being hit by the radiator, hood, or fender, or they may be crushed by being run over by the wheels. Hip and rib fractures and hepatic and splenic lacerations are frequently encountered in severely wounded pedestrians. *Head injuries* are common and are often due to crushing or secondary impact. Skull fractures and intracranial bleeding are common.

INJURIES TO OCCUPANTS:

Injuries to occupants depend mainly on the rate of deceleration or acceleration of the parts of the body. The *impact force* in number of G's (the force of gravity) is equal to $0.034\, v^2/d$, where v is the velocity of the vehicle in feet per second and d is the stopping distance in feet. *Ejection from the vehicle* during or after the initial deceleration usually increases the number and severity of injuries, and *ejected passengers receive fatal injuries five times as often as those who are not thrown from a vehicle.* Seat belts reduce the incidence of ejection and subsequent injuries. However, an improperly placed seat belt may result in severe intra-abdominal injury, such as splenic rupture [11]. *Acceleration injuries* are most often due to impact at the rear of the vehicle, and the typical type of injury (the whiplash) is discussed on page 205. *Deceleration injuries* are most common in the head and chest.

Driver injuries

Drivers often suffer severe rib cage distortion by being thrown against the steering wheel; rib fractures and lacerations of the lungs, heart, and/or liver are frequent, with little evidence of external chest injury in many cases.

Front-seat passenger injuries

In *front-seat passengers* the force of impact may be taken up mainly by the head, which strikes the roof or windshield, and the hands, which grasp the dashboard. In such cases the cervical vertebrae may be injured, fracture of the odontoid process, and/or rotatory subluxation of the first cervical upon the second cervical vertebra occurring not uncommonly. Severe or fatal spinal cord damage may be produced. When the head strikes the windshield and a knee is thrown against the dashboard, compression fractures of vertebrae are common, especially in the lower thoracic and upper lumbar regions. Forceful impact of a knee against the dashboard may result in a fracture of the patella or the femur above or within the condyle. Thrusting the foot against the floorboard may produce a fracture in the lower third of the tibia and/or fibula; an "explosion fracture" of the ankle in which the talus smashes into the distal end of the tibia; a fracture or dislocation of the talus; and occasionally fracture of the femur or pelvis. Chest and/or abdominal injuries may be suffered from impact against the windshield, dashboard, or door.

Rear-seat passenger injuries

Rear-seat passengers receive injuries to the head and vertebral column when the former strikes the roof, backrest of the front seat, or windshield; to the chest and abdomen by being thrown against the front seat or a door; and to the lower extremities when the feet are thrust against the floor or front seat.

Other injuries

The incidence of *lacerations due to broken glass* has been reduced by the use of safety glass, but severe and even fatal injuries are still common from fragments of windshield and window glass. A few vehicular accident deaths are due to drowning, electrocution by high tension wires, and burns.

3. The Battered-Child Syndrome

The *battered-child syndrome* [12, 13] is characterized by severe physical abuse of a young child, usually administered by a parent. It is often unrecognized because injuries are inflicted over a period of time, and a history of assault is seldom obtained. The mortality rate is about 10 percent, and *permanent brain injury* is suffered in another 25 percent of cases. Most of the children are below 3 years of age. Besides evidence of multiple traumata the child shows general evidence of neglect. The *adults involved* are characterized as immature and quick to react with violent aggression. They are frequently alcoholics and/or sexually promiscuous. Many suffered similar attacks in their own childhood. The battered infant or child is usually an unwanted one. The *most important diagnostic feature* is a striking discrepancy between the physical findings and the history supplied by the parents. The injuries are quite variable and sometimes mimic hemorrhagic diatheses, neurologic disorders, or nutritional deficiencies such as scurvy. Subdural hematoma, with or without skull fracture, is a common finding. Subcutaneous hemorrhages of various ages due to contusion are frequently noted. *The diagnosis is usually established by the radiologic finding of multiple bone fractures in different stages of healing.* Subperiosteal calcification secondary to hemorrhage is often seen.

4. Mechanical Intracranial and Intraspinal Injuries

INTRACRANIAL INJURIES:

The brain is well protected against injury by many anatomic elements. The *hair and scalp* tend to cushion blows, and the *marked mobility of the head* frequently enables it to dodge injury or decrease the force of impact. The *domed contour of the skull* causes many blows to glance off. The *skull is elastic* because of its dome shape and the organic content of its bones. The relatively thin *cranial vault is reinforced by a series of bony buttresses* which tend to direct fracture lines to the base of the skull and dissipate them. The *dura* gives added protection to the brain, and the *falx cerebri and tentorium cerebelli* mitigate against excessive jarring of the brain.

General features

Intracranial injuries may occur with or without fracture of the skull; about 25 percent of fatal head injuries occur without a skull fracture. The *mortality rate* in severe head injuries is about 50 percent, but the overall mortality for acute head injuries is less than 10 percent. *Important factors in fatal cases of head trauma* are extensive and multiple cerebral damage, shock, asphyxia, concomitant trauma or disease, and infection [14]. In about 50 percent of *fatal blunt-force head injuries* death is due to secondary involvement of vital areas of the brain – the midbrain, posterior hypothalamus, and medulla oblongata [15]. Edema of these areas is found in half such cases, and hemorrhage and necrosis are present in the rest. *Failure of respiration* is the usual cause of death when vital brain areas are damaged.

Coup injury

Contrecoup injury

Coup injury is a contusion or laceration of the brain occurring beneath the area of impact on the scalp. It is caused by the impact of a moving object on the stationary head or by striking the head against a sharp object such as a table edge or open drawer. *Contrecoup injury* is a type of contusion or laceration which occurs when the head is in motion and the momentum of impact momentarily throws the brain forcibly against the skull opposite the point of impact [16]. Thus, a fall on the back of the head results in contrecoup lesions at the tips of the frontal and temporal lobes where the brain is forced against the irregular bone of the anterior and middle cranial fossae. A fall on the top of the head may produce contrecoup lesions in the corpus callosum and hippocampal gyri. Coup or contrecoup injuries occur only rarely in the occipital lobes.

Types of head injury

Cranial and intracranial injury has been divided into three types: (1) injury to the skull and brain by impact of a moving object on the head, (2) compression of the skull between two relatively broad surfaces, and (3) impact of the moving head against an immobile object [17].

Injury to the brain and skull by the impact of a moving object on the head occurs in industrial accidents and criminal assaults. When the *impact* is *due to a relatively large object with a slow velocity,* a locally depressed skull fracture with secondary brain damage such as contusion or laceration may result. When the *injury* is *due to penetration of the skull and brain by a pointed instrument with a slow velocity,* as in a stab wound with an ice pick, cerebral laceration occurs and post-traumatic epilepsy is common due to the development of a glial scar. When the *impact* is *due to a sharp-edged instrument,* an incised wound with a splitting fracture at either end may develop. When the *impact* is that *of a small object with a high velocity,* such as a bullet or flying wooden or metal fragment, the skull and brain wound may be tangential, penetrating, or perforating (through and through). There are a cone of destruction due to cerebral laceration and secondary tracts due to accelerated bone fragments. *In all injuries caused by the impact of moving objects on the head, no significant gross brain damage occurs unless the skull is fractured.*

Compression of the skull between two relatively broad surfaces occurs during delivery when the fetal head is compressed between forceps blades, subdural hemorrhage being the most common result, and in *crushing head injuries* in children and adults. In crushing injuries skull fractures are usually at right angles to the direction of compression *(meridional fractures).*

The most common types of cranial and intracranial injuries are due to impact of the moving head against an immobile or relatively immobile object and occur in automobile accidents and falls. They are almost never due to direct assault. In such injuries subdural hematoma, subarachnoid hemorrhage, cerebral contusion, and intracerebral hemorrhage may develop through the coup-contrecoup mechanism. *Contrecoup injuries occur exclusively when the head is in motion,* at which time the brain tends to lag behind the moving skull. When the skull is abruptly stopped by impact against an immobile object, the lagging brain is struck by the wall of the skull opposite to the area of impact. The pole of the brain diametrically opposed to the point of impact is contused by striking a bony prominence during a gliding motion initiated by the impact. A secondary wave then flows back in the opposite direction toward the impact site, and this may thrust the brain surface there against a bony prominence and produce *coup injury.* The smooth bony surface over the occipital lobe accounts for the absence of contusion there. A shearing stress around the rostrum of the corpus callosum as it is thrust into the opening beneath the falx cerebri may account for secondary injury in this region. When a person strikes the side of the head flatly against an immobile object, the contrecoup lesion is always more severe than the coup one.

Cerebral contusion

Cerebral contusion [18, 19] is due to the momentary pressing of the skull against the meninges and brain at the time of impact. It may be coup or contrecoup in type. Multiple contusions of varying ages are common in chronic alcoholics. Early there are characteristic *hemorrhages arranged in parallel rows at the peaks of the gyri.* Such hemorrhages occur at the moment of impact and are found in persons who die immediately. Later *contusion necrosis* produces a triangular defect with the base peripherally. Such necrosis is due to impact waves of high magnitude. *Old contusions* appear as trenchlike defects at the tips of convolutions.

Cerebral laceration

Cerebral laceration is the tearing of brain tissue due to a depressed skull fracture, penetrating or bullet wound, or sudden torsion of the brain from the impact of an object against the skull. Traumatic hemorrhage is common. The lesion also may be contrecoup in type.

Punch drunk

Punch drunk is a chronic brain syndrome in boxers, who develop mental confusion and uncertainty of equilibrium. Multiple petechial hemorrhages, usually old and pink, are found throughout the cerebrum at postmortem examination. These punctate hemorrhages are probably due to breaks at the capillovenular junctions. Intracranial pressure waves set up by impacts against the skull raises the venous pressure above the corresponding arteriolar pressure temporarily with a reversal in blood flow and rupture of the relatively weak capillovenous junctions [20].

Cerebral concussion

Cerebral concussion is a transient clinical state characterized by the instantaneous onset of paralytic and other central nervous system symptoms following a head injury. *Concussion is more severe in injuries in which the head is in motion* (falls, automobile accidents) than when it is stationary at the moment of impact. Vibration waves are set up by the impact and pass over and through the brain. The cranial vault receives the impact first, so that *motor areas,* especially the more superficial foci controlling the lower extremities, are affected early, producing weakness. The *labyrinth* is often involved to produce vertigo and a loss of balance. If the *upper brain stem* is affected, there is a loss of consciousness. Shock and death may result from severe concussion with involvement of the *medulla.* If the shock waves expend themselves in the cerebrospinal fluid system, focal *subependymal (Duret's) hemorrhages* are found in the floor of the fourth ventricle. There is evidence that *coma in concussion* is due to blocking of sensory responses in the reticular formation in the midbrain which are essential for consciousness [21].

The acute stage of concussion is followed by the stage of *cerebral irritability,* which may last for a long period *(postconcussion syndrome).* In adults this is characterized by headaches, dizziness, and irritability, while in children personality alterations, such as increased aggressiveness or recessiveness and antisocial behavior, are very common [22]. About 15 percent of such children develop convulsions or enuresis.

The *pathologic findings in fatal cerebral concussion* are inconspicuous. In some cases petechiae are scattered through the brain. These may lead to foci of gliosis. Brain injury without overt structural damage, as in concussion, may be due to the violent force-driven development of bubble-like cavities within fluid accompanied by a high-potential electric discharge within the brain [23]. Brain injury with structural damage is explained, according to this theory, by the violent collapse of such fluid cavities in the brain.

Epidural hemorrhage:

Epidural (extradural) hemorrhage [24] is usually due to fracture, most commonly of the greater wing of the sphenoid bone, in the region where the *anterior branch of the middle meningeal artery* courses through the bone. The posterior branch is also a frequent source of hemorrhage. A few cases are due to bleeding from meningeal or dural venous sinuses or from emissary veins. With venous bleeding the onset of symptoms is sometimes delayed for 1 to 3 weeks. The *hemorrhage is arterial* in over 90 percent of the cases and requires immediate surgical treatment. Classically the patient is knocked unconscious at the time of injury, regains consciousness and has a *lucid* interval, then becomes comatose again as the hemorrhage increases in size. However, the lucid interval is often absent. There is commonly an ipsilateral dilated, fixed pupil due to pressure on the oculomotor nerve as it courses through the superior orbital fissure. The *mortality rate* is about 30 percent.

pathologic changes

A firm clot is usually found overlying the outer dural surface. If several days have elapsed between the time of the trauma and surgical removal of the clot or death, fibroblasts from the dura penetrate the coagulum superficially. The underlying brain is indented and hemorrhagic and it may show cortical softening due to compression of the venous drainage *(venous infarction).*

Acute subdural hemorrhage

Acute subdural hemorrhage occurs in almost all head injuries of any severity due to the stretching and/or tearing of the dura mater and arachnoid membrane. Small rents in arteries or veins lead to varying degrees of hemorrhage. This bleeding is rarely of clinical significance and is usually overshadowed by the concomitant cerebral damage. Occasionally a clot large enough to cause cerebral compression may form within a few hours or days. The relationship of acute subdural hemorrhage to chronic subdural hematoma is not entirely clarified, but it is likely that the latter is the end result of unrecognized acute bleeding beneath the dura mater.

Subdural hematoma:

Chronic subdural hematoma results from *rupture of a small or large bridging vein* crossing the subdural space from the arachnoid membrane to the dura mater.

The largest are due to rupture of the great vein of Galen behind the corpus callosum. Occasionally an arachnoid vein may rupture. *Trauma to the head,* sometimes of an apparently trivial nature, *is the underlying cause. Spinal subdural hematoma* may be produced by a fall on the buttocks. Subdural bleeding is especially common in alcoholics because of their proneness to head injuries from falls, arachnoidal edema, and the hemorrhagic tendency secondary to hepatic damage. *Clinically* symptoms appear 3 to 6 weeks after the injury when the clot is organized. They include headache, confusion, somnolence, and coma. There may be tenderness over the region of the clot. The cerebrospinal fluid is under increased pressure and is clear or xanthochromic. *Cerebral angiography* shows displacement of the terminal branches of the middle cerebral artery away from the surface of the skull in cases of subdural hematoma in the frontoparietal region.

pathologic changes

Following the injury, a clot forms in the subdural space loosely attached to the dura and arachnoid. Within 24 hours proliferation of fibrous tissue from the dura begins, and in 3 to 4 weeks the clot is covered by fibrous tissue, forming a thin sac (the *neomembrane*). The sac is filled with dark brown fluid or clotted blood due to bleeding from giant capillaries. The older concept of enlargement by imbibition of fluid through the membrane as the osmotic pressure within the sac increases is no longer widely held. A slowly enlarging hematoma may attain a volume one-tenth that of the brain before clinical signs of increased intracranial pressure develop, and a volume of at least 40 ml. is necessary for significant cerebral compression [25]. The underlying cerebral cortex is indented by the expanding mass, but it can regain its usual contour if the clot is evacuated. As the hematoma enlarges, it produces venous stasis deep in the underlying white matter with resulting cerebral edema and infarction. *Microscopically* perivenular demyelinization and gliosis are seen. If the hematoma is not removed, *death,* usually due to brain stem hemorrhage caused by mesencephalic compression or to medullary compression, eventuates.

Subarachnoid hemorrhage

Subarachnoid hemorrhage is the most common type of intracranial bleeding due to trauma. It *is usually associated with cerebral or cerebellar contusion or laceration,* and traumatic subarachnoid hemorrhage frequently occurs over the occipital lobes and cerebellum. Blood in the subarachnoid space acts as an irritant and causes a moderate meningeal inflammatory reaction. The blood often disappears completely in persons who survive. *Nontraumatic subarachnoid hemorrhage* is usually due to rupture of a berry aneurysm of a branch of the circle of Willis, but may be "spontaneous" due to rupture of an apparently normal subarachnoid vessel. Subarachnoid hemorrhage also occurs in carbon monoxide poisoning, acute cerebral congestion due to strangling or status epilepticus, and hemorrhagic diatheses.

Pulsating exophthalmos

Pulsating exophthalmos is uncommon and is due to an arteriovenous fistula between the carotid artery and the cavernous sinus following a fracture of the base of the skull. The transmission of the arterial pulse through the sinus and ophthalmic vein produces the pulsating protrusion of the ipsilateral eye.

Bullet wounds

Intracranial bullet wounds [26] are much more frequent in men than women and are suicidally inflicted in over half the cases. In about 25 percent there is a *perforating wound,* the bullet passing entirely through the head and leaving both entry and exit wounds. The rest are *penetrating wounds,* the bullet being lodged in the brain or the skull or scalp away from its site of entrance. *Bullet wound tracks* in the brain are single in about 80 percent of cases, but two or more tracks may be produced by one bullet due to ricochet off the skull opposite the entry site or tangential skidding along the skull. Therefore, in a perforating wound the exit site may not be opposite the point of entry. Bullet wound tracks are about the size of the diameter of the bullet, except when a larger piece of skull bone is propelled through the canal ahead of a bullet or when permanent cavitation is produced by a high-velocity missile. The track shows relatively little hemorrhage in patients dying within an hour of the shooting. *Old wound tracks* become cystic and enlarged due to resorption of necrotic brain tissue. *Remote contusions* are common away from the wound track, especially *in the cerebellar tonsils.* These are due to impact of the contused area of the brain against the skull, falx cerebri, or tentorium cerebelli at the moment of injury. The entire brain is enlarged at the moment of passage of a bullet through it, because of temporary cavitation along the wound track. The cerebellar tonsils are slammed against the walls of the foramen magnum, causing subarachnoid and intratonsillar hemorrhage in many cases. *Edema of the entire brain* due to hypoxia often occurs following bullet wounds. The *cause of death* in fatal cases is injury to the respiratory center due to compression of the medulla oblongata in the foramen magnum either at the moment of impact or later when increased intracranial pressure develops due to cerebral edema and hemorrhage.

SPINAL CORD INJURIES

Spinal cord injuries are most commonly due to fractures, dislocations, or subluxations of the vertebrae. In the cervical region these may be due to *whiplash injury*. Penetrating and bullet wounds occasionally cause trauma to the spinal cord. A number of cases of spinal cord compression due to acute flexion of the cervical vertebrae in persons using trampolines have occurred [27]. Severe injury to the spinal cord produces motor and/or sensory paralysis below the level of the lesion. *Pathologic changes and reactions* in the cord are similar to those in the brain. *Hematomyelia* is a hemorrhage into the cord and is due to trauma. The hemorrhage may extend for long distances up and down the gray matter due to antecedent softening. Rarely the hemorrhage is repaired by gliosis, but most cases end fatally.

NEUROGLIAL REACTION TO INJURY

All three glial elements – microglial cells, oligodendrocytes, and astrocytes – take part in the reaction to injury. The astrocytes and oligodendrocytes together make up the *neuroglia. Microglial cells* are mesodermal in origin and are part of the reticuloendothelial system. Their function is phagocytic. In and about areas of central nervous system injury with necrosis, the microglia transform from small cells with fine branching processes into swollen, rounded, phagocytic scavenger cells (compound granular cells, *Gitterzellen),* the cell cytoplasm becoming filled with large and small fat globules (disintegrating myelin). The microglial cells transport the ingested myelin to nearby vessels, discharging it there. *Oligodendrocytes* are derived from the neuroectoderm and are small cells with few processes. They appear to play a part in the preservation of myelin, being analogous to the peripheral Schwann sheath cells. In areas of central nervous system injury they rapidly swell and become vacuolated. *Astrocytes* are neuroectodermal in origin and are large cells with numerous processes, one of which is attached to a small vessel as a vascular footplate (sucker foot). In foci of injury the astrocytes are destroyed, but those in the surrounding regions proliferate and form a dense fibrillar network. Thus the defect is filled in by *gliosis* within a few days if it is not too large.

ASPHYXIA AND DROWNING

1. *Asphyxia*

ASPHYXIA:

Asphyxia is characterized by the struggle to breathe against some type of interference with respiratory movements. Anoxia, cyanosis, and carbon dioxide accumulation rapidly ensue. The respiratory center is stimulated, and attempts at breathing are rapid and tumultuous. The *causes* of asphyxia include any obstruction to the air passages such as smothering, strangling, gagging, hanging, a foreign body in the trachea, diphtheritic membrane, laryngeal edema, or compression of the chest. If the cause of the obstruction is not quickly removed, there is marked cyanosis and congestion of the head and neck. Veins may burst under the greatly increased pressure. In certain cases there may be fractures of the tracheal cartilages, edema of the larynx, or contusions of the subcutaneous tissues of the neck. *Hanging* produces an inverted-V type of contusion line on the front and sides of the neck, whereas *ligature strangulation* causes a circular contusion around the neck. In cases of hanging, the contusion line is usually higher than in those of ligature strangulation. The contusions may be patterned according to the object employed for hanging or strangulation. In *manual strangulation* fingernail scratches are often present on the neck skin. In about 90 percent of cases of sudden asphyxia from a variety of causes, *pulmonary edema* is found [28]. The amount of edema fluid varies from slight to massive and is patchily distributed throughout the lungs. The edema fluid is usually stringy or granular in appearance. Congestion is prominent in asphyxia due to strangulation.

Traumatic asphyxia

Traumatic asphyxia follows violent thoracic compression, such as crushing between two vehicles. There is a deep cyanosis of the upper thorax anteriorly and of the neck, the head, and the interscapular triangle posteriorly. Numerous small hemorrhages occur throughout the muscles and tissues of the neck. The veins of the head and neck are tremendously distended. *Traumatic asphyxia is due to compression of the superior vena cava.*

2. *Drowning*

DROWNING:

Drowning is a special type of asphyxia in which ventilation of air is blocked by spasm of the larynx (10 percent) or by filling of the lungs with water (90 percent). In the former there is pulmonary congestion and edema; in the latter the lungs are filled with a frothy fluid. Pulmonary edema occurs in both freshwater and saltwater drowning, and it may be massive in cases of drowning in chlorinated fresh water [29]. A few drowning deaths are caused by the vagovagal reflex set off by sudden immersion in cold water with stimulation of the vagus by water in the nasopharynx; cardiac standstill is produced. In cases of drowning in which the lungs are filled with water, there is an initial glottic spasm, during which copious amounts of water are swallowed, overdistending the stomach. Vomiting follows, the glottis relaxes, and gasping inspirations draw great amounts of water into the lungs. Most cases of drowning occur in nonswimmers or inexperienced swimmers, but occasional cases involve experienced swimmers, especially due to the development of unconsciousness during underwater swimming. This is due to the hyperventilation practiced by such swimmers prior to entering the water [30]. During voluntary overbreathing, the partial pressure of carbon dioxide (P_{CO_2}) in the blood is decreased and body stores of carbon dioxide are depleted. It is probable that, while swimming under water, sufficient hypoxia may develop to cause loss of consciousness before the blood P_{CO_2} attains levels which would produce an overwhelming urge to breathe and cause the swimmer to surface. Exercise appears to increase the subject's tolerance to developing hypercapnia.

Death due to drowning

In persons drowning in fresh water [31], *death* usually occurs in 2 to 4 minutes. It *results from ventricular fibrillation,* which is due to an extreme rise in the serum potassium concentration to as high as 8 milliequivalents per liter, caused by the release of potassium ions from erythrocytes by hemolysis produced by hemodilution. The latter is caused by the absorption of hypotonic water into the bloodstream in the lungs. Within 3 minutes after submersion the body fluids are 70 percent aspirated fresh water in experimental animals. That the abrupt marked increase in blood volume due to absorption of water may overload and cause the failure of an already hypoxic myocardium has been proposed as an important factor in freshwater drowning deaths [32].

In cases of drowning in salt water, death typically occurs in 6 to 7 minutes *due to myocardial anoxia.* A sudden rise in the serum magnesium level may be a factor in the cardiac standstill.

If water enters the lungs before the heart stops, the salt content of the blood is altered. With sea (salt) water the amount of sodium chloride in blood from the left ventricle will be greater than in blood from the right ventricle. With fresh water, the reverse is true. This is known as the *Gettler test;* its validity has been questioned. In all cases of drowning in which water enters the lungs before cardiac action ceases, the *specific gravity of the* left atrial *plasma* is less than that of the right atrial plasma, due to hemodilution in the pulmonary capillaries [33]. The *measurement of total solids in the right and left atrial blood* by means of a refractometric TS (total solids) meter is of value in the diagnosis of drowning, especially in fresh water [34]. Because of hemodilution the total solids per unit volume in left heart blood is less than in that from the right heart in freshwater drowning.

Diatoms up to 30μ in diameter may be disseminated via the bloodstream, to the liver, kidneys, brain, and bone marrow in cases of drowning. In badly decomposed bodies microscopic plankton may be found in the bone marrow following nitric acid digestion. The presence of diatoms in the lungs alone is not reliable evidence of drowning unless they are widely disseminated in both lungs [35].

TRAUMA DUE TO HEAT

The body is far more sensitive to an increase than a decrease in its temperature. An elevation of 5°C. (9°F.) above normal tissue temperature is injurious. The higher the temperature, the shorter is the duration required for cell death.

1. Thermal Burn

THERMAL BURN:

Thermal burn (local hyperthermia) is an injury produced by heat and usually involving the skin. *Cutaneous burns* may be divided into three degrees according to their severity. A *first-degree burn* is characterized by erythema without significant epidermal alteration; a *second-degree burn* is typified by vesicle formation and destruction of the epidermis with little or no irreversible damage to the dermis; and a *third-degree burn* is one in which there is dermal damage extensive enough to interfere with epidermal regeneration.

Local pathologic changes

Pathologically the earliest evidence of thermal injury is dilatation of capillaries and other small vessels. If endothelial injury occurs, there is an increase in capillary permeability, and *edema* follows. Fluid may collect beneath the epidermis, causing *vesiculation.* The earliest cellular change in the epidermis and dermis is a redistribution of the nuclear fluid and solids. This is followed by nuclear swelling caused by the imbibition of fluid. Rupture of the nuclear membrane leads to karyorrhexis or pyknosis. The cytoplasm becomes granular and later coagulates. Collagenous fibers have the appearance of a gel. *Thermally destroyed tissue* evokes an aseptic acute inflammatory response and acts as a foreign body. *Infection* is common at burn sites because of the occurrence of a break in the skin barrier together with the presence of a protein-rich edema fluid.

Systemic effects

Systemic effects of cutaneous burns may be due to pain, plasma loss, and the absorption of toxic breakdown products from damaged cells. These effects include:

1. *Primary* (neurogenic) *shock.*

2. *Secondary shock.* This may be due to plasma loss at the burned surface and/or the absorption of vasotoxic substances. The marked *hemoconcentration* may lead to phlebothrombosis in the extremities. Small thromboses in gastric and duodenal vessels may be the cause of the acute ulcers *(Curling's ulcers)* which occur in the stomach and duodenum.

3. *Intravascular hemolysis.* Hemoglobin is released, and this, together with the accompanying shock, may produce hypoxic nephrosis.

Infection of burn site

In patients with severe and extensive burns, infection of the burn site and septicemia due to gram-negative organisms have become frequent. Pseudomonas aeruginosa is the most common infecting organism, and pseudomonas infection was a contributing factor in 35 percent of the deaths in fatal burns in one series [36]. *Escherichia coli* and *Proteus* and *Klebsiella-Aerobacter* species are also common burn invaders. *Staphylococcus aureus* and fungi, such as *Candida albicans* and *Mucor* species, are isolated in some fatal infections. *Pseudomonas burn infections and septicemia* typically occur about 2 weeks after the burn in patients who have had extensive antibiotic therapy, especially for staphylococcal infections. Leukopenia and hypothermia are frequently noted in septicemia with pseudomonas and other gram-negative bacterial infections. In pseudomonas infection the organisms proliferate beneath the eschar over burned areas, and the zone between the eschar and underlying dermis or subcutaneous tissue becomes intensely infiltrated with neutrophils. Purplish black pockets develop in and beneath the eschar due to hemorrhage and necrosis.

Autopsy findings

Autopsy findings in deaths from burns, aside from the local effects of the burn, include visceral congestion and edema, especially of the lungs, due to shock; cloudy swelling in the liver and kidneys; acute (Curling's) ulcers of the stomach and duodenum; adrenal cortical degeneration; subendocardial and epicardial hemorrhages; and hypoxic nephrosis or bilateral cortical necrosis of the kidneys. In many fatal burns due to fire the *inhalation of smoke, hot air, particulate matter, and flame produces severe lung lesions* [37]. These may be the major cause of death. The changes include acute tracheobronchitis and bronchiolitis, intra-alveolar hemorrhage, focal atelectasis, and bronchopneumonia. The bronchopneumonia occurs in about half of fatal burns in which the patient survives longer than 2 days.

Staphylococcus aureus and gram-negative bacteria are the most common causative organisms.

Death during a fire

Death during a fire is recognized by the presence of carbon monoxide in concentration above 5 percent in the blood, the presence of particles of soot in the respiratory tract, and true vesicles of the skin. Blood carbon monoxide values in burned bodies should be corrected by use of the hematocrit and hemoglobin levels to eliminate errors due to postmortem changes. Blood alcohol and barbiturate levels should also be determined, and the body should be x-rayed for evidence of trauma. In a burned body, contractions of the muscles caused by heat produce a characteristic *"pugilistic attitude,"* which resembles the position of a fighter defending himself. Muscle contraction may cause fractures of the bones of the extremities. *Most deaths during fires are accidental,* and few are due to burn effects. The *cause of death* is usually carbon monoxide poisoning, coronary artery disease with a low carbon monoxide level, or fatty metamorphosis of the liver (in alcoholics). Suicides are rare by burning except in the insane. Homicide by burning is usually confined to infants and the aged. Many times, however, a dead or dying person may be burned to conceal the true cause of death or the identity of the victim. *Artifacts* caused by burning may simulate skull fractures, due to boiling of the brain with steam production, and extradural or subdural hematoma, due to the oozing of blood and shrinkage of the brain. *Fire fractures* are extruded, never depressed, and are usually multilinear.

2. Heat stroke

HEAT STROKE

Heat stroke (systemic hyperthermia) is due to an environmental temperature which overwhelms the temperature-regulating mechanism of the body. The skin is very hot, and the body temperature may reach 42.5°C. (108.5°F.). The victim may become unconscious rapidly *(heat apoplexy)* or gradually. Death seldom occurs in a healthy person. In *fatal cases* there is usually an associated disease such as coronary sclerosis. The *hemorrhages* in heat stroke may be due to fibrinolysis and hypofibrinogenemia plus increased capillary fragility [38]. Hypoprothrombinemia has also been reported in heat stroke. The *pathologic changes* [39] include petechial hemorrhages in the skin and mucosa, and hyperemia and even small hemorrhages in the brain. Congestion and edema are present in the lungs. Focal necroses and fragmentation of myocardial fibers are common. In the kidneys there is occasionally a distal convoluted tubular epithelial degeneration with hemoglobin casts *(hypoxic nephrosis).* The plasma potassium level may be markedly elevated due to the release of potassium from thermally damaged erythrocytes. After death, rapid and marked rigor mortis and decomposition occur.

3. Heat Exhaustion

HEAT EXHAUSTION

Heat exhaustion is produced by an environmental temperature which severely strains the temperature-regulating mechanism of the body. *Clinically* there are weakness, pallor, stupor, and a decreased blood pressure due to peripheral vascular collapse. The oral temperature is low, and the skin is cold. *Muscle cramps (heat cramps)* often occur in heat exhaustion due to the depletion of body salt by excessive sweating.

TRAUMA DUE TO COLD

1. *Frostbite*

FROST-BITE:

Frostbite (local cold injury, local hypothermia) is due to prolonged exposure of a body part to a freezing or near-freezing temperature. Chilling of the tissues decreases the metabolic activity of the cells. *Cell death occurs when there is intracellular ice formation or infarction due to plugging of small blood vessels.* Injury to the endothelium of small blood vessels leads to edema and plugging of the vessels with tightly packed erythrocytes. The process may lead to wet or dry gangrene of the part.

The type and duration of exposure to or contact with freezing temperatures are the most important factors in determining the extent of *frostbite injury* [40]. Touching cold metal, especially when the skin is wet, is the most dangerous type of contact, the skin often being torn off when it is pulled away. The combination of wind and cold is much more serious as a freezing factor than cold air alone. The reduction of atmospheric pressure at high altitudes has little effect on the susceptibility to frostbite. *Factors which predispose to frostbite* in mountain climbers and others *at high altitudes,* other than the very cold temperature, are loss of judgment due to cerebral hypoxia, loss of huge quantities of body heat through the lungs by panting and overexertion, impairment of shivering as a heat-producing mechanism, and difficulty of providing the increased caloric needs of the body by the intake of food. Frostbite rarely occurs in healthy individuals who are standing still and adequately clothed. Its development is usually associated with fatigue, a storm, or an accident. Frostbite frequently occurs in exposed individuals who are intoxicated with alcohol. This is probably due to peripheral vasodilation with loss of body heat stores through the skin.

Frostbite is almost always limited to an extremity or to the chin, cheeks, nose, and ears. This is due to the *capillary shunt mechanism* in the peripheral areas of the body which sends the blood directly from arterioles to venules in order to maintain the core temperature of the vital organs of the body. The tissues in areas in which the capillary circulation is decreased or absent soon freeze, ice crystals forming between the cells. Water is drawn from the cells, dehydrating them. Such crystals develop within the cells on exposure to extremely intense cold, and the formation of intracellular ice crystals produces rapid cell death.

Superficial frostbite

Superficial frostbite involves only the skin, which becomes white and waxy early. *Rewarmed frostbitten areas* are a mottled blue or purple, and swollen. In more severe cases vesicles and bullae develop in the epidermis in 24 to 36 hours. These gradually dry up and become black. The epidermis peels off, and the involved area remains red and very sensitive to cold for a long time.

Chilblains

Chilblains is a relatively mild and reversible form of superficial frostbite. It is due to exposure to not too severe cold or to cold with a high humidity. The involved skin is dark blue, and on warming it remains blue, swells, and becomes painful. After some days the epidermis peels off.

Deep frostbite

Deep frostbite involves the skin, subcutaneous tissue, and deep tissues, even bone. Huge bullae develop within 3 to 7 days. The involved areas become blue, purple, or gray. The bullae eventually dry up, blacken, and slough off. *Unless such cases are rapidly rewarmed, portions of the affected tissue are lost.* In 1 to 2 weeks the most distal portion either becomes black and shriveled *(dry gangrene),* or, if infection has occurred, it becomes soft, swollen, and reddish black *(wet gangrene).*

2. *Systemic Hypothermia*

SYSTEMIC HYPOTHERMIA

In *systemic hypothermia (freezing),* coma ensues once cold has broken through the body's temperature-controlling mechanism. Death results from a sufficiently low body temperature. The circulation fails at about 21°C. (70°F.). Most freezings in the United States occur in abandoned infants and in alcoholics. *Pathologic changes* are nonspecific and resemble those of shock. Moderate right heart dilatation and pulmonary edema are found. Lobar pneumonia is common in those living long enough to develop it. In patients exposed to prolonged *therapeutic hypothermia* at about 30°C. (86°F.), pneumonitis and pulmonary atelectasis may occur [41]. Gastric ulceration and hemorrhage also develop in patients under hypothermia, due to a stress reaction or to an increased hematocrit caused by the transfer of plasma water into erythrocytes. In the latter case, thrombosis may occur in small gastric vessels and lead to infarction and ulceration.

TRAUMA DUE TO LIGHT

The shorter the wave length of light rays, the lesser is the penetration and the greater the irritation. Ultraviolet rays, with a wave length less than 3800 angstroms, are the most irritating; *infrared rays,* with a wave length greater than 8000 angstroms, are the most penetrating.

SUNBURN

Sunburn is due mainly to the ultraviolet rays of the spectrum with wave lengths between 2950 and 3250 angstroms, and the mechanism of injury appears to be photochemical in nature. The early sensation of heat and erythema are due to infrared rays, but the ultimate changes are independent of the heat of the sunlight. The *skin and systemic changes* are essentially the same as in other types of first- or second-degree burns. Tanning is produced by an increase in melanin in the epidermis and dermis. *Certain drugs,* such as sulfonamides, barbiturates, chlorpromazine, promethazine, chlorothiazide, and demethylchlortetracycline, *may sensitize the skin to sunlight* with the production of a dermatitis in which papules, vesicles, and/or wheals appear in the skin. This unexplained phenomenon also occurs in certain diseases such as porphyria, lupus erythematosus, and pellagra.

SKIN LESIONS RELATED TO SUNLIGHT

Some skin lesions are directly related to sunlight. *Senile (solar) keratoses* are thickened patches of the skin on the face and hands of persons exposed to sunlight most of the time, such as farmers and sailors. The lesions are premalignant. *Xeroderma pigmentosum* is a rare congenital hypersensitivity to light. Erythema, increased pigmentation, and warty elevations appear in the skin in childhood. The lesions are premalignant, with epidermoid carcinoma or melanocarcinoma frequently developing. *Porphyria* is a rare congenital metabolic disturbance in some forms of which hematoporphyrins in the blood act as sensitizers to light. The skin is sensitive, vesicles appearing on slight exposure to sunlight. The bones become pigmented red, and the urine turns red on exposure to light. Exposure of the patient to intense light may cause convulsions and even death.

EFFECTS OF LASER RADIATION

Laser (light amplification by the stimulated emission of radiation) *irradiation* [42] is used in the treatment of retinal detachment and is being tested experimentally for a number of purposes. Most lasers function in the red or infrared bands of the light spectrum, so that *the principal biologic effects are due to heat.* Retinal burns are readily induced by laser irradiation. Sharply demarcated, punched-out third-degree skin burns with surrounding vesiculation occur in experimental animals exposed to a laser beam, and carcinoma in situ has developed in the skin of a human volunteer. Visceral perforations due to heat have occurred in experimental animals when the abdomen has been irradiated with a laser beam. Pigment cells are selectively destroyed in tissue cultures exposed to laser beams, and dividing cells are arrested in prophase temporarily.

TRAUMA DUE TO ELECTRIC ENERGY

1. Electric Injury

ELECTRIC INJURY:

For *trauma* to occur *due to electric energy* it is necessary for a part of the body to lie between two conductors in such a way as to complete an electric circuit. The electric current follows the path of least resistance through the body, often being conducted via the blood and cerebrospinal fluid according to the classic theory. However, a 60-cycle alternating current may pass through an animal body along the shortest path between contacts, regardless of intervening anatomic structures. The *harmful effects of an electric current* include cell death by heat or electrolysis, stimulation of powerful muscle contractions, and inhibition of vital centers such as the cardiac and respiratory centers of the medulla. The *nature and severity of the harmful effects* depend on:

1. *Type of electric current.* Within the range of electric currents to which humans are ordinarily exposed, an alternating current is more dangerous than a direct current. Currents of high frequency (above 200 cycles per second) and faradic (induced) currents rarely produce electric injury.

2. *Amount of current.* This is determined by the formula $C = V/R$, where C is the current in amperes, V is the potential in volts, and R is the resistance of the body in ohms.

3. *Path of the current through the body.* A current which passes through the brain or through the left side of the body is more dangerous than a current of equal magnitude which is limited to the extremities or passes through the right side of the body.

4. *Duration of the flow of current.* The amount of heat generated increases directly with time, and the probability of irreversible cell damage also increases with time.

Pathologic changes

The *mark of entry* of an electric current is a round or oblong, rosette-like or linear, gray, white, or yellow elevation of the skin. In the center there is a small crater-like depression. Microscopically the epidermal markings are obliterated. *Burns occur at the points of entry and exit of the current,* especially at the exit which is usually on the feet. The burn is dry and ischemic at first, but after a day hyperemia and edema appear. Small cavities appear in the epidermis; then sloughing of the skin and ulceration occur. The systemic effects are like those of other burns. The amount of heat produced and hence the capacity to cause a burn is calculated by the formula $H = C^2R/4.187$, where H is the heat produced in gram-calories per second. Burns are common from metallic conductors which have been rendered extremely hot by short circuits, but such burns are not electrothermal. Currents of 110 volts rarely produce burns unless there is protracted contact. *Soft tissues present less resistance to the passage of electric currents than bone*, so that a current which enters one arm and leaves through the trunk or the lower extremities will produce greater damage at the elbow, where there is the least soft tissue, than at any place except the points of entry and exit.

Causes of death

Death from electric energy is usually due to respiratory or cardiac failure. If death from electrocution is instantaneous, as in legal executions, no pathologic changes aside from burns at areas of contact are found. In *legal electrocutions* the actual cause of death is a rapid increase of body temperature (up to 140°F.) to a level that causes coagulation of protein.

2. Lightning Injury

LIGHTNING INJURY

Lightning [43] produces results similar to those caused by an electric current. The morphologic changes are surprisingly slight, since a lightning bolt has millions of volts and a current of about 20,000 amperes. Characteristic *current markings* or *lightning figures* (peculiar arborescent red lines on the skin) about a small, deep burn are found at the sites of entrance and exit of the current. Unconsciousness usually is caused by a lightning stroke, and apnea due to medullary paralysis is common. The heart undergoes a violent ventricular contraction at the time of the stroke, then there is a slow relaxation. A regular bradycardia then develops. There is no ventricular fibrillation. *Death* is due to myocardial anoxia and occurs several minutes after the lightning stroke.

TRAUMA DUE TO MICROWAVE RADIATION

MICROWAVES

Microwaves lie between the infrared and radio wave bands on the electromagnetic spectrum, with frequencies from 1000 to more than 30,000 megacycles per second and wave lengths from 30 cm. to less than 1 cm. The waves are produced by special tubes such as the magnetron and klystron. *Radar* (from radio detection and ranging) is a detecting apparatus using microwaves. *Maser* is microwave amplification by stimulated emission of radiation. The *allowable exposure* to microwaves in terms of power density is 10 to 100 milliwatts per square centimeter of body surface.

MICROWAVE INJURY: Thermal effects

The *pathologic effects of exposure to microwaves are due to the deep penetration of the tissues by the waves and the development of high tissue temperatures.* The degree of temperature increase depends on the specific tissues exposed and the efficiency of their heat-eliminating mechanism, the intensity of the radiation, the frequency of the radiation, and the duration of exposure. The heat from microwaves is thought to be due mainly to the dipolarity of water in the blood and tissues. In a person exposed to the direct beam of a radar transmitter within 10 feet of the antenna, an intolerable sensation of heat in the abdomen developed in less than a minute [44]. Severe pain, vomiting, and shock ensued. Death occurred in 24 hours. *Pathologic findings* included a sanguineopurulent peritoneal exudate, ulceration and perforation of the jejunum, hemorrhage and edema of the small intestine, and hemorrhagic infarcts of the spleen. Similar changes have been produced in experimental animals exposed to microwave radiation.

Non-thermal effects

Nonthermal effects of microwaves include the production of *lenticular cataracts* in man and experimental animals as well as mitotic arrest, depression of lymphocyte formation, tubular and interstitial damage in the testes, and decreased erythrocyte survival time in animals. These effects occur in the low-frequency microwave range, and they may be due to the reorientation of molecular components in the cells of affected tissues.

TRAUMA DUE TO IONIZING RADIATION

IONIZING RADIATION:

Ionizing radiation consists of that part of the electromagnetic spectrum (x-rays and gamma rays) and certain types of particulate radiation (alpha and beta particles, neutrons, deuterons, and protons) which carry sufficient energy to produce ionization in materials into which they are absorbed. *Alpha particles* consist of 2 protons and 2 neutrons (helium nucleus); *beta particles* are high-speed electrons, and beta rays are streams of such electrons; *gamma rays* have extremely short wave lengths, being shorter than x-rays. *Alpha particles and beta rays are absorbed by the skin; gamma rays penetrate the deeper tissues. Ionizing radiations act mainly on cell nuclei,* and cells are more vulnerable during mitosis than when at rest. In general, *the radiosensitivity of cells is proportional to the rapidity with which they reproduce and inversely proportional to the degree of their differentiation.* The effects of ionizing radiation on the animal body are genetic and somatic. The *genetic effects* are mutations, mainly due to gene deletions, similar to those occurring spontaneously. The *somatic effects* may be acute or chronic and localized or general, depending on the amount and rate of radiation exposure and the amount of the body exposed.

Measurement

The *unit of measurement for ionizing radiation* is the *roentgen* (R), the amount of x-radiation or gamma radiation that produces in 1 cc. of air sufficient ions to carry 1 electrostatic unit of positive or negative charge. A *rad (radiation absorbed dose)* is a unit of radiation absorbed by tissue and is equivalent to 100 ergs per gram. With x-rays 1 R of exposure will produce about 1 rad of absorbed dose in soft tissue. A *rem (radiation equivalent for man)* is the amount of any form of ionizing radiation which will produce approximately the biologic effect of 1 R of x-rays. For x-rays 1 rem is equivalent to 1 rad.

ACUTE RADIATION SICKNESS

Acute radiation sickness occurs in individuals whose whole bodies have absorbed over 100 rems. *Clinically* nausea, vomiting, diarrhea, and severe mental depression develop within a few hours after exposure and usually clear within 48 hours in nonfatal cases. The mortality rate reaches 50 percent with 450 rems, and almost all persons receiving 600 rems die. There are *no specific pathologic changes in acute radiation death. Grossly* widespread hemorrhages are found. *Microscopically* lymph nodes show lymphocytic degeneration and disappearance with reticular hyperplasia. Mature lymphocytes fragment and undergo dissolution. The spleen undergoes changes similar to those in lymph nodes, together with acute subendothelial hyalin deposition in the arterioles. In the gastrointestinal tract there are acute epithelial sloughing due to loss of intercellular cohesion, edema, and hemorrhages. Mitotic division is halted in crypt cells so that there is no replacement of the lost surface epithelium [45]. Fluid transudes across the bare surface into the intestinal lumen, leading to diarrhea, electrolyte imbalance, and hemoconcentration. Depletion of cortical lipids and degeneration of the zona glomerulosa are found in the adrenals. The lungs show congestion and edema, hemorrhage, and pneumonitis with little neutrophilic response.

RADIATION BURNS

Radiation burns appear after a latent period of about 2 weeks. All degrees of burns may appear from hyperemia to ulceration. The subcutaneous tissue and even the muscles may be involved. Healing is slow and scarring is marked. *Epidermoid carcinoma is common in old radiation burns.*

RADIATION DERMATITIS

Radiation dermatitis is due to frequent exposure to small doses of radiation. The *pathologic changes* include patches of atrophy and hyperkeratosis, hyperpigmentation, telangiectases, and splitting of the nails. Fingers and toes may be lost. *Microscopically* the changes are secondary to vascular damage. The capillaries are telangiectatic. In arterioles, and to a lesser extent in venules, there is a thickening of the intima, with marked narrowing or occlusion of the vessels. Thromboses are common. The dermis shows a dense, acellular fibrosis. The epidermis is thickened, with elongated rete pegs. Foci of epidermoid carcinoma are common. Similar changes occur in irradiated mucosa, such as that of the cervix uteri.

INTERNAL EFFECTS

Internal effects of ionizing radiation are due to ingestion of radioactive material, as in watch dial workers, or to extensive bombardment of the tissues. In patients who receive radiation therapy to the chest wall, mediastinum, or lung, as for carcinoma of the breast, lymphoma, or bronchogenic carcinoma, *radiation pneumonitis* sometimes occurs [46]. Within 1 or many months after exposure a fibrin-rich exudate accumulates within the alveoli in the involved portion of the lung, and fibrin membranes line the alveolar walls. After 6 to 24 months a proliferative phase develops. *Grossly* the exposed segment of lung becomes pinkish tan and firm. *Microscopically* alveolar septal and interstitial fibrosis is found. Radium, thorium, strontium 90, and other radioactive elements are stored in the bones, causing aplastic anemia, osteogenic sarcoma, and leukemia. In the mandible there is bone destruction similar to that found in phosphorus poisoning, with bacterial infections at the tooth roots and loss of teeth.

DELAYED EFFECTS

Delayed effects of ionizing radiation [47] include epidermoid carcinoma of the skin in about 25 percent of cases of chronic radiation dermatitis, basal cell carcinoma of the skin, leukemia, aplastic anemia, thrombocytopenia, thyroid carcinoma in children following thymic irradiation, bronchogenic carcinoma, osteogenic sarcoma, fibrosarcoma, endometrial carcinoma and carcinosarcoma, lenticular cataracts, and intra-uterine developmental defects.

TRAUMA DUE TO ATOMIC ENERGY

ATOMIC BOMB EXPLOSION:

The injuries caused by atomic explosions [48] *are due to the blast, the intense heat, and the radioactivity released.* The *radiation* released by the fission of uranium and plutonium is almost entirely made up of highly penetrative gamma rays. *The degree and type of injury in atomic explosions depends on the distance from the hypocenter of the explosion to the body.* Persons directly beneath or near the hypocenter at Hiroshima and Nagasaki were killed instantaneously by the blast and/or heat. The blast caused trauma by *air blast* with visceral ruptures and especially by flying objects and falling buildings. Many of the victims showed multiple fractures, but these were rare among survivors. The *burns* were of the *flash type,* an enormous temperature existing momentarily (2000°C.). Persons farther from the hypocenter showed varying effects of blast injury and burns.

Radiation effects were apparent within a few days or later. Survivors exposed to *very large amounts of radiation* developed marked hyperthermia, prostration, and anorexia, and died in a few days. In those exposed to *large amounts of radiation,* the male germinal, lymphopoietic, granulocytopoietic, and erythropoietic cells were most severely affected. The principal effects appeared in 2 to 3 weeks as aspermatogenesis, agranulocytosis, thrombocytopenia, and anemia. The last three effects were due to *bone marrow suppression.* Many of these patients died of *overwhelming infections or hemorrhages.* Among survivors who were exposed to heavy radiation there has been a definitely increased incidence of thyroid carcinoma [49] and leukemia. The latter differs from naturally occurring cases of leukemia in that the survival period after the clinical onset of acute and chronic myelogenous leukemia has been shorter in persons exposed within 1400 meters of the hypocenter of the atomic explosion as compared to nonexposed persons; and diffuse myelofibrosis has been more common in exposed than in nonexposed persons with chronic myelogenous leukemia [50]. Studies of the hexosamine: collagen ratio in the skin and aorta of persons exposed to atomic radiation as compared to controls indicate *accelerated aging* in the exposed group [51]. *Microcephaly* occurred rather frequently in fetuses of less than 4 months gestation exposed in utero to irradiation [52].

Ocular effects

Persons looking at an atomic or nuclear fireball can suffer instantaneous *chorioretinal burns,* due to near infrared waves. This effect is *similar to eclipse blindness,* in which chorioretinal burns are caused by looking directly at the sun for a long period of time. There is a small burn with perforation of the retina and choroid in the area on which the fireball image is focused on the retina. *Ionizing radiation is absorbed by all ocular tissues.* The most serious effects are on the lens, which is avascular and cannot dissipate the radiation. *Radiation cataracts* are due to beta rays and neutrons and develop in the posterior lens capsule.

THERMONUCLEAR EXPLOSION

The *effects of a hydrogen bomb (thermonuclear) explosion* would be the same as those described for atomic bomb explosion, but on a more massive scale. The *blast and heat effects* would result from both the thermonuclear explosion and the atomic explosion used to trigger it. The *radioactivity* would result from the triggering atomic explosion and neutrons. *Blast effects* would be caused by a direct (incident) blast wave coming directly or diagonally downward from the fireball, a reflected wave coming up from the ground, and a severe earthquake-like ground shock. The ground shock would be most severe with a surface explosion and would be followed by hurricane-like winds ("drag"). Intrafireball temperatures reach millions of degrees, so that anything within the fireball radius would be vaporized. Even though the extremely high temperatures have a very short duration, thermal damage would occur over a broader area than the blast destruction. *Fires* ignited by the heat would be spread over an extensive area by the high winds of the "drag." A *fire storm* might last for several hours with ground temperatures of about 800°C. (1400°F.). Atmospheric oxygen would be exhausted by the fires, and lethal concentrations of carbon monoxide would accumulate. The *radiation* would consist of gamma rays and neutrons, and within 18 hours lethal doses (over 1000 R may be spread as much as 100 miles from the explosion site by winds. It is estimated that over 90 percent of casualties from a thermonuclear explosion would be due to radioactive fallout.

TRAUMA DUE TO CHANGES IN ATMOSPHERIC PRESSURE

EFFECTS OF ATMOSPHERIC PRESSURE CHANGES:

The *effects of changes in atmospheric pressure* depend on the direction and magnitude of the change, the rate of change, and the duration of change.

Human beings tolerate an increase better than a decrease in atmospheric pressure of the same magnitude. Air pressure can be tripled (45 pounds per square inch) without apparent harm, but a reduction to one-half the normal pressure (to 7.5 pounds per square inch) may cause death from anoxia.

Aero-embolism

The rate of change of pressure is very important. A *too rapid decrease in pressure,* whether from high to normal or from normal to low, releases nitrogen and carbon dioxide bubbles from solution in the plasma. *Aeroembolism,* with occlusion of capillaries in the brain and spinal cord, occurs. Numerous small infarcts result. *Fat embolism* in the lungs also occurs, possibly due to rupture of sinusoid walls by gas bubbles in fatty bone marrow [53]. Expansion of air in the paranasal sinuses may cause pain and in the middle ear may rupture the tympanic membrane. The syndrome caused by a too rapid decrease in atmospheric pressure is known as *caisson disease, decompression sickness, bends, staggers,* or *diver's palsy. Clinically* there are headache, vertigo, dyspnea, muscle pains, and paralyses. In the *chokes,* which is due to aeroembolism in the pulmonary vessels, there are chest pain, choking sensations, and cyanosis. *Autopsy findings in fatal cases of decompression sickness* [54] include aeroembolism to the right atrium, congestion and edema of the lungs, gas bubbles in large pulmonary arteries, fatty metamorphosis of the liver, and a few gas bubbles within cerebral blood vessels. These bubbles are about 80 percent nitrogen and 15 to 20 percent carbon dioxide, with a trace of oxygen.

Decompression sickness

DIVING SYNDROMES

Pathologic changes in divers, other than decompression sickness, include:

1. *Aerotitis media.* This is due to obstruction of the eustachian tube so that there is no equalization of pressure within the middle ear, a relative vacuum forming there. The tympanic membrane is pushed inward with congestion or hemorrhage of the drum or bleeding into the middle ear.

2. *Aerosinusitis,* with sinus pain and hemorrhage due to blocking of the ostia.

3. *Aerodontalgia* due to tiny air pockets behind tooth fillings.

4. *Squeeze effects* due to the increasing pressure under water as the depth increases (0.445 pounds per square inch per foot of descent).

5. *Drowning.*

6. *Nitrogen narcosis* (rapture of the deep). This is related to the increased amount of nitrogen dissolved in the blood under pressure and may be due to solution of nitrogen in cerebral lipids to produce anesthesia. The diver feels dizzy and acts as though he is inebriated.

7. *Oxygen poisoning.* This is related to the increased amount of oxygen dissolved in the plasma under increased pressure and is characterized by tingling sensations, visual and auditory disturbances, confusion, nausea, vertigo, muscle twitching, and convulsions.

8. *Rupture of alveoli* ("lung burst") due to the expansion of air within them during an ascent in which the breath is held. This may produce *mediastinal emphysema, pneumothorax,* and/or *air embolism.* In air embolism, tearing of veins in the massively expanded lungs leads to the presence of several liters of air in the

left atrium and ventricle [55]. *Cerebral air embolism* may also occur. These accidents are more common among skin divers, who often use a Self-Contained Underwater Breathing Apparatus (SCUBA) [56], but most types also occur in "hard-hat" divers with diving suits.

BLAST INJURY

The *effects of a too rapid increase in pressure* are best exemplified by *blast injury* [57]. Disruptive effects are produced by very sudden and marked changes in pressure due to explosions. In blast injury the *primary effects* are due to the blast pressure which produces damage mainly in the air-containing areas of the body. The *secondary effects* are due to flying missiles, and *tertiary effects* are caused by the motion of the victim initiated by the blast. There also may be miscellaneous effects, such as those due to burns from fires set by the explosion. With conventional explosives a blast pressure of 7 to 15 psi (pounds per square inch) causes *rupture of the tympanic membrane.* Pressures above 80 psi cause *internal blast injury,* and a blast pressure over 200 psi causes death. A *nuclear blast* lasts longer and would cause injuries at less than 80 psi and death at less than 200 psi. At overpressures of 5 psi, building and automobile destruction occurs, and low-velocity missiles are created. The *pulmonary lacerations* which are common in *air blast injuries* cause alveolar rupture and intra-alveolar hemorrhage. In *immersion blast,* water may be blown through the anus and rupture the colon or small intestine. *Solid blast injuries* occur by transmission of the blast waves through solid structures. Internal injury may occur without surface trauma.

PROLONGED EXPOSURE

Prolonged exposure to a moderately high pressure is not injurious. *Prolonged exposure to a low pressure* leads to the development of polycythemia, increased blood volume and hemoglobin, and hyperplasia of the bone marrow. In children born and raised at altitudes above 12,000 feet the ratio of left and right ventricular weights (Hermann-Wilson index), which normally attains the value characteristic of adults at the age of 4 months, indicates a definite right ventricular hypertrophy. In such children the hypertrophy is mainly in the basal portion of the right ventricle [58].

ALTITUDE SICKNESS

Altitude or mountain sickness (acute pulmonary edema of high altitude) [59] occurs suddenly in skiers, mountain climbers, and soldiers not totally acclimatized to heights over 9000 feet in the absence of heart disease. It also occurs in natives or others adapted to living at high altitudes upon returning from a stay of days or weeks in the lowlands. The *cause* is uncertain, but may be a sudden rise in pulmonary arterial pressure with shifting of blood from the systemic to the pulmonary circulation. The edema may be rapidly fatal, although most cases recover. At autopsy the lungs are quite heavy due to marked intra-alveolar edema with numerous hyaline membranes [60]. Intra-alveolar hemorrhages are common. Some cases show a secondary bronchopneumonia.

PHYSIOLOGIC AND PATHOLOGIC EFFECTS OF HYPERGRAVIC AND HYPOGRAVIC STATES

HYPERGRAVIC AND HYPOGRAVIC STATES

Hypergravic and hypogravic states [61, 62] have become the subjects of intensive investigation with the dawning of the Space Age. Much has yet to be learned, but as data have been accumulated it has become increasingly clear that the problems of sustaining human and other higher animal life in space are enormous and extremely complex. These problems can be divided into three phases: launch, orbit, and reentry.

LAUNCH EFFECTS:

Hypergravic effects during launching are imparted by the forces involved in the firing of the ballistic missile which propels the manned capsule into space. The large liquid-fuel first-stage rocket used has a slow increase in acceleration up to a peak of less than 10 G. Following a momentary or brief coasting period, second-stage rocket firing, with characteristics like that of the first-stage firing, occurs. These *launching (lift-off) accelerations are well within tolerable limits,* since man can tolerate 8 G exposures for about 90 seconds, and the burning time of these rockets is usually less than 1 minute after the attainment of 4 G accelerations.

Boost accelerations

The *effects of boost accelerations* are minimized by positioning the space passenger in the capsule so that the long axis of his body is perpendicular to the direction of flight *(forward acceleration).* With such positioning man can tolerate more than 16 G briefly without protective suiting and without the blackout or unconsciousness that is common with *headward acceleration* because of the profound inertial effects on the cardiovascular system in the upright position (impairment of venous return to the heart and decreased cardiac output) even at thrusts of 4 G [63]. The *effects of high-magnitude forward acceleration* include severe chest pain, dyspnea, and progressive decreases in vital capacity and tidal volume. The supine position is preferable to the prone state. Chimpanzees exposed to 40 transverse G for 60 seconds in the fully supine position suffered relatively little damage as compared to subjects in partially supine or prone positions [64]. In both groups lesions were mainly vascular, with intra-alveolar hemorrhages, and edema and hemorrhages in the periorbital tissues, urinary bladder, and restraint sites. *Escape* in case of rocket and/or guidance system failure is a difficult problem, since deceleration forces above 40 G may affect the capsule.

ORBIT EFFECTS: Hypogravic effects

Hypogravic effects come into play during the period of orbiting or other space flight free of the gravitional field of the earth or its moon or another planet. This *period of zero gravity,* during which the space passenger is weightless, lasts from about 90 minutes to days or longer. Thus far astronauts have found weightlessness to be fairly innocuous. At least one lost spatial orientation during darkness in his spacecraft due to effects of weightlessness on vestibular function [65]. Following longer flights there has been a *tendency to postural hypotension* following return to earth. On prolonged flights of several weeks or months muscle atrophy and demineralization of bone with hypercalcemia due to immobilization may present problems. *Nongravitational problems* in space travel include provision of an adequate oxygen and food supply, disposal of body wastes, and exposure to radiation.

Radiation in space

Radiation at high altitudes and in space [66, 67] consists of cosmic rays, protons, electrons, and x-rays. *Cosmic rays* have extremely short wave lengths and stupendous energy potentials; heavy primary cosmic rays, which are 80 percent protons, 19 percent alpha particles, and 1 percent nuclei of elements of atomic number greater than 2, have energies between 10^9 and 10^{18} electron volts per particle. *Protons* in space arise from the decay of cosmic ray neutrons "backscattered" from the earth's atmosphere and from the solar wind (ionized hydrogen ejected from the sun). The intensity of proton beams fluctuates with solar activity and their contact with magnetic fields. High-intensity radiation fields, of which the best known are the *Van Allen belts,* are present at altitudes beyond 50 miles above the earth. The inner Van Allen ring is from 1400 to 3400 miles above the equator, and the outer belt begins at 8000 and extends to 12,000 miles. The intensity of radiation in these regions precludes sustained flight through them because of the heavy total body radiation that would be received and the effects of exposure on the skin and especially the lenses of the eyes. *Radiation-induced lenticular cataracts* are common after exposure to neutrons and/or protons. Heavy radiation can be avoided by rapid traversal of the belts, exit via polar routes, or shielding. In regard to shielding, an added problem arises in that when the charged electrons and protons impact on matter, x-rays are formed and become a new radiation menace. However, minimal x-ray production can be achieved by using metals of low atomic number, such as beryllium, in the shield.

REENTRY EFFECTS

Hypergravic effects during reentry are mainly those of deceleration. The entire capsule or the seat is rotated 180° prior to reentry so that the *decleration forces* are applied in the same direction as were the acceleration forces during launching. For purposes of stabilization, the vehicle is spinning. Maximum *tolerance for spin* is attained with the heart as the center of rotation, 80 rpm being tolerated for 100 seconds in the absence of additional deceleration forces. Upon entering the earth's atmosphere, the capsule is subject to heat due to friction and may tumble. Upon reorienting itself, it swings through arcs of constantly decreasing amplitude and increasing frequency. The G forces sustained during this period depend on the distance of the passenger from the capsule's center of gravity and the frequency and amplitude of oscillation. As it nears the earth, the vehicle begins a straight-line fall. This is broken by use of a parachute, and the capsule lands in a net, on land or in water. The *final impact* must be regulated so as not to exceed human tolerance, which is above 50 G applied at 500 G per second for less than 0.2 second, or about 40 G applied at 1500 G per second for less than 0.2 second.

REFERENCES

1. Adelson, L. Recent progress in forensic pathology. *J. Forensic Sci.* 4:250, 1959.
2. Frankel, C. J. Medical-legal aspects of injuries to the neck. *J.A.M.A.* 169:216, 1959.
3. Silliphant, W. M., and Beyer, J. C. Wound ballistics. *Milit. Med.* 117:238, 1955.
4. Steinberg, B. Gunshot wounds. *A.M.A. Arch. Path.* 59:263, 1955.
5. Light, F. W., Jr. Gunshot wounds of entrance and exit in experimental animals. *J. Trauma* 3:120, 1963.
6. Adelson, L. A microscopic study of dermal gunshot wounds. *Amer. J. Clin. Path.* 35:393, 1961.
7. Spitz, W. U., Petty, C. S., and Fisher, R. S. Physical activity until collapse following fatal injury by firearms and sharp pointed weapons. *J. Forensic Sci.* 6:290, 1961.
8. Guerin, P. F. Shotgun wounds. *J. Forensic Sci.* 5:294, 1960.
9. Eckert, W. G., Kemmerer, W. T., and Chetta, N. J. The traumatic pathology of traffic accidents. *J. Forensic Sci.* 4:309, 1959.
10. McFarland, R. A. The epidemiology of motor vehicle accidents. *J.A.M.A.* 180:289, 1962.
11. Cocke, W. M., and Meyer, K. K. Splenic rupture due to improper placement of automobile safety belt. *J.A.M.A.* 183:693, 1963.
12. Kempe, C. H., Silverman, F. N., Steele, B. F., Droegemueller, W., and Silver, H. K. The battered-child syndrome. *J.A.M.A.* 181:17, 1962.
13. Fontana, V. J., Donovan, D., and Wong, R. J. The "maltreatment syndrome" in children. *New Eng. J. Med.* 269:1389, 1963.

14. Ulin, A. W., Olsen, A. K., and Martin, W. L. Factors determining mortality in patients with acute head injury. *J.A.M.A.* 157:496, 1955.
15. Freytag, E. Autopsy findings in head injuries from blunt forces. *Arch. Path.* (Chicago) 75:402, 1963.
16. Courville, C. B. Coup-contrecoup mechanism of craniocerebral injuries. *Arch. Surg.* 45:19, 1942.
17. Courville, C. B. Forensic neuropathology. II. Mechanisms of craniocerebral injury and their medicolegal significance. *J. Forensic Sci.* 7:1, 1962.
18. Lindenberg, R., and Freytag, E. The mechanism of cerebral contusions. *A.M.A. Arch. Path.* 69:440, 1960.
19. Lindenberg, R., and Freytag, E. Morphology of cortical contusions. *A.M.A. Arch. Path.* 63:23, 1957.
20. Angrist, A. A physical explanation of intracerebral hemorrhages in head trauma. Paper read at the 2d International Meeting on Forensic Pathology and Medicine, New York, Sept. 20, 1960.
21. Ward, A. A., Jr. Physiological basis of concussion. *J. Neurosurg.* 15:129, 1958.
22. Dillon, H., and Leopold, R. L. Children and the post-concussion syndrome. *J.A.M.A.* 175:86, 1961.
23. Gross, A. G. A new theory on the dynamics of brain concussion and brain injury. *J. Neurosurg.* 15:548, 1958.
24. McKissock, W., Taylor, J. C., Bloom, W. H., and Till, K. Extradural haematoma. *Lancet* 2:167, 1960.
25. Aronson, S. M. The pathogenesis of subdural hematoma. Paper read at the 2d International Meeting on Forensic Pathology and Medicine, New York, Sept. 20, 1960.
26. Freytag, E. Autopsy findings in head injuries from firearms. *Arch. Path.* (Chicago) 76:215, 1963.
27. Ellis, W. G., Green, D., Holzaepfel, N. R., and Sahs, A. L. The trampoline and serious neurological disorders. *J.A.M.A.* 174:1673, 1960.
28. Swann, H. E. Occurrence of pulmonary edema in sudden asphyxial deaths. *A.M.A. Arch. Path.* 69:557, 1960.
29. Modell, J. H. Resuscitation after aspiration of chlorinated fresh water. *J.A.M.A.* 185:651, 1963.
30. Craig, A. B. Underwater swimming and loss of consciousness. *J.A.M.A.* 176:255, 1961.
31. Swann, H. G., and Spafford, N. R. Body salt and water changes during fresh and sea water drowning. *Texas Rep. Biol. Med.* 9:356, 1951.
32. Spitz, W. U., and Blanke, R. V. Mechanism of death in fresh-water drowning. *Arch. Path.* (Chicago) 71:71, 1961.
33. Freimuth, H. C., and Swann, H. E., Jr. Plasma specific gravity changes in sudden deaths. *A.M.A. Arch. Path.* 59:214, 1955.
34. Chiaraviglio, E. D. C., and Wolf, A. V. Diagnosis of drowning. Use of TS meter, osmometer, and chloridimeter. *Arch. Path.* (Chicago) 75:337, 1963.
35. Adelson, L. Recent advances in forensic pathology. *J. Forensic Sci.* 4:250, 1959.
36. Rabin, E. R., Graber, C. D., Vogel, E. H., Finkelstein, R. A., and Tumbusch, W. A. Fatal pseudomonas infection in burned patients. *New Eng. J. Med.* 265:1225, 1961.
37. Sochor, F. M., and Mallory, G. K. Lung lesions in patients dying of burns *Arch. Path.* (Chicago) 75:303, 1963.
38. Shibolet, S., Fisher, S., Gillat, T., Bank, H., and Heller, H. Fibrinolysis and hemorrhages in fatal heatstroke. *New Eng. J. Med.* 266:169, 1962.

39. Malamud, N., Haymaker, W., and Custer, R. P. Heat stroke. *Milit. Surg.* 99:397, 1946.
40. Washburn, B. Frostbite. *New Eng. J. Med.* 266:974, 1962.
41. Smith, R. M., and Stetson, J. B. Therapeutic hypothermia. *New Eng. J. Med.* 265:1097, 1147, 1961.
42. Litwin, M. S., and Glew, D. H. The biological effects of laser radiation. *J.A.M.A.* 187:842, 1964.
43. Ravitch, M. A., Lane, R., Safar, P., Steichen, F. M., and Knowles, P. Lightning stroke. *New Eng. J. Med.* 264:36, 1961.
44. McLaughlin, J. T. Tissue destruction and death from microwave radiation (Radar). *Calif. Med.* 86:336, 1957.
45. Smith, J. C. The pathogenesis of focal somatic irradiation injury. *Amer. J. Clin. Path.* 41:609, 1964.
46. Jennings, F. L., and Arden, A. Development of radiation pneumonitis. *Arch. Path.* (Chicago) 74:351, 1962.
47. Tullis, J. L. Delayed effects of ionizing radiations in man. *A.M.A. Arch. Path.* 66:403, 1958.
48. Liebow, A. A., Warren, S., and DeCoursey, E. Pathology of atomic bomb casualties. *Amer. J. Path.* 25:853, 1949.
49. Socolow, E. L., Hashizume, A., Neriishi, S., and Nitani, R. Thyroid carcinoma in man after exposure to ionizing radiation. A summary of the findings in Hiroshima and Nagasaki. *New Eng. J. Med.* 268:406, 1963.
50. Anderson, R. E., Yamamoto, T., Yamada, A., and Will, D. W. Autopsy study of leukemia in Hiroshima. *Arch. Path.* (Chicago) 78:618, 1964.
51. Anderson, R. E. Aging in Hiroshima atomic bomb survivors. *Arch. Path.* (Chicago) 79:1, 1965.
52. Hollingsworth, J. W. Delayed radiation effects in survivors of the atomic bombings. *New Eng. J. Med.* 263:481, 1960.
53. Haymaker, W., and Johnston, A. D. Pathology of decompression sickness. *Milit. Med.* 117:285, 1955.
54. Sillery, R. J. Decompression sickness. *A.M.A. Arch. Path.* 66:241, 1958.
55. Butterfield, D. E., Mack, J. D., and Majno, G. Skin diving. *New Eng. J. Med.* 269:255, 1963.
56. Duffner, G. J. Scuba diving injuries. *J.A.M.A.* 175:375, 1961.
57. Cohen, H., and Biskind, G. R. Pathologic aspects of atmospheric blast injuries in man. *Arch. Path.* 42:12, 1946.
58. Recavarren, S., and Arias-Stella, J. Topography of right ventricular hypertrophy in children native to high altitude. *Amer. J. Path.* 41:467, 1962.
59. Nayak, N. C., Roy, S., and Narayanan, T. K. Pathologic features of altitude sickness. *Amer. J. Path.* 45:381, 1964.
60. Arias-Stella, J., and Kruger, H. Pathology of high altitude pulmonary edema. *Arch. Path.* (Chicago) 76:147, 1963.
61. Di Giovanni, C., Jr., and Chambers, R. M. Physiologic and psychologic aspects of the gravity spectrum. *New Eng. J. Med.* 270:35, 88, 134, 1964.
62. Ward, J. E. Physiological aspects of hypergravic and hypogravic states. Application to space flight. *J.A.M.A.* 172:665, 1960.
63. Steiner, S. H., Mueller, G. C. E., and Taylor, J. L., Jr. Hemodynamic changes during forward acceleration. *Aerospace Med.* 31:907, 1960.
64. Stoll, A. M., and Mosely, J. D. Physiologic and pathologic effects in chimpanzees during prolonged exposure to 40 transverse G. *J. Aviation Med.* 29:575, 1958.
65. Wagner, B. M. Bioastronautics. Man in the space environment. *Arch. Path.* (Chicago) 78:454, 1964.

66. Langham, W. H. Implications of space radiations in manned space flights. *Aerospace Med.* 30:410, 1959.
67. Schaefer, H. J. Tissue ionization dosages in proton radiation fields in space. *Aerospace Med.* 31:807, 1960.

GENERAL REFERENCES

Courville, C. B. *Forensic Neuropathology.* Mundelein, Ill.: Callaghan, 1964, pp. 15–152. (The result of long experience and experimentation in trauma involving the nervous system.)

Gonzales, T. A., Vance, M., Helpern, M., and Umberger, C. J. *Legal Medicine: Pathology and Toxicology* (2d ed.). New York: Appleton-Century-Crofts, 1954, pp. 157–493, 523–554. (An authoritative presentation of most types of injuries due to physical agents.)

Moritz, A. R. *The Pathology of Trauma* (2d ed.). Philadelphia: Lea & Febiger, 1954. (A thorough discussion limited to mechanical injuries.)

10 INJURIES DUE TO CHEMICAL AGENTS

POISONS

A *poison* is a substance which, when it has been introduced into or upon the body and is absorbed into the bloodstream, by its chemical action is capable of seriously affecting health or destroying life. In general, less than 50 gm. of the substance must produce such effects for it to be considered a poison. *Toxicology* is the science which treats of poisons. Many valuable drugs act as poisons when doses much larger than the therapeutic ones are used; such examples are discussed in the appropriate parts of this section on Poisons. Toxic effects of drugs in therapeutic doses are treated under Untoward Effects of Therapeutic Agents later in this chapter.

Poisons may be *classified according to physiologic action as corrosives* (the chief action is a local destruction of tissue, e.g., the strong acids and alkalis); *irritants* (the most characteristic effects are gastrointestinal irritation, e.g., arsenic, phosphorus, croton oil); and *neurotoxics* (the toxic action is exerted on the central nervous system, e.g., alcohol, strychnine, carbon monoxide, morphine). They may also be *classified according to origin as gaseous, inorganic, alkaloidal, nonalkaloidal organic, and food poisons.*

Poisoning may be suicidal, homicidal, or accidental, so that toxicology is of great medicolegal importance. There are about 10,000 fatal poisonings annually in the United States. Of these, 55 percent are accidental, 44 percent suicidal, and 1 percent homicidal. About 1500 poison deaths occur in children, many being due to salicylates or kerosene. Ethyl alcohol, carbon monoxide, barbiturates, and heavy metals are the most frequently encountered poisons in adults.

1. Gaseous Poisons

Except for carbon monoxide poisoning, deaths from *toxic gases* are usually accidental. The general findings in cases of gaseous poisoning are signs of acute asphyxia and cyanosis. In any suspected cases, samples of the atmosphere should be collected in evacuated airtight gas tubes for analysis.

OXYGEN

Oxygen, ordinarily the sustainer of life, can produce pathologic changes in persons exposed to 100% concentrations at atmospheric pressure for as little as 24 hours [1]. Lesions are common in patients requiring mechanical ventilation *(respirator lung syndrome).* They develop progressively reduced vital capacity and increasing hypoxia. Pulmonary insufficiency is the usual cause of death. At *autopsy* the lungs are heavy and beefy. In the early *exudative phase* there are congestion with edema fluid, hemorrhage, fibrin, and hyaline membranes within the alveoli. The later *proliferative phase* shows severe intra-alveolar edema, septal fibroblastic proliferation, and prominence of alveolar lining cells. High oxygen concentrations produce retrolental fibroplasia in premature infants. *Oxygen at high pressures* (3 atmospheres or higher, as in hyperbaric therapy) may induce grand mal convulsions [1a].

CARBON MON-OXIDE:

Carbon monoxide (CO) is the most common gaseous poison. Suicidal and homicidal poisonings are usually by manufactured illuminating gas and automobile exhausts. Accidental deaths are commonly due to defective gas or charcoal stoves, gas refrigerators, or smoldering fires. *Air concentrations* above 0.1 percent carbon monoxide are dangerous; 0.35 percent is fatal in less than 1 hour. *In fatal poisonings the blood is 30 to 80 percent saturated with carbon monoxide,* about half the cases showing 70 to 80 percent saturation. *Inhaled carbon monoxide combines with hemoglobin in the blood to form cherry red carboxyhemoglobin.* The affinity of hemoglobin for carbon monoxide is about 210 times that for oxygen. Carboxyhemoglobin is extremely stable, and carbon monoxide can be identified in the blood in decomposed and embalmed bodies.

Acute poisoning

In *acute carbon monoxide poisoning* [2] the conscious patient complains of headache, weakness, dizziness, dimness of vision, nausea, and vomiting. Proteinuria is frequent but is usually transient. The body temperature frequently falls due to a decrease in metabolic rate. There is sometimes an increase in the blood sugar level with glycosuria. Transient or permanent blindness may result from prolonged hypoxia with degenerative changes in the optic nerve or optic thalamus. At 30 to 50 percent air saturation, *coma with intermittent convulsions* develops. The face, blood, and viscera are cherry red. If the patient lives for several days, a bilateral necrosis of the lenticular nuclei, especially the globus pallidus, may occur. This is probably due to ischemia, from small thromboses. Erythema of the hands and feet is common, and blebs and bullae, 0.5 to 20 cm. in diameter, may appear on the skin of the trunk, face, and extremities. Serous fluid separates the dermis and epidermis, and there is an acute inflammatory reaction. These lesions may be mistaken for burns. Gangrene of a foot or lower leg occurs rarely due to vascular occlusion and hypoxia.

Relapsing and chronic poisoning

Relapsing carbon monoxide poisoning may occur in patients who have shown apparent recovery. Confusion followed by coma is characteristic. Foci of necrosis are found in the cerebral subcortical white matter. *Chronic carbon monoxide poisoning* occurs in taxi drivers and garage attendants, whose blood may contain up to 10 percent carboxyhemoglobin. Some constantly exposed persons develop polycythemia. Irreversible changes may occur in the bone marrow, such as hyperplasia, as well as fatty metamorphosis of the liver and heart and degeneration of the ganglion cells of the brain. Visual hallucinations sometimes occur in chronic carbon monoxide poisoning. Permanent hearing loss is rare. The sense of smell may be lost or perverted.

CARBON DIOXIDE

Carbon dioxide (CO_2) is normally present in the atmosphere (0.03 percent by volume). Carbon dioxide concentrations of 0.1 to 1 percent produce lassitude and headache, and 8 to 10 percent may cause death by asphyxia, due to lack of oxygen. Such deaths are accidental. The *pathologic findings* are those of anoxia, and include petechial hemorrhages in the pericardium, pleurae, and galea of the scalp.

INDUSTRIAL GASES:

Hydrogen sulfide (H_2S), sulfur dioxide (SO_2), nitric oxide (NO), nitrogen dioxide (NO_2), chlorine (Cl_2), and ammonia (NH_3) are industrial hazards. In addition to displacement of oxygen by these gases, all are powerful irritants to the respiratory tract. Hydrogen sulfide in concentrations above 0.1 percent can produce very rapid death by paralysis of the medullary respiratory center.

Pathologic changes

If an exposed individual survives the immediate effects, within a few hours there is *massive edema of the lungs,* followed by infiltration of the alveoli by polymorphonuclear leukocytes and deposition of fibrin. The bronchial walls are swollen and hyperemic, and the bronchial epithelium is desquamated. The fluid in the alveolar spaces may coagulate to form *hyaline "asphyxial" membranes.* Within a few days secondary bacterial infection may be superimposed. In fatal *hydrogen sulfide poisoning* there may be a greenish cyanosis and greenish discoloration of the blood, cerebrum, and other viscera [2a]. A strong odor of rotten eggs is present about the body.

Nitrogen dioxide

Nitrogen dioxide (NO_2) is an insidious poison gas. *Poisoning* is caused by the breakage of carboys containing nitric acid, exposure to welding operations, and exposure to burning x-ray films or explosives. It also occurs among silo workers *(silo-filler's disease)* [3] due to the reduction of nitrates in corn to nitrous acid (HNO_2) during silage. The HNO_2 breaks down to NO_2 and NO (nitric oxide), the latter being oxidized to NO_2. Nitrogen dioxide may be inhaled without immediate irritation. Hours or even days later severe congestion and edema develop along with an acute tracheobronchitis. Nodular or miliary densities appear on x-ray. Bronchopneumonia or interstitial pneumonitis may ensue. Rarely an organizing bronchiolitis obliterans occurs due to the "healing" of focal necrotic lesions.

WAR GASES

Gases used in warfare are of five general types: (1) *tear gases* (chloracetophenone, brombenzyl cyanide, and O-chlorobenzalmalononitrile) which produce a transient inflammation of the conjunctivae; (2) *sneeze gases* (sternutators) (diphenylchlorarsine and diphenylaminochlorarsine), which produce inflammation in the nose and pharynx; (3) *choking gases* (chlorine and phosgene); (4) *blister gases* (mustard gas and lewisite); and (5) *blood and nerve poisons* (hydrocyanic acid, carbon monoxide, and cholinesterase inhibitors).

With *choking gases (lung irritants)* the lips, ears, fingers, and dependent parts are dusky and livid. Serosanguineous pleural fluid is found, and there are petechiae in the pleura. The trachea and bronchi are filled with pink frothy fluid. The lungs are bulky. In persons dying in the first few hours the alveoli and bronchioles are filled with edema fluid. Later fibrin and polymorphonuclear leukocytes appear, and the bronchial and alveolar epithelium is desquamated. A bronchopneumonia is present in those surviving for 2 to 4 days.

Blister gases (vesicants) produce edema of the dermis, vesicles in the epidermis and at the epidermo-dermal junction, and necrosis of the epidermis. The vesicles contain fibrin and polymorphonuclear leukocytes. The bronchi are filled with fibrinopurulent exudate, and the mucosa is purple, necrosis of the wall often extending to the cartilage plates. The lungs are voluminous. There is marked congestion, and the alveoli are filled with erythrocytes, edema fluid, and polymorphonuclear leukocytes. Foci of bronchopneumonia are found. The tear gas, l-chloracetophenone, is the active ingredient in chemical mace. Sprayed on the skin, l-chloracetophenone causes an erythematous contact dermatitis in sensitive persons [3a].

2. Corrosives

ACID CORROSIVES

Acid corrosives include the mineral acids (hydrochloric, sulfuric, and nitric acids), some organic acids (oxalic, acetic, and formic acids), and salts with a strongly acidic and a weak basic radical, such as silver nitrate and zinc chloride. Corrosive acids are usually ingested accidentally or with suicidal intent. Acid burns on the skin are often accidental, but may result from assault, the acid being thrown in the face. Occasionally corrosive acids are employed in attempted abortions, severe burns being produced on the vulva and in the vagina.

The *local actions of a corrosive acid* are extraction of water, coagulation of protein to form an acid albuminate, and formation of acid hematin from hemoglobin. These effects are seen on the skin, about the lips, and in the mouth, pharynx, and esophagus. There is usually erosion or ulceration. *Swallowed dilute or weak acids* irritate the gastric mucosa, throwing the rugae into folds and producing a bright red barred pattern at the tips of the folds; erosions and ulcerations are frequent. *Microscopically* there is an intense acute inflammatory reaction at the tips of the rugate folds. *Swallowed concentrated strong acids* char the gastric mucosa, turning it brown or black (yellow with nitric acid). This process is known as *carbonization* and is due to the withdrawal of water from the tissue and production of acid hematin from the blood. The mucosa may be widely ulcerated or the wall may perforate, leading to a chemical peritonitis. The acid may enter the duodenum and produce similar effects. *Ingested acid may be regurgitated to enter the air passages* and cause an acute inflammatory reaction in the larynx, trachea, and bronchi. Corrosive acids may produce *death by shock* from their local actions. Ingested acids may be absorbed to produce acidosis and fatty changes in the liver and kidneys. In cases of regurgitation, death may be by laryngeal spasm or edema or by bronchopneumonia. *Stenosis of the esophagus or stomach* may follow acid ingestion by several weeks or months.

HALOGENS:

The *halogens* include chlorine, bromine, iodine, and fluorine. Pathologically they act like corrosive acids. *Chlorine,* a yellow-green gas dangerous to life in 1:50,000,000 concentrations, has been discussed with the gaseous poisons.

Bromine

Bromine, a reddish brown, pungent liquid, may be inhaled as vapors (producing an acute laryngotracheobronchitis and pulmonary edema) or ingested (causing corrosion and brownish discoloration of the gastric mucosa). Bromine is converted to sodium bromide in the body. Sodium or potassium bromide, if used as a sedative, may cause coma and death in large doses or produce *chronic bromidism* with prolonged use. In this the body chlorides are largely replaced by bromides. Pustules appear on the skin, and subcutaneous nodules may form *(nodose bromoderma).* Mental changes and muscular weakness are common.

Iodine

Iodine is usually ingested accidentally or suicidally as tincture of iodine. Brown stains or burns are common about the lips. The gastric mucosa is corroded. Absorbed iodine produces degenerative changes in the renal tubular epithelium. Prolonged use of iodine in susceptible individuals leads to *iodism,* with a skin rash, anemia, and emaciation.

Fluorine

Fluorine is the most active member of the halogen group. *Hydrofluoric acid,* used in engraving and fertilizers, causes severe, painful skin burns. It is corrosive if inhaled or ingested. *Sodium fluoride* is used in rat and roach poisons (these are usually dyed blue); when ingested it produces a *massive hemorrhagic inflammatory reaction throughout the gastrointestinal tract.* If the fluoride is absorbed before death, renal tubular epithelial degeneration is produced, and calcium fluoride is excreted because of the affinity of fluoride ions for calcium ions. Tetany and convulsions may occur before death because of this loss of calcium. *Organic fluoride compounds,* such as sodium fluoracetate (1080) and fluorethynol, are used in rodenticides and are very toxic, causing changes similar to those produced by sodium fluoride. *Chronic fluoride poisoning* causes mottling of the enamel, thickening of bone trabeculae, and anemia.

ALKALINE CORROSIVES

Alkaline corrosives include potassium, sodium, and ammonium hydroxides, and lye (a mixture of sodium hydroxide and sodium carbonate). Their action on the body is to form alkaline albuminates and soaps with cell protoplasm, and alkaline hematin with hemoglobin. The *pathologic lesions* are similar to those with acid corrosives, but alkaline corrosives produce tissue liquefaction and penetrate deeply. Therefore, they typically cause greater tissue damage and subsequent scarring than do acid corrosives. *Strictures of the esophagus or pylorus* are especially common in those who survive the acute effects of the ingestion of lye. Strong caustic alkalis are sometimes used by murderers to obliterate the corpse; it may be converted to a soapy liquid mass with only a few bones remaining.

ORGANIC CORROSIVES

Organic corrosives include phenol (carbolic acid), cresol, Lysol, formaldehyde, and acetaldehyde. *Lysol* is a 50 percent solution of cresols in potassium-saponified linseed oil and is very alkaline. Organic corrosives coagulate (fix) the cellular protein and eventually produce necrosis. Poisoning by them is usually accidental or suicidal. The *general pathologic findings* are brown corrosive patches about the mouth, coagulation necrosis of the gastric mucosa, visceral congestion, and renal tubular epithelial degeneration. The cresols in Lysol have an affinity for the cerebral lipids. *Lysol* used as a douche may produce corrosive lesions in the vagina. *Cresols* may also produce hemolysis. With *phenol poisoning* the urine is typically smoky and grayish green.

3. *Metallic Poisons*

Metallic poisons cause their principal effects on the parenchymatous organs after absorption, although some are escharotic or corrosive locally on the skin and mucous membranes. Most reactions to metals or metallic compounds are delayed except in high doses. The metals are absorbed in the stomach and excreted in the cecum, so that *cecal inflammation is highly suggestive of metal poisoning.*

ARSENIC:

Arsenic is nontoxic in the metallic state. However, its organic and inorganic compounds are highly poisonous. *Inorganic arsenic compounds* were formerly extensively used for homicidal purposes. These compounds are protoplasmic poisons. Today inorganic arsenic is usually ingested accidentally as arsenic trioxide in rat poisons and tree and garden sprays. Four types of poisoning occur:

1. *Acute paralytic form.* This type is due to ingestion of large quantities. Death occurs within 24 hours due to medullary center depression. Such cases are often suicidal.

2. *Gastrointestinal form,* which is characterized by diarrhea, abdominal cramps, vomiting, delirium, oliguria, dehydration, and death in a few days. Pathologic findings include a congested and edematous gastric and intestinal mucosa. The mucosa may be stained yellow by the formation of arsenic trisulfide. These changes are due to the excretion of arsenic through the gastrointestinal tract rather than to a direct corrosive action. In a few days fatty changes appear in the heart, liver, and kidneys.

3. *Subacute form,* due to small repeated doses, is characterized by gastrointestinal hemorrhages, hepatic necrosis, and renal tubular degeneration.

4. *Chronic form,* which is often homicidal. Hyperpigmentation of the skin with hyperkeratosis occurs. Palisading of basal cells of the epidermis is found. The palms and soles may be involved. In 2 to 3 weeks white striae grow across the nails *(Nee lines).* Mental changes and peripheral nerve palsies occur. A patchy segmental demyelinization (of Gombault) occurs in involved sensory and motor fibers. At death relatively small amounts of arsenic may be present in the tissues.

Organic arsenicals

Organic arsenic compounds include trivalent arsenicals, such as arsphenamine, formerly widely used in luetic therapy, and pentavalent arsenicals, such as tryparsamide, used in trypanosomal disease therapy. *Toxic effects* are usually subacute or chronic and include exfoliative dermatitis, hepatic necrosis, and aplastic anemia.

ANTIMONY

Antimony compounds are toxic. Most poisonings are accidental and are due to antimony chloride ($SbCl_3$) or tartar emetic ($KSbOC_4H_4O_6$). The pathologic effects are similar to those produced by arsenic compounds.

MERCURY

Mercury forms mercuric (bivalent) and mercurous (univalent) salts, the latter being less soluble and less toxic than the former. *Mercurous chloride* (calomel) is relatively nontoxic unless it is converted to mercuric chloride in the body. *Organic mercurial compounds,* such as merbromin (Mercurochrome) and thimerosal (Merthiolate), are only slightly toxic, but have caused poisoning occasionally. Some individuals, particularly those on mercurial diuretics, may store relatively large amounts of mercury in the kidneys without toxic effects. *Mercuric chloride* (corrosive sublimate) is the most toxic mercury compound. It is often marketed for antiseptic purposes as dark blue, coffin-shaped tablets. Suicides are common by this means. Shortly after ingestion there is vomiting, with severe cramps. Later a bloody diarrhea and oliguria develop. *Pathologic changes* include corrosive lesions in the mouth, pharynx, and esophagus due to direct irritation by the tablets. Similar changes are found in the vagina when mercuric chloride tablets are used as an abortifacient. The gastric rugae are thrown into folds, and the mucosa forms a silver-gray slough. A similar pseudomembrane is produced in the vagina by mercuric chloride solutions. An acute hemorrhagic colitis is common due to excretion of part of the absorbed mercuric chloride. The *most characteristic change* is the severe degeneration and necrosis, with acute calcification, in the proximal convoluted tubular epithelium. The kidneys are grossly pale and swollen.

BISMUTH

Bismuth compounds are occasionally the cause of accidental poisoning, especially the subcarbonate and subsalicylate. *Acute poisoning* is characterized by a necrotizing colitis and necrosis of the renal tubular epithelium, similar to the changes seen in mercury poisoning. *Nuclear acid-fast inclusion bodies are present in the renal tubular epithelium* [4]. *Chronic poisoning* produces a grayish blue pigmentation of the skin and gums, as well as of the mucous membranes in the colon and elsewhere.

LEAD: Acute poisoning

Lead is poisonous as the metal and its compounds. It is excreted via the urine and feces, and these are commonly used for lead determinations. *Acute lead poisoning* is usually suicidal or accidental. It may result from the ingestion of a large amount of a lead salt or repeated ingestion of small amounts, the effects being cumulative. Some cases have been due to inhalation of the fumes from burning lead storage battery casings. *Acute gastrointestinal symptoms* include a metallic taste in the mouth, retching or vomiting, and bloody or black diarrhea (the latter due to the black lead sulfide formed). Muscle cramps are also common. *Pathologic findings* are hemorrhagic gastritis and colitis, the mucosal surfaces often being covered by a black or gray crust.

Chronic poisoning:

Chronic lead poisoning (plumbism) is much more common than the acute form. It is frequent among painters and children. The latter eat lead-containing paint as a form of pica. *Clinically* there are weight loss, anemia (with basophilic stippling of red cells), colic, a bluish black lead line in the gums at the base of the teeth, and peripheral palsies. Wrist and foot drops are common.

pathologic changes

Pathologic changes are nonspecific. *Massive edema of the brain* is frequent in children *(lead encephalopathy)*. Myelin degeneration and astrocytic gliosis are found in the white matter. Lead encephalopathy usually develops suddenly in the summer months in children 2 to 4 years old. This propensity for occurrence during the summer may be due to the effects of increased sunlight on circulating porphyrins [5]. A patchy segmental demyelinization (of Gombault) develops in involved motor nerves in *lead neuropathy*. Acid-fast *intranuclear inclusion bodies in proximal convoluted renal tubular epithelial cells* are Feulgen-positive and may or may not contain deoxyribonucleic acid (DNA) [6]. In experimental poisoning the inclusions appear first after 1 month. They begin as a small electron-dense zone halfway between the nucleolus and the nuclear membrane. As the inclusion enlarges, it displaces the nucleolus and becomes centrally located within the nucleus. The mitochondria of some inclusion-containing cells are swollen and rounded. *Increased urinary coproporphyrin* is a recognized feature of lead poisoning [7]. It has been suggested that lead inhibits iron utilization in heme synthesis in erythroblasts, resulting in porphyrin precursor accumulation. Rarely acute intermittent porphyria is associated with lead poisoning. Grayish retinal stippling about the optic disk may be seen on ophthalmoscopic examination. A *lead line* in bones appears on x-ray as a zone of increased density at the epiphyses in children. The *gum line* is due to the deposition of lead sulfide around small submucosal blood vessels. The lead is stored in bones, liver, kidneys, brain, and muscles, in decreasing order of concentration.

Versenate nephrosis

The *specific treatment of lead poisoning is versenate* (disodium calcium ethylenediamine tetra-acetic acid), which acts as a chelating agent, binding heavy metals, especially lead, in soluble, nonionized complexes which are excreted in the urine (over 90 percent). An *acute versenate nephrosis* [8] has been reported in a few cases. The kidneys are pale and swollen, and microscopically there is an acute proximal convoluted tubular epithelial necrosis with vacuolization of the distal convoluted tubular epithelium. Focal glomerular tuft necrosis and hyalin droplets within glomerular epithelial cells are also found.

NICKEL

Nickel is an uncommon cause of poisoning. Workers with the metal may develop a widespread nodular eczema *(nickel itch).* The inhalation of *nickel carbonyl* ($NiCO_4$) causes dyspnea, cyanosis, vomiting, and dilatation of the pupils. In dogs exposed to *nickel carbonyl dust* [9], congestion is found in the wall of the lower trachea and major bronchi. The bronchi are filled with thick, blood-streaked mucus. The lungs show extensive foci of consolidation, especially in the lower lobe. *Microscopically* congestion and edema and alveolar septal and epithelial cellular swelling are found after 2 days. Fibroblastic proliferation and bronchial leukocytic infiltration begin on the third day. Within 5 days the alveolar epithelial cells show nuclear atypism and vacuolization.

CHROMIUM

Chromium salts, such as potassium dichromate or chromate, and *chromic acid* are occasionally ingested suicidally or accidentally. Fatal cases are rare. The salts are escharotic and produce ulcers in the mouth, pharynx, and esophagus. The gastric mucosa is inflamed, greenish gray or greenish brown, and stiffened due to the coagulation of protein. Fatty changes develop in the liver, kidneys, and heart. The viscera may be bluish gray, and the blood is brown due to methemoglobin formation. Industrially the *inhalation of chromium salts* produces ulceration of the respiratory mucosa. The incidence of bronchogenic carcinoma is significantly high in chromate workers. Inhalation of *chromic acid* has produced hepatocytic necrosis and bile stasis, resulting in jaundice. *Skin contact with the salts* causes chronic ulcers, especially about the fingernails.

IRON

Iron salts, such as ferrous sulfate or ferric chloride, are occasional causes of acute poisoning when taken as an abortifacient or accidentally by children. They are gastrointestinal irritants and in fatal cases cause sloughing of the gastric mucosa which is greenish black or brown. Periportal hemorrhages and necrosis are found in the liver, and methemoglobin is sometimes formed. The feces are black. It has been postulated that the iron combines with sulfhydryl groups, thus interfering with oxidation.

ZINC

Zinc salts, by accidental or suicidal ingestion, produce congestion, necrosis, and ulceration of the upper alimentary tract. *Zinc stearate dusting powders* have caused occasional deaths in infants, possibly due to inhalation. *Fungicides containing zinc chloride* may cause escharotic (sloughing) ulcers on the skin. In industry, *"spelter chills," "brass-founder's ague,"* and *"brazier's disease"* probably are caused by inhalation of zinc fumes or dust. Throat irritation, painful cough, weakness, muscle pains, and chills develop. Recovery occurs in a few hours.

COPPER

Copper is not toxic as a metal, but its salts, especially copper sulfate (blue vitriol), occasionally cause fatal poisoning. Most cases are suicidal. The gastric mucosa is corroded, and covered with a dry, green or reddish brown crust. Ulcers may be found in the intestine. Fatty changes occur in the liver. The formation of hematin may darken the color of the blood.

CADMIUM AND BERYLLIUM

Cadmium and beryllium fumes cause a pneumonitis and pulmonary fibrosis, respectively, in workers with these metals. These conditions are discussed in Chapter 19 with the other pneumoconioses.

VANADIUM

Vanadium is used in the manufacture of dyes and steel alloys. Workers exposed to dusts and fumes of vanadium compounds, especially the trioxide (V_2O_3), may develop a chronic syndrome known as *vanadiumism.* They have nausea, diarrhea, anemia, cachexia, a nonproductive cough, and hematuria. In fatal cases pulmonary congestion, gastrointestinal inflammation, and renal hemorrhages are found.

THAL-LIUM

Thallium is a heavy metal used in some rat poisons as thallium sulfate, in fungicides, and in depilatory creams. *Acute thallium poisoning* [10] is characterized by gastrointestinal hemorrhage, vomiting, diarrhea or constipation, delirium, convulsions or tremors, paresthesias, and coma. Death due to respiratory paralysis may occur in a few days. Acute inflammation and mucosal blackening (due to thallium sulfide) are found in the mouth, stomach, and small intestine. *Chronic poisoning* is due to the storage of thallium in the bones, muscles, and brain. *Epilation* (falling out of the hair) due to a toxic effect on hair follicles leads to *alopecia.* White transverse bands appear in the nails, and a bluish gum line develops after about a month. Optic atrophy may result from anterior optic or retrobulbar neuritis.

GOLD

Gold compounds used in therapy sometimes cause toxic reactions. The most consistent *pathologic findings* are cloudy swelling and necrosis of the renal epithelium, central necrosis of the liver, and ulcerative enteritis and colitis. *Chrysiasis* is the permanent pigmentation of the skin caused by parenteral use of gold preparations.

MAN-GANESE

Manganese compounds occasionally cause poisoning. *Potassium permanganate* may be ingested for suicidal purposes, causing a corrosive gastroenteritis with a brownish black mucosal crust. *Chronic manganese poisoning* is industrial due to the inhalation of dust. It causes parkinsonism, due to degenerative changes in the basal ganglia, or "manganese pneumonia," which may be fatal.

SODIUM CHLO-RIDE

Sodium chloride is toxic in high concentrations, the lethal dose being estimated as about 3 gm. per kilogram of body weight in adults. A number of infants in a hospital nursery suffered fatal *acute salt poisoning* [11] in 1962 when sodium chloride was inadvertently introduced into their formula. Autopsy findings included dehydration shrinkage of the renal convoluted tubules which were surrounded by a zone of clear hyperosmolar fluid within the tubular basement membrane; subarachnoid and intraventricular hemorrhage due to rupture of ballooned capillaries; sinus thrombosis, especially in the sagittal sinus; capillary thrombosis and petechial hemorrhages with microinfarction in the cerebral white matter; and a suppurative and hemorrhagic pneumonitis centered around blood vessels, especially those which had undergone a necrotizing arteritis.

4. Nonmetallic Inorganic Poisons

PHOS-PHORUS:

Phosphorus is more toxic in the white or yellow form than in the allotropic red form. It is a protoplasmic poison and interferes with cell oxidation. Poisoning is suicidal or accidental, the latter especially in children, who eat the tips of lucifer matches or rat poison containing phosphorus. *Acute poisoning* produces rapid death by medullary depression, or there may be severe nausea and vomiting, without corrosion of the gastric mucosa. *Subacute poisoning* is typified by fatty metamorphosis of the liver and severe hepatic necrosis, with leucine and tyrosine in the urine. The liver necrosis typically begins peripherally in the lobules, but it is often diffuse by the time of death. Fatty changes are marked in the heart and kidneys. These patients survive 4 to 14 days. *Chronic poisoning* is industrial and is typified by necrosis of the mandible (phossy jaw).

Organic phosphorus compounds

Organic phosphorus compounds are now used in insecticides. Among these are tetraethyl pyrophosphate (TEPP), diethyl *p*-nitrophenyl thiophosphate (parathion), and the only moderately toxic malathion. Their toxic effects are potentiated in patients taking phenothiazides [12]. *The compounds inhibit cholinesterase,* producing lacrimation, salivation, sweating, bronchoconstriction, and miosis *(muscarine-like effects).* They also produce *nicotine-like effects,* such as flushing, throbbing of the head, and heart block. *The erythrocyte cholinesterase activity is markedly reduced. Histochemically* a decreased cholinesterase activity in the motor end-plates in intercostal muscles can be demonstrated in fatal cases [13]. The *therapy* is high doses of *atropine sulfate* intravenously. *Pralidoximes* are also of value, especially in parathion poisoning.

BORIC ACID

Boric acid and borax occasionally cause toxic effects due to absorption when used as lavages and as drying powders for diaper rash. Eczematoid lesions or exfoliative dermatitis occurs, and there are renal tubular epithelial degenerative changes.

SELENIUM

Selenium is used in the therapy of dandruff and industrially. The *selenium sulfide* used in shampoos and dandruff treatments is barely absorbed by the intact scalp; however, any open scalp lesion provides an opportunity for toxic assimilation of the compound. Selenium may be absorbed in toxic amounts through the skin, producing a garlic odor on the breath, vomiting, and slight anemia. The *garlic-breath odor* is due to the formation of volatile methylselenite [14]. Selenium compounds may also produce an eczematoid dermatitis which may be made worse by exposure to sunlight. The toxic effects of *tellurium* are similar.

TELLURIUM

NITRITES

Nitrites occasionally are severely toxic. *Sodium nitrite* is used to color meat and as a pickling agent. The allowable residue in meats is 0.01 percent. In excess it produces vasodilation by relaxing smooth muscle, gastrointestinal irritation with nausea and vomiting, cold perspiration, vertigo, headache, cyanosis, tachycardia, decrease in blood pressure, methemoglobinemia, and coma. Large doses cause gastric hemorrhage, diarrhea, and tonic convulsions.

5. *Volatile Organic Poisons*

METHYL ALCOHOL

Methyl alcohol is imbibed either knowingly or mistakenly for ethyl alcohol. It produces a severe gastritis and in some cases a focal or diffuse acute pancreatitis. The odor of alcohol is present. *Blindness from optic atrophy* may occur. There is edema of the retina with degeneration of the ganglion cells.

ETHYL ALCOHOL:

Acute alcoholism

Ethyl alcohol in excess acts as a poison. The cases of *acute poisoning* are often due to other organic compounds mixed with ethyl alcohol, as in "smoke," the term used for various paint removers, varnish and lacquer thinners, and antifreeze mixtures which contain isopropyl alcohol, methyl alcohol, acetone, and/or ethylene glycol, as well as or instead of ethyl alcohol. *Acute poisoning* causes a severe gastritis, fatty metamorphosis of the liver, and edema of the brain. The fatty changes result from increased triglyceride formation within hepatocytes, excessive mobilization of free fatty acids from fat deposits, and probably peroxidation of hepatic lipids [15]. An acute pancreatitis occasionally occurs during a heavy drinking bout. Aspiration of gastric contents during vomiting episodes is common. In some cases of acute alcoholism, cytoplasmic vacuolization of rubriblasts (proerythroblasts) has been observed in the bone marrow [16]. This vacuolization is similar to that found in chloramphenicol bone marrow toxicity. The vacuoles in acute alcoholism may be related to the absence in erythrocytes of alcohol dehydrogenase, which is essential for the initial metabolism of alcohol.

Chronic alcoholism

Chronic alcoholism may produce fatty changes in the liver, kidneys, and heart; atrophy of the seminiferous tubules; cerebral edema; and decreased resistance which may lead to lobar pneumonia or bronchopneumonia. *Fat embolism* from the liver to the lungs and brain is common and may be the cause of death in about 25 percent of the cases with fatty livers. The latter are grossly fatty and show large lipid-containing cysts. The fat appears to be suddenly released from the cysts into the hepatic sinusoids, probably due to increased intrahepatic pressure from slight trauma over the liver [17]. Repeated episodes of fat embolism to the brain over long periods leads to slight to moderate cerebral and cerebellar atrophy, with loss of pyramidal, basal ganglia, and Purkinje cells; loss of myelin, especially in the outer cerebral cortex; Virchow-Robin space widening; and perivascular hemorrhages [18]. Decreased cellularity and loosening are often noted in the granular layer of the cerebellum. Delirium tremens, Korsakoff's syndrome (amnesia and confabulation, often with severe lower extremity pain, tenderness, and slight weakness), vitamin deficiencies, and portal cirrhosis of the liver are commonly associated with chronic alcoholism.

ISOPROPYL ALCOHOL

Isopropyl alcohol (rubbing alcohol), despite its ready availability, is a rare cause of severe or fatal poisoning [19]. It is usually ingested accidentally or as a substitute for ethyl alcohol. *Clinically* isopropyl alcohol poisoning is characterized by deep coma with hyporeflexia or areflexia. Acetonuria is always found because of the conversion of about 15 percent of ingested isopropanol to acetone. There appears to be either an absorption ceiling for isopropyl alcohol or a rapid excretion and detoxification above a critical level, because the blood level in fatal cases seldom rises above 150 mg. per 100 ml. Isopropanol is about twice as toxic as ethyl alcohol, and *death is due to central nervous system depression. Pathologic findings* are minimal and nonspecific. In persons dying after several days there are hemorrhagic gastritis and hypoxic nephrosis with hemoglobin casts in renal tubules.

ETHYLENE GLYCOL

Ethylene glycol is a constituent of antifreeze mixtures. It is usually imbibed mistakenly for ethyl alcohol or by alcoholic prisoners. The lethal dose is about 100 ml. The toxicity of ethylene glycol may be due to one or more of the intermediate compounds found in its degradation – glycoaldehyde, glycolic acid, and glyoxylic acid [20]. *Autopsy findings* [21] include swollen, pale kidneys, with fan-shaped or wheat sheaf-shaped crystals of calcium oxalate seen best in polarized light in the tubular epithelium and lumina. In those surviving 4 to 5 days hydropic changes occur in the renal tubular epithelium and hepatic parenchymal cells.

DIETHYLENE GLYCOL

Diethylene glycol is about twice as toxic as ethylene glycol. A number of cases of poisoning occurred in 1937 when this compound was used as a solvent in elixir of sulfanilamide. *Clinically* anuria develops rapidly. *Pathologic findings* include an enlarged pale liver with fatty and severe hydropic changes, especially in the centrolobular cells, and pale, swollen kidneys with marked hydropic changes in the tubular epithelium. No calcium oxalate crystals are found.

CHLOROFORM

Chloroform may cause death by central nervous system paralysis during anesthesia or by cholemia later. *Death from anesthesia* produces no specific changes. *Delayed chloroform poisoning* causes a severe fatty metamorphosis of the liver, kidneys, and heart. Diffuse hepatic necrosis may occur.

CARBON TETRACHLORIDE

Carbon tetrachloride may be inhaled by cleaning-plant workers or ingested, particularly by children and alcoholics. Carbon tetrachloride produces an *acute hepatic necrosis* [22]. The toxic action may be due to the peroxidative degeneration of lipids in the endoplasmic reticulum of hepatocytes [23]. *Prolonged repeated exposures* may lead to toxic cirrhosis of the liver. Acute fatty changes also appear in the heart and kidneys. Leucine and tyrosine crystals may appear in the renal tubules. *Death may be anesthetic* (within a few minutes), *hepatic* (2 to 3 days), *or renal* (10 to 14 days). *Most deaths are renal* in nature. After 8 to 10 days a uremic pneumonitis with hyaline membranes may occur. The membranes are probably due to an outpouring of a fibrin-rich fluid into the alveoli as part of the uremia [24].

CYANIDES

Cyanides are among the most potent poisons known. Hydrocyanic acid (HCN) is a volatile liquid with a low boiling point. Its fumes are used to fumigate buildings and ships. Potassium cyanide and sodium cyanide are present in silver polishes, electroplating chemicals, and white shoe polish. They are commonly used for suicides and homicides. Children may ingest them accidentally. They are converted to hydrocyanic acid by the gastric acid. In *fatal cases* death is often rapid due to paralysis of the medullary respiratory centers. The *cyanides interfere with cellular oxidation by blocking the cytochrome oxidase system. At autopsy the odor of bitter almond* is prominent. The viscera are congested. The blood remains fluid and is often bright red.

VOLATILE AROMATIC COMPOUNDS:

Volatile aromatic poisons include benzene, nitrobenzene, aniline, amphetamine, pyridine, naphthalene, camphor, gasoline, and kerosene. *Amphetamine* and *dextroamphetamine* capsules (speed) may be ingested to produce trips; toxic effects are hyperirritability, insomnia, delirium, palpitations, and gastrointestinal symptoms. A few fatal cases have occurred.

Benzene

Benzene may cause poisoning by industrial inhalation of fumes or by suicidal ingestion. In *acute poisoning* the respiratory or gastrointestinal mucosa (depending on the route of entry) shows marked reddening, edema, and hemorrhages. The brain is edematous, and the blood is dark red and remains fluid after death. *Chronic poisoning* is due to prolonged exposure to the fumes or to therapeutic use of benzene. Bone marrow activity is severely depressed, with the development of aplastic anemia, agranulocytosis, and thrombocytopenia. Multiple hemorrhages are common, and fatty changes occur in the liver, kidneys, and heart. A periostitis and osteomyelitis of the maxilla, with a loss of teeth, may develop. Occasional cases of stem cell or acute myelogenous leukemia have occurred in workers occupationally exposed to benzene.

Nitrobenzene

Nitrobenzene is a protoplasmic poison which causes death by central nervous system depression. The most striking finding in fatal cases of nitrobenzene poisoning is the *chocolate brown color of the blood due to the formation of methemoglobin and nitrobenzene hemoglobin.* A strong odor of *bitter almond* is also noted.

Aniline

The toxic effects of *aniline* are similar to those of nitrobenzene.

Naphthalene

Naphthalene is used extensively as a moth repellent and in dye manufacture. A staggering gait, vomiting, and abdominal and urinary tract pain are the characteristic signs and symptoms. *Hemolytic anemia* may develop. It is due to a metabolite of naphthalene, α-naphthol. Jaundice and hemoglobinuria may follow, the urine being port wine in color. *Autopsy findings* include gastrointestinal inflammation, fatty changes in the liver, and pigment casts in the renal tubules.

Camphor

Camphor may be ingested by children in medications and moth balls. Occasionally toxic amounts of camphor have been absorbed by infants from clothing. The *clinical picture* resembles acute alcoholism, but convulsions may ensue. *Death* is due to paralysis of the medullary vital centers. The odor of camphor is present on the breath and the viscera.

Gasoline and kerosene

Gasoline and kerosene are common causes of poisoning in children, kerosene being the most frequent poison in children under 5 years. The mortality is about 5 percent. These petroleum products are irritating to the pharyngeal, esophageal, gastric, and small intestinal mucosa, which becomes edematous and may be ulcerated. A *pneumonitis,* which is probably due to aspiration of the hydrocarbons into the lungs, commonly develops. This is typically bilateral and basal, with multiple, small, poorly defined patches of severe intra-alveolar edema and acute inflammation. Later the lesions tend to coalesce, and secondary bacterial infection may occur. *Clinically* there are nausea and vomiting, abdominal cramps, coughing and choking (the ingested hydrocarbon can be smelled on the breath), tachypnea, cyanosis, signs of basal consolidation, tachycardia, fever, and drowsiness or even coma.

Glue-sniffing

Glue-sniffing, the purposeful inhalation of the vapors of plastic cements, is a major problem among older children and adolescents [25]. The plastic and model cements vary somewhat in composition, but all contain *highly volatile organic solvents* such as benzene, toluene, xylene, carbon tetrachloride, chloroform, ethylene dichloride, acetone and other ketones, amyl, ethyl, and butyl acetates, tricresyl phosphate, and various alcohols. The contents of tubes are usually squeezed into a handkerchief or other cloth and held up to the nose and mouth. The vapors produce a "jag," with exhilaration, excitement, a staggering gait, and slurred speech. The *effects are similar to those of ethyl alcohol.* After about 30 minutes the child becomes drowsy, stuporous, and even unconscious. *Tolerance* to the solvents develops in *chronic glue-sniffers.* The inhalations are habit-forming, but true addiction does not develop. Chromosome breaks in leukocytes and hepatic damage with abnormal liver biopsies and high alkaline phosphatase levels have been found in glue-sniffers [25a].

THESAUROSIS

A number of cases of *thesaurosis (storage disease) involving the lungs* may have resulted from the inhalation of hair sprays containing macromolecular resins such as polyvinylpyrrolidone [26]. Death has occurred in several cases. Chest films have shown a fuzzy or irregular nodular bilateral pulmonary infiltrate with moderate hilar adenopathy. Discontinuance of use of the hair spray has led to prompt regression of the radiologic changes. In the lungs there is an acute diffuse interstitial fibrosis very similar to that of the Hamman-Rich syndrome. Interstitial fibrosis, alveolar epithelial hyperplasia, numerous intra-alveolar macrophages containing PAS-positive cytoplasmic granules, and a sparsity of neutrophils and lymphocytes are found. In the hilar lymph nodes the changes vary from slight reticuloendothelial hyperplasia to sarcoid-like granulomata.

POLYMER-FUME FEVER

Polymer-fume fever occurs in industrial workers exposed to the fumes of tetrafluoroethylene polymers (Teflon, Fluon) [27]. When such polymers are heated to temperatures above 300°C., the inhaled fumes produce an influenza-like syndrome with chills, fever, malaise, chest tightness, shortness of breath, cough, and headache. Some cases are attributed to smoking cigarettes contaminated with polymer-fume dust. Long-chain fluorocarbon breakdown products cause the toxic effects. The *pathologic changes* are unknown.

6. Nonvolatile, Nonalkaloidal Organic Poisons

BARBITURATES

Barbiturates are derivatives of barbituric acid and are used therapeutically as sedatives and hypnotics. *Overdoses cause death by paralysis of the respiratory center. Poisoning* by barbiturates may be accidental, homicidal, or suicidal. Use of barbiturates for suicidal purposes is increasing in frequency. Many deaths occur during acute alcoholism, the two poisons having a synergistic central nervous system depressant effect. In general, the barbiturates cause toxic symptoms at five to 10 times the oral therapeutic dose and are fatal at 12 times this dose. The incidence of *acute barbiturate intoxication* [28] is constantly increasing. There are over 1000 deaths due to barbiturate poisoning in the United States annually. Barbiturate intoxication is over twice as common in women as men. The most important complication is *aspiration bronchopneumonia,* which occurs in about 10 percent of the cases. Cardiac arrhythmia appears in over 5 percent. A *mortality rate* of about 5 percent has remained constant for many years in acute barbiturate poisoning. *Pathologic findings* in deaths due to barbiturate poisoning are nonspecific and include congestion and edema of the lungs, liver, kidneys, and brain. Bronchopneumonia is found in those who survive for a few days. In those surviving for several days there may be a bilateral symmetric necrosis of the globus pallidus.

SALICYLATES

Salicylates are very common causes of accidental poisoning in children who ingest aspirin tablets or methyl salicylate. Occasional suicides are due to salicylates. The lethal dose is variable. *Pathologic findings* in poisoning by methyl salicylate are congestion and acute inflammation of the gastric and intestinal mucosa, submucosal renal pelvic hemorrhages, visceral congestion, and the *odor of oil of wintergreen* throughout the body. In *poisoning by aspirin (acetylsalicylic acid)* there is erosion of the gastric mucosa and visceral congestion. *Chronic salicylate poisoning (salicylism)* is characterized by mental depression, anorexia, renal irritation, and a skin eruption.

HEXACHLOROPHENE

Hexachlorophene [29] is a component of certain antiseptic detergents such as pHisoHex. It is *a chlorinated bis-phenolic compound.* Ingestion of hexachlorophene-containing detergent has usually occurred accidentally in hospitals by mistaking the compound for milk of magnesia. Following ingestion there are nausea, vomiting, abdominal cramps, and diarrhea. Shock due to peripheral vascular collapse may ensue. Hexachlorophene appears to react mainly as a *gastrointestinal irritant.* The fatal dose in man is 5 to 10 mg. of hexachlorophene, which is present in a 3 percent concentration in antiseptic detergents.

7. Alkaloidal Poisons

NICOTINE

Nicotine is the principal alkaloid in tobacco leaves. Poisoning may be suicidal, homicidal, or accidental, by the ingestion of tobacco or of insecticides containing nicotine. Nicotine first excites, then depresses the central nervous system. *Death* is due to medullary depression and a specific curare-like action on the respiratory muscles. The lethal dose is 3 to 4 drops of the alkaloid. Only hydrocyanic acid produces a more rapid death. *Pathologic findings* include marked visceral congestion and dark, fluid blood.

OPIATES:

Morphine and codeine

Opium is the dried milky exudate of the unripe capsules of the poppy. It contains 20 alkaloids, of which the most important are morphine, codeine, thebaine, and papaverine. *Morphine* is the most toxic of the opium alkaloids. It depresses the cerebrum, then the medulla. It may stimulate the cord, causing tetanoid convulsions. The lethal dose in nonaddicts is 1 to 6 grains (65 to 390 mg.). *Codeine* is less toxic than morphine. Its effects are similar. *Pathologic findings* in acute morphine poisoning include visceral congestion, cyanosis, and dark, fluid blood. The pupils are typically contracted, but may be dilated. *Heroin* is a synthetic morphine derivative. Its action and pathologic effects are like those of morphine. It is rapidly destroyed in the body and thus is difficult to detect. Addicts, especially "mainliners" who use a common spoon, eye dropper, and needle for intravenous injections, often develop *bacteremia and acute bacterial endocarditis.* Occasionally mycotemia, especially candidial infection, occurs. Chronic hepatic dysfunction is common among heroin addicts, presumably due to serum hepatitis virus transmitted by the use of common utensils [30]. Heroin

BELLADONNA ALKALOIDS

Atropine, scopolamine, and hyoscyamine are related alkaloids; all block the muscarinic action of acetylcholine in the parasympathetic system. Atropine is the most toxic, its lethal dose being about 3 mg. In cases of poisoning there is first an excited phase, with dry throat, dilated pupils, hallucinations, delirium, choreiform movements, and convulsions. The *skin* is flushed and may show a deep red eruption. Just before death, a paralytic phase ensues. *Death* is by medullary failure. *Pathologic findings* are visceral congestion and faint signs of the red skin eruption.

STRYCHNINE

Strychnine is a powerful central nervous system stimulant which causes *tetanoid convulsions* in toxic amounts. Poisoning is usually suicidal, but many cases are accidental, and a few are homicidal. The *pathologic changes* are nonspecific. Rigor mortis occurs shortly after death and may persist for days. The body may be in opisthotonos.

8. "Food" Poisons

MILK SICKNESS

Milk sickness [31] in man is due to the ingestion of milk from cows which have fed on certain poisonous plants (white snakeroot, rayless goldenrod) and are suffering from *trembles.* The toxic substance is *tremetol.* The mortality is about 10 percent. *Pathologic changes* are severe fatty metamorphosis, especially in the liver, with petechiae and ecchymoses in all tissues.

POISON HEMLOCK

Poison hemlock (Conium maculatum), also known as the common or spotted hemlock or as spotted cowbane, is a member of the parsley family. All parts of the plants are poisonous, especially the unripe fruit. The toxic principles are the alkaloids *D-coniine* (α-n-propyl-piperidine) and *γ-coniceine. Coniine,* which *has a curare-like action,* gives the plant the odor of mouse urine. In persons, usually children, accidentally eating the plant there are nausea and vomiting; excessive salivation; dysphagia; pupillary dilatation; ptosis; loss of visual accommodation; thickening of speech; diminution in hearing; drowsiness; muscle fibrillation and tremors, with mild convulsions; muscle weakness, beginning in the lower extremities, with progressive loss of muscle control and even paralysis; clear intellect; bradycardia early, with late tachycardia; and tachypnea early, with later weak, slow, shallow, and irregular breathing. *Death* is due to respiratory muscle paralysis and medullary respiratory center depression. It may occur within ½ to 3 hours after ingestion. The *postmortem findings* are severe visceral congestion. Parts of the plant may be recognizable in the gastric contents. *Water hemlock (Cicuta virosa* or *maculata),* also called spotted cowbane, is poisonous, especially the roots. The toxic agent is *cicutoxin,* the action of which is *similar to* that of *strychnine.*

FAVISM

Favism is due to the ingestion of broadbeans *(Vicia faba)* in sensitive individuals. Within a few days there is an *acute hemolytic anemia in persons with an inherited deficiency of glucose-6-phosphate dehydrogenase in erythrocytes.* Jaundice, hemoglobinuria, hepatomegaly, and splenomegaly develop. The acute illness lasts 3 to 4 days; the mortality rate is about 10 percent.

LATHYRISM

Lathyrism (lupinosis) is due to the ingestion of chick peas *(Lathyrus savitus* or *L. cicera)* in India and southern Europe. A toxic compound in the peas causes leg weakness, spastic paraplegia, girdle paresthesias, lumbar pain, and tremors. *Experimental lathyrism* in rats has become a valuable research method. Garden sweet peas *(L. oderatus)* produce multiple mesenchymal disorders including hernias, dissecting aneurysms, kyphoscoliosis, tooth degeneration, corneal opacities, and delayed wound healing. The toxic compound in *L. oderatus* is *β-aminoproprionitrile* (BAPN). Similar changes can be produced by α-aminoacetonitrile. Related lesions are not produced in humans.

NUTMEG POISONING

Nutmeg poisoning [32] is caused by the ingestion of 5 gm. or more of nutmeg to induce menstruation or abortion or to produce effects like alcoholic intoxication. The *toxic principle* is *myristicin* (5-allyl-1-methoxy-2,3-methylenedioxybenzene). There are burning abdominal pain, excitement, and fear of impending death, followed by coma, shock, and acidosis, usually with complete recovery in 24 hours.

MUSHROOM POISONING: *Amanita phalloides* poisoning

Mushroom poisoning (mycetismus) is usually due to *Amanita phalloides* (90 percent of the cases), most of the other cases being due to *Amanita muscaria. Poisoning by Amanita phalloides* and its phenotypes (such as *A. brunnescens)* is of the choleriform type, the toxins being phalloidine and amanitine. *Clinically* there are sudden severe abdominal pain, nausea, vomiting, and diarrhea. Dehydration is marked, and jaundice appears in 2 to 3 days. Mortality is about 60 percent. Death is generally on the fifth to eighth day. *Pathologic findings* are fatty changes in the heart, liver, kidneys, and muscles, submucosal hemorrhages in the stomach and intestine, and fluidity of the blood.

***Amanita muscaria* poisoning**

Poisoning by *Amanita muscaria* is *neurotoxic* (mycetismus nervosus). Death is uncommon. In Russia the extract is used in beverages as an intoxicant. The *pharmacologic effects* are due to muscarine which stimulates smooth muscle and gland cells as acetylcholine does. The mushroom also contains bufotenin (n-n-dimethylserotonin). *Clinically* there are excessive salivation, lacrimation, sweating, dyspnea, confusion, hallucinations, and contracted pupils. If death occurs, it is by medullary depression.

9. Insecticides

Insecticides are growing in importance as poisons because of their increasingly widespread use. Poisoning may be by *ingestion* or *inhalation.* Sprayed fruit and vegetables occasionally are the sources of the poison. Insecticides containing organic phosphates and nicotine have been discussed.

ROTENONE PYRETHRUM DDT

Rotenone is found in derris root. In toxic amounts it stimulates the vomiting center in the medulla, then later depresses the medulla. *Pyrethrum* is an extract of soy bean or sesame oil. The pyrethrins are only slightly toxic, but have caused death by medullary depression. Household preparations of pyrethrum are toxic mainly due to the *kerosene solvent. DDT (dichlorodiphenyltrichlorethane)* is only slightly toxic. When large amounts are ingested there is an excited, convulsive phase followed by central nervous system depression and coma. *Pathologic findings* include central zonal hepatic necrosis and renal tubular epithelial degeneration. *Chlordane* (octachlorotetrahydromethanoindane) is toxic to the skin (spraying), respiratory tract (inhalation), and gastrointestinal tract (ingestion). It has caused several accidental and suicidal deaths. *Autopsy findings* [33] include pulmonary edema, bronchopneumonia, congestion and edema of the gastrointestinal mucosa and viscera, and multiple petechial hemorrhages in the brain, myocardium, and urinary bladder.

CHLORDANE

UNTOWARD EFFECTS OF THERAPEUTIC AGENTS

With the tremendous increase in the number of highly effective and often lifesaving therapeutic agents which have been introduced during the past 30 years, drug reactions have become fairly common. Fortunately most of these are mild, but some are serious and even fatal. The patient who has a significant drug reaction is much like the man about whom Carl Sandburg wrote in *The People, Yes,* "I took so much medicine that I was sick a long time after I got well."

1. Sulfonamides

Sulfonamides [34] may produce injury by mechanical means, direct cytotoxic effects, or hypersensitivity. An excessive concentration of sulfonamide crystals in the urine may result in precipitation of crystalline or amorphous material in the renal calyces or pelvis or in a ureter. Mechanical ureteral obstruction may result. Crystalluria is related to the urinary concentration and solubility of sulfonamide compounds and rarely occurs with the derivatives in use today. The rare cases of aplastic anemia which have been attributed to sulfamethoxypyridazine, sulfisoxazole, and other sulfonamides are probably due to a direct myelotoxic effect. *Hypersensitivity reactions* are numerous; they include *drug fever,* which develops between the seventh and 10th day of therapy in 2 to 5 percent of patients on a variety of sulfonamides; *serum sickness,* which may appear after 3 to 17 days of therapy; *anaphylactic reactions,* which sometimes occur in previously sensitized individuals; *skin rashes,* which usually develop during the first week of therapy and may be urticarial, purpuric, scarlatinal, or morbilliform, or an exfoliative dermatitis or photosensitivity reaction, and which occur in about 2 percent of patients on sulfisoxazole; periarteritis nodosa rarely; a few cases of fatal "hypersensitivity" myocarditis which have been attributed to sulfamethoxypyridazine; acute diffuse interstitial nephritis; and *blood dyscrasias.* Among the blood dyscrasias are *acute hemolytic anemia,* which is most commonly associated with sulfonilamide and sulfapyridine; occasional cases have occurred with sulfisoxazole and sulfamethoxypyridazine. Some cases represent a primaquine-type hemolysis (see page 252). Agranulocytosis is due to hypersensitivity with leukocyte agglutinin formation, but a direct myelotoxic effect may also be involved. There is a maturation arrest at the myeloblast stage. It occurs in about 0.1 percent of patients on sulfadiazine, and occasional cases develop with sulfisoxazole, sulfamethoxypyridazine, sulfapyridine, and sulfathiazole. Occasional cases of thrombocytopenic purpura have been associated with sulfamethoxypyridazine and sulfisoxazole due to formation of antiplatelet antibodies. Hepatic injury occurs in less than 0.1 percent of patients on sulfonamides and may vary from intrahepatic cholestasis to massive necrosis.

2. Antibiotics

Mild to overwhelming *mycotic infections,* especially due to *Candida albicans,* are fairly common in patients on prolonged antibiotic therapy, due to suppression of bacterial growth.

PENICILLIN

Penicillin ranks first among drugs in incidence of allergic responses, hypersensitivity reactions occurring in about 3 percent of patients. These are due to a combination of penicillenic acid or another metabolite with protein to form an antigenic penicilloyl-protein complex [35]. *Urticaria* is the most frequent form; exfoliative dermatitis, angioneurotic edema, serum sickness, and periarteritis nodosa also occur. *Fatal anaphylaxis* develops in about one in 3 million doses. A few cases of Coombs test-positive hemolytic anemia have occurred following the prolonged administration of high doses of penicillin [36]. In these cases circulating antipenicillin antibody is present in the serum and coats the erythrocytes. An interstitial nephritis has developed in patients taking *methcillin* (dimethoxyphenyl penicillin) [36a]. Clinically there are fever, eosinophilia, hematuria, and proteinuria. Renal biopsies reveal infiltration of the interstitial tissue by eosinophils, lymphocytes, and macrophages. Tubular epithelial degeneration is also found. The glomeruli appear normal.

TETRACYCLINES

Permanent yellow to brownish yellow *staining of the teeth* has been reported in a high percentage of children under 10 years of age receiving prolonged chlortetracycline, oxytetracycline, and tetracycline therapy. The compounds are incorporated in the teeth as a calcium orthophosphate complex and cause a focal inhibition of calcification and enamel hypoplasia [37]. The teeth of fetuses may be affected in utero when mothers take *tetracyclines* after the third month of pregnancy [38]. Severe and even fatal fatty metamorphosis of the liver has occurred in several pregnant women with pyelonephritis treated with high doses of tetracyclines, especially when given intravenously [39]. *Tetracycline degradation products* (anhydrotetracycline and epianhydrotetracycline) may cause a reversible *Fanconi-like syndrome* with acidosis, proteinuria, glycosuria, aminoaciduria, and hyperphosphaturia [40]. Kidney biopsies reveal cytoplasmic vacuolization and hyalin droplets in the convoluted tubular epithelium, especially in the distal portions. The vacuoles may be due to potassium loss. A case simulating disseminated lupus erythematosus, with photosensitivity, aminoaciduria, proteinuria, hematuria, and pyuria, has been attributed to degraded tetracycline [41]. In about 5 percent of patients taking *demethylchlortetracycline* a *photosensitivity reaction* occurs in the skin with an exaggerated erythema on exposure to sunlight or an ultraviolet lamp [42].

CHLORAMPHENICOL

An often fatal *aplastic anemia* has been reported frequently in patients using *chloramphenicol.* It is attributed to the marrow toxicity of the nitrobenzene radical in the molecular structure of chloramphenicol, although this has been disputed [43]. Reversible vacuolization of marrow erythroid cells is observed in early cases. There is evidence of some suppression of erythrocyte production in about 30 percent of patients on chloramphenicol. Thrombocytopenia has been reported rarely with this drug.

ERYTHROMYCIN

In patients taking *erythromycin,* a macrolide ester, a maculopapular *skin rash* develops in less than 0.2 percent. A cholestatic hepatitis (intrahepatic cholestasis) has occurred in association with erythromycin estolate [44]. There is periportal infiltration with eosinophils, neutrophils, and lymphocytes in liver biopsies.

OLEANDOMYCIN

Clinical jaundice develops in less than 5 percent of patients on erythromycin. Cholestatic hepatitis with jaundice also occurs in about 5 percent of patients on *triacetyloleandomycin* [45]. Liver biopsies reveal bile thrombi, periportal mononuclear cell infiltration, and hepatocellular degeneration. Over 10 percent of patients on this drug for more than 10 days show evidence of hepatitis without jaundice.

NEOMYCIN

In some patients receiving large doses of *neomycin,* a nonabsorbable oral antibiotic, a *malabsorption syndrome* resembling sprue develops [46]. A nephropathy with focal foamy cytoplasmic vacuolation of the convoluted tubular epithelium appears in a few patients on large doses [47]. *Hearing loss* due to outer cochlear hair cell damage has occurred in patients on neomycin or kanamycin with renal failure.

NITROFURANTOIN

Hypersensitivity reactions to *nitrofurantoin* include a few cases of anaphylactoid reactions and pulmonary infiltration and pleural effusion with eosinophilia [48]. A primaquine-type hemolytic anemia, sometimes with megaloblastic dyspoiesis, develops occasionally [49]. A peripheral polyneuropathy with paresthesias, weakness, and sensory impairment in the extremities has been reported in patients on nitrofurantoin [50]. Acute fibrinous pericarditis has developed in several patients taking *psicofuranine,* a purine nucleoside analogue [51].

3. Drugs Used in the Therapy of Tuberculosis and Fungus Infections

STREPTOMYCIN

ISONIAZID

Hypersensitivity reactions are more common in patients taking streptomycin than dihydrostreptomycin. They include eosinophilia, urticaria, and skin rashes. *Vestibular damage* with vertigo, tinnitus, and deafness occurs in some patients on *streptomycin.* Necrosis of the inferior vestibular and ventral cochlear nuclei is sometimes found. Vestibular changes are less common and deafness more frequent with *dihydrostreptomycin* [52], occurring in about 1 percent of patients. Hearing loss has occurred in children of mothers who received streptomycin during pregnancy [53]. Thrombocytopenia has occurred rarely in patients on streptomycin. In a few cases taking *isoniazid (isonicotinic acid hydrazide), hepatic damage* with jaundice has occurred. There have been rare cases of fatal massive hepatic necrosis [54]; this is more common with the related compound iproniazid.

AMPHOTERICIN

GRISEOFULVIN

Amphotericin B occasionally causes acute renal tubular epithelial necrosis with early deposition of calcium in damaged tubules [55]. A normocytic, normochromic *anemia,* probably due to suppression of erythrocyte production, is fairly common [56]. Occasional patients taking *griseofulvin* have developed severe angioneurotic edema, urticaria (including cold urticaria), or a photosensitivity-induced maculopapular skin rash [57].

4. Antimalarial Drugs

QUININE

QUINACRINE

Reactions to *quinine* include *cinchonism,* characterized by ringing in the ears and visual disturbances (diplopia, disturbed color perception, blurring, and night blindness); acute *hemolytic anemia;* thrombocytopenia due to antiplatelet antibody formation occasionally; and hypoprothrombinemia rarely. Over 50 percent of persons receiving *quinacrine* (Atabrine) for over a week develop a lemon *yellow skin pigmentation.* Eczematoid, exfoliative, and contact dermatitis appears in less than 1 percent of patients. Hepatic necrosis has developed occasionally.

CHLORO-QUINE

Chloroquine, a 4-aminoquinoline compound, occasionally causes visual disturbances such as blurring, halos due to corneal edema, scotomata, and nyctalopia. These disturbances are reversible except for *retinal changes* [58], which occur in about 3 percent of the cases. In these the macular area is consistently involved. There is destruction of rods and cones with migration of pigment from the pigment epithelium to the inner nuclear layer. The foveal cones are preserved, accounting for the preservation of visual acuity. With peripheral retinal destruction the retinal arterioles become narrowed or obliterated. The chloroquine accumulates in melanin-containing cells of the eye, and some cases of peripheral pigmentary changes resemble retinitis pigmentosa. Posterior subcapsular lens opacities sometimes appear. Other reactions to chloroquine include a few cases of nerve deafness after prolonged therapy, loss of hair pigmentation and focal alopecia, and leukopenia. Chloroquine, as well as primaquine and diaminodiphenyl sulfone, provokes methemoglobinemia in patients with a deficiency of nicotinamide adenine dinucleotide methemoglobin reductase in erythrocytes [58a].

PAMA-QUINE AND PRIMA-QUINE

Among patients on *pamaquine and primaquine,* 8-aminoquinoline compounds, an acute *hemolytic anemia* occurs in those with a *deficiency of glucose-6-phosphate dehydrogenase* (G-6-PD) in their erythrocytes [59]. Such cells have a low content of reduced glutathione, and the production of reduced triphosphopyridine nucleotide and methemoglobin is impaired. Heinz bodies appear in erythrocytes early during the hemolytic crises. (See also page 286.)

5. Analgesics and Antirheumatic Drugs

ACETYL-SALICYL-IC ACID

ACETO-PHENET-IDIN

AMINO-PYRDINE

PHENYL-BUTAZONL

PHENAZO-PYRIDINE

Reactions to *acetylsalicylic acid (aspirin)* include occasional hypersensitivity reactions such as angioneurotic edema, urticaria, skin rashes, and asthma; primaquine-type hemolytic anemia rarely; and hypoprothrombinemia with massive doses. In persons taking prolonged excessive doses of *acetophenetidin* there have been numerous cases of renal papillary necrosis [60] and chronic interstitial nephritis with fibrosis and a slight lymphocytic infiltrate [61]. A primaquine-type hemolytic anemia occasionally develops. *Aminopyrine* produces agranulocytosis due to maturation arrest of granulocytes in the bone marrow and development of antileukocyte antibodies. Reactions to *phenylbutazone* include reactivation of peptic gastric or duodenal ulcer with hemorrhage or perforation in several cases; acute tubular necrosis with renal failure in a few cases [62]; and agranulocytosis, thrombocytopenia, or aplastic anemia occasionally. With *phenazopyridine* a hemolytic anemia with Heinz body formation and methemoglobinemia rarely develop [63].

6. Anticonvulsants

DIPHENYL-HYDAN-TOIN

Gingival hyperplasia develops in about 50 percent of patients on prolonged *diphenylhydantoin* therapy. Pyroninophilic bodies consisting of protein containing ribonucleic acid and similar to ones found in lupus erythematosus are present in the gingivae [64]. The gums are enlarged, especially over the anterior teeth. The mucosa shows parakeratosis and acanthosis with rete peg elongation. There are capillary proliferation and lymphocytic infiltration in the densely collagenous submucosa. *Other reactions* to diphenylhydantoin include a few cases of hepatic necrosis; megaloblastic anemia responsive to folic acid therapy; agranulocytosis; and a *lymphoma-like syndrome* with lymphadenopathy due to lymphoid and reticular hyperplasia and eosinophilic infiltration. In the lymphoma-like syndrome the changes may simulate Hodgkin's granuloma or lymphosarcoma [65]. Circulating antibodies against diphenylhydantoin have been detected by the basophilic degranulation test in these cases [66]. Agranulocytosis and the lymphoma-like syndrome also occur occasionally with *methylphenylethyl hydantoin. Trimethadione* therapy has been associated with occasional cases of nephrotic syndrome with glomerular epithelial foot process fusion [67]. In patients on *phenylacetylurea,* liver damage varying from slight hepatocellular degeneration to fatal massive necrosis may occur [68]. Thrombocytopenia occurs rarely with phenylacetylurea therapy.

TRIMETHADIONE

PHENYLACETYLUREA

7. Anesthetics

Among patients anesthetized with *halothane* a number of cases of fatal, predominantly centrolobular *hepatic necrosis* associated with fatty metamorphosis have occurred [69]. The necrosis may be due to an impurity, dichlorohexafluorobutene [70].

HALOTHANE

8. Ataraxic (Psychosoplegic) Drugs (Tranquilizers)

PHENOTHIAZINES:

The *phenothiazine derivatives* are classified as aliphatic derivatives (chlorpromazine, promazine, and trifluopromazine), piperidine derivatives (mepazine and thioridazine), and piperazine derivatives (prochlorperazine, trifluoperazine, and perphenazine). *Extrapyramidal effects* are most commonly associated with the piperazine derivatives. They include a classic Parkinson syndrome; akathisia (uncontrollable restlessness); and a dystonic (tetanoid) syndrome with face and jaw muscle spasms, oculogyric crises, and shoulder girdle muscle twitching [71]. The signs clear on withdrawal of the drug used. *Autonomic effects* are mainly anticholinergic and include paralytic ileus and bladder paralysis with mepazine and chlorpromazine, and aggravation of glaucoma due to the mydriatic effect of mepazine. *Cholestatic hepatitis* with obstructive jaundice occurs in 1 to 2 percent of patients on chlorpromazine [72] and occasionally with mepazine, promazine, prochlorperazine, and trifluoperazine. It is a hypersensitivity reaction. Bile thrombi are found in distended canaliculi, granular bile pigment is present in the cytoplasm of hepatocytes, and there is a periportal infiltration with lymphocytes and eosinophils. Rarely massive hepatic necrosis has occurred with chlorpromazine and prochlorperazine [73].

Extrapyramidal effects

Autonomic effects

Hepatic effects

Endocrine effects include spontaneous or induced lactation in up to 25 percent of nonpregnant women on phenothiazines such as trifluoperazine, thioridazine, chlorpromazine, and prochlorperazine [74]; breast engorgement in lactating women on chlorpromazine; gynecomastia, menstrual irregularities, and false positive pregnancy tests with chlorpromazine and prochlorperazine. Among the *blood dyscrasias,* agranulocytosis has occurred rarely with promazine, chlorpromazine, trifluopromazine, mepazine, thioridazine, and prochlorperazine; thrombocytopenic purpura and hemolytic or aplastic anemia develop very rarely. *Photosensitivity with purplish skin pigmentation* has occurred in patients on prolonged high doses of chlorpromazine, promazine, prochlorperazine, and mepazine [75]. *Lenticular opacities* have developed with prolonged phenothiazine therapy [76]. A potentiation of poisoning by organic phosphorus compounds has been noted in patients taking promazine [77] and in animals on chlorpromazine experimentally. A number of cases of *sudden and unexpected death* have occurred among psychiatric patients receiving phenothiazines. The most frequent mechanism of such deaths is cardiac arrhythmia. In a number of the cases

Endocrine effects

Blood dyscrasias

Skin pigmentation

Sudden deaths

abundant acid mucopolysaccharide is found about arterioles subendocardially in the region of the right and left atrial and ventricular conduction bundles [78]. Foci of myocardial degeneration are found nearby.

CHLOR-DIAZE-POXIDE

Reactions to *chlordiazepoxide* include agranulocytosis due to antileukocyte antibody formation rarely; menstrual irregularities, such as delay in or failure of ovulation and premature or delayed bleeding, frequently [79]; and ataxia.

9. Antidepressant Drugs

HYDRA-ZIDE DERIVA-TIVES

Hepatic necrosis with jaundice has occurred often in patients on *iproniazid* and less commonly in those taking *phenipramine* and *β-phenylisopropylhydrazine.* The incidence of *iproniazid hepatitis* has been roughly 1 percent, and the mortality rate about 15 percent. A hypernoradrenalinemia may occur with the toxic doses of β-phenylethylhydrazine *(phenelzine),* a monoamine oxidase inhibitor. Elevated blood epinephrine and norepinephrine levels and increased urinary secretion of vanilyl mandelic acid and catecholamines are found [80].

IMI-PRAMINE

TRANYL-CYPRO-MINE

Reactions to *imipramine,* a dibenzazepine derivative, include agranulocytosis in several cases; cholestatic jaundice in a number of patients; a mild Parkinson-like syndrome with tremors and dysarthria rarely, and epileptiform convulsions occasionally. In several patients taking *tranylcypromine and other monoamine oxidase inhibitors,* attacks of forceful heartbeat, headache, and hypertension, with rare deaths due to intracerebral hemorrhage, have occurred following meals, especially the ingestion of cheese. These are due to potentiation of the pressor effects of tyramine in cheeses and wine [81]. A case of nonfatal hepatic necrosis simulating viral hepatitis has been reported in a patient taking tranylcypromine [82].

10. Sedative and Hypnotic Drugs

MEPRO-BAMATE

Meprobamate has been associated with development of a *fixed drug eruption* consisting of pruritic, round or oval, erythematous, 2 to 10 cm. plaques which later become hyperpigmented. The eruption occurs in the same areas on readministration of the drug. It also occurs with *carisoprodol* (isopropyl meprobamate) [83] and occasionally with phenolphthalein, barbiturates, iodides, mercurials, acetylsalicylic acid, and quinine. *Other reactions* to meprobamate include purpuric, erythematous maculopapular, vesicular, or pustular skin rashes; urticaria or anaphylactoid reaction rarely; and aplastic anemia, thrombocytopenia, and agranulocytosis (due to antileukocyte antibody formation) rarely.

THALIDO-MIDE

Several thousand infants born of mothers who used *thalidomide* early in pregnancy (28th through 42nd days of gestation) were born with *phocomelia* (seal extremities) [84]. There was a failure of development of the long bones of one or more extremities. Embryonic death, increased abortions, or multiple congenital anomalies are produced experimentally by administering thalidomide in early pregnancy in animals [85].

11. Muscle Relaxants

ZOXAZOL-AMINE

Several cases of hepatic necrosis with a few deaths have occurred in patients on *zoxazolamine* [86].

12. Hypoglycemic Drugs

CHLORPROPAMIDE · TOLBUTAMIDE · PHENFORMIN

Chlorpropamide, a sulfonylurea, has been associated with hypoglycemic reactions in overdoses; cholestatic hepatitis with obstructive jaundice in a few cases; agranulocytosis [87] and thrombocytopenia (due to antiplatelet antibody formation) rarely; and a skin reaction in about 5 percent of patients (pruritus, maculopapular rash, photosensitivity eruption, or exfoliative dermatitis). Reactions to *tolbutamide,* also a sulfonylurea, include hypoglycemic reactions with overdoses, in elderly diabetics [88] and in patients being treated for Parkinson's disease [89]; aplastic anemia [90] and thrombocytopenia rarely; cholestatic hepatitis [91] rarely; goiter with hyperthyroidism due to the interference with the biosynthesis of thyroxine by the sulfonylureas; and photosensitivity dermatitis. In patients on *phenformin,* a biguanide, severe ketoacidosis or lactic acidosis may develop, especially in patients with chronic renal disease [92].

13. Diuretics

ACETAZOLAMIDE · CHLOROTHIAZIDE

Among patients on *acetazolamide,* a sulfonamide, agranulocytosis and thrombocytopenia (due to antiplatelet antibody formation) develop rarely. *Chlorothiazide,* an aromatic sulfonamide, may precipitate *thiazide diabetes* (the stimulation of latent diabetes or aggravation of existing diabetes mellitus) by an unknown mechanism [93]. There is a direct toxic effect on the pancreas in animals. A direct inhibition of islet cells and alteration of peripheral insulin by protein binding have been proposed as explanations of thiazide diabetes. Acute or chronic pancreatitis has occurred in a few patients taking chlorothiazide or *hydrochlorothiazide. Other reactions* to chlorothiazide include the production of impending hepatic coma in patients with cirrhosis by elevation of the blood ammonia level; cholestatic hepatitis rarely; acute gouty arthritis due to the development of hyperuricemia because of interference with the tubular secretion of uric acid [94]; agranulocytosis; and thrombocytopenic purpura (due to antiplatelet antibody formation) rarely. Thrombocytopenia has occurred in several newborn infants whose mothers used thiazides during pregnancy [95]. A pruritic lichen planus-like eruption and an erythematous photosensitivity dermatitis have developed in a few patients taking thiazides. Ulceration, stenosis, and perforation of the small intestine have occurred with *enteric coated potassium chloride combined with thiazides,* due to the local effects of high concentrations of potassium [96, 97]. The lesion develops in the middle and distal jejunum and ileum and is usually single. The serosa is thickened and depressed, especially on the antimesenteric region. There is a marked narrowing of the lumen in a segment 1 to 2.5 cm. long. An annular ulcer is often present in the stenotic segment. Microscopically the ulcer shows acute and chronic inflammation. The submucosa has undergone fibrous thickening, and submucosal hemorrhage is frequent. In the adjacent mesentery the arteries may show intimal thickening due to edema and fibroblastic proliferation, and the veins reveal medial fibromuscular hypertrophy. The vascular lumina are narrowed.

CHLORTHALIDONE · SPIRONOLACTONE

Among patients on *chlorthalidone,* agranulocytosis and pancytopenia have developed rarely and acute hemorrhagic pancreatitis has been reported. *Spironolactone,* an aldosterone blocking agent, may produce gynecomastia after prolonged use [98].

14. Antihypertensive, Antiserotonin, and Cholesterol-Inhibiting Drugs

HYDRALAZINE

PROCAINAMIDE

Several patients taking *hydralazine* have developed a *syndrome like lupus erythematosus* with widespread fibrinoid necrosis of collagen [99]. Similar changes have been induced by *procainamide,* a cardiac depressant [100]. Both drugs have been associated with the development of agranulocytosis rarely, with the formation of antileukocyte antibodies in patients on hydralazine. In a few persons taking *hexamethonium,* intra-alveolar interstitial pulmonary fibrosis has developed [101]. A few cases of hemolytic anemia have been reported in persons taking *methyldopa* [102].

METHYSERGIDE

A number of cases of *retroperitoneal fibrosis* have developed in patients on *methysergide,* an antiserotonin agent [103]. Early changes are a lymphocytic infiltration of retroperitoneal fat followed by a plasmocytic infiltration and fibroblastic proliferation. The walls of small retroperitoneal veins and arteries are infiltrated by lymphocytes, plasmocytes, and sometimes eosinophils. The vessels show intimal thickening and luminal narrowing or obliteration. A few cases of pulmonary, pleural, aortic, and cardiac valvular fibrosis have been reported in patients on methysergide.

TRIPARANOL

Several patients taking *triparanol* developed anterior capsular lenticular *cataracts* before use of this cholesterol-inhibiting drug was discontinued [104].

15. Vasopressor Agents

LEVARTERENOL

Ischemic necrosis of the small intestine and colon has occurred in patients in shock in whom *levarterenol or other vasopressor amine* has been used [105].

16. Drugs Used in Anemia Therapy

COBALTOUS SALTS

IRON-DEXTRAN

The use of *cobaltous salts* alone or with ferrous sulfate has led to the development of thyroid hyperplasia with hypothyroidism in several cases, due to the inhibition of enzymes involved in oxidation and binding of inorganic iodine by cobalt. Among patients using *iron-dextran complex* a few leukemoid reactions have occurred, and there have been occasional anaphylactoid reactions

17. Drugs Used in Hyperthyroidism Therapy

PROPYLTHIOURACIL

METHIMAZOLE

Reactions to *propylthiouracil* include agranulocytosis due to hypersensitivity with formation of antileukocyte antibodies rarely [106], hypoprothrombinemia occasionally [107], cholestatic hepatitis in a few cases, skin pigmentation, and alopecia. Patients taking *methimazole* have developed agranulocytosis and thrombocytopenia rarely and cholestatic hepatitis in a few cases.

18. Steroid Hormones

ADRENAL CORTICOSTEROIDS: Ocular effects

Activation of tuberculosis

A number of toxic reactions have been attributed to *adrenal corticosteroids.* Posterior subcapsular lenticular *cataract* develops in about 40 percent of patients with rheumatoid arthritis on long-term steroid therapy [108]. Few patients have severe visual impairment. Topical ophthalmic preparations containing corticosteroids may cause increased intraocular pressure with prolonged use and perforation of a cornea thinned by disease. The incidence of mycotic keratitis is increased by the use of such preparations. *Activation of latent or inactive tuberculous lesions* due to suppression of tuberculoprotein allergy and body defense mechanisms has frequently occurred in patients using corticosteroids. Epithelial proliferation in pulmonary alveoli and bronchioles with bronchiolar squamous metaplasia has occurred in several patients on cortisone therapy [109]. *Formation or reactivation of a peptic ulcer* of the stomach or duodenum has occurred many times [110]. *Acute pancreatitis* with peripancreatic fat necrosis also occurs in patients on steroid therapy [111].

Peptic ulcer

Endocrine effects include thyrotoxicosis rarely in patients on prolonged, high-dosage steroid therapy [112], and Cushing's syndrome, diabetes mellitus, osteoporosis with increased tendency to fracture, and hirsutism in women with long-term therapy. Aseptic necrosis of the femoral head due to retardation of the normal repair of wear and tear has occurred [113], and a Charcot-like arthropathy has developed following intra-articular steroid injections. *Pseudotumor cerebri,* with headache, nausea, vomiting, and papilledema, has appeared in patients on prolonged steroid therapy [114]. Agranulocytosis due to antileukocyte antibody formation has rarely occurred with the use of dexamethasone. *Severe infections* caused by fungi, protozoa, bacteria, and viruses, due to the suppression of antigen-antibody responses, anti-inflammatory effects, and delayed wound healing have frequently occurred in patients on steroid therapy, and widespread hematogenous dissemination is common in such cases. Many of the untoward effects associated with corticosteroids may also be produced by the use of *adrenocorticotropic hormone (ACTH).*

Endocrine effects

Infections

NOR-ETHYNODREL

Among women using *norethynodrel alone or in combination with methyl ethinyl estradiol (mestranol),* numerous cases of *thromboembolism* have been reported with pulmonary embolism in about 25 percent and death in less than 10 percent [115, 116]. About half these patients had predisposing lesions for thrombosis. Distinctive lesions have been found in arteries and veins in which thrombosis has occurred [117]. There are endothelial hyperplasia with the formation of papillary projections and fibrous intimal thickening in small pulmonary arteries.

The increased risk of thromboembolism in women taking oral contraceptives is evidently due to the estrogens in them. Platelet reactivity to adenosine diphosphate is enhanced by the administration of estrogens [117a]. The increased tendency to thrombosis also appears to be related to decreased fibrinolysis. Decreased antithrombin III activity and elevated plasminogen levels, which have been correlated with decreased fibrinolysis, have been found in women taking oral contraceptives [117b].

Two types of *change* have been described *in the uterine cervix* of women on antiovulants [117c]. These are squamous metaplasia of the endocervical mucosa and hyperplasia of the endocervical glands. Atypical squamous and columnar cervical cells are found by exfoliative cytology in a small number of women on estrogen-progestogen compounds [117d]. A pseudodecidual reaction occurs in the endometrium of women using the oral contraceptive *norethynodrel.* Sometimes marked *lobular hyperplasia* occurs in the breasts of some women on oral contraceptives. The question as to the possible relationship of the use of antiovulants to the development of mammary carcinoma remains unanswered [117e]. There is an increased incidence of *vulvovaginitis* due to *Candida albicans* in women using norethynodrel with mestranol [118]. A number of *ocular changes* have been reported in women taking norethynodrel and/or norethindrone [119]. These include central retinal vein thrombosis, thrombosis of several retinal arterial branches, posterior cyclitis with papilledema, optic neuritis, and retrobulbar neuritis. *Skin lesions* which develop include chloasma (hyperpigmentation of the forehead and cheeks) [119a], photosensitivity [119b], and alopecia (falling out of the hair) during the use of or after the discontinuance of oral contraceptives [119c].

NOR-ETHIN-DRONE

When *norethindrone* is used during the 10th to 16th weeks of pregnancy, *masculinization of female fetuses* with clitoral hypertrophy and partial fusion of the labia has been produced. Cholestatic jaundice has occurred in a few women using norethindrone in combinations [120]. Liver biopsies have shown bile thrombi in centrolobular canaliculi. With electron microscopy these canaliculi are dilated and have a few small microvilli.

ANDRO-GENS

Norethandrolone [121], *methyltestosterone, and methandrostenolone* sometimes produce *intrahepatic cholestasis.* In such cases the bile canaliculi are dilated and contain bile thrombi. Bile pigment is present within hepatocytes and Kupffer cells. Centrolobular hepatocytes may show degenerative changes.

19. Cancer Chemotherapeutic Drugs

ALKYLAT-ING AGENTS

The *polyfunctional alkylating agents* include methyl bis (β-chloroethyl) amine, chlorambucil, cyclophosphamide, triethylene melamine, triethylene thiophosphoramide, and busulfan. These compounds inhibit cell division and seriously damage dividing cells. The most severe toxic effect is *bone marrow depression* with leukopenia or agranulocytosis and thrombocytopenia. This occurs frequently, especially with high doses. *Alopecia* occurs in about 25 percent of patients on cyclophosphamide.

ANTI-METABO-LITES

The *antimetabolites* temporarily block the anabolic pathway for nucleic acid synthesis. The *folic acid antagonists* are 4-aminopteroyl glutamic acid and 4-amino-10-N-methylpteroyl glutamic acid. These cause bone marrow depression with leukopenia or agranulocytosis and thrombocytopenia frequently, megaloblastosis of the bone marrow due to interference with folic acid metabolism, oral and gastrointestinal ulcers frequently, and extensive hepatic fibrosis occasionally in children [122]. *6-Mercaptopurine* produces bone marrow depression in high doses, and several cases of hepatic necrosis have resulted from its use [123]. *5-Fluorouracil* produces bone marrow depression with leukopenia or agranulocytosis and thrombocytopenia after 8 to 10 days, stomatitis with ulcers frequently, and alopecia in up to 30 percent of the cases. *Vincaleukoblastine* causes bone marrow depression, with granulocytopenia typically more marked than thrombocytopenia; stomatitis in about 5 percent of cases; and alopecia in about 2.5 percent. Experimentally, increased fetal mortality and multiple congenital malformations are produced by its administration in early pregnancy in animals [124].

RADIO-ACTIVE ISOTOPES

Bone marrow depression occurs with the use of the *radioactive isotopes* iodine-131 (^{131}I), phosphorus-32, and gold-198, and myxedema and renal damage are produced by ^{131}I.

OTHER AGENTS

Urethane produces bone marrow depression, as does *desacetylmethylcolchicine,* which also is sometimes associated with alopecia. *Actinomycin D* causes a bone marrow depression in which thrombocytopenia is more marked than granulocytopenia, alopecia, stomatitis, and dermatitis in previously irradiated areas. *Mitomycin C* produces severe bone marrow depression with leukopenia or agranulocytosis and thrombocytopenia.

20. Types of Drug Reactions

Hemolytic anemia

Primaquine-type, associated with a deficiency of glucose-6-phosphate dehydrogenase in erythrocytes

- Primaquine
- Pamaquine
- Sulfanilamide
- Sulfapyridine
- Sulfisoxazole
- Sulfamethoxypyridazine
- Nitrofurantoin
- Acetylsalicylic acid
- Acetophenetidin
- Menadione
- Phenylhydrazine

Penicillin
Quinine
Quinidine
Stibophen
Methylphenylethyl hydantoin
Methyldopa

Aplastic anemia

Numerous cases

- Chloramphenicol
- Phenylbutazone
- Benzene
- Nitrogen mustards

Occasional or rare cases

- Sulfamethoxypyridazine
- Sulfisoxazole
- Other sulfonamides
- Ristocetin
- Streptomycin
- Quinacrine
- Quinidine
- Aminopyrine
- Diphenylhydantoin
- Methylphenylethyl hydantoin
- Trimethadione
- Chlorpromazine
- Promazine
- Trifluopromazine
- Prochlorperazine
- Mepazine
- Tolbutamide
- Promethazine
- Tripellennamine
- Methimazole
- Potassium chlorate
- Gold salts

Agranulocytosis

Numerous cases

- Polyfunctional alkylating agents (nitrogen mustards, triethylene melamine, thio TEPA)
- Antimetabolites
- Urethane
- *Sulfadiazine
- *Aminopyrine

Occasional or rare cases

- Sulfisoxazole
- Sulfamethoxypyridazine
- *Sulfathiazole
- *Sulfapyridine
- Amodiaquine
- Phenylbutazone
- Oxyphenbutazone
- *Gold salts
- *Chlordiazepoxide
- Imipramine
- *Meprobamate
- Tripelennamine
- Chlorpropamide
- Acetazolamide
- Chlorothiazide
- Hydrochlorothiazide
- Chlorthalidone
- Diphenylhydantoin

*Cause of immunoleukopenia due to development of antileukocyte antibodies [125].

Agranulocytosis, Occasional or rare cases (Cont.)

- Methylphenylethyl hydantoin
- Trimethadione
- Chlorpromazine
- Promazine
- Trifluopromazine
- Mepazine
- Thioridazine
- *Hydralazine
- Procainamide
- *Tolazoline
- Potassium chlorate
- *Propylthiouracil
- Methimazole
- *Dexamethasone
- Actinomycin D
- Penicillamine

Thrombocytopenia

Numerous cases

- †Quinidine
- Polyfunctional alkylating agents
- Antimetabolites
- Urethane

Occasional or rare cases

- †Sulfamethoxypyridazine
- †Sulfisoxazole
- Streptomycin
- Chloramphenicol
- †Quinine
- Phenylbutazone
- Oxyphenbutazone
- Methylphenylethyl hydantoin
- Phenylacetylurea
- Meprobamate
- †Chlorpropamide
- Tolbutamide
- †Acetazolamide
- †Chlorothiazide
- †Hydrochlorothiazide
- Methimazole
- †Diphenhydramine
- †Chlorpheniramine
- Actinomycin D
- Mitomycin C

Cholestatic hepatitis [126, 127]

Numerous cases

- Sulfonamides
- Erythromycin estolate
- Triacetyloleandomycin
- Chlorpromazine
- Norethandrolone

Occasional or rare cases

- *p*-Aminosalicylic acid
- Carbarsone
- Promazine
- Mepazine
- Prochlorperazine
- Trifluoperazine
- Imipramine
- Ectylurea
- Chlorpropamide
- Tolbutamide
- Chlorothiazide
- Propylthiouracil
- Methimazole
- Methyl testosterone

Hepatic necrosis [126, 127]

Numerous cases

- Iproniazid
- Pyrazinamide
- Carbon tetrachloride

*Cause of immunoleukopenia due to development of antileukocyte antibodies [125].

†Cause of immunothrombocytopenia due to formation of antiplatelet antibodies [125].

Occasional or rare cases	
Sulfonamides	Halothane
Isoniazid	Chlorpromazine
Quinacrine	Zoxazolamine
Phenylacetylurea	Cincophen
Diphenylhydantoin	6-Mercaptopurine

Anaphylactic or anaphylactoid reactions [128]

Numerous cases	
Penicillin	Thiamine
Vaccines, antitoxins, toxoids	Mercurial diuretics
Occasional cases with fatalities	
Acetylsalicylic acid	Cortisone
Trimethadione	ACTH
Occasional or rare nonfatal cases	
Sulfonamides	Probenecid
Chlortetracycline	Amodiaquine
Demethylchlortetracycline	Meperidine
Vancomycin	Meprobamate
Novobiocin	Diphenhydramine
Nitrofurantoin	Iron dextran
Streptomycin	Chymotrypsin
p-Aminosalicylic acid	Cincophen

Photosensitivity reactions [129]

Sulfonamides	Mepazine
Demethylchlortetracycline (PT)	Promethazine
Griseofulvin	Chlorpropamide (PT)
Chlorpromazine (PT, PA)	Tolbutamide (PT)
Promazine	Chlorothiazide (PT, PA)
Prochlorperazine	Hydrochlorothiazide (PT, PA)

Phototoxicity (PT) may occur with the first exposure to the drug and involves a high percentage of patients using it. The skin reaction is characterized by erythema and hyperpigmentation.

Photoallergic response (PA) requires previous exposure to the drug and involves only a small percentage of patients taking it. The skin reactions include erythema, urticaria, papular rash, and eczema.

REFERENCES

1. Nash, G., Blennerhassett, J. B., and Pontoppidan, H. Pulmonary lesions associated with oxygen therapy and artificial ventilation. *New Eng. J. Med.* 276:368, 1967.

1a. Balentine, J. D. Pathologic effects of exposure to high oxygen tensions. *New Eng. J. Med.* 275:1038, 1966.

2. Rowan, T., and Coleman, F. C. Carbon monoxide poisoning. *J. Forensic Sci.* 7:103, 1962.

2a. Adelson, L., and Sunshine, I. Fatal hydrogen sulfide intoxication. *Arch. Path.* (Chicago) 81:375, 1966.

3. Delaney, L. T., Jr., Schmidt, H. W., and Stroebel, C. F. Silo-filler's disease. *Proc. Mayo Clin.* 31:189, 1956.

3a. Penneys, N. S., Israel, R. M., and Indgin, S. M. Contact dermatitis due to l-chloroacetophenone and chemical mace. *New Eng. J. Med.* 281:413, 1969.
4. Beaver, D. L., and Burr, R. E. Bismuth inclusions in the human kidney. *Arch. Path.* (Chicago) 76:89, 1963.
5. Hass, G. M., Brown, D. V. L., Eisenstein, R., and Hemmens, A. Relations between lead poisoning in rabbit and man. *Amer. J. Path.* 45:691, 1964.
6. Beaver, D. L. The ultrastructure of the kidney in lead intoxication with particular reference to intranuclear inclusions. *Amer. J. Path.* 39:195, 1961.
7. Galambos, J. T., and Dowda, F. W. Lead poisoning and porphyria. *Amer. J. Med.* 27:803, 1959.
8. Reuber, M. D., and Bradley, J. E. Acute versenate nephrosis. *J.A.M.A.* 174:263, 1960.
9. Sunderman, F. W., Range, C. L., Sunderman, F. W., Jr., Donnelly, A. J., and Lucyszyn, G. W. Nickel poisoning. XII. Metabolic and pathologic changes in acute pneumonitis from nickel carbonyl. *Amer. J. Clin. Path.* 36:477, 1961.
10. Reed, D., Crawley, J., Faro, S. N., Pieper, S. J., and Kurland, L. T. Thallotoxicosis. *J.A.M.A.* 183:516, 1963.
11. Elton, N. W., Elton, W. J., and Nazareno, J. P. Pathology of acute salt poisoning in infants. *Amer. J. Clin. Path.* 39:252, 1963.
12. Arterberry, J. D., Bonifaci, R. W., Nash, E. W., and Quinby, G. E. Potentiation of phosphorus insecticides by phenothiazine derivatives. *J.A.M.A.* 182:848, 1962.
13. Petty, C. S. Histochemical proof of organic phosphate poisoning. *A.M.A. Arch. Path.* 66:458, 1958.
14. Ransone, J. W., Scott, N. M., Jr., and Knoblock, E. C. Selenium sulfide intoxication. *New Eng. J. Med.* 264:384, 1961.
15. Di Luzio, N. R. A mechanism of the acute ethanol-induced fatty liver and the modification of liver injury by antioxidants. *Lab. Invest.* 15:50, 1966.
16. McCurdy, P. R., Pierce, L. E., and Rath, C. E. Abnormal bone-marrow morphology in acute alcoholism. *New Eng. J. Med.* 266:505, 1962.
17. Durlacher, S. H., Meier, J. R., Fisher, R. S., and Lovitt, W. V., Jr. Sudden death due to pulmonary fat embolism in chronic alcoholics with fatty livers. *J. Forensic Sci.* 4:215, 1959.
18. Lynch, M. J. G. Brain lesions in chronic alcoholism. *A.M.A. Arch. Path.* 69:342, 1960.
19. Adelson, L. Fatal intoxication with isopropyl alcohol (rubbing alcohol). *Amer. J. Clin. Path.* 38:144, 1962.
20. Bove, K. E. Ethylene glycol toxicity. *Amer. J. Clin. Path.* 45:46, 1966.
21. Smith, D. E. Morphological lesions due to acute and subacute poisoning with antifreeze (ethylene glycol). *A.M.A. Arch. Path.* 51:423, 1951.
22. Jennings, R. B. Fatal fulminant acute carbon tetrachloride poisoning. *A.M.A. Arch. Path.* 59:269, 1955.
23. Recknagel, R. O., and Ghoshal, A. K. Lipoperoxidation as a vector in carbon tetrachloride hepatotoxicity. *Lab. Invest.* 15:132, 1966.
24. Umiker, W., and Pearce, J. Nature and genesis of pulmonary alterations in carbon tetrachloride poisoning. *A.M.A. Arch. Path.* 55:203, 1953.
25. Glaser, H. H., and Massengale, O. N. Glue-sniffing. Deliberate inhalation of vaporized plastic cements. *J.A.M.A.* 181:300, 1962.
25a. Ryley, T., Malcolm, A., Sereny, G., Smart, R., and Weiler, R. Glue-sniffing may alter chromosomes. *J.A.M.A.* 207:1441, 1969.
26. Bergmann, M., Flance, J., Cruz, P. T., Klam, N., Aronson, P. R., Joshi, R. A., and Blumenthal, H. T. Thesaurosis due to inhalation of hair spray. *New Eng. J. Med.* 266:750, 1962.

27. Lewis, C. E., and Kerby, G. R. An epidemic of polymer-fume fever. *J.A.M.A.* 191:375, 1965.
28. Dobos, J. K., Phillips, J., and Covo, G. A. Acute barbiturate intoxication. *J.A.M.A.* 176:268, 1961.
29. Wear, J. B., Jr., Shanahan, R., and Ratliff, R. K. Toxicity of ingested hexachlorophene. *J.A.M.A.* 181:587, 1962.
30. Potter, H. P., Jr., Cohen, N. N., and Norris, R. F. Chronic hepatic dysfunction in heroin addicts. *J.A.M.A.* 174:2049, 1960.
31. Hartmann, A. F., Sr., Hartmann, A. F., Jr., Purkerson, M. L., and Wesley, M. E. Tremetol poisoning – not yet extinct. *J.A.M.A.* 185:706, 1963.
32. Payne, R. B. Nutmeg intoxication. *New Eng. J. Med.* 269:36, 1963.
33. Derbes, V. J., Dent, J. H., Forrest, W. W., and Johnson, M. F. Fatal chlordane poisoning. *J.A.M.A.* 158:1367, 1955.
34. Weinstein, L., Madoff, M. A., and Samet, C. M. The sulfonamides. *New Eng. J. Med.* 263:952, 1960.
35. Van Arsdel, P. P., Jr., O'Rourke, T. K., Horan, J. D., and Kumasaka, Y. Serum hemagglutinating antibodies in penicillin allergy. *J.A.M.A.* 185:584, 1963.
36. Petz, L. D., and Fudenberg, H. H. Coombs-positive hemolytic anemia caused by penicillin administration. *New Eng. J. Med.* 274:171, 1966.
36a. Baldwin, D. S., Levine, B. B., McCluskey, R. T., and Gallo, G. R. Renal failure and interstitial nephritis due to penicillin and methcillin. *New Eng. J. Med.* 279:1245, 1968.
37. Witkop, C. J., Jr., and Wolf, R. O. Hypoplasia and intrinsic staining of enamel following tetracycline therapy. *J.A.M.A.* 185:1008, 1963.
38. Kline, A. H., Blattner, R. J., and Lunin, M. Transplacental effect of tetracyclines on teeth. *J.A.M.A.* 188:178, 1964.
39. Schultz, J. C., Adamson, J. S., Jr., Workman, W. W., and Norman, T. D. Fatal liver disease after intravenous administration of tetracycline in high dosage. *New Eng. J. Med.* 269:999, 1963.
40. Mavromatis, F. Tetracycline nephropathy. *J.A.M.A.* 193:191, 1965.
41. Sulkowski, S. R., and Haserick, J. R. Simulated systemic lupus erythematosus from degraded tetracycline. *J.A.M.A.* 189:152, 1964.
42. Saslaw, S. Demethylchlortetracycline phototoxicity. *New Eng. J. Med.* 264:1301, 1961.
43. McCurdy, P. R. Chloramphenicol bone marrow toxicity. *J.A.M.A.* 176:588, 1961.
44. Gilbert, F. I., Jr. Cholestatic hepatitis caused by esters of erythromycin and oleandomycin. *J.A.M.A.* 182:1048, 1962.
45. Ticktin, H. E., and Zimmerman, H. J. Hepatic dysfunction and jaundice in patients receiving triacetyloleandomycin. *New Eng. J. Med.* 267:964, 1962.
46. Jacobson, E. D., and Faloon, W. W. Malabsorptive effects of neomycin in commonly used doses. *J.A.M.A.* 175:187, 1961.
47. Greenberg, L. H., and Momary, H. Audiotoxicity and nephrotoxicity due to orally administered neomycin. *J.A.M.A.* 194:827, 1965.
48. Robinson, B. R. Pleuropulmonary reaction to nitrofurantoin. *J.A.M.A.* 189:239, 1964.
49. Pritchard, J. A., Scott, D. E., and Mason, R. A. Severe anemia with hemolysis and megaloblastic erythropoiesis. *J.A.M.A.* 194:457, 1966.
50. Rubinstein, C. J. Peripheral polyneuropathy caused by nitrofurantoin. *J.A.M.A.* 187:647, 1964.
51. Costa, G., Holland, J. F., and Pickren, J. W. Acute pericarditis produced by psicofuranine, a nucleoside analogue. *New Eng. J. Med.* 265:1143, 1961.

52. Heck, W. E., Hinshaw, H. C., and Parsons, H. G. Auditory ototoxicity in tuberculosis patients treated with dihydrostreptomycin. *J.A.M.A.* 186:18, 1963.
53. Robinson, G. C., and Cambon, K. G. Hearing loss in infants of tuberculous mothers treated with streptomycin during pregnancy. *New Eng. J. Med.* 271:949, 1964.
54. Cohen, R., Kalser, M. H., and Thomson, R. V. Fatal hepatic necrosis secondary to isoniazid therapy. *J.A.M.A.* 176:877, 1961.
55. Wertlake, P. T., Butler, W. T., Hill, G. J., and Utz, J. P. Nephrotoxic tubular damage and calcium deposition following amphotericin B therapy. *Amer. J. Path.* 43:449, 1963.
56. Brandriss, M. W., Wolff, S. M., Moores, R., and Stohlman, F., Jr. Anemia induced by amphotericin B. *J.A.M.A.* 189:663, 1964.
57. Cheng, T. S. Cold urticaria and photosensitivity due to griseofulvin. *J.A.M.A.* 193:848, 1965.
58. Bernstein, H. N., and Ginsberg, J. The pathology of chloroquine retinopathy. *Arch. Ophthal.* (Chicago) 71:238, 1964.
58a. Cohen, R. J., Sachs, J. R., Wicker, D. J., and Conrad, M. E. Methemoglobinemia provoked by malarial chemoprophylaxis in Vietnam. *New Eng. J. Med.* 279:1127, 1968.
59. Kellermeyer, R. W., Tarlov, A. R., Brewer, G. J., Carson, P. E., and Alving, A. S. Hemolytic effect of therapeutic drugs. Clinical considerations of the primaquine-type hemolysis. *J.A.M.A.* 180:388, 1962.
60. Maisel, J. C., and Priest, R. E. Fatal phenacetin nephritis. *Arch. Path.* (Chicago) 77:646, 1964.
61. Reynolds, T. B., and Edmondson, H. A. Chronic renal disease and heavy use of analgesics. *J.A.M.A.* 184:435, 1963.
62. Richardson, J. H., and Alderfer, H. H. Acute renal failure caused by phenylbutazone. *New Eng. J. Med.* 268:809, 1963.
63. Greenberg, M. S., and Wong, H. Methemoglobinemia and Heinz body hemolytic anemia due to phenazopyridine hydrochloride. *New Eng. J. Med.* 271:431, 1964.
64. Ramon, Y., Ziprkowski, L., and Goldring, D. Pyrininophilic bodies in the gingivae. *Amer. J. Clin. Path.* 38:507, 1962.
65. Saltzstein, S. L., and Ackerman, L. V. Lymphadenopathy induced by anticonvulsant drugs and mimicking clinically and pathologically malignant lymphomas. *Cancer* 12:164, 1959.
66. Robinson, D. S., MacDonald, M. G., and Hobin, F. P. Sodium diphenylhydantoin reaction with evidence of circulating antibodies. *J.A.M.A.* 192:171, 1965.
67. Sinks, L. F., Parker, E. C., and Boulware, J. R. Trimethadione nephrosis. *Amer. J. Dis. Child.* 105:196, 1963.
68. Pfaff, J., Jr., and Forbeck, D. L. Toxicity associated with Phenurone. *J. Forensic Sci.* 6:134, 1961.
69. Lindenbaum, J., and Leifer, E. Hepatic necrosis associated with halothane anesthesia. *New Eng. J. Med.* 268:525, 1963.
70. Cohen, E. N., Bellville, J. W., Budzikiewicz, H., and Williams, D. H. Impurity in halothane anesthetics. *Science* 141:899, 1963.
71. Scime, I. A., and Tallant, E. J. Tetanus-like reactions to prochlorperazine (Compazine). *J.A.M.A.* 171:1813, 1959.
72. Lindsay, S., and Skahen, R. Jaundice during chlorpromazine (Thorazine) therapy. *A.M.A. Arch. Path.* 61:84, 1956.
73. McFarland, R. B. Fatal drug reaction associated with prochlorperazine (Compazine). *Amer. J. Clin. Path.* 40:284, 1963.

74. Hooper, J. H., Jr., Welch, V. C., and Shackelford, R. T. Abnormal lactation associated with tranquilizing drug therapy. *J.A.M.A.* 178:506, 1961.
75. Satanove, A. Pigmentation due to phenothiazines in high and prolonged dosage. *J.A.M.A.* 191:263, 1965.
76. Barsa, J. A., Newton, J. C., and Saunders, J. C. Lenticular and corneal opacities during phenothiazine therapy. *J.A.M.A.* 193:10, 1965.
77. Arterberry, J. D., Bonifaci, R. W., Nash, E. W., and Quinby, G. E. Potentiation of phosphorus insecticides by phenothiazine derivatives. *J.A.M.A.* 182:848, 1962.
78. Richardson, H. L., Graupner, K. I., and Richardson, M. E. Intramyocardial lesions in patients dying suddenly and unexpectedly. *J.A.M.A.* 195:254, 1966.
79. Whitelaw, M. J. Menstrual irregularities associated with use of methaminodiazepoxide. *J.A.M.A.* 175:400, 1961.
80. Solberg, C. O. Phenelzine intoxication. *J.A.M.A.* 177:572, 1961.
81. Horwitz, D., Lovenberg, W., Engelman, K., and Sjoerdsma, A. Monoamine oxidase inhibitors, tyramine, and cheese. *J.A.M.A.* 188:1108, 1964.
82. Brandt, C., and Hoffbauer, F. W. Liver injury associated with tranylcypromine therapy. *J.A.M.A.* 188:752, 1964.
83. Honeycutt, W. M., and Curtis, A. C. Fixed drug eruption to carisoprodol and cross reaction to meprobamate. *J.A.M.A.* 180:691, 1962.
84. Taussig, H. B. A study of the German outbreak of phocomelia. The thalidomide syndrome. *J.A.M.A.* 180:1106, 1962.
85. DiPaolo, J. A. Congenital malformation in strain A mice. Its experimental production by thalidomide. *J.A.M.A.* 183:139, 1963.
86. Eisenstadt, H. B., and Elster, B. B. Zoxazolamine hepatitis. *J.A.M.A.* 176:847, 1961.
87. Stein, J. H., Hamilton, H. E., and Sheets, R. F. Agranulocytosis caused by chlorpropamide. *Arch. Intern. Med.* (Chicago) 113:186, 1964.
88. Gardner, P., Goodner, C. J., and Dowling, J. T. Severe hypoglycemia in elderly patients receiving therapeutic doses of tolbutamide. *J.A.M.A.* 186:991, 1963.
89. Cherner, R., Groppe, C. W., Jr., and Rupp, J. J. Prolonged tolbutamide-induced hypoglycemia. *J.A.M.A.* 185:883, 1963.
90. Chapman, I., and Cheung, W. H. Pancytopenia associated with tolbutamide therapy. *J.A.M.A.* 186:595, 1963.
91. McMahon, T. F. Cholestatic jaundice, liver decompensation, and shock resulting from tolbutamide. *Med. Ann. D. C.* 32:509, 1963.
92. Tranquada, R. E., Bernstein, S., and Martin, H. E. Irreversible lactic acidosis associated with phenformin therapy. *J.A.M.A.* 184:37, 1963.
93. Wolff, F. W., Parmley, W. W., White, K., and Okun, R. Drug-induced diabetes. Diabetogenic activity of long-term administration of benzothiadiazines. *J.A.M.A.* 185:568, 1963.
94. Aronoff, A. Acute gouty arthritis precipitated by chlorothiazide. *New Eng. J. Med.* 262:767, 1960.
95. Rodriguez, S. U., Leikin, S. L., and Hiller, M. C. Neonatal thrombocytopenia associated with ante-partum administration of thiazide drugs. *New Eng. J. Med.* 270:881, 1964.
96. Allen, A. C., Boley, S. J., Schultz, L., and Schwartz, S. Potassium-induced lesions of the small bowel. II. Pathology and pathogenesis. *J.A.M.A.* 193:1001, 1965.
97. Boley, S. J., Schultz, L., Krieger, H., Schwartz, S., Elguezabal, A., and Allen, A. C. Experimental evaluation of thiazides and potassium as a cause of small-bowel ulcer. *J.A.M.A.* 192:763, 1965.

98. Mann, N. M. Gynecomastia during therapy with spironolactone. *J.A.M.A.* 184:778, 1963.
99. Heine, W. I., and Friedman, H. Hydralazine lupus syndrome associated with a possible antihydralazine antibody. *J.A.M.A.* 182:726, 1962.
100. Kaplan, J. M., Wachtel, H. L., Czarnecki, S. W., and Sampson, J. J. Lupus-like illness precipitated by procainamide hydrochloride. *J.A.M.A.* 192:444, 1965.
101. Doniach, I., Morrison, B., and Steiner, R. E. Lung changes during hexamethonium therapy for hypertension. *Brit. Heart J.* 16:101, 1954.
102. Cahal, D. A. Methyldopa and haemolytic anemia (Letter to the Editor). *Lancet* 1:201, 1966.
103. Graham, J. R., Suby, H. I., LeCompte, P. R., and Sadowsky, N. L. Fibrotic disorders associated with methysergide therapy for headache. *New Eng. J. Med.* 274:360, 1966.
104. Laughlin, R. C., and Carey, T. F. Cataracts in patients treated with triparanol. *J.A.M.A.* 181:339, 1962.
105. Haber, M. H., Brown, W. T., and Schneider, K. A. Ischemic necrosis of multiple organs in prolonged shock. *J.A.M.A.* 183:1107, 1963.
106. Walzer, R. A., and Einbinder, J. Immunoleukopenia as an aspect of hypersensitivity to propylthiouracil. *J.A.M.A.* 184:743, 1963.
107. Gilbert, D. K. Hypoprothrombinemia as a complication of propylthiouracil. *J.A.M.A.* 189:855, 1964.
108. Black, R. L., Oglesby, R. B., von Sallmann, L., and Bunim, J. J. Posterior subcapsular cataracts induced by corticosteroids in patients with rheumatoid arthritis. *J.A.M.A.* 174:166, 1960.
109. Berkheiser, S. W. Epithelial proliferation of the lung associated with cortisone administration. *Cancer* 16:1354, 1963.
110. Robert, A., and Nezamis, J. E. Histopathology of steroid-induced ulcers. An experimental study in the rat. *Arch. Path.* (Chicago) 77:407, 1964.
111. Schreier, R. W., and Bulger, R. J. Steroid-induced pancreatitis. *J.A.M.A.* 194:564, 1965.
112. Brown, D. M., and Lowman, J. T. Thyrotoxicosis occurring in two patients on prolonged high doses of steroids. *New Eng. J. Med.* 270:278, 1964.
113. Boksenbaum, M., and Mendelson, C. G. Aseptic necrosis of the femoral head associated with steroid therapy. *J.A.M.A.* 184:262, 1963.
114. Walker, A. E., and Adamkiewicz, J. J. Pseudotumor cerebri associated with prolonged corticosteroid therapy. *J.A.M.A.* 188:779, 1964.
115. Reed, D. L., and Coon, W. W. Thromboembolism in patients receiving progestational drugs. *New Eng. J. Med.* 269:622, 1963.
116. Schatz, I. J., Smith, R. F., Breneman, G. M., and Bower, G. C. Thromboembolic disease associated with norethynodrel. *J.A.M.A.* 188:493, 1964.
117. Irey, N. S., Manion, W. C., and Taylor, H. B. Vascular lesions in women taking oral contraceptives. *Arch. Path.* (Chicago) 89:1, 1970.
117a. Elkeles, R. S., Hampton, J. R., and Mitchell, J. R. A. Effect of estrogens on human platelet behavior. *Lancet* 2:315, 1968.
117b. Peterson, R. A., Krull, P. E., Finley, P., and Ettinger, M. G. Changes in antithrombin III and plasminogen induced by oral contraceptives. *Amer. J. Clin. Path.* 53:468, 1970.
117c. Kyriakos, M., Kempson, R. I., and Konikov, N. F. A clinical and pathologic study of endocervical lesions associated with oral contraceptives. *Cancer* 22:99, 1968.
117d. Kline, T. S., Holland, M., and Wemple, D. Atypical cytology with contraceptive hormone medication. *Amer. J. Clin. Path.* 53:215, 1970.

117e. Hertz, R. The problem of possible effects of oral contraceptives on cancer of the breast. *Cancer* 24:1140, 1969.
118. Porter, P. S., and Lyle, J. S. Yeast vulvovaginitis due to oral contraceptives. *Arch. Derm.* (Chicago) 93:402, 1966.
119. Walsh, F. B., Clark, D. B., Thompson, R. S., and Nicholson, D. H. Oral contraceptives and neuro-ophthalmologic interest. *Arch. Ophthal.* (Chicago) 74:628, 1965.
119a. Resnik, S. Melasma induced by oral contraceptive drugs. *J.A.M.A.* 199:601, 1967.
119b. Erickson, L. R., and Peterka, E. S. Sunlight sensitivity from oral contraceptives. *J.A.M.A.* 203:980, 1968.
119c. Cormia, F. E. Alopecia from oral contraceptives. *J.A.M.A.* 201:635, 1967.
120. Larsson-Cohn, U., and Stenram, U. Jaundice during treatment with oral contraceptive agents. *J.A.M.A.* 193:422, 1965.
121. Gilbert, E. F., DaSilva, A. Q., and Queen, D. M. Intrahepatic cholestasis with fatal termination following norethandrolone therapy. *J.A.M.A.* 185:538, 1963.
122. Hutter, R. V. P., Shipkey, F. H., Tan, C. T. C., Murphy, M. L., and Chowdhury, M. Hepatic fibrosis in children with leukemia. A complication of therapy. *Cancer* 13:288, 1960.
123. Einhorn, M., and Davidsohn, I. Hepatotoxicity of mercaptopurine. *J.A.M.A.* 188:802, 1964.
124. Ferm, V. H. Congenital malformations in hamster embryos after treatment with vinblastine and vincristine. *Science* 141:426, 1963.
125. Tullis, J. L. Leukocyte and thrombocyte antibodies. *J.A.M.A.* 180:958, 1962.
126. Popper, H., and Schaffner, F. Drug-induced hepatic injury. *Ann. Intern. Med.* 51:1230, 1959.
127. Schaffner, F. Iatrogenic jaundice. *J.A.M.A.* 174:1690, 1960.
128. Kern, R. A. Anaphylactic drug reactions. *J.A.M.A.* 179:19, 1962.
129. Sams, W. M. Photosensitizing therapeutic agents. *J.A.M.A.* 174:2043, 1960.

GENERAL REFERENCES

Gonzales, T. A., Vance, M., Helpern, M., and Umberger, C. J. *Legal Medicine: Pathology and Toxicology* (2d ed.). New York: Appleton-Century-Crofts, 1954, pp. 690–902. (An expert presentation of the pathologic aspects of poisoning.)

Camps, F. E. (Ed.) *Gradwohl's Legal Medicine* (2d ed.). Baltimore: Williams & Wilkins, 1968, pp. 553–689. (An authoritative and well-illustrated discussion of the legal and medical aspects of poisons.)

11 DISTURBANCES OF PIGMENT METABOLISM

IRON AND HEMOGLOBIN METABOLISM [1]

IRON METABOLISM

Of the usual daily intake of about 15 mg. of iron, only about 1.5 mg. is absorbed, almost entirely in the duodenum. The *mechanism of iron absorption* is incompletely understood, but there appears to be a *mucosal block* which limits the amount absorbed to the amount needed by the body. Iron is absorbed in its ferrous state. In the duodenal mucosal cells some iron is oxidized to the ferric form and combines with a protein, apoferritin, to form *ferritin.* Other iron enters the bloodstream in its reduced ferrous state. It combines with a β_1-globulin, siderophilin or transferrin, again changing to the ferric form. The normal *serum iron level* is 50 to 180 mcg. (micrograms) per 100 ml. of blood, and the serum iron binding capacity is 300 to 360 mcg. per 100 ml. The *total body iron* is 4 to 5 gm. Excess iron above that incorporated into hemoglobin and present unbound in the plasma is stored in the tissues as ferritin. About 0.5 gm. is deposited in the liver. As iron is needed, it is returned to the bloodstream. About 1 mg. of iron is lost daily in shed epithelial cells containing the mineral. In women iron is excreted in menstrual blood (about 300 mg. annually) and in milk. Otherwise the human body has no normal route for the excretion of iron.

HEMOGLOBIN METABOLISM

Hemoglobin is the oxygen-bearing component of erythrocytes. It contains 0.335 percent iron; its molecular weight is about 68,000. Hemoglobin is a combination of a pigment complex (heme) and a protein (globin), heme being a ferrous complex of protoporphyrin IX. There are four molecules of heme to one of globin. Porphyrins are the basic respiratory pigments of most living forms. In the adult male the *normal hemoglobin content* of whole blood is 13 to 16 gm. per 100 ml.; in women it is 12 to 14 gm. Normally there is 2 to 5 mg. of hemoglobin per 100 ml. of plasma, and the level may reach 200 to 500 mg. per 100 ml. in severe hemolytic anemias. *Hemoglobinuria* begins at a plasma level of 135 mg. per 100 ml. Once begun, it continues until the level drops to 30 to 50 mg. per 100 ml. Plasma hemoglobin is bound to haptoglobin, an α_2-globulin, to form a molecule too large to pass through the renal glomerular capillary. Thus the plasma hemoglobin must exceed the haptoglobin level before hemoglobinuria begins [2]. The reticuloendothelial cells of the spleen, liver, lymph nodes, bone marrow, and elsewhere effect the breakdown of free hemoglobin to bilirubin. The *main pigments of hemoglobin breakdown* are hemosiderin, hematoidin–bilirubin, and hematin (an abnormal breakdown product).

1. Hemosiderin

HEMO-SIDERIN

Hemosiderin is a brownish granular pigment formed when excessive amounts of hemoglobin are deposited in the tissues, as in a hemorrhage. It is deposited intracellularly as fine crystals and consists of a high proportion of ferric hydroxide polymers (35 percent) bound to apoferritin. It contains loosely bound ferric iron which gives a positive Prussian blue reaction with potassium ferrocyanide and HCl, forming ferric ferrocyanide. Normally there are small amounts of hemosiderin in the liver and spleen from the breakdown of hemoglobin by the reticuloendothelial cells.

Hemosiderosis:

Excessive hemosiderin deposition *(hemosiderosis)* occurs in the tissues in hemorrhages (local hemosiderosis); hemolytic anemias, such as sickle cell anemia; pernicious (megaloblastic) anemia; chronic passive congestion; multiple blood transfusions (transfusional siderosis) [3]; and massive oral or parenteral iron therapy.

pathologic changes

In the spleen hemosiderin is deposited in the phagocytic cells of the red pulp and sinusoids. Hemosiderin deposits of marked degrees may be associated with fibrotic nodules in the spleen in Banti's disease, sickle cell anemia, and other congestive splenomegalies. Connective tissue fibers are encrusted with iron-containing pigments. In the liver, hemosiderin appears mainly in the Kupffer cells, but is also present in hepatocytes. Long-standing deposition produces fibrosis, as in congestive and pigmentary cirrhosis. In the kidneys it is deposited in the tubular epithelium, and in the *lungs* the pigment is found in macrophages in the alveolar spaces (heart-failure cells). Pigment deposition also occurs in the lymph nodes, bone marrow, adrenal cortex, and thyroid gland in transfusional hemosiderosis.

Primary hemochromatosis:

Primary (endogenous) hemochromatosis [4] is a rare disturbance of iron pigment metabolism, usually occurring in middle-aged males. Some cases are heredofamilial. It is characterized by excessive hemosiderin pigmentation of the skin and viscera, especially the liver and pancreas, associated with fibrosis. The *cause* appears to be an inborn defect in the duodenal mucosa; absorption of a greatly increased amount of iron results. The total body iron may reach 50 gm., over 10 times the normal amount.

clinical features

The *clinical picture* depends on the sites and degree of involvement. The principal features are bronzing of the skin, signs of diabetes mellitus (polyuria, polydipsia, polyphagia, and glycosuria), and signs of pigmentary cirrhosis of the liver (ascites, hemorrhages, hepatomegaly, and venous changes). The so-called *bronze diabetes* is usually mild but may be insulin-resistant.

pathologic changes

In the skin, hemosiderin deposits occur in the dermis about sweat glands, and there is also an increase in melanin deposition in the epidermis. The pancreas is usually slightly enlarged, firm, and deeply pigmented. Large deposits of hemosiderin and yellowish lipofuscin pigment are found in the acinar and duct epithelial cells, islets of Langerhans, and interstitial tissue. Fatty infiltration and fibrosis are common. The liver is usually enlarged, rusty red or ochre in color, and nodular. The lobules are separated by dense fibrous tissue *(pigmentary cirrhosis)*. The fibrosis begins in the portal areas, and the fibrous bands about hepatic lobules tend to be broad. *Hemosiderin* and scanty amounts of *hemofuscin are found mainly in the hepatic parenchymal cells,* with lesser amounts in the Kupffer cells and bile ductule epithelium. Fat is present in the hepatocytes only during alcoholic bouts and episodes of poor nutrition. In about 7 percent of the cases of pigmentary cirrhosis a hepatocarcinoma develops. Liver biopsies show that after 40 to 60 phlebotomies, in each of which 500 ml. of blood is withdrawn, about 75 percent of the liver iron is removed [5]. After 90 phlebotomies about 95 percent of the liver iron is gone. Only a slight decrease in fibrosis is noted following multiple phlebotomies. The spleen is often enlarged to over twice its normal size (average weight, 400 gm.), and is firm and deep purple. It is markedly congested due to the portal hypertension associated with the hepatic cirrhosis. Only small amounts of hemosiderin are present, mainly in the capsule, trabeculae, and blood vessel walls. Significant amounts of hemosiderin are deposited in the myocardial fibers and may contribute to the development of cardiac failure. Hemosiderin is also found in the epithelial cells of the thyroid, parathyroid, anterior pituitary, salivary, and lacrimal glands, and of the stomach and duodenum.

Secondary hemochromatosis:

Secondary (exogenous) hemochromatosis occurs in cases of chronic refractory anemia, especially in those receiving multiple blood transfusions [6] and prolonged intravenous or oral iron therapy. Over 200 transfusions of 500 ml. each are usually necessary to produce hemochromatosis. Each pint of blood contains about 250 mg. of iron. This rare form of hemochromatosis occurs at any age and in males and females about equally. *Clinically* skin pigmentation occurs in about half the cases, but diabetes mellitus and full-blown hepatic cirrhosis are rare.

pathologic changes

In contrast to primary hemochromatosis, in the secondary form *hemosiderin pigment is deposited mainly in reticuloendothelial cells,* with a lesser involvement of epithelial cells. Major deposits are in the liver (principally in the Kupffer cells), spleen, lymph nodes, bone marrow, and adrenal cortex, especially in the zona glomerulosa. Hemofuscin deposition does not occur. The hepatic fibrosis is usually slight, but in a few cases broad bands of fibrosis develop.

Bantu hemochromatosis

Bantu hemochromatosis [7] occurs among the Bantus of South Africa, especially the men. It is apparently due to the ingestion of very large amounts of iron daily in their food and fermented alcoholic beverages. The excessive *hemosiderin deposits are mainly in reticuloendothelial cells* of the liver and spleen. In advanced cases epithelial cells of the liver, pancreas, and thyroid gland are involved, and the hepatic cirrhosis is indistinguishable from that of primary hemochromatosis. The cirrhosis probably results from the effects of the heavy iron deposits, excessive alcoholic intake, and poor nutrition.

2. *Hematoidin and Bilirubin*

HEMATOIDIN AND BILIRUBIN:

Hematoidin and bilirubin are closely related or identical chemically. These pigments do not contain iron. *Hematoidin* is formed in tissue from hemoglobin, especially when oxygen tension is low, as in an infarct or hemorrhage. Hematoidin appears extracellularly as brown rhombic crystals or amorphous burrs. *Bilirubin* is the ultimate breakdown product of hemoglobin by reticuloendothelial cells. It appears as amorphous yellow granules or sheaves of crystals and is Prussian blue-negative and Gmelin test-positive.

Bilirubin metabolism

The *mechanism of bilirubin metabolism* [8] begins in reticuloendothelial cells with an oxidative opening of the α-methene bridge of the porphyrin ring. This produces verdohemoglobin, a biliverdin-iron globin. Biliverdin is transformed to bilirubin in the reticuloendothelial cells and this is transported to the liver as a bilirubin-albumin complex. In the liver the bilirubin-protein complex is dissociated at the hepatocytic plasma membrane, and the bilirubin is converted to bilirubin monoglucuronide and diglucuronide by reaction with uridine diphosphoglucuronic acid. This reaction is mediated by the enzymes uridine diphosphoglucuronic acid dehydrogenase and glucuronyl transferase. Soluble bilirubin diglucuronide enters the bile canaliculi and is excreted in the bile. Monoglucuronide conjugation also occurs extrahepatically. From 10 to 15 percent of bilirubin is not conjugated to glucuronides; about half of this is converted to bilirubin sulfate.

Bile formation

Electron microscopy has clarified to some extent the exact *anatomic pathway of bile formation in the liver* [9]. The hepatic sinusoidal endothelium forms an incomplete lining separating the sinusoidal blood from the hepatocytes. The endothelium is interrupted by spaces or pores measuring up to 2μ in diameter. These spaces allow the passage of all blood elements, except the cellular ones, from the sinusoidal lumen to the space of Disse. There is no basement membrane in the wall; thus the hepatic cells are bathed continually in a fluid with all noncellular blood constituents. The *hepatic cell membranes* have numerous fine villous projections which increase their surface contact with this protein-rich fluid. Many small pinocytotic cytoplasmic vesicles are formed beneath the cell membrane bordering on the space of Disse, and there is evidence of the imbibition of fluid and fine particles in this region. It is by such an energy-consuming mechanism that bilirubin unbound from serum albumin is taken into the hepatocytes.

Bile canaliculi

The *bile canaliculi* are enlargements of the interhepatocellular space lined only by hepatic cell membranes from which numerous microvilli project. Electron-dense particles aggregate in groups around the bile canaliculi and are frequently incorporated within Golgi substance, which is most prominent in the cytoplasmic region adjacent to the canaliculus (peribiliary cytoplasm). *Glucuronyl transferase activity* is associated with the microsomes of the endoplasmic reticulum. Glucuronide-conjugated bilirubin, cholesterol, alkaline phosphatase, bile salts, and other bile constituents cross the hepatocytic membrane into the canaliculus by an energy-consuming secretory mechanism, so that they are present in high concentration in the bile. Bile constituents such as sodium, potassium, and chloride, which are present in blood and bile in equal concentrations, apparently reach the bile canaliculus through the narrow interhepatocellular spaces which are actually extensions of the space of Disse.

Urobilinogen

In the intestine bilirubin is reduced by the action of bacteria to colorless mesobilirubinogen which is converted to the colorless chromogens, *d*-urobilinogen and stercobilinogen (urobilinogen). Oxidation transforms these into urobilins, the brown pigments of feces. Most *urobilinogen* is excreted in the feces as such or as urobilin. The rest is absorbed and carried to the liver, whence it is mainly excreted in the bile. Small amounts are excreted in the urine.

van den Bergh reaction

The *van den Bergh reaction* is a valuable laboratory method in cases of disturbances in bilirubin metabolism. Bilirubin diglucuronide reacts immediately with diazotized sulfanilic acid (Ehrlich's diazo reagent), and so is known as *direct-reacting bilirubin.* The diglucuronide is easily dissociated from serum proteins, to which it is loosely bound, dialyzes easily, and appears in the urine when it is present in a significant amount in the plasma. On the other hand, bilirubin bound to serum protein and unconjugated with glucuronic acid does not react with Ehrlich's diazo reagent unless it is brought into solution by alcohol *(indirect-reacting bilirubin).*

3. Jaundice

Jaundice (icterus) is a condition in which there are hyperbilirubinemia and deposition of bile pigments in the tissues. *Clinically* there is a yellow, orange, or green discoloration of the skin, sclerae, and mucous membranes. The tears and cerebrospinal fluid are usually not discolored in jaundiced patients.

MECHANISMS [10]:

Jaundice may be produced by any of the following *mechanisms:* (1) increased bilirubin load; (2) disturbance in bilirubin transport; (3) disturbance of bilirubin conjugation; and (4) disturbance of bilirubin excretion.

Increased bilirubin load: hemolytic jaundice

Jaundice resulting from an excessive bilirubin load occurs in the hemolytic anemias and in shunt hyperbilirubinemia. In hemolytic states the amount of hemoglobin released from erythrocytes is increased from the normal 6 gm. daily to as much as 45 gm. The normal liver can excrete large amounts of bilirubin. However, in *hemolytic jaundice* there is some hepatocellular damage. This results from accompanying anemia and possibly from the effects of the elevated serum hemoglobin level. In hemolytic jaundice the urine and fecal urobilinogen content is markedly increased, because even though not all the excess bilirubin can be metabolized by the liver, greatly increased amounts are excreted in the bile. This leads to increased urobilinogen formation in the intestine and the presence of elevated amounts in the feces and urine.

shunt hyperbilirubinemia

Primary shunt hyperbilirubinemia [11] is a rare, familial form of jaundice. It is due to an excessive production of bilirubin unrelated to the breakdown of circulating erythrocytes. The finding of erythroid hyperplasia (increased numbers of erythrocyte precursors) in the bone marrow in such cases suggests that the excess bilirubin derives from marrow erythrocytes and/or their precursors either by cell destruction or by direct bilirubin synthesis from heme. Patients with shunt hyperbilirubinemia have an increase in indirect-reacting serum bilirubin and in urine and fecal urobilinogen. Normally about 15 percent of bile pigments are derived from sources other than the breakdown of heme in circulating erythrocytes.

Bilirubin transport disturbance

In *Gilbert's disease* (constitutional hepatic dysfunction) [12], the cause of the jaundice may be a defect in bilirubin transport from the serum to the site of conjugation within hepatocytes. This familial disorder is probably transmitted as an autosomal dominant. It is characterized by the development of icterus in adolescents or adults, with indirect serum bilirubin levels that may rise to 18 mg. per 100 ml., but usually are not over 3 mg. per 100 ml. There is no neurologic involvement. Some patients have low levels of glucuronyl transferase activity.

Bilirubin conjugation disturbance

Jaundice resulting from disturbance in bilirubin conjugation occurs in physiologic jaundice in the newborn, breast-milk jaundice, and the Crigler-Najjar syndrome. In the immature hepatic cells of the *newborn,* a deficiency of glucuronyl transferase produces jaundice due to defective bilirubin conjugation. *Breast-milk jaundice* [13] occurs in breast-fed infants during the second to fourth week of life. It is due to the inhibition of glucuronyl transferase by the steroid, pregnane-3, α-20, β-diol, in human milk. The jaundice clears after cessation of breast feeding. *Congenital familial nonhemolytic jaundice with kernicterus (Crigler-Najjar syndrome)* is due to a congenital deficiency or absence of glucuronyl transferase activity. Type 1 is inherited as an autosomal recessive and is severe. The hepatic cells are unable to conjugate bilirubin, menthol, salicylates, or tetrahydrocortisone. It usually occurs in Jewish infants, and icterus, with persistent indirect serum bilirubin levels from 20 to 45 mg. per 100 ml., appears shortly after birth. The bile is almost colorless, and the fecal urobilinogen level is very low. Kernicterus develops, and most of the infants die within 1 year. Type 2 is probably transmitted as an autosomal dominant with variable expressivity. Some bilirubin conjugation occurs, and serum bilirubin levels run between 8 and 22 mg. per 100 ml. Kernicterus does not develop.

Bilirubin excretion disturbance: Dubin-Johnson syndrome

Disturbance of bilirubin excretion may occur within the liver or extrahepatically. *Intrahepatic excretory disturbances* occur in the Dubin-Johnson and Rotor syndromes, cholestatic drug jaundice, benign recurrent intrahepatic cholestasis, inspissated bile syndrome, viral hepatitis (see Chapter 7), and primary biliary cirrhosis. *Chronic idiopathic jaundice (Dubin-Johnson syndrome)* [14] is characterized by chronic or intermittent jaundice in adolescents or young adults, with little loss of hepatic function and an excellent prognosis. *Clinically* the patients complain of right upper quadrant or epigastric pain. Both direct and indirect serum bilirubin levels are elevated, the total bilirubin being as high as 6 mg. per 100 ml. There are slight abnormalities in cephalin flocculation and thymol turbidity tests. Bromsulphalein retention is frequently noted. Serum protein, alkaline phosphatase, and cholesterol levels, and prothrombin activity are normal. There is a consistent failure to visualize the gallbladder on cholecystography, presumably due to inability of the liver to excrete the test dyes. In cases subjected to laparotomy, the liver has been described as smooth and dark brown, dark green, or black. *Microscopically liver biopsies have shown coarsely granular, amorphous brown pigment within hepatocytes,* especially in the centrolobular zones. Otherwise the liver is normal. *Electron microscopy* reveals that the pigment is deposited within lysosomes and that the bile canaliculi are normal [15]. The exact nature of the pigment is unknown, but it contains catecholamines. Its deposition within hepatocytes is probably due to an inborn secretory defect within hepatocytes involving bilirubin diglucuronide, catecholamines, bromsulphalein, and dyes used in cholecystography.

Rotor syndrome

The *Rotor syndrome* is a chronic familial nonhemolytic jaundice with an elevated direct serum bilirubin level and without abnormal pigment in the liver [16].

cholestatic jaundice

Cholestatic drug jaundice may be of the chlorpromazine type, which is allergic in nature, or of the testosterone type. Among the drugs causing cholestasis are sulfonamides, erythromycin estolate, certain phenothiazine derivatives, chlorothiazide, norethandrolone, and methyltestosterone. In both forms electron microscopy has revealed alterations in the microvilli of bile canaliculi, which are obstructed by bile thrombi. *Cholestatic jaundice of pregnancy* [17] may be related to the elevated estrogen level during gestation. It is characterized by jaundice, itching, nausea, occasional vomiting, and right upper quadrant tenderness. Liver biopsies show intracanalicular bile plugs and slight hepatocytic necrosis.

recurrent intrahepatic cholestasis

Benign recurrent intrahepatic cholestasis [18] is a rare idiopathic disorder characterized by repeated episodes of jaundice associated with pruritus, dark urine, clay-colored feces, and weight loss. The serum bilirubin level is markedly increased, especially the direct fraction, as is the alkaline phosphatase level. The attacks begin in childhood or adolescence and usually last several weeks. There is no apparent impairment of liver function between periods of jaundice. *Liver biopsies* during icteric episodes have shown *marked bile stasis within intralobular canaliculi,* minimal hepatocytic necrosis, and a moderate periportal lymphocytic infiltrate. Similar changes have been described in *benign postoperative intrahepatic cholestasis* [19].

other excretion disturbances

The *inspissated bile syndrome* occurs in infants with severe erythroblastosis fetalis. The bile is viscid and obstructs the canaliculi and bile ductules. *Extrahepatic biliary obstruction* produces *posthepatic (obstructive) jaundice* (page 276).

CLASSIFICATIONS:

Jaundice may be classified as: (1) retention or regurgitation jaundice (Rich); (2) hemolytic, parenchymatous, or obstructive (McNee); or (3) prehepatic, hepatic (hepatocellular or hepatocanalicular), or posthepatic (Ducci).

Retention jaundice

In *retention jaundice* the defect in bilirubin metabolism lies in the inability of the liver cells to remove an increased, or sometimes normal, amount of bile pigment from the blood. It is due to hypoxia of hepatic cells from anemia (usually hemolytic); chronic passive congestion of the liver rarely; a disturbance of bilirubin transport within the liver; and defective bilirubin conjugation due to immaturity of the liver cells in the newborn infant, or to a developmental deficiency of glucuronyl transferase. In retention jaundice the elevated serum bilirubin level is mainly of the indirect (unconjugated) type.

Regurgitation jaundice

Regurgitation jaundice is due to a leakage or regurgitation of bile pigment into the bloodstream. It may be caused by increased intrabiliary pressure with actual disruption of bile capillaries or by increased permeability of damaged bile canaliculi. This in turn is caused by necrosis of hepatic cells, which swell to compress the bile canaliculi and plug them with debris, and by obstruction of the extrahepatic bile passages. In regurgitation jaundice the serum bilirubin is mainly conjugated and direct-reacting.

Prehepatic jaundice

Prehepatic jaundice is actually hepatogenous. Although the etiologic hyperbilirubinemia is due to a sudden hemolysis, the jaundice results from the inability of the liver cells to remove the increased amount of circulating bilirubin. The cause of this inability is hypoxia of the hepatic cells. Prehepatic jaundice may occur in (1) hemolytic anemia (congenital and acquired hemolytic jaundice, sickle cell anemia, Mediterranean anemia, and erythroblastosis fetalis), (2) hemoglobinurias (mismatched transfusions, paroxysmal hemoglobinuria), and (3) fever associated with hemolysis (hemolytic septicemia and malaria, especially blackwater fever). The elevated serum bilirubin is largely indirect-reacting.

Hepatic (hepatogenous) jaundice:

Intrahepatic (hepatogenous) jaundice may be hepatocellular and/or hepatocanalicular in origin. In the *hepatocellular type* the icterus is due to a defect in hepatic cell functions of converting bilirubin to bilirubin diglucuronide and excreting the bilirubin. In the *hepatocanalicular type* the cause is damage to or obstruction of the fine intrahepatic biliary passages. Most cases of hepatogenous jaundice are mixed, because in a disease process producing hepatocytic necrosis, swelling of the affected cells often obstructs the bile canaliculi and small ducts by compression. The serum bilirubin in hepatogenous jaundice is usually mainly indirect-reacting, but it is both indirect and direct and gives a biphasic van den Bergh reaction.

hepatocellular jaundice

Hepatocellular jaundice is caused by: (1) hypoxia due to hemolytic processes; (2) immaturity of the liver cells in the newborn infant *(icterus neonatorum);* (3) a deficiency or inhibition of glucuronyl transferase; (4) chronic passive congestion of the liver (rarely); and (5) necrosis of liver cells due to severe and prolonged hypoxia, poisons (chloroform, carbon tetrachloride, phosphorus), viral hepatitis, yellow fever, leptospirosis, and congenital syphilis. In icterus due to causes listed in (5) there is hepatocanalicular damage and/or obstruction, so that the jaundice is mixed in these cases.

hepato-canalicular jaundice

Hepatocanalicular jaundice is caused by (1) necrosis of liver cells – see (5) under hepatocellular jaundice; and (2) certain drugs, such as chlorpromazine and methyltestosterone.

Post-hepatic jaundice

Posthepatic (obstructive) jaundice is due to obstruction of the extrahepatic tree (hepatic or common bile duct) and may be caused by: (1) plugging of the lumen by calculi (stones), parasites, or neoplasm; (2) stricture of the lumen due to a congenital defect, inflammation, or neoplasm; and (3) external compression due to an inflammatory, parasitic, or neoplastic mass. The serum bilirubin is mainly direct-reacting in posthepatic jaundice.

LABORATORY DATA

The *laboratory differentiation* of hepatogenous jaundice and posthepatic (obstructive) jaundice is shown in Table 11-1. *Laboratory findings are often variable in jaundice,* especially in cases due to parenchymatous hepatic damage because of the mixture of retentive and regurgitative elements in the production of the jaundice. In posthepatic jaundice, the damming back of bile will eventually damage hepatic cells and produce a mixed type of icterus.

TABLE 11-1. Laboratory Differentiation of Hepatogenous and Posthepatic (Obstructive) Jaundice

Test	Hepatogenous jaundice	Posthepatic (obstructive) jaundice
Serum albumin	Decreased	Normal
Serum globulin	Elevated	Normal
Cephalin flocculation	Positive	Negative
Thymol turbidity	Positive	Negative
Serum alkaline phosphatase	Less than 10 Bodansky units	More than 10 Bodansky units
Serum cholesterol	Decreased	Increased
Serum cholesterol esters	Decreased	Normal or slightly increased
van den Bergh reaction	Mainly indirect	Mainly direct
Prothrombin time	Increased (little change with intravenous vitamin K)	Increased (relieved by intravenous vitamin K)
Urine urobilinogen	Increased (in the hemolytic types)	Absent with complete obstruction
Urine bilirubin	Absent	Present
Urine bile salts	Absent	Present
Fecal urobilinogen	Increased (in the hemolytic types)	Decreased or absent (feces often clay-colored)

EFFECTS OF JAUNDICE: Kernicterus

Bilirubin retention causes little effect except for discoloration. However, high concentrations of indirect-reacting bilirubin are toxic to the central nervous system, especially in the newborn infant. The *kernicterus* of the hemolytic anemia, erythroblastosis fetalis, is a bilirubin encephalopathy. The thrusting of enormously increased amounts of bilirubin upon the immature hepatic cells of the newborn leads to the accumulation of large amounts of unconjugated bilirubin in the serum. The lipid-soluble albumin-bound bilirubin passes the immature blood-brain barrier of the newborn. The pigment damages ganglion cells, especially in the basal ganglia, which are stained yellow. Several *extraneural lesions associated with kernicterus* have been described [20]. In the kidneys, necrosis of the medullary pyramids *(papillary necrosis)* may be striking. Changes vary from desquamation of degenerated collecting tubular epithelium to severe tubular and peritubular necrosis with heavy neutrophilic infiltration. In severe cases the medullary pyramids are very congested, and there is a concentration of bilirubin pigment *("bilirubin infarcts")*. In the adrenal gland, focal necrosis with a neutrophilic infiltrate may occur in the fetal cortex. In the mucous glands of the mouth and upper respiratory tract and occasionally in the salivary glands, the gland lumina and ducts are dilated and filled with necrotic epithelial cellular debris. Similar changes occur in the mucosal epithelium and Brunner's glands of the gastrointestinal tract. The splenic malpighian corpuscles may undergo slight to "explosive" lymphocytic necrosis. Completely necrotic lymph follicles simulate microabscesses. *The lesions parallel the distribution of bilirubin crystals in the tissues,* the most striking correlation between necrosis and pigmentation being in the renal medulla. Unconjugated bilirubin and partially conjugated bilirubin monoglucuronide are responsible for the cellular toxicity.

Cholemic nephrosis

The *effects of jaundice on the kidneys* include *cholemic (icteric) nephrosis,* caused by severe icterus. *Grossly* the kidneys are swollen and green or brown due to bile staining. *Microscopically* numerous yellow or golden brown *bilirubin pigment casts are found in the lumina of distal convoluted and collecting tubules.* The tubular epithelium shows cloudy swelling or more severe degenerative changes. The exact mechanism of the tubular damage is not known. The soluble bilirubin diglucuronide, which may be excreted by the tubular epithelium, is not toxic. The condition develops more commonly in regurgitative jaundice, so that bile salts have been implicated. Severe hepatic damage may produce an abnormal aminoaciduria, and experimentally renal tubular damage can be caused by serine, cystine, lysine, arginine, aspartic acid, histidine, and tryptophan. Perhaps an abnormal increase in one or more of these acids is irritating to the tubular epithelium. No change is seen in the glomeruli by light microscopy, but electron microscopy reveals small black granules in the thickened basement membrane and mesangial matrix [21]. The epithelial foot processes are fused.

Pruritus

Malabsorption

The *regurgitation of bile salts* (sodium glycocholate and sodium taurocholate) may produce *pruritus* (itching) and *bradycardia* (slow cardiac rate). It is also possible that some toxic agent, normally detoxified by the liver, causes these effects. The *absence of bile salts from the intestine* causes steatorrhea, since fats and cholesterol are not well absorbed, and a bleeding tendency due to nonabsorption of vitamin K.

4. Hematin

HEMATIN:

Hematin is not a normal breakdown product of hemoglobin. It appears in some hemolytic crises and rapidly combines with blood protein to form methemalbumin. It appears in the tissues as brownish pigment resembling hemosiderin. Hematin is Prussian blue-negative (its iron is firmly bound). It may appear in the renal tubules in massive hemoglobinuria, such as transfusion reactions, due to the action of the acid in the urine on the hemoglobin.

Malarial pigment

Malarial pigment is closely related to hematin. It is Prussian blue-negative. Massive amounts of brown pigment are found in the reticuloendothelial cells of the liver and spleen. It is split by reticuloendothelial cells into hemosiderin and bilirubin. *Schistosomal pigment* is practically identical in composition and distribution to malarial pigment.

5. Hematoporphyrins

Hematoporphyrins are iron-free pigments normally present in minute amounts in the blood and urine. They appear in higher concentrations in the porphyrias, in which there is excessive formation of uroporphyrins and coproporphyrins.

PORPHYRIAS: Erythropoietic porphyria

The *porphyrias* [22] are due to defects in porphyrin metabolism. *Congenital erythropoietic porphyria* results from a rare, recessively transmitted metabolic error within normoblasts in the bone marrow. Abnormal concentration of porphyrins are detectable within the normoblasts by fluorescence microscopy. A prominent part of this disorder is a *photosensitivity dermatitis.* Early lesions are pemphigoid vesicles or bullae on skin surfaces exposed to sunlight. The skin is most sensitive to light wave lengths in the near ultraviolet band (about 4000 angstroms). With the passage of years, scarring leads to mutilations such as a loss of fingers and tips of the nose and ears, and to ectropion (an outward turning of the eyelids with exposure of the eyes). Dentine and cortical bone may be red or reddish brown due to porphyrin deposition. The urine may be burgundy red due to urophyrin I and coproporphyrin I excretion. A hemolytic anemia is often associated with erythropoietic porphyria.

Erythropoietic protoporphyria

Erythropoietic protoporphyria [23] is probably transmitted as a dominant but often appears in partial form clinically. Fully developed cases show increased erythrocyte, plasma, and fecal protoporphyrin levels. The urinary porphyrin content is not elevated. A photosensitivity dermatitis may occur. In light-exposed areas the skin show periodic acid-Schiff (PAS)-positive hyaline material surrounding capillaries in the superficial dermis. In the liver, pigment containing red, fluorescent protoporphyrin is found within bile canaliculi and interlobular bile ducts [24]. Gallstones containing poorly soluble protoporphyrin may be found.

Hepatic porphyria:

Hepatic porphyria is much more common than the erythropoietic form. It appears as (1) acute intermittent porphyria, which is inherited as a mendelian dominant; (2) porphyria cutanea tarda, in which there is a late onset of photosensitive skin lesions; (3) mixed hepatic porphyria; and (4) a latent form (paraporphyria).

acute intermittent hepatic porphyria

In *acute intermittent hepatic porphyria,* uroporphyrins and coproporphyrins are excreted in the urine and feces in increased amounts, along with the porphyrin precursors, porphobilinogen and δ-amino levulinic acid. This disorder occurs more often in females than males. Barbiturates, alcohol, and exposure to oil-base paint or sunlight may precipitate the neuropsychiatric signs. *Clinically* there are psychiatric symptoms in about 60 percent of the cases (catatonic excitement, hallucinations); bulbar signs in 20 percent (dysphagia, diplopia, anisocoria [unequal pupils], and dysarthria); convulsions; peripheral nerve palsies; frequent abdominal, chest, or back pain; obstipation; dysuria, burgundy wine-colored urine occasionally, and an offensive urine odor; and a malar flush with a butterfly pattern. The *pathologic changes* are nonspecific degeneration in the neurons of cranial nerve nuclei, the anterior horns, and the sympathetic ganglia. Liver biopsies reveal large amounts of porphyrin precursors and variable amounts of porphyrins.

porphyria cutanea tarda

Porphyria cutanea tarda [25] is chronic and is characterized by a marked elevation of urinary uroporphyrin, a lesser increase in urinary coproporphyrin, and normal or slightly elevated fecal porphyrin levels. It occurs in persons with chronic liver diseases due to alcoholism, hemochromatosis, drug reactions, and hepatocarcinoma. A number of cases have followed exposure to crop dusting with the fungicide hexachlorbenzene. In some patients the disease appears to be hereditary. The increased uroporphyrin and coproporphyrin production is attributed to alterations in oxidation-reduction reactions in the liver. Skin lesions are due to the photosensitizing effects of uroporphyrin; they include erythema, vesicles, bullae, and patches of depigmentation. The changes in the liver are varied and include portal, postnecrotic, and pigmentary cirrhosis, and hepatocarcinoma.

Information on the porphyrias is summarized in Table 11-2 (page 280).

MELANIN METABOLISM

MELANIN:

Melanin [26] is a brownish black pigment forming the normal coloring material of the skin, the iris and choroid of the eye, the medulla and zona reticularis of the adrenal glands, and certain parts of the central nervous system. In the skin it is produced by melanocytes, branched secretory cells of the basal layer of the epidermis thought to be specialized nerve endings derived from the ectoderm of the neural crest. The melanocytes of the retinal pigment epithelium arise in the outer layer of the optic cup. Because of their clear cytoplasm, melanocytes are called cellules claires. These cells are *dopa-positive,* even when they contain no visible pigment; i.e., they contain the melanin precursor, dihydroxyphenylalanine (dopa), which reacts with appropriate reagents to form a black pigment within the cells. *Melanophores* are pigment-bearing cells of the dermis and are dopa-negative. They phagocytize pigment and carry it into the superficial dermis. The amount of melanin in the skin varies in different races and individuals, although the number and distribution of melanocytes appears to be the same in all races of man.

Chemistry

Melanin is a biochrome of high molecular weight which is formed by the enzymatic oxidation of tyrosine within melanocyte organelles, the melanosomes. The copper-containing enzyme *tyrosinase* catalyzes the hydroxylation of tyrosine to dihydroxyphenylalanine and the oxidation of the latter to dopaquinone. Zinc ions catalyze the oxidation of dopachrome to 5,6-dihydroxyindole, which is then converted to tyrosine-melanin. Combination of this with protein produces melanoprotein. As this light brown pigment accumulates within melanosomes, the latter become melanin granules. These are argyrophilic but do not stain with reagents used to demonstrate iron-containing pigments. Melanin darkens on exposure to ultraviolet light; the *function* of melanin is to be an

TABLE 11-2. The Porphyrias

Type	Inheritance	Defect	Photosensitivity	Urine porphyrins	Fecal porphyrins	Special features
Erythropoietic porphyria	Recessive	Abnormal porphyrin concentrations in normoblasts	Vesicles and bullae with later scarring and mutilation	Increased uro- and coproporphyrin I	—	Hemolytic anemia; dentine and bone may be stained red
Erythropoietic protoporphyria	Dominant	Increased protoporphyrin production in bone marrow	May occur	Not elevated	Increased protoporphyrin	Fluorescent protoporphyrin found in liver; gallstones may form
Acute intermittent hepatic porphyria	Dominant	Excessive porphyrin production in liver	None	Increased uro- and coproporphyrins and porphobilinogen	Increased uro- and coproporphyrins and porphobilinogen	Occurs in females more than males; attacks precipitated by barbiturates, alcohol, or sunlight; neuropsychiatric manifestations
Porphyria cutanea tarda	Appears to be hereditary in some cases	Increased porphyrin production in liver	Late – erythema, vesicles, bullae, and depigmentation	Marked increase in uroporphyrin, lesser elevation of coproporphyrin	Normal or slight increase in uro- and coproporphyrin	Occurs in patients with portal, postnecrotic, or pigmentary cirrhosis, or hepatocarcinoma; some cases have followed exposure to fungicide, hexachlorbenzene

epidermal and retinal sunlight-absorbing shield. Melanin *metabolism* is controlled by the melanocyte-stimulating hormones (alpha and beta MSH) (intermedin) from the pars intermedia of the pituitary gland, and to a lesser extent by adrenocorticotropic hormone (ACTH). However, these compounds are not essential for normal melanin pigmentation.

Increased melanin pigmentation

Pathologic increases in melanin pigmentation occur in many states. In *Addison's disease* there is bronzing of the skin, especially in those areas exposed to sunlight or in those already heavily pigmented. Addison's disease is due to the destruction of the adrenal cortices by tuberculosis, cancer, or idiopathic atrophy. The bronzing of the skin is due to an increase in melanin. The increased pigmentation is probably due to increased melanocytic activity stimulated by the secretion of MSH and ACTH by the hypophysis. Normally adrenal cortical hormones depress MSH and ACTH secretion. *Other disease states* demonstrating increased melanin pigmentation are: hemochromatosis (with iron pigments); multiple neurofibromatosis (café au lait spots); fibrous dysplasia of bone (Albright's syndrome); pregnancy; ACTH-producing neoplasms and ACTH therapy; tuberculosis; cachexia (patchy hyperpigmentation); urticaria pigmentosa; bite of a louse (punctate hyperpigmentation); ephelis (freckle); lentigo (a small, dark brown skin spot due to excessive melanin production by an increased number of melanocytes); junctional nevus; compound nevus; intradermal nevus; blue nevus; Mongolian spot; and melanocarcinoma. The *pigment cell neoplasms* are discussed on page 787.

Decreased melanin pigmentation

Decreased melanin pigmentation occurs in: albinism (congenital deficiency or absence of melanin), vitiligo or leukoderma (patchy areas of depigmentation), burn or wound scars, pinta (irregular or patchy areas of depigmentation), and leprosy (due to nerve involvement).

Melanosis coli

Melanosis coli is a brown or black discoloration of the mucosa of the appendix and large intestine due to a melanin-like pigment held in macrophages. It ends sharply at the ileocecal valve. Pigment is also present in the submucosa and mesenteric lymph nodes. Melanosis coli is found in about 10 percent of autopsies on elderly persons. It may be due to fecal stasis resulting from chronic constipation or partial colonic obstruction. These lead to absorption of protein breakdown products which are converted to pigment by a tyrosinase-like enzyme. Melanosis coli is especially common in patients with chronic constipation who use cascara sagrada as a laxative. This compound contains an anthraquinone which may be converted to a melanin-like pigment in the bowel wall.

Ochronosis:

Ochronosis [27] in its endogenous form is a rare, recessively transmitted, congenital disorder of melanin-like pigmentation due to an inborn error in tyrosine metabolism. Homogentisic acid oxidase is absent in the liver and kidneys of patients with ochronosis. Homogentisic acid (an intermediate in the oxidation of tyrosine) is not oxidized, so that it accumulates in the extracellular fluid. The compound is selectively deposited in cartilage, which becomes ochre-colored or black due to melanin-like pigment. Deposits within synovia produce *ochronotic arthritis,* and involvement of the intervertebral disks may result in an ankylosing spondylitis with development of a "poker spine." *Prostatic calculi* are commonly formed. In the kidneys an *ochronotic nephrosis* may occur, with melanin-like pigment deposit in, and swelling or necrosis of, the proximal convoluted tubular epithelium. The kidneys are dark brown, and brown or black pigment casts are found in the tubular lumina. There is an *alkaptonuria.* The urine becomes brownish black on standing or after the addition of alkali, due to the presence of homogentisic acid.

exogenous ochronosis

Exogenous ochronosis is caused by the absorption of phenol from ulcers or wounds dressed for a prolonged period with phenol solution or ointment, or with picric acid (trinitrophenol). It is very rare today.

LIPOCHROME METABOLISM

LIPO-CHROMES

Lipochrome pigments are yellowish and soluble in fat solvents. They do not take the usual fat stains and are normally present in the corpus luteum, testes, adrenal cortex, ganglion cells, and fat. They are wear-and-tear pigments and increase with age. In *brown atrophy of the heart* the pigments which appear at the nuclear poles of the myocardial fibers (Abnutzung pigment) may be lipochromes or hemoglobin derivatives; however, they are insoluble in fat solvents. *Carotene* is probably related to the lipochromes. *Ceroid* is a greenish yellow, acid-fast, fluorescent lipoidal pigment. It is probably a polymer of peroxides of unsaturated fatty acids. It stains with fat stains but is not soluble in the lipid solvents. It is seen in the hepatic cells in experimental cirrhosis, in macrophages throughout the body, in the adrenal cortex, and in the ovaries.

THE ANEMIAS

ANEMIA: Causes

Anemia is a decrease below normal in the number of circulating erythrocytes and hemoglobin per unit volume of the blood. It *may be caused* by external or internal *loss of blood* from the vascular tree (hemorrhage); by *excessive destruction of erythrocytes* within the vascular system (hemolytic anemias, hemoglobinurias); *or* by *decreased erythropoiesis in the bone marrow* due to a nutritional deficiency (iron, vitamin B_{12}), a deficiency of erythropoietin, toxic inhibition of the marrow (aplastic anemia), or displacement of erythropoietic cells by neoplastic ones.

Classification by erythrocyte size and shape

Anemias may be characterized by changes in erythrocyte size and shape and in the hemoglobin concentration. In *microcytic anemia* the erythrocyte diameter is below the normal 7.5μ and the mean corpuscular volume is less than normal, whereas in *macrocytic anemia* the cell diameter and mean corpuscular volume are above the normal values. In *hypochromic anemia* the mean corpuscular hemoglobin and the mean corpuscular hemoglobin concentration are below normal. Anemia due to hemorrhage is *normocytic* (i.e., there is no alteration in cell size or shape) unless iron stores are depleted.

Abnormal hemoglobins

Some anemias are due to the presence of *abnormal hemoglobin* in the erythrocytes [28]. Normal adult hemoglobin is labeled A, and that of the fetus is F. *Hemoglobin A* consists of two pairs of peptide chains, α and β. The chains contain 141 amino acids in a definite sequence; the β chain sequence begins with valine-histidine-leucine-threonine-proline-glutamic acid-glutamic acid-lysine and runs through 146 amino acids. *Hemoglobin F* has the same α chains; in its γ chains, glycine replaces the terminal valine of the β chains. *Abnormal hemoglobins* S, C through Q, and others have been reported. Their occurrence in the blood is genetically determined. In *hemoglobin C* lysine replaces the first glutamic acid in the β chain sequence. *Hemoglobin S* differs from the normal type only in the replacement of this glutamic acid by valine in the β chain. Hemoglobins S and C are present in individuals with sickle cell anemia or with the sickling trait. C and F are present in rare cases of combined sickle cell and Mediterranean anemias. M is a methemoglobin.

DEFINITIONS:

Some terms relating to anemia are defined below [29].

Anisocytosis

Anisocytosis is an abnormal variation in the size of erythrocytes (normal range, 6.2 to 8.2μ in diameter). It may occur in any severe anemia, but is most marked in the macrocytic anemias.

Autoantibodies

Autoantibodies react with the patient's own erythrocytes and with the erythrocytes of other persons of the same blood group. They occur as warm or cold autoagglutinins or autohemolysins and may be complete or incomplete. Autoantibodies are present in auto-immune hemolytic anemias and some hemoglobinurias. Their development is paradoxic and poorly understood.

Basophilic stippling

Basophilic stippling (punctate basophilia) is the presence of fine or coarse granules of blue-staining material containing ribonucleic acid in the cytoplasm of young erythrocytes. The granules are aggregates of ribosomes of reticulocytes. Basophilic stippling is commonly seen in the anemia of lead poisoning.

Cabot rings

Cabot rings are round basophilic loops found in the cytoplasm of immature erythrocytes, especially in pernicious anemia. The rings are thought to be artifacts.

Coombs' test: direct test

Coombs' test is a method for the detection of antibodies on erythrocytes or in the serum. The *direct antiglobulin test* detects the presence of incomplete antibodies fixed to the surface of erythrocytes but incapable of producing agglutination in vitro. Coombs' antiglobulin serum is prepared by immunizing rabbits against human globulin or serum. The direct Coombs test is performed by exposing the patient's washed erythrocytes directly to the antiglobulin serum. It is usually positive in auto-immune hemolytic anemia, erythroblastosis fetalis, and paroxysmal cold hemoglobinuria. The test is negative in hemolytic diseases due to intracorpuscular defects.

indirect test

The *indirect antiglobulin test* detects the presence of antibodies in the serum after the patient's erythrocytes have been saturated. Normal erythrocytes of a known genotype are first exposed to the serum suspected of containing antibodies and then to antiglobulin serum. If antibodies from the serum are fixed on the erythrocytes, the latter will be agglutinated by the antiglobulin serum. The indirect Coombs test is usually positive in severe erythroblastosis fetalis, and may be positive or negative in auto-immune hemolytic anemia.

Elliptocytosis

Elliptocytosis (ovalocytosis) is a congenital abnormality in the shape of erythrocytes, the cells being oval, rod-shaped, or sausage-shaped. Elliptocyte precursors through the reticulocyte have a normal shape. The condition is sometimes prominent in thalassemia.

Heinz bodies

Heinz bodies are small, spherical or ovoid, refractile inclusions occurring singly or multiply in injured erythrocytes in cases of erythroblastosis fetalis and hemolytic anemias due to toxic agents [30]. The bodies represent precipitation of denatured hemoglobin. They are insoluble and make the erythrocytes less flexible than normal, so that they are readily trapped and lysed in the spleen.

Howell-Jolly bodies

Howell-Jolly bodies are spherical chromatin remnants of the normoblast nucleus. They are common in erythrocytes in severe anemias and following splenectomy.

Isoantibodies

Isoantibodies are naturally occurring antibodies (the anti-A and anti-B blood group antibodies in serum) and immune antibodies formed by immunization against the A, B, Rh, MNS, and other blood groups by mismatched transfusions or transplacentally. Iso-immune hemolytic diseases include hemolytic reactions to serologically incompatible blood transfusions, and erythroblastosis fetalis.

MCH
MCHC
MCV

Mean corpuscular hemoglobin (MCH) is determined by multiplying the hemoglobin in grams per 100 ml. by 10 and dividing by the erythrocyte count in millions. The normal MCH is 27 to 32 micromicrograms per cell. The *mean corpuscular hemoglobin concentration* (MCHC) is the result of multiplying the hemoglobin in grams per 100 ml. by 100 and dividing by the hematocrit. Normal values are 32 to 36 percent. The *mean corpuscular volume* (MCV) is calculated by dividing 10 times the hematocrit by the erythrocyte count in millions, the normal value being 82 to 92 cubic microns.

Meniscocytes

Meniscocytes (drepanocytes) are crescent-shaped erythrocytes characteristic of sickle cell anemia. Their shape is due to the insolubility of hemoglobin S in its deoxygenated form. Doubly refractile masses of rodlike particles (tactoids) are produced, deforming the erythrocytes.

Osmotic fragility

Osmotic fragility refers to the concentration range of hypotonic saline (a water solution containing less than 0.85 percent sodium chloride) within which lysis of erythrocytes occurs. With normal red cells, hemolysis begins at 0.44 percent and is complete at 0.32 percent saline. The osmotic fragility is markedly increased in spherocytes. In congenital spherocytosis, lysis begins at 0.68 percent and is complete at 0.46 percent. It is increased to a lesser degree in several other types of hemolytic anemia, although in sickle cell anemia the osmotic fragility of the erythrocytes is decreased, lysis beginning at 0.36 percent and being complete in a 0.20 percent saline solution.

Pappenheimer bodies

Pappenheimer bodies (siderotic granules) are purplish coccoid granules found at the periphery of erythrocytes in anemias due to impaired heme synthesis *(sideroachrestic* anemias). The granules contain iron in ferritin.

Poikilocytosis

Poikilocytosis is the presence of erythrocytes showing major abnormalities in shape. It is prominent in pernicious anemia.

Reticulocytes

Reticulocytes are young erythrocytes which contain granules and filaments (substantia granulofilamentosa) of basophilic substance (ribonucleic acid and protoporphyrin). Normally 0.5 to 1.5 percent of circulating red cells are reticulocytes. These cells increase in number in the peripheral blood during erythropoietic hyperactivity, such as in chronic blood loss, hemolytic anemias, and pernicious anemia (during therapy).

Spherocytes

Spherocytes are erythrocytes with a spheroid shape and a small diameter. Their presence is characteristic of a number of hemolytic anemias, especially congenital spherocytic anemia. Spherocyte precursors are not rounded. The spheroid shape is the result of an alteration in the cell surface due to either an intrinsic defect or an antigen-antibody reaction there. Spherocytes show an increased osmotic fragility because their spheroid shape renders them liable to rupture on slight swelling. The cells appear to be destroyed fairly rapidly in the spleen.

Target cells

Target cells (leptocytes, platycytes) are flatter than normal erythrocytes. A central hemoglobin condensation gives target cells a dark center and periphery, with an intervening lighter zone. The flat shape affords these cells a decreased osmotic fragility. They occur in hemolytic anemias, especially thalassemia, sicklemia, and hemoglobin C disease.

CLINICAL FEATURES

The *general clinical characteristics* of severe anemia are weakness, pallor (the skin may have a lemon yellow or greenish color), brittleness of the nails, dyspnea, tachycardia, systolic cardiac murmurs, congestive heart failure, headaches, tinnitus, vertigo, paresthesias, amenorrhea, slight fever (marked elevations in hemolytic crises), and splenomegaly. Most of these changes are caused by the hypoxia due to deficient oxygen delivery to the affected tissues.

CLASSIFICATION

Based on etiology, anemias can be classified into seven major groups.

I. *Anemias due to external or internal loss of blood*
II. *Anemias due to excessive destruction of erythrocytes (hemolytic anemias)*
    A. Hereditary forms
        1. Congenital spherocytic anemia
        2. Hereditary nonspherocytic anemias
        3. Elliptocytic (ovalocytic) anemia
        4. Sickle cell anemia (a hemoglobinopathy)
        5. Thalassemia (a hemoglobinopathy)
        6. Paroxysmal nocturnal and march hemoglobinuria
    B. Acquired forms
        1. Acquired auto-immune hemolytic anemia
        2. Acquired iso-immune hemolytic anemias
            a. Due to ABO blood group incompatibility
            b. Due to Rh incompatibility (erythroblastosis fetalis)
        3. Paroxysmal cold hemoglobinuria
        4. Hemolytic anemias due to infectious agents
        5. Hemolytic anemias due to drugs or chemicals
        6. Hemolytic anemias due to physical agents
            a. Mechanical hemolytic anemia
        7. Hemolytic anemias due to unknown causes
III. *Anemias due to deficiencies*
    A. Iron-deficiency anemia
    B. Pyridoxine-responsive anemia
    C. Vitamin B_{12}-deficiency anemias (megaloblastic anemias)
        1. Pernicious anemia
    D. Folic acid-deficiency anemia
    E. Erythropoietin-deficiency anemia
IV. *Anemias due to marrow inhibition (aplastic anemia)*
    A. Aplastic anemia due to ionizing radiation
    B. Aplastic anemia due to drugs and chemicals
    C. Pure red cell agenesis associated with thymoma
V. *Anemias due to marrow replacement*
    A. Anemia associated with leukemia and plasmocytic myeloma
    B. Anemia associated with metastatic carcinoma
    C. Anemia associated with lipidoses
    D. Anemia associated with myelofibrosis
VI. *Anemias due to defective heme synthesis*
    A. Sideroblastic anemia
    B. Anemia of erythropoietic porphyria
VII. *Anemias due to hypersplenism* (splènic anemia, Banti's syndrome)

1. Anemias Due to Hemorrhage

Anemia may result from acute or chronic blood loss. In a nonfatal sudden hemorrhage of up to 1500 ml., the anemia is of short duration. During the period of erythrocyte replacement the new cells are sometimes hypochromic. *Chronic blood loss* may occur with bleeding hemorrhoids, hookworm infestation, peptic ulcer of the stomach or duodenum, ulcerative carcinoma of the stomach, small intestine, or colon, ulcerative colitis, and hemorrhagic diatheses. The anemia is normochromic until body iron stores are depleted; then it becomes hypochromic. In the *bone marrow* following significant acute or chronic blood loss, erythroid hyperplasia is found.

2. Hemolytic Anemias

Anemias due to excessive erythrocyte destruction (hemolytic anemias) may be due to inherited intrinsic defects in the erythrocytes, to acquired auto-immune or iso-immune antibodies which react with antigens on the erythrocyte surfaces, or to certain hemolytic venoms, toxins, chemicals, and drugs. Inherited defects are present in, for example, congenital spherocytic anemia, hereditary nonspherocytic anemia, sickle cell anemia, and thalassemia; acquired antibodies cause, among others, auto-immune hemolytic anemia and erythroblastosis fetalis (discussed on page 368).

SPHEROCYTOSIS:

Congenital spherocytic anemia is inherited as a mendelian dominant. *Clinically* there are hemolytic crises with jaundice, fever, splenomegaly, spherocytosis, and an increased fragility of erythrocytes in hypotonic saline. The Coombs test is positive in only 20 percent of the cases. Nearly all these patients improve following splenectomy.

Pathologic changes

The *spleen* weighs 500 to 1500 gm. In a hemolytic attack it has a dark reddish purple outer and cut surface. *Microscopically* there are enormous numbers of erythrocytes in the pulp with relatively empty sinusoids; a prominence of the endothelial cells, especially the nuclei, of the sinusoids; normal-sized, spread-out follicles; and an absence of or small amounts of blood pigments. The bone marrow is hyperplastic.

HEREDITARY NONSPHEROCYTIC HEMOLYTIC ANEMIAS:

In the *hereditary nonspherocytic hemolytic anemias* the erythrocytic defect is not always known. Anemia is often present at birth. In the peripheral blood, oval and elliptical erythrocytes, anisocytosis, and poikilocytosis are noted. Osmotic fragility is normal, but the *erythrocyte life span is markedly reduced.* The serum bilirubin may be as high as 5 mg. per 100 ml., almost entirely indirect-reacting. Splenectomy is less effective in hereditary nonspherocytic hemolytic anemia than in the spherocytic form. The *spleen* is usually enlarged to 200 to 300 gm. *Microscopically* it shows distinct sinusoids without prominent endothelial cells. The red pulp is congested, but not to the extent seen in spherocytic anemia.

Due to pyruvate kinase deficiency

In some cases a *deficiency of erythrocytic pyruvate kinase,* inherited as a mendelian recessive, is found [31]. These patients frequently have severe anemia, which is exacerbated by stress and infections. Macrocytes and acanthocytes (erythrocytes with spurlike projections) may be found in the peripheral blood.

Due to G-6-PD deficiency

Glucose-6-phosphate dehydrogenase (G-6-PD) deficiency in erythrocytes [32] is transmitted as a sex-linked characteristic. Full expression of the trait appears in males and homozygous females. Among heterozygous females expressivity is variable. The deficiency is present in over 10 percent of Negroes in the United States and is common among Sardinians, Greeks, and Sephardic Jews. About 2 percent of persons with G-6-PD deficiency have a chronic hemolytic anemia without any demonstrable challenge, but in most such individuals the anemia is induced by a drug, an infection, or the ingestion of fava beans (favism). An *acute hemolytic anemia* occurs in G-6-PD-deficiency patients upon the use of pamaquine, primaquine, sulfonamides, acetophenetidin, nitrofurantoin, and menadione, or the ingestion of fava beans or naphthalene. Only aged erythrocytes are destroyed, and the anemia is self-limited even if the drug is continued. Inability of the erythrocytes to maintain reduced glutathione probably makes them vulnerable to oxidative stresses induced by the challenging agents. During the acute hemolytic phase the patient has jaundice, hemoglobinemia, and hemoglobinuria, and Heinz bodies are present within erythrocytes.

Due to other deficiencies

Rare cases of *hereditary hemolytic anemia* due to deficiencies of the enzymes hexokinase, phosphoglycerate kinase, adenosine triphosphatase, 6-phosphogluconate dehydrogenase, triosephosphate isomerase, glutathione synthetase, glutathione peroxidase, and glutathione reductase in erythrocytes have been described [33].

ELLIPTOCYTIC ANEMIA

Elliptocytic (ovalocytic) hemolytic anemia occurs in only slightly more than 10 percent of persons who have inherited the trait of elliptocytosis as a mendelian dominant. With or without anemia the blood of individuals with this trait may contain up to 90 percent elliptical or oval erythrocytes after the age of 3 months. This form of hemolytic anemia varies from mild to marked. Jaundice and splenomegaly may be present. Normal-shaped reticulocytes are found in the peripheral blood. Osmotic fragility of the elliptocytes is usually normal, and the direct Coombs test is negative.

SICKLE CELL ANEMIA:

Sickle cell (drepanocytic, Herrick's) *anemia* (meniscocytosis) is a hemolytic anemia of Negroes characterized by sickling of the red cells under reduced oxygen tension. The *sickling trait* is transmitted as an incomplete dominant and is due to the formation of an abnormal hemoglobin (sickle cell or type S hemoglobin). Another abnormal hemoglobin (type C) is often found with the type S hemoglobin in cases of sicklemia *(C-variant of sickle cell disease)*, and rarely hemoglobin D is present in sickle cell anemia (hemoglobin S-D disease). Only 1 in 40 of the 9 percent of American Negroes who show the sickling trait has clinical sickle cell anemia. Those with the trait are heterozygous in regard to the sickling dominant, and those with the disease are homozygous (i.e., the dominant was present in both parents). In persons with sickle cell anemia the erythrocytes are resistant to infection with the plasmodia which cause malaria.

Clinical features:

Signs of sickle cell anemia do not appear before the third month of life, by which time type S hemoglobin has significantly replaced type F. From infancy on, patients with sickle cell anemia have increased erythrocyte destruction, jaundice with a serum bilirubin level from 1 to 6 mg. per 100 ml., and increased urine and fecal urobilinogen levels. After a number of years, continued hemolysis leads to the development of hemosiderosis and bilirubin stones in the gallbladder. The disease is punctuated by *sickle cell crises. Vascular occlusive crises* may be due to local or generalized capillary stasis; venous thrombosis; and pulmonary thrombotic, bone marrow, or fat embolism. Focal capillary stasis may produce the hand and foot syndrome, in which these extremities are swollen, warm, and painful; recurrent febrile crises marked by bone and joint pains,

vascular occlusive crises

abdominal cramps, hepatomegaly, leukocytosis, and metabolic acidosis; hepatic crises with regurgitative jaundice; and priapism. The painful and febrile crises occur most commonly in children and appear to be triggered by infections, cold, and hypoxia. Pulmonary embolism is more common in adults than children. It is especially frequent during pregnancy and parturition. *Hematologic crises* may be aplastic or hemolytic in type. *Aplastic crises* result from bone marrow injury due to infection, drugs, or other causes of erythroid cellular injury. During such crises the patient shows weakness, dizziness, and signs of cardiac failure. Some patients show leukopenia and thrombocytopenia besides a profound anemia. *Hemolytic crises* are caused by infections, drugs, or other factors which induce increased erythrocytic destruction. The patient suffers a precipitous drop in the erythrocyte count and increased jaundice with elevated serum bilirubin and urine and fecal urobilinogen levels. In long-term cases of sickle cell anemia, leg ulcers are common. Skull films have a "hair-on-end" appearance due to the arrangement of diploic trabeculations as medial striations; the diploic space is widened due to marrow hyperplasia.

aplastic crises

hemolytic crises

Pathologic changes [34]:

Focal capillary stasis due to localized sickling may produce aseptic necrosis in *bones,* particularly the heads of the femur and humerus, the tibia, and the fibula. The *spleen,* which is usually enlarged early in the disease, suffers numerous infarcts with fibrous replacement or cystic degeneration. After many years it becomes very small, fibrous, and loaded with hemosiderin pigment. In the *liver* large amounts of hemosiderin pigment are found within Kupffer cells and hepatocytes. In patients with *sickle cell hepatopathy* (hepatic crisis with regurgitative jaundice), the sinusoids are engorged with sickled erythrocytes, and there is mainly centrolobular hepatocytic necrosis. After repeated episodes a postnecrotic cirrhosis may develop in the liver. The most common *kidney* lesion is papillary necrosis, most often in the left upper calyces. Erythrocytic sickling in arterioles and capillaries leads to infarction and sloughing of the tips of papillae. The resultant ulcers heal by fibrous scarring. Tubular epithelial degeneration and peritubular capillary engorgement and hemorrhage are frequently found. Iron-containing pigment deposits are found in tubular epithelial cells and glomerular mesangial cells [35]. Infarction and gangrene of the *small intestine* occasionally occur. Priapism results from meniscocytic engorgement of the cavernous sinuses of the penis. Small infarcts may appear in the brain, especially in the gray matter of the cerebral cortex. The cortical capillaries and meningeal veins are packed with sickled erythrocytes. Peripheral *retinal infarcts* occur due to capillary sickling and vasospasm. Retinal arterioles and venules become dilated and tortuous. The bulbar conjunctiva is pale, and the entrapment of sickled red cells in dilated vessels forms corkscrew-shaped, comma-shaped, or sausage-shaped sacculations.

generalized capillary stasis

Generalized capillary stasis is associated with sudden death in patients with sickle cell anemia and sickle cell trait. Capillary stuffing with sickled erythrocytes is found throughout the body. *Venous thrombosis* in cases of sickle cell anemia is found in splenic, portal, pelvic, extremity, and meningeal veins and dural sinuses. *Pulmonary emboli* composed of aggregates of meniscocytes, platelets, and leukocytes entangled in fibrin are typically small and do not cause pulmonary infarction. *Pulmonary fat and bone marrow embolism* results from focal necrosis of bone marrow and release of its elements into the bloodstream. Fat embolism is more common in patients with sickle cell trait and hemoglobin S-C disease than in those with sickle cell anemia. This is because the marrow contains fewer cells and more fat in the first two conditions than in the last. Capillaries of the brain and renal glomeruli may be blocked by fat emboli. Except during

venous thrombosis

pulmonary embolism

aplastic crises the *bone marrow* in sickle cell anemia reveals moderate to marked erythroid hyperplasia. In cases surviving for a number of years, moderate to extensive *hemosiderin deposits* are present, besides in the liver and spleen, in the lymph nodes, bone marrow, thryoid gland, lungs, myocardium, and kidney. Black, multifaceted calcium bilirubinate gallstones commonly form in the gallbladder.

bone marrow

hemosiderosis

THALASSEMIA

Thalassemia (Mediterranean or Cooley's anemia) is a hereditary hypochromic, microcytic anemia occurring predominantly in children of Italian and Greek heritage. Type F hemoglobin is usually present in larger amounts, and hemoglobin A_2, which normally constitutes about 2 percent of the hemoglobin, is sometimes increased in patients with thalassemia. The trait is transmitted as a mendelian recessive. Children in whom the trait is homozygous develop a severe and often lethal anemia *(thalassemia major)*. In those who are heterozygous, a mild form of the disease is found *(thalassemia minor)*. In thalassemia, flat target cells and elliptocytes are common in smears of the peripheral blood. The *spleen* becomes enlarged, weighing up to 1000 to 1500 gm., and may show foci of extramedullary hematopoiesis. Similar foci are found in lymph nodes. They consist of clumps of erythroid precursors and megakaryocytes. *Skeletal rarefactions,* especially in the skull, give a mongoloid appearance. There is a fullness of the cranial and malar bones due to enlargement of the marrow space. The *bone marrow* reveals erythroid hyperplasia. The skin may be yellow due to jaundice. Generalized hemosiderosis and even secondary hemochromatosis occur in some cases due to repeated hemolysis and blood transfusions [36].

The hereditary paroxysmal hemoglobulinurias will be discussed, together with the acquired forms, on page 290.

ACQUIRED HEMOLYTIC ANEMIAS:

Acquired hemolytic anemia is due to chemical or bacterial agents, malarial parasites, excessive heat (burns or heat stroke), circulating autohemolysins, or unknown causes. Among the known causes are certain snake venoms, primaquine, acetophenetidin, and sulfonamides. Drug-induced hemolytic anemias are discussed in Chapter 10. In acquired hemolytic anemia, spherocytosis may or may not be present. Hemolysis appears to result from a decrease in the tensile strength of the membrane of the erythrocyte in some acquired hemolytic anemias. In the primaquine drug-induced type it is associated with a deficiency of glucose-6-phosphate dehydrogenase in the sensitive erythrocytes. A few of the acquired hemolytic anemias will be discussed here in more detail.

Auto-immune hemolytic anemia

Auto-immune hemolytic anemia (AHA) [37] is caused by the development of an autohemolysin and/or an autohemagglutinin in the serum. The Coombs test is positive, demonstrating the presence of absorbed abnormal globulin on the surface of erythrocytes. In about 30 percent of the patients the anemia is associated with leukemia or a lymphoma, and AHA also develops in patients with other malignant neoplasms or collagen diseases. Only about 50 percent of these patients improve after splenectomy. About 40 percent of the patients with AHA show spherocytosis, and about 30 percent show increased osmotic fragility. The changes in the *spleen* are similar to those found in congenital spherocytic anemia, except that hemosiderosis is severe and congestion of the pulp with relatively empty sinusoids is found in only about 30 percent of cases of AHA.

Mechanical hemolytic anemia

Mechanically induced hemolytic anemia has occurred in several patients following insertion of intracardiac prostheses during open-heart surgery [38]. The erythrocytes appear to be mechanically injured by pounding against the unendothelialized surfaces of the prostheses used to correct valvular and septal defects. Hemolytic anemia has also occurred rarely in cases of calcific aortic and mitral stenosis. The hemolysis results from trauma to erythrocytes caused by the calcified heart valves. Erythrocytes with segments broken out and helmet-shaped cells are found in the *peripheral blood* in mechanical hemolytic anemia. The *bone marrow* shows erythroid hyperplasia. An auto-immune mechanism, with formation of an erythrocyte autoantibody due to mechanical damage or to the multiple blood transfusions given during such surgery, has been postulated as the basis for this form of hemolytic anemia [39].

PAROXYSMAL HEMOGLOBINURIA

Paroxysmal hemoglobinuria is characterized by sudden attacks of hemoglobinuria with fever and chills. *Precipitating factors* include syphilis, exposure to cold, and long marches among soldiers *(march hemoglobinuria)*. *Paroxysmal cold hemoglobinuria* is an acquired auto-immune reaction due to the presence of the Donath-Landsteiner hemolysin or of a cold agglutinin in the patient's serum. Following exposure to cold the patient develops a chill and fever, muscle aches, abdominal pain, and prostration. Reddish brown or black urine is passed for a few hours. This hemoglobinuria results from an acute hemolysis which may be slight, moderate, or massive. The direct Coombs test is positive during the acute attack. *Paroxysmal nocturnal hemoglobinuria* (PNH) [40] (Marchiafava-Micheli syndrome) is an uncommon inherited disorder characterized by episodes of hemoglobinuria usually occurring during sleep. Following such an episode the morning urine is red or brown. The hemoglobinuria is due to hemolysis of erythrocytes precipitated by a lowering of the blood pH caused by carbon dioxide retention during sleep. A deficiency of acetylcholinesterase is present in the stroma of erythrocytes in cases of PNH [41]. The disorder appears most often in the 20 to 40 year age group. It is superimposed on a chronic hemolytic anemia, and some patients develop a pancytopenia. *Pathologic changes* include hemosiderosis of the liver, spleen, lymph nodes, and kidneys. *Venous and,* less commonly, *arterial thrombosis* occur in the mesenteric, hepatic, and cerebral vessels. Infarction of the intestine, liver, and cerebrum sometimes results.

3. Anemias Due to Deficiencies

IRON-DEFICIENCY ANEMIA:

Iron-deficiency anemia ("tired blood") is caused by a chronic loss of blood due to an inadequate intake of iron, or to interference with assimilation of iron in the small intestine. The plasma iron content is decreased, usually to less than 35 mcg. per 100 ml.; the total plasma iron-binding capacity is increased. The anemia is *hypochromic,* the MCHC being 25 to 30 percent, and *microcytic,* the MCV being 55 to 75 cubic microns. In the peripheral smear the erythrocytes are small, pale, and often elongated or elliptical.

Pathologic changes

In severe anemia fatty metamorphosis is found in the *heart, liver,* and *kidneys.* The bone marrow is hyperplastic, about 50 percent of its cells being normoblasts. No stainable iron is present in the marrow.

PYRIDOXINE-RESPONSIVE ANEMIA

Pyridoxine-responsive anemia [42] is a rare hypochromic, microcytic anemia which, as its name indicates, promptly responds to vitamin B_6 (pyridoxine) therapy. Pyridoxal-5-phosphate derived from pyridoxine acts as a coenzyme in the synthesis of δ-aminolevulinic acid, a precursor of protoporphyrin. Almost all cases of this form of anemia have appeared in males. An hereditary or acquired enzyme defect may underlie the development of the anemia. Pyridoxine deficiency alone does not cause it. In pyridoxine-responsive anemia the liver and spleen are enlarged. Microscopically the liver shows excessive iron deposits in hepatocytes and Kupffer cells, minimal fatty metamorphosis, and portal fibrosis [43]. These changes are indistinguishable from those of primary hemochromatosis. The bone marrow shows normoblastic hyperplasia. The anemia is of moderate to severe degree. The erythrocyte life span is decreased, serum iron is elevated, and bone marrow iron content is increased.

PERNICIOUS ANEMIA:

Pernicious anemia (Addison's anemia) is a megaloblastic anemia which is characterized *clinically* by remissions and exacerbations, lemon yellow skin, achlorhydria and often paresthesias, spasticity, and loss of vibratory sensation. A similar anemia occurs in infestation with *Diphyllobothrium latum.* Megaloblastic anemia may also develop in pregnancy, the puerperium, infancy, hepatic disease, regional ileitis, and sprue, as well as following gastrectomy.

Pathologic physiology

In pernicious anemia there is deficient absorption of vitamin B_{12} (cyanocobalamin, *extrinsic factor, erythrocyte-maturing factor)* due to the absence or deficiency in the gastric juice of the *intrinsic factor* [44], which is normally secreted by the gastric mucosa. The intrinsic factor normally combines with vitamin B_{12} to effect its absorption in the ileum. About 40 percent of patients with pernicious anemia have serum autoantibodies against human intrinsic factor. *Folic acid* (pteroyl glutamic acid), another member of the vitamin B complex, is also a stimulus to erythrocyte maturation. Macrocytic anemia may result from a folic acid deficiency.

Blood picture

In an *untreated relapse* the erythrocyte count is 0.5 to 3 million per cubic millimeter with numerous macrocytes (erythrocytes 8 to 8.5μ in diameter). The MCV is usually over 100 cubic microns and the MCH is above normal, but the MCHC stays below 36 percent. The erythrocytes show anisocytosis and poikilocytosis. Typically, less than 1 percent of the erythrocytes are reticulocytes. Howell-Jolly bodies and Cabot rings are often found. Leukopenia (4000 to 5000 white blood cells per cubic millimeter) is usual, and there may be a "shift to the right" with large, six- or seven-segmented neutrophils (macropolycytes). A moderate thrombocytopenia also occurs, but purpura is not common. In the *bone marrow* there is an erythroid hyperplasia, with about equal numbers of megaloblasts and normoblasts. The myelocytes contain few granules, and the megakaryocytes are frequently large and agranular. With *effective therapy* the megaloblasts disappear from the bone marrow within 1 to 2 days, only normoblasts being present. In the peripheral blood the reticulocyte count increases and polychromatophilia is seen.

Pathologic changes

During a relapse the *bone marrow* is red and cellular, being composed of megaloblasts and normoblasts. Before the onset of a *clinical remission* the megaloblasts decrease in number and more mature forms appear. In full remission the bone marrow is normal. The liver and spleen are moderately enlarged and firm. The cut surfaces may be a rust brown. The Kupffer cells and splenic pulp are loaded with hemosiderin. In *untreated cases* of pernicious anemia the *fundus of the stomach* has a thin, semiopaque mucosa. The gastric glands are decreased in number and are cystic, the parietal cells being almost entirely absent. The interstitial tissue is increased in amount and infiltrated by lymphocytes. Similar, but less marked, changes are seen in the pyloric part of the stomach. *Small intestinal biopsies* reveal decreased numbers of mitoses in crypt epithelial cells, both cytoplasmic and nuclear enlargement of epithelial cells, and shortening of villi [45]. The *spinal cord* may be smaller than normal, especially in the regions of the dorsal and lateral columns. The posterior columns and the direct and indirect pyramidal tracts show degeneration of myelin and axis cylinders (subacute combined degeneration of the spinal cord). The *heart* may be dilated and hypertrophied, weighing 400 to 600 gm. The myocardium is pale and fatty. The *lymph nodes* are enlarged and contain hemosiderin deposits.

Effects of therapy

Liver extract or folic acid brings about remission of the megaloblastic hyperplasia of the bone marrow. *Folic acid* has no effect on the cord changes. *Parenteral vitamin* B_{12} *therapy* causes remission of the anemia and other symptoms. The small intestinal mucosa returns to normal in about 2 months.

ERYTHROPOIETIN-DEFICIENCY ANEMIA

Erythropoietin is a substance which is probably secreted by the granular cells of the renal juxtaglomerular apparatus and which stimulates the differentiation of bone marrow stem cells into erythroid precursors [46]. Its secretion is controlled by the oxygen content of renal arterial blood. In many types of anemia increased levels of erythropoietin have been found in the plasma and urine of patients, presumably due to the decreased oxygen content of the arterial blood. While *erythropoietin-deficiency anemia* has not been recognized as an entity, it is likely that decreased erythropoietin production by the damaged kidneys plays an important role in the pathogenesis of the *anemia of chronic renal disease.* Other factors, such as bone marrow depression by toxic metabolic products retained in the body during renal failure and hemolysis, probably also play a role in the development of this condition. The degree of anemia is roughly parallel to the extent and duration of the renal damage. The anemia is normocytic and may become profound in the late stages of renal failure. In the bone marrow, normoblastic hypoplasia, normal cellularity, or erythroid hyperplasia may be found.

4. Anemias Due to Marrow Inhibition (Aplastic Anemia)

APLASTIC ANEMIA:

Aplastic anemia (aregenerative anemia) is characterized by a marked decrease in or lack of erythropoietic as well as granulopoietic and megakaryocytic activity in the bone marrow due to toxic inhibition. It may be produced by certain chemicals and drugs (benzene, nitrogen mustards, sulfonamides, chloramphenicol, phenylbutazone, gold salts, urethane), physical agents (ionizing radiation), and unknown causes. *Congenital aplastic* (Diamond-Blackfan) *anemia* usually appears at the age of 2 to 3 months, is characterized by a severe anemia and slight leukopenia, and is idiopathic. *Familial aplastic anemia* occurs in children and is sometimes associated with the Fanconi syndrome. In the latter cases there are pancytopenia, mental retardation, and congenital anomalies such as dwarfism, microcephaly, gonadal and genital hypoplasia, and microphthalmia. Aplastic crises or marrow exhaustion may occur in the hemolytic anemias. Pure *red cell agenesis* (deficient erythropoiesis) without suppression of granulocytic and thrombocytic development may be associated with a thymoma, usually of the spindle cell type [47].

Blood picture

There is a marked reduction in the number of erythrocytes, leukocytes (often less than 1000 per cubic millimeter), and platelets in the peripheral blood. In pure red cell agenesis, only the number of erythrocytes is decreased.

Pathologic changes

The *bone marrow* picture varies from moderate hematopoiesis to complete replacement of the marrow by fat, fibrous tissue, or a gelatinous material. In pure red cell agenesis the marrow is normocellular, shows little or no erythropoietic activity, and contains lymphocytes with scanty basophilic cytoplasm. In the *oral mucosa,* gangrenous ulcers occur, with an acute inflammatory reaction showing few polymorphonuclear leukocytes. Foci of *extramedullary hematopoiesis* may develop in the liver, spleen, and lymph nodes. *Hemosiderosis* occurs in the liver, spleen, lymph nodes, and other organs because of the multiple blood transfusions often necessary in the therapy of the refractory anemia. Some cases of idiopathic aplastic anemia with widespread myelofibrosis (fibrosis of the bone marrow) eventuate in a myeloproliferative syndrome and develop agnogenic myeloid metaplasia, myelogenous leukemia, polycythemia, or thrombocytosis by neoplastic proliferation of foci of extramedullary hematopoiesis.

5. Anemias Due to Marrow Replacement (Myelophthisic Anemia)

MYELOPHTHISIC ANEMIA

Myelophthisic anemia is due to the extensive replacement of the bone marrow by (1) neoplastic growth such as multiple myeloma, leukemia, and metastatic carcinoma from the breast, prostate gland, kidneys, lungs, or thyroid glands, (2) lipid storage in reticuloendothelial cells (Hand-Schüller-Christian, Niemann-Pick, and Gaucher's disease), or (3) myelofibrosis (fibrous replacement of the marrow). *Extramedullary hematopoiesis* in the spleen and elsewhere may be prominent.

6. Anemias Due to Defective Heme Synthesis

SIDEROBLASTIC ANEMIA

Sideroblastic anemia is a rare, refractory anemia which appears to be due to abnormal heme synthesis in the bone marrow, possibly in the combination of protoporphyrin and iron [48]. There is a moderate to severe *hypochromic* anemia. The serum iron level is elevated, and large amounts of iron are present in the bone marrow and liver. Stainable iron is found within erythrocytes as siderotic granules, erythroblasts *(sideroblasts),* and macrophages in the bone marrow. Electron microscopy shows iron concentrated within erythroblast mitochondria [49], which are probably the site of hemoglobin formation. Most of the iron in the bone marrow is present in ferritin. The marrow shows an erythroid hyperplasia. Some patients who have survived for a number of years have developed a terminal acute leukemia or bone marrow aplasia [50].

ANEMIA IN ERYTHROPOIETIC PORPHYRIA

In *erythropoietic porphyria,* which is due to an inherited defect in porphyrin metabolism, a hemolytic anemia often occurs. Erythropoietic porphyria is discussed on page 278.

7. Anemias Due to Hypersplenism

SPLENIC ANEMIA:

Splenic anemia (Banti's syndrome) is characterized clinically by splenomegaly, anemia, leukopenia, thrombocytopenia, ascites, and hemorrhage from esophageal varices. The *basic cause* is excessive destruction of blood cells in the spleen or depression of the bone marrow by splenic hormonal secretion secondary to marked and prolonged congestion of the spleen (hypersplenism). In most cases this is due to (1) increased pressure in the splenic vein, which in turn may be caused by portal hypertension in cirrhosis of the liver; (2) cavernomatous transformation of the portal vein; (3) schistosomiasis; (4) thrombosis of the splenic vein; or (5) pressure on the vein from an aneurysm of the splenic artery.

Pathologic changes

Grossly the *spleen* weighs 500 to 1000 gm., although spleens weighing over 6000 gm. have occurred. The capsule is thickened. The cut surface is dry, fibrotic, and beefy. Tiny brown spots *(siderotic nodules, Gamna-Gandy bodies)* dot the cut surface. *Microscopically* dilatation of the sinusoids is marked. Hemorrhages in the pulp are frequent. Older cases show fibrosis by reticular proliferation. The Gamna-Gandy bodies consist of hypha-like filaments on which iron pigments are encrusted. Bamboo cane-like, pale green crystals are found, as well as intracellular and extracellular hemosiderin deposits. Splenic vein changes may be primary or secondary and include thrombosis, phlebosclerosis, endophlebitis, and calcification. The liver often shows portal cirrhosis. Esophageal varices develop through dilatation of collateral venous channels in the gastrosplenic ligament. Rupture of a varix may produce fatal hemorrhage.

EXOGENOUS PIGMENTS

Exogenous pigments may be inhaled, ingested, or injected into the body. The *inhaled pigments,* such as carbon dust (anthracosis), are discussed in the Pneumoconioses in Chapter 19.

ARGYRIA

Argyria is a permanent ashen gray discoloration of the skin and conjunctivae due to the precipitation of silver as an albuminate. The deposition of silver follows its prolonged use as medicinal salts or as argyrol nose drops. Silver is sometimes deposited as black pigment in the basement membranes of glomeruli and in the intestinal wall. There are no functional effects. In the skin silver is deposited mainly in the basement membranes surrounding eccrine sweat glands. By electron microscopy the metal appears as electron-dense bodies arranged in concentric rings in the basement membranes [51].

CAROTENE PIGMENT

Carotene pigment is occasionally dissolved in the lipids of epidermal keratin and the subcutaneous fat in sufficient amounts to give the skin a yellow color. This has occurred in individuals who eat large amounts of carrots.

TATTOOS

Tattoo pigments are injected into the skin for ornamental purposes by means of a needle. Tattoos with carbon, India ink, vermillion, and Prussian blue are permanent, while those with cinnabar, cochineal, aniline dyes, and ordinary ink fade with time. In occasional cases of serum hepatitis the virus is injected by a tattoo needle. Microscopically in tattoos granules of pigment are found between collagen fibers and clustered about blood vessels in the superficial dermis. Some pigment may be within the cytoplasm of macrophages.

THOROTRAST

Thorotrast (colloidal thorium dioxide) was injected as a contrast medium for angiography (outlining blood vessels by x-ray) and pyelography (outlining the renal pelves and ureters by x-ray) from about 1925 to 1948. Thorium is a heavy radioactive metal which emits alpha particles mainly. The intravenously or intra-arterially injected Thorotrast was deposited in the *liver* within the cytoplasm of parenchymal cells and enlarged Kupffer cells as granular, grayish brown pigment. In the *spleen* it was deposited diffusely in the red and white pulp, both extracellularly and within phagocytic reticuloendothelial cells. Similar deposits occurred in the *bone marrow.* Many reports of lesions attributed to thorium poisoning (due to the radioactivity) have been published. The lesions have usually developed after a lag period of 3 to 22 years following the use of Thorotrast [52]. They include hyaline thickening of the capsule of the liver and spleen, hemangioendothelial sarcoma of the liver and spleen, hepatocarcinoma, cholangiocarcinoma, granulomata in the renal pelvis, fibrosarcoma of the kidney, epidermoid carcinoma in a maxillary sinus, fibrosarcoma at the injection site, and aplastic anemia.

REFERENCES

1. Smith, J. C. Heme pigment metabolism: A clinicopathologic spectrum. *Med. Ann. D.C.* 37:353, 1968.
2. Allison, A. C., and apRees, W. Binding of haemoglobin to plasma proteins (haptoglobin): Its bearing on "renal threshold" for haemoglobin and aetiology of haemoglobinuria. *Brit. Med. J.* 2:1137, 1957.
3. Dubin, I. N. Idiopathic hemochromatosis and transfusion siderosis. *Amer. J. Clin. Path.* 25:514, 1955.
4. Kleckner, M. S., Kark, R. M., Baker, L. A., Chapman, A. Z., Kaplan, E., and Moore, T. J. Clinical features, pathology, and therapy of hemochromatosis. *J.A.M.A.* 157:1471, 1955.
5. Block, M., Moore, G., Wasi, P., and Haiby, G. Histogenesis of the hepatic lesion in primary hemochromatosis with consideration of the pseudo-iron deficient state produced by phlebotomies. *Amer. J. Path.* 47:89, 1965.
6. Morningstar, W. A. Exogenous hemochromatosis. *A.M.A. Arch. Path.* 59:355, 1955.
7. Bothwell, T. O., Abrahams, C., Bradlow, B. A., and Charlton, R. W. Idiopathic and Bantu hemochromatosis. *Arch. Path.* (Chicago) 79:163, 1965.
8. Gartner, L. M., and Arias, I. M. Formation, transport, metabolism and excretion of bilirubin. *New Eng. J. Med.* 280:1339, 1969.
9. Biava, C. G. Studies on cholestasis: A re-evaluation of the fine structure of normal human bile canaliculi. *Lab. Invest.* 13:840, 1964.
10. Sherlock, S. Jaundice. *Brit. Med. J.* 1:1359, 1962.
11. Israels, L. G., and Zipursky, A. Primary shunt hyperbilirubinaemia. *Nature* (London) 193:73, 1962.
12. Powell, L. W., Hemingway, E., Billing, B. H., and Sherlock, S. Idiopathic unconjugated hyperbilirubinemia (Gilbert's syndrome). *New Eng. J. Med.* 277:1108, 1967.
13. Stiehm, E. R., and Ryan, J. Breast milk jaundice. *Amer. J. Dis. Child.* 109:212, 1965.
14. Dubin, I. N., and Johnson, F. B. Chronic idiopathic jaundice with unidentified pigment in liver cells. *Medicine* (Balt.) 33:155, 1954.
15. Toker, C., and Trevino, N. Hepatic ultrastructure in chronic idiopathic jaundice. *Arch. Path.* (Chicago) 80:453, 1965.
16. Arias, I. M. Studies of chronic familial nonhemolytic jaundice with conjugated bilirubin in the serum with and without an unidentified pigment in the liver cells. *Amer. J. Med.* 31:510, 1961.
17. Kreek, M. J., Weser, E., Sleisenger, M. H., and Jeffries, G. H. Idiopathic cholestasis of pregnancy. *New Eng. J. Med.* 277:1391, 1967.
18. Schapiro, R. H., and Isselbacher, K. J. Benign recurrent intrahepatic cholestasis, *New Eng. J. Med.* 268:708, 1963.
19. Schmid, M., Hefti, M. L., Gattiker, R., Kistler, H. J., and Senning, A. Benign postoperative intrahepatic cholestasis. *New Eng. J. Med.* 272:545, 1965.
20. Bernstein, J., and Landing, B. H. Extraneural lesions associated with neonatal hyperbilirubinemia and kernicterus. *Amer. J. Path.* 40:371, 1962.
21. Sakaguchi, H., Dachs, H., Grishman, E., and Churg, J. Renal glomerulus in obstructive jaundice. *Arch. Path.* (Chicago) 79:512, 1965.
22. Tschudy, D. P. Biochemical lesions in porphyria. *J.A.M.A.* 191:718, 1965.
23. Harber, L. C., Fleischer, A. S., and Baer, R. L. Erythropoietic protoporphyria and photohemolysis. *J.A.M.A.* 189:191, 1964.
24. Cripps, D. J., and Scheuer, P. J. Hepatobiliary changes in erythropoietic protoporphyria. *Arch. Path.* (Chicago) 80:500, 1965.

25. Huang, S., Mengel, C. E., and Polt, S. S. Hepatic porphyria. *Arch. Path.* (Chicago) 79:394, 1965.
26. Fitzpatrick, T. B., Seiji, M., and McCugan, A. D. Melanin pigmentation. *New Eng. J. Med.* 265:328, 374, 430, 1961.
27. Lichtenstein, L., and Kaplan, L. Hereditary ochronosis. *Amer. J. Path.* 30:99, 1954.
28. Hill, R. L. The abnormal human hemoglobins. *Lab. Invest.* 10:1012, 1962.
29. Barnei, A., Jr. Erythrocytic inclusions: Their diagnostic significance and pathology. *J.A.M.A.* 198:151, 1966.
30. Necheles, T. F., and Allen, D. M. Heinz-body anemias. *New Eng. J. Med.* 280:203, 1969.
31. Oski, F. A., Nathan, D. G., Sidel, V. W., and Diamond, L. K. Extreme hemolysis and red-cell distortion in erythrocyte pyruvate kinase deficiency. *New Eng. J. Med.* 270:1023, 1964.
32. Beutler, E. Glucose-6-phosphate dehydrogenase deficiency. *Amer. J. Clin. Path.* 47:303, 1967.
33. Fairbanks, V. F., and Fernandez, M. N. The identification of metabolic errors associated with hemolytic anemia. *J.A.M.A.* 208:316, 1969.
34. Diggs, L. W. Sickle cell crises. *Amer. J. Clin. Path.* 44:1, 1965.
35. McCoy, R. C. Ultrastructural alterations in the kidney of patients with sickle cell disease and the nephrotic syndrome. *Lab. Invest.* 21:85, 1969.
36. Ellis, J. T., Schulman, I., and Smith, C. H. Generalized siderosis with fibrosis of liver and pancreas in Cooley's (Mediterranean) anemia. *Amer. J. Path.* 30:287, 1954.
37. Rappaport, H., and Crosby, W. H. Auto-immune hemolytic anemia. *Amer. J. Path.* 33:429, 1957.
38. De Cesare, W., Rath, C., and Hufnagel, C. Hemolytic anemia of mechanical origin with aortic-valve prosthesis. *New Eng. J. Med.* 272:1045, 1965.
39. Pirofsky, B., Sutherland, D. W., Starr, A., and Griswold, H. E. Hemolytic anemia complicating aortic-valve surgery. *New Eng. J. Med.* 272:235, 1965.
40. Gaither, J. C. Paroxysmal nocturnal hemoglobinuria. *New Eng. J. Med.* 265:421, 1961.
41. Auditore, J. V., Hartmann, R. C., Flexner, J. M., and Balchum, O. J. The erythrocyte acetylcholinesterase enzyme in paroxysmal nocturnal hemoglobinuria. *A.M.A. Arch. Path.* 69:534, 1960.
42. Bottomley, S. S. Pyridoxine-responsive anemia. *J.A.M.A.* 180:653, 1962.
43. Hathway, D., Harris, J. W., and Stenger, R. J. Histopathology of the liver in pyridoxine-responsive anemia. *Arch. Path.* (Chicago) 83:175, 1967.
44. Herbert, V., and Castle, W. B. Intrinsic factor. *New Eng. J. Med.* 270:1181, 1964.
45. Foroozan, P., and Trier, J. S. Mucosa of the small intestine in pernicious anemia. *New Eng. J. Med.* 277:553, 1967.
46. Stohlman, F., Jr. The kidney and erythropoiesis. *New Eng. J. Med.* 279:1437, 1968.
47. Schmid, J. R., Kiely, J. M., Harrison, E. G., Jr., Bayrd, E. D., and Pease, G. L. Thymoma associated with pure red-cell agenesis. *Cancer* 18:216, 1965.
48. Bell, R. E., and Shewchuck, H. W. Refractory normoblastic anemia with sideroblasts in the bone marrow. *Amer. J. Clin. Path.* 35:338, 1961.
49. Sorenson, G. D. Electron microscopic observations of bone marrow from patients with sideroblastic anemia. *Amer. J. Path.* 40:297, 1962.
50. Brittin, G. M., Stohlman, F., Jr., and Tanaka, Y. A primary sideroblastic anemia terminating in bone marrow aplasia. *Amer. J. Clin. Path.* 50:467, 1968.

51. Prose, P. H. An electron microscopic study of human generalized argyria. *Amer. J. Path.* 42:293, 1963.
52. Baserga, R., Yokoo, H., and Henegar, G. C. Thorotrast-induced cancer in man. *Cancer* 13:1021, 1960.

GENERAL REFERENCES

Ingelfinger, F. J. The liver. In Sodeman, W. A. (Ed.), *Pathologic Physiology* (4th ed.). Philadelphia: Saunders, 1967, pp. 672–680. (A discussion of the mechanisms of jaundice.)

Miale, J. B. *Laboratory Medicine – Hematology* (3d ed.). St. Louis: Mosby, 1967. (An imaginative approach to the anemias as well as a thorough treatment of the erythrocyte.)

Wintrobe, M. M. *Clinical Hematology* (6th ed.). Philadelphia: Lea & Febiger, 1967. (A standard and authoritative textbook on blood diseases.)

12 GENERAL DISORDERS OF NUTRITION AND GROWTH

NUTRITIONAL DISTURBANCES

1. Starvation and Related States

Definitions

Starvation is the prostrate physical state resulting from a prolonged complete lack of nourishment. *Inanition* is a state of physical exhaustion due to a prolonged lack of food. *Emaciation* is a physical state in which there is severe wasting of the body flesh; *marasmus* is a progressive emaciation, especially in infants. *Cachexia* is a general state of ill health and wasting, especially of the skeletal muscles, due to poor nutrition.

Causes

The *causes* of starvation and other malnutrition states include: (1) unavailability of sufficient food to sustain life or adequate nutrition; (2) failure to ingest sufficient food because of either anorexia (lack of appetite) or psychiatric reasons; (3) failure to absorb sufficient food from the intestinal tract because of disease; and (4) chronic debilitating diseases such as tuberculosis and cancer.

Pathologic physiology

In the starvation state the body reacts to make maximal use of adipose tissue as an energy source and to maintain protein reserves [1]. Glucose is excluded from tissues which can use free fatty acids as fuel. By means of the Cori cycle, glucose formed by the energy released by the oxidation of fat is shuttled to peripheral glycolytic tissues, such as erythrocytes and leukocytes. The glucose is converted to lactate and pyruvate, which is carried to the liver and remade into glucose. The brain spares glucose by using β-hydroxybutyrate and acetoacetate for energy. Eventually, however, in prolonged starvation, body stores of fat, protein, and glucose will be drawn on so heavily that wasting results.

Pathologic changes

In *starvation,* and to a lesser extent in the related states, there is a general atrophy involving numerous body tissues. The central nervous system, bones, and heart show lesser degrees of wasting than do other tissues. The fat depots are depleted, the fat cells within them becoming small *(fetalization of fat).* With marked depletion the fat is yellowish brown and translucent. The fat cells are collapsed and separated by a protein-poor fluid *(serous atrophy of fat).* The mobilization of fat from the depots may lead to *fatty metamorphosis of the liver.* Later the liver becomes quite small with tiny hepatocytes. In far-advanced malnutrition states, tissue proteins are catabolized, producing severe *muscle wasting.* A *granulofatty degeneration occurs in skeletal muscle in severe cachexia* [2]. The degree of degenerative change is variable and is not directly related to the overall weight loss. The muscle fibers are moderately to markedly shrunken and have a round or prismatic shape on cross section. Later the fibers degenerate. In all marked nutritional disturbances lymphoid tissue is depleted, and testicular or ovarian atrophy leads to aspermatogenesis or anovogenesis. The plasma proteins, especially albumin, may fall to a level so low that the plasma osmotic pressure drops and allows fluid to escape into the tissues *(nutritional edema). Signs of multiple vitamin deficiencies* are common in starvation states.

2. Kwashiorkor

KWASHIORKOR:

Kwashiorkor is a protein deficiency occurring in infants after weaning. It is usually seen in the underdeveloped areas of the world and especially in African natives. It is caused by the extremely low protein diet. In *marasmic kwashiorkor* [3] there is a combined severe protein and caloric deficiency.

Clinical features

Clinically kwashiorkor is characterized by failure to grow, a skin rash (especially on the axillary folds, inguinal regions, and buttocks), graying or reddening of the hair due to loss of pigment, edema (which may become generalized), diarrhea, steatorrhea, apathy, anemia, and signs of vitamin deficiencies. The *hair* becomes dry, thin, straight, brittle, and depigmented and may fall out spontaneously. When periods of malnutrition alternate with relatively adequate dietary intake, depigmented bands appear in the hair *("flag sign"). Laboratory findings* include decreased values for serum proteins (usually less than 4 gm. per 100 ml.) – the decreases are mainly in the albumin fraction, serum cholesterol, alkaline phosphatase, amylase and lipase, and blood urea nitrogen. The mortality rate is 40 to 80 percent.

Pathologic changes

The liver is enlarged and shows marked fatty metamorphosis. Hepatic fibrosis does not occur in uncomplicated cases of kwashiorkor, but occasionally a nutritional type of cirrhosis develops. In the pancreas and parotid glands, atrophy of many acinar cells occurs, with subsequent fibrosis. The small intestinal wall may become so atrophic as to be nearly transparent. The thyroid acini are small and lined by cuboidal epithelium. The skeletal muscles are atrophic and show varying degrees of loss of cross striations. The skin lesions are hyperkeratotic and hyperpigmented plaques which slough off to leave a "crazy pavement" pattern of depigmentation.

3. Vitamin Deficiencies

AVITAMINOSES:

Avitaminoses are caused by an absence or deficiency of one or more vitamins – the exogenous organic catalysts which are effective in minute amounts and are essential for the maintenance of the normal structure and function of cells, and whose biologic actions are intrinsically related to intracellular enzyme systems. *Vitamin deficiencies* may be due to: inadequate intake, digestion, absorption, and/or utilization; an increased requirement (as in pregnancy or during lactation); and/or an excessive loss by excretion. Vitamin deficiency results in primary changes, caused by metabolic disturbances in the tissues or organs physiologically served by the vitamin involved, and secondary effects (inanition, organ atrophy, and arrest of growth) on the body as a whole.

Avitaminosis A:

Vitamin A is a fat-soluble and fat solvent-soluble higher alcohol derived from carotenes. It is essential for epithelial cell integrity and the synthesis of rhodopsin (visual purple).

pathologic changes

The *basic lesion* is a squamous metaplasia of columnar and transitional epithelium *(keratinizing metaplasia)*. This occurs in the conjunctivae, nasal mucosa, paranasal sinuses, salivary glands, respiratory tree, pancreas, renal pelves, ureters, and uterus. *Follicular hyperkeratosis* occurs in the skin, keratin plugging of hair follicles and sebaceous gland atrophy being found. In the respiratory tree, blockage of bronchi and bronchioles by desquamated epithelial cells may lead to bronchiectasis (a permanent dilatation of bronchi). *Xerophthalmia* is a late lesion in which the cornea becomes dried, keratinized, ulcerated, and infected. It is due to plugging of the lacrimal gland ducts by keratotic debris. *Bitot's spots* are localized areas of xerosis (abnormal dryness of the conjunctiva). *Nyctalopia (night blindness)* is due to exhaustion of the visual purple in the retina, the lack of vitamin A interfering with its regeneration.

Avitaminosis D (rickets, osteomalacia):

Vitamin D includes several fat solvent-soluble sterols such as activated ergosterol (calciferol, D_2) and 7-dehydrocholesterol (D_3). The latter is formed in the skin by the action of ultraviolet light on its provitamin. Vitamin D enhances the absorption of calcium and phosphorus from the intestine and activates alkaline phosphatase in the bones, kidneys, and intestine.

clinical features

Clinically rickets is a disease of infancy and early childhood characterized by anemia, splenomegaly, flabby muscles, knock-knees, bowlegs, and poor formation of the teeth. The soft *femora* bend outward, the *tibiae,* forward. Kyphosis, scoliosis, and lumbar lordosis may develop due to defective calcification of the vertebrae. *Pigeon breast* (prominence of the sternum), *rachitic rosary* (a row of knobs at the costochondral junctions), and *bossing* (rounded eminences) *of the frontal and parietal bones* are common and are due to excessive osteoid formation. *Harrison's groove* appears at the costal margins below the pigeon breast due to the pull of the diaphragm. The serum calcium and phosphorus levels may be low. *Osteomalacia* occurs in adults, especially in women during pregnancy.

pathologic changes

The *basic lesion in rickets* is an abundant formation of osteoid tissue which fails to calcify. The bones, especially the epiphyses, are soft. The epiphyses widen longitudinally and laterally and are irregular. *Microscopically* the first changes are an absence of the layer of clear cells on the diaphyseal side of the epiphyseal cartilage plus the absence of an ingrowth of capillaries. The matrix between the degenerated cartilage cells does not become calcified. Cartilage cells are not arranged in rows, and the zone of proliferating cartilage may become 10 times the normal width. Prolongations go into the metaphysis, giving an irregularity to the epiphyseal line. In the zone of preparatory calcification no calcium is laid down. The broad zone of osteoid tissue resembles bone morphologically, but contains little or no calcium salts. Osteoid tissue extends into the perichondrium, causing thickenings. In the *healing process* there is an active calcification of osteoid tissue, and some of the thickening is resorbed. In *osteomalacia* decalcification of the bones occurs, especially in the lumbar vertebrae, pelvis, and leg bones. Compressions and bowing may occur.

Avitaminosis E:

Vitamin E includes four fat-soluble and fat solvent-soluble oils (tocopherols) which are antioxidant, preserving readily oxidizable vitamins and unsaturated fatty acids in the food, and are essential for normal reproduction in many lower animals. *Changes* in avitaminosis E *in man* are minor. In severe deficiencies, ceroid deposition in smooth muscle cells and decreased tolerance of erythrocyte membranes to oxidants, without evidence of hemolysis, have been observed [4]. In male mice there is a degeneration of the seminiferous tubular epithelium.

In female mice, degeneration of the placenta with death and resorption of the fetus occurs.

Avitaminosis K: *Vitamin K* includes two fat solvent-soluble naphthoquinones as well as several synthetic forms, one of which, menadione (K_3), is several times more active than the natural compounds. Vitamin K_1 is ingested in food, and vitamin K_2 is synthesized by intestinal bacteria. Vitamin K is essential for the synthesis of prothrombin in the liver. Serum prothrombin conversion accelerator (factor VII), Christmas factor (factor IX), and the Stuart factor (factor X) are also dependent on vitamin K. Deficiencies of vitamin K occur in obstructive jaundice, because of nonabsorption due to a lack of bile, and in the newborn infant, due to the absence of intestinal bacteria.

pathologic changes: There is *hemorrhage or inadequate clotting.* The former varies from petechiae to large hematomata. Hemorrhages occur commonly in the skin, muscles, gastrointestinal tract, urinary tract, and brain. Avitaminosis K is the most common cause of cerebral hemorrhage in the newborn infant, especially in association with birth trauma.

Avitaminosis B_1: *Vitamin B_1 (thiamine)* is water-soluble. It is an acetylcholine antagonist pharmacologically and plays a role in the normal function of nervous tissue. Vitamin B_1 is essential for the maintenance of a good appetite and gastrointestinal tonus. Thiamine pyrophosphate (TPP, cocarboxylase) takes part in oxidative decarboxylations leading to carbon dioxide formation. In thiamine deficiency the intracellular citric acid cycle is interfered with due to the absence of cocarboxylase. Methylglyoxal, which accumulates because of failure of utilization of pyruvate, may be toxic to the myocardium and produce the acute failure in Shöshin beriberi.

clinical features: *Clinically* thiamine deficiency may occur as an isolated *polyneuritis,* beriberi, or Wernicke's disease. In *beriberi* there is a peripheral neuritis characterized by loss of ankle and knee reflexes early, decrease in vibratory and position sensation in the feet, muscular weakness beginning in the feet, and calf and thigh pain. In *beriberi heart disease* the symptoms are exertional dyspnea, palpitations, cardiac enlargement, and signs of heart failure. *Wet beriberi* is characterized by anasarca. *Shöshin beriberi* [5] is a fulminant form of beriberi heart disease characterized by acute cardiovascular collapse and death within several hours. There are severe dyspnea, precordial pain, restlessness, anxiety, "stocking-glove" cyanosis of the hands and feet, cardiomegaly due to dilatation, hepatomegaly, and peripheral edema. Shöshin beriberi occurs in diets low in protein and fat and high in carbohydrate and occurs in the United States mainly in chronic alcoholics. *Wernicke's encephalopathy* usually occurs in chronic alcoholics; these patients show mental confusion, extraocular muscle palsies, and ataxia, plus signs of beriberi.

pathologic changes: In the *peripheral nerves,* myelin degeneration, fragmentation of axis cylinders, and even Wallerian degeneration may occur. There are degenerative changes in the motor cells of the anterior horn and sensory cells of the posterior root ganglia. The *muscles* supplied by involved nerves and nerve cells become atrophic. In *beriberi heart disease* there are cardiac *hypertrophy and dilatation,* especially *of the right atrium and ventricle.* The myocardium is edematous and infiltrated by lymphocytes. The muscle fibers show cloudy swelling and hydropic and fatty degeneration. In *wet beriberi* there is widespread edema of the subcutaneous tissues with effusions into the serous cavities due to cardiac failure and hypoproteinemia. Acute pulmonary edema is found in *Shöshin beriberi.* In *Wernicke's encephalopathy* there are lesions in the thalamus, hypothalamus, mamillary bodies, and nuclei of cranial nerves III, IV, VI, VIII (vestibular nerve), and X. In these lesions there is degeneration of ganglion cells, with surrounding hemorrhage. A slight glial reaction occurs, with formation of gitter cells (lipid-vacuolated microglial cells). The condition has been called *superior hemorrhagic polioencephalitis,* but it is not an inflammation.

Avitaminosis B_2

Vitamin B_2 (riboflavin) is a water-soluble vitamin which, combined as mononucleotides or dinucleotides, acts as a coenzyme. This coenzyme takes part in the production of important flavoprotein enzymes, such as succinic dehydrogenase. Riboflavin in retinal pigment participates in light adaptation. Pure riboflavin deficiencies are rare, since multiple B-complex deficiencies are usually associated. Attributed to *ariboflavinosis* are scaly erosions at the corners of the mouth *(cheilosis),* desquamations at the sides of the nose, photophobia, itching and burning of the eyes, and dimness of vision. The ocular symptoms are due to *invasion of the cornea by capillaries* from the limbic plexus producing corneal opacities, a late manifestation of the deficiency.

Avitaminosis P. P. (pellagra):

Nicotinamide is soluble in hot water; it is a component of coenzyme I (diphosphopyridine nucleotide, DPN) and coenzyme II (triphosphopyridine nucleotide, TPN). These coenzymes are dehydrogenases. *Nicotinic acid (niacin, P. P. [pellagra-preventing] factor)* is a vasodilator.

clinical features

Clinically pellagra is the disease entity produced by a niacin deficiency. It is characterized by symmetric hyperpigmentation and erythema of the skin of exposed parts of the body, followed by desquamation, and by diarrhea and mental disturbances.

pathologic changes

The *skin* is red and edematous. *Microscopically* there is marked hyperkeratosis, and granules of melanin pigment are found throughout the epidermis. The dermis is edematous and infiltrated with lymphocytes; its blood vessels are dilated. Similar changes are found in the *tongue* and *buccal mucosa.* In the *intestinal tract* there is submucosal lymphocytic infiltration. Atrophy and cystic dilatation of the crypts of Lieberkühn and of the mucinous glands of the colon *(colitis cystica superficialis)* are characteristic. The *brain* shows edema and loss of ganglion cells late in the course of the disease. Focal demyelinization of the lateral and posterior columns of the spinal cord and of nerve roots and peripheral nerves may occur.

Avitaminosis B_6:

Pyridoxine hydrochloride (vitamin B_6) is water-soluble. It is essential for complete tryptophan metabolism and takes part in fat and fatty acid metabolism. As pyridoxal-5-phosphate it acts as a coenzyme in the decarboxylation of certain amino acids. Clinical deficiencies are rare in man.

pathologic changes

The most common lesion is a *seborrheic dermatitis* about the eyes, in the eyebrows, and at the angles of the mouth. There are scaly, reddened plaques showing hyperkeratosis and hair follicle plugging. A *cheilosis* similar to that seen in ariboflavinosis also may appear. *Pyridoxine-responsive anemia* is discussed on page 290.

Other B-complex avitaminoses

Avitaminoses due to B_{12} (cyanocobalamin) and folic acid deficiencies are discussed with the anemias on page 291. Those due to deficiencies of other members of the B complex (pantothenic acid, biotin, inositol, and *p*-aminobenzoic acid) are uncommonly encountered clinically in man.

Avitaminosis C (scurvy, scorbutus):

Vitamin C (ascorbic acid) is water-soluble; it is essential for the development of intercellular substances such as collagen, reticulum, dentine, and bone matrix. Because of this, it plays an important part in tooth and bone formation, callus production in fracture repair, and wound healing. Ascorbic acid is needed for the maintenance of normal capillary permeability. It may play a role in the production of adrenal cortical hormones.

clinical features

Clinically scurvy is characterized by weakness, soft, spongy gums which bleed easily, looseness of the teeth which may fall out, joint tenderness, and multiple hemorrhages. Capillary fragility is increased. *Infantile scurvy* (Barlow's disease) is the form most often seen today. It usually appears in the latter half of the first year. Bone lesions predominate, and subperiosteal hemorrhages are so exquisitely tender that the child screams when touched.

pathologic changes

The *basic lesion* is the inability of connective tissue to produce and maintain intercellular substances (collagen, bone matrix, dentine, cartilage, and nonepithelial cement substances, including that of the vascular endothelium). Weakening of blood vessel walls leads to hemorrhages in the skin, mucous membranes, muscles, and lungs, under the periosteum, and into joints. *Bone growth* comes to a standstill and absorption continues, so that the bones become rarefied and fragile. The *bone lesion is a disturbance of ossification.* At the epiphyseal line the normal line of ossification is broadened and becomes dense. Bone fragments are scattered about, and hemorrhages are frequent. *Microscopically* there is little cartilaginous or bony matrix. Osteoblasts become spindle-shaped, proliferate, and form a thick cellular layer between bone and periosteum, with little matrix. Hemorrhagic areas are present.

4. *Hypervitaminoses*

HYPERVITAMINOSES:

Hypervitaminoses are clinical states due to an excessive intake of one or more vitamins as a fad, by mistake, or as a result of overexuberant vitamin therapy.

Hypervitaminosis A

Hypervitaminosis A in its *acute form* occurs from eating the liver of polar bears or other Arctic animals. There are abdominal pain, nausea and vomiting, severe headache, dizziness, and irritability followed by a strong desire to sleep. Within a day or two the skin peels. The *chronic form* occurs in persons taking over 50,000 units of vitamin A daily for over a year and is characterized by intermittent bone and joint pain, fatigue, insomnia, hair loss, dryness and fissuring of the lips, anorexia, weight loss, and desquamation and dusky hyperpigmentation of the skin. In children *cortical hyperostosis* (overgrowth of bone cortex) *and thinning of the epiphyseal cartilage of long bones* may occur [6]. *Premature ossification of the epiphyseal plate* causes failure of the bone to reach normal length. Vitamin A intoxication may also cause *pseudotumor cerebri* [7], especially in overweight adolescent girls receiving daily doses of over 100,000 units for several months as treatment for acne. Pseudotumor cerebri, as the name implies, mimics many of the signs of a brain tumor. There is increased intracranial pressure with headache and papilledema (a bulging forward of the optic nerve heads in the fundi of the eyes). In prolonged and severe cases blindness results from optic atrophy. Other signs of chronic hypervitaminosis A are present; these and the papilledema and increased intracranial pressure subside after withdrawal from vitamin A therapy. Experimentally numerous *congenital defects in mammals* can be induced by administration of large amounts of vitamin A during pregnancy [8]. Individuals ingesting huge amounts of carrots, tomato juice, and other foods containing large amounts of carotene will develop *carotenemia* (the presence of excessive amounts of carotene in the blood) and the harmless *accumulation of yellow carotene pigment in the skin.*

Hypervitaminosis D

Hypervitaminosis D is characterized by an elevated blood calcium level, decreased phosphorus level, and *widespread metastatic calcification* (the deposition of salts of calcium removed from bones in the renal tubules, lungs, and gastric mucosa). In the kidneys the hypercalcemia leads to impaired calcium binding or transport by mitochondria and mitochondrial swelling in the proximal convoluted tubular epithelial cells [9]. These changes are followed by the deposition of calcium in mitochondria, cytoplasmic vacuoles, and the basement membrane. Metastatic calcification together with osteosclerosis occurs in *infantile hypercalcemia* [10], which is probably due to an inborn defect in the breakdown of vitamin D in the body. *Renal stones* have resulted from prolonged and excessive use of vitamin D. Dihydrotachysterol, a derivative of irradiated ergosterol which is not a form of vitamin D but is pharmacologically similar, readily produces hypercalcemia.

Hypervitaminosis K

Excessive doses of vitamin K in children are associated with an increased incidence of hemolytic anemia, hyperbilirubinemia, and kernicterus (yellowing of the basal ganglia and other parts of the brain due to deposition of excessive amounts of bilirubin pigment). Rarely a severe hemolysis has resulted from intravenous administration of *phytonadione* (Mephyton).

B-complex hypervitaminoses

Thiamine administered intravenously has on rare occasions produced acute circulatory failure. Anaphylaxis occasionally occurs in patients sensitized to repeated thiamine injections. A hyperthyroidism-like syndrome (irritability, intolerance to heat, tachycardia) has been reported in patients on prolonged and excessive thiamine therapy. *Nicotinic acid* in excessive doses produces a selective vasodilation, urticaria, nausea, and vomiting; intravenous administration may cause circulatory collapse or anaphylaxis. *Nicotinamide* is not toxic, nor is *riboflavin.*

Vitamin C has no known toxicity even in very large doses.

DISTURBANCES OF GROWTH AND CELL DIFFERENTIATION

Growth occurs by the multiplication of cells. Within an animal or plant species the cells have a limited power of multiplication. *Cell differentiation* is antagonistic to growth, since cell division and cell function are not possible at the same time. The more highly differentiated cells proportionately lose their power of reproduction. The body cells can be classified as follows [11]:

I. Intermitotics
   A. Vegetative intermitotics (e.g., primitive blood cells)
   B. Differentiating intermitotics (e.g., cells of the stratum spinosum, secondary spermatocytes)
II. Postmitotics – cells which ordinarily age and die without giving birth to daughter cells

A. Reverting postmitotics – cells which can on urgent demand revert to the intermitotic state (e.g., smooth muscle cells, renal tubular epithelium)
B. Fixed postmitotics (e.g., neurons)

1. Congenital Malformations and Anomalies

Congenital malformations [12] are gross structural defects present at birth. Microscopic malformations, inborn errors of metabolism, or physiologic disturbance present at birth are included in the broader term *congenital anomalies.* One or more significant congenital malformation is found in 2 to 3 percent of all liveborn infants, and the incidence of congenital malformations appears to be increasing. The *causes* of congenital malformations and anomalies can be classified as genetic, chromosomal, and environmental.

CAUSES:

Genetic defects

Malformations with a genetic basis are directly traceable to a gene or genes inherited from one or both parents or a sporadic mutant gene. Such genes may be dominant or recessive. Achondroplastic dwarfism is transmitted by a dominant gene; cystic fibrosis of the pancreas is caused by a recessive gene. In some defects the mode of inheritance varies, appearing to be dominant in some families and recessive or sex-linked recessive in others. Recessive genes can manifest themselves in carriers, and persons may carry a dominant gene without showing its effects, due to low penetrance of the gene. A genetic malformation produced by a particular gene may range in severity from slight to marked, such a gene being said to have *variable expressivity.* One or more of the features of a syndrome of malformations typically inherited as a unit *(pleiotrophy)* may be absent or variable. Finally, many congenital malformations have a significant genetic background although they are not inherited in any well-defined pattern. Such defects appear in a higher percentage in the family of the patient than in the general population. Cheiloschisis (cleft lip), anathoschisis (cleft palate), and club foot belong in this category of malformations *inherited in a "nonmendelian" manner,* which makes up the largest group of genetically determined malformations in man.

Chromosomal abnormalities:

Recently tremendous interest has arisen in the group of *malformations associated with chromosomal abnormalities* [13, 14]. The 44 autosomes and 2 sex chromosomes of human cells are arranged in descending order of size and grouped as follows in the Denver nomenclature: group A (autosomes 1, 2, and 3); group B (autosomes 4 and 5); group C (autosomes 6 through 12 and the X sex chromosome); group D (autosomes 13, 14, and 15); group E (autosomes 16, 17, and 18); group F (autosomes 19 and 20); and group G (autosomes 21 and 22 and the Y sex chromosome). The normal female sex chromosome pairing is XX, and the male pairing is XY.

Chromosomal abnormalities may occur by failure of a chromatid pair to separate prior to polar migration in the dividing cell *(nondisjunction);* fracture of at least two chromatids during gametogenesis and reunion of the fragments with incorrect chromosomes *(translocation);* fracture of a chromatid during meiosis with failure of a fragment to reunite *(deletion);* fracture with upside-down reattachment of the fragment *(inversion);* fracture with adherence of a fragment to a chromosome which carries the same loci (specific gene sites) as those present in the fragment *(duplication, partial trisomy);* and development of a chromosome with genetically identical arms on either side of the centromere *(isochromosome formation).* Resulting abnormalities may be in the number of chromosomes in body cells *(aneuploidy, trisomy),* in the structure of the chromosomes, or in both.

Chromosomal defects may not always result in obvious developmental abnormalities.

The *causes of chromosomal abnormalities* are largely unknown. *Factors significantly associated* with such changes include *advanced maternal age* (except in Turner's syndrome); *congenital rubella* [15]; *maternal use of lysergic acid diethylamide* (LSD) [16]; *exposure of the parents to ionizing radiation or radiomimetic drugs* such as nitrogen mustard; and the *existence of a chromosomal abnormality in a parent* (the parental abnormality need not be similar to that occurring in the offspring). High doses of *cyclamates and cyclohexylamine,* a cyclamate breakdown product, produce chromosomal breaks in vitro in human leukocytes and tissue culture cells [17]. Chromosomal abnormalities are commonly found in the fetuses of *spontaneous abortions.* Some, such as trisomy 6-12 and trisomy 16, have not been reported during extrauterine life and appear to be lethal.

gonadal dysgenesis

In classic *Turner's syndrome (ovarian dysgenesis)* there are only 45 chromosomes, 1 sex chromosome being absent (XO). This syndrome includes bilateral ovarian agenesis, infantile genitalia, short stature, webbed neck, high arched palate, cardiovascular and renal defects, and cubitus vulgus (an outward deviation of the extended forearm). Variant chromosomal patterns in Turner's syndrome include $X^{\vee}$, in which there are gonadal but not somatic defects; X_{π}; XX_1; XO/XX; and XO/XY. In the rare *familial XY gonadal dysgenesis* [18] the patients are phenotypic females with uteri and gonadal streaks. In the *XXX (superfemale) syndrome* a high incidence of mental defect occurs in women with normal fertility. In *Klinefelter's syndrome* (testicular dysgenesis) (page 617) there are 47 chromosomes due to the presence of an additional X sex chromosome (XXY). The features include atrophy of the testicular tubules with persistence of the interstitial cells and gynecomastia (enlargement of the male breasts). A number of mosaic variations have been reported in testicular dysgenesis. In the *YY syndrome* the sex chromosomal pattern is XYY or XXYY. These patterns are seen in tall, chromatin-positive, mentally defective, aggressive, often criminal, males.

3/B translocation syndrome

The *3/B translocation syndrome* [19] is familial. The chromosomal abnormality is a translocation of a 3 chromosome and a group B (4-5) chromosome. About 40 percent of the offspring of female carriers are affected. Multiple congenital anomalies are present, such as cleft lip and palate, proptosis of the eyelid, ocular colobomata, interventricular and interatrial septal defects, renal hypoplasia, and muscular hypotonia.

cri-du-chat syndrome

In the *cri-du-chat syndrome* there is a deletion of most of the short arm of a B chromosome, probably 5. The infant shows a round face, microcephaly, micrognathia, and a mewing cry due to a faulty laryngeal development.

trisomy syndromes

The *group D trisomy syndrome* (Patau's syndrome) [20], in which there are 7 instead of 6 autosomes in the 13-15 group, is characterized by bilateral microphthalmia with retinal dysplasia, harelip, cleft palate, polydactyly (the presence of extra digits), trigger thumb (one which clicks at the metacarpophalangeal joint), interventricular septal defect, capillary hemangiomata, arhinencephaly, and cerebral and cerebellar defects. Anomalous nuclear projections are frequently present in neutrophils and eosinophils of infants with D_1 trisomy [21]. The level of fetal hemoglobin remains high, and hemoglobin A_2 is low beyond the neonatal period [22]. A high maternal age is frequently found.

In *Group E (17-18) trisomy* (Edwards' syndrome) [23] an extra autosome is present on one of these chromosomes. The affected infants have an elongated gestational period, but have low birth weights. Most cases die in early infancy. The *trisomy 18 syndrome* usually occurs in females and is characterized by mental retardation; flexion and deviation of the fingers; low-set, malformed ears; micrognathia (small jaw); a poorly ossified, short sternum; diaphragmatic hernia; diastasis recti (a defect in the rectus abdominalis muscle) or periumbilical hernia; limited hip abduction; muscular hypotonia at birth with later hypertonia; cardiac and renal malformations, especially patent ductus arteriosus; rocker bottom foot or pes equinovarus; and a prominent occiput.

mongolism

In *mongolism (Down's syndrome)* (see page 670) there are typically 47 chromosomes due to trisomy on autosome 21 or by reciprocal translocation involving this autosome. Some cases of mongolism have 46, 48, or 49 chromosomes. The infant has a small brain with defective gyri and a reduced number of neurons; slanting eyes; white flecks in the irides; fat cheeks and back of the neck; a protruding tongue; short thumbs; square palms with a simian line; markedly hypotonic musculature; and cardiac defects, especially persistent atrioventricular ostium ("mongol heart"). Acute or subacute leukemia occurs commonly (mongoloid-leukemic syndrome).

monosomy G

Complete monosomy G (21-22) [24], theoretically considered incompatible with life, has been found in a 5-year-old mentally retarded girl. She has wide-set, downward-slanting eyes; a small mouth; flared nostrils; and small, low-set ears. She walks with assistance, dragging the left foot. There is a positive left Babinski.

chromosomal abnormalities in malignancies [25]

In over 95 percent of cases of *chronic myelogenous leukemia* an abnormally small acrocentric chromosome *(Philadelphia or Ph^1 chromosome)* of the pair 21-22 is consistently found in the leukemic cells. About half a long arm is deleted, leaving 45½ chromosomes. In acute stem cell and acute myelogenous leukemia, various chromosomal abnormalities have been reported, including the presence of the Ph^1 chromosome. In *chronic lymphatic leukemia* most patients have a normal karyotype. However, some cases display absence or marked shortening of the short arms of chromosome 21 in lymphocytes and epidermal cells. This is the *Christchurch or Ch^1 chromosome.* It has also been found in a mongoloid child with erythremic myelosis eventuating in acute myeloblastic leukemia [26]. Aneuploidy is found in cases of *acute lymphoblastic leukemia,* the cells being hyperdiploid with more than 100 chromosomes each. The *Melbourne or M^1 chromosome* is a chromosome 17 or 18 with deleted short arms. It is found in lymphocytes in patients with Hodgkin's disease or follicular lymphoma.

Environmental factors:

Among the *environmental factors responsible for congenital malformations,* embryonic infection with the *rubella virus* is the best established. Among liveborn children of women who contracted rubella during the first trimester of pregnancy almost 20 percent are found to have congenital malformations; fetal death occurs in about 15 percent of such pregnancies. The incidence and degree of the teratogenicity (capability of producing fetal malformations) varies according to the period of maternal infection, being higher the earlier in gestation infection occurs. Rubella in the first month of pregnancy produces defects in about 25 percent of the liveborn children; in the second month, about 20 percent; and in the third month, about 10 percent. *Cardiac and ocular defects* are more common when rubella develops in the first 2 months of pregnancy, and *auditory defects* when infection is in the second and third months. About 0.5 percent of all births are congenitally deformed or abnormal because of rubella infection, and maternal rubella causes a risk for the fetus of death or defective development in 1:2 to 1:3 cases. Unfortunately maternal immunity to or protection against rubella by means of gamma globulin or convalescent serum does not necessarily protect the embryo against the teratogenic effects of the virus.

Prenatal infection with the salivary-gland virus of cytomegalic-inclusion disease causes congenital hydrocephalus (enlargement of the head due to accumulation of cerebrospinal fluid in the ventricles), microcephaly, microgyria, and porencephaly. Congenital malformations have been noted in cases of *maternal Asian influenza,* but these are probably related to the high fever and intensive drug therapy rather than to teratogenic effects of the virus. Studies on maternal infections during early pregnancy by the viruses of mumps, chickenpox, poliomyelitis, rubeola, and ECHO virus type 9 have shown no relationship to the development of congenital malformations. Fetal infection with the protozoan cause of toxoplasmosis produces congenital hydrocephalus, microcephaly, microphthalmos (abnormally small eyes), and cerebral calcification.

abortifacients and therapeutic agents

Unsuccessful attempted abortion during early pregnancy occasionally leads to the development of congenital malformation. *Quinine* has been implicated in the development of congenital deafness. The *folic acid antagonist, 4-aminopteroylglutamic acid,* used in attempted therapeutic abortions, has been associated with the development of anencephaly, meningocele, hydrocephalus, and cleft lip and palate. Conversely, congenital malformations may result from *attempts to avert abortion.* Cases of habitual or threatened abortion treated during pregnancy with oral *synthetic progesterone* have resulted in fetal *masculinization of female infants,* with enlargement of the clitoris and partial fusion of the labial folds. Several therapeutic agents have been indicted in the development of congenital malformations. *Thalidomide* used in early pregnancy caused a tragically high number of cases of *phocomelia* [27], in which the bones of the upper extremity are defective or absent and the hands or rudimentary fingers are developed like those in the flippers of a seal. *Tolbutamide,* used in the treatment of maternal diabetes, and *busulfan,* employed in maternal leukemia, have been reported as producing congenital defects rarely. The use of large doses of *cortisone* in early pregnancy has been related to the development of cleft palate in two infants.

maternal metabolic disorders

Maternal diabetes is associated with an increased incidence of congenital malformations. With the exception of *maternal iodine deficiency* which leads to cretinism, maternal nutritional deficiencies are not directly related to congenital malformations. *Maternal auto-immunization to thyroglobulin* with the production of antithyroid antibodies may be a cause of cretinism in the absence of iodine deficiency.

ionizing radiation

X-radiation and other types of ionizing radiation are notoriously teratogenic. The *use of x-rays* diagnostically or therapeutically *during pregnancy* has caused microcephaly, spina bifida, cleft palate, and club foot, and has been implicated in the development of leukemia in early childhood. In *pregnant women exposed to atomic bomb explosions* a high incidence of microcephaly and mental retardation has been noted in the offspring. Besides the direct teratogenic effects on the fetus by ionizing radiation there is the danger of *production of mutations in germ cells* which are capable of producing congenital malformations through many generations. Such mutations are induced by relatively small radiation doses. The mimicking of a genetically determined malformation such as microcepha by an environmental agent such as irradiation is known as *phenocopy*.

fetal hypoxia

The role of *fetal hypoxia* as a cause of congenital defects is questionable since children born at relatively high altitudes and those born of mothers with cyanotic cardiovascular disorders show no increased incidence of malformations, although their birth weights are somewhat lower than normal. However, gross malformations have resulted in animals from induced fetal hypoxia [28].

TERATA:

Monsters (terata) are grossly malformed fetuses with an excess or deficiency of parts. They may be classified as follows:

I. Monosomatous – a single fetus involved
   A. Pantosomatous – the whole or nearly the whole body involved
   B. Merosomatous – only a part of the body involved (These are discussed with the specific system involved.)
   C. Heterotopic – only the arrangement of the parts of the body altered

II. Polysomatous – two or more fetuses involved
   A. Twins joined by their umbilical vessels
   B. Twins joined more or less completely (double monsters)
      1. Symmetrically joined
      2. Asymmetrically joined

Panto-somatous terata

Microsomia (true dwarfism) is an abnormal, symmetric, and proportionate smallness of all parts of the body. It is due to a pituitary deficiency. *Macrosomia* (gigantism) is the reverse of microsomia, all parts of the body being excessively large. It is common when the mother is diabetic.

Hetero-topic terata

Situs inversus, a partial or complete transposition of the viscera, is due to an abnormal rotation to the left during embryonic life. *Dextrocardia* is the transposition of the heart to the right side of the body and is frequently associated with other cardiac anomalies.

Poly-somatous terata

Double monster is a united set of twins. *Symmetric double monsters* are called *Siamese twins.* They occur in about 1 in 50,000 births and are more common in females than males by over 2 to 1. The two bodies may be joined at different anatomic points in different sets. In *craniopagus* the fusion is in the head region; in *thoracopagus,* the thoracic regions; in *cephalothoracopagus,* the head and thoracic region; in *xiphopagus,* at the xiphoid process; and in *ischiopagus,* the pelvic region. *Dicephalus* is a two-headed monster.

Among *asymmetric double monsters (unequal twins), allantoidoangiopagus* is a placental parasite, the rudimentary twin being attached to the fetus by the umbilical vessels. The rudimentary twin may be amorphous or acardiac. In *parasitic fetus* the development of one twin is arrested, and it attaches to the other, becoming a *parasitic craniopagus, parasitic thoracopagus, parasitic ischiopagus, epignathus* (attached at the mandible), or a *sacral teratoma.* The parasite may be fairly well developed *(fetus in fetu)* or a mere jumble of tissues, as in the *congenital teratoma.* The latter may also be included within the body in the mediastinum.

Other malformations are discussed under the system involved.

2. Agenesis, Aplasia, and Hypoplasia

Agenesis is the failure of development of the anlage of a part, so that it is completely lacking. *Aplasia* is an almost complete lack of development of a part, so that proper form and structure are not acquired. *Hypoplasia* is a lack of development of a part to full or mature size.

3. Hyperplasia

HYPER-PLASIA

Hyperplasia is an increase in the number of cells of a part. It merges with the process of neoplasia (tumor formation). Hyperplasia may occur in response to chronic irritation (as in lymphoid tissue) or to endocrine stimulation, or it may be compensatory. It is present in certain viral diseases, such as verruca vulgaris. It occurs in reverting postmitotic and in intermitotic cells. The *liver* has great powers of compensatory hyperplasia. The remaining *thyroid* tissue may become hyperplastic when part of it is removed. The *bone marrow* is hyperplastic when there is an increased demand for blood. The *prostate* often becomes hyperplastic in men over 45, probably due to a relative hyperestrinism.

4. Hypertrophy

HYPER-TROPHY

Hypertrophy is an increase in the size of individual cells or fibers so that an organ is enlarged. There is no increase in the number of cells or fibers. True hypertrophy occurs in response to some demand for increased function. *Physiologic hypertrophy* occurs apart from disease; examples are the pregnant uterus (in which the muscle fibers are lengthened 10 times and broadened four times) and the muscles of athletes or laborers (e.g., a blacksmith's arm). *Adaptive hypertrophy* occurs in hollow viscera when the outlet is partly obstructed, the wall becoming thickened from enlargement of the muscle fibers; examples are the left ventricle in aortic stenosis, the stomach in pyloric stenosis, and the urinary bladder in urethral obstruction. *Compensatory hypertrophy* is an increase in size to make up for a loss in tissue, especially in paired organs such as the kidney. Thus, when one kidney is removed, the elements of the other (glomeruli and tubules) enlarge. The kidney also shows compensatory hyperplasia when its paired organ becomes atrophic or is excised.

5. Atrophy

ATROPHY:

Atrophy is an acquired decrease in size of a portion of the body, an organ, a tissue, or individual cells. The term is applied only when full size was once present, so that atrophy must be distinguished from hypoplasia, aplasia, and agenesis. In atrophy the reduction in size in a part may be due to a decrease in the number of its structural units or in the size of the individual units, or both.

Cause

Atrophy is caused by a change or disturbance in cell metabolism. Most often the change is due to interference with cell nutrition, either from an absence of nutritive elements or from an inability of the cell to absorb or metabolize nutrients. The *basic chemical mechanism* is probably increased intracellular proteolytic enzyme (cathepsin) activity due to a decreased pH resulting from anoxia.

Pathologic changes

The unspecialized connective tissues are less affected than parenchymal cells, so that the former often appear relatively increased. Besides, there is frequently fibrous or fatty replacement of lost elements. *Increased pigmentation* is common within atrophic cells, especially in the myocardium *(Abnutzung or wear-and-tear pigment).*

Types:

Physiologic atrophy includes those examples which are not pathologic, such as that of the thymus after puberty, of the inner zone of the adrenal cortex in infancy, or of the uterus and ovaries at the menopause. *Starvation* (inanition) *atrophy* has been discussed on page 299.

senile atrophy

Senile atrophy results broadly from aging, but the causes of such atrophy vary according to the tissues involved. Many changes are due to a *local decrease in blood supply,* as in senile atrophy of the brain, in which the gyri are narrowed and the sulci and ventricles widened. Loss of ganglion cells and gliosis are microscopic findings. *Changes in endocrine influence* cause atrophy in certain organs, such as the breasts and uterus. Such *endocrine atrophy* also occurs in the thyroid and adrenal glands, ovaries, and other organs controlled by the anterior pituitary in hypopituitary cachexia (Simmonds' disease). A *decrease in growth stimuli* leads to involution of lymphoid tissue. *Irreversible chemical changes* are responsible for the degeneration of elastic tissue in aging.

disuse atrophy

Disuse atrophy is local, resulting from inactivity of an organ or tissue. Forced inactivity of a muscle commonly leads to a reduced size. Neurotropic atrophy is due to muscle paralysis from destruction of its motor neurons, as in poliomyelitis. Bones also soon atrophy from disuse, as when a limb is immobilized in a cast; the bones become porous, with a decreased calcium content. Glandular organs, such as the pancreas, atrophy following occlusion of their ducts.

pressure atrophy

Pressure atrophy results from prolonged or continuous pressure on a localized area or cell group. Pressure interferes with the vascular and lymphatic supply, preventing cell nutrition. Such pressure may result from an expanding neoplasm (solid or cystic), amyloid deposition, an aneurysm, or hydronephrosis.

overwork atrophy

Overwork atrophy is uncommon, increased functional demand usually producing hypertrophy. Overwork atrophy may occur in muscles used constantly occupationally and in the accessory respiratory muscles in severe emphysema.

6. *Metaplasia*

META-PLASIA:

Metaplasia is a form of abnormal regeneration in which a type of cell different from that normally found in a given location is produced. It results from the regaining of the embryonal potentiality of cells to form different types of cells, and it occurs under certain conditions (chronic inflammation, vitamin A deficiency, and neoplasia). Metaplasia is principally found in epithelial and connective tissue. Epithelial cells can produce only other epithelial types of cells, and connective tissue cells, other connective tissue types of cells. Metaplasia occurs through the multiplication of cells such that the resulting new cells are of a different type than the parent cells. In general, cells of greater differentiation are replaced by cells of a less differentiated type.

Epithelial metaplasia

Epithelial metaplasia usually consists of the replacement of columnar epithelium by stratified squamous epithelium. *Chronic inflammation* may produce metaplasia in the bronchi, gallbladder, renal pelves (transitional to squamous epithelium), or prolapsed uterus. *Vitamin A deficiency* leads to extensive epithelial metaplasia of the respiratory tract, eyes, salivary glands, pancreas, and renal pelves.

Connective tissue metaplasia

Connective tissue metaplasia occurs mainly in areas of *chronic inflammation,* especially where there has been necrosis and calcification. Heterotopic bone is formed by fibroblasts which assume the character of osteoblasts. Bone trabeculae, often surrounding bone marrow, are formed. The mechanism is not known, but it appears to be some fault in the chemical organizers.

Endothelial metaplasia

Endothelial (mesothelial) metaplasia occurs when serosal surfaces are chronically irritated, the flat cells becoming cuboidal, columnar, or stratified. Gland-like spaces may be formed.

False metaplasia

False metaplasia occurs when the appearance of cells is altered by forces from without, as the flattening of columnar or cuboidal lining cells of a cyst by the fluid pressure or as the distortion and compression of cells in a rapidly growing neoplasm.

7. *Anaplasia*

ANAPLASIA

Anaplasia is the reversion of a more highly to a less highly differentiated (more primitive) cell form. It must not be confused with metaplasia which is an adaptation to recognizable environmental changes. Anaplasia is most commonly found in neoplastic cells.

REFERENCES

1. Cahill, G. F., Jr. Starvation in man. *New Eng. J. Med.* 282:668, 1970.
2. Marin, O. S. M., and Denny-Brown, D. Changes in skeletal muscle associated with cachexia. *Amer. J. Path.* 41:23, 1962.
3. Scrimshaw, N. S., and Béhar, M. Protein malnutrition in young children. *Science* 133:2039, 1961.
4. Binder, J. H., Herting, D. C., Hurst, V., Finch, S. C., and Spiro, H. M. Tocopherol deficiency in man. *New Eng. J. Med.* 273:1289, 1965.
5. Wolf, P. L., and Levin, M. B. Shōshin beriberi. *New Eng. J. Med.* 262:1302, 1960.
6. Pease, C. N. Focal retardation and arrestment of growth of bones due to vitamin A intoxication. *J.A.M.A.* 182:980, 1962.
7. Morrice, G., Jr., Havener, W. H., and Kapetansky, F. Vitamin A intoxication as a cause of pseudotumor cerebri. *J.A.M.A.* 173:1802, 1960.
8. Kalter, H., and Warkany, J. Experimental production of congenital malformations in strains of inbred mice by maternal treatment with hypervitaminosis A. *Amer. J. Path.* 38:1, 1961.
9. Scarpelli, D. G. Experimental nephrocalcinosis: A biochemical and morphologic study. *Lab. Invest.* 14:123, 1965.
10. Wilkerson, J. A. Idiopathic infantile hypercalcemia, with subcutaneous fat necrosis. *Amer. J. Clin. Path.* 41:390, 1964.
11. Finerty, J. C., and Cowdry, E. V. Cells and their behavior. In Anderson, W. A. D. (Ed.), *Pathology* (5th ed.). St. Louis: Mosby, 1966, p. 1.
12. Warkany, J., and Kalter, H. Congenital malformations. *New Eng. J. Med.* 265:993, 1046, 1961.

13. Eggen, R. R. Cytogenetics: Review of recent advances in a new field of clinical pathology. *Amer. J. Clin. Path.* 39:3, 1963.
14. Rowley, J. D. Cytogenetics in clinical medicine. *J.A.M.A.* 207:914, 1969.
15. Nusbacher, J., Hirschhorn, K., and Cooper, L. Z. Chromosomal abnormalities in congenital rubella. *New Eng. J. Med.* 276:1409, 1967.
16. Hsu, L. Y., Strauss, L., and Hirschhorn, K. Chromosome abnormality in offspring of LSD user. *J.A.M.A.* 211:987, 1970.
17. Stone, D., Lamson, E., Chang, Y. S., and Pickering, K. W. Cytogenetic effects of cyclamates on human cells in vitro. *Science* 164:568, 1969.
18. Sternberg, W. H., Barclay, D. L., and Kloepfer, H. W. Familial XY gonadal dysgenesis. *New Eng. J. Med.* 278:695, 1968.
19. Walzer, S., Favara, B., Ming, P. L., and Gerald, P. S. A new translocation syndrome (3/B). *New Eng. J. Med.* 275:290, 1966.
20. Patau, K., Smith, D. W., Therman, E., Inhorn, S. L., and Wagner, H. P. Multiple congenital anomaly caused by an extra autosome. *Lancet* 1:790, 1960.
21. Lutzner, M. A., and Hecht, F. Nuclear anomalies of the neutrophil in a chromosomal triplication: The D_1 (13-15) trisomy syndrome. *Lab. Invest.* 15:597, 1966.
22. Wilson, M. G., Schroeder, W. A., Graves, D. A., and Kach, V. D. Hemoglobin variations in D-trisomy syndrome. *New Eng. J. Med.* 277:953, 1967.
23. Uchida, I. A., Bowman, J. M., and Wang, H. C. The 18-trisomy syndrome. *New Eng. J. Med.* 266:1198, 1962.
24. Al-Aish, M. S., de la Cruz, F., Goldsmith, L. A., Volpe, J., Mella, G., and Robinson, J. C. Autosomal monosomy in man. *New Eng. J. Med.* 277:777, 1967.
25. Gottlieb, S. K. Chromosomal abnormalities in certain human malignancies. *J.A.M.A.* 209:1063, 1969.
26. Juberg, R. C., and Jones, B. The Christchurch chromosome (Gp-). *New Eng. J. Med.* 282:292, 1970.
27. Taussig, H. B. A study of the German outbreak of phocomelia: The thalidomide syndrome. *J.A.M.A.* 180:1106, 1962.
28. Ingalls, T. H., and Philbrook, F. R. Monstrosities induced by hypoxia. *New Eng. J. Med.* 259:558, 1958.

GENERAL REFERENCES

Arey, L. B. *Developmental Anatomy* (7th ed.). Philadelphia: Saunders, 1965. (A highly regarded textbook and laboratory manual of embryology.)

Follis, R. H., Jr. *Deficiency Disease.* Springfield, Ill.: Thomas, 1958.

Potter, E. L. *Pathology of the Fetus and the Newborn* (2d ed.). Chicago: Year Book, 1961, pp. 155–170, 203–233. (An authoritative discussion of malformations in general and of conjoined twins.)

13 HEREDITARY DISEASES

GENETICS – GENERAL CONSIDERATIONS

Inherited traits

Inherited traits are transmitted from one generation to the next by their representation in the *chromosomes* of the sex cell (spermatozoon or ovum). The hereditary material in the chromosomes is *deoxyribonucleic acid* (DNA). The molecular arrangement of DNA provides the chemical basis for inheritance of traits, i.e., the composition of the *genes.* Each genetic trait is represented by two genes *(alleles),* one derived from each parent. If the two alleles are identical, the individual is *homozygous* for that particular trait, if they are different, he is *heterozygous.*

Most known inherited traits are not diseases, but merely contribute to the physical individuality (e.g., height, body build, color of hair or eyes, contour of face, dental pattern). Some inherited traits, such as blood group or the ability to taste phenylthiocarbamide, are evident only by special tests. Even when there is no manifest hereditary disease, the altered molecular pattern of the chromosomes will modify the enzyme pattern involved in biochemical processes and may influence the course of acquired diseases, thus accounting for the individual variation in the clinical pattern of diseases. The unexpected finding that certain genetic markers like the blood groups occur with greater frequency in certain diseases (duodenal ulcer in group O individuals and gastric carcinoma in group A) suggests that *susceptibility* to certain diseases may be genetically determined.

Mutation

According to the chemical concept of heredity, a permanent, genetically transmitted variation (i.e., a *genetic mutation*) occurs when there is an alteration in the molecular arrangement of the DNA of the chromosomes of the sex cells. Mutations develop following *irradiation* by x-rays and other forms of radiant energy. They may result from replication errors or mutagenic chemicals in *embryonic life.* Although we usually think of genetic mutations as being harmful, they may be beneficial, resulting in *adaptation* to an unfavorable environment.

Genotype and phenotype

The *genotype,* or genetic constitution of the individual, is the sum total of the inherited traits, some of which are manifest and some not manifest but capable of being transmitted. The *phenotype* consists only of those inherited traits which are manifest in the individual.

Dominant gene

An *autosomal dominant gene* is expressed in each generation, affects the two sexes equally, and is usually heterozygous. Homozygotes generally demonstrate a stronger manifestation of the trait than heterozygotes. Examples of disorders transmitted by dominant genes are achondroplastic dwarfism, osteogenesis imperfecta, Huntington's chorea, neurofibromatosis, and renal glycosuria.

Recessive gene

An *autosomal recessive gene* is expressed only in homozygotes. The two sexes are equally affected. All children of two affected parents show the trait, and 1 in 4 children of two normal heterozygotes is affected. Examples of disorders transmitted by recessive genes are albinism, cystic fibrosis of the pancreas, galactosemia, and polycystic kidneys.

Sex-linked gene

A *sex-linked gene* is located on the X sex chromosome. A female may be homozygous with one allele on each X. A male can only be hemizygous. *Sex-linked dominant genes* are rare. Heterozygous mothers transmit such traits to sons and daughters equally. Hemizygous affected fathers transmit them only to their daughters. A *sex-linked recessive gene* is expressed phenotypically only in a male or homozygous female. Hemizygous fathers do not transmit such a trait, but their daughters are heterozygous carriers. The latter then transmit the trait to half their sons, and half their daughters are carriers. Affected females are the daughters of carrier females and affected males. Examples of sex-linked hereditary diseases are hemophilia, Christmas disease, glucose-6-phosphate dehydrogenase deficiency, and some cases of gargoylism.

Lethal traits

Lethal traits cause the death of the affected homozygous individuals in utero or during infancy. They are, of course, recessive traits, else the line of their transmission would disappear. It is likely that certain cases of abortion or infertility are actually instances of lethal traits. Slightly less serious are the *sublethals* which cause death of the individual, usually before the reproductive period; examples are osteogenesis imperfecta, amaurotic familial idiocy (Tay-Sachs disease), xeroderma pigmentosum, and epiloia (tuberous sclerosis).

Sports

Diseases that are usually inherited may appear de novo in an individual and subsequently appear in his family. These *sports* have been explained on the basis of mutation in spermatozoa or ova, induced by some new harmful influence.

Multi-organ defects

Occasionally *abnormalities of several organs* are associated in a genetic pattern, as epiloia, in which a peculiar nodular gliosis of the brain (tuberous sclerosis) is often associated with an acne-like skin eruption (adenoma sebaceum) and hamartomas of the heart and kidney; this may mean that the determining genes are located in close proximity in the chromosomes.

Types of hereditary disease: blood

Hemophilia is a sex-linked hereditary defect in blood coagulation. Sickle cell anemia is a hemolytic anemia of Negroes due to a molecular abnormality in the hemoglobin. Mediterranean anemia (thalassemia) is a hemolytic anemia of peoples of Greek and Italian origin, inherited as a simple recessive trait.

metabolism

Diabetes mellitus, agammaglobulinemia, lipoid storage diseases, gout, and undoubtedly many other metabolic disorders have a genetic component, but in most of these the trait has not been precisely defined.

skeleton

Multiple cartilagenous exostoses, chondrodystrophy, and brachydactyly are inherited as simple dominant traits; they are not sex-linked.

Progressive muscular dystrophy, pseudohypertrophic muscular dystrophy, Friedreich's ataxia, and hepatolenticular degeneration (Wilson's disease) are inherited, mostly as recessive traits, but variably. neuro-muscular

Ichthyosis congenita is transmitted as a lethal recessive trait. Xeroderma pigmentosum is a sublethal recessive trait; multiple skin carcinomas develop in exposed skin surfaces. Albinism is usually a recessive trait, often associated with inherited eye disease. skin

Color blindness, coloboma of the iris, retinitis pigmentosa, and retinoblastoma are examples of eye diseases that are genetically determined. eye

Many hereditary diseases are discussed elsewhere. Those in which there is a congenital deficiency of a coagulation factor are treated in Chapter 2; the hemoglobinopathies and porphyrias in Chapter 11; neurologic diseases in Chapter 26; and individual disorders as indicated in the index. Chromosomal abnormalities are discussed on page 306. In general, only those disorders which are not covered elsewhere are included in the remainder of this chapter.

HEREDITARY ENZYME DEFECTS

1. Disturbances in Amino Acid Metabolism

Phenylketonuria (PKU, phenylpyruvic oligophrenia) occurs about once in 10,000 births and in 1 percent of mental defectives. It is transmitted by a rare recessive gene. There is a *block in the conversion of phenylalanine to tyrosine due to a deficiency of phenylalanine hydroxylase.* Phenylalanine accumulates in the blood and cerebrospinal fluid. The excess is converted to phenylpyruvic acid, and this in turn is changed to other aromatic acids. In an unknown way the phenylalanine in excess, or one of its products, damages neurons, producing mental deficiency, convulsions, and EEG changes. The intelligence quotient is usually less than 30. Children with phenylketonuria are often blue-eyed blondes, the light skin and eye pigmentation being due to decreased melanin pigmentation. PHENYL-KETO-NURIA

Tyrosinosis [1] is very rare. Transmission is by an autosomal recessive. Large amounts of *p*-hydroxyphenylpyruvic acid are excreted, apparently due to *absence of* p-*hydroxyphenylpyruvic oxidase.* Hepatomegaly and splenomegaly appear early in infancy. Death due to postnecrotic cirrhosis and hepatic failure may occur in early childhood. TYRO-SINOSIS

Ochronosis (alkaptonuria) is usually transmitted by an autosomal recessive gene, 1 in 4 children in a family being affected. A few cases are transmitted by a simple dominant. There is a *deficiency of homogentisic acid oxidase,* so that the conversion of homogentisic acid to maleylacetoacetate is blocked. Black melanin-like pigments deposited in the sclerae, ear and nasal cartilages, and tendons appear in the second or third decade. Ochronotic arthritis develops by middle age, especially in the spine. This enzymatic defect is compatible with long life. Ochronosis is also discussed on page 281. OCHRO-NOSIS

Albinism is a generalized or localized decrease or absence of melanin pigment formation. In *universal albinism* melanin is absent in hair, skin, uvea, and retina. ALBI-NISM:

Generalized albinism is similar, except that melanin is present in the iris and sometimes in the skin. Both types are transmitted as an autosomal recessive. The albinism is due to the *absence of tyrosinase* in melanocytes, which are present in normal numbers. The conversion of tyrosine to dihydroxyphenylalanine quinone is blocked. Patients have white or pale yellow hair, red pupils, and pink or bluish irides. They are usually subnormal mentally.

Partial albinism

Partial albinism is due to the absence of pigment in certain parts of the body. *Piebald albinism* and *white forelock* with skin spotting are transmitted as autosomal dominants. *Ocular albinism,* in which there is an absence of retinal pigment, is a sex-linked recessive trait in males. Heterozygous carriers show a stippled chocolate-brown macular pigmentation.

MAPLE SYRUP URINE DISEASE

Maple syrup urine disease [2] is transmitted as a recessive. On the third to fifth day of life, signs appear. These are absence of the Moro reflex, irregular jerky respirations, spasticity, and opisthotonos. The urine has the odor of maple syrup. Its cause is a *deficiency of branched-chain ketoacid decarboxylase.* Valine, leucine, and isoleucine are markedly increased and threonine, serine, and alanine are decreased in the blood and urine. The defect lies in the oxidative decarboxylation of branch-chained amino acids. Death occurs within a few weeks or months. At autopsy the brain is edematous and shows gliosis and defective myelinization in the white matter.

ISOVALERIC ACIDEMIA

Isovaleric acidemia [3] is a disorder of leucine metabolism caused by a *deficiency of isovaleryl-CoA dehydrogenase.* The short-chain fatty isovaleric acid, a leucine metabolite, accumulates in body fluids. *Clinically* the affected children have periodic episodes of acidosis and coma, with intensification of an offensive body odor characteristic of isovaleric acid. There is also slight mental retardation.

HYPERVALINEMIA

Hypervalinemia [4] is due to a *deficiency of valine transaminase.* Vomiting, failure to gain weight normally, and mental retardation appear in infancy. The hereditary pattern is unknown.

ORNITHINE CYCLE DISTURBANCES

Disturbances of the ornithine cycle include *hypoammonemia* associated with ornithine transcarbamylase deficiency, in which the conversion of ornithine to citrulline is blocked; citrullinuria; argininosuccinic aciduria; and lysine intolerance. In *citrullinuria* there is a deficiency of the enzyme which converts citrulline to argininosuccinic acid, so that there is an increase of the former in plasma, urine, and cerebrospinal fluid. A marked mental defect is present. *Argininosuccinic aciduria* is probably transmitted as a recessive and is due to a deficiency of argininosuccinase. There is a block in the conversion of argininosuccinic acid to arginine. The former is present in high levels in the urine and cerebrospinal fluid. Clinically there are mental retardation, convulsions, and brittle nails and hair. In *lysine intolerance,* vomiting and coma, with elevated serum lysine and ammonia and blood urea nitrogen, develop shortly after birth. Lysine inhibits arginase activity, so that urea formation is slow.

METHIONINE METABOLISM DISTURBANCES:

Normally methionine is converted to homocysteine by demethylation, and then combination with serine produces cystathionine. *Disturbances of methionine metabolism* are homocystinuria and cystathioninuria.

Homocystinuria

Homocystinuria [5] is due to a *deficiency of hepatic cystathionine synthetase,* so that homocystine builds up in the blood and overflows into the urine. Its heredity is unknown. Clinically there are severe mental retardation (the intelligence quotient may be less than 30), ectopia lentis, fine hair, bone changes, and thromboembolism. *Pathologic changes* include focal necrosis and gliosis in the brain; degeneration of the zonular ligaments of the lens; fatty metamorphosis of the liver; arachnodactyly, osteoporosis, or pectus excavatum; elastic degeneration and patchy fibrosis of arteries [6]; and arterial thrombosis and embolism with infarction.

Cystathio-ninuria

Cystathioninuria is rare, and its heredity is unknown. There is a *deficiency of the hepatic enzymes cystathionase and homoserine dehydratase.* The conversion of cystathionine to cystine and homoserine is blocked so that cystathionine accumulates in tissues and is excreted in the urine. Mental retardation is severe. Cystathioninuria occurs with other defects such as iminoglycinuria [7], phenylketonuria, and nephrogenic diabetes insipidus.

HISTIDI-NEMIA

Histidinemia [8] is probably transmitted as an autosomal recessive and appears to be due to a *deficiency of histidase.* The conversion of histidine to urocanic acid is blocked, and there is an increased concentration of histidine in blood and urine. The urine may give a false positive ferric chloride test for phenylketonuria. Mental and/or speech retardation occurs.

HYPER-GLY-CINEMIA

Hyperglycinemia is apparently due to *absence of an enzyme for conversion of glycine to serine.* The level of glycine is increased in blood and urine. Clinically there are episodes of vomiting, dehydration, and ketosis; decreased serum gamma globulin, with multiple infections; neutropenia and thrombocytopenia; and retardation of development.

HYPER-PRO-LINEMIA

Hyperprolinemia [9] is probably due to a *deficiency of proline dehydrogenase* so that there is a block in the conversion of proline to pyrroline-5-carboxylic acid. The blood and urine levels of proline are increased. There are mental retardation, convulsions, hearing loss, and renal hypoplasia.

HYDROXY-PRO-LINEMIA

Hydroxyprolinemia results from a *deficiency of hydroxyproline oxidase.* A marked increase of hydroxyproline is found in serum and urine. There is severe mental retardation.

HYPER-SARCO-SINEMIA

Hypersarcosinemia [10] is a rare metabolic disorder characterized by increased levels of sarcosine in the blood and urine. Its genetic pattern is unclear. The cause is assumed to be a *deficiency of sarcosine dehydrogenase,* so that the conversion of sarcosine to glycine is blocked. *Clinically* there are tremors, muscle weakness, and moderate mental retardation.

CARNO-SINEMIA

Carnosinemia [11] is rare and is presumed to be due to a *deficiency of carnosinase.* There is a failure of hydrolysis of carnosine (β-alanyl histidine) to β-alanine and histidine, so that carnosine levels in the blood and urine are elevated. Increased levels persist in some patients even when meat and other dietary sources of carnosine are withheld; therefore carnosine must be released from skeletal muscle. High concentrations of homocarnosine are found in the cerebrospinal fluid. *Clinically* twitching and convulsions begin in infancy. There is severe physical and mental retardation. Similar clinical features plus somnolence were present in an infant in whom hyper-β-alaninemia and markedly elevated urine levels of β-alanine, β-amino-isobutyric acid, and taurine were found [12]. Abnormal amounts of γ-aminobutyric acid were present in body fluids. Increased tissue carnosine concentrations were found post mortem. It is postulated that a *deficiency of β-alanine-α-ketoglutarate transaminase* leads to accumulation of β-alanine, with consequent increased carnosine production.

ORGANIC ACIDURIA

Organic aciduria (Lowe's syndrome) is probably transmitted as a sex-linked intermediate trait. All cases have occurred in males, but heterozygous females may develop lenticular cataracts. Its cause is unknown. There are marked aminoaciduria, proteinuria, alkaline urine, and decreased ammonia excretions. Affected children show "snowflake" cortical lenticular cataracts, glaucoma, moderate to marked mental and physical retardation, decreased muscle tone, a high-pitched cry, and signs of rickets.

2. Disturbances in Carbohydrate Metabolism

PENTOSURIA

Pentosuria (*l*-xyloketosuria) is transmitted by an autosomal recessive gene. It is probably due to a *deficiency of* the mitochondrial enzyme *NADP-xylitol dehydrogenase.* The conversion of *l*-xylulose to *d*-xylulose is blocked, so that the former accumulates in the urine. The condition occurs in healthy individuals following the eating of large amounts of fruits and berries, as well as in some patients with muscular dystrophy. There is no clinical manifestation.

FRUCTOSURIA

Essential fructosuria is extremely rare and is transmitted as a recessive. It is probably the result of a *deficiency of hepatic fructokinase.* There is usually no clinical manifestation.

FRUCTOSE INTOLERANCE

Hereditary fructose intolerance (aldolase deficiency) is transmitted as an autosomal recessive. It is due to a *deficiency of hepatic aldolase.* When the patient ingests fructose in fruits or cane sugar, nausea, vomiting, substernal pain, excessive sweating, tremors, coma, and convulsions develop. With continued eating of such foods, hepatic cirrhosis and mental retardation may appear. There is prolonged fructosemia with hypoglycemia. The blood sugar may fall as low as 10 mg. per 100 ml.

GALACTOSEMIA

Galactosemia [13] is rare and is transmitted by an autosomal recessive. It is *due to a deficiency of galactose-1-phosphate-uridyl transferase needed for one step in the conversion of galactose to glucose.* After a few days of milk ingestion, the infant vomits, fails to gain weight, and develops hepatomegaly. Jaundice is common, and ascites and edema may occur. After several months mental retardation and lenticular cataracts appear. Except for the mental defect the changes are largely reversible on a galactose-free diet. In fatal cases the liver shows severe fatty metamorphosis. There may be a pseudoglandular transformation of hepatocytes with giant cell formation [14]. In the brain, loss of neurons and gliosis may develop in the cerebral cortex, basal ganglia, dentate nucleus of the cerebellum, and olivary nuclei of the medulla.

GLYCOGEN STORAGE DISEASES:

Glycogen storage diseases [15] are congenital and familial disorders typified by the deposition of large amounts of glycogen in the tissues because of specific enzyme defects.

Type I (von Gierke's disease)

Type I glycogen storage disease (von Gierke's disease) [16] is probably transmitted by an autosomal recessive gene. *Its cause is a deficiency of glucose-6-phosphatase,* so that the conversion of glucose-6-phosphate to glucose is blocked. Hepatomegaly develops in the first year. Later weight loss, vomiting, marked hypoglycemia, convulsions, and coma develop. The response of the blood sugar to epinephrine injection is slight or absent. Large amounts of glycogen are deposited in the liver and kidneys.

Type II (Pompe's disease)

Type II (generalized glycogen storage disease, Pompe's disease) [17] is probably transmitted as a rare recessive gene. It is *due to a deficiency of α (1 → 4)-glucosidase* (acid maltase). Signs, such as failure to gain weight, periods of cyanosis and dyspnea, and globular heart on x-ray, and left-axis deviation on ECG, appear in early infancy. The heart is two to five times its normal weight. The myocardial fibers are filled with glycogen, which is also found in skeletal and smooth muscle fibers and may appear in almost any tissue. In the liver the hepatocytes are somewhat enlarged and stain palely. The nuclei are central in position. By electron microscopy glycogen is both dispersed through the cytoplasm and packed within lysosomes. In the kidneys lysosomal glycogen is found in glomerular epithelial and mesangial cells and in the epithelium of distal convoluted and collecting tubules [18].

Type III (Forbes' disease)

Type III glycogenosis (limit dextrinosis, Forbes' disease) is *due to a deficiency of the debrancher enzyme, amylo-1,6-glucosidase* and/or oligo-(1,4 → 1,4)-glucantransferase. The mode of transmission is unknown. Progressive hepatomegaly develops in childhood. Retarded growth, a doll-like facies, and fasting hypoglycemia are also present. Liver biopsies show hepatocytes filled with glycogen and slight periportal fibrosis. In *skeletal muscle,* glycogen is deposited in sarcolemmal outpouchings and, to a lesser degree, within muscle fibers. Electron microscopy demonstrates glycogen deposits beneath the sarcolemmal membrane, between myofibrils, and between I and A band filaments [19]. Cardiac muscle fibers contain glycogen deposits. The amount of glycogen which accumulates in skeletal and cardiac muscle does not disturb their functioning.

Type IV (Andersen's disease)

Type IV (amylopectinosis, Andersen's disease) [20] is apparently *due to a deficiency of the brancher enzyme, amylo-(1,4 → 1,6)-transglucosidase or* α-1,4-glucan; α-1,4-glucan 6-glycosyl transferase [21]. Signs appear in late infancy or early childhood. There are edema, ascites, hemorrhages, and abnormal hepatic function tests. The blood sugar is normal. Death occurs by the age of 10 years. The liver shows a finely nodular cirrhosis with large amounts of glycogen in the hepatocytes. The reticuloendothelial cells in the spleen, lymph nodes, and intestinal lymph follicles are filled with glycogen. The glycogen in this disorder is sticky and precipitates slowly.

Type V (McArdle's syndrome)

Type V (glycogen storage disease of skeletal muscle, McArdle's syndrome) [22] is probably transmitted by a rare recessive. There is a *deficiency of myophosphorylase.* The child develops progressive weakness, dysphagia, regurgitation, macroglossia, cardiomegaly, and hepatomegaly. On biopsy the skeletal muscles are full of glycogen.

Type VI (Hers' disease)

Type VI (hepatophosphorylase deficiency glycogenosis, Hers' disease) is due to a *deficiency of phosphorylase in the liver and in leukocytes.* Myophosphorylase is normal.

Types VII, VIII, and IX

Type VII glycogenosis is due to a deficiency of muscle phosphofructokinase, and *Type VIII* by a deficiency or inhibition of muscle phosphohexoisomerase. Both forms are very rare. In *Type IX* there is a deficiency of hepatic phosphorylase kinase; it is similar to *Type VI.*

3. Disturbances in Lipid Metabolism

FABRY'S DISEASE

Fabry's disease (angiokeratoma corporis diffusum universale) [23] is a rare disorder of glycolipid metabolism. It is transmitted by a sex-linked gene with variable penetrance in the heterozygous female. The cause is a *deficiency of ceramidetrihexosidase* which catalyzes the cleavage of galactose from ceramidetrihexoside. As a result two closely related glycolipids are deposited in the endothelium, smooth muscle cells, and fibroblasts of blood vessels in the skin, heart, kidneys, gastrointestinal tract, and central nervous system. The predominant lipid is ceramidetrihexoside. In affected males, leukocytes are totally deficient in α-galactosidase; in female carriers there is a decrease of this enzyme [24]. *Clinically* there are multiple purple macules and papules around the umbilicus and on the lips, scrotum, and buttocks; corneal opacities, cataracts, and retinal edema; episodes of fever and burning pain in the extremities; anemia; and death in the fourth or fifth decade of life, usually due to renal failure.

GENERALIZED GANGLIOSIDOSIS

Generalized gangliosidosis [25] is probably transmitted as an autosomal recessive. Its cause is a *deficiency of β-galactosidase.* Because of this, ganglioside GM_1 accumulates and is deposited in cerebral neurons and reticuloendothelial cells of the liver, spleen, and elsewhere. A mucopolysaccharide, probably keratan sulfate, is also deposited in the liver and spleen [26]. Cerebral degeneration is progressive, and death usually occurs by the age of 2 years.

HURLER'S SYNDROME

A *β-galactosidase deficiency* is also present in *Hurler's syndrome,* types 1 to 3 [27]. In Hurler's syndrome (lipochondrodystrophy, gargoylism) there are excessive deposits of gangliosides GM_1, GM_2, and GM_3 in the cerebrum, and chondroitin sulfate B and heparitin sulfate in the liver, spleen, kidneys, and other viscera. Liver biopsies show varisized discrete vacuoles in hepatocytes and Kupffer cells [28]. Yellowish brown droplets fill the Kupffer cells with osmium stains. Skin biopsies reveal cytoplasmic vacuoles in stratum malpighii cells, fibroblasts, macrophages, and Schwann cells [29]. In both the liver and skin the vacuoles represent sites of mucopolysaccharide deposits. It is puzzling that while most cases of Hurler's syndrome are transmitted by an autosomal recessive gene, type 2 is a sex-linked recessive trait. Children with gargoylism are often dwarfed. The head is enlarged, and the eyes wide apart. There is diffuse or focal corneal clouding. The skin is coarse and dry. The neck is short, and the head looks as though it sits directly on the thorax. There is kyphosis. The abdomen is protuberant due to enlargement of the liver and spleen. A flexion deformity of the extremities is common. Frequently mental retardation and deafness are found.

REFSUM'S DISEASE

Refsum's disease (heredopathia atactica polyneuritiformis) [30] is transmitted as an autosomal recessive. The branched-chain fatty phytanic acid accumulates in tissues due to a *deficiency of phytanic acid hydroxylating enzyme.* The clinical features are related mainly to involvement of the nervous system.

4. Miscellaneous Enzyme Defects

PRIMARY HYPEROXALURIA

Primary hyperoxaluria (oxalosis) is a rare disorder of glyoxylate metabolism. It is usually transmitted as an autosomal recessive trait. *Type 1, glycolic aciduria,* is due to a *deficiency of 2-oxo-glutarate:glyoxylate carboligase.* The less common *type 2, glyceric aciduria* [31], results from a *deficiency of D-glyceric dehydrogenase.* In primary hyperoxaluria there are elevated urine concentrations of oxalic and glycolic or glyceric acids, calcium oxalate renal stone formation, pyelonephritis, hypertension, and death due to renal failure by adolescence. Calcium oxalate crystals are found in the kidneys, myocardium, media of small arteries, testes, and bones.

XANTHINURIA

Xanthinuria [32] is characterized by a marked excess of urinary xanthine and the subsequent formation of xanthine stones in the renal pelves. The trait is transmitted as an autosomal dominant. A *deficiency of xanthine oxidase* is the cause.

PRIMARY HYPERURICEMIA

The pathogenesis of *gout* (see page 762) is incompletely understood. Hyperuricemia is inherited as an autosomal dominant, but only a small fraction of persons with elevated serum uric acid levels develop clinical gout. It has been proposed that *primary hyperuricemia* results from overproduction of uric acid due to a *deficiency of hypoxanthine-guanine phosphoribosyl transferase.* A complete absence of this enzyme is found in children with a neurologic disorder associated with a disturbance of purine metabolism [33]. The syndrome is inherited as a sex-linked trait. Affected boys show choreoathetosis (purposeless movements), spasticity, mental retardation, and loss of fingertips. There are elevated serum and urine levels of uric acid, and increased concentrations of the oxypurines, hypoxanthine and xanthine, in the cerebrospinal fluid.

LYSOSOMAL ACID PHOSPHATASE DEFICIENCY

A *deficiency of lysosomal acid phosphatase* has been found in brain, liver, spleen, kidneys, and fibroblasts in an infant [34]. The associated clinical features were vomiting, lethargy, decreased muscle tone, opisthotonos, and death. The liver was enlarged. Microscopically, enlarged hepatocytes showed cytoplasmic vacuoles which stained for lipids. Similar changes were found in renal tubular epithelial cells. In the brain there was focal neuronal degeneration. The disorder was evidently inherited as an autosomal recessive.

HYPOPHOSPHATASIA

Hypophosphatasia is characterized by signs of severe rickets despite adequate administration of vitamin D. It is due to a *deficiency of alkaline phosphatase.* The condition is apparently transmitted as an autosomal recessive.

ADRENOGENITAL SYNDROMES

Type I (adrenal hyperplasia with virilism) is apparently transmitted as an autosomal recessive gene. The disorder is more common in girls than boys. It is due to a *deficiency of 21-hydroxylase,* so that there is a block in the conversion of 17-hydroxyprogesterone to compound S, an intermediate in cortisol formation. The resulting cortisol deficiency leads to increased anterior pituitary production of ACTH. The latter causes excessive androgen secretion by the hyperplastic zona reticularis of the adrenal cortex. In girls there is pseudohermaphroditism with enlargement of the clitoris and persistence of the urogenital sinus. In boys the penis becomes enlarged, and pubic, axillary, and facial hair appears. The testes remain small and undeveloped. In both sexes there is marked acceleration of body height. Urinary 17-ketosteroids are increased.

Type II (adrenal hyperplasia with hypertension) is due to *11-hydroxylase deficiency.* There is a block in the conversion of compound S to cortisol. Hypertension develops in childhood and is occasionally severe enough to cause cardiac failure or cerebral hemorrhage. The hypertension is evidently related to increased desoxycorticosterone production by the adrenal cortex. The hereditary pattern of transmission is unclear.

Type III (adrenal hyperplasia with electrolyte disturbances) is apparently transmitted as a rare recessive gene. It has been attributed to profound 21-hydroxylase deficiency. There is no cortisol formation, and aldosterone production is decreased. Affected infants are irritable and anorexic. Vomiting and weight loss ensue. The serum sodium level is low, and the potassium level is elevated. Death may occur in infancy due to salt loss and dehydration or to hyperkalemia. The zona glomerulosa may be absent in the adrenal glands.

Type IV (3-β-hydroxysteroid dehydrogenase deficiency) results in a block in the conversion of pregnenolone to progesterone. Male infants are born with hypospadias and failure of development of the external genitalia. Females have labial fusion and enlargement of the clitoris. Death usually occurs within a few months due to electrolyte disturbances.

17-Hydroxylase deficiency syndrome [35] consists of hypertension, hyperkalemia, primary amenorrhea, and failure of development of secondary sex characteristics in a young adult. There is a block between progesterone and 17-hydroxyprogesterone and as a result, progesterone is found in excess. Due to elevated ACTH secretion, the adrenals produce increased amounts of corticosterone and desoxycorticosterone.

OTHER ENZYME DEFECTS

A number of *enzyme defects* are discussed elsewhere. Crigler-Najjar syndrome is described on page 273; hemolytic anemias due to deficiencies of glucose-6-phosphate dehydrogenase and other enzymes, page 286; Gaucher's disease, page 389; Niemann-Pick disease, page 389; and metachromatic leukodystrophy, page 691.

DISTURBANCES IN TRANSPORT MECHANISMS

HARTNUP DISEASE

H (Hartnup) disease [36] is probably transmitted by an autosomal recessive. There is a *defective transport of tryptophan across the renal proximal convoluted tubular epithelium.* Absorption of tryptophan by the small intestinal mucosa is incomplete. The transformation of tryptophan into formyl-kynurenine is blocked. Kynurenine is a nicotinic acid precursor. *Clinically* there are an erythematous, raw, weeping, pellagra-like rash; ataxia; nystagmus; tremors; mental retardation; marked aminoaciduria; and an increased urinary indole compound excretion.

CYSTINURIA

Cystinuria is characterized by *defective renal transport of cystine, lysine, arginine, and ornithine* – all dibasic amino acids. Two types of cystinuria are transmitted by different autosomal recessive genes. In both, homozygous patients show large amounts of all four amino acids in the urine and tend to develop cystine stones. In Type I, heterozygous carriers have no urinary abnormalities. In Type II, heterozygous patients have increased levels of only cystine and lysine in the urine. Plasma levels of all four amino acids are normal or low in cystinuria. A defect in their reabsorption leads to high concentrations in the urine. The precipitation of cystine crystals produces a cystine stone in the renal pelvis.

CYSTINOSIS

Cystinosis occurs in the Fanconi syndrome (see page 592). It is associated with multiple defects in renal transport in this syndrome. The disorder is transmitted by an autosomal recessive gene. Cystine is deposited in the liver, spleen, kidneys, lymph nodes, bone marrow, and eyes, mainly within reticuloendothelial cells. The cause of the cystine deposition is unknown.

RENAL GLYCOSURIA

Renal glycosuria is transmitted as an autosomal dominant. There is glucose in the urine despite a normal blood sugar. The condition is benign, and no patient is known to have developed diabetes mellitus. There is an inborn *defect in the renal transport mechanism for glucose,* so that there is a failure of the normal almost complete reabsorption of glucose from the proximal convoluted tubules.

NEPHROGENIC DIABETES INSIPIDUS

Nephrogenic diabetes insipidus is transmitted as an autosomal dominant with decreased penetrance and expressivity in females. There is an inborn failure of the renal tubules to absorb water due to their nonresponsivity to antidiuretic hormone. A large volume of dilute urine is excreted daily beginning in infancy. There is severe thirst, and dehydration and fever are frequent. Unexplained mental retardation and failure to develop physically also occur.

LEUKOCYTE ABNORMALITIES

PELGER ANOMALY

The *Pelger-Huët anomaly* [37] is characterized by a high percentage of neutrophils with two lobes. These often have a pince-nez appearance with a narrow nuclear bridge between the lobes. Sex chromatin is not seen in neutrophils of affected females. This common and benign trait is transmitted as an autosomal dominant.

MAY-HEGGLIN ANOMALY

In the *May-Hegglin anomaly* [38], which is transmitted as an autosomal dominant, there is a cytoplasmic accumulation of ribonucleic acid in neutrophils. The platelets are large and poorly granulated. No clinical manifestations are noted.

CHEDIAK-HIGASHI DISEASE

Chediak-Higashi syndrome [39] is inherited as an autosomal recessive. The cause is unknown, but the disease appears to be a generalized abnormality of unit membrane-bound organelles, such as lysosomes. A similar disorder occurs in mink [40] and cattle. The syndrome becomes clinically apparent at from 1 to 8 years of age with partial albinism due to pigmentary dilution, photophobia, lymphadenopathy, hepatosplenomegaly, and decreased resistance to infections. Death typically occurs by the age of 15 years due to infection or development of a malignant lymphoma. Large cytoplasmic granules are present in leukocytes; with Giemsa stains the granules are red in lymphocytes and greenish gray in neutrophils. In the skin, hair, and uvea, melanin pigment is present in clumps of large granules. The liver shows focal necrosis and a periportal infiltration of lymphocytes and other mononuclear cells. In the spleen, normal and atypical lymphocytes are seen in the follicles. Foci of extramedullary hematopoiesis are present. In the bone marrow, normal cell production is decreased due to an infiltration of lymphocytes and macrophages. In a case in whom a lymphoma develops there is an extensive infiltration of the liver, spleen, kidneys, lymph nodes, bone marrow, and brain with immature lymphocytes and reticulum cells. Virus-like particles have been found in the peripheral leukocytes of patients with the lymphoma associated with Chediak-Higashi syndrome.

REFERENCES

1. Gentz, J., Jagenburg, R., and Jetterström, R. Tyrosinemia. *J. Pediat.* 66:670, 1965.

2. Lonsdale, D., and Barber, D. H. Maple-syrup-urine disease. *New Eng. J. Med.* 271:1338, 1964.
3. Budd, M. A., Tanata, K., Holmes, L. B., Efron, M., Crawford, J. D., and Isselbacher, K. J. Isovaleric acidemia. *New Eng. J. Med.* 277:321, 1967.
4. Dancis, J., Hutzler, J., Tada, K., Wada, Y., Morikawa, T., and Arakawa, T. Hypervalinemia: Defect in valine transamination. *Pediatrics* 39:813, 1967.
5. Schimke, R. N., McKusick, V. A., Huang, T., and Pollack, A. D. Homocystinuria. *J.A.M.A.* 193:711, 1965.
6. McCully, K. S. Vascular pathology of homocysteinemia: Implications for the pathogenesis of arteriosclerosis. *Amer. J. Path.* 56:111, 1969.
7. Whelan, D. T., and Scriver, C. R. Cystathioninuria and renal iminoglycinuria in a pedigree. *New Eng. J. Med.* 278:924, 1968.
8. Ghadimi, H., Partington, M. W., and Hunter, A. A familial disturbance of histidine metabolism. *New Eng. J. Med.* 265:221, 1961.
9. Schafer, I. A., Scriver, C. R., and Efron, M. L. Familial hyperprolinemia, cerebral dysfunction and renal anomalies occurring in a family with hereditary nephropathy and deafness. *New Eng. J. Med.* 267:51, 1962.
10. Gerritsen, T., and Waisman, H. A. Hypersarcosinemia, new error of metabolism. *Fed. Proc.* 24:470, 1965.
11. Perry, T. L., Hansen, S., Tischler, B., Bunting, R., and Berry, K. Carnosinemia. *New Eng. J. Med.* 277:1219, 1967.
12. Scriver, C. R., Pueschel, S., and Davies, E. Hyper-β-alaninemia associated with β-aminoaciduria and γ-aminobutyricaciduria, somnolence and seizures. *New Eng. J. Med.* 274:635, 1966.
13. Hansen, R. G. Hereditary galactosemia. *J.A.M.A.* 208:2077, 1969.
14. Suzuki, H., Gilbert, E. F., Anido, V., Jones, B., and Klingberg, W. G. Galactosemia. *Arch. Path.* (Chicago) 82:602, 1966.
15. Sidbury, J. B., Jr., and Heick, H. M. C. Glycogen storage diseases. *Southern Med. J.* 61:915, 1968.
16. Field, R. A. The glycogenoses: von Gierke's disease, acid maltase deficiency, and liver glycogen phosphorylase deficiency. *Amer. J. Clin. Path.* 50:20, 1968.
17. Hug, G., and Schubert, W. K. Glycogenosis type II. *Arch. Path.* (Chicago) 84:141, 1967.
18. Witzleben, C. L. Renal cortical tubular glycogen localization in glycogenosis type II (Pompe's disease). *Lab. Invest.* 20:424, 1969.
19. Neustein, H. B. Fine structure of skeletal muscle in type III glycogenosis. *Arch. Path.* (Chicago) 88:130, 1969.
20. Holleman, L. W. J., van der Haar, J. A., and de Vaan, G. A. M. Type IV glycogenosis. *Lab. Invest.* 15:357, 1966.
21. Reed, G. B., Jr., Dixon, J. F. P., Neustein, H. B., Donnell, G. N., and Landing, B. H. Type IV glycogenosis. *Lab. Invest.* 19:546, 1968.
22. Pearson, C. M. Glycogen metabolism and storage disease of types III, IV, and V. *Amer. J. Clin. Path.* 50:29, 1968.
23. Bagdade, J. D., Parker, F., Ways, P. O., Morgan, T. E., Lagunoff, D., and Eidelman, S. Fabry's disease. *Lab. Invest.* 18:681, 1968.
24. Kint, J. A. Fabry's disease: Alpha-galactosidase deficiency. *Science* 167:1268, 1970.
25. Okada, S., and O'Brien, J. S. Generalized gangliosidosis: Beta-galactosidase deficiency. *Science* 160:1002, 1968.
26. Suzuki, K. Cerebral G_{M1}-gangliosidosis: Chemical pathology of visceral organs. *Science* 159:1471, 1968.

27. Ho, M. W., and O'Brien, J. S. Hurler's syndrome: Deficiency of a specific beta galactosidase isoenzyme. *Science* 165:611, 1969.
28. Callahan, W. P., Hackett, R. L., and Lorincz, A. E. New observations by light microscopy on liver histology in the Hurler's syndrome. *Arch. Path.* (Chicago) 83:507, 1967.
29. DeCloux, R. J., and Friederici, H. H. R. Ultrastructural studies of the skin in Hurler' syndrome. *Arch. Path.* (Chicago) 88:350, 1969.
30. Steinberg, D., Herndon, J. H., Jr., Uhlendorf, B. W., Mize, C. E., Avigan, J., and Milne, G. W. A. Refsum's disease: Nature of the enzyme defect. *Science* 156:1740, 1967.
31. Williams, H. E., and Smith, L. H., Jr. L-glyceric aciduria. A new genetic variant of primary hyperoxaluria. *New Eng. J. Med.* 278:233, 1968.
32. Watts, R. W. E., Engelman, K., Klinenberg, J. R., Seegmiller, J. E., and Sjoerdsma, A. Enzyme defect in a case of xanthinuria. *Nature* (London) 201:395, 1964.
33. Rosenbloom, F. M., Kelley, W. N., Miller, J., Henderson, J. F., and Seegmiller, J. E. Inherited disorder of purine metabolism. *J.A.M.A.* 202:175, 1967.
34. Nadler, H. L., and Egan, T.. J. Deficiency of lysosomal acid phosphatase. *New Eng. J. Med.* 282:302, 1970.
35. Goldsmith, O., Solomon, D. H., and Horton, R. Hypogonadism and mineralocorticoid excess. The 17-hydroxylase deficiency syndrome. *New Eng. J. Med.* 277:673, 1967.
36. Pomeroy, J., Efron, M. L., Dayman, J., and Hoefnagel, D. Hartnup disorder in a New England family. *New Eng. J. Med.* 278:1214, 1968.
37. Skendzel, L. P., and Hoffman, G. C. The Pelger anomaly of leukocytes. *Amer. J. Clin. Path.* 37:294, 1962.
38. Wassmuth, D. R., Hamilton, H. E., and Sheets, R. F. May-Hegglin anomaly. *J.A.M.A.* 183:737, 1963.
39. Bedoya, V., Grimley, P. M., and Duque, O. Chediak-Higashi syndrome. *Arch. Path.* (Chicago) 88:340, 1969.
40. Windhorst, D. B., White, J. G., Zellickson, A. S., Clawson, C. C., Dent, P. B., Pollara, B., and Good, R. A. The Chediak-Higashi anomaly and the Aleutian trait in mink: Homologous defects of lysosomal structure. *Ann. N.Y. Acad. Sci.* 155:818, 1968.

GENERAL REFERENCES

Hsia, D. Y. *Inborn Errors of Metabolism* (2d ed.), Part I. Chicago: Year Book, 1966.

Thompson, J. S., and Thompson, M. W. *Genetics in Medicine.* Philadelphia: Saunders, 1966.

14 INTRODUCTION TO NEOPLASMS

J. Chandler Smith, M.D.*

GENERAL CONSIDERATIONS

1. Definitions

Some terms relating to neoplasms are defined below. Definitions

Neoplasm. A focal autonomous new growth having no useful function.

Tumor. Any neoplasm; previously a swelling from any cause (obsolete).

Benign. The property, of a neoplasm, of noninvasiveness; the neoplasm remains localized.

Malignancy. The property, of a neoplasm, of marginal invasion, relentless growth, and distant spread with a lethal effect.

Cancer. Any malignant neoplasm.

Carcinogenic. A tendency to cause cancer.

Sarcoma. A malignant neoplasm arising from connective tissue cells.

Carcinoma. A malignant neoplasm arising from epithelial cells.

Primary tumor. A malignant neoplasm that occurs first and from which metastases subsequently arise.

Secondary tumor. A contiguous extension of primary tumor to an adjacent organ or structure, or distant metastases from the primary site.

Metastatic tumor. A secondary malignant growth that originates from a primary tumor and is separated from it.

Oncology. The study of neoplasia.

*Professor of Pathology, The George Washington University School of Medicine, Washington, D.C.

2. The Nature of Neoplasia

Neoplasia is the process of tumor formation. It is one of the most important of all pathologic processes, accounting for disability, prolonged and often extreme discomfort, economic adversity, and death at all ages and in considerable numbers. More than 52 million Americans now living will eventually have cancer.

What is a tumor?

The word *tumor* in ancient times meant swelling regardless of the cause so that it encompassed non-neoplastic lesions such as inflammations, cysts, and hyperplasias. In its modern connotation, it *refers to the process of neoplasia alone.* Tumors differ from normal tissues more in degree than in kind so that a strict definition of the word is not altogether possible. Nevertheless, Willis [1] ventures the following, "A tumor is an abnormal mass of tissue, the growth of which exceeds and is uncoordinated with that of the normal tissues, and persists in the same excessive manner after cessation of the stimuli that evoked the change." The tissue of a tumor is ordinarily lacking in normal histologic pattern and is therefore abnormal; the growth proceeds to the detriment of the host rather than as a reparative consequence of a preceding injury, and the growth continues after the agent stimulating its onset is withdrawn. Thus a tumor is an *uncontrolled growth of abnormal tissue that is harmful to the host.*

Behavior of tumor cells

The pathologic process of neoplasia is most usefully considered from the standpoint of the behavior of the tumor cells. The two main categories are indicated by the words *benign* and *malignant.* Benign neoplasms do not invade adjacent tissue, do not spread to distant sites, and are the cause of localized effects. In contrast, malignant tumors invade normal tissue, spread elsewhere in the body, and cause death by local and disseminated effects. Benign tumors are much more common than malignant tumors and they tend to arise at an earlier age and to enlarge at a slower rate. In addition, benign tumors are cured by total excision, whereas malignant tumors are often incurable because of spread outside the resectable region.

Characteristics of benign tumors

Certain gross and microscopic features indicate whether a tumor is benign or malignant. *Grossly* benign tumors are characterized by sharply circumscribed margins that are often encapsulated, by central portions that tend to remain solid and viable, and by a texture that is uniformly soft or resilient. The *microscopic feature* is the resemblance of benign tumor cells to normal cells so that while the tissue pattern is altered and ordinarily easily distinguished from normal, the individual cells are often not. Thus nuclear size and staining, as well as cell size and shape, mimic the normal, and mitotic figures are both scarce in number and normal in configuration. Benign behavior, however, should not be taken to mean that such tumors are necessarily innocuous. They are slowly growing, usually solid masses that block ducts, dam up secretions, compress vessels, and impinge on nerves and other solid structures. They may thus be the *cause of pressure atrophy, ischemic necrosis, bacterial infection, and stagnation of fluid in dilated chambers.* They may also ulcerate and bleed briskly. In these ways the effects of benign tumors may be serious and even life-threatening. Total excision is curative.

Characteristics of malignant tumors

Malignant tumors are characterized *grossly* by serrated margins due to irregular invasion of adjacent tissues, by foci of necrosis in the central portions, and by a hard consistency. These features strongly indicate the diagnosis of malignancy on gross inspection alone. *Microscopically* the malignant tumor is characterized by a pronounced distortion of tissue pattern, by necrosis and often hemorrhage in the central parts, and by leukocytic infiltration especially about the invasive margins. In addition, the most conspicuous changes are variation in cell size and shape; variation in nuclear size, shape, and staining qualities; and increase in frequency of mitotic figures, some or many of which may be tripolar or otherwise abnormal. These microscopic alterations collectively are known as *anaplasia;* they connote malignant behavior of the tumor cells. The histologic pattern thus departs substantially from normal, and the gross and microscopic features indicate the malignant behavior of the lesion.

Benign vs. malignant

It is to be emphasized that the distinction between benign and malignant is not always possible since *intermediate stages exist.* Also, benign tumors may undergo malignant transformation, and the tissue during this period of transition may show equivocal gross and microscopic changes. Such transformation is occasionally seen in the muscle tumors of the uterine wall, and frequently in the polypoid tumors of the colonic mucosa.

A proof of malignancy is the development of discrete tumor nodules in parts of the body separated from the primary site. This phenomenon, called *metastasis,* is due to the detachment of tumor cell clusters from the site of origin and their transport in the lymph or bloodstreams to other tissues, especially the liver and lungs. While this phenomenon is proof of malignancy, the *absence of metastasis does not establish benign behavior.* Basal cell carcinomas of the skin, for example, and gliomas of the brain, are malignant tumors that invade and destroy adjacent tissue but rarely spread away from the primary site. The two strongest evidences of malignancy are therefore invasion of adjacent tissues and metastasis to distant sites. These properties are indicated in Table 14-1.

TABLE 14-1. Contrast of Benign and Malignant Tumors

Characteristic	Benign tumor	Malignant tumor
Gross		
Margin	Smooth, often encapsulated	Rough and serrated, without capsule
Center	Resilient, soft, and viable	Firm and nonresilient, with focal necrosis
Microscopic		
Tissue pattern	Often resembles normal	Usually departs sharply from normal
Adjacent tissue	Compressed	Invaded
Basement membranes	Intact	Disrupted
Blood and lymph vessels	Intact	Invaded
Cells	Normal size and shape	Usually large, often irregular
Nuclei	Normal size and staining	Large, usually hyperchromatic
Clinical		
Rate of growth	Slow	Rapid
Metastasis	None	Usual
Effects	Local	Local and disseminated

3. Nomenclature

Tumors may be named according to their composition, cause, or portion of the body from which they arose. Of these, composition is the most useful. Benign tumors are indicated by the suffix *oma* affixed to the name of the tissue comprising the lesion. Thus benign tumors of fibrous and adipose tissue are called fibromas and lipomas, respectively. There are also neuromas, chondromas, osteomas, leiomyomas, rhabdomyomas, and myxomas.

Classes of cancer: carcinoma

Malignant tumors are collectively known as cancers; they are divided into two classes: *those arising from epithelial cells,* which are called *carcinomas,* and *those arising from mesenchymal tissues* (exclusive of the lymphopoietic system), which are called *sarcomas.* The word *carcinoma* is ordinarily preceded by the name of the cell of origin so that squamous cell carcinoma, transitional cell carcinoma, and adenocarcinoma are common terms. Descriptive modifiers are also used; hence oat cell carcinoma, colloid carcinoma, and medullary carcinoma. Oat cell is not a preferred term; it refers to a uniformly small cell cancer originating in the bronchial mucosa. *Colloid carcinomas* are characterized by large lakes of mucin which give the tumor a glistening sticky cut surface and a special histologic appearance. They occur in the colon and rectum, and occasionally in the breast. *Medullary carcinomas* are composed of solid epithelial masses and hence tend to have uniformly soft, fleshy cut surfaces. In contrast to these soft cancers, most malignant epithelial tumors stimulate the formation of fibrous connective tissue and it is this property that accounts for the characteristic firm, nonresilient cut surface. The connective tissue-stimulating effect is called *desmoplasia.* When the connective tissue is abundant, and the cut surface is hard, the tumor is referred to as *scirrhous.* The formation of glands is also indicated by the prefix *adeno.* Thus scirrhous adenocarcinoma is a fibrotic malignant epithelial neoplasm that produces glandlike structures.

In addition to these modifiers, special terminology has been added to indicate the degree of *differentiation* of the tumor, i.e., its *degree of resemblance to the tissue from which it arose.* Thus for carcinomas of squamous type, the presence of intercellular bridges, cytoplasmic keratin, and layered arrangement has been noted, and for carcinomas of gland-bearing surfaces such as the colon or breast, the fidelity with which the glands of the normal tissue are simulated becomes part of the modifying aspect. Both reveal a high degree of differentiation. The purpose of this is to correlate the degree of differentiation with the prognosis since in a general way high differentiation connotes slow growth, late metastasis, and improved prospects for cure. Nevertheless, most malignant tumors disclose varying degrees of differentiation, and such a small part of the total bulk of the tumor is examined microscopically that this practice has had limited success. It is therefore perhaps sufficient to express this feature only as undifferentiated carcinoma, or partially or well-differentiated squamous cell or adenocarcinoma. Carcinoma simplex is a term of diminishing use that equates with undifferentiated carcinoma. It should be noted that "undifferentiated" precludes identifying the tissue pattern, so that "undifferentiated squamous cell carcinoma" or "undifferentiated adenocarcinoma" are contradictions of terminology.

sarcoma

The cancers arising in mesenchymal tissues are called *sarcomas. Sarcomas occur much less frequently than carcinomas, they tend to arise at a slightly earlier age, and they tend to be highly malignant.* The terminology for sarcomas varies with descriptive words – e.g., spindle cell sarcoma, round cell sarcoma – and with words indicating the cell or tissue of origin, such as osteogenic sarcoma, chondrosarcoma, and reticulum cell sarcoma. Modifiers indicating the degree of differentiation are ordinarily not used in the terminology of sarcomas.

lymphoma

Malignant tumors of the lymphohematopoietic system are sarcomatous in nature since they arise from mesenchymal tissues, but they differ from the other mesodermal cancers in that the tumor cells often circulate in large numbers in the bloodstream, as in the leukemias, and *multicentric sites of origin rather than metastatic dissemination from a primary site are thought to occur.* For the tumors of lymphoid tissue, the generic word is *lymphoma.* The suffix would seem to indicate that the lymphomas are benign tumors; they are not benign, however, and so are often and collectively known as the *malignant lymphomas.* Even this term, however, is not altogether satisfactory because it implies the existence of a benign class of lymphoma, which does not exist; all the lymphomas are malignant.

4. Classification of Neoplasms

I. Neoplasms of connective tissue
   A. Benign: fibroma, lipoma, myxoma, chondroma, osteoma, leiomyoma, rhabdomyoma
   B. Malignant: same stem with *-sarcoma* substituted for *-oma*
II. Neoplasms of epithelium
   A. Squamous and transitional epithelium
      1. Benign: papilloma
      2. Malignant: epidermoid carcinoma, basal cell carcinoma, transitional cell carcinoma
   B. Glandular epithelium
      1. Benign: adenoma
      2. Malignant: adenocarcinoma
   C. Special
      1. Of chorionic epithelium
         a. Benign: hydatidiform mole
         b. Malignant: choriocarcinoma or chorioepithelioma
      2. Miscellaneous
         a. Usually benign, of dental structures: adamantinoma
         b. A special malignant neoplasm of the kidney (hypernephroma), and others
III. Neoplasms of blood vessels
   A. Benign: hemangioma, lymphangioma
   B. Malignant: hemangiosarcoma or hemangioendothelioma, lymphangiosarcoma, lymphangioendothelioma
IV. Neoplasms of the nervous system
   A. Of meninges or ependyma, usually "benign": meningioma, ependymoma
   B. Of glial tissue proper: gliomas of several types, most of which are malignant
V. Neoplasms of mixed tissue origin
   A. From embryonic cells of unlimited capacity for differentiation: teratoma, usually malignant
   B. From embryonic cells with unusual but limited capacity for differentiation: mixed neoplasms
VI. Neoplasms of miscellaneous or unknown tissue origin
   A. Of hemopoietic tissues

1. Benign: nonexistent
2. Malignant: lymphosarcoma, Hodgkin's disease, leukemia, multiple myeloma

B. Pigmented neoplasms
1. Benign: pigmented nevus
2. Malignant: malignant melanoma

C. Others

5. Prevalence of Cancer

It was estimated that in 1970, 960,000 Americans would be treated for cancer, 625,000 new cases would be diagnosed, and 330,000 patients would die of this disease [2]. That is more than *900 deaths per day.* It is one out of every six deaths in 1970. Moreover, if present trends continue, *one of every four persons now living will develop the disease.* Cancer is expected in the future to affect two of every three families in America. Cancer was second only to cardiovascular disease as the most frequent cause of death in the United States in 1967 [2]. When it is realized that these figures relate only to the malignant component of the neoplastic process, and that benign tumors, although less important, are more frequent than malignant tumors, the magnitude of the total process of neoplasia can be seen to be very large.

Distribution by site and sex

The distribution of malignant tumors within the body is of much interest since certain structures frequently give rise to tumors, and others show no such tendency. Table 14-2 reveals the estimated cancer deaths in 1970 by site and sex. *The most frequent cancer sites in the male are the lung, colon, and prostate,* while *in the female the breast, colon, and uterus are especially prone to malignant neoplasia.* In addition, the *lymphomas are common in both sexes.*

Distribution by age

There are fewer cancer deaths per 100,000 population in the age group of 10 to 14 years than in any other 5-year period. Above this age period the rate rises steadily with each 5-year period, including the group 85 and over. But the death rate from all other causes is accelerated also, so that the *probability* of dying of cancer begins to decline after 35 in the female and after 55 in the male.

When expressed as a percentage of all deaths, *cancer deaths reach the peak at age 45 to 49 in the female and 60 to 64 in the male.* This difference is due in part to the large number of deaths from heart disease in males age 40 to 60.

There are more deaths from cancer during the *first 5 years of life* than during any subsequent 5-year period until age 25. This is chiefly because of the frequency of *leukemia* in this group.

From age 25 to 55, more women than men die of cancer in each age group; this is due to the high frequency of cancer of the breast and uterine cervix during this period. Nevertheless, when all age groups are considered, total cancer deaths in males slightly exceed total cancer deaths in females. The ratio in 1970 is 55 men to 45 women. *One-fourth of all cancer deaths occur during the peak decade of 60 to 69 years.*

Morbidity vs. mortality

The difference between the *morbidity* and *mortality* rates of various cancers should be noted. A cancer that is very slowly progressive (as most skin cancer) or very amenable to treatment (as cancer of the lip) will have a much higher morbidity than mortality rate.

TABLE 14-2. Estimated Cancer Deaths by Site and Sex, 1970

Site	Males	Females	Total
All malignant neoplasms	180,000	150,000	330,000
Buccal cavity and pharynx	5,100	1,850	6,950
Esophagus	4,600	1,500	6,100
Stomach	9,300	6,300	15,600
Colon and rectum	22,300	23,500	45,800
Liver, biliary passages	4,700	5,200	9,900
Pancreas	10,400	7,800	18,200
Larynx	2,550	350	2,900
Lung	51,200	10,500	61,700
Breast	250	30,100	30,350
Prostate	17,000	–	17,000
Uterus	–	12,900	12,900
Ovary	–	9,900	9,900
Kidney	3,900	2,400	6,300
Urinary bladder	6,100	2,800	8,900
Skin	3,000	2,100	5,100
Brain and nerves	4,600	3,300	7,900
Thyroid	350	700	1,050
Bone	1,100	800	1,900
Leukemia	8,400	6,300	14,700
Lymphomas	9,950	7,965	17,900
Other	11,250	10,250	21,500

From American Cancer Society [2].

Geographic variation

It should not be presumed that the relative frequency of cancer at the various sites shown in Table 14-2 is geographically uniform. Indeed, the sharp variation in cancer incidence in different countries bears importantly on the questions of heredity and environmental factors in the causation of cancer. Carcinoma of the stomach, for example, has undergone an abrupt decline in America, whereas it is extremely common in Russia, Chile, Iceland, and Japan [3]. Carcinoma of the nasopharynx, uncommon in America, is 10 to 50 times more common in Asia than elsewhere in the world [4]. In Japan lymphocytic leukemia is vanishingly scarce, whereas cancers of the breast, colon, and prostate are remarkably uncommon. In America all these kinds of cancer are common. It is not altogether clear why these differences exist, but *environmental factors are highly suspect* [5].

COURSE OF THE DISEASE, DIAGNOSIS, TREATMENT

1. *Effects of Tumors*

BENIGN TUMORS: Pressure atrophy

The effects of tumors depend on whether they are persistently invasive and hence malignant, or indefinitely localized and thus *benign*. In the latter instance, *pressure effects* are conspicuous; the circumscribed growth pushes against adjacent structures which as a result undergo pressure atrophy. The skin over a subcutaneous fibroma, for example, becomes raised, thin, and shiny. Occasionally it may ulcerate but more commonly it remains indolent for a long period. Pressure on nerves is a cause of *pain. Ulceration* is attended by *infection,* and *hemorrhage* from ulcerated surfaces is common. The leiomyoma of the gastric wall frequently ulcerates over the mucosal surface, and hemorrhage may be massive. When benign growths are large, the central portions may undergo degeneration as in the "carneous" or red softening that takes place in fibromyomas of the myometrium. *Frank necrosis, however, except in the largest tumors, is not frequent.* The effects of benign tumors thus tend to be localized to the sites of growth and consist for the most part of pressure effects and less frequently of hemorrhage and infection with acute inflammation. Benign tumors of the *endocrine organs* may cause *systemic effects* by the excess hormones produced.

Hemorrhage and infection

MALIGNANT TUMORS: Invasion, necrosis

Malignant tumors have both local and distant effects. Since the tumor cells are invasive, the site of origin becomes indurated as edema, hyperemia, and inflammation accompany the infiltrative process. The progress of the lesion is more rapid than with benign growths, and ulceration is common when skin or mucosal surface is affected. Thus bronchi are eroded, intestinal mucosa ulcerates, and skin surfaces break down with bleeding that is occasionally brisk but usually slight and more or less constant. Hemoptysis, occult blood in the stool, occasionally melena, and unexplained anemia reflect this. Necrosis is especially common in the central portions of malignant tumors and this is often true even when the lesion is small. With ulceration and necrosis, infection is frequent. An ulcerated, indurated, gradually progressive "sore" is a cardinal clinical sign of malignant disease, especially when it occurs on a cancer-prone surface such as the exposed skin of the face or the lower lip, the site of a preexisting nevus, or on the uterine cervix. The same events take place in internal structures, where there is the additional possibility of fistula formation. Thus cancer of the esophagus may erode into the trachea or bronchus to form a tracheo-esophageal or bronchoesophageal fistula, cancer of the cervix may extend into the rectum to form a rectovaginal fistula, and cancer of the prostate may extend into the urinary bladder to cause ulceration and hemorrhage from that site. Compressed or invaded veins may become thrombosed. *Invasion, ulceration, necrosis, thrombosis, and attachment to adjacent structures with fistula formation are the principal local effects of malignant tumors.*

Metastasis:

Distant effects of malignant tumors are both localized and systemic. *Localized effects are due to metastases* which are discrete tumor cell clusters that arise at sites distant from the primary cancer. The mechanism of this phenomenon is the *embolization of the blood and lymph* so that aggressive cells at the margins of the primary tumor extend into capillaries and are swept by the vascular current to other sites. Embolization does not guarantee metastasis, however, and the conditions necessary for metastatic growth are not altogether known. Nevertheless, there are two large vascular sieves through which the blood passes, i.e., the *hepatic sinusoids* and the *pulmonary capillaries,* and it is at these two sites that metastatic implants are especially common. The functional reserve of both these organs is so great, however, that detectable impairment of hepatic or pulmonary function is not evident clinically unless the metastatic process is either diffuse or extremely widespread [6].

Lymphatic spread may occur either by cell propagation along lymphatic channels or by embolism within the lymphatic vessels. In either instance the secondary growths appear in the *regional lymph nodes.* By this avenue neoplastic cells may eventually reach the thoracic duct and then extend along it in the direction of flow, finally seeding the lungs with cell emboli. If neoplasm obstructs the large lymphatic ducts, lymph flow reverses itself and retrograde metastasis may occur. Carcinomas generally have a tendency to spread by lymphatics.

distribution of metastases

The distribution of metastases is a function of both time and site of origin. In general, the longer the time after origin of the primary cancer, the wider is the distribution of metastases. It is for this reason that the prospect of cure by surgical extirpation of the primary site cannot be improved by delaying the operative procedure since eradication of all tumor appears to be the requirement of cure. Tissues frequently affected by metastatic disease in addition to *lungs, liver, and lymph nodes* include especially the *kidneys, bone, adrenals, and brain.* In addition, involvement by direct extension to serosal surfaces is common so that wide implantation of tumor cells on pleura and peritoneum, often with the accumulation of much fluid, is frequent in the later stage of malignant disease.

pattern of metastases

With respect to site, certain general rules tend to be followed. For example, carcinoma of the colon regularly spreads to mesenteric lymph nodes and to the liver. Carcinoma of the lung metastasizes to liver, bone, brain, and especially to adrenals. Metastatic involvement of the spleen is infrequent regardless of the source, although it is often involved by lymphomas, including Hodgkin's disease, which are regarded as cancers with multicentric sites of origin. Primary tumors of the brain tend to remain localized within the skull although the tumor cells from gliomas may be released into the cerebrospinal fluid. This is most frequent with medulloblastomas, and in that instance the diagnosis may be established by cytologic examination of the spinal fluid.

mechanism of metastasis

The phenomenon of *metastasis is largely due,* according to Coman [7, 8], *to* three factors: (1) a *localized deficiency of calcium* which correlates with a decreased adherence of adjacent tumor cells, (2) an *ameboid activity* on the part *of the detached cells,* and (3) a *spreading factor* such as hyaluronidase that is perhaps produced by the tumor cells. This combination of factors is presumed to account for the detachment of cells from the advancing margins of the cancer and for penetration of them into vascular channels. Transit to other sites is achieved by venous, arterial, and lymphatic embolization. Less frequently penetration of serosal surfaces takes place with seeding of pleura or peritoneum. In these instances the serosa-lined cavity may fill with hemorrhagic transudate, probably from blocked lymphatic drainage, or with mucoid material produced by the tumor cells. Less frequently the tumor cells stimulate fibrous tissue formation that seals the serous space and fixes the viscera to the parietal surfaces.

It is not entirely clear why metastases are frequent in lungs, liver, bones, kidneys, and adrenals, and infrequent in such tissues as spleen and skeletal muscle. Explanations include localization due to mechanical factors of blood flow, and local chemical conditions that are favorable to metastatic growth at selected sites. In experimental studies, Coman and colleagues [8] followed the distribution of tumor cells injected into the hearts of rabbits, and subsequently noted the occurrence of metastases in various tissues. They found that when the tumor cell emboli were arrested in arterioles, metastases were infrequent, and *when the tumor cells progressed on to capillaries, metastatic growth was common.* They concluded from this that once the tumor cells progress to capillaries, mechanical factors alone are sufficient to explain the distribution of the secondary growths.

Systemic effects

Systemic effects are also due to cancer although the mechanism is not entirely clear. Loss of weight and regression of appetite are early signs. As the tumor progresses, these become pronounced, and emaciation and cachexia are conspicuous in the late period of the illness. Laboratory findings associated with these clinical effects include especially anemia and depletion of serum proteins. It is possible that *absorption of toxic materials from necrotic tumor* contributes to deterioration of a systemic nature.

2. *Diagnosis of Cancer*

Various *clinical features* are suggestive of the diagnosis of cancer. They include weakness, anorexia, loss of weight, and depletion of energy that are insidious in onset and progressive in a gradual and relentless way. Suspicion is heightened when these are associated with the physical findings of a slowly enlarging mass or an ulcer at a cancer-bearing site.

Radiographic examination

More often physical examination is not helpful in the early part of the clinical illness because the primary site is internal. Two adjuncts to diagnosis are then useful – *radiographic and laboratory examinations.* These often fail to certify the diagnosis but strongly corroborate the clinical suspicion. A variety of techniques are helpful, including chest x-rays, contrast studies of the digestive tract, scan of various organs with injected radioactive isotopes, biochemical studies of the blood for evidence of organ dysfunction, and the use of gas as in pneumoencephalography to detect displacement of the ventricular system of the brain.

Tissue examination

While all these may make the clinical diagnosis of cancer virtually certain, *tissue examination is generally necessary to establish the diagnosis. The most reliable procedure is biopsy* in which a small portion of the lesion is excised, fixed, stained, and examined under the microscope by a pathologist. Somewhat less certain is needle biopsy in which the tissue is treated in the same way. The volume of tissue is so small, however, that alteration of tissue pattern may be difficult to discern, or the needle may fail to penetrate nodules of tumor so that the specimen consists of a cylinder of normal tissue. The method is nevertheless often successful in diagnosing primary cancer of the prostate and metastatic cancer of the liver. Recently it has become possible to treat venous blood in such a way that circulating cancer cells may be identified. The tumor cells are two to six times larger than leukocytes and display large nuclei, hyperchromatism, and multinucleation. It has been found that a larger number of tumor cells circulate at an earlier time than had previously been suspected; in a study of 547 patients with cancer, circulating tumor cells were found in about 20 percent in the first examination of a 20 ml. sample of blood [9]. It is, of course, necessary to distinguish circulating tumor cells from megakaryocytes, endothelial cells, and atypical leukocytes. The method is still being investigated and is not yet in general routine use.

Cytologic screening

While these procedures often establish the diagnosis of cancer, none is suitable for the screening of large numbers of patients and the detection of malignant disease at its inception. This is of critical importance since clinically evident malignant tumors are often incurable because of metastatic spread, while unsuspected tumors are often treatable while cure is still possible. Cytologic examination of exfoliated cells is thus extremely useful. Moreover, some common malignant tumors arise on surfaces from which specimens can be easily taken. The method is especially appropriate for monitoring the uterine cervix, large bronchi, and cells floating in aspirated pleural effusions and ascitic fluid. Examination must be performed by pathologists and technologists specially trained in these techniques.

The finding of large, irregular, or hyperchromatic nuclei in desquamated cells raises the suspicion of malignant disease and indicates the advisability of biopsy. It is to be emphasized that *cytologic findings may justify further procedures, but ordinarily do not suffice for the diagnosis of cancer.*

Dysplasia-neoplasia transition

With the technique of cytologic screening came the realization that cancers pass through incipient stages, often of long duration, before becoming frankly invasive. This stage, in which the individual cells are anaplastic in appearance but penetration of the basement membranes and invasion of the subjacent tissue has not yet occurred, is known as *carcinoma in situ. This condition is usually found about a decade prior to the detection of invasive cancer* of the uterine cervix and suggests that this transition period lasts about 10 years before frank carcinoma develops [10]. Ablative therapy at this stage of malignant transformation is curative. It should be mentioned, however, that the diagnosis of carcinoma in situ is somewhat subjective, and care must be exercised in crediting cure to lesions of uncertain progression. This matter is fraught with difficulty because cases of carcinoma in situ must be distinguished from precancerous conditions, some of which are known to regress spontaneously [11, 12].

Biochemical examination

The procedures mentioned do not complete the contribution of the laboratory to the diagnosis of cancer. Certain biochemical changes are also utilized. For example, *choriocarcinoma* is accompanied by a high concentration of *chorionic gonadotropin* in the serum, and the decline of this substance in the blood after the removal of the uterus is indicative of cure while persistence of an elevated blood level is suggestive of metastatic disease. Much more commonly the diagnosis of *metastatic carcinoma of liver* is a clinical question. The epithelial cells of the biliary tract secrete the enzyme *alkaline phosphatase,* and when metastatic nodules obstruct the flow of bile, even in only parts of the liver, increased serum levels of this enzyme are seen. Normal cells and malignant epithelial tumor cells of the *prostate* produce the enzyme *acid phosphatase* which usually escapes in the pathway of secretions of the gland, i.e., through the urethra. With cancerous invasion of paraprostatic tissue, and especially with metastasis to bone, the circulating level undergoes a sharp rise and is accordingly useful in the diagnosis of metastatic disease from this site. An additional example is the presence of *5-hydroxytryptamine* (serotonin) in the blood in cases of *metastatic carcinoid.* (Details of these diagnostic features are given under the systems in which these tumors arise.) It is thus evident that the laboratory provides especially useful techniques for certifying the diagnosis of cancer, for establishing the precise kind of cancer, and for following the progress of the malignant disease.

3. Treatment of Cancer

Objectives of treatment

The treatment of patients with cancer has two main *objectives: cure* and the amelioration of distress. The latter is called *palliation,* and it is the objective when cure is no longer possible. *Cure is accomplished by ablation or destruction of all the malignant cells.* This may be done by *surgical extirpation* as with cancer of the breast, or with *radiation therapy* as with cancer of the uterine cervix. Sometimes the two methods are combined with one preceding the other in either order. No matter what technique is used, however, elimination of all the cancer cells is the goal, and it is presumed that this is the requirement of cure.

The diagnosis of primary cancer does not reveal whether tumor cells have spread by direct invasion to nonresectable structures or whether metastasis has taken place to distant sites. It is nevertheless evident that with the passage of time one or both of these will occur, and when that happens, cure will usually no longer be possible. In awareness of this, the principle of treatment is the *eradication of all tumor from the largest amount of expendable tissue at the earliest moment.* Or, conversely, it may be stated that the *result of treatment cannot be improved by delaying the application of treatment, or by decreasing the amount of tissue from which all tumor is ablated.* The treatment may be too radical, of course, and in realization of this a limitation is necessary. The principle is thus refined to state that the treatment should not be so radical as to jeopardize the recovery of the patient, nor so simple as to allow recurrence because of failure to ablate tumor from expendable tissue. Within these limits, which must be judged separately for every case, lies the highest prospect of cure. The principle of curative treatment is discussed by Smith [13].

Principle of treatment

Palliation

When metastatic disease is known to be present, or when the tumor has spread into nonresectable tissue, the purpose of therapy becomes palliation rather than cure. For this, radiation and drug therapy are mainly relied on. *Radiation impounds energy randomly into cells* and the effect of this is to damage and distort the connections between molecules. *This is especially important in the DNA molecules of the nuclei.* When the intricate process of mitotic division occurs, that damage impedes the divisional process. Since malignant tumor cells divide more rapidly than normal cells, these cells are more vulnerable to irradiation; hence a selective effect is achieved. Certain tumors are especially responsive to radiation; they are in general those cancers whose cells are undergoing most frequent mitoses and those that are composed primarily of lymphoid tissue. The latter example is not based on a high divisional rate for the lymphoid cells; the reason for the special sensitivity of lymphoid tissue to radiation is not known. Examples of high radiation sensitivity are the undifferentiated carcinoma of the lung, neuroblastoma of the adrenal, retinoblastoma of the eye, and the malignant lymphomas, especially those of lymphocytic type. In addition, Hodgkin's disease, particularly when localized, is effectively suppressed by radiation therapy. The results are regarded as the equivalent of cure, although some tumor always persists so that cure by this method is never really achieved.

The *chemotherapy* of cancer is developing rapidly with increasing numbers of antitumor agents being identified. The principal ones fall into five categories – hormones, alkylating agents, antimetabolites, plant alkyloids, and antibiotics [14]. With *hormones* and with *plant alkyloids,* an environment is created that suppresses tumor cell growth although the precise mechanism is not clear. The *alkylating agents* appear to crosslink the strands of DNA in the nuclei of cells so that the mitotic divisional process is impaired. It is thus radiomimetic in its effect. The *antimetabolites* block the production of DNA by incorporating abnormal molecules into the nuclei of the rapidly dividing tumor cells. The *antibiotics* also appear to block DNA production, but by the mechanism of inhibiting an enzyme needed for the synthesis of transfer RNA, which in turn is needed for the synthesis of DNA. Examples of these agents and some tumors affected by them are shown in Table 14-3. Since most of the chemotherapeutic agents operate through inhibition of DNA synthesis or impairment of mitotic division, it may be seen that the tumors especially responsive to them are those characterized by rapid cell growth.

4. Results Without and With Treatment

Without treatment

Patients with cancer who are not treated almost invariably die from the effects of the tumor. The duration of life after the time of diagnosis, however, may be

TABLE 14-3. Anticancer Chemotherapeutic Agents

Class	Drug	Disease
Hormones	Estrogen	Cancer of prostate
	Cortisone	Leukemia
Alkylating agents	Nitrogen mustard	Hodgkin's disease
	Cyclophosphamide	Leukemia
Antimetabolites	6-Mercaptopurine	Leukemia
	5-Fluorouracil	Leukemia
	Methotrexate	Choriocarcinoma
Plant alkyloids	Vincristine	Lymphomas
	Vinblastine	Lymphomas
Antibiotics	Dactinomycin	Choriocarcinoma, Wilms' tumor

prolonged [15]. In his study of 100 cases of untreated cancer of the breast, Daland [16] found that 22 were alive after 5 years and 5 were alive after 10 years. The converse of this is that 78 died of cancer within 5 years, and 95 within 10 years. All the patients eventually succumbed to metastatic disease. Thus it is seen that the *outlook without treatment is essentially hopeless.*

With treatment

The objective of treatment is the eradication of all tumor cells since it is presumed that even a single viable cancer cell will multiply and eventually cause recurrence of the disease. This is expected from the experimental evidence that a single leukemic cell injected into a normal mouse eventually causes a lethal leukemic state in that animal [17]. Except for choriocarcinoma of the endometrium which has perhaps been cured by antimetabolites, there are only two presently known methods that are capable of achieving cure, alone or in combination, i.e., radiation and extirpative surgery. The cancers most amenable to these methods are those that are superficial and accessible to early recognition and prompt treatment. Best results are accordingly found with cancers of the skin, lip, buccal mucosa, breast, uterine cervix, and endometrium.

When the cancers are deep, the same methods may be appropriate but the results are worse because (1) the tumors are not clinically evident in the early stage, (2) spread outside the treatable field often occurs before the diagnosis is made, or (3) vital structures adjacent to the tumor cannot be sacrificed by the method of treatment. Cancers of the lungs, stomach, and pancreas, for example, are thus attended by relatively poor results.

The result of treatment is expressed by the rate of survival, and the periods for tally are customarily 5 and 10 years. If no recurrence of the disease is evident 5 years after treatment, the outlook is hopeful and the prospect is good that all tumor has been ablated. At 10 years, cure is usually presumed and the prognosis from that time forward is often no different from that of comparable persons without malignant disease.

Accomplishment of treatment

The accomplishment of the method of treatment is the eradication of tumor from a certain volume of tissue. For simple mastectomy, for example, that volume is the amputated breast, and for radical mastectomy it is the breast plus the pectoral muscles and the axillary contents including the lymph nodes. With

Cause of recurrence

radiation therapy the tissue volume is defined by the radius of the cancerocidal effect whether it applies to the breast, the endometrial cavity, or the external uterine cervix. Whether a given patient survives and is cured, or succumbs sometime later from metastatic disease, depends on whether tumor cells have spread outside the resectable tissue in the case of surgical treatment, or outside the cancerocidal radius of the x-rays or gamma rays in the case of radiation therapy. In either of these events, cure is ordinarily no longer possible. The indication that tumor has spread beyond the treatable field is the presence of tumor at the periphery of the resected specimen or in the lymph nodes adjacent to the margins of the excised tissue. *Whenever this finding is made, the prospect of cure is substantially reduced.* The outlook for the patient is thus largely revealed by the distribution of the tumor cells in the treated tissue, and this is disclosed by pathologic study when a resected specimen is available for examination.

Tumor cell distribution

The factors that are associated with tumor cell distribution prior to therapy, and hence determine the curability of cancer, are especially the *promptness with which the patient seeks medical attention for a sign or symptom,* and *the earliness with which the tumor cells spread away from the site of origin.* Only the former factor can be affected by the patient, and it is accordingly important that the signs and symptoms of malignant disease be given the widest public notice so that well patients are encouraged to undergo physical examination for cancer detection at regular intervals. The second factor is the *aggressiveness of the cancer cells.* That is an inherent property of the individual tumor. The reason for variations in aggressiveness in tumors of different kinds, and in different tumors of the same kind, is simply not known. The term that dignifies this area of ignorance is *biologic predeterminism* [18]. Those cancers that are characterized by rapid invasive growth and early metastasis are accordingly attended by the lowest rates of survival. In general, sarcomas and undifferentiated carcinomas behave in this way, while epithelial tumors that closely resemble the normal tissue from which they arose, and are hence well differentiated, tend to grow more slowly and spread less rapidly.

Treatment evaluation:

From the foregoing it is evident that the *result of treatment will be due to two factors – the volume of tissue cleared of tumor by the method of treatment, and the distribution of the tumor cells with respect to that volume at the time of treatment.* The latter is always uncertain from clinical examination of the patient. In order to compare different methods of treatment, however, it is necessary to control the variable of tumor cell distribution so that comparability within the groups is achieved.

staging

This is done by *grouping patients according to arbitrary stages of the disease,* i.e., according to the extent of tumor cell spread. For example, stage I for cervical cancer consists of those cases in which the tumor appears localized to the cervical tissue; in stage II the tumor cells are thought to be spread to the parametrium, in stage III the infiltration has extended to the pelvic wall, and in stage IV the cancer involves the urinary bladder or the rectum or has extended outside the true pelvis. Similar schemes for the staging of tumor cell distribution are utilized for cancers of the breast and colon. These schemes allow the results of treatment to be compared between groups of cases of the same stage. Comparability is not entirely achieved by these plans, however, because the practice of staging, which is based on clinical estimation, is not altogether accurate. Moreover, the difference in the accomplishment of comparable methods of treatment is often slight. It is for these two reasons that identification of the superior method of treatment by a comparison of survival rates is especially difficult [19, 20]. Realization that the accomplishment of the method is the volume of tissue ablated of tumor, by whatever means, and the rate of survival is the proportion of patients in whom all the tumor lay within the tissue ablated, facilitates interpretation of the results of different methods of treatment. Despite these matters, however, the practice of clinical staging of cancer is useful, and the principal benefit is to indicate in a general way the prognosis for the patient.

grading

In addition to staging, the *grading of cancer has also been used for the purpose of indicating the prospects for cure.* Grading requires histologic examination and expresses the degree of differentiation of the tumor in the diagnosis. Well-differentiated carcinomas, i.e., those closely resembling the normal tissue of origin, are generally less rapidly invasive than poorly differentiated cancers in which anaplasia is pronounced and differentiation is slight. Although several schemes are available for such grading, especially for cancer of the uterine cervix, only limited usefulness has been achieved because the histologic pattern varies within different portions of the same tumor, and the extent of spread of the neoplasm is not reflected in the degree of differentiation of the lesion. Nevertheless, in a general way it may be said that the higher the differentiation of the tumor, the less aggressive it is expected to be and the better the prospects for a favorable result.

Expectations

The prospect for cure varies so much with the site of origin of the tumors that prognosis for individual cancers will be included under the section on neoplasia within the various anatomic systems. When metastasis has occurred, or when the malignancy is multicentric as with the lymphomas, palliation is the highest expectation of treatment. For such lesions, radiation and drug therapy are the methods of choice. While cure cannot yet be claimed for the anticancer drugs (except perhaps for choriocarcinoma) or for radiation (except for superficial cancers), much progress is nevertheless being made, the prolongation of life is being regularly achieved, and remissions for extended periods are being recorded for patients with such rapidly growing cancers as acute leukemia, Burkitt's lymphoma, and Wilms' tumor [14].

5. *Causes*

The cause of some cancers is established, and in others a causative agent is highly suspect. The known causes of cancer include *hereditary defects, ionizing radiation, chemical carcinogens,* and *living agents.*

Heredity

Hereditary defects are presumably due to randomly acquired mutations. Three conditions associated with malignant tumor formation are clearly inherited, two as dominant genes. They are retinoblastoma of the eye, familial polyposis of the colon, and xeroderma pigmentosum of the skin; all are uncommon.

Retinoblastoma arises in infancy, usually before the age of 2, and is ordinarily unilateral. While most cases are sporadic, a familial pattern for others is well known [21]. In the latter, a single dominant gene, not always achieving expression, seems to be at fault. In *polyposis coli,* the mucosa of the entire colon is studded with hundreds of adenomas of different sizes. This condition is transmitted as a dominant gene carried by either parent [22]. A unique feature is that the adenomas are not present at birth and do not develop until adolescence. The condition is of particular importance because one or more of the adenomas regularly undergoes malignant transformation several years after the clinical onset of the disease. Total colectomy is thus required for prophylactic treatment. A third inherited condition is *xeroderma pigmentosum* in which the skin is extremely sensitive to solar radiation. Beginning in early life the skin shows widespread freckling, keratosis, telangiectasia, and papilloma formation. Sometime later, and especially in areas exposed to sunlight, malignant transformation takes place and carcinomas, sarcomas, or melanoblastomas form. Unlike the previously described conditions, xeroderma pigmentosum is inherited as a simple recessive character [23]. In some other and more common cancers, such as of breast, uterus, and prostate, a familial incidence higher than that of the general population has been discerned [24].

Ionizing radiation

Ionizing radiation also causes cancer. While it is not common, and the mechanism is not clear, two features nevertheless stand out: *a relatively high dose and a relatively long time are required for the process to take place.* When these conditions exist, a wide variety of malignant tumors may arise, the kind depending especially on the tissue exposed, the intensity of the ionization, and the duration of the exposure.

For some time after the discovery of x-rays in 1895, it was not realized that exposure was harmful. Radiation workers of those days therefore worked without shielding, and years later an especially common effect was atrophy and fibrosis of the skin of the hands, with subsequent contraction, ulceration, and the formation of squamous cell carcinomas. Radiation carcinogenesis also became apparent in the high incidence of *carcinoma of the lung in the pitchblende miners* of central Europe. The mines were unventilated, the dust contained radioelements, and these were inhaled over long exposure times. Radon, an alpha emitter, was one of the offending agents, and from 44 to 75 percent of the pitchblende miners eventually developed malignant disease [25]. Particularly tragic is the American experience of *watch-dial painters* who moistened the tips of their paint brushes with their lips. The brushes were dipped in radium paint, the paint was thus absorbed, and the radium was sequestered especially in bone. Years later, osteogenic sarcomas arose in many of these workers [26].

Medical efforts have also contributed to the examples of radiation carcinogenesis. It was previously standard practice to *treat enlargement of the thymus and hyperplasia of the lymphoid tissue about the nasopharynx with ionizing radiation.* Years later it was discovered that the incidence of carcinoma of the thyroid is higher in the irradiated patients than in a comparable segment of the nonradiated population [27]. Another medical example was the *use of Thorotrast,* a radiopaque material used for contrast studies of the biliary and other systems. Thorotrast contains thorium dioxide which is taken up by the reticuloendothelial system and retained indefinitely. Years after intravenous injection of this material, which emits alpha radiation, endothelial sarcomas of the liver and carcinomas of bile duct and hepatic cell types arose [28]. An additional and most convincing medical example occurred with the use of radiation for the *treatment of ankylosing spondylitis* which was popular for a time in England. High doses were used and subsequently, after a period of several years, an increased incidence of myelogenous leukemia occurred in these patients [29].

It might thus be foreseeable that the *irradiation exposures incident to the atom bombing in Japan would also be attended by an increased incidence of leukemia.* This did occur; the cases were mostly myelogenous in type, the frequency increased with proximity to the epicenter, and the peak incidence occurred approximately 4 to 8 years after the time of exposure and subsequently subsided [30]. Projecting that experience further, inquiry was made as to whether leukemia is more common in radiologists than in physicians in other specialties. The evidence indicates an incidence of *leukemia in American radiologists that is substantially higher than that in the general male population or in medical specialists not engaged in the field of radiology* [31]. Altogether these examples certify the carcinogenic effect of ionizing radiation. The mechanism of this effect is not precisely known, although disruptions at critical sites in the nuclei of cells are presumed to be causative.

While the case for ionizing radiation as a carcinogenic agent is clear, it is not to be overlooked that radiation of lower energy also has a somewhat similar effect. For example, sunlight with its ultraviolet component causes squamous cell carcinoma of exposed tissue, especially the lower lip and skin of the face. Those employed in outdoor occupations such as sailors and farmers are especially prone.

Chemical carcinogens

Chemical agents also cause cancer. The first report of this was by Potts in 1775 who observed a high incidence of scrotal cancer in chimney sweeps. Soot was the suspect material. In 1915 confirmation was provided by Yamagiwa [32] who produced cancer of the skin by applying coal tar repeatedly to the ears of rabbits. This was the *first experimental production of cancer by a chemical agent.* Subsequent investigations revealed that the *carcinogenic materials in coal tar are especially benzpyrene, methylcholanthrene, and derivatives of anthracene.* Of these, the first two are particularly potent, and *benzpyrene is the most important,* being present in soot, smoked fish and meats, and cigarette smoke. These hydrocarbons in experimental application cause carcinomas and sarcomas in visceral tissues and on skin surfaces depending on whether they are applied, ingested, or injected. The cholanthrene hydrocarbons are of particular interest because of their structural resemblance to normal biologic materials, i.e., sterols and bile salts. They thus suggest the possibility of carcinogenic substances being produced in the body.

The carcinogenic properties of hydrocarbons are also of importance because of the magnitude of *cigarette smoking.* In 1955, 68 percent of men and 32 percent of women in America over 18 years of age regularly smoked cigarettes [33]. The popularity of this practice, until recently, has continued upward. For example, cigarette consumption per person over 15 years of age in America was 138 per year in 1910, 3322 in 1950, and 3986 by 1962. Cigarette smoke contains a tar that is carcinogenic; painted on the backs of mice, it produces papillomas and squamous cell carcinomas [34]. In the United States the number of deaths due to *cancer of the lung* rose from about 6500 in 1942 to 45,000 in 1967. Moreover, *death rates* are higher for smokers than nonsmokers, and the rates correlate with the number of cigarettes smoked. For men smoking 10 cigarettes per day, the death rate from all causes is 40 percent greater than for nonsmokers; at 10 to 19 cigarettes per day, the rate is 70 percent greater, and at 40 or more cigarettes per day, the death rate is 120 percent greater than that of nonsmokers. In comparison, it is of interest that the smoking of fewer than 5 cigars per day does not raise the death rate, nor does pipe smoking even though as many as 10 pipefuls are smoked per day for as long as 20 years.

In 1932 the *azo dyes* were found to have the selective effect of producing benign and malignant *tumors of the liver.* The most potent of these was dimethylaminoazobenzene, known more commonly as butter yellow. This disclosure was of much importance because the dye was used at one time to impart the color of butter to margarine. The *aromatic amines* are also known to be carcinogenic, and no matter how applied, one of them, 2-naphthylamine, selectively causes cancer of the urinary bladder. Occupational exposure was thus a risk of the aniline dye industry. The parent structures of these three classes of organic molecules are shown in the figure.

Polycyclic hydrocarbons

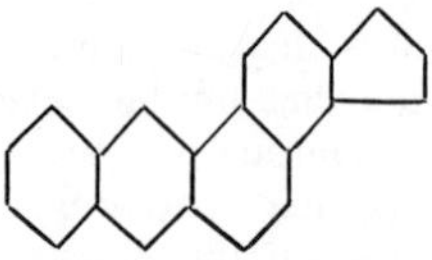

benzpyrene 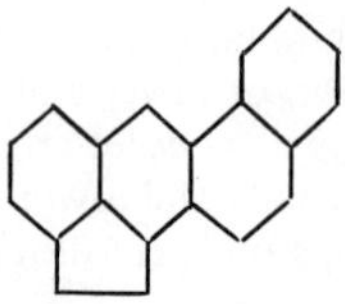　　cholanthrene 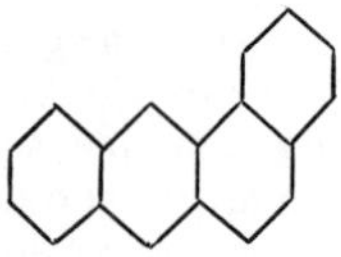　　benzanthracene

Azo dye

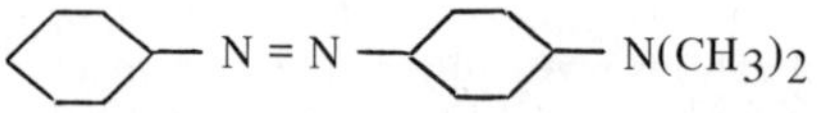

$N = N$ — $N(CH_3)_2$

dimethylaminoazobenzene (butter yellow)

Aromatic amine

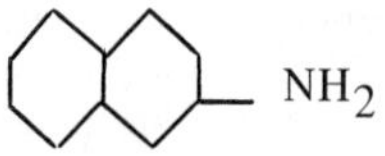

NH_2

2-naphthylamine

Molecular structure of chemical carcinogens.

In addition, several other chemical agents are known to be carcinogenic. Examples include *arsenic* which induces papillomas and carcinomas of the skin, *asbestos* which is suspected of causing mesothelioma of the pleura, and *beryllium salts* which cause skeletal sarcomas in rabbits. More recently *plastics and metal foils, especially silver,* have been found experimentally to produce malignant tumors. The subject is reviewed by Bischoff and Bryson [35]. Thus the list of carcinogenic agents continues to grow. It is nevertheless to be understood that some of the examples pertain only to the experimental animal rather than to man, and others are present in the human environment only in vanishingly small amounts. The place and importance of chemical agents in the etiology of human cancer is far from settled.

Living agents

With respect to living agents, *viruses* have held the principal role. No virus is yet established as a cause of human cancer, but the evidence from experimental studies strongly suggests that some human malignant tumors are so caused, and that more than one virus may be carcinogenic for humans. It is evident that proof of this is extremely difficult since humans can hardly be used as test models, and the coexistence of a virus and a malignant tumor does not certify that the former is the cause of the latter. In addition, as Rowe [36] points out, Koch's postulates are not easily met because of the ordinarily long interval between the period of virus multiplication in the body and the time of tumor formation. Finally, some viruses known to be tumorigenic are not consistently so. The problem of establishing cause is thus complex.

In 1910 Peyton Rous [37] discovered that a virus causes sarcomas in fowls. Some years later, in 1932, Shope [38] isolated a viral agent from fibromas and papillomas of rabbits. A third pivotal discovery was made by Bittner [39]. It had been presumed that the high incidence of mammary carcinoma in certain strains of mice was an inherited legacy passed from mothers to offspring. Bittner found, however, that when the weanling mice were breast-fed by nontumorigenic strains, the mammary cancers failed to occur. In this way it was learned that a carcinogenic subcellular agent was passing to the offspring through the breast milk of the mother. These three early investigations are the foundation of the interest in the viral cause of human cancers. Since that time, viral causes of several kinds of tumors have been isolated for several species of animals.

The most important known tumor viruses are listed in Table 14-4. It is of interest that no properties so far recognized set these organisms apart from

TABLE 14-4. The Most Important Known Tumor Viruses

Group	Virus	Host	Tumorigenicity
Papovavirus	Polyoma	Mouse	Natural
	Simian vacuolating	Monkey	Artificial
Adenovirus	12, 18, 7	Human, mouse, rat	Artificial
Poxvirus	Fibroma	Rabbit	Natural
Myxovirus-like	Leukemia	Mouse	Natural
	Leukosis	Chicken	Natural
	Mammary	Mouse	Natural

nontumorigenic viruses. Moreover, not all members of any group are tumorigenic. The papovaviruses and adenoviruses contain DNA and replicate in the nucleus of the infested cell, the poxviruses contain DNA and replicate in the cytoplasm, and the myxovirus-like agents contain RNA and attach to the membranes of the affected cells [36]. Duryee and co-workers [40] have shown cytologic and histochemical similarities between virus-induced neoplasms in frogs and spontaneous neoplasms in humans.

In connection with the possibility of a viral-induced human cancer, Burkitt [41] has described a lesion regarded as a malignant lymphoma that is common in Africa and presents unusual epidemiologic features. These include a high prevalence in children, a unique geographic distribution, and an independence from racial selectivity. In addition, the condition occurs at altitudes under 5000 feet, at places with temperatures above 60°F., and in areas in which the rainfall exceeds 20 inches per year. At such sites, man-biting mosquitoes are plentiful and are known to be carriers of viral diseases. These features give weight to the possibility that the tumor is vector-borne, possibly by mosquitoes, and that the agent, if it is infective, may be a virus.

Other living agents are associated with tumor formation although a direct causal relationship is not established. *Bacterial infections,* for example, especially when associated with chronic draining sinuses, may be complicated by tumor formation in the lining cells of the sinus tract. Certain *parasitic ova* are also associated with cancer – *Schistosoma haematobium* with carcinoma of the urinary bladder, *S. mansoni* with cancer of the colon, and *S. japonicum* and *Clonorchis sinesis* with cancer of the liver. More recently, *aflatoxin,* a metabolic product of the fungus *Aspergillus flavum,* has been found to be a potent hepatocarcinogen, and, in addition, it is found in relatively high concentration in the diet of Africans where the incidence of liver cell cancer is especially high [42].

6. Proposed Mechanisms of Cancer Formation

The mechanism of cancer formation is a separate consideration from the cause of cancer. While mechanisms are not altogether understood, a variety of stimulating proposals have been advanced. An early concept was that of Warburg [43]. who believed that the process of malignant transformation involved a *change from normal cellular respiration with oxygen consumption to a dependency on fermentation for the generation of cellular energy.* Warburg proposed that this adaptation takes place gradually, requires several generations, and causes a more aggressive cellular growth pattern that is manifested by tumor formation. A principal evidence for this is that much more lactic acid is produced by cancer cells than by normal cells. The cause of this defect is now attributed to a malfunction of the mitochondria in the tumor cells [44].

Shortly after the suggestion of Warburg, Osgood [45] pointed out that under normal conditions when a cell divides, one member remains immature to divide again while the other matures, functions, and eventually dies without dividing. Since the intermitotic period for the reproducing cell is proportional to the life span of the mature cell, renewal and depletion are in balance and the total number of cells in the population remains constant. Osgood proposed that a *decrease in the intermitotic period* would account for an arithmetic increase in the cell number and represent benign neoplasia, while an alteration causing both cells to remain immature would provide for a logarithmic increase in cell number and represent malignant neoplasia. He suggested that mutations might be the cause of both these changes.

Failla [46] proposed that normal cells produce an *antiproliferating agent* and that when a mutation affects the gene controlling this agent, the substance is no longer produced. In that event the cell divides without limit and becomes malignant. A tumor arises, however, only when the adjacent normal cells fail to produce sufficient antiproliferating agent and the tumor cells reach a sufficient mass to overwhelm the inhibitory effect at the margins of the new growth.

More recently Pitot [47] has considered neoplasia in terms of *cell differentiation.* He has pointed out that messenger RNA templates become stabilized as the cell differentiates and becomes mature. He suggests that in neoplasia a carcinogen may alter the stability of certain messenger RNA templates, giving rise to a new state of differentiation that includes a selective growth advantage for those cells. The importance of this suggestion is that it provides for a mechanism of neoplasia that does not require a genomic change in the nucleus of the affected cell.

Whether the critical step occurs in the nucleus, on an RNA template, or on a cell membrane, it is clear that the precise mechanism of neoplastic transformation, if it is indeed a single mechanism, is not yet precisely defined.

NEOPLASMS NOT RESTRICTED TO A SINGLE ORGAN SYSTEM

The discussion of neoplasms of the individual organs is presented with the pathology of the organ systems. Those neoplasms which are not restricted to a single organ system – as neoplasms arising in fibrous connective tissue or in surface epithelium – are now considered.

1. Neoplasms Arising From Fibrous Connective Tissue

BENIGN: Fibroma

The classic *benign tumor* arising *from fibrous connective tissue* is the *fibroma.* The most common *sites* for the fibroma are the subcutaneous tissues and the fascial planes between muscles of the extremities; less commonly fibromas occur in ovaries, bones, and parenchymatous viscera. *Grossly* these neoplasms are usually distinctly encapsulated, rolling about easily in the tissues because of their lack of attachment. They are firm and rubbery. On section they have a white, moist, glistening appearance. Sometimes the cut surface has a sticky or slippery feel, due to mucinous degeneration. *Microscopically* the characteristic cells are fibroblasts. Their spindle-shaped nuclei are separated by wavy connective tissue fibrils.

The fibroma has little tendency to become malignant.

Variants of fibroma

Several variants of the fibroma are commonly recognized. The *myxoma,* which seems to be simply a fibroma with extensive mucinous degeneration, occurs in the soft tissues of the extremities of elderly persons, usually as a deep-seated fusiform mass between muscles. *Desmoid* or *desmoid tumor* is the fibroma which appears in women during the course of pregnancy, usually in the abdominal wall and particularly in the sheath of the rectus abdominis muscle. It sometimes grows with alarming rapidity. The *dermatofibroma protuberans* is a firm, rounded fibroma bulging above the skin. The *neurofibroma* (neurilemmoma, neurinoma) is a common benign fibrous tissue tumor formed from the sheath of Schwann of a peripheral nerve, and usually revealed as a subcutaneous nodule (see Chapter 26). So-called *fibroids* of the uterus actually arise from smooth muscle and are considered under that heading. A pseudotumor, often referred to as *palmar* or *plantar fibromatosis,* is a flat, bandlike formation of fibrous connective tissue that occurs in the palmar or plantar fascia and causes contraction of the tendons of the fingers or toes. It is a diffuse process of unknown cause, not a distinct neoplasm. A *keloid* is a nodular fibrous growth that develops in a skin scar following accidental injury or surgery. It is common in the Negro, rare in members of other races. Its cause is unknown; it is thought not to be a true neoplasm.

MALIGNANT: Fibrosarcoma

The *malignant neoplasm of fibrous tissue* is known as the *fibrosarcoma.* It is the classic malignant tumor of the soft tissues of the extremities. While not common in any location, its most frequent *sites* are the fascia between the muscles of an extremity, the chest wall, the retroperitoneal tissues, subcutaneous tissues, and periosteum. Rarely fibrosarcomas arise in the fibrous tissue stroma of a visceral organ, such as the prostate, lungs, or stomach. *Grossly* it is unencapsulated, and often shows scattered yellow areas of necrosis or reddish foci of hemorrhage. The less cellular, and usually less malignant, forms of the neoplasm are somewhat firmer. *Microscopically* the softest neoplasms of this type are composed almost entirely of cell nuclei, and have insignificant amounts of connective tissue fibrils. In the firmer fibrosarcomas the cells have relatively more cytoplasm, the neoplasm approaching the histologic appearance of the fibroma. There is no separate supporting stroma in this neoplasm, blood vessels are thin-walled, and neoplastic cells are adjacent to the vessels and may in fact line vessels. Bizarre atypical cell forms, multinucleated giant cells, and atypical mitotic figures are commonly seen, especially in the more malignant forms of fibrosarcoma.

Natural history of fibrosarcoma

The fibrosarcomas range from the lowest to the highest grades of malignancy. The lowest-grade fibrosarcomas, as revealed by a regular cell pattern of almost adult fibroblasts, are slowly growing tumors, occurring usually after middle life. They may remain local for years before invading veins and metastasizing to the lungs. Generous surgical excision will result in cure in many of these well-differentiated neoplasms. At the other end of the scale of malignancy are the high-grade fibrosarcomas, composed of cells with large spindle-shaped nuclei and scant cytoplasm. These neoplasms occur chiefly in children or young adults and grow rapidly, invading veins and metastasizing early, chiefly to the lungs.

Variants of fibrosarcoma

In the elderly person the fibrosarcoma often undergoes mucoid degeneration, giving a moist, even cystic appearance to the cut surface. This variant, known as the *myxosarcoma* or the *fibromyxosarcoma,* usually grows slowly, recurring locally after excision but metastasizing late. The *malignant schwannoma* is the malignant tumor of the fibrous sheath of peripheral nerves, and is the malignant equivalent of the neurofibroma; this tumor is considered in more detail in Chapter 26. The fibrous tumor of the serous membranes known as *fibrous mesothelioma* is rare, seen more often in the pleura than in the pericardium or peritoneum. It tends to seed over the serosal surface, restricting the movement of the contained viscera, forming dense adhesions. Metastasis is late and rather unusual (see Chapter 19).

2. Neoplasms Arising From Adipose Tissue

BENIGN: Lipoma

The *benign neoplasm* arising in *adipose tissue,* the *lipoma,* is a very common tumor. Its most frequent *sites* are the subcutaneous tissues of the neck, shoulders, and back, but it may be found beneath the skin anywhere, in the mesentery, or in the retroperitoneal tissues. Rarely lipomas occur in the submucosa of the stomach or intestines. The *gross* appearance of a lipoma is almost always characteristic; it is soft, and presents a well-defined capsule which separates it from the adipose tissue in which it is usually embedded. The cut surface is distinctly yellow and glistening, resembling normal subcutaneous fat. *Microscopically* the lipoma resembles normal adult adipose tissue in all respects, and cannot be distinguished from it unless the section includes the capsule.

Subcutaneous lipomas tend to remain benign throughout life, but occasionally the retroperitoneal or mesenteric lipomas become malignant.

Xanthoma

The *xanthoma* is a controversial lesion, considered by some to be a variant of the lipoma, but there is serious doubt whether it is a true neoplasm, an inflammatory swelling, or a manifestation of disturbed lipid metabolism. (Many patients with xanthomas show a high value for serum cholesterol.) The most common *sites* for xanthomas are about the joints, particularly the finger joints, where they are commonly attached to tendon sheaths; rarely xanthomas are encountered in the bones, meninges, or lungs. *Grossly* xanthomas are firmer than lipomas, and they are not always encapsulated. The cut surface has a distinctly yellow color. *Microscopically* the xanthoma is composed of mononuclear cells, fibroblasts, and occasional giant cells. The mononuclear cells contain tiny fat droplets, giving the cytoplasm a foamy appearance in paraffin sections. The Touton giant cell, which is characteristic of the xanthoma, is smaller than the Langhans giant cell and has a peripheral ring of nuclei. There is no known malignant neoplasm corresponding to the xanthoma.

Variants of lipoma

The *hibernoma* is a rare fatty tumor occurring chiefly about the neck and shoulders, and resembling the so-called hibernating gland of bears and certain other animals. Occasionally abnormal but unencapsulated collections of fat occur in one breast or in the neck, producing the condition known as *lipomatosis;* these masses are ordinarily considered non-neoplastic. *Adiposis dolorosa* (Dercum's disease) is a poorly understood disease manifest by painful fatty swellings. Occasionally an abdominal hernia, especially at the umbilicus, may contain adipose tissue from the omentum and be confused with a lipoma.

MALIGNANT: Liposarcoma

The malignant *liposarcoma* is a relatively rare tumor. It may occur in adipose tissue anywhere but its most common *sites* are in the lower extremities and in the retroperitoneal or mesenteric tissues. *Grossly* it is soft and unencapsulated, usually being indistinguishable from fibrosarcoma, but sometimes it has a yellowish gray appearance suggesting modified fat. *Microscopically* it contains immature fibroblasts, embryonic fat, and occasional large, branching stellate cells, the lipoblasts. These can be shown to contain neutral fat in their cytoplasm if frozen sections are prepared and stained with Sudan III or Scarlet R. (Tumor cells of other origin may contain neutral fat as a result of cell degeneration; the demonstration of cytoplasmic fat is therefore not diagnostic of liposarcoma.)

Liposarcomas infiltrate and spread in about the same way as do fibrosarcomas, but in our experience metastasis is usually later and less widespread than with fibrosarcomas.

3. *Neoplasms Arising From Smooth Muscle*

BENIGN: Leiomyoma

Benign tumors of *smooth muscle origin – leiomyomas* – are extremely common. The most frequent *site* is the uterus (see Chapter 24), followed by the stomach and esophagus; rarely leiomyomas are encountered in the dermis, presumably derived from the arrectores pilorum muscles, or possibly from the muscle coats of blood vessels. *Grossly* leiomyomas are slowly growing tumors, sometimes reaching the size of a man's head. They are well encapsulated, and the cut surface has a glistening, grayish white, whorled appearance. Secondary changes (infarction, mucinous degeneration liquefaction and cyst formation, calcification, and even ossification) may occur as a result of ischemia. *Microscopically* the leiomyoma is composed of smooth muscle cells – elongated or spindle-shaped cells with prominent nuclei and fibrillar cytoplasm. These fibrils run in all directions, intertwining with each other.

MALIGNANT: Leiomyosarcoma

Sometimes the leiomyoma takes on more rapid growth and assumes the character of a malignant tumor, but this probably occurs in no more than 2 to 3 percent of the cases. The *leiomyosarcoma* occurs in the same *sites* as its benign counterpart – chiefly the uterus or gastrointestinal tract. *Grossly* it may have a semblance of a capsule, especially if it began as a benign tumor, but often there is no capsule. The neoplasm is usually soft and brainlike, and tends to show areas of necrosis and hemorrhage. *Microscopically* leiomyosarcoma may be indistinguishable from fibrosarcoma, even when differential stains are employed. Bizarre nuclear forms and multinucleated giant cells are somewhat more common in the muscle tumor than in fibrosarcoma. It is sometimes difficult to distinguish the leiomyosarcoma from the benign leiomyoma, especially when the latter shows the growth stimulus that results from pregnancy. Mitosis counts per calculated volume of tissue are sometimes used to aid in the differentiation. The *natural history* of the leiomyosarcoma is usually one of slow local growth and spread to adjacent tissues, followed later by venous invasion and pulmonary metastases.

4. Neoplasms Arising From Striated Muscle

BENIGN: Rhabdomyoma

The *benign tumor* of *voluntary muscles,* the *rhabdomyoma,* occurs very rarely. It is most commonly seen as a *congenital neoplasm* involving the myocardium in the condition known as epiloia (see Chapter 13), in which other types of benign tumors occur in the brain and kidneys. Rhabdomyoma is most unusual in voluntary muscles themselves. A related neoplasm, whose status is not clearly established, is the *granular cell myoblastoma,* a benign tumor that occurs chiefly in the tongue, but also in subcutaneous sites where voluntary muscles are found. This tumor may be recognized microscopically by nests of large cells with finely granular cytoplasm, lying between bundles of normal-appearing striated muscle fibers. Some believe that this tumor arises from peripheral nerves rather than from voluntary muscles.

MALIGNANT: Rhabdomyosarcoma

The *rhabdomyosarcoma,* although also rare, is somewhat more common than its benign counterpart. It may occur in pure form in the muscles of the extremities, or more commonly as a part of a complex mesodermal tumor of the uterus or kidneys. The characteristic *rhabdomyoblasts* are large, often multinucleated cells with intensely eosinophilic cytoplasm, often stretching out in long ribbon-like processes. Cross striations can be found in the cytoplasmic processes if carefully searched for. More rarely alveolar and embryonal forms occur [48], showing little resemblance to muscle cells. The rhabdomyosarcoma is a rapidly progressive tumor in most instances. Death usually results from pulmonary metastasis within a year or two of onset. Lymph node metastases also occur in about half the cases – a finding at variance with the usual experience with sarcomas as a group.

5. Neoplasms of Mixed Mesenchymal Origin

Occasionally several types of connective tissues become neoplastic in a part at the same time, giving rise to *complex tumors.* Thus a neoplasm consisting of *fibrous and fatty tissues* and of *blood vessels* may form a local mass deep in the flesh of an extremity. Such tumors are sometimes known as *mesenchymomas.* Since this term is occasionally used for malignant neoplasms of the same mixed origin, one should modify the term, speaking of benign or malignant mesenchymomas. Strange malignant tumors of this type, occasionally mixed with neoplastic epithelial elements, sometimes occur in the uterus (see Chapter 24). In other instances mesenchymal tissues may be intermixed with ectodermal or endodermal elements to give rise to truly complex tumors known as teratomas. Sometimes the tissues of a teratoma may present such a range of variation as to be confused with a deformed twin attached to the host (see Chapter 16).

6. Neoplasms of Surface Epithelium

The *benign tumor* of *squamous epithelium* is the *papilloma;* the term is also

BENIGN: Squamous papilloma

applied to benign neoplasms arising from surfaces covered with transitional or columnar epithelium. The squamous papilloma is one of the most common neoplasms; the ordinary wart of the *skin of the hands* (verruca vulgaris) is the classic example. Other common sites for the *squamous papilloma* are the *buccal mucosa, larynx,* and *external genitalia. Grossly* these neoplasms project above the epithelial surface in a branching, cauliflower pattern, usually 0.5 to 1 cm. in height. *Microscopically* the neoplasm has a fibrous and vascular stalk covered over abundantly with well-differentiated epithelial cells; the resulting growth closely resembles a head of cauliflower. The papilloma of the skin surface is dry and firm, sometimes even hornlike, because of its heavy cornified layer; generally the papilloma of a mucous surface is soft, since the keratinous layer is usually poorly developed in a mucous membrane.

Papillomas of transitional and columnar epithelium

Papillomas may also arise from the *transitional epithelium* of the *urinary bladder, ureter,* and *renal pelvis,* from the *columnar epithelium* lining the *colon, gallbladder, uterine cervix,* and *ducts of glandular organs* such as the breast, and from the *cells lining neoplastic cysts,* as of the ovaries, pancreas, or thyroid gland. In each of these instances they grow out from the epithelial surface, into a preformed space. *Grossly* these tumors are often smaller and more delicate and fernlike than the papillomas of squamous epithelium, but they show the same branching pattern. *Microscopically* the fibrous and vascular stalk is covered over with the type of epithelium characteristic of the location.

Malignant potentiality

True squamous papillomas, especially those of the skin, rarely became malignant, but the papillomas of the urinary tract, colon, and mammary ducts are more apt to do so. Each of these neoplasms is considered in more detail in the chapter dealing with the corresponding organ system.

MALIGNANT: Epidermoid carcinoma

The *malignant neoplasm* common to all surfaces covered with *squamous epithelium* is the *epidermoid carcinoma.* Its usual *sites* are *skin, lip, buccal mucosa, esophagus, larynx, bronchi* (where its development is preceded by squamous metaplasia of the ciliated epithelial lining), and *uterine cervix. Grossly* this neoplasm begins as a slight thickening of the skin or mucosal surface; later this may become ulcerated in the center, leaving raised indurated edges. The lesion tends to bleed easily and will not heal. Usually there is only slight elevation of the surface; most of the growth is downward, into the deeper tissues. *Microscopically* the first evident change is an increase in the size of the cell nuclei in relation to the amount of cytoplasm. These large, dark-staining nuclei are scattered throughout the thickness of the epidermis, obliterating the normal cell layers. At this earliest stage there is no penetration of the basement membrane and the neoplasm is said to be *preinvasive,* or *carcinoma in situ.* Later the neoplastic epithelial cells penetrate the normal basement membranes and infiltrate the deeper tissues. The grading of malignant neoplasms, discussed briefly on page 343, is widely used in the pathologic evaluation of epidermoid carcinomas. In the least malignant (grade I) neoplasms of this series, each nest of cells contains a laminated keratinous mass (pearly body) indicating good cell maturation; in the most malignant cases (grade IV) there is no keratin and the neoplastic cells consist largely of nuclei and show numerous mitoses. *Spread* is characteristically by the lymphatics to the regional lymph nodes; distant metastasis is a relatively late occurrence in epidermoid carcinomas.

Basal cell carcinoma

The other malignant neoplasm arising from squamous epithelium, the *basal cell carcinoma,* occurs only in the *skin;* it is not found on mucosal surfaces such as the buccal mucosa, larynx, or vagina. This neoplasm is considered in detail in Chapter 29.

7. Neoplasms of Secretory Epithelium

BENIGN: Adenoma

The *benign neoplasm* of *secretory epithelium* is the *adenoma.* It occurs characteristically either in the substance of a glandular organ (as the *breast, thyroid, adrenal, kidney, pancreas*) or in a secreting mucous membrane *(colon, stomach, bronchus).* When it occurs in a mucous membrane, it is thought to arise from the mucous glands lying beneath the epithelial surface. *Grossly* such a neoplasm elevates the covering epithelium and bulges into the lumen of the organ in *polypoid* form. In the colon (the most common site) the mucosal nodule is pulled in the direction of the fecal stream by the milking peristaltic action, and often comes to have an elongated stalk *(pedicle). Microscopically* adenomatous polyps consist of many small epithelial glands growing in a mass on the end of a fibrous stalk (see Chapter 20). An adenoma growing within a glandular organ such as the breast is usually characterized *grossly* by a well-defined capsule which separates it from the normal tissues. *Microscopically* well-differentiated epithelial glands are seen, separated by a variable amount of fibrous tissue.

Variants of adenoma

In some adenomas the fibrous tissue is abundant and seems to be an important part of the growth, as in *fibroadenomas* of the breast. Sometimes the epithelium of an adenoma continues to secrete within the confines of its capsule, in which case a cyst may be formed, as in *cystadenomas* of the ovaries or pancreas. In benign cystic adenomatous neoplasms of this type, it is common for papillary epithelial growths to arise from the cyst wall and project into the cavity. This gives the more complex *papillary cystadenoma,* which is a common neoplasm of the ovary.

MALIGNANT: Adenocarcinoma

The *malignant neoplasm* arising from *secretory epithelium* is the *adenocarcinoma.* As with its benign counterpart, the adenocarcinoma may arise either from the epithelium of a glandular organ such as the *breast, thyroid,* or *pancreas,* or from the secretory glands of a mucous membrane, such as the *colon, stomach,* or *endometrium.* In the latter type there is often a polypoid projection into the lumen *grossly,* but this is usually broad-based (sessile) rather than pedunculated, and shows atypical glandular epithelium penetrating the bowel wall. An adenocarcinoma of a glandular organ grows as an unencapsulated nodular mass with finger-like projections of malignant epithelial cells extending into the surrounding tissues. In both forms of adenocarcinoma, *spread* is characteristically by *lymphatic channels* to the regional lymph nodes. Hematogenous dissemination is also common in these neoplasms, resulting in metastases to distant organs, especially liver, lungs, brain, and bones.

Variants of adenocarcinoma

A number of subvarieties of adenocarcinoma are described. The *scirrhous carcinoma* is a very firm adenocarcinoma consisting of relatively few neoplastic cells growing in an abundant fibrous stroma; it is a common form of breast cancer. The *medullary* or *encephaloid carcinoma* is an adenocarcinoma of soft, brainlike consistency, due to the fact that it is made up almost entirely of neoplastic cells, with relatively little stroma. Tumors with these features are common in the breast and stomach. The *mucinous carcinoma,* also known as mucoid or colloid carcinoma, is an adenocarcinoma in which the neoplastic cells continue to secrete mucin, even as they infiltrate the tissues away from a mucosal surface. This neoplasm, common in the stomach and colon, is characterized grossly by a translucent appearance and sticky feel, and microscopically by small pools of mucin within the substance of the tumor. The adenocarcinomas of the various organ systems are discussed in detail under those systems.

REFERENCES

1. Willis, R. A. *Pathology of Tumours* (4th ed.). New York: Appleton-Century-Crofts, 1967.
2. *1970 Cancer Facts and Figures.* New York: American Cancer Society, 1969.
3. Wynder, E. L. On the epidemiology of gastric cancer. In Shivas, A. A. (Ed.), *Racial and Geographical Factors in Tumour Incidence.* Edinburgh: Edinburgh University Press, 1967, pp. 37–65.
4. Shanmugaratnam, K. Nasopharyngeal carcinoma in Asia. In Shivas, A. A. (Ed.), *Racial and Geographical Factors in Tumour Incidence.* Edinburgh: Edinburgh University Press, 1967, pp. 169–188.
5. Shivas, A. A. (Ed.). *Racial and Geographical Factors in Tumour Incidence.* Edinburgh: Edinburgh University Press, 1967.
6. Smith, J. C. Diffuse intrasinusoidal metastatic cancer of the liver. *Ann. Intern. Med.* 54:104, 1961.
7. Coman, D. R. Mechanism of the invasiveness of cancer. *Science* 105:347, 1947.
8. Coman, D. R., DeLong, R. P., and McCutcheon, M. Studies on the mechanism of metastasis. The distribution of tumors in various organs in relation to the distribution of arterial emboli. *Cancer Res.* 11:648, 1951.
9. Pruitt, J. C., Hilberg, A. W., Morehead, R. P., and Mengoli, H. F. Quantitative study of malignant cells in local and peripheral circulating blood. *Surg. Gynec. Obstet.* 114:179, 1962.
10. Graham, J. B., Sotto, L. S. J., and Paloucek, F. B. *Carcinoma of the Cervix.* Philadelphia: Saunders, 1962.
11. Lewis, G. C., Wentz, W. B., and Jaffe, R. M. *New Concepts in Gynecological Oncology.* Philadelphia: Davis, 1966, p. 48.
12. Petersen, O., and Wiklund, E. Further studies on the spontaneous course of cervical precancerous conditions. *Acta Radiol.* (Stockholm) 188 (Suppl.):210, 1959.
13. Smith, J. C. The principles and evaluation of curative cancer therapy. *J. Mich. Med. Soc.* 57:546, 1958.
14. *Progress Against Cancer, 1969.* A report of the National Advisory Cancer Council. Washington: U.S. Dept. of Health, Education, and Welfare, 1969.
15. Shimkin, M. B. Duration of life in untreated cancer. *Cancer* 4:1, 1951.
16. Daland, E. M. Untreated cancer of the breast. *Surg. Gynec. Obstet.* 44:264, 1927.
17. Furth, J., and Kahn, M. C. The transmission of leukemia in mice with a single cell. *Amer. J. Cancer* 31:276, 1937.
18. MacDonald, I. Biologic predeterminism in human cancer. *Surg. Gynec. Obstet.* 92:443, 1951.
19. Smith, J. C. The inadequacy of survival rates in the evaluation of cancer therapy. *Surg. Gynec. Obstet.* 103:307, 1956.
20. Smith, J. C. The importance of a premise. *Surg. Gynec. Obstet.* 126:117, 1968.
21. Francois, J. *Ophthalmic Genetics.* Progress in Medical Genetics, vol. 2. New York: Grune & Stratton, 1962, p. 331.

22. Dukes, C. E. Familial intestinal polyposis. *Ann. Eugen.* 17:1, 1952.
23. Cockayne, E. A. *Inherited Abnormalities of the Skin and Its Appendages.* London: Milford, 1933, p. 93.
24. Gorer, P. A. Cancer: Statistical and Diagnostic Pitfalls. In Sorsby, A. (Ed.), *Clinical Genetics.* London: Butterworth, 1953, p. 558.
25. Upton, A. C. The dose-response relation in radiation-induced cancer. *Cancer Res.* 21:717, 1961.
26. Aub, J. C., Evans, R. D., Hempelmann, L. H., and Martland, H. C. The late effects of internally deposited radioactive materials in man. *Medicine* 31:221, 1952.
27. Saenger, E. L., Silverman, F. N., Sterling, T. D., and Turner, M. E. Neoplasia following therapeutic irradiation for benign conditions in childhood. *Radiology* 74:889, 1960.
28. Baserga, R., Yokoo, H., and Henegar, G. C. Thorotrast-induced cancer in man. *Cancer* 13:1021, 1960.
29. Court-Brown, W. M., and Abbatt, J. D. The incidence of leukemia in ankylosing spondylitis treated with x-rays. A preliminary report. *Lancet* 1:1283, 1955.
30. Heyssel, R., Brill, A. B., Woodbury, L. A., Nishimura, E. T., Ghose, T., and Yamasaki, M. Leukemia in Hiroshima atom bomb survivors. *Blood* 15:313, 1960.
31. Hempelmann, L. H. Epidemiological studies of leukemia in persons exposed to ionizing radiation. *Cancer Res.* 20:18, 1960.
32. Yamagiwa, K. Pathogenesis of cancer. *J. Cancer Res.* 3:1, 1918.
33. Terry, L. L. *Smoking and Health.* Progress in Clinical Cancer, vol. 1. New York: Grune & Stratton, 1965, p. 538.
34. Bock, F. G., Moore, G. E., and Clark, P. C. Carcinogenic activity of cigarette smoke condensate. III. Biological activity of refined tar from several types of cigarettes. *J. Nat. Cancer Inst.* 34:481, 1965.
35. Bischoff, F., and Bryson, G. Carcinogenesis through solid state surfaces. *Progr. Exp. Tumor Res.* 5:85, 1964.
36. Rowe, W. P. A survey of the tumor virus problem from an epidemiologic standpoint. *Cancer Res.* 25:1271, 1965.
37. Rous, P. Transmission of a malignant growth by means of a cell-free filtrate. *J.A.M.A.* 56:198, 1911.
38. Shope, R. E. Transmissable tumor-like condition in rabbits. *J. Exp. Med.* 56:793, 1932.
39. Bittner, J. J. Some possible effects of nursing on mammary gland tumor incidence in mice. *Science* 84:162, 1936.
40. Duryee, W. R., Long, M. E., Taylor, H. C., Jr., McKelway, W. P., and Ehrmann, R. L. Human and amphibian neoplasms compared. *Science* 131:276, 1960.
41. Burkitt, D. A sarcoma involving the jaws in African children. *Brit. J. Surg.* 46:218, 1958.
42. Alpert, M. E., and Davidson, C. S. Mycotoxins. A possible cause of primary carcinoma of the liver. *Amer. J. Med.* 46:325, 1969.
43. Warburg, O. On the origin of cancer cells. *Science* 123:309, 1956.
44. Wallach, D. F. H. Generalized membrane defects in cancer. *New Eng. J. Med.* 280:761, 1969.
45. Osgood, E. E. A unifying concept of the etiology of the leukemias, lymphomas, and cancers. *J. Nat. Cancer Inst.* 18:155, 1957.
46. Failla, G. The aging process and cancerogenesis. *Ann. N.Y. Acad. Sci.* 71:1124, 1958.

47. Pitot, H. C. Some aspects of the development biology of neoplasia. *Cancer Res.* 28:1880, 1968.
48. Horn, R. C., and Enterline, H. T. Rhabdomyosarcoma: A clinico-pathologic study and classification of 39 cases. *Cancer* 11:181, 1958.

15 DISEASES RELATED TO PREGNANCY

1. General Considerations

Any disease – diabetes, tuberculosis, cancer, heart disease, etc. – may occur during pregnancy and complicate its course. Most diseases occurring during pregnancy increase the frequency of intra-uterine fetal death; a few diseases, especially rheumatoid arthritis, may go into remission during pregnancy. The diseases under consideration in this chapter are those which are particularly apt to occur during pregnancy, or have a particular significance when they occur during pregnancy. The abnormalities of the placenta and umbilical cord are also included here.

Biochemical and physiologic changes

A number of important physiologic alterations occur during pregnancy [1]. Of these, the alterations in hormone secretion are among the most striking. *Gonadotropins,* presumably of pituitary and placental origin, can be detected in the serum and urine a few days after the first missed menstrual period; they increase rapidly, reaching their maximum concentration early in the second month. This hormone is the basis for the biologic tests for pregnancy. The gonadotropins are believed to cause persistence of the corpus luteum and otherwise play a role in the development of the fetus. *Progesterone,* formed first in the corpus luteum and later in the placenta, is believed to maintain the endometrium, permitting implantation and growth of the embryo. *Estrogen* and progesterone stimulate the growth of the breasts by inciting hyperplasia of the acinar epithelium. *Steroids* closely resembling ACTH are elaborated by the placenta. *Plasma volume* increases by about 25 percent during the course of pregnancy, rising sharply near the end of the second trimester. One effect of this increase is to dilute the cellular elements, thus lowering the hemoglobin by about 2 gm. per 100 ml., on the average. A similar dilution effect is often noted in blood chemical values.

2. Toxemia of Pregnancy

Clinical features

Toxemia of pregnancy is usually manifest by one or more of the following: *proteinuria, hypertension, visual impairment,* or *edema.* In the most seriously affected patients, there may also be *convulsions;* this marks the disease known as *eclampsia.* With serious cases without convulsions the disease is referred to as preeclampsia, implying that convulsions will occur if the condition remains untreated. *Premature labor* is an important clinical feature of the toxemias, due to the increased uterine contractility resulting from an increased secretion of pituitary oxytocin [2]. The increase in tonus and in contractions of the uterus is said to cause a reduction of the maternal blood flow in the placenta, and may also account for the increased tendency toward abruption of the placenta *(abruptio placentae)* in toxemia. These two factors, both of which would promote fetal anoxia, may account for the *high fetal mortality* in toxemia of pregnancy.

Cause

The immediate *cause* of toxemia remains unknown. In some way severe renal ischemia is triggered. The glomerular filtration rate is decreased. Since the changes are reversible in the kidneys, it is likely that renal vasospasm is responsible for them. Retinal vasospasm is regularly observed in toxemia of pregnancy. Preeclampsia has been induced experimentally in pregnant rats by administering desoxycorticosterone, sodium chloride, and renin [3]. An eclampsia-like disorder has also been produced in pregnant rats by a Vitamin E-deficient diet [4], but there is no evidence that this is a factor in human eclampsia.

Pathologic changes

The lesions are almost always confined to the liver and kidneys, and in some cases there may be almost no demonstrable changes. The *liver* is enlarged, soft, and yellow and has hemorrhages in the capsule and parenchyma. Microscopically there are scattered areas of necrosis, which may be peripheral or in any portion of the lobule. In occasional cases the necrosis is extreme. The *kidneys* are swollen and may show petechial hemorrhages. Microscopic changes are noted in the glomeruli (thickening of capillary basement membranes, intravascular thrombosis) and in the tubules (epithelial swelling and degeneration). Electron microscopy on renal biopsies reveals swelling and vacuolization of the glomerular endothelium [5]. Abundant secretory granules are found in the juxtaglomerular cells, indicating active renin secretion.

3. Bilateral Cortical Necrosis of the Kidneys

Most cases of this extremely rare disease occur during pregnancy. There is complete necrosis, resembling infarction, involving the cortex of both kidneys, including the columns of Bertin, but leaving the pyramids unaffected. It is considered in detail in Chapter 22.

4. Infections During Pregnancy and the Puerperium

Infectious diseases

The importance of *maternal rubella* during the first trimester of pregnancy has been indicated in Chapter 7. *Maternal syphilis* is of great importance, since the fetus is apt to be seriously injured unless treatment is given early in pregnancy (see Chapter 6).

Urinary tract infections

Urinary tract infections tend to occur during the latter part of pregnancy, and are probably related to distortion of the urinary tract by the enlarging uterus. Enteric or pyogenic bacteria are usually responsible. The infection usually involves the pelvis and parenchyma of the kidney (pyelonephritis). The pathologic changes are the same as those found in pyelonephritis in the nonpregnant patient, and are considered in Chapter 22.

Uterus infections

Puerperal infections usually begin locally in the reproductive tract, chiefly the uterus *(puerperal endometritis)*. They are much more frequent after abortions than after delivery at term. Criminal abortion is often the background. Bacteria invade the large vascular sinuses readily, cause *septic thrombosis of the pelvic veins,* and often septic embolism of the lungs; thus there may be bacteremia, septicemia, or pyemia in *puerperal sepsis.* Enteric organisms, pyogenic cocci, or even anaerobic saprophytes may be the cause of infection.

Breast infections

Breast infections occur during lactation, and are usually a result of cracking of the nipples with invasion of the tissues by bacteria from the skin. Infection spreads along the duct system, fascial planes, and lymphatics. *Breast abscess,* requiring surgical drainage, is the most serious form, but minor degrees of *mastitis* are more frequent.

5. Abnormal Sites of Placental Implantation

Normal implantation

Usually the ovum is fertilized near the lateral end of the uterine tube. The fertilized ovum then migrates within the lumen of the tube to the uterus, where it embeds itself in the endometrium which has been prepared by the hormones to receive it. Its usual site of implantation is the upper portion of the uterine cavity, either anteriorly or posteriorly.

Ectopic pregnancy: sites

Sometimes the normal migration of the ovum is prevented by a stricture or other abnormality of the uterine tube. Under these circumstances most embryos are unable to attach themselves to the mother and they die without causing any symptoms. Sometimes the embryo finds circumstances suitable for its development outside the uterine cavity, in which case the pregnancy is said to be ectopic. *Tubal pregnancy* is the most common form of ectopic pregnancy; it occurs about once in 300 pregnancies. The burrowing trophoblast usually erodes and ruptures the tube early in pregnancy. Sometimes *tubal abortion* occurs, the fetus being extruded from the lateral end of the tube into the abdominal cavity. *Interstitial pregnancy* is implantation in a cornu of the uterus in the interstitial portion of the uterine tube. Its course is similar to that of tubal pregnancy. *"Abdominal" pregnancy,* i.e., peritoneal pregnancy, may result either from direct implantation of the fertilized ovum upon the peritoneum or from extrusion of the fetus of a tubal pregnancy into the abdominal cavity. *Ovarian pregnancy* may be a result of aberrant endometrial tissue in the ovary (endometriosis) providing a satisfactory site for growth of the pregnancy. It is extremely rare.

outcome

Seldom does pregnancy go to term under any of these circumstances. Sometimes the fetus dies at an early age, probably as a result of inadequate oxygenation. Calcium may then be deposited in the tissues of the dead fetus, producing a *lithopedion,* and the placenta may be converted to scar tissue. More commonly the erosive character of the trophoblast leads to sudden intraperitoneal *hemorrhage* early in pregnancy. Prompt blood replacement and corrective surgery are required to save the mother; the fetus is too young to survive. In those rare cases where pregnancy goes to term, delivery by the vaginal route is obviously impossible. Even with cesarean section there is great danger of hemorrhage as the placenta separates.

Placenta praevia

In about 1 of 200 pregnancies the placenta is implanted too low on the uterine wall. The stretching of the lower uterine segment in the last trimester may then cause tearing or separation of the placenta. Occasionally the placenta may cover the internal os of the uterus, making normal delivery virtually impossible. Both central and marginal placenta praevia cause a *high fetal mortality* from anoxia. They also cause *maternal hemorrhage,* and, if uncorrected, maternal death.

6. Abnormalities of the Placenta

Abnormal form

There is considerable variation in the *shape of the placenta and its membranes.* These abnormalities are probably largely dependent upon abnormal placement of the placenta. When two or three lobes of more or less equal size are present, it is spoken of as a *bipartite or tripartite placenta;* these have no real clinical significance. When a small lobe is appreciably separated from the main placental mass, it is called a *succenturiate* (accessory) *lobe;* this may sometimes be left behind after delivery and cause continued hemorrhage. Occasionally the placenta has an elevated inrolled edge at the periphery, more or less completely encircling it. This is the *circumvallate placenta,* a condition associated with an increased likelihood of intra-uterine fetal death, probably due to fetal anoxia since the umbilical cord is sometimes compressed beneath the ring.

Abnormal origin of cord

The *umbilical cord* is normally inserted somewhere near the center of the fetal surface of the placenta, but sometimes the cord is attached eccentrically or even at the very edge of the placental mass (marginal attachment). Rarely the placental vessels converge to form the cord in the membranes entirely outside the placental mass. This *velamentous* origin of the cord carries some danger for the fetus; if the rupture of the amniotic sac occurs through the region of these vessels, as in *vasa praevia,* it may cause fetal death from exsanguination. (Note that the blood loss is fetal, not maternal.)

Abnormal size

The placenta grows with pregnancy, being about one-seventh the weight of the fetus at term. An abnormally *large increase in placental size* may be due to syphilis, erythroblastosis, hydatidiform mole, or unknown conditions; each of these is considered in more detail elsewhere.

Placental infarcts

Placental infarcts are extremely common; they are usually not important as a cause of fetal death, since the size of the placenta provides a large margin of safety. Infarcts are usually marginal and result from interference with the maternal blood supply. Recent infarcts are usually red, older ones white or even hyalinized.

Syphilitic placentitis

When pregnancy occurs during active *syphilitic infection* of the mother, both the placenta and the fetus are usually affected. The placenta is usually larger than normal, and quite pale and firm because of fibrosis of the villi. Great numbers of spirochetes may be demonstrable in the placenta with Levaditi's staining method. The treponema may also pass to the fetus to produce congenital syphilis (see Chapter 6).

7. Abnormalities of Placental Separation

Premature separation

Normally the placenta separates spontaneously from the uterine wall after the infant is born. Usually about 250 ml. of blood is lost. Sometimes the placenta separates partially or completely before the fetus is born, resulting in excessive maternal bleeding and often in fetal anoxia and fetal death. *Premature separation* of the placenta, also called *abruptio placentae,* occurs more commonly in toxic than in normal mothers. Sometimes the hemorrhage extends diffusely into the myometrium and broad ligaments from the placental site *(uteroplacental apoplexy* or *Couvelaire uterus).* In abruptio placentae, there is often hypofibrinogenemia, but it is not clear whether this is cause or effect. In the era before blood and fibrinogen were available, death from exsanguination was a common outcome in such cases.

Sometimes the placenta does not come away from the uterine wall promptly and completely after delivery. In such cases there may be *continued uterine hemorrhage,* and often *infection* as well. Sometimes the difficulty is due to atony of the uterus or to abnormalities of the uterine wall such as leiomyomata.

Incomplete separation

In other mothers, due perhaps to preceding disease, there is no decidua interposed between the villi and the myometrium. In these women the villi extend directly into the vascular sinuses of the myometrium. The condition, known as placenta accreta, usually comes to light as a result of continued hemorrhage after delivery. Curettage usually is required to remove the dense scarred area in which myometrium and organized placental tissue are merged.

Placenta accreta

8. *Abnormalities of the Umbilical Cord*

Most of the abnormalities of the umbilical cord are mechanical and result in interference with blood flow in the cord. The cord may *prolapse* ahead of the fetus, in which case it may be compressed between the presenting part and the cervix. The cord may be *twisted* about the neck of the fetus as a result of intrauterine activity of the fetus. Occasionally an overhand *knot* is formed in the cord. These complications, more common with twins than with single pregnancies, may cause fetal asphyxia and death.

Strangulation

Rarely, in certain extreme fetal deformities, there may be only one umbilical artery. Varicosities of the umbilical vein are sometimes seen. Cysts are sometimes observed at the fetal end of the cord, arising either from the omphalomesenteric duct or from the urachus.

Other abnormalities

9. *Multiple Pregnancies*

Multiple pregnancy is an uncommon condition (but not a disease!) of pregnancy. Twins occur in 1.61 percent, triplets in 0.01189 percent, and quadruplets in 0.00203 percent of all pregnancies in the United States. Multiple pregnancies may be either monovular (33 percent), with identical individuals, or polyovular (67 percent), with fraternal individuals. The differentiation can usually, but not always, be made by examining the placental membranes. There have been a number of instances of high multiple pregnancies (quintuplets, sextuplets, septuplets) in women using pituitary gonadotropin or clomiphene because of earlier infertility [6].

10. *Abnormalities of Amniotic Fluid*

In early pregnancy it appears that amniotic fluid is formed by transudation from the amnion. Later it consists largely of *fetal urine.* Obviously there must be a means to eliminate the excess fluid from the amniotic sac. On the basis of the abnormalities of amniotic fluid accumulation, it appears that amniotic fluid must be swallowed by the fetus and absorbed from its gastrointestinal tract. Presumably the fluid is, in part, passed back to the mother via the placenta, and in part reexcreted in the fetal urine. Normally a fine balance is maintained between formation and absorption, so that the quantity of amniotic fluid remains reasonably constant at about 500 ml. for the last few weeks of pregnancy. Either an increase or a decrease in the amount of fluid usually signifies an abnormal pregnancy.

Normal formation and absorption

Polyhydramnios

Any significant increase in the amount of amniotic fluid (1000 ml. or more) is termed *polyhydramnios.* This may occur in *multiple pregnancies.* A marked degree of polyhydramnios is usually noted in association with fetal *anencephaly.* Perhaps in these cases cerebrospinal fluid is secreted into the amniotic sac along with fetal urine. In fetal disorders interfering with absorption from the gastrointestinal tract, such as *esophageal or duodenal atresia,* polyhydramnios is commonly noted. In one case in our files sudden, painful accumulation of amniotic fluid occurred, apparently coincidental with the development of high intestinal obstruction due to strangulated hernia in the fetus. Polyhydramnios is commonly noted in association with *maternal diabetes;* although the explanation is not entirely clear, it seems likely that it is due to fetal diuresis under the influence of the mother's diabetogenic hormone. *Erythroblastosis fetalis* is often associated with an excess of amniotic fluid, but the explanation is not known.

Oligohydramnios

A decrease or absence of amniotic fluid *(oligohydramnios)* is much rarer than an excess. This is generally due to failure of fetal urine formation, as in *bilateral renal agenesis.* In cases of complete *urethral obstruction,* the amniotic sac may be dry while the urinary bladder and ureters are greatly distended with urine.

Cloudy amniotic fluid

Normally the amniotic fluid is clear and watery or faintly straw-colored. It becomes cloudy in the presence of *infection of the sac,* or when *meconium* is passed into the sac in utero. Meconium in the fluid means that the anal sphincter of the fetus has relaxed, and is evidence of fetal distress, usually from anoxia.

11. Abnormalities Related to Labor

Abnormalities of position or presentation, or of the forces of labor, may make labor prolonged or difficult. Lacerations of the cervix, perineum, urinary bladder, or rectum sometimes result.

Rupture of the uterus

Rarely rupture of the uterus occurs during labor. This may be due to unusually difficult labor (as with cephalopelvic disproportion), to an area of weakness in the uterine wall (as following previous myomectomy or cesarean section), or to faulty obstetric practice (as injudicious use of forceps or of oxytocic agents). The rupture usually occurs in the lower portion of the uterus, most often laterally or obliquely; it may tear the large veins or arteries in this area, resulting in sudden massive hemorrhage.

Amniotic fluid embolism

On rare occasions amniotic fluid may enter the maternal circulation during delivery and cause sudden maternal collapse. In fatal cases squamous epithelial cells derived from the baby's vernix caseosa can sometimes be found in the mother's pulmonary arterioles. Afibrinogenemia and serious uterine hemorrhage occur in some women who survive amniotic fluid embolism. This condition has been discussed on page 44.

12. Neoplasms During Pregnancy [7]

Vascular tumors *(chorioangiomata)* are occasionally encountered as firm encapsulated masses protruding from the fetal surface of the placenta. They have no known endocrine or other effect upon either the fetus or the mother.

Chorionic epithelium

Of much greater importance are the neoplasms of the chorionic epithelium. These tumors, arising from fetal trophoblasts, invade maternal tissues. The normal trophoblast normally invades maternal tissues, particularly the vascular sinuses of the endometrium, in order to attach the chorionic villi (fetal) to the uterine wall (maternal). Normally this invasiveness is limited to the uterus, and is lost with the shedding of the placenta at the end of labor.

Hydatid mole

Since the destructive and malignant neoplasms of chorionic epithelium often arise from *hydatidiform moles,* this condition is considered first. A hydatidiform mole occurs once in about 2500 pregnancies. Considered by some to be a neoplasm, it is considered by others to be degenerative. The swelling of the villi is due to the imbalance between the fetal and maternal circulation that results when the fetal circulation fails, usually as a result of fetal death. Clinically the first manifestation of the presence of a mole is often the excessively *rapid growth* of the uterus due to growth of the placental mass. This is usually followed, at about the third to the fifth month of pregnancy, by *uterine bleeding* or *abortion.* Placental tissue passed at this time may show a *characteristic gross appearance:* the villi, instead of being delicate and stringy, are cystic and grapelike. In other cases the diagnosis may not be grossly evident. *Microscopically* the mole shows the cystic, almost avascular villi together with irregular clumps of large, often multinucleated, syncytial cells like the cells of a malignant neoplasm. If continued uterine bleeding and persistently positive tests for pregnancy necessitate curettage, the resulting specimen usually shows that similar cells extend into the myometrium and even into the walls of the uterine sinuses. If the patient continues to bleed for several weeks after the curettage, this suggests the possibility of choriocarcinoma. About 2 percent of all hydatid moles develop into choriocarcinoma, and over 10 percent become chorioadenoma destruens.

Choriocarcinoma

Choriocarcinoma is an extremely rare neoplasm, much rarer than the emphasis sometimes given it would indicate. In about half the cases it arises in women with a hydatid mole; the remainder of the cases are about equally divided between abortions and full-term pregnancy. Choriocarcinoma usually occurs in the uterus, but it may occur at the site of an ectopic pregnancy. *Grossly* the uterus containing a choriocarcinoma shows *shaggy, fleshy hemorrhagic masses* filling the uterine cavity and extending into the myometrium. *Microscopically* the neoplasm is composed of clusters of large, extremely bizarre, often multinucleated *giant cells,* extending into the myometrium and often filling the vascular sinuses. Necrosis and hemorrhage are seen, both in the tumor masses and in the myometrium. Chorionic villi as such are not a feature of the neoplasm. The course of choriocarcinoma is almost unpredictable. Sometimes it is first suspected when multiple nodules are seen in the radiograph of the chest a year or more after a presumably normal pregnancy. Very rarely both the primary neoplasm and the metastases have disappeared spontaneously. Usually the tumor *spreads locally* to the vagina and parametrium, *invades the veins,* and *metastasizes to the lungs, liver,* and *brain.* Usually the tumor cells continue to manufacture *gonadotropic hormone* in both the primary growth and the metastases; urine diluted 1:100 will often still give a positive biologic test for pregnancy. Multiple bilateral cysts of the ovary, often 6 to 10 cm. in diameter, usually are present in patients with choriocarcinoma, and, for that matter, in patients with benign hydatidiform mole; the significance of the ovarian cysts is not clear. Rarely choriocarcinoma may arise in a *teratomatous neoplasm,* without relation to placental tissue.

Chorioadenoma destruens

Chorioadenoma destruens is another rare neoplasm arising from chorionic epithelium. It is *locally invasive and destructive* but does not ordinarily metastasize. It is seen as a discrete, rounded, fleshy hemorrhagic mass, generally in the lower portion of the uterus. *Microscopically* it consists of chorionic villi covered with active trophoblastic cells, infiltrating in a local area marked off sharply from surrounding unaffected myometrium.

Other neoplasms

The chorionic neoplasms discussed above are the only tumors specifically arising from the state of pregnancy. Certain other neoplasms affect, or are affected by, pregnancy. Thus certain common benign tumors of the reproductive organs (leiomyomata of the uterus, cystic tumors of the ovaries) may interfere with normal placental implantation, prevent the development of the embryo, cause abortion, or interfere with the course of labor. The desmoid tumor (fibroma) of the abdominal wall is usually first noted during pregnancy.

Rarely do malignant neoplasms in the mother metastasize to the placenta; metastasis to the fetus is almost unknown [8].

REFERENCES

1. Macy, I. G. Metabolic and biochemical changes in normal pregnancy. *J.A.M.A.* 168:2265, 1958.
2. Caldeyro-Barcia, R. Quoted in *Physiology of Prematurity: Transactions of the First Conference.* New York: Josiah Macy, Jr. Foundation, 1957.
3. Masson, G. M. C., Corcoran, A. C., and Page, I. H. Renal and vascular lesions elicited by "renin" in rats with desoxycorticosterone hypertension. *A.M.A. Arch. Path.* 53:217, 1952.
4. Stamler, F. W. Fatal eclamptic disease of pregnant rats fed anti-vitamin E stress diet. *Amer. J. Path.* 35:1207, 1959.
5. Fisher, E. R., Pardo, V., Paul, R., and Hayashi, T. T. Ultrastructural studies in hypertension. IV. Toxemia of pregnancy. *Amer. J. Path.* 55:109, 1969.
6. Cameron, A. H., Robson, E. B., Wade-Evans, T., and Wingham, J. Septuplet conception: Placental and zygosity studies. *J. Obstet. Gynaec. Brit. Comm.* 76:692, 1969.
7. Hertig, A. T., and Mansell, H. Tumors of the female sex organs. 1. Hydatidiform mole and choriocarcinoma. Section IX, Fascicle 33, in *Atlas of Tumor Pathology.* Washington: Armed Forces Institute of Pathology, 1956.
8. Potter, J. F., and Schoeneman, M. Metastasis of maternal cancer to the placenta and fetus. *Cancer* 25:380, 1970.

GENERAL REFERENCES

Novak, E. R., and Woodruff, J. D. *Gynecologic and Obstetric Pathology* (6th ed.). Philadelphia: Saunders, 1967, pp. 432–450, 473–574.

Potter, E. L. *Pathology of the Fetus and the Newborn* (2d ed.). Chicago: Year Book, 1961.

16 DISEASES PECULIAR TO THE FETUS AND NEWBORN INFANT; NEOPLASMS OF INFANCY AND CHILDHOOD

DISEASES PECULIAR TO THE FETUS AND NEWBORN INFANT

1. Infant and Perinatal Mortality Statistics

Infant deaths

Infant deaths occurring "just before, during, and just after the process of birth are all associated with the same biologic process" [1] and should be considered together. The term *perinatal* is often applied to this total period. Improvements in nutrition, housing, sanitation, and the treatment of infectious diseases have caused a marked reduction in the mortality of older infants, but there has been relatively *little improvement in the perinatal mortality,* which is less affected by environmental factors [2].

Perinatal deaths

The *chief cause of death during the first week of life is prematurity* (37 percent); *anoxia* and abnormalities of pulmonary ventilation are second (26 percent), with *birth injuries* third (10 percent) and *congenital malformations* fourth (9 percent) [1].

Abortion or stillbirth

Many of the diseases discussed in this chapter may cause death of the fetus either before or after delivery. If death occurs in utero, labor usually begins a few days thereafter, resulting in abortion or stillbirth. (The difference between abortion and stillbirth is somewhat arbitrary and is determined by state law. A pregnancy terminating *before 5 months gestation* is usually considered an *abortion* and need not be reported as a birth. *After* that period it is considered a *stillbirth* and must be reported to the health authorities.)

2. Diseases That Develop in Utero (Fetal or Antenatal)

Anoxia or asphyxia

Interference with fetal oxygenation is the most common cause of intra-uterine death and of death during labor. Anoxia may be due to abnormalities of the *placenta,* such as premature separation or placenta praevia; to abnormalities of the umbilical *cord,* such as prolapse, knots, or entanglement; or to *maternal anoxia,* as from excessive sedation, etc. Fetal mortality is greater in multiple than in single pregnancies, probably due to disorders of the cord. Disproportion of the fetus to the birth canal also increases the likelihood of compression of the cord and fetal death from anoxia.

Maternal diseases

Toxemia of pregnancy predisposes to premature separation of the placenta and causes fetal death via anoxia. *Maternal diabetes* is usually associated with a large fetus, and the fetal death rate is increased. Heart disease, tuberculosis, and cancer in the mother often contribute to fetal death.

Anomalies

Congenital malformations (cardiac, respiratory, gastrointestinal, hepatic, genitourinary, skeletal, nervous) may cause intra-uterine death, but more commonly cause *neonatal death* or death later in infancy. *Monsters* (major fetal malformations, externally manifest) may be due to genetic mutations or to injury of the embryo at an early stage of development, as by anoxia or infection. The most important congenital abnormalities are described under the organ system affected.

Infections

Although the embryo may be damaged as a result of *maternal infections* during early pregnancy, especially German measles, the *fully formed fetus is rarely affected.* There are rare reports of viral infections developing in utero; these undoubtedly reach the fetus via the circulation from the mother. Bacterial infections of the fetus in utero are somewhat more common and may be transmitted from the infected mother by the placental circulation, as in syphilis. During prolonged labor, with the cervix open, the birth canal may become infected from the outside, resulting in fetal pneumonia. Certain infectious diseases (toxoplasmosis, inclusion disease) may be contracted by the fetus in utero without the mother showing any evidence of infection.

Erythroblastosis fetalis:

Erythroblastosis fetalis is a most remarkable disease, especially in its theoretical aspects. It is a *chronic hemolytic disease,* due to an *incompatibility* in genetically transmitted factors. It is not a hereditary disease in the ordinary sense of the word: no ancestor has the disease; the afflicted infant may recover; and if so, his offspring need not be affected. In this disease the fetal red blood cells are destroyed by a *maternal agglutinin* interacting in the fetus with a *fetal agglutinogen* which has been inherited from the father.

Rh theory

The usual agglutinogen in erythroblastosis is the *Rh factor,* so named from the Rhesus monkey; this antigen is present on the red cells of all Rhesus monkeys, and on the red cells of about 85 percent of Americans. The red cells of patients having this agglutinogen are clumped by the specific agglutinin (anti-Rh); such patients are known as *Rh positive.* Patients are said to be *Rh negative* if their red cells are not clumped by anti-Rh serum. The Rh factor is a *dominant* trait; an individual who is heterozygous for this genetic factor will test out as Rh positive. There are actually three different blood agglutinogens in the Rh set (Rh_0, Rh_1, and Rh_2), and these may occur in various combinations. These subgroups are also designated D, C, and E, respectively. If the fetus and mother both have this trait (Rh positive), or both lack it (Rh negative), or if the mother has it (Rh positive) and the fetus lacks it (Rh negative), no harm results. If the mother is Rh negative and has an Rh-positive husband (as is the case in about 13 percent of all marriages), the possibility exists for fetal erythroblastosis; nevertheless, less than 0.5 percent of all matings give rise to erythroblastosis. The difference is due in part to *heterozygosity* of the father, in part to other factors, known and unknown. Rarely a fetal-maternal incompatibility in *ABO blood groups* may cause fetal erythroblastosis, but this form is seldom fatal.

maternal sensitization

The only apparent way by which the mother can develop antibodies against the fetal Rh agglutinogen is for fetal red cells to leak into the maternal circulation, thus sensitizing her, i.e., causing the formation of anti-Rh substances in her blood plasma. If there is an ABO incompatibility as well, the mother's naturally occurring antibodies will destroy the fetal red cells before maternal sensitization to Rh can develop, according to Levine [3]. (Note that anti-Rh is not naturally occurring in Rh-negative individuals, as is the case with the agglutinins to the major blood groups – see Chapter 4.) Even when the mother becomes sensitized, she shows no sign of illness and she remains Rh negative. However, these anti-Rh substances diffuse through the placental barrier and enter the fetal circulation. There they coat the fetus' Rh-positive red cells, causing their *intravascular hemolysis.*

successive pregnancies

Usually it takes one or two pregnancies with an Rh-positive fetus, or one transfusion of Rh-positive blood, to sensitize the mother. Hence, *erythroblastosis usually appears in the second or later pregnancies,* rarely in the first. If the father is homozygous, erythroblastosis is usually noted in successive infants after the first in which it appears. If he is heterozygous, approximately half the offspring are affected after the first. In each affected fetus after the first, the disease is usually worse than in the preceding erythroblastotic fetus.

manifestations

In mild cases the disease may be demonstrable only by laboratory test: Coombs' antiglobulin serum will reveal the maternal antibody coating the infant's red cells. In moderately severe cases there will be jaundice (apparent a few hours after birth), anemia, or edema. In severe cases fetal death occurs in utero.

Pathologic changes

The tissue changes are essentially similar to those in the other hemolytic anemias or in incompatible blood transfusions. The *blood* picture is one of anemia; there are large numbers of nucleated red cells (hence the name *erythroblastosis*) both in blood smears and in tissue sections. The *placenta, liver,* and *spleen* are large; enlargement of the placenta is due to edema, whereas *extramedullary erythropoiesis* is the chief cause for the enlargement of the liver and spleen. The kidneys are large and pale and the tubules show epithelial degeneration and heme casts. The brain (in infants living some hours) shows marked icteric tinting of the basal ganglia (kernicterus). This results in degeneration of ganglion cells; in those infants who survive, it produces neurologic disorders with or without mental retardation.

clinicopathologic picture of Rh

In practice, the mother's Rh and blood group are determined early in her first pregnancy. If she is Rh positive, nothing further is done, but if she is Rh negative, the husband's blood is also tested. If the husband is also Rh negative, there need be no further concern, but if he is Rh positive, the possibility of fetal erythroblastosis exists. If this possibility exists, the mother is tested at intervals during pregnancy to see if *anti-Rh substances* are being formed. If they are not present in the mother's blood, it may be that the fetus is Rh negative; this would mean that the father was heterozygous. If anti-Rh substances are present, there is a strong likelihood that the fetus will have erythroblastosis, and arrangements are made in advance for immediate postnatal determinations of *bilirubin* on the baby and for exchange transfusions. Erythroblastotic infants can often be saved, and spared all harmful manifestations, by prompt *exchange transfusion with Rh-negative blood.* (Why is Rh-negative blood used if the fetus is Rh positive? Because maternal anti-Rh substances are present in the fetal circulation and will destroy transfused Rh-positive cells just as they destroy the fetus' own Rh-positive cells. After a time the maternal antibodies will disappear from the fetus, and Rh-positive blood can be used for any subsequent transfusions that may be needed.)

Other diseases

Congenital neoplasms (see later section in this chapter) and *hereditary diseases* (see Chapter 13) also begin in utero; because of their importance they are considered as separate topics, however.

3. Diseases That Develop During Labor (Intranatal) or During the Neonatal Period

The *most common cause of intranatal death is interference with oxygenation,* due to the same causes as were listed under antenatal deaths. Live-born infants that are damaged by anoxia in utero may die soon after birth, or, if they survive, may show mental derangement or paralysis. The following causes of fetal death or injury are in addition to *anoxia.*

Birth trauma

According to Potter [4], "The passage through the birth canal is the most hazardous experience to which the ordinary individual is ever subjected." *Head injury* is less frequent with natural cephalic delivery than with any other type of delivery. Skull fractures occur rarely; intracranial hemorrhage, due to laceration of the dural membranes, is more common and usually results from excessive molding of the head during labor. This may tear the tentorium cerebelli or the falx cerebri, causing disruption of the large vascular sinuses in these membranes, and subdural hemorrhage. *Spinal cord injury* is rare but may result from fracture or separation of the vertebrae. Injuries of the *liver* and *adrenal glands,* with massive hemorrhage, may be observed, especially following breech deliveries. Pressure from improperly applied forceps may cause *nerve injury* and *paralysis.* Brachial plexus paralysis *(Erb's palsy)* may result from lateral traction during breech delivery. *Fractures* of the clavicle, and less often of the humerus and femur, may occur.

Infections

Ophthalmia neonatorum, or gonorrheal conjunctivitis of the newborn infant, is usually due to contamination of the eyes during passage through the infected birth canal, and to failure to apply proper prophylactic measures. Contamination of the stump of the cord may cause *omphalitis* (inflammation of the navel), which may be complicated by fatal septicemia. *Clostridium infections* of the umbilical cord may occur. *Pneumonia* may be contracted during passage through the birth canal or from attempts at resuscitation. *Thrush,* a mouth infection due to *Candida albicans,* is common in debilitated infants. Epidemics, chiefly of bacterial *enteritis* or of *skin infections,* occur occasionally in hospital nurseries and may be very difficult to eradicate.

Hyaline membrane disease

Hyaline membrane disease of the lungs is frequently found at autopsy in *infants dying 24 to 48 hours after birth,* and especially in premature infants. Alveoli and bronchioles show a *hyaline eosinophilic membrane lining the air spaces.* There are relatively few leukocytes. The condition is discussed in detail on page 478.

Fibroplasia

Retrolental fibroplasia signifies a *detachment of the retina,* usually occurring several weeks after birth, especially in cases of premature birth. It is usually bilateral and causes *blindness.* The condition is due to *excessive use of oxygen* during the neonatal period. Retrolental fibroplasia is discussed in detail on page 811.

4. Prematurity

Definition

An infant is said to be premature if its birth weight is less than 2500 gm. (5½ pounds), regardless of the length of gestation.

Frequency and importance

Prematurity ranks high among the causes of death and is by far the *most important cause of death during the neonatal period.* It accounts for about 30 percent of all deaths under 1 year of age.

Causes of prematurity

The causes of prematurity in the infant are, of course, the causes of premature labor in the mother, and as such are largely *unknown.* Among the known causes are maternal disease, such as *toxemia, premature separation of the placenta,* and *cervical incompetence.* Mothers of premature infants tend to be older and to have had previous abortions and stillbirths. Multiple pregnancy is a cause of prematurity.

Causes of death

Infants weighing less than 1500 gm. often show no abnormalities at autopsy and are judged to be inadequately developed for extra-uterine survival, even under ideal circumstances. Inability to ventilate the lungs is probably the basic fault, due either to lack of development of the lungs or to lack of respiratory force. Except for this factor, and the somewhat greater incidence of hyaline membrane disease in the premature infant, the causes of death in the premature are the same as those in the mature infant.

5. Placental Dysfunction (Postmaturity Syndrome)

Placental dysfunction is believed to be a cause of stillbirths after gestation of 300 days or more. The fetus is said to outgrow the placenta, and the fetus eventually may die in utero before the onset of labor, apparently from increasing anoxia.

NEOPLASMS OF INFANCY AND CHILDHOOD

1. General Concepts

Most neoplasms of early childhood are probably *congenital in origin,* although they often are not recognized until some time after birth. Early symptoms may be extremely vague and variable; a visible swelling is often the first sign. Neoplasms of the skin are commonly evident at birth; most of these are benign, although they often continue to grow as long as the infant grows. Internal neoplasms are less frequently evident at birth and are more likely to be malignant.

2. Statistical Data

Cancer mortality in childhood

The death rate from neoplastic diseases is higher for the age period from birth to 5 years than for any subsequent 5-year period until age 25. Although the quoted figures vary, it seems that neoplastic diseases (including, of course, leukemia) are *second only to accidents* as causes of death in children from 2 to 12 years of age. (Deaths occurring between birth and 2 years are largely due to the complications of delivery, prematurity, congenital malformations, etc.) A few years ago the infectious diseases outnumbered neoplasms in this age group, but, in those parts of the world where good medical care is readily available, most infectious diseases have yielded to preventive and therapeutic measures.

Types of cancer in childhood

Connective tissue cancers, i.e., *sarcomas,* make up a much larger proportion of the malignant neoplasms of childhood than of later life. In addition to this difference in predominant cell type, there are also important differences in the organ distribution of the primary cancers in childhood as compared with those in adults. In children, cancers of the neural, hemopoietic, and urinary systems predominate, whereas in adults cancers of the alimentary, reproductive, and respiratory systems are most numerous. The *relative frequency* of the most common malignant neoplasms causing death during ages 0 to 15 years is as follows:

Cancer Deaths in Infancy and Childhood	Percentage
Leukemia and malignant lymphomas	60
Neoplasms of the central nervous system	23
Neoplasms of the kidney	5
Neoplasms of bone	4
Neoplasms of the eye	2
Miscellaneous cancers	6
	100

3. Leukemia and Malignant Lymphomas

Leukemia causes more deaths before age 5 than it does in any 5-year period thereafter until age 60 to 64. The leukemia of childhood is usually *acute* and more often *lymphoblastic* than myeloblastic. Males are more often affected than females. Although temporarily responsive to therapy in many instances, death usually occurs within 1 year of onset. Purpura, anemia, fever, and swellings are common manifestations. For unknown reasons, mongolism is often noted in those infants manifesting leukemia shortly after birth.

Of the fatal malignant lymphomas of childhood, all of which are discussed in detail in Chapter 17, *lymphoblastoma* is the most frequent type; it is more common after age 5 than before. Its course is the same as that in adults and adolescents. *Burkitt's tumor* is an undifferentiated malignant lymphoma which occurs predominantly in children.

4. Neoplasms of the Central Nervous System

Cancer of the nervous system, constituting about 23 percent of all cancer deaths in childhood, causes more deaths before age 5 than in any following 5-year period until age 40 to 44. Tumors of the brain are much more frequent than tumors of the spinal cord. *Brain tumors* of childhood commonly arise *below the tentorium.* As they enlarge, they tend to compress the aqueduct of Sylvius, producing interference with the circulation of cerebrospinal fluid and *hydrocephalus.* If the fontanelles have not closed, they will tend to bulge. Brain tumors do not metastasize outside the central nervous system. As with brain tumors of adults, most brain tumors of childhood are believed to arise from the supporting tissue (glia) rather than from parenchymal cells (see Chapter 26).

Medulloblastoma

Medulloblastoma, a highly malignant neoplasm, is almost exclusively a tumor of childhood. It usually arises in the *posterior cranial fossa* and extends by local invasion; in addition it may seed over the meninges, giving rise to secondary tumors at some distance, even in the spinal cord. *Microscopically* the tumor cells are small and hyperchromatic; often they look like lymphocytes because of their scant cytoplasm.

Astrocytoma

Astrocytoma is perhaps *more frequent* than the medulloblastoma but is not characteristically a tumor of childhood; most astrocytomas occur in later life. These tumors are *slow-growing* and often *cystic;* the tumor may be a small nubbin bulging into a cyst. *Microscopically* the component cells are elongated and show branching fibrillar cytoplasmic extensions, best demonstrated with gold chloride stains.

Ependymoma

Ependymoma is presumably derived from the *lining cells of the ventricular system.* They are often located in the fourth ventricle, causing *hydrocephalus* early. *Microscopically* they are composed of cells which closely resemble epithelium, often arranged in nests, or lining small cystic spaces, or forming a papillary mass.

Craniopharyngioma

Craniopharyngioma is a rather complex tumor derived from embryonic elements in the region of the *pituitary* gland. It is often *cystic.*

5. Cancer of the Kidney

Cancers of the kidneys cause about 5 percent of all cancer deaths during the age period 0 to 15 years. Most of these neoplasms are unilateral; they are probably prenatal in origin. They cause more deaths before age 5 than during any subsequent 5-year period until age 45 to 49.

Wilms' tumor

The characteristic renal neoplasm of childhood is the *embryoma,* more generally known as *Wilms' tumor* (see Chapter 22). In some instances occurrence of this tumor seems to run in families. Symptoms are usually minimal; a palpable mass is the first sign. The tumor is encapsulated until late in its course; it then invades the renal pelvis and renal veins and metastasizes to distant organs, chiefly the lungs. Rough examination of the patient is believed to cause the dissemination of neoplastic cells, and should be avoided. These tumors are mesodermic in origin, arising from the metanephric blastema. *Microscopically* two or more cell types are usually seen: (1) embryonic epithelium, generally forming imperfect tubules, and (2) embryonic fibrous connective tissue growing as sarcoma. The tumor sometimes responds favorably to x-ray irradiation.

6. Cancer of Bone

Bone sarcoma accounts for about 4 percent of all cancer deaths before age 15. Its frequency rises further during the age period 15 to 19, accounting for 14 percent of all cancer deaths in this age group. The usual type of bone tumor in childhood is the *osteogenic sarcoma,* but Ewing's tumor, periosteal sarcoma, and chondrosarcoma also occur (see Chapter 28).

7. Cancer of the Eye

Although the total number of cases is small at any age, there are more deaths from malignant neoplasms of the eye under age 5 than in any subsequent 5-year period throughout life.

Retinoblastoma

The childhood eye tumor, the *retinoblastoma,* is distinctive; it does not occur in later life. The tumor often affects *both eyes,* although commonly appearing first in one. Siblings are frequently affected. There can be little doubt that a tendency to the development of this tumor is *inherited.* First manifestations are related to *vision.* As vision fails, the poor eye tends not to focus, producing a form of *strabismus.* After growing for a while in the bulb, the tumor cells penetrate to the loose tissues of the orbit and spread into the cranial cavity along the optic nerve. Contrary to neoplasms of the brain proper, systemic *metastases* may occur with retinoblastoma. Microscopically the characteristic cell is slightly elongated, resembling somewhat the rods and cones of the retina. These cells tend to arrange themselves in radial fashion about a clear space, resulting in *rosettes.* (Retinoblastoma is also discussed in Chapter 30.)

8. Miscellaneous Cancers

The remaining malignant neoplasms of childhood are a mixed group accounting for about 6 percent of all cancer deaths before age 15. In this group are several interesting, although rare, tumors.

Neuroblastoma

The *neuroblastoma* is usually encountered as a *retroperitoneal tumor* of infancy. It may spread to bones, including the skull, or to liver and other viscera. Very rarely the neuroblastoma regresses, either spontaneously or as a result of therapy (x-ray, vitamin B_{12}). Occasionally as it regresses its component cells seem to mature to those of a benign tumor, the ganglioneuroma. When metastasis occurs to the skull, the x-ray appearance is characteristic (see Chapter 26).

Thyroid cancer

Thyroid carcinoma rarely causes death in childhood, although it is not uncommon for it to be first manifest in this age period. Cancer of the thyroid gland tends to be a slowly growing neoplasm at all ages (see Chapter 27) and this is particularly true in children. In a number of instances thyroid cancer has developed at an early age following irradiation of the mediastinum and neck because of thymic enlargement.

Teratomas comprise a small portion of the neoplasms in this group, but since they are not always malignant and since they also occur in later life, they are considered under a separate heading in this chapter.

9. Benign Neoplasms

Many benign neoplasms are evident at birth, since they commonly affect the *skin* or *superficial soft tissues.*

Hemangioma

Hemangiomas are the most common neoplasms in newborn infants. Although microscopically some of these are very cellular, justifying the designation *hemangioendothelioma,* those present at birth rarely prove to be malignant [3]. The skin is the tissue most commonly affected (see Chapter 29), but hemangiomas may also occur in the liver, brain, retina, and bones.

Lymphangioma

Lymphangiomas often resemble local areas of edema. Larger cystic lymphangiomas, often called *hygromas,* commonly cause massive swellings, as in the neck, extremities, or buttocks.

Nevi

Pigmented *nevi,* sometimes having a rough verrucous surface, occur in the skin of the trunk or extremities (see Chapter 29).

Polyposis

Intestinal polyposis may occur as a hereditary disorder of the colon; there is a strong tendency to the development of *colonic cancer.*

Epiloia is a rare hereditary disorder in which benign neoplasms of several organ systems occur (see Chapter 26).

Certain *cystic tumors* related to teratomas are described in the section following.

10. Teratomas

Definitions

A *teratoma* is a neoplasm composed of multiple tissues foreign to the organ or part. A *cystic teratoma* is a cystic neoplasm showing chiefly tissues of ectodermal origin, but often having derivatives of the other germ layers as well; *dermoid cyst* is a widely used synonym for cystic teratoma but is a less specific term.

Origin

Although many teratomas are not recognized until the *third decade,* most are believed to have their origin in *embryonic life.* In some instances, especially in the newborn infant, the appearance suggests an *included twin,* similar to "Siamese twins." (Note the derivation of the word *teratoma: terato-,* monster; *-oma,* tumor.) Teratomas may arise from displaced embryonic tissue, or the chemical organizers or growth hormones of early embryonic life may be at fault. The teratomas of adult life are believed by many to arise from totipotent sex cells of ovary or testis, as a result of parthenogenesis.

Location

Most teratomas of the newborn infant and of childhood are located in the *midline:* base of skull, neck, mediastinum, retroperitoneal tissues, sacrococcygeal area. The teratomas of later life may be slowly growing tumors present since birth. and in the locations just given, but more commonly are found in the *gonads,* especially in the ovaries (see Chapter 24).

Gross and microscopic appearance

These neoplasms may be either *cystic* or *solid,* or may have cystic and solid areas intermingled. Microscopically the appearance is extremely varied. The cystic areas correspond to secretory or desquamative cell elements, i.e., *glandular* or *squamous epithelium.* Fat, fibrous tissue, muscle, cartilage, bone, nails, teeth, hair and hair follicles, sweat and sebaceous glands, ciliated, cuboidal, or squamous epithelium may be mingled in total disarray or organized so as to resemble vaguely a fetal part. Any tissue of the body may be present. In addition, some teratomas contain embryonic elements, including malignant trophoblastic cells (choriocarcinoma). In such cases, even in the male, the formation of chorionic gonadotropin may be sufficient to give a positive pregnancy test (see Chapter 15).

Course

Some teratomas are completely benign, others highly malignant; the course can be predicted by the degree of anaplasia of the component cells. Teratomas present at birth are usually benign, although they may kill by crowding vital structures. Teratomas of the testes are usually malignant, those containing trophoblastic tissue being especially so (see Chapter 23).

11. Other Neoplasms of Complex Structure

The neoplasms included in this group – hamartoma, choristoma, mesenchymoma, and "mixed" tumor – are usually benign; in fact, in some ways they resemble congenital malformations more than true neoplasms. Thus a *hamartoma (hamart-,* defect; *-oma,* tumor) is a complex tumor in which one or more tissue elements, normal to the organ, are abnormally mixed and overgrown; a hamartoma of the lung may consist of an unorganized conglomeration of well-differentiated cartilage, connective tissue, and ciliated epithelium, occupying a part of one lobe and displacing normal structures. A *choristoma* is an organized growth of normal cells in some organ where such cells would not normally occur; a choristoma of the intestine may consist simply of a mass of aberrant pancreatic tissue. A *mesenchymoma* is a neoplasm consisting of several different forms of connective tissue, intermingled with each other; malignant mesenchymomas may also occur (see Chapter 14). *"Mixed" tumor* is a confused term, generally applied to a benign salivary gland neoplasm having both epithelial and connective tissue elements.

REFERENCES

1. Baumgartner, L., and Pakter, J. Challenge of fetal loss, prematurity, and infant mortality – assessing the local situation. *J.A.M.A.* 167:936, 1958.
2. Verhoestraete, L. J., and Puffer, R. R. Challenge of fetal loss, prematurity and infant mortality – a world view. *J.A.M.A.* 167:950, 1958.
3. Levine, P. The protective action of ABO incompatibility on Rh isoimmunization and Rh hemolytic disease – theoretical and clinical implications. *J. Med. Educ.* 34:418, 1959.
4. Potter, E. L. *Pathology of the Fetus and the Newborn* (2d ed.). Chicago: Year Book, 1961.

17 THE HEMIC AND LYMPHATIC SYSTEM

1. Introduction

Anatomy

The cells of the hemic and lymphatic system are either (1) *fixed,* such as the cells lining the sinuses of the spleen, lymph nodes, bone marrow, liver, and adrenal cortex, or (2) *circulating,* such as the cells of the blood and the histiocytes of connective tissue.

Physiology: fixed elements

The *fixed tissue elements* are the parent cells of the circulating elements, and have many functions, not all of which are yet understood: *hemopoiesis, destruction of overage and defective cells* in the blood, *salvage* of certain materials for further use, and *manufacture of antibodies.*

circulating elements

The *circulating elements* are the mobile forces of the system. The *erythrocytes* act primarily in the transport of oxygen and carbon dioxide. The *leukocytes* have multiple functions: they are attracted to local areas of tissue injury, where they aid in the destruction and removal of bacteria by phagocytosis; they also take part in repair and regeneration after injury. The *phagocytic cells,* especially the monocytes, participate in the absorption of lipids and other substances from the intestine, and serve as scavenger cells in the tracheobronchial tree. Other circulating cells, especially the *platelets,* play a part in blood coagulation.

Blood picture

Since the cell elements of the blood are formed largely in the bone marrow and destroyed largely in the spleen, the *blood picture* at any time is the resultant of these two functions of the fixed portion of the system.

2. General Aspects of Diseases of the System

Infections

Both the fixed and circulating elements participate in most of the diseases of the hemic and lymphatic system, but often the two parts are affected differently. In *acute infections,* the circulating cells participate actively in the struggle with the infecting agents at the site of inflammation; the fixed cells, especially the leukoblastic cells of the bone marrow, serve as "bench strength" for the contest, undergoing active hyperplasia in order to supply new circulating cells. In *chronic infections,* the causative agent may be carried into the fixed tissues in the cytoplasm of the circulating cells. By this Trojan-horse tactic, *Mycobacterium tuberculosis, Histoplasma capsulatum,* and *Leishmania donovani* may be transported to the reticuloendothelial cells of the liver, spleen, lymph nodes, and bone marrow.

Storage diseases

The *storage diseases* affect chiefly the fixed elements: certain foreign chemical agents *(dextran, acacia, thorium dioxide)* and certain abnormal metabolic products *(amyloid, phospholipids, cystine)* may accumulate and remain permanently in the reticuloendothelial cells of the liver and spleen, causing enlargement of these organs, and sometimes interfering with their normal functions.

Neoplasms

In the *neoplastic diseases* of the system *(leukemia, multiple myeloma, polycythemia vera, Hodgkin's disease, lymphosarcoma),* it is the fixed elements that are primarily affected, although the neoplastic cells commonly spill over into the blood, as in leukemia.

3. Leukemia

Nature and causes

Leukemia is a neoplastic proliferation of the leukoblastic tissue – in the layman's words, cancer of the blood. As with other cancers, it may have diverse causes. Virus-like particles have been found in leukemic cells in lymph nodes and bone marrow in some cases of leukemia [1]. Leukemia has been produced experimentally by cell-free filtrates (in chickens), by roentgen irradiation (in mice), and by carcinogenic hydrocarbons (in mice). It has appeared in human beings following excessive doses of radiant energy, as in the survivors of Hiroshima and Nagasaki, in pioneer radiologists inadequately protected from x-rays, in children irradiated in the mother's uterus, and in patients treated with radiation (such as for spondylitis).

Relationship of bone marrow and blood

In most cases of leukemia there is an increase in the number of circulating leukocytes corresponding to the overproduction of neoplastic white cells in the bone marrow. When the number of circulating cells is greatly increased, the blood sometimes becomes visibly altered, the "white blood" – leukemia – of Virchow, who first described the condition. When there is no significant increase in the number of circulating white cells but immature white cells are present in the blood, the disease is sometimes referred to as *subleukemic leukemia.* When leukemic changes are evident in the bone marrow but the circulating white cells are neither immature nor increased in number, the condition is usually referred to as *aleukemic leukemia.* In the last two instances this state may be a temporary phase in the course of the disease or, more rarely, the disease may be subleukemic or aleukemic throughout its course.

Leukemia and the myeloproliferative disorders

Leukemia, like other malignant neoplasms, usually follows a relentless course to death. Occasionally a condition indistinguishable from leukemia is seen as a transient phase in a disorder of the blood and bone marrow that ranges widely in its manifestations from aplastic anemia to polycythemia and from thrombocytopenia to thrombocythemia. We have seen an example of this variation in an orchard worker using arsenic-containing fungicides, and another in a shoe salesman exposed intermittently over a number of years to irradiation from a fluoroscope-like machine formerly used in the fitting of shoes. In such cases the bone marrow is often reduced in cellularity or obliterated by sclerotic changes. New foci of extramedullary hemopoiesis resembling leukemic infiltration may develop in the liver and spleen, causing enlargement of these organs. Immature red and white cells may appear in the peripheral blood. Miale [2], following Dameshek, discusses the *myeloproliferative disorders* in some detail, and notes that it may sometimes be impossible to distinguish between the hyperplastic and neoplastic affections of the hemopoietic tissues.

Clinically a distinction is usually made between *acute* and *chronic* leukemia. The former occurs chiefly in children and young adults; there is almost complete replacement of bone marrow and circulating leukocytes by primitive forms of the white cell; the disease terminates fatally, usually within a year or less. Chronic leukemia occurs chiefly in later adult life; the cells of the bone marrow and blood more nearly resemble adult cells; the course of the disease is more protracted but extremely variable.

Clinical forms: acute and chronic

In *lymphocytic (lymphatic, lymphoblastic) leukemia* the affected cells are the lymphocyte and its precursor, the lymphoblasts. The acute form of the disease, characterized by extremely immature cells in the blood and bone marrow, severe anemia, thrombocytopenia, purpura, fever, tumor-like masses in the skin and a fulminating course, accounts for most cases of leukemia in infants and children. The chronic form is variable; in the elderly person it may be a relatively benign condition lasting many years and producing few symptoms.

Cell types: lymphocytic

In *myelocytic (myeloid, myelogenous, myeloblastic) leukemia* the affected cells are the granulocyte and its precursors, the myelocyte and myeloblast. Neutrophilic granulocytes usually predominate; rarely the eosinophilic, or more rarely the basophilic, granulocytes may be numerous. Both acute and chronic forms affect all age groups but the acute form is more numerous in childhood.

myelocytic

Monocytic leukemia is a somewhat controversial type, since many cases so diagnosed terminate as a myelocytic leukemia. The affected cells are the monocyte and its precursor, the monoblast. The *histiocytic leukemia* described by some authors is probably a variant of this group. Young adults are chiefly affected. Mouth lesions are common and severe.

monocytic

Stem cell leukemia (blast cell, unclassified) is a type of leukemia that may include few or many cases, depending upon the skill and self-assurance of the observer. The leukemic cells are so immature that they cannot be classified even with the help of Goodpasture's peroxidase stain. Such cases are almost always acute.

stem cell

Certain pathologic changes are more or less common to all cell types of leukemia.

Pathologic changes:

The *functioning bone marrow* is greatly extended at the expense of the fatty marrow. The marrow becomes *soft* and *pinkish red,* sometimes seeming almost purulent. In acute forms the neoplastic cells may permeate the bone cortex and elevate the periosteum; this change may be observed on x-ray. Microscopically the leukemic cells displace all other elements of the marrow.

bone marrow

The *blood* usually shows characteristic changes. In most cases the total *leukocyte count is elevated,* ranging from 50,000 to 300,000 per cubic millimeter. Occasionally, chiefly in cases of chronic myelocytic leukemia, the leukocyte count may be over a million cells per cubic millimeter. At such times the circulating leukocytes are usually fairly mature and the blood platelets may be increased. In aleukemic leukemia, and after therapy in patients having an elevated leukocyte count, the white cells may number 1000 or less per cubic millimeter, the atypical cells almost entirely disappearing from the blood. *Anemia* and *thrombocytopenia* are common and often severe in acute leukemia and in

blood

aleukemic leukemia; in chronic leukemia these changes are less noteworthy. The *leukemic cells* may be recognized in the differential blood smear by their large size, large nuclei, prominent nucleoli, and lack of cytoplasmic granules. These immature cells are often quite fragile; many are broken up in the preparation of the smear, giving "basket" forms of distorted nuclei.

Occasionally an extremely high leukocyte count – 100,000 or even more per cubic millimeter – occurs in the absence of leukemia. These *leukemoid reactions* are transient, occur chiefly in children, and are usually related to infection or blood destruction. Sometimes cytochemical methods may be helpful in distinguishing leukemoid reactions from true leukemia.

lymph nodes

Lymph node enlargement may occur in any form of leukemia but is most striking in *lymphatic* leukemia; occasionally in myelogenous leukemia the lymph nodes are not enlarged at all. The lymph nodes are soft and often hemorrhagic in acute leukemia; they are usually firmer and grayer in chronic forms.

spleen

The *spleen* is *enlarged* in most forms of leukemia, especially in the myelogenous form, in which the spleen may weigh up to 10,000 gm.; more commonly it weighs 600 to 1000 gm. and is firm, dark, and relatively dry. *Infarcts* are common, due presumably to a thrombotic tendency resulting from increased blood viscosity. Microscopically, in addition to the leukemic cells, there are usually foci of myeloid metaplasia, i.e., islands of hemopoietic tissue forming red cells and megakaryocytes as well as leukemic cells. This metaplasia occurs in the spleen in any condition in which the blood-forming elements are crowded out of the bone marrow.

liver, kidneys

The *liver* and *kidneys* are usually *enlarged,* with *white* or *gray* markings in the parenchyma due to leukemic cell infiltration. In myelogenous leukemia the infiltration is usually in streaks, whereas in lymphatic leukemia it is more focal, suggesting lymph follicles.

other organs

The *skin, gingiva, omentum, intestines, meninges, orbit, brain,* and other tissues often show leukemic infiltrates, particularly in acute leukemia. These often develop as tumor masses, sometimes greenish *(chloroma),* more often brawny and reddish brown. Perhaps the sequence of events in such cases is: (1) thrombocytopenia, due to the leukemic cells crowding the platelet precursors out of the marrow; (2) hemorrhage into the tissues; (3) multiplication of leukemic cells in the area where they have been spilled by hemorrhage, resulting in (4) local tumor masses composed of leukemic cells and elements of old blood.

Clinical features: acute

In acute leukemia, especially in children, *purpura* is often the presenting symptom. Thrombocytopenia is the usual explanation given for the hemorrhage, but some additional coagulation defect related to prothrombin undoubtedly exists. Paradoxically *thrombosis* and *infarction* sometimes occur instead of hemorrhage. These may affect any organ, particularly the spleen.

chronic

In chronic leukemia, the symptoms are vague and general: fatigue, pallor, and loss of weight. Their cause can usually be assigned to *anemia.* Symptoms may also be localized to specific areas, due to leukemic infiltration of organs or tissues: dragging pain in the left upper quadrant of the abdomen from *splenic enlargement; lymph node swellings* in the neck, axillae, or groin: *bone pain* from elevation of the periosteum by leukemic infiltrates; and *skin nodules.*

Many cases of leukemia are discovered as a result of a routine blood study carried out because of suspected anemia or infections. (Infections often usher in leukemia, especially the acute form.)

Mode of death

In acute leukemia, death usually results from *hemorrhage,* as in the gastrointestinal tract or brain. In chronic leukemia, patients may survive many years, often succumbing to unrelated conditions or to *infections.* Some agents used in the treatment of leukemia, such as nitrogen mustard, radioactive phosphorus, and whole-body irradiation, may produce extreme leukopenia, following which fatal infections often develop. *Fungus infections* such as cryptococcosis and candidiasis occur frequently. (In leukemic patients the inflammatory reaction is often quite different from that usually seen: exudates may consist largely of immature cells, or in aleukemic leukemia there may be almost no cell response to infection.)

4. Multiple Myeloma

Though often classified under bone neoplasms, *multiple myeloma* is primarily a tumor of marrow elements. It is rare in people under 50 years of age. In most instances the lesions are widespread and involve *many bones,* hence multiple. Rarely a solitary myeloma or plasmacytoma occurs; this neoplasm usually occurs in bone, but occasionally the upper respiratory tract or other soft tissues are affected. Sometimes the solitary myeloma develops later into multiple myeloma.

Pathologic changes: bones

Multiple myeloma chiefly affects the flat bones *(ribs, skull, sternum, vertebrae).* Rounded *punched-out* areas of cortical bone destruction give the characteristic picture on x-ray. The bone destruction is due to the expanding mass of plasma cells in the underlying marrow. Rarely multiple myeloma is revealed on x-ray as a diffuse *osteoporosis* rather than as multiple lytic lesions. *Fractures* may occur, especially if weight-bearing bones such as the vertebrae are affected.

bone marrow

The normal bone marrow is usually crowded out by soft gelatinous masses composed of *plasma cells,* many of which are *atypical* and *immature.* Plasma cells may be identified in smears made from bone marrow aspirate. Occasionally plasma cells may be found in the peripheral blood. Very rarely plasma cell leukemia occurs; these may actually be instances of lymphocytic leukemia (the close relationship between lymphocytes and plasma cells is noted on page 59).

kidney

Kidney lesions are inconstant, but may be diagnostic when they occur. The Bence Jones protein may precipitate as *casts in the renal tubules.* A *foreign body reaction* consisting of giant cells and lymphocytes may occur about the precipitate; there may be extensive damage of the interstitial tissue and tubules, the glomeruli being unaffected. Renal failure and uremia rarely occur.

other organs

Other organs show lesions infrequently. Plasma cell masses resembling metastases may on rare occasions appear in the liver and other viscera, but usually multiple myeloma remains *confined to bone.* As a result of the crowding out of the normal bone marrow by the myeloma cells, foci of *myeloid metaplasia* are often established in the spleen, liver, and lymph nodes, resulting in enlargement of these organs. Rarely primary or *idiopathic amyloidosis* (see Chapter 4) occurs.

Clinical features

Pain, fractures, and symptoms of compression of the spinal cord or nerve roots are common and are due to bone destruction; *weakness* and other constitutional symptoms are due to anemia, which may be extreme.

Laboratory findings

Anemia and *leukocytosis* result from bone marrow replacement. Chemical changes in multiple myeloma are extremely important, and often of diagnostic value. An *abnormal plasma protein,* not precisely the same in every instance, appears in the gamma globulin fraction. (A relationship between plasma cell proliferations and the gamma globulins was noted in Chapter 4.) In about half the cases of multiple myeloma an abnormal protein *(Bence Jones protein)* appears in the urine; it appears as a cloud when the urine is warmed, disappears on boiling, and reappears on cooling. An apparently identical protein is sometimes found in leukemia and other diseases. *Blood calcium* is inconstantly elevated, but seldom to the extent of causing metastatic calcification or urinary calculi. The increased gamma globulin causes an *increased sedimentation rate, rouleaux* formation, and consequent *difficulty in blood typing.* Isoagglutinins and increased blood hemolysis are commonly noted.

5. *Waldenström's Macroglobulinemia*

Clinical features

Waldenström's macroglobulinemia occurs most commonly in men from 50 to 70 years of age. *Clinically* it is characterized by weight loss, unusual susceptibility to infection, gum and gastrointestinal bleeding, epistaxis, hepatic and splenic enlargement, lymphadenopathy, thrombocytopenia, and anemia. Cardiac failure may result from increased viscosity of the blood. About 10 percent of the patients have Bence Jones protein in their urine. The SIA water test is usually positive; i.e., when a drop of serum is placed in water it turns milky. An M spot appears on paper electrophoresis. Clotting factors are deficient, and the erythrocyte sedimentation rate is often markedly elevated. Ultracentrifugation demonstrates sedimentation constants in the 19 to 20 S (Svedberg unit) range or above.

Pathologic changes

Generalized bone demineralization is usually found. *Microscopically* there are diffuse infiltrates of lymphoid plasmocytes in the bone marrow, lymph nodes, and spleen, and, less constantly, in the liver, kidneys, adrenals, pancreas, and brain [3]. The lymphoid plasmocyte has an eccentric round to oval nucleus and ample cytoplasm, sometimes with a clear zone about the nucleus. Periodic acid Schiff-stain positive material is present in the cytoplasm and nucleus. That in the nucleus is probably hexose-rich γ-macroglobulin. In the *Bing-Neel syndrome* there is a diffuse infiltration of the Virchow-Robin spaces in the brain with lymphocytes, plasmocytes, and lymphoid plasmocytes. Renal biopsies and kidney sections may show amyloidosis or large deposits on the endothelial side of the glomerular basement membrane [4]. Immunofluorescence indicates these deposits consist of IgM.

6. *Polycythemia Vera*

This rare disease is a *neoplastic proliferation of the erythroblastic tissues,* comparable in many ways to leukemia, and in fact frequently terminating as myelogenous leukemia. Symptoms (flushed skin, bloodshot conjunctivae, headaches) are due to the *increased red cell count* (often 8 to 12 million per cubic millimeter), hemoglobin content, and cell volume, and the increased blood viscosity resulting therefrom. Blood *platelets are increased* in this condition, and there is a great tendency toward venous and arterial *thrombosis.* The *bone marrow shows marked hyperplasia* of all the cell elements. Polycythemia vera must be distinguished from secondary polycythemia, a theoretically reversible, non-neoplastic condition resulting from prolonged anoxia, as with congenital heart disease or chronic emphysema.

7. *Hodgkin's Disease*

Hodgkin's disease is usually fatal and involves especially the lymph nodes, but also the spleen, liver, and bone marrow, and sometimes other organs. Its cause is unknown; it is generally considered to be a *neoplastic process,* but it has several features of a *granuloma.*

Relationship to other lymphomas

Most pathologists feel justified in differentiating between Hodgkin's disease and the other neoplastic processes affecting lymph nodes. Custer and Bernhard [5], however, on the basis of a large experience, came to the conclusion that the various forms of Hodgkin's disease, chronic lymphatic leukemia, and lymphosarcoma represent a single malignant mesenchymal neoplasm, differing only in the degree or stage of differentiation and in the number of lymphocytes in the blood. They reported a series of cases in which the histologic pattern varied at different times in the same patient, and even in different portions of the same lymph node at the same time.

Forms: paragranuloma

Jackson and Parker [6] recommended that cases of Hodgkin's disease be divided into three groups: paragranuloma, granuloma, and sarcoma. *Hodgkin's paragranuloma* is a *relatively benign* disease. Its usual manifestation is *cervical lymph node enlargement.* The bones and viscera are rarely involved. In the affected lymph nodes, lymphocytes predominate; Reed-Sternberg cells and eosinophils are present but not numerous. Necrosis and fibrosis are absent. About half the patients recover completely; about a quarter of the cases persist relatively unchanged, and a quarter gradually convert to Hodgkin's granuloma. (The use of the term *Hodgkin's paragranuloma* is open to criticism since the name *Hodgkin's* carries a malignant connotation to most clinicians. If the histologic changes in a given lymph node indicate a favorable outcome, the noncommittal term *hyperplastic lymphadenitis* is probably more appropriate.)

granuloma

Hodgkin's granuloma is the *common form* of the disease and is the form meant when the term *Hodgkin's disease* is used without qualification. It is slightly more common in males, and shows its peak incidence in the third decade, but occurs at all ages. This form of the disease is described in more detail in following sections.

sarcoma

Hodgkin's sarcoma occurs in an *older age group* (50 to 70 years) than the other two forms and shows no sex preference. It is rarely observed as a transition from the other two forms, and may well be *more closely related to reticulum cell sarcoma* than to the classic Hodgkin's disease. Its most common site of origin is the *retroperitoneal lymph nodes,* and the first symptom is usually pain. The affected nodes are enlarged and soft, frequently necrotic. Microscopically there is less pleomorphism than in the other forms of Hodgkin's disease. Large cells with abundant cytoplasm are numerous, but typical Reed-Sternberg cells must be present to make the diagnosis. The course of Hodgkin's sarcoma is that of a *highly malignant neoplasm.*

Pathologic changes in Hodgkin's granuloma: lymph nodes

Lymph nodes are affected in almost every case of Hodgkin's disease. The first group of nodes affected is usually the cervical, but axillary, mediastinal, retroperitoneal, and inguinal nodes are commonly affected also. Involved nodes are globular, rubbery, nontender, and usually discrete. On section the nodes are grayish white and moist, and show scattered yellow areas of necrosis. Microscopically the normal pattern of follicles and sinuses is replaced by a *diffuse, characteristically pleomorphic infiltrate.* Plasma cells, lymphocytes, eosinophils, and neutrophils are common, but the most characteristic cell is the *Reed-Sternberg giant cell.* These cells, also known as Dorothy Reed cells, are 12 to 40μ in diameter, irregular in shape, and have an abundant cytoplasm, which may be either slightly basophilic or slightly acidophilic. Usually there are two or more nuclei, often symmetrically arranged like mirror images, giving an owl-eye appearance. The nuclei may be lobulated or indented, and usually the nucleoli are prominent. Necrotic foci containing a number of neutrophils are noted in some nodes affected by Hodgkin's disease, but are absent in others. Fibrosis is also variable; it may be increased by radiation therapy.

other organs

Of the other organs the *spleen* is probably most often affected (75 percent of fatal cases). There is *general enlargement* of the spleen plus, in most instances, *focal gray lesions* in which the microscopic picture is like that in the lymph nodes. *Liver enlargement* is only slightly less frequent; it shows small nodules and streaks similar to the focal splenic lesions. The bones are involved in about half the fatal cases, the vertebrae in particular being affected. The lungs may show streaks of "Hodgkin's tissue" radiating into the parenchyma from enlarged mediastinal nodes. The gastrointestinal tract and kidneys are occasionally affected. Nervous system involvement is rare.

Clinical features in Hodgkin's granuloma

Among the most common symptoms are *lymph node enlargement, pain* (from involvement of bone, nerve, or viscera), recurring episodes of *fever* (Pel-Ebstein fever), and *weakness.* The symptoms and signs may resemble almost any disease of any organ: cough, fever, and pleural effusion are common in cases with mediastinal node involvement, suggesting pulmonary tuberculosis; abdominal pain, fever, and diarrhea may occur in cases in which the mesenteric nodes are affected, and may suggest chronic pancreatitis; right upper quadrant abdominal pain and jaundice may suggest gallbladder disease when the nodes at the hilum of the liver are involved. For unknown reasons, itching of the skin is a common symptom; ordinarily the skin shows no evidence of infiltration by Hodgkin's tissue. Hemolytic anemia occurs fairly frequently, but the blood picture is so variable that it is never diagnostic. *Lymph node biopsy* is the usual method by which the diagnosis is made.

Prognosis in Hodgkin's granuloma

The course of the disease is almost uniformly fatal, but every experienced pathologist has in his records a few cases of apparent cure or spontaneous recovery. In most of these patients only the cervical lymph nodes were affected at the time of diagnosis. The lymph node swelling may subside temporarily under x-ray or nitrogen mustard therapy, but in our experience this form of treatment seldom results in cure. Usually there is a series of relapses and remissions lasting from a few months to a number of years; 30 months from the onset of symptoms to death is about average. Death is usually a result of involvement of a vital organ, or of intercurrent infection.

8. Lymphosarcoma

Neoplasms designated as lymphosarcomas may be indistinguishable from Hodgkin's disease clinically and grossly, but microscopically they are distinctive in that they lack the pleomorphism of Hodgkin's disease, showing instead a single-cell strain of neoplasm. The term *malignant lymphoma* is often used as a clinical diagnosis to cover the entire group of diseases, i.e., the various forms of Hodgkin's disease and lymphosarcoma.

Types

Four apparently related neoplasms are often grouped together as lymphosarcomas. These are *lymphocytoma, lymphoblastoma, follicular lymphoblastoma,* and *reticulum cell sarcoma.* Custer and Bernhard [5] say: "These terms are useful, but only to designate the predominating histologic pattern of a lymphoma at the time of a particular examination." The *lymphocytoma* consists of relatively uniform round cells almost indistinguishable individually from normal lymphocytes, but blotting out the normal node structure by their monotony. It is somewhat less malignant in its course than the *lymphoblastoma,* which is composed of larger, more anaplastic cells resembling the lymphoblast, the precursor of the lymphocyte. (Occasionally a case of lymphocytoma or lymphoblastoma will show the blood picture of lymphatic leukemia terminally, emphasizing the close relationship between these diseases.) *Follicular lymphoblastoma* (Brill-Symmers disease) is the *least malignant* of the neoplasms in this group, often lasting 5 to 20 years. There is an increase in the size and number of the lymph follicles, compressing the sinuses and distorting the architecture. The component cells are small lymphocytes, relatively well differentiated. *Reticulum cell sarcoma,* the *most malignant* neoplasm in this group, is considered by many to be identical with Hodgkin's sarcoma. It is composed of large cells with abundant acidophilic cytoplasm. Reticulin fibers are intimately arranged about the individual cells, and this feature, demonstrable only by silver stains, is diagnostic when present. Fairly often this tumor is manifest as a neoplasm of the stomach or intestines, these organs usually being involved in continuity with the regional lymph nodes.

Sites of involvement

All neoplasms in this group ordinarily seem to arise in one group of lymph nodes and to spread directly to an adjoining group. *Cervical, mesenteric, retroperitoneal,* and *mediastinal nodes* are commonly involved. In some instances these neoplasms may be primary in tissue other than ordinary lymph nodes, especially in the tonsils, Peyer's patches of the intestine, and spleen. Occasionally a neoplasm indistinguishable from one or another of this group will appear to be primary in the liver, bone marrow, skin, or even uterus or brain; in such cases one must assume that it originates in histiocytes, which occur in all organs.

Related conditions

There remain a number of miscellaneous related neoplasms. The *lymphoepithelioma* is a highly malignant neoplasm usually primary in tonsillar tissue, where lymphatic elements and squamous epithelium are closely intermingled. It resembles the reticulum cell sarcoma in many of its features. *Mycosis fungoides* is a brawny, plaquelike thickening of the skin associated with severe itching, sometimes followed years later by malignant lymphoma of the lymph nodes and viscera. Its cause is unknown; it bears no relation to mycotic infections. Although the term *benign lymphoma* is sometimes used clinically, it seems that the only condition possibly suited to this term is the *lymphoid polyp* of the rectum. This is a submucosal growth of well-differentiated lymphoid tissue, usually projecting as a polyp into the lumen of the lower bowel, where it may be seen on routine proctoscopic examination. It is not a true neoplasm.

9. Burkitt's Tumor

Burkitt's tumor is an undifferentiated malignant lymphoma which occurs predominantly in children. Originally identified in Africa, the neoplasm is found in many parts of the world. There is epidemiologic and morphologic evidence that the tumor is caused by a virus. It is endemic in mosquito-ridden, high-rainfall regions of Africa, and virus-like particles have been found in neoplastic cells [7].

Clinical features

Clinically tumor masses appear suddenly and grow rapidly, most commonly in the jaws, abdomen, and retroperitoneal soft tissues. Paraplegia, due to infarction of the lower thoracic portion of the spinal cord or to direct compression of the cord by meningeal involvement with the neoplasm, is sometimes the presenting sign. The outcome is typically death within a few weeks or months in untreated cases. However, in patients treated with cyclophosphamide the tumor masses have disappeared.

Pathologic changes

The *most frequent sites* of tumor involvement are the abdominal and pelvic viscera, retroperitoneal soft tissues, facial bones, salivary and thyroid glands, cranial nerves, and meninges. In girls and women, bilateral ovarian infiltration is characteristic, as are bilateral breast tumors in young women. Involvement of lymph nodes, spleen, and bone marrow is uncommon. *Grossly* the tumor masses are usually discrete, solid, and nodular. They may attain a large size. *Microscopically* [8] there is a monotonous proliferation of poorly differentiated lymphoreticular cells varying from 10 to 25μ in diameter. These cells have a round or oval nucleus with shallow indentations and large nucleoli. Many nuclei show mitotic activity. There is a moderate amount of strongly basophilic cytoplasm which contains several tiny vacuoles. Special stains reveal lipid droplets. Scattered amid the sheets of neoplastic cells are macrophages with abundant cytoplasm containing tumor cell remnants. These macrophages produce a *"starry sky" pattern* within the neoplasm.

10. Metastatic Neoplasms of Lymph Nodes

Metastatic neoplasms of lymph nodes far outnumber the primary neoplasms. Most of the metastatic neoplasms are of epithelial origin, i.e., *carcinoma.* Since in most cases the primary neoplasm, as of breast or lip, is known to exist for some time before the metastasis appears, there is usually no difficulty in identifying the nature of the process. Sometimes, however, a patient is seen who has neoplastic involvement of several groups of nodes, as determined by physical examination and x-ray study, but the primary site is undetermined. Such a case may represent an extremely difficult diagnostic problem. The authors have attempted to help with this problem by a statistical study of their autopsy experience. Tabulation has been made of all metastases found at autopsy in 868 patients dying with malignant neoplastic diseases. From these data the relative frequency of metastasis from each primary site to each group of lymph nodes has been calculated, the data for males and females having been kept separate for greater usefulness. These tables are presented here as Tables 17-1 and 17-2.

11. Storage Diseases

Storage tendency of the system

The cells of the hemic and lymphatic system are hoarders; any particulate matter available to them is taken into the cytoplasm and may be stored indefinitely. This tendency is a reflection of one of the important normal functions of the system, namely, the *conservation of iron* derived from the breakdown of overage erythrocytes. In a similar way, cells of the system pick up *malarial pigment* and hold it for years; we have seen the pigment at autopsy in elderly persons who had not been known to have malaria since childhood. In *hemochromatosis* (see Chapter 11), large quantities of iron are stored in the system – sufficient at times to permit the ready visualization of the liver on a radiograph.

Thorium

At one time diagnostic use was made of this storage trait of the reticuloendothelial system. If *thorium dioxide* is injected intravenously into a patient, it is

TABLE 17-1. Computer Table for Aid in Diagnosis of Lymph Node Neoplasms in the Male

Lymph node region affected	Site or type of primary neoplasm																
	Leukemia	Malignant lymphoma	Lung and bronchus	Buccal mucosa and tongue	Stomach	Pancreas	Colon and rectum	Oropharynx and esophagus	Larynx	Skin (melanoma)	Prostate	Urinary bladder	Salivary glands	Thyroid gland	Kidney	Male breast	Miscellaneous
Cervical	10	17	17	13	5	2	3	3	6	4	3	2	3	1	1	2	4
Axillary	19	35	13	6	3	0	0	0	0	13	0	0	0	0	0	6	0
Thoracic	6	14	37	4	6	5	5	2	3	4	3	2	2	1	5	0	4
Mesenteric	7	17	16	0	11	14	14	2	3	4	2	0	0	1	2	0	9
Retroperitoneal	8	22	9	1	5	11	14	1	3	4	5	4	1	0	6	1	4
Inguinal	32	47	0	0	0	0	0	0	0	16	5	0	0	0	0	0	0

*Based on autopsy data in 394 male patients who died with malignant neoplasms in the George Washington University Hospital, 1948–1957.

†In using this table, begin with the lymph nodes which are known to be involved. Let us assume that, in a male patient (see Table 17-2 for females), the cervical nodes are enlarged and the chest x-ray shows that the mediastinal nodes are also enlarged. Find these categories on the left and follow across, noting the headings corresponding to the largest numbers on the two lines. The largest number opposite "Cervical" is 17 and is found under "Lymphoma" and also under "Lung and bronchus." The largest number opposite "Thoracic" is 37 and is found under "Lung and bronchus." The sum of the numbers under "Lung and bronchus" (17 plus 37 = 54) is larger than the sum under "Lymphoma" (17 plus 14 = 31). Hence the most likely neoplasm in a male showing enlargement of these two groups of nodes is a bronchogenic carcinoma. Note that if the inguinal nodes had also been enlarged, the likelihood would have shifted to lymphoma.

TABLE 17-2. Computer Table for Aid in Diagnosis of Lymph Node Neoplasms in the Female*†

Lymph node region affected	Site or type of primary neoplasm																	
	Leukemia	Malignant lymphoma	Breast	Lung and bronchus	Colon and rectum	Uterine cervix	Uterine fundus	Ovary	Stomach	Kidney	Urinary bladder	Pancreas	Gallbladder and bile ducts	Buccal mucosa and tongue	Skin (melanoma)	Thyroid gland	Liver	Vulva	Miscellaneous
Cervical	6	14	48	5	2	3	2	3	2	0	2	0	0	3	5	3	2	0	2
Axillary	3	13	72	0	0	0	0	2	0	0	0	2	0	2	3	2	2	0	0
Thoracic	5	10	52	6	2	5	2	6	2	0	0	1	0	0	4	1	2	0	3
Mesenteric	3	13	33	3	10	8	3	7	4	2	1	1	3	1	3	1	1	0	2
Retroperitoneal	4	10	27	2	7	19	3	11	1	3	3	1	3	1	3	1	1	1	2
Inguinal	15	46	0	0	0	15	0	0	0	0	0	0	0	8	8	0	0	8	0

*Based on autopsy data in 474 female patients who died with malignant neoplasms in the George Washington University Hospital, 1948–1957.

†The instructions for use of Table 17-1 apply. The great frequency of involvement of the different lymph node groups in females dying with carcinoma of the breast is clearly shown. When this table is used for a diagnostic problem and one is reasonably certain that the tumor scoring highest (for example, "Breast") is *not* present, obviously the tumor corresponding to the next highest sum becomes the most likely.

rapidly removed from the circulation and stored in the cytoplasm of the Kupffer cells of the liver and the endothelial cells of the spleen, where it remains for life. Radiographs of the abdomen taken after such an injection reveal the size and contour of the liver and spleen clearly, and will reveal abscesses and neoplastic masses which displace the normal tissues. Untoward complications of this storage of a radioactive substance developed, however, and led to abandonment of the procedure. The authors have seen both aplastic anemia and primary endothelioma of the spleen following the use of thorium in this way.

Storage diseases

In certain infectious and metabolic disorders, the storage trait results in diseases of the hemic and lymphatic system. *Histoplasma* and certain *protozoa* accumulate in the fixed elements of this system and produce their clinical manifestations (see Chapter 8). In Chapter 4 it is noted how *amyloid* may be stored in the reticuloendothelial system. There remain for consideration here certain rare metabolic diseases in which storage of some metabolic byproduct occurs in these organs.

Lipoid storage diseases:

The lipoid storage diseases (lipoidoses, reticuloendothelial granulomas) are the most important storage diseases of this system. In all these, *lipid substances accumulate in the cytoplasm of the fixed cells of the system, causing swelling and vacuolization. Splenomegaly* and *hepatomegaly* are common to all. The individual diseases are distinguished from each other by chemical identification of the specific lipid deposited in the spleen.

Gaucher's disease

Gaucher's disease (pronounced go-shay), presumably an *inherited* disorder, is due to the accumulation of the glucocerebroside, D-glucosyl-N-acylsphingosine. This substance, which cannot be demonstrated by ordinary fat stains, causes a great *ballooning of the cells* which contain it (Gaucher's cells). The spleen may be greatly enlarged and there may be leukopenia from the resulting hypersplenism. Severe anemia, and even distortion of the bones themselves, may result from the accumulation of masses of these cells in the bone marrow. The disease is usually first manifest in childhood and causes death in a few years.

Niemann-Pick disease

Niemann-Pick disease occurs in *infants* and is generally fatal before the third year. It is *familial,* affecting particularly *Jewish females.* The lipid is *sphingomyelin,* which stains with ordinary fat stains. *Vacuolated endothelial cells* are widely distributed in the body and may sometimes be detected on blood smears. Blindness and idiocy sometimes occur, due to lipid deposits in the retina and in ganglion cells of the brain.

Tay-Sachs disease

When blindness and idiocy occur, Niemann-Pick disease may be indistinguishable clinically from Tay-Sachs disease, also known as *amaurotic familial idiocy.* The latter is a *familial* disease which occurs in *Jewish infants* and shows deposits of *lecithin* in *ganglion cells of the brain,* followed by scarring (gliosis). Amaurosis *(blindness)* is due to changes in the macula and optic nerve. The alterations in the macula are evident on ophthalmoscopic examination as the *cherry-red spot,* which is diagnostic. Apparently the reticuloendothelial cells are not involved in most cases of Tay-Sachs disease, but combined forms of this disease and Niemann-Pick disease are said to occur.

Hand-Schüller-Christian disease

Even more complex in its interrelationships is Hand-Schüller-Christian disease. In this rare chronic disease, chiefly of *young adults, cholesterol and its esters* are deposited in phagocytic cells. The most extensive deposits occur in bone, especially in the bones of the base of the skull and of the face, where defects can often be demonstrated by x-ray. These destructive bone lesions may involve the sella turcica and secondarily the pituitary gland, causing diabetes insipidus; or the temporal bones and auditory nerve, causing deafness; or the bones of the orbit, causing protrusion of the eyes (exophthalmos). Spleen, lymph nodes, and lungs are less frequently involved. In the affected areas there are eosinophils and plasma cells along with the phagocytes containing lipid. This mixture of cell types results in a lesion which suggests a granuloma. Some investigators consider that this disease is in fact an inflammatory process rather than a metabolic disease, and point out a certain resemblance to eosinophilic granuloma of bone and Letterer-Siwe disease. *Eosinophilic granuloma of bone* is a solitary lesion composed of histiocytes and eosinophils, often healing spontaneously. *Letterer-Siwe disease,* also known as nonlipid reticuloendotheliosis, is a *rapidly fatal febrile disease* of unknown cause; it is characterized by focal granulomatous lesions in lymph nodes, spleen, and bone marrow of infants. Histologically these three diseases may resemble each other, and the chemical features, which one would expect to be distinctive, are not always predictable.

12. Inflammatory Diseases of Lymph Nodes

Lymph node enlargement

Most diseases of the lymph nodes, whether inflammatory or neoplastic, are manifest by *enlargement.* Lymph node enlargement is always an important *objective symptom or sign.* Infection accounts for most instances of lymph node enlargement in children; in adults node enlargement is more ominous, since it is often due to neoplasm. Normal lymph nodes are flat and bean-shaped and generally not palpable; however, in an occasional thin, apparently healthy person they can be felt, especially in the groin. Abnormal nodes are generally enlarged, rounded, and easily palpable. They may be hard, soft, or even fluctuant; tender or not; discrete or matted.

Generalized enlargement

When lymph node enlargement is generalized, a systemic disease must be suspected, usually either infectious or neoplastic. Of the infectious processes, *rubella* is the most common cause in children, while *syphilis, tuberculosis,* and *brucellosis* probably lead the list in adults. Of the neoplastic processes, *leukemia* leads the list at all ages. Malignant lymphoma and metastatic carcinoma sometimes show generalized lymph node enlargement late in their course, but earlier, enlargement is generally regional. It has been reported that generalized lymph node enlargement may also occur in response to certain drugs (see Chapter 10).

Localized enlargement

Localized or *regional lymph node enlargement has regional significance.* The cause is usually to be found in the region drained by the enlarged nodes, and may be either an infectious or a neoplastic process. Of the infectious processes, the following are the most important, by regions: *anterior cervical* – tonsilitis, upper respiratory and dental infections, and infectious mononucleosis; *posterior cervical* – scalp infections; *axillary* – infections of the breast and upper extremity, including in the latter tularemia and cat-scratch disease; *mesenteric* – mesenteric adenitis (see page 391) and intestinal infections, including typhoid fever; *inguinal* – lymphopathia venereum and chancroid. (Care must be exercised to distinguish regional lymph node enlargement from cysts, neoplasms, and nonlymphoid lesions occurring in the same part of the body, such as salivary gland tumors or thyroid nodules in the neck, and femoral hernia or undescended testicle in the groin.)

Acute lymphadenitis

In acute inflammation of a lymph node, the node becomes *enlarged, soft, tender,* and sometimes *fluctuant.* The enlargement is due to hyperplasia of the cell elements and accumulation of the inflammatory exudate. Fluctuation in acute lymphadenitis usually means pyogenic infection and abscess; it is common in the axilla and groin.

Infectious mononucleosis

Infectious mononucleosis is a *mildly contagious disease* affecting *adolescents* and *young adults.* It is probably caused by the herpesvirus-like Epstein-Barr (EB) virus. The disease is usually manifest by *sore throat, fever, swelling of the cervical lymph nodes,* and sometimes splenomegaly. The blood leukocytes usually number 10,000 to 20,000 per cubic millimeter, and *immature cells,* probably lymphoblasts, are commonly noted in the blood smear; similar cells are also seen in the sinuses of the lymph nodes. Such cases have on occasion been confused with acute leukemia. After several weeks' illness with mononucleosis, a *heterophil antibody* appears in the serum, capable of agglutinating sheep's red blood cells. The Paul-Bunnell test, used to demonstrate this antibody, is not absolutely specific for mononucleosis, but if guinea pig kidney or some other substance is used to absorb the occasional interfering antibodies (Davidsohn differential test), the test assumes diagnostic significance. The disease is usually mild, terminating spontaneously after a few weeks, but in some instances it is quite severe, even fatal. *Hepatitis* is an important complication. Massive intraperitoneal hemorrhage due to spontaneous rupture of the spleen has occurred occasionally. The spleen may show a rather characteristic lesion microscopically, consisting of infiltration of the capsule and trabeculae by the immature lymphocytes.

Mesenteric adenitis

Acute mesenteric lymphadenitis is a poorly understood condition of unknown cause, occurring chiefly in *children.* Symptoms may be indistinguishable from *acute appendicitis,* but there is usually no leukocytosis. The mesenteric and retroperitoneal nodes are greatly swollen and soft. Microscopically the nodes show a nonspecific acute inflammatory reaction.

Chronic lymphadenitis

Persistent enlargement of lymph nodes should always make one suspicious of *neoplasm,* especially when it occurs in the adult; however, it may be due to *chronic infection* or to *unknown causes.* In chronic infections the enlargement is due to hyperplasia of the follicles and reticulum cells of the sinuses, and to some extent to an exudation of inflammatory cells in the sinuses. Specific types of chronic lymphadenitis are as follows:

Tuberculous lymphadenitis may be cervical, mediastinal, or mesenteric, depending upon the avenue of entry of the bacilli and other factors. It is a manifestation of primary infection (see Chapter 6), and the lesion is characteristically caseous; when hypersensitivity supervenes, the caseous focus may liquefy, forming a "cold abscess." This may rupture into a bronchus in the case of mediastinal node involvement, or onto the skin in the case of a cervical node.

Boeck's sarcoid is an important granulomatous lesion of lymph nodes, especially mediastinal, but also cervical and mesenteric. The lesions resemble tuberculosis, with focal collections of epithelioid cells and giant cells, but there is no necrosis and acid-fast bacilli are absent. (See Chapter 6.)

Cat-scratch disease is a granulomatous lesion chiefly of the axillary lymph nodes, showing focal areas of necrosis and epithelioid cell proliferation resembling tuberculosis. It is believed to be a chlamydial infection. (See Chapter 7.) A skin test, using an antigen prepared from lymph node material, is confirmatory.

Lymphogranuloma venereum causes a chronic suppurative lymphadenitis in the inguinal nodes, chiefly in males (see Chapter 23). It is a virus infection of venereal origin, confirmed by the Frei test. In females, lymphatic drainage is posterior, and rectal stricture is a common sequel (see Chapter 24).

Brucellosis, syphilis, lupus erythematosus, and *erythema nodosum* cause generalized lymphadenitis, but cannot be definitely identified histologically.

Dermatopathic lymphadenitis is a chronic nonspecific hyperplasia of the reticulum cells and follicles, causing enlargement of nodes draining areas of skin ulceration due to any cause. Melanin pigment and neutral fat are commonly noted in the phagocytic cells.

13. Diseases of the Spleen

The spleen is a poorly understood organ that is not essential to life; its removal is usually followed by mild but persistent leukocytosis and thrombocytosis but there are no serious after-effects. The normal spleen is not palpable; it must be enlarged to a weight of about 500 gm. (normal weight about 150 gm.) before it can be felt under the costal border. *Most diseases of the spleen cause some degree of enlargement of the organ,* but not always to such an extent as to render it palpable. Diseases affecting the spleen usually also involve the lymph nodes; most of these diseases have been considered in other sections of this chapter.

Causes of splenomegaly

Among the important causes of splenic enlargement are the following:

1. *Acute splenic tumor,* occurring in certain acute infectious diseases such as typhoid fever. The sinuses are engorged with inflammatory cells and "sludged blood."

2. *Leukemia,* all forms. The sinuses are engorged with leukemic cells.

3. *Congestive splenomegaly,* such as in portal hypertension, including cirrhosis of the liver, Banti's syndrome (splenic anemia), and portal vein thrombosis, rarely in congestive heart failure. The sinuses are stuffed with normal blood elements.

4. *Secondary amyloidosis,* as in chronic destructive diseases of the lungs, bones, and joints. The amyloid material is deposited in the walls of the splenic sinuses or in the follicles.

5. *Hodgkin's disease.* The parenchyma is infiltrated with "Hodgkin's tissue," like that in the lymph nodes.

6. *Lymphosarcoma,* including all of the various forms. The parenchyma is infiltrated by neoplastic cells.

7. *Metastatic neoplasms* from any source may involve the spleen, although this organ is much less often invaded than the liver, lymph nodes, and most other organs. New growths are established resembling the parent neoplasm.

8. *Lipoid storage diseases* (Gaucher's, Niemann-Pick, etc.). The sinuses are stuffed with the lipid-laden phagocytes.

9. *Histoplasmosis, leishmaniasis, tuberculosis, brucellosis,* and other chronic

bacterial, fungus, and protozoan diseases. There is proliferation of reticuloendothelial cells and formation of granulomatous lesions.

10. *Hypersplenism* in its various or combined forms, associated with excessive destruction of the various cells of the blood. There is engorgement of the sinuses with normal blood elements, sometimes erythrophagocytosis, but usually no pathognomonic finding. (Included under this heading are the acquired hemolytic anemias, leukopenias, and thrombocytopenias, generally of unknown cause, but sometimes secondary to neoplasms, infections, or drugs.)

11. *Various anemias* in which myelofibrosis or bone marrow replacement leads to myeloid metaplasia of the spleen. Ectopic foci of hemopoietic tissue are found throughout the splenic pulp.

12. *Lupus erythematosus.* Collagen deposits are found about small vessels and in their walls, and there is hyperplasia of reticuloendothelial cells.

13. Certain hereditary blood diseases associated with abnormal forms of erythrocytes *(sickle cell anemia, Cooley's anemia, spherocytic anemia).* There are variable changes, including marked congestion of the pulp cords, fibrosis, and myeloid metaplasia (see Chapter 11).

Miscellaneous diseases of the spleen

Rarely the spleen is affected by a disease process resulting in some structural alteration other than enlargement. *Cysts* are rare and may be congenital or acquired; acquired cysts may be due to *Echinococcus* disease or more commonly to the liquefaction of massive infarcts. *Atrophy and fibrosis* are seen following recurrent infarction and are characteristic of late states of sickle cell anemia. *Accessory spleens* tend to appear in any condition causing splenic enlargement; they are usually found in the region of the hilum of the spleen.

REFERENCES

1. Murphy, W. H., Ertel, I. J., and Zarafonetis, C. J. D. Virus studies of human leukemia. *Cancer* 18:1329, 1965.
2. Miale, J. B. *Laboratory Medicine – Hematology* (3d ed.). St. Louis: Mosby, 1967. (The myeloproliferative disorders are exceptionally well presented.)
3. Dutcher, T. F., and Fahey, J. L. Histopathology of macroglobulinemia of Waldenström. *J. Nat. Cancer Inst.* 22:887, 1959.
4. Morel-Moroger, L., Basch, A., Danon, F., Verroust, P., and Riche, G. Pathology of the kidney in Waldenström's macroglobulinemia. *New Eng. J. Med.* 283:123, 1970.
5. Custer, R. P., and Bernhard, W. G. The interrelationship of Hodgkin's disease and other lymphatic tumors. *Amer. J. Med. Sci.* 216:625, 1948. (A valuable study based upon the large collection of cases in the Armed Forces Institute of Pathology, Washington, D.C.)
6. Jackson, H., and Parker, F. *Hodgkin's Disease and Allied Disorders.* New York: Oxford University Press, 1947.
7. Bell, T. M. Viruses associated with Burkitt's tumor. *Progr. Med. Virol.* 9:1, 1967.
8. Berard, C., O'Conor, G. T., Thomas, L. B., and Torloni, H. Histopathological definition of Burkitt's tumor. *Bull. W.H.O.* 40:601, 1969.

GENERAL REFERENCE

Amromin, G. D. *Pathology of Leukemia.* New York: Hoeber, 1968.

18 THE CARDIOVASCULAR SYSTEM

CARDIOVASCULAR DISEASES IN GENERAL

1. Introduction

Definition

The cardiovascular diseases include *all the organic and functional disorders of the heart and great vessels,* if one uses the term in its broadest sense. However, not all blood vessel diseases are covered under this heading: arterial or venous diseases that are essentially limited to a single organ system (e.g., the brain) are considered under that system rather than here.

Mortality from cardiovascular diseases:

Diseases of the cardiovascular system account for about *55 percent of all deaths* at the present time (see Table 18-1). It has not always been thus: in 1900 only 20 percent of all deaths were due to cardiovascular diseases. The increase is due chiefly to the aging of the population; the death rate from cardiovascular diseases is particularly high in the older age groups. The control of infectious diseases by sanitary measures and antibiotics has caused the noninfectious diseases to move up on the lists, especially the diseases of later life – heart disease and cancer. When adjusted for the age of the population, it appears that the *incidence of heart disease may actually be falling* [1]. Thus the rise in the *relative* frequency of heart disease is not alarming; it does, however, present a challenge to the medical profession.

white and nonwhite

In general, death rates from cardiovascular diseases are slightly *higher in whites than in nonwhites* (534.6 to 462.6 per 100,000), presumably due to the greater average age at death in whites. Significant variations in this overall ratio occur in certain specific cardiovascular diseases. Thus *arteriosclerotic heart disease,* including coronary artery disease, has a death rate per 100,000 of 303.3 in whites and 175.3 in nonwhites. *Hypertensive heart disease* has a death rate of 28.1 per 100,000 in whites as compared to 64.1 in nonwhites. These differences are undoubtedly due to the difference in incidence of one or more of the causative factors of these diseases as they operate in whites and nonwhites.

by age groups

Deaths from cardiovascular diseases have a striking correlation with *age* (see Table 18-2). Under 1 year of age, death rate from these diseases is 12.9 per 100,000 in that age group, and these deaths are chiefly from *congenital malformations.* In the age group 1 to 9 years, the death rate from heart disease falls to its lowest level, 1.9 per 100,000; most of these deaths are also due to

TABLE 18-1. Major Causes of Death in the United States

Cause	Number of deaths	Percentage of all deaths
Cardiovascular diseases	994,747	54.8
Neoplasms	290,267	16.0
Accidents	100,669	5.6
Pneumonia and influenza	70,761	3.8
Prematurity, and other diseases peculiar to infancy	62,688	3.5
Tuberculosis, all forms	9,311	0.5
All other causes	285,106	15.7
Totals	1,813,549	99.9

Calculated from mortality tables, *Vital Statistics of U.S.*, 1963.

Table 18-2. Age Distribution of Deaths from Cardiovascular Diseases

Age group	Total deaths from cardiovascular diseases	Total deaths from all causes	Cardio-vascular deaths as percentage of all deaths	Death rate from cardiovascular diseases*
Under 1 year	524	103,390	0.5	12.9
1– 9 years	390	25,622	1.6	1.9
10–19 years	1,421	21,422	6.7	4.3
20–29 years	3,172	29,732	10.7	13.9
30–39 years	12,104	48,110	25.2	50.5
40–49 years	44,119	110,259	40.0	190.7
50–59 years	107,853	219,403	49.1	574.5
60–69 years	206,440	360,406	57.3	1,534.0
70–79 years	312,809	478,711	65.3	3,861.4
80 and over	305,274	415,866	73.4	11,913.1
All ages	994,797	1,813,549	54.8	527.6

Calculated from mortality tables, *Vital Statistics of U.S.*, 1963.
*Rate per 100,000 estimated midyear population in specified group.

congenital heart disease. After the decade 20 to 29, the incidence of cardiovascular diseases *rises about 10 percent with each decade,* accounting in large part for the progressive increase in total deaths as aging occurs.

geographic differences

Death rates from cardiovascular diseases show a significant variation from country to country, and also, in some instances, within a given country. These *geographic differences* persist when the figures are corrected to eliminate extraneous factors related to race and age at death. Thus the death rate from cardiovascular diseases among white males age 45 to 64 in the United States is more than twice that seen in males of the same age in The Netherlands. Cardiovascular death rates generally are *highest in the United States, Finland, and Australia,* in that order, and *lowest in The Netherlands, Sweden, Italy, Switzerland, and Norway,* among nations reporting their mortality data to the World Health Organization for the years 1958 to 1960 [1]. These differences are probably chiefly due to *environmental factors,* but *genetic factors* may also be involved, as well as differences in the methods of reporting deaths. Among environmental factors, *diet* usually gets the most attention, especially in relation to coronary artery disease. Increasing attention is also being given to variations in *trace minerals,* especially *cadmium,* in the drinking water [2] and in the air [3].

Morbidity

Morbidity, i.e., the incidence of heart disease among the living, is known only for small samples of the population. According to data collected by the American Heart Association [1], there were, in 1960 to 1962, some 14,621,000 persons in the U.S. age 18 to 79 who had definite heart disease, and 12,979,000 additional persons with suspected heart disease. These figures include an estimated 17,401,000 persons with hypertension.

2. *Manifestations of Cardiovascular Disease*

Work of the heart

The normal work load of the heart, when calculated for the average life span, is truly remarkable. At 72 systoles per minute and an average ejection of about 65 ml. per systole, it is evident that the *heart pumps about 58 barrels of blood per day,* even at rest! The normal heart can increase its output temporarily by 300 to 400 percent, and in one accustomed to heavy exercise, as the trained athlete, this work load may be increased on demand by as much as 500 percent [4]

Cardiac reserve

When coronary circulation is good and nutritional reserves are adequate, the *heart can compensate for extreme increases in work load provided they are temporary. The normal heart ordinarily does not fail.* When there is within the heart some factor inducing strain – as a leaking heart valve – or impairing oxygenation of the myocardium – as sclerotic narrowing of the coronary arteries or severe anemia – the heart may be unable to compensate for even minor increases in work load. Under such circumstances, after varying degrees of exertion, there may be excessive fatigue, cough, dyspnea, or substernal oppression. If circumstances continue to deteriorate, one or another of the following complications may ensue: *sudden death, congestive heart failure, cardiogenic shock,* or *cardiac cachexia.*

Sudden death

While death from heart disease is often said to be sudden, rarely is it without warning. Usually there are *premonitory symptoms and signs,* and in most instances the patient is known to have heart disease. In such cases death may be due to the sudden onset of some serious *abnormality of cardiac rhythm* (heart block or ventricular fibrillation), to the *occlusion of one coronary artery* by thrombosis when the others are narrowed by sclerotic changes, to the *rupture of an aneurysm,* to *pulmonary* or *cerebral embolism,* or the like.

Congestive heart failure

When the heart fails gradually, two mechanisms probably come into play, both leading to *congestion* and *edema* of the viscera and dependent parts of the body. The first mechanism – *backward failure* of the heart – occurs when a ventricle becomes unable to eject blood in adequate quantity during systole: a "dam in the stream" develops, blood accumulates in the corresponding atrium, venous pressure rises, and there is a loss of fluid and electrolytes into the tissues due to simple hydrostatic pressure. The other mechanism, known as *forward failure,* is explained as follows: when the left ventricle becomes unable to eject blood in adequate quantity, the tissues are deprived of their normal circulation and tissue hypoxia results, leading to increased capillary permeability, salt and water retention, and hence edema (see Chapter 2).

Cardiogenic shock

Sometimes the body reacts to cardiac inadequacy by a neurovascular crisis known as cardiogenic shock: an acute, severe *hypotensive episode* resulting in marked *diminution of cardiac output.* This form of shock occurs frequently in myocardial infarction, and may be noted in conjunction with any level of venous pressure. As with other forms of shock, cardiac shock tends to become irreversible after a few hours.

Cardiac cachexia

With chronic heart failure it is common for significant *loss of weight* to occur if fluid accumulation is discounted. This state of cachexia is especially noted in individuals who have had several bouts of congestive heart failure. Multiple factors are believed to act in the causation of this syndrome [5], but the chief factor is believed to be *tissue hypoxia* from forward failure. Hypometabolism and loss of interest in food are also believed to contribute to the wasting.

3. *Heart Failure*

Definition

Heart failure is said to occur when the *heart is unable to pump blood* at a rate sufficient to meet the requirements of the tissues.

Causes:

While many complex factors affecting muscle structure and chemistry and fluid dynamics are involved in the question of heart failure [6], the picture can be summed up as follows. Heart failure results from: (1) conditions which so affect the heart as to make it *unable to perform its normal work load,* (2) conditions which cause a *persistent increase in the work load of the heart,* or (3) some *combination* of the first two factors.

impaired cardiac function

Conditions which impair the heart's ability to carry out its normal functions include: *impaired coronary circulation, disease of the heart muscle, impaired venous filling of the heart, interference with impulse formation or propagation,* and *reduced oxygen-carrying capacity of the blood.*

increased work load

Conditions which cause an increase in the heart's work load, other than temporary increases due to exercise or excitement, include: *increased arterial resistance* (systemic or pulmonary hypertension), *disease of the heart valves* either congenital or acquired, *abnormal communications* between the right and left sides of the heart or between the systemic and pulmonic arterial systems, *increased metabolic demands,* and, occasionally, *decreased arterial resistance* (high-output failure).

Left- and right-sided heart failure

It is customary and convenient to separate left from right ventricular failure, although realizing that neither can long exist in pure form since continuation of the one inevitably leads to the other. *Left ventricular failure* results in distention of the left atrium, engorgement of the pulmonary veins, and transudation of fluid into the alveoli, i.e., pulmonary edema. *Right ventricular failure* results in distention of the right atrium, distention of the cervical veins, engorgement of the superior and inferior venae cavae, congestion of the liver, and peripheral edema.

Left ventricular strain: causes

The following cardiovascular disorders interfere with the emptying of the left ventricle, causing overstretching of its muscle fibers and eventually left ventricular hypertrophy:

1. *Systemic hypertension.* In hypertension the diastolic pressure in the aorta is high, hence increased force of ventricular contraction is required in order to open the aortic valve.

2. *Aortic stenosis.* In this condition the cusps of the aortic valve are unduly rigid, thus interfering with systolic ejection from the left ventricle and giving an effect similar to that seen with hypertension. Narrowing of the orifice is also often a feature of aortic stenosis; this requires a prolongation of systole in order to achieve the same stroke output, and hence adds further to the strain upon the left ventricle.

3. *Aortic insufficiency.* In this condition the valve leaks, and blood from the aorta flows back into the left ventricle during diastole. In order to maintain the circulation in the presence of aortic insufficiency, a greater amount of blood than normal must be expelled from the left ventricle with each systole.

4. *Systemic arteriovenous aneurysm or fistula.* In this condition a communication exists between the high-pressure arterial system and the low-pressure venous system, hence blood spills off into the veins with each systole. The effect is much the same as with aortic insufficiency, since increased left ventricular output is required with each systole in order to keep the blood moving.

5. *Persistent ductus arteriosus* or *interventricular septal defect* causes the same effect as arteriovenous fistula, due to spillage of blood from the high-pressure systemic circulation into the low-pressure pulmonic system.

6. *Aortic aneurysm* usually causes no significant cardiac strain, but occasionally the vis a tergo is so dissipated in a large aneurysm that increased systolic output is required to maintain the circulation.

effects

Increased thickness of the left ventricular wall and *pulmonary edema,* often with pleural effusion, are the basic pathologic findings common to all forms of left ventricular strain. The usual symptoms are *dyspnea, orthopnea,* or *cough,* and sometimes *paroxysmal nocturnal dyspnea.* Foamy pink fluid may exude from the nose or mouth in severe cases. Physical findings include *dullness at the base* of each lung, or posteriorly in the case of the bed patient, and *moist bubbling rales* in the same areas. The heart radiograph usually shows the heart enlarged downward and to the left, giving a boot-shaped contour. The electrocardiogram shows left axis deviation.

Right ventricular strain: causes

Certain other cardiovascular disorders *interfere with the emptying of the right ventricle* and cause *right ventricular hypertrophy.* These disorders, and their mode of action, follow:

1. *Pulmonary hypertension.* As with systemic hypertension, an increased ventricular contraction is required in pulmonary hypertension in order to open the pulmonic valve.

2. *Pulmonic stenosis* provides the same handicap to the right ventricle that aortic stenosis does to the left.

3. *Pulmonic insufficiency* – a rare lesion in pure form – is strictly comparable in its effects to aortic insufficiency, a relatively common lesion.

4. *Pulmonary arteriovenous aneurysm or fistula* results in spilling of blood from the higher-pressure pulmonary artery to the lower-pressure pulmonary vein, and an effect similar to that in pulmonic valve insufficiency.

effects

Increased thickness of the right ventricular wall, liver enlargement, and *edema of the lower extremities* are pathologic findings common to all forms of right ventricular strain. The usual symptoms are *cyanosis* (from peripheral stasis and inadequate pulmonary blood flow), *pain in the right upper quadrant of the abdomen, ascites,* and *edema of the legs.* Physical signs include *edema, enlargement of the liver, increased venous pressure,* and *clubbing of the fingers.* There may be *secondary polycythemia* or *erythrocytosis.* The heart radiograph shows a broadening of the heart shadow, especially a prominence of the upper portion of the left border; the latter finding is apparently due to hypertrophy of the pulmonary conus. The electrocardiogram shows right axis deviation. The term *cor pulmonale* is commonly applied to all cases of right ventricular strain, but more especially to those grouped under the heading of pulmonary hypertension.

Myocardial strain, generally

When myocardial abnormalities occur, they commonly affect the walls of both ventricles and produce mixed manifestations and effects. These include *coronary artery disease,* with or without infarction; *metabolic disorders,* as fatty degeneration, amyloid or glycogen infiltration, or myxedema; *inflammatory diseases* such as rheumatic fever, lupus erythematosus, nonspecific myocarditis, sarcoid, and the like.

"Functional heart disease"

Functional disturbances of the heart may at times show mixed manifestations of right- and left-sided heart failure; there are usually *no demonstrable lesions in the heart itself.* Included are abnormalities of cardiac rhythm, fluid overload from intravenous therapy, severe anemia, thiamine deficiency, and hyperthyroidism.

Defects of diastolic filling

Syndromes suggesting cardiac failure are sometimes seen when the heart does not fill normally during diastole: for example, when pericardial effusion compresses the heart from the outside, when calcified pericardial tissue restricts the motion of the heart, when the superior or inferior vena cava is blocked by a thrombus or neoplasm, or when shock limits the return of blood to the heart.

Pathologic physiology:

The measure of an effective circulation is whether or not the oxygen needs of the body are being met. All living tissues require oxygen, in proportion to their metabolic activity. When these needs are not met, corrective forces come into play. When the demands for oxygen are local, i.e., confined to a single organ or part, they may be met temporarily by a local increase in blood flow resulting from selective vasodilatation, presumably mediated through the *kallikrein-kinin system* (see Chapter 3). If the oxygen demand is local but persistent, as in chronic inflammatory processes, *new blood vessels develop,* resulting in greatly increased blood flow in the part. If the demand for oxygen increases further and becomes generalized, as with prolonged violent exercise or increased metabolic activity, a *systemic response* is required. The O_2-CO_2 chemoreceptors are activated, resulting in greater depth and rapidity of respiration, and at the same time the heart rate increases so as to increase systemic blood flow. This increased blood flow is brought about by two major mechanisms [4]: (1) the so-called *Starling mechanism,* by which *increased return of blood to the heart* results in an *increased stroke-volume output,* and (2) *increase in heart rate.* These two mechanisms together are able to satisfy most ordinary or physiologic requirements for oxygen.

myocardial effects

When the heart's work load is persistently increased above its level of tolerance, *dilatation of the affected chamber(s)* occurs, due to stretching of individual muscle fibers. Apparently this stretching is associated with increased protein synthesis [7], resulting in increased mass of the muscle fiber *(hypertrophy).* Hypertrophy occurs with amazing rapidity: within 2 days after production of constriction of the pulmonary artery in cats, the weight of the right ventricular myocardium was doubled [7]. However, contractility per unit of mass remains depressed: only the increased mass permits the continued performance of the heart's work. The cause of the depressed contractility is probably a combination of chemical factors, most of which are unknown. Two factors that are believed to operate are: (1) *reduction of the heart's ability to utilize fatty acids* for energy metabolism, and (2) a *depression of the enzyme, ADPase,* which normally liberates the energy for the contractile process [7].

autonomic effects

In addition to these strictly myocardial effects of heart failure, the function of the sympathetic nervous system is affected [7]. In heart failure the *synthesis of cardiac norepinephrine,* essential for the regulation of cardiac contractility, heart rate, and peripheral vascular tone, *is seriously depressed.* In addition, *constriction of peripheral arteries and veins occurs,* providing *more blood* for those organs which have a high metabolic requirement at rest, especially the heart and the brain, and *returning more blood to the heart* so that the Starling mechanism for increasing cardiac output can continue to be operative.

renal-adrenal effects

An important *homeostatic mechanism* that is active in congestive heart failure has to do with variations in blood volume, and in salt and water movement in the body. This mechanism is believed to operate about as follows [8]: As congestive heart failure develops, there is progressive *reduction in renal blood flow and in glomerular filtration.* This incites an *increase in output of renin* by the *juxtaglomerular cells* of the afferent arterioles of the renal glomeruli. The increased renin, acting upon the zona glomerulosa of the adrenal cortex via a complicated series of enzyme interactions, causes an *increased output of aldosterone.* The increase in circulating aldosterone causes an *increased reabsorption of sodium* in the renal tubules. Sodium retention is followed by *water retention,* resulting in an *increase in circulating blood volume.* Theoretically the increased blood volume results in *increased blood pressure and improved blood flow to the kidney,* thus increasing glomerular filtration, reducing the output of renin, and restoring the system to normal. However, when heart failure is severe, most of the retained water resulting from sodium retention passes into the tissue spaces as *edema,* and into the serous cavities to form *effusions,* thus preventing the restoration of normal renal blood flow.

Symptoms

Symptoms in congestive heart failure parallel disturbed function, and are added one upon the other. *Increased hypoxia* is manifest first by *dyspnea* on exertion, later by dyspnea at rest, finally by *orthopnea. Dysfunction of the sympathetic nervous system* is manifest by *tachycardia* and *cool, moist skin.* The *failing ventricle,* whether right or left or combined, results in *increased venous pressure* and eventually *edema,* either peripheral or pulmonary or both. Finally, as *serious reduction in cardiac output* develops, there is *impaired blood flow to the various organ systems,* resulting in their *dysfunction,* perhaps manifest by hypotension, diminished urine output, mental confusion, anorexia, jaundice, extreme weakness and cachexia, and finally death.

4. Classification of Cardiovascular Diseases

There are several classifications of cardiovascular diseases, each designed to serve a particular purpose. For the student of pathology a *combined etiologic-pathologic classification* seems to be easiest to understand. The practicing physician would add to this a *physiologic classification* expressing the type of rhythm (atrial fibrillation, heart block, etc.), and the medicolegal expert would probably add a classification indicating the *degree of functional impairment* (class I – cardiac patient without limitation of activity, class IV – cardiac patient with symptoms at rest).

The classification used here, and based upon postmortem studies, is as follows:

Congenital anomalies of the heart and great vessels
Rheumatic heart disease
Endocarditis, myocarditis, and pericarditis
Arteriosclerosis
Hypertension and hypertensive cardiovascular disease
Coronary artery disease and myocardial infarction: ischemic heart disease
Cardiovascular syphilis
Aneurysms
Cor pulmonale
Metabolic heart disease
Neoplasms of the heart
Peripheral vascular diseases

CONGENITAL ANOMALIES OF THE HEART AND GREAT VESSELS

1. Basic Concepts

Embryology

When the human fetus is *3 weeks old,* the heart is a simple tube. Increased rate of cardiac growth beginning at about that time results in a looping of the tube to the right within the pericardium. By the *eighth week* all major developmental changes have occurred: *cephalad movement of the venous end* of the tube, *partition of the heart* into right and left sides and into atria and ventricles, *partition of the bulbus cordis* into aorta and pulmonary artery, and *development of valve cusps and rings.* For the remainder of intra-uterine life the heart and great vessels undergo simple enlargement, in keeping with the growth of the fetus as a whole.

Circulatory changes at birth

The fetal circulation differs from that of the infant after birth in many ways but especially in that the *placenta is the organ of gaseous exchange prior to birth,* while the *lungs take over this function after birth.* Thus major blood flow in the fetus is through the placenta with minimal and unimportant blood flow through the lungs. It is estimated that, just before birth, 70 percent of the partially oxygenated blood put out by the right ventricle *bypasses the lungs* [9]. The *foramen ovale* and its thick upper margin deflect blood from the inferior vena cava into the left atrium to supply the head with a rich saturation of oxygen, and the *ductus arteriosus* diverts blood from the pulmonary artery into the thoracic aorta. Shortly after birth, with the cessation of the placental circulation and the expansion of the lungs, *resistance in the pulmonary vascular bed is markedly reduced,* resulting in a reversal of blood flow in the ductus. *Within a few minutes after birth, pulmonary blood flow increases threefold to tenfold.* After a short period of adjustment the ductus arteriosus is functionally closed, first by constriction, later by obliterative fibrosis. If intracardiac anomalies such as atresia of the pulmonic orifice exist, the alterations described in the ductus will not occur. Blood flow in the ductus may continue from aorta to pulmonary artery, and may in fact be lifesaving for a time.

Patho-genesis [10]:

Three *mechanisms for the development of congenital cardiovascular anomalies* are generally considered possible: (1) *genetic,* (2) *environmental,* and (3) *developmental arrest;* the older concept that cardiovascular anomalies may be a sequel of fetal endocarditis has been largely abandoned.

genetic factors

According to Jackson [10], there is approximately a *threefold increase in the incidence of congenital heart disease among siblings of a child with congenital heart disease,* as compared to the random occurrence. Concordance, i.e., the occurrence of the same type of lesion in the sibling as in the prepositus, is less frequent. There is apparently *no greater frequency of congenital heart disease in the twin* of a child with such disease than in non-twin siblings. Parental consanguinity is frequently noted in patients with *dextrocardia.* Some families appear to have a significantly greater number of cases than would be expected by chance, particularly instances of *persistent ductus arteriosus* and *atrial septal defect.* Congenital heart disease is occasionally found in a patient having evidence of a *syndrome governed by a single autosomal gene.* Thus in *Marfan's disease,* and certain other diseases in which there is a genetically determined *biochemical abnormality of connective tissues, aortic aneurysms* may occur as a result of the connective tissue defect. In addition, cardiovascular anomalies have been found frequently in individuals with *chromosomal defects.* In *trisomy 21* (Down's syndrome), cardiovascular anomalies occur in about 40 percent of the cases, persistent common atrioventricular canal being the most common lesion. In a series of 32 cases of *trisomy 13–15* collected by Warkany et al. [11], there were 27 instances of cardiovascular anomalies, and in a series of 84 cases of *trisomy 18,* 83 had cardiovascular anomalies; in both these groups ventricular septal defects and persistent ductus arteriosus were the most frequent lesions. On the other hand, several studies of chromosomal patterns in patients known to have cardiovascular anomalies have shown a *low incidence of chromosomal defects.* Emerit and associates [12] concluded that chromosomal aberrations were responsible for no more than 3 to 5 percent of his cases of congenital heart disease.

environ-mental factors

Among environmental factors causing cardiac anomalies, *virus infections, drugs, hypoxia,* and *metabolic disorders* have been cited. About 2 to 4 percent of all cases of congenital heart disease are associated with *maternal rubella.* In one series of infants with the so-called congenital rubella syndrome, as many as 67 percent showed evidence of congenital heart disease, chiefly *persistent ductus arteriosus* but also *ventricular septal defect.* Certain knowledge of maternal rubella infection during the first 8 weeks of pregnancy is commonly considered to be an indication for therapeutic abortion. Maternal infection with *Coxsackie B virus* has been suggested [13] as a cause of congenital heart disease on serologic evidence. Of the several *drugs taken during pregnancy* that have been studied, *thalidomide* is the only one known to be associated with cardiovascular anomalies in the offspring. While lesions were varied in the thalidomide cases, *hypoplasia and coarctation of the aorta,* and other *anomalies of the great vessels* were most frequently noted. Experimentally *hypoxia* in pregnant rats may produce congenital heart disease, and *pregnancy at high altitude* (Peru) has been charged with causing congenital heart disease, particularly *persistent ductus.* In the *infantile hypercalcemia syndrome,* associated with mental retardation and facial deformity but of unknown cause, supravalvular aortic stenosis and other cardiovascular defects may occur. In almost all instances in which congenital cardiovascular anomalies have resulted from environmental factors, the *causative agent appears to have been active during the period of rapid evolution of the fetal heart from a simple tube,* i.e., between the third and the eighth weeks of gestation.

developmental arrest

As the term is used here, developmental arrest includes disturbances of any of the processes in cardiac development: growth itself, differentiation, migration, septation, and fusion. It seems unlikely that developmental arrest is actually a different mechanism from genetic and environmental factors in the causation of congenital cardiac anomalies, since both of these probably also act by arresting development. These two sets of factors simply cannot be proved to be active in the great majority of cases of cardiovascular anomalies, and some other designation must therefore be used for the large group in which no cause can be identified.

Frequency

Cardiac malformations are probably *not important in the causation of fetal death,* since the several interconnections between the fetal pulmonic and systemic circuits provide adequate oxygen to vital areas, even if serious atresias or other defects exist. The autopsy incidence of cardiac anomalies is lower among stillborn fetuses than in infants born alive [9]. It has been estimated [10] that the *overall incidence of significant congenital heart lesions is about 6 per 1000 births.* The prevalence of congenital heart disease among schoolchildren has been reported as between 1.4 and 6.0 per 1000 in different series [14]. There is no evidence of increased incidence in any particular national, racial, or socioeconomic group, or in either sex [14].

Manifestations

Congenital anomalies of the heart and great vessels may be manifest in a variety of ways. Some, especially those associated with significant right-to-left shunting, are manifest by *cyanosis* as a result of reduced pulmonary blood flow and impaired oxygenation of the blood. Some provide the basis for *bacterial endocarditis.* Many are manifest by *heart murmurs,* which may be first detected at birth, in later childhood, or even in adult life; in some instances the murmur is the only clinical sign present. Some are associated with *heart failure.* Minor forms, such as right aortic arch or certain forms of atrial septal defect, are quite compatible with normal life without the production of any symptoms or signs, being discovered only incidentally at autopsy.

Outcome

Congenital heart disease is a serious affliction. Infants with the most extreme defects die during the neonatal period. It has been estimated [15] that, of children born alive with congenital heart lesions, *20 percent are dead by the end of the first week,* an additional *10 to 20 percent by the end of the first month,* and a *total of 60 to 70 percent by the age of 10 years.* These statistics antedate open-heart surgery; it is likely that current experience would be more favorable.

2. *Anomalies of Position*

Total absence of the heart is apparently compatible with intra-uterine survival only in the case of twins, and then only if the defective twin receives its blood from the umbilical artery of the intact twin. In such instances the defective twin is usually an ovoid mass, without externally evident head or extremities (holocardius amorphus); the intact twin is healthy and tends to survive. *Dextrocardia* may occur as a solitary defect or, more commonly, in association with a reversed position of the liver and intestines (situs inversus). Pulmonary suppuration (abscess, bronchiectasis) may be associated with this condition (Kartagener's syndrome). *Displacement of the heart,* due to diaphragmatic hernia or incomplete closure of the chest anteriorly, may also occur.

3. Septal Defects

Simple abnormalities of the septum, i.e., without other cardiac defects, are *common,* and the milder forms are compatible with a relatively normal life. Extracardiac defects such as harelip or cleft palate are commonly associated with septal defects [16].

Interatrial defects

The most common septal defect is one between the right and left atria; it may be either of two types, an *ostium primum defect* or an *ostium secundum defect.* The former, caused by a failure of fusion of the septum primum with the atrioventricular canal cushion, is low on the interatrial septum and may in fact involve the two atrioventricular valve rings, converting them into a single ring. Usually much less significant is the ostium secundum defect, also known as *persistent foramen ovale.* Apparently due to a failure in proper development of the septum secundum, this defect is high above the valve rings and is often functionally closed by an endocardial flap, even when anatomically patent. Systolic *murmurs* are sometimes heard in cases of atrial septal defects, but they are extremely variable and may be absent.

Interventricular defects

Interventricular septal defects are among the most common congenital cardiac malformations, and may occur *alone or as part of a combined lesion* such as the tetralogy of Fallot. The defect commonly occurs in the membranous portion of the septum just below the aortic valve and is usually small – in fact, spontaneous closure of such defects have been reported. A harsh systolic murmur is often noted.

Effects

With interatrial and, more particularly, with interventricular septal defects there is usually *some degree of left-to-right shunt* after birth, increasing pulmonary blood flow and pulmonary arterial pressure. Ordinarily there is *no cyanosis* unless right ventricular failure, respiratory infection, or a bout of coughing occurs; at such times the pressures may be so altered that the direction of the shunt is reversed, i.e., right to left, resulting in cyanosis.

4. Combined Lesions

Valvular defects

Congenital valvular defects are rarely found except in association with septal lesions. Presumably the valvular lesions cause high pressures in the corresponding cardiac chambers, preventing the closure of the normal septal openings of embryonic life. *Congenital pulmonic stenosis or atresia* results in a reduction of pulmonary blood flow and therefore impairs oxygenation of the blood. In such instances the ductus arteriosus usually remains patent and gives some measure of relief. *Congenital aortic atresia* or stenosis, which may be associated with congenital mitral stenosis and rudimentary left ventricle, presents special problems because of the location of the coronary ostia. The condition can be suspected at autopsy when the ascending limb of the aortic arch is noted to be smaller than the descending limb: blood from the persistent ductus arteriosus flows in reverse direction in the transverse portion of the arch. *Mitral stenosis* has been described as a congenital lesion and may occur in conjunction with persistent interatrial septal defect (Lutembacher's syndrome).

Tetralogy of Fallot

The best known, and probably the most common, of the major combined cardiac lesions is the *tetralogy of Fallot.* Of the four defects, the most significant is the narrowing of the outflow tract from the right ventricle *(pulmonic stenosis);* this results in high pressure in the right ventricle, causing *right ventricular hypertrophy,* and preventing closure of the *interventricular septal defect.* Much less evident is the fourth defect of the tetralogy, *dextroposition of the aorta:* the aorta arises more or less over the septum, receiving blood from both left and right ventricles, blood from the latter via the septal defect. In this combination of lesions, cyanosis is usually present from birth ("blue baby") due to inadequate oxygenation of the blood as a result of diminished pulmonary blood flow. Clubbing of the fingers and polycythemia are also commonly noted. Oddly, a child with this affliction seems to be more comfortable when squatting than when standing.

Eisenmenger's complex

Eisenmenger's complex consists of an *interventricular septal defect* plus *right ventricular hypertrophy* and *displacement of the aorta to the right* – in other words, the tetralogy of Fallot minus pulmonic stenosis. Pulmonary blood flow is excessive because of the septal defect, and this may lead in time to pulmonary hypertension, right ventricular failure, reversal of the shunt, and cyanosis.

5. Anomalies of the Great Vessels

Transposition of the great arteries

Transposition of the aorta and pulmonary artery, i.e., the *aorta arising from the right ventricle* and the *pulmonary artery arising from the left ventricle,* is a most serious congenital anomaly: mortality is 85 percent in the first 6 months of life [17]. Survival is possible only in those instances in which both left-to-right and right-to-left shunts exist or are provided shortly after birth. Cyanosis is usually present at birth.

Taussig-Bing anomaly

Related to transposition of the great arteries, the Taussig-Bing anomaly has been defined [18] as *origin of both the aorta and pulmonary artery from the right ventricle,* the pulmonary artery in relation to a ventricular septal defect while the aorta is not. Several variations are described. In Lev's series the age of the oldest patient at death was 20 years.

Persistent ductus arteriosus

Persistence of the ductus arteriosus after birth is probably usually a result of an *intrinsic abnormality in the ductus* itself [10], except perhaps when there is an associated lesion such as aortic atresia which causes unusual pressure differences between the two ends of the ductus. *Rubella infection in early pregnancy* is commonly associated with persistent ductus. *Blood is usually shunted from the aorta to the pulmonary artery,* resulting in a low diastolic pressure in the systemic circulation and a wide pulse pressure. Often there is a loud, more or less continuous murmur *("machinery murmur"),* sometimes noted by the nursing mother as a purring sound, but there is usually *little cardiac embarrassment* during early life unless other lesions are also present. The increased pulmonary blood flow gradually causes pulmonary hypertension, resulting eventually in reversal of the shunt; cyanosis usually becomes evident at this time. Subacute bacterial endocarditis may develop within the persistent vessel.

A narrowing of the aorta, commonly called coarctation, may occur at *either of two sites: just proximal to the ligamentum arteriosum,* in which case it is known as the *infantile type,* or *just distal to the ligamentum,* known as the *juvenile type.* The former is usually associated with persistence of the ductus while the latter is often associated with a *great increase in the collateral arterial circulation of the thorax.* Regardless of its site, the effect of coarctation is *diminished blood flow below the constriction.* The blood pressure in the arms is elevated while that in the legs is lower than normal. Hypertension during adolescence should always make one look for the signs of coarctation, such as increased collateral circulation and notching of the ribs on x-ray. Coarctation of the aorta

Persistent right aortic arch, instead of the left as normal, ordinarily causes no difficulty per se, but the ligamentum arteriosus may then pass behind the trachea and esophagus forming a *vascular ring* which compresses these structures, causing difficulty in swallowing. The condition can be corrected by surgical division of the ligamentum. Right aortic arch

6. Importance of the Pulmonary Circulation

The crucial aspect of all forms of congenital heart disease is the question of the *adequacy of the pulmonary circulation and the oxygenation of blood* [9]. *Decreased pulmonary blood flow* is seen with pulmonic stenosis, with most cases of tetralogy of Fallot, and with transposition of the great arteries, accounting for *cyanosis shortly after birth. Increased pulmonary flow* occurs whenever there is a significant left-to-right shunt, whether due to interatrial or interventricular septal defect or to persistent ductus arteriosus. This sometimes leads to *pulmonary edema in the infant,* but more commonly symptoms do not occur until some months or years after birth. With the persistence of a left-to-right shunt, changes occur in the small pulmonary arteries: thrombosis, hyalinization, and fibrosis, resulting in a progressive reduction of the pulmonary vascular bed and in pulmonary hypertension. These changes, and the associated right ventricular strain, usually require 5 to 10 years to develop. It is important that these facts be appreciated and that corrective surgery be done before irreversible sclerotic changes develop in the pulmonary arterial tree.

RHEUMATIC HEART DISEASE

1. Rheumatic Fever

The term *rheumatick fever* was apparently first used by Haygarth in 1805 to differentiate certain cases of acute rheumatism from chronic aching and painful disorders of the extremities. In 1812 Wells reported that the heart was affected in certain cases of acute rheumatism. The valvular nature of this involvement was noted by Bouillaud in 1837. The present concept of rheumatic fever is essentially that of a *recurring febrile illness, more frequent in children than in adults, having a tendency to involve the heart and the joints.* History [19]

Many different bacteria have been isolated from the throat, blood, joints, and heart valves during rheumatic fever, but *none with any regularity,* and the same organisms are encountered with nearly the same frequency in the same tissues in nonspecific respiratory infections. Cause:

streptococcus

Group A streptococci are encountered somewhat more frequently than other bacteria and are *generally believed to be causally related;* the data have recently been reviewed in an editorial in *Lancet* [20]. Epidemiologic studies show that *rheumatic fever and streptococcal infections follow much the same pattern,* and have been declining, both in frequency and in severity. Patients with rheumatic fever show a high frequency of *streptococcal antibodies* in their sera. *Antibiotic therapy* that is used to prevent recurrences of streptococcal infections is also effective in preventing recurrences of rheumatic fever. Failure to find streptococci regularly in the lesions of rheumatic fever, and the inability to induce comparable lesions experimentally with any of the known products of the streptococcus, have been the main stumbling blocks to the wholehearted acceptance of the theory of streptococcal etiology. It has now been shown that certain *antibodies against strains of group A beta-hemolytic streptococci are also capable of reacting against components of human myocardial fibers and of heart valves,* and that corresponding cross-reacting auto-antibodies are to be *found in the serum of patients with rheumatic fever.* These antibodies also react with other organisms on occasion. It may well be that in the future other antigens giving similar cross reactions will be identified and that these agents may also on occasion incite the symptoms known as rheumatic fever.

other factors

Although there are still many unanswered questions, the following *predisposing factors* for rheumatic fever are well recognized: (1) *age* – children aged 6 to 9 are particularly susceptible; (2) *season* – the disease is more common in the winter and spring months; (3) *heredity* – certain families seem to have greater susceptibility than others; (4) *nutrition and housing* – the disease is most frequent in low income groups; (5) *climate* – rheumatic fever is more frequent in colder, mountainous districts, although cases also occur in the tropics.

Pathogenesis

In most instances the clinical syndrome of rheumatic fever follows an infection due to streptococcus group A. Usually the *streptococcal infection* (sore throat, scarlet fever) subsides, and about 2 to 4 weeks later there is *recurrence of fever,* often with *migratory joint pain and swelling.* In more severe cases the heart action is rapid and violent, and there may be *precordial pain* and perhaps mild *heart failure. Leukocytosis* and an *increased erythrocyte sedimentation rate* are commonly noted. Involuntary muscle movements (Sydenham's *chorea,* St. Vitus' dance), *subcutaneous nodules,* and skin rashes (especially *erythema marginatum)* occur in some cases. These varied manifestations – the *rheumatic fever syndrome* – are generally believed to be due to an *antigen-antibody reaction* comparable to serum sickness. The streptococcus or its products is generally believed to be the antigen. *"Rheumatic activity"* is said to persist clinically as long as any of these manifestations continue, even if there is no evidence of continuing streptococcal infection.

Pathologic changes: general

Rheumatic fever is sometimes referred to as a *connective tissue disease,* although all connective tissues are certainly not equally affected. Lesions of rheumatic fever have been described in many organs, including the brain, joints, skin, aorta, lungs, pleura, and peritoneum. The heart is the organ in which the most distinctive lesions occur, however, and the *pathology of rheumatic fever is fundamentally a study of the cardiac lesions.*

endocarditis

The earliest visible lesions are on the *heart valves,* and particularly on the mitral valve. Tiny warty deposits, composed of fibrin, platelets, a few red cells, and leukocytes, are laid down in a row corresponding to the line of closure of the heart valves. These *verrucae* are firmly attached; there is no tendency toward fragmentation and embolism. Following single attacks there may be complete healing of the verrucae, without deformity. In other cases these exudative lesions are invaded at their base by fibroblasts; there is *agglutination of the valve cusps* at their commissures, and *thickening and rigidity* of the leaflets. With recurrences there is renewed exudation, followed again by organization and further deformity. *Residual damage after rheumatic fever is a result of this deformity.* Thickening, fusion, and shortening of the chordae tendineae of the mitral valve lead to *mitral insufficiency, giving a systolic apical murmur;* rigidity and fusion of the cusps lead to *mitral stenosis, giving a presystolic or late diastolic murmur. Mitral stenosis is the classic residual lesion after recurring rheumatic fever.* The aortic, tricuspid, and pulmonic valves may also be affected (stenosis or insufficiency), the frequency being in the order given. Verrucae are also sometimes noted on the endocardium of the left atrium (MacCallum's patch).

myocarditis

During the active febrile phase of rheumatic fever the *myocardium is usually involved.* Here the *Aschoff bodies* (nodules) are best seen. Sometimes there is also a somewhat diffuse cellular reaction. Aschoff bodies occur along the course of small vessels and are most numerous in the myocardium of the left ventricle. The Aschoff body is a focal lesion of microscopic size consisting of fragments of muscle fibers, and strands of collagen and fibrinoid material, intermingled with cells having one or more nuclei which apparently represent attempts at muscle cell regeneration. Lymphocytes, plasma cells, fibroblasts, and occasionally neutrophils are present also. The fact that most of the elements of the Aschoff body are derived from muscle cells has been emphasized effectively by Murphy [21]. This correlates with the evidence derived from fluorescent microscopy, showing that *gamma globulins* presumably derived from circulating auto-antibodies, *react directly with the muscle cell* [22]. This disruption of myocardial fibers probably accounts for the alterations in the electrocardiogram and for the myocardial failure which sometimes occur during acute rheumatic fever. During the febrile phase of the disease, murmurs are believed due to relaxation of the valve rings, not to actual disease of the valves. In most instances the Aschoff body heals completely; sometimes there is a tiny residual scar, usually without functional effect.

significance of Aschoff nodules

Aschoff bodies are found in the myocardium in about half (32 to 87 percent, according to different observers) the fatal cases which are considered clinically to be rheumatic fever [23]. Similar focal myocardial lesions have been described in other conditions, as in typhoid fever, scarlet fever, syphilis, meningococcal infections, brucellosis, serum sickness, and following therapy with sulfonamide drugs. Similar lesions have been produced in the hearts of experimental animals by the injection of living or dead streptococci, tubercle bacilli, dysentery organisms, foreign serum, and egg albumin. Nevertheless it is generally held that *neither "true" Aschoff nodules nor the clinical picture of rheumatic fever has ever been produced in animals by experimental means.* Thus, although the Aschoff body is generally considered to be *pathognomonic for rheumatic fever,* there is some *reason to question its specificity as evidence of streptococcal infection.* Perhaps any agent attacking the muscle cell directly may produce Aschoff bodies.

Lesions similar to Aschoff bodies are sometimes noted in the pericardium, heart valves, and synovium, but the lesions in these tissues are more exudative than is the Aschoff body in the myocardium.

pericarditis

Acute pericarditis occurs in about 10 percent of cases of acute rheumatic fever. There is a *serofibrinous inflammation* of the pericardium, but without distinctive features; a *friction rub* may be noted clinically. With healing there may be a few synechiae, but the residual effect is usually not serious. It is unlikely that constrictive pericarditis, which may be crippling, is due to rheumatic fever.

extracardiac lesions

Rheumatic lesions in other viscera are rarely distinctive, although the *subcutaneous nodule,* with its central area of fibrinoid necrosis and surrounding zone of epithelioid cells, is fairly characteristic.

Outcome:

Bland and Jones [24] conducted a monumental investigation of the outcome following rheumatic fever. They traced for 20 years 1000 consecutive patients on whom a diagnosis of rheumatic fever or rheumatic heart disease was made between the years 1921 and 1931. The *average age at the time of diagnosis was 8 years.*

life expectancy

One hundred and twelve patients (11.2 percent) died within 5 years after the first visit, 90 died within the next 5 years, and 99 died during the following 10 years. Thus the *total mortality in the 20 years following diagnosis was 30.1 percent.*

residual heart disease

The great majority, probably 284, of the 301 patients dying during the 20-year period died of rheumatic heart disease or related conditions. To these should be added 302 patients who showed signs of heart disease at the end of the 20 years. Thus 586 patients *(58.6 percent) had permanent cardiac damage following rheumatic fever.* (It was noted that signs of well-defined rheumatic heart disease, observed at the first visit, *disappeared* completely in 108 patients during the 20-year period. On the other hand, signs of valvular disease *appeared later* in 44 percent of 347 patients originally thought to be free of cardiac involvement.)

disability

Of the 699 patients surviving 20 years after the diagnosis of rheumatic fever was made, there were 555 showing none-to-slight limitation of activity, 133 showing moderate limitation, and 6 showing marked limitation.

mode of death

The causes of death in the 301 patients dying during the period of study were as follows: rheumatic fever or congestive heart failure, grouped together, 77 percent; bacterial endocarditis, 10 percent; sudden or unexpected death, 3 percent; cerebral embolism, 1 percent; uncertain causes, 3 percent; unrelated to heart disease, 6 percent.

The current outlook should be much better. Streptococcal infections appear to have been much milder since about 1950, and the incidence and severity of rheumatic fever seem to have been correspondingly less; antibiotics are available that are effective in the control of streptococcal infections; open-heart surgery is prolonging the lives and reducing the suffering of patients with residual valvular disease.

2. *Residual Cardiac Lesions After Rheumatic Fever*

Gross stigmata

It is customary to accept *almost any form of distortion, thickening,* or *agglutination of the mitral valve* as definite evidence of prior rheumatic fever. When other valves are involved and the mitral valve is unaffected, other evidence of prior rheumatic fever must be sought in the heart. The following are generally accepted as evidence of prior rheumatic fever: *thickening and shortening of chordae tendineae,* in the absence of definite changes in the valve cusps; *pericardial adhesions* not otherwise accounted for; and *thickening and wrinkling of the endocardium of the left atrium.*

Micro-scopic stigmata

The following are the usual microscopic criteria for the identification of residual heart lesions as rheumatic, arranged in the order of their dependability: *Aschoff bodies* in the myocardium; *fibrinoid necrosis* and elastic tissue alterations adjacent to small blood vessels, but without significant cell exudate; inflammation of the walls of small arteries – *rheumatic arteritis;* increased *vascularization of the endocardium,* particularly of the valve cusps; and *increase in cardiac histiocytes* in the interstitial tissue.

It must be recognized that much of our "knowledge" about rheumatic fever is based on meager evidence [19]. Since a causative agent cannot be demonstrated in the lesions, and since rheumatic fever cannot be recognized by any chemical, serologic, bacteriologic, or other test, we have no certain means of distinguishing rheumatic fever from other diseases which may resemble it. In the final analysis, the "rheumatic stigmata" listed above are evidence of prior inflammation, but are not evidence that this inflammation was due to any specific agent, bacterial or otherwise.

3. Anatomic Forms of Valvular Heart Disease

Although valvular heart disease constitutes only about 2.5 percent of all cases of fatal cardiovascular disease, its importance in clinical practice, and especially in young people, is greater than this figure would indicate. *The chief clinical evidence of valvular heart disease is the heart murmur.* Murmurs are easy to hear but it requires great skill to interpret them correctly. The clinical interpretation is significantly wrong in about 20 percent of cases, as determined by autopsy data.

MITRAL STENOSIS: Pathologic changes

Mitral stenosis is the classic residual valvular lesion after recurrent rheumatic fever. The stenosis is due to *thickening* and *rigidity* of the cusps, and *agglutination* of the cusps at the commissures. Both sexes are equally affected.

Functional effect

Functionally there is interference with filling of the left ventricle, hence reduction of left ventricular output during systole. In addition, there are *hypertrophy and dilatation of the left atrium* (demonstrable as a filling defect in the esophagus after swallowing barium paste), *engorgement of the pulmonary circulation* (pulmonary hypertension), and *right ventricular hypertrophy. Fibrosis of the lungs,* sometimes called brown induration because of the associated hemosiderin pigment, further aggravates the respiratory embarrassment. *Recurrent pulmonary infarction* is frequent, usually due to emboli arising in the leg veins where thrombosis develops as a result of stasis. Thrombosis may occur in the left atrial appendix, especially when atrial fibrillation develops. This may occasionally result in embolism in the systemic circulation. Some degree of mitral insufficiency is usually present: the valve is too rigid to close completely.

Signs

Presystolic crescendo murmur, with or without thrill, maximum near the apex is the principal sign. This may be lost when atrial fibrillation – a common complication – develops. The electrocardiogram usually shows *right ventricular strain.* The findings by chest x-ray show *prominence of the pulmonary conus* and broadening of the heart shadow.

MITRAL INSUFFICIENCY: Pathologic changes

Mitral insufficiency is a very common clinical diagnosis, but difficult to recognize at necropsy except in association with mitral stenosis. *Shortening of the chordae tendineae* or dilatation of the left ventricle (as in heart failure from any cause) may hold the mitral orifice open during ventricular systole. Rupture of a papillary muscle or of the chordae tendineae may permit the valve to flap back into the atrium in ventricular systole.

Functional effect

The effect of mitral insufficiency is a leakage of blood from the left ventricle back into the left atrium during systole, thereby reducing the systolic output into the aorta; hypertrophy and dilatation of both the left atrium and the left ventricle result.

Signs

A *systolic apical murmur* is the usual sign of mitral insufficiency; in many instances the distinction from a "functional" murmur is impossible or arbitrary. The electrocardiogram usually shows some degree of left ventricular strain. The findings by chest x-ray are not distinctive.

AORTIC STENOSIS: Pathologic changes

Aortic stenosis is, among the valvular heart diseases, *second in importance only to mitral stenosis.* In some instances the cusps are thickened and agglutinated at their commissures, but are not nodular or distorted. More often the cusps show *nodular calcified masses,* distorting the commissures, narrowing the orifice, and rendering the cusps more rigid. In some instances the valve destruction produces some degree of insufficiency as well. In calcific aortic valve disease the male to female ratio is about 3 or 4 to 1. Age at death is usually about 60 years; aortic stenosis is rarely encountered at autopsy before age 40. The mitral valve is also affected in about one-third of the cases. Most authorities consider calcific aortic stenosis to be a result either of *rheumatic fever* or of a degenerative process comparable to *atherosclerosis.* However, there is much evidence that it may be a sequel of *chronic bacterial endocarditis,* specifically *brucellar endocarditis* [25].

Functional effect

The effect of aortic stenosis is to interfere with the systolic ejection of blood from the left ventricle. Marked *hypertrophy of the left ventricle* results. Congestive heart failure is the usual termination. Some degree of coronary insufficiency is common as heart failure develops; this may cause *anginal pain* and be confused with myocardial infarction. *Sudden death* without prior symptoms is sometimes observed; this may be due to heart block (the conduction bundle may be compressed by the calcified masses at the base of the aortic valve) or to the sudden onset of coronary insufficiency when left ventricular failure begins. Adam-Stokes *syncopal attacks* are commonly observed in patients with aortic stenosis.

Signs

A *systolic murmur and thrill in the aortic area,* transmitted into the neck, are characteristic but are not always present. Pulsus parvus et tardus is the classic pulse finding, reflecting the low pulse pressure, but it too is frequently missing. Pulse tracings show a low amplitude and prolonged ventricular ejection. Conduction defects, including *complete heart block,* are commonly observed on the electrocardiogram. The chest radiograph shows the *boot-shaped heart* of left ventricular hypertrophy. In some cases calcified masses can be identified in the heart valves because of their dancing motion during fluoroscopy.

AORTIC INSUFFICIENCY: Pathologic changes

Aortic insufficiency may be due to *extension of an inflammatory reaction from the aorta,* with shortening and rolling of the cusps and widening of the commissures, as in *syphilis;* to *thickening and retraction of the cusps,* as in *rheumatic fever;* to congenital or acquired *dilatation of the aortic valve ring,* as in Marfan's disease or aneurysm; or to *nodular calcific lesions* of the cusps, like those seen in calcific aortic stenosis except that the orifice is held rigidly open. Rarely a tear in the aortic wall at a commissure (see section on Dissecting Aneurysms) may lower one cusp below its mates, permitting insufficiency.

Functional effect

The effect of aortic insufficiency is to add a great burden to the left ventricle, since it must force out a greater than normal quantity of blood with each systole in order to compensate for the valvular leakage. Marked *hypertrophy of the left ventricle* results. Sudden death may occur, especially when syphilis is the cause, since the syphilitic fibrosis of the adjacent aortic wall may narrow the ostia of the coronary arteries.

Signs

A *diastolic murmur is noted in the aortic area* in aortic insufficiency. If the leakage is at all large, there will be signs of extremely *wide pulse pressure:* dancing arteries, capillary pulse in the fingers, pulsating arteries in eye grounds, and pistol-shot sounds over the femoral arteries. Pulse tracings show high rise and abrupt fallaway. The systolic blood pressure is usually normal or slightly elevated whereas the diastolic is generally quite low (10 to 40 mm. of mercury). Left ventricular strain may be noted on the electrocardiogram. The chest radiograph shows boot-shaped enlargement of the left ventricle.

PULMONIC STENOSIS: Pathologic changes

Pulmonic stenosis is usually *part of a combined congenital defect.* Occasionally this orifice may be involved in rheumatic fever, especially when the mitral and aortic valves are also affected. Certain recent observations suggest that pulmonic stenosis may, very rarely, be part of a metabolic disorder associated with hepatic metastasis from a malignant carcinoid tumor of the intestines. The valve cusps are agglutinated at the commissures, and the orifice is narrowed.

Effects

The effect of pulmonic stenosis is chiefly upon the *right ventricle,* which becomes hypertrophied and dilated. *Pulmonary blood flow is reduced. Cyanosis* and *clubbing of the fingers* are common.

Signs

Systolic murmur and thrill may be noted in the pulmonic area. If surgery is to be undertaken, detailed studies, including cardiac catheterization with direct determination of pressures and of oxygen saturation of the blood, may be necessary to determine whether combined lesions exist.

PULMONIC INSUFFICIENCY

Pulmonic insufficiency is a *very rare lesion* in pure form, and is uncommon even in combination with other valve lesions. Its effects are *comparable to those of aortic insufficiency,* including dancing arterial shadows at the hili of the lungs on fluoroscopy.

TRICUSPID DISEASE

Tricuspid stenosis or insufficiency is rarely seen, but may occur in combination with rheumatic disease of the other valves. With insufficiency the systolic impulse from the right ventricle may be transmitted backward and appear in the veins of the neck or as a painful, pulsating liver. (This must not be confused with the epigastric pulsation often noted normally in slender, nervous individuals.)

SURGERY FOR VALVULAR HEART DISEASE

The prognosis and management of cases of chronic valvular heart disease has changed greatly and for the better in recent years. With the *heart-lung machine* supporting life, the cardiac surgeon can *explore the interior of the heart,* and *repair damaged valves* where this is indicated, or, in selected cases, *excise the valve and replace it with a prosthesis.* As the result of experience, indications for surgery have been greatly refined, surgical techniques have been improved, patient monitoring has minimized postoperative hazards, and *surgical mortality has been greatly reduced.* Thousands of patients who in former years would have been destined to cardiac invalidism and early death, have now been restored to an active, productive life.

ENDOCARDITIS, MYOCARDITIS, AND PERICARDITIS

1. Nonbacterial Endocarditis

Three forms of nonbacterial endocarditis are usually recognized: (1) *rheumatic (verrucous) endocarditis* (see preceding section), (2) *Libman-Sacks endocarditis* of disseminated lupus erythematosus (see Chapter 4), and (3) *thrombotic endocarditis (endocardiosis).* The last of these, endocardiosis, has generally been supposed to be an incidental autopsy finding in elderly or debilitated patients, without clinical significance, but Angrist and Oka [26] believe that the process may be much more significant. Sterile valvular thrombi often occur as *part of a general thrombotic process.* As Angrist and Oka suggest, it seems likely that these valvular thrombi may contain bacteria if the underlying disease process is one associated with bacteremia. Our own experience lends support to this point of view.

2. Acute Bacterial Endocarditis

Terminology

While the separation of *acute* from *subacute* endocarditis is somewhat arbitrary because of the extensive overlap between the two groups, it still seems to serve a useful purpose in that the incidence of preexisting heart disease is different in the two groups and the outlook is somewhat different. Acute endocarditis is sometimes fungal in origin, hence the term *bacterial* is also subject to question. We shall, however, follow the time-honored terminology.

Causes

Acute endocarditis is usually said to occur as a complication of a bacterial infection in some other part of the body (such as pneumonia, osteomyelitis, puerperal endometritis, or gonorrheal salpingitis), and the causative agent is usually given as *Diplococcus pneumoniae,* staphylococcus, beta-hemolytic streptococcus, or *Neisseria intracellularis.* In the authors' experience the picture has changed somewhat in the last few years as a result of the antibiotic therapy used to combat these serious infections. Most recent cases of acute bacterial endocarditis seen by the authors have *developed in hospitalized patients under therapy for some chronic disease* such as urologic infections or rheumatoid arthritis. Many of the patients have been receiving *steroids* as well as *antibiotics,* and in many instances the organisms recovered on blood culture have been *antibiotic resistant.* As others have noted [27], we have also seen an increasing number of patients in whom "main-line" *drug addiction* was the major underlying cause. The frequency of rheumatic heart disease as a predisposing factor has also become less important; perhaps this accounts for the older age of the patients affected today with bacterial endocarditis.

Pathologic changes

The *mitral and aortic valves* are most commonly affected, especially if these valves are already abnormal, as from rheumatic fever or a congenital defect. Normal valves may also be affected. If the tricuspid or pulmonic valve is involved, either *N. intracellularis* or a *fungus* is apt to be the causative agent, and if the latter, drug addiction should be suspected. The affected valve usually shows evidence of *extensive destruction,* often with *perforation. Vegetations* are usually massive and friable. The lytic action of the bacterial and leukocytic enzymes results in frequent, often massive, *emboli.* Emboli usually contain pyogenic bacteria and hence may cause abscesses where they lodge. Mycotic aneurysms sometimes occur at points of lodgement of bacterial emboli; these may rupture, causing fatal hemorrhage.

Clinical features

The illness is usually characterized by a *septic course* lasting days or weeks. Murmurs are usually present after a few days, and may change in timing, pitch, and intensity from day to day, due to progressive destruction of the valve cusps. Recovery may occur with early and specific antibiotic therapy. When death occurs, it is usually a result of heart failure or embolism.

3. Subacute Bacterial Endocarditis (Endocarditis Lenta)

Cause

Subacute bacterial endocarditis is usually a *slowly developing febrile illness.* In most instances the avenue of entry of the infecting organism is not evident, although it is generally assumed to be the upper respiratory tract. Occasionally onset is preceded by *dental extraction, cystoscopy,* or some other type of manipulation; in such cases it is usually assumed that *bacteremia* occurred at the time of the manipulation but this is seldom established. The causative agent is usually a *nonpyogenic organism;* the alpha-hemolytic group of streptococci *(S. viridans)* is found in about 85 percent of the cases, *S. fecalis* (enterococcus) in 10 percent, and less frequently *Hemophilus influenza, Brucella,* or various fungi.

Pathologic changes

This disease occurs as a late *complication of valvular heart disease,* usually *rheumatic* (about 90 percent) or *congenital* (about 10 percent). *Normal valves are rarely affected.* The frequency of involvement of valves is in the following order, corresponding to the frequency of valvular lesions after rheumatic fever: mitral, mitral and aortic combined, aortic, and tricuspid. When congenital defects account for the localization of the lesion, the vegetations are usually formed directly on the defect, as in a patent ductus arteriosus, on the edge of the orifice in interventricular septal defects, or on bicuspid aortic valves. The affected valve shows *evidence of previous rheumatic disease* in most cases: fibrosis, thickening, and agglutination of the cusps. In addition, small, firm, greenish vegetations composed of fibrin, a few leukocytes, and bacteria are attached to the surface of the valves. The organisms tend to cause a slow dissolution of the vegetations, small bits breaking off at a time. Valve destruction and perforation may occur, but these are less frequent than in acute bacterial endocarditis. The myocardium often shows minute exudative lesions (Bracht-Wächter lesions), presumably due to embolism. *Infarcts* are found in various organs. Although the emboli may contain bacteria, the organisms are nonpyogenic and the resulting infarcts do not suppurate. The renal lesion, *focal embolic glomerulonephritis,* is marked by multiple tiny emboli within the glomerular tuft, causing many minute hemorrhages ("flea-bitten" kidney).

Blood cultures

Since the bacteria in the valvular lesions are often covered over by fibrin, blood cultures are not constantly positive, although they are usually positive at some time during the course of the illness. In suspected cases, blood cultures should be repeated frequently until a positive culture is obtained, so that the *sensitivity of the organism to the various antibiotics* can be determined.

Clinical features

The most outstanding clinical manifestations in subacute bacterial endocarditis are those resulting from *embolism.* Cerebral embolism sometimes causes *sudden death.* Multiple emboli to the kidneys may cause recurrent *hematuria* and rarely *uremia.* Embolism to the spleen is common and may cause *pain on respiration. Sudden blindness* in one eye may occur as a result of embolism to the central artery of the retina. *Petechiae* in the skin, retina (Roth's spots), conjunctivae, and buccal mucosa are usually found if searched for carefully; the patient does not usually note their occurrence. The course is generally protracted, usually of several months' duration, often with periods of apyrexia alternating with periods of low-grade fever. In most cases *heart murmurs* are heard throughout the course of the illness, usually changing slightly from day to day. *Anemia* is common and may be severe; occasionally it is the outstanding objective finding. Either leukocytosis or leukopenia may occur. *Splenomegaly* is common.

Outcome

With appropriate antibiotic therapy, cure of the infection can be accomplished in about half the cases. However, the heart valves suffer permanent added damage, and this may lead to later death from heart failure. Thus there are three serious features to subacute bacterial endocarditis: *infection, embolism,* and *cardiac damage.*

4. *Myocarditis and Related Disorders*

Definition

When the term *myocarditis* is properly used, it signifies *inflammation of the myocardium.* The term is, however, sometimes used in a less accurate sense. Thus *toxic myocarditis* is used to indicate a state of degeneration of the muscle fibers; it may occur in diphtheria and certain other febrile illnesses. *Chronic myocarditis* is sometimes incorrectly used to designate a state of fibrosis of the myocardium, such as may follow coronary artery disease. The subject of myocardial diseases has been thoroughly reviewed by Mattingly [28].

Types

The following are the most important types of true myocarditis:

1. *Rheumatic myocarditis* is presumably the most common, and occurs during the course of acute rheumatic fever (see earlier section of this chapter).

2. *Fiedler's myocarditis* is a rare, subacute inflammatory condition of the myocardium in which giant cells are conspicuous. Although its etiology is unknown, it appears to be a sequel of respiratory infections. Fluorescent antibody studies suggest that it may be a complication of *Coxsackie B virus* infections [29]. The diagnosis is rarely made during life.

3. *Granulomatous myocarditis* is sometimes seen in fatal cases of *Boeck's sarcoid.* There are giant cells and epithelioid cells, as in sarcoid lesions of other organs. In other instances, granulomatous interstitial myocarditis may be a result of *protozoan infection* (South American trypanosomiasis or Chagas' disease), or perhaps of *hypersensitivity states.*

4. Milder forms of *interstitial myocarditis,* characterized by focal collections of lymphocytes and monocytes about small vessels, may be seen in fatal cases of many *infectious diseases,* including influenza, varicella, leptospirosis, diphtheria, scarlet fever, and brucellosis. Presumably the transient nonspecific changes in the electrocardiogram seen in such cases are a result of myocarditis.

5. *Suppurative myocarditis* is a manifestation of pyemia, especially that due to the staphylococcus.

6. A chronic, sclerosing form of *endomyocarditis* called *endocardial fibroelastosis,* seen occasionally in infants, is currently suspect of being a manifestation of intra-uterine (i.e., maternal) infection by the *mumps virus* [30].

Certain other forms of myocardial disorders are considered under a subsequent heading, Metabolic Heart Disease.

5. *Acute Pericarditis*

Cause

Acute pericarditis is usually a complication of infection of some other organ. Thus *suppurative pericarditis* is usually a complication of bacteremia, as in lobar pneumonia, osteomyelitis, lung abscess, etc.; *tuberculous pericarditis* is usually due to spread to the pericardial sac from adjacent tuberculous lymph nodes; *rheumatic pericarditis* may occur along with rheumatic endocarditis and myocarditis; a *nonbacterial pericarditis* often occurs in uremia (unknown cause), in myocardial infarction, in metastatic tumors of the pericardium, in trauma to the chest wall, and in viral infections, especially Coxsackie B.

Clinical features

Clinically pericarditis is usually manifest by *chest pain,* often radiating to shoulders, arms, or neck, and by *dyspnea.* In rapidly developing effusions there may be interference with diastolic filling of the chambers, and death due to *cardiac tamponade.* A *friction rub,* due presumably to roughening of the two serous membranes by fibrin deposits, is commonly heard in *dry* or *fibrinous pericarditis;* it tends to disappear as fluid accumulates. X-ray cannot ordinarily reveal pericardial fluid accumulations of less than 300 ml. The electrocardiogram will often reveal pericardial effusion by low amplitude and other changes.

Pathologic changes

The pathologic features vary from case to case, depending upon the cause and duration of the process. In *acute pericarditis due to pyogenic bacteria,* the fluid is frankly purulent. In *nonspecific pericarditis* and in *pericarditis due to rheumatic fever,* the fluid is sterile, usually slightly cloudy, and contains little fibrin. In *tuberculous pericarditis* there may be frank caseation necrosis of the involved tissues and a thick layer of fibrin may collect, or there may be a blood-tinged effusion. In *pericarditis due to neoplasm,* tumor nodules are usually seen and the fluid may be grossly bloody. In *pericarditis due to myocardial infarction,* fibrin is commonly deposited over the necrotic area of the myocardium. In *uremic pericarditis* a dry fibrinous exudate is usual.

6. *Chronic Pericarditis*

Adhesions of minor degree are often encountered between the two layers of the pericardium, usually without symptoms having been recorded during life. When pericardial adhesions are dense, and particularly when they are associated with dense *mediastinal, pleural,* and *chest wall adhesions,* they may produce heart failure. Such conditions are presumably a sequel of active pericarditis, but often there is no history of antecedent disease. Sometimes adhesions may be so dense that *retraction of the chest wall* is noted with each systole (Broadbent's sign). *Constrictive pericarditis* (Pick's disease) is a crippling disease, sometimes a sequel of mediastinal tuberculosis. It occurs chiefly in males, the average age being 40 years [31]. *Dense scar tissue,* often with a heavy layer of *calcium* frosting, may surround the ventricles, atria, or great vessels as an unyielding band. As a result the heart chambers may be *unable to dilate* to receive blood during diastole. *Clinically* dyspnea, ankle edema, and especially abdominal swelling due to peritoneal effusion are the chief symptoms; distention of the cervical veins, hepatomegaly, high venous pressure, and a reduction of cardiac output are the chief signs. Surgical removal of the constricting bands may cure the condition completely.

7. Hemopericardium

Hemorrhage into the pericardial sac may be a result of *trauma, rupture of the heart or aorta, neoplasm of the heart,* or *inflammatory disease.* Even when due to rupture of the heart or of an aneurysm of the intrapericardial portion of the aorta, death is ordinarily not immediate since adhesions between the two layers of the pericardium tend to delay the accumulation of blood. In a matter of hours there may develop an interference with diastolic filling of the heart, a condition known as *cardiac tamponade,* which will cause death. In the case of *penetrating wounds* of the heart, whether from a broken rib in a crushing injury of the chest or from knife or bullet wounds, there is necessarily a tear in the parietal as well as the visceral pericardium. This permits blood in the pericardial sac to escape into the pleural sac, minimizing the chances of tamponade but making death from *exsanguination* likely. If recovery does occur in such a case, there may be extensive pericardial and mediastinal *adhesions.* When blood accumulates slowly in the pericardial sac, or when the amount of blood in the sac is small, as is usually the case with contusions, neoplasms, or inflammatory diseases, the clinical picture may be indistinguishable from pericarditis.

ARTERIOSCLEROSIS

Definitions

Arteriosclerosis is the name given to a group of diseases of the arteries manifest by thickening and hardening of their walls. The group includes arteriolar sclerosis, atherosclerosis, and medial sclerosis. In the first of these, *arteriolar sclerosis,* the smallest arterioles are affected, showing thickening of their muscle coats, a result of increased blood pressure *(hypertension).* In *atherosclerosis* the large muscular arteries – aorta, coronaries, cerebrals – are involved, and show calcified plaques in the intima, with a tendency to *thrombus* formation and to *rupture* (hemorrhage). *Medial sclerosis* is the least important of the three; the *calcium deposits in the media* that are characteristic of the condition ordinarily do not cause any narrowing of the lumen or weakening of the wall. As a class, the group are considered to be *"wear-and-tear" diseases:* they become much more common with advancing years.

1. Arteriolar Sclerosis

Arteriolar sclerosis (also known as arteriolosclerosis) is a form of arteriosclerosis characterized by *thickening of the walls and narrowing of the lumen of the arterioles,* and *often associated with hypertension.* The vessels affected include the *afferent arterioles of the kidneys* (nephrosclerosis: see Chapter 22), the *central arterioles of the splenic follicles,* the *arterioles of the retina,* and the *intimate vasculature of the viscera.* The arteriolar changes are generally believed to be a *result of hypertension,* usually of the idiopathic (essential) type; some observers consider the arteriolar lesions to be the cause rather than the result of hypertension, but this seems unlikely because of the findings on renal biopsy in early cases of hypertensive disease. *In benign essential hypertension,* acellular eosinophilic material (polysaccharide) is found in the walls of the arterioles; this material, plus hypertrophy of the muscular coat, results in thickening of the walls at the expense of the lumen. *In malignant hypertension,* some of the arterioles show, in addition, a smudgy eosinophilic necrosis of their walls, often resulting in thrombosis or hemorrhage. The *effect* of arteriolar sclerosis is to sustain the hypertension and make it irreversible. Thus it maintains a *bursting force* within the vessels. If the arterial tree is weakened at any point, particularly by atherosclerosis, the vessel may *rupture* under this pressure.

2. Atherosclerosis

Frequency

Atherosclerosis is the *most common and the most important form of arteriosclerosis.* Some degree of atherosclerosis is found at necropsy in persons of all ages, but it increases in severity and extent with *advancing years.* In early adult life it is much more common in the male than the female. After the menopause the rate rises in the female, so that male and female are about equally affected. *Coronary atherosclerosis and its complications are directly responsible for 55 percent of all deaths due to cardiovascular diseases,* and in combination with hypertension is probably indirectly responsible for an additional third [1].

Vessels affected

The large and medium-sized arteries of the greater circulation, especially the *aorta,* the *coronary* and *cerebral arteries,* and the *arteries of the lower extremities,* are chiefly affected. The pulmonary arteries and the veins are rarely affected. In affected arteries, atheromatous plaques are generally heaviest about the mouths of vessels and at points of bifurcation.

Cause: cholesterol

The cause of atherosclerosis is almost certainly cholesterol or the physicochemical form in which cholesterol occurs in blood plasma, namely the lipoproteins. The evidence for this conclusion is varied and so abundant as to be almost overwhelming. It can be summarized as follows: (1) *cholesterol is abundant in the lesions* of atherosclerosis in the artery walls; (2) *atherosclerosis can be produced experimentally in animals by feeding cholesterol;* (3) atherosclerosis is common in those *population groups* (U.S., Europe) *characterized by high blood levels of cholesterol* and rare in groups (China, central Africa) characterized by low levels; (4) in a given population group, those *individuals having high blood levels of cholesterol* are much more prone to develop atherosclerosis than are those having low blood levels; (5) in a given population group, the frequency of atherosclerosis will vary from time to time in relation to changes in *diet that are associated with changes in blood cholesterol;* (6) in a given population group, the incidence of atherosclerosis increases with the age of the individual up to about age 55 and remains relatively constant thereafter, *paralleling the increase of blood cholesterol with age;* (7) individuals having *metabolic disorders characterized by high blood levels of cholesterol* (familial hypercholesterolemia, hypothyroidism) are much more prone to develop atherosclerosis than are those having metabolic disorders characterized by low blood levels of cholesterol (hyperthyroidism, liver diseases). Friedman [32] has gone so far as to state that individuals with moderate hypercholesterolemia (250 to 350 mg. per 100 ml.) are three to five times more likely to develop "vascular accidents" than are individuals with cholesterol values below 250 mg. per 100 ml., that individuals with cholesterol values above 350 mg. per 100 ml. "almost never escape from prematurely occurring vascular accidents," and that individuals with persistent cholesterol values above 500 mg. per 100 ml. "might justly be considered as seriously ill as a patient harboring a malignant neoplasm."

blood lipoproteins

The data quoted above relative to cholesterol do not take into account certain important facts, however. *Cholesterol does not exist in the serum in free form* but in combination with serum phospholipids, triglycerides, and certain protein moieties, i.e., *as lipoproteins,* the actual composition of which varies from person to person. The question naturally arises as to whether the *concentration* of cholesterol is more or less important than the *physicochemical form* in which cholesterol exists. On the basis of either ultracentrifugation or paper electrophoresis, the *blood lipoproteins can be separated into several groups.* Brown [33] reports that those lipoproteins of lowest density yield 87 percent triglycerides and 4 percent cholesterol, whereas other important lipoproteins of somewhat greater density yield 10 percent triglycerides and 50 percent cholesterol. Serum determinations of triglycerides and of cholesterol give little indication of whether or not hyperlipoproteinemia is present, or, if so, which type. Cases of hyperlipoproteinemia have been divided into *five types* by Frederickson and co-workers [34], depending upon the types of lipoprotein which constitute the major proportion of the whole. Distribution of these types in the population is believed to be *determined primarily by inheritance,* based upon enzyme differences, and secondarily by the occurrence or nonoccurrence of certain *disease states such as diabetes mellitus.* Frederickson's types II, III, and IV are the ones most commonly associated with early and severe atherosclerosis. Type II includes familial hypercholesterolemia in which nodular xanthomas occur in tendons. Type IV occurs particularly in association with obesity, diabetes, and gout; affected patients often show xanthomas of the skin. Readers are referred to Frederickson's original articles for further details of his various types, which have more relevance to therapy than to basic pathology.

summary

The refinements of physical chemistry referred to above do not alter the basic point: *differences in the incidence of atherosclerosis in population groups are chiefly a result of differences in diet.* Diets rich in eggs, butter, and animal fat are more atherogenic than are diets consisting chiefly of vegetables, rice, and fish. In individual cases the development of atherosclerosis is determined by multiple factors, including inherited differences, diet, intercurrent disease. *Blood cholesterol remains the single most generally useful and used chemical determination for the detection of proneness to atherosclerosis* in the individual, i.e., as part of health evaluation.

Pathogenesis: theories

Granted that cholesterol complexes are somehow at fault, just how does the process begin? Two different *theories* are currently debated: (1) the plaque is formed by the influx and trapping of lipoprotein within cells of the arterial wall, as a result of hyperlipemia, injury of the arterial wall, and hypoxia [35]; (2) the plaque represents a hyalinized thrombus, formed on the intima as a result of local and systemic factors. This second theory was originally proposed by Rokitansky and recently revived by Duguid and others [36, 37, 38]; hypercholesterolemia is deemed to play its part by increasing the tendency for the blood to coagulate, by inhibiting fibrinolysis, leaving a relatively insoluble deposit to be incorporated into the residual fibrous plaque. The lipids probably play an additional role by *attracting calcium ions* into the plaque.

opinions

The author's (TMP) concept of the pathogenesis of atherosclerosis, based upon gross and microscopic study of autopsy material, is as follows: the *initiating lesion is probably a crack or fissure in the intima* of the artery, resulting from the effects of wear and tear. *Loss of elasticity of intimal tissues due to aging* probably precedes the development of these cracks, which then occur as a result of more or less normal physical forces: slight distortion of the coronary arteries must occur with each systole and with each breath, and similar changes undoubtedly occur in other arteries as a result of changes of position and other muscular movements.

Once the crack or fissure has occurred, *platelets fill in the defect,* and *fibrin forms,* enmeshing a few red and white blood cells. (Careful inspection of the aortic intima at autopsy often reveals small, elongated flat thrombi, if they are not wiped off by an overzealous assistant.) The shape of the thrombus is determined by the movement of the bloodstream over it; perhaps its size is determined by these same forces plus certain inherent *"coagulability factors"* in the blood, especially its cholesterol content. *Fibrinolysis* now comes into play to reduce the size of the thrombus somewhat, making it conform to the curvature of the vessel and to the rheologic forces. In the meantime, *connective tissue cells derived from the subintimal tissues at the base of the original cleft grow into the thrombus* and attach it more firmly to the vessel wall; *endothelial cells cover over* the flattened, organized thrombus. At this stage a small collection of red cells, platelets, and fibrin, elongated in one direction to conform to the original intimal cleft, lies embedded in the intima and covered over with endothelium. Macrophages and their enzymes act upon these elements, red cells are lysed releasing the lipid fraction from the capsules of the cells, and this lipid fraction plus that derived from plasma undergoes further chemical change. Iron derived from hemoglobin is present in early lesions. The final result is a *tiny streak of lipid material* in the intima as seen grossly, and a *collection of foam cells* and perhaps *a few cholesterol crystals embedded in hyaline connective tissue* microscopically. This portion of the vessel wall is now even less elastic than the normally aging tissues about it, and subsequent cracks are apt to occur at its juncture with these tissues. The process thereby is repeated, resulting in larger clefts, larger thrombi, and enlargement of the plaque.

These *larger plaques tend to attract calcium* into their substance by the process of dystrophic calcification. The calcium is deposited in a thin, eggshell-like layer, conforming to the curvature of the vessel where it lies. When calcium is added in sufficient amount, it brings two new features to the plaque: it is *hard and totally inelastic,* hence the underlying media tends to become somewhat atrophic and weakened as systolic pressure pounds upon it. Secondly, the *edge of the calcified plaque is ragged and sharp.* It seems quite likely that the plaque, when subject to such forces as compression or twisting, would tend to tear adjacent tissues, admitting blood beneath the plaque. Depending upon the size of the vessel affected and the direction of the forces involved, a *new and larger thrombus* may form, *closing the vessel,* or the *elevated plaque may itself close a small artery* (such as a coronary) effectively.

local factors

While the sequence of events as given above is somewhat conjectural, all the things described have been seen repeatedly in necropsy tissues. Certainly thrombosis and atherosclerosis are two parts to the one problem. Certainly also it is not enough to emphasize systemic factors in atherosclerosis – *local factors must be important* to account for the characteristic locations of the plaques and accompanying thrombi: coronary arteries are more often affected than any other vessels of their size because the coronary arteries are subject to more motion than any other arteries; in the coronary arteries the lesions are more common in the proximal portion than elsewhere because this is the specific portion of the coronary arteries that is kinked and twisted most; the abdominal aorta is more prone to atheromatous lesions and thrombosis than the thoracic aorta because the abdominal aorta is more exposed to changes in pressure and position than the thoracic aorta is; in the abdominal aorta the lesions occur most conspicuously about the mouths of the lumbar arteries because these are the points of greatest fixation of the aorta and therefore subject to greatest tensions; systemic arteries are more subject to these lesions than are the pulmonary arteries because pressures in the systemic arteries are greater. Another observation that has led us to believe that thrombosis is the primary event: we have seen lesions quite identical to *atheroma on the pleural surface of the diaphragm,* following by some months the occurrence of hemothorax. Hence collections of blood cells and fibrin can be incorporated into connective tissues, and cholesterol crystals can be formed from such materials.

Pathology

No matter what may be the mechanisms for the inception of the atherosclerotic plaque, the following are its distinctive features. Minimal lesions of atherosclerosis are evident grossly as narrow, *yellow, subintimal streaks,* or as *elevated hyaline plaques.* Microscopically there are swelling, hyalinization, and fibrosis of the ground substance of the intima and subintima; the presence of fine droplets of lipid in the subintimal tissues, and sometimes in foam cells or lipophages, may be noted. In larger lesions these lipid masses coalesce, intervening tissues disintegrate and even liquefy, and cholesterol crystals appear; at this stage the lesion is soft, reddish brown, and elevated above the surrounding intima, and may be spoken of as an *atheroma.* Atheromatous ulcers and surface thrombi are common, and *calcium* is deposited in the lesions. *New capillaries* enter the area, apparently arising directly from the lumen of the vessel affected; these capillaries are said to be the source of minute hemorrhages in the lesions.

Effects

In large arteries, such as the *aorta,* these atheromatous lesions cause no significant narrowing of the lumen. In the *cerebral* or *coronary* arteries or the arteries of the *extremities,* there is narrowing of the lumen by the atheromatous plaques; *ischemia* of the affected part often follows. In arteries of any size the *vessel is weakened* at the site of the atheroma, resulting in thinning of the wall and *predisposing to rupture and hemorrhage.* The roughened intima also *predisposes to thrombus formation;* such a thrombus may be relatively unimportant in the aorta or femoral arteries, but it may completely occlude an artery already narrowed by atheromatous plaques, such as a coronary or cerebral artery or an artery of the extremities.

Clinical features

The clinical manifestations in atherosclerosis are dependent upon the effects of the atheromatous plaque itself (i.e., narrowing of the arterial lumen and ischemia of the affected part), and upon the local developments in the atheromatous lesion (hemorrhage or thrombosis). Ischemia is usually manifested by a *gradual impairment of function,* while hemorrhage or thrombosis is usually revealed by *sudden catastrophic symptoms* related to the affected part. In the chief arterial systems the usual manifestations are as follows:

1. *Cerebral.* Gradual ischemia leads to cerebral atrophy, mental retardation, and senility; catastrophe may be intracranial hemorrhage, or thrombosis and infarction.

2. *Coronary.* Gradual ischemia leads to angina pectoris or myocardial failure, or both; catastrophe is manifest usually as coronary thrombosis, rarely as rupture and hemorrhage.

3. *Aorta and common iliacs.* Gradual encroachment upon the lumen rarely leads to localizing symptoms, presumably because of the large size of the aorta; occasionally, when thrombosis is added, the Leriche syndrome results: weakness of the legs, pain in the legs on walking, atrophy of the muscles of the thighs and buttocks, and sexual impotence. Catastrophe is usually manifested by rupture of an atherosclerotic aneurysm of the aorta, with exsanguination.

4. *Subclavians.* Gradual reduction in the lumen of the vessels is associated with weakness and numbness in the arm, sometimes vertigo and pain. With complete occlusion these symptoms are simply more severe. Pulse may be weak or absent ("pulseless disease"), and blood pressure may be low or unobtainable in the affected arm.

5. *Carotids* (Takayasu's disease). With gradual ischemia there may be vertigo, diplopia, and headaches. With complete occlusion these symptoms are emphasized and ocular symptoms become conspicuous: diplopia, flashing lights (photopsia), and even blindness; convulsions may also be noted.

6. *Femorals and popliteals.* Gradual ischemia leads to muscular weakness, "intermittent claudication," and atrophy; catastrophe is usually evident as thrombosis and gangrene, but rupture and hemorrhage from aneurysm may occur.

Atherosclerosis and hypertension

Hypertension and atherosclerosis tend to occur in the same patient, but the two diseases are generally believed to be distinct. Hypertension may be a stress factor leading to preliminary changes in the intima of the artery, permitting atheromas to form. That blood pressure is related to atherosclerosis is suggested by several facts: (1) atheromas are rare in the pulmonary artery under ordinary circumstances, but develop in patients showing pulmonary hypertension; (2) in patients with coarctation of the aorta, atherosclerosis tends to occur in the vessels of the head and upper extremities where the blood pressure is high but not in the vessels of the lower extremities where the blood pressure is low.

3. Medial Sclerosis (Mönckeberg's Sclerosis)

Medial sclerosis is a form of arteriosclerosis commonly occurring in the medium-sized arteries (radials, tibials, splenic) and is characterized by elongation and tortuosity of the vessels. Its precise *cause* is unknown, but it appears to be a *deterioration of tissues due to aging.* The media of the artery is primarily affected; the elastic layer is usually frayed and destroyed and calcium deposits occur chiefly in relation to this layer. With the loss of elasticity of the vessel wall, the *artery stretches and becomes tortuous.* The medial deposits do not cause narrowing of the lumen, weakening of the wall, or predisposition to hemorrhage or thrombosis. Hence medial sclerosis produces no apparent clinical effects, in spite of the very striking alteration in the gross, microscopic, and x-ray appearance of the vessel. When there are clinical manifestations of arterial disease in such patients, they are usually due to the *coincident occurrence of atherosclerosis of the intima;* the two processes are thought to be unrelated. Hypertension is also generally believed to be unrelated to medial sclerosis. In many cases the systolic blood pressure appears to be elevated as ordinarily measured, but this is probably due to the difficulty with which the "pipestem" arteries are compressed by the cuff rather than to an actual increase of the systolic pressure in the lumen. The diastolic pressure is commonly normal.

HYPERTENSION AND HYPERTENSIVE CARDIOVASCULAR DISEASE

1. Basic Considerations

Definition

Hypertension signifies a persistent elevation of the blood pressure, or, otherwise stated, an increased resistance to blood flow. When the term is used without further qualification, *systemic hypertension,* i.e., in the major circulation, is usually intended; *pulmonary hypertension* and *portal hypertension* are also important pathologic concepts and clinical entities. For the systemic circuit, it is generally accepted that a patient is hypertensive if the systolic blood pressure is persistently above 140 mm. of mercury or the diastolic blood pressure is above 90 mm. of mercury. Blood pressure tends to *increase moderately with age,* but the rule-of-thumb that the systolic blood pressure is 100 plus the patient's age is a bit too general. Falsely high readings by the conventional method may be obtained in obese persons or in those with advanced sclerosis of the brachial arteries.

Frequency

The frequency of hypertensive cardiovascular disease is determined in large part by the definition of terms, as given above. Since hypertensive disease and arteriosclerosis often act in combination to cause death from cerebral hemorrhage or thrombosis, myocardial infarction, and cardiac and renal failure, it is almost impossible to separate one from the other in mortality statistics; one or the other of these two diseases, or the two acting in combination, are said to account for about 90 percent of all deaths from cardiovascular disease [1]. Insofar as the two can be separated, however, it appears that the *death rate from hypertension and hypertensive heart disease has been falling* steadily and significantly in the last 30 years in the United States.

Pathology

The characteristic lesions of hypertensive cardiovascular disease are *largely confined to the arterioles* and were described in the earlier section on Arteriolar Sclerosis. In most cases the organs showing these arteriolar changes are reduced in size as a result of ischemic atrophy.

2. *Causes of Hypertension*

Essential hypertension

In about 90 percent of the cases of hypertensive cardiovascular disease, no definite cause for hypertension can be identified: these make up the group known as primary or essential hypertension. Many theories have been proposed to explain cases in this indefinite group. Conn [39] insists that some 20 percent of the group are instances of *primary aldosteronism* due to a small aldosterone-secreting adrenal tumor, and that patients in this group are curable by excision of the tumor; this would, of course, remove these cases from the "essential" classification. The experience of Laragh et al. [40] is quite at variance with that of Conn. Schroeder [41], who has been studying the role of trace metals in the etiology of cardiovascular diseases for a number of years, has suggested that *cadmium* may be to blame. The theory is attractive, since cadmium is known to be *present in the kidneys of hypertensive patients* in increased concentration, *is capable of producing hypertension in rats,* and occurs in *higher concentration in water and air* in those geographic areas having a high mortality from heart disease than in areas having a low mortality from these diseases. The cadmium evidence has been summarized by Carroll [42]. *Excessive salt intake* has also been incriminated [43].

The following factors, while not directly causative, are believed to predispose to essential hypertension: (1) *hereditary* – if both parents are hypertensive, the chances are great that the offspring will be hypertensive; (2) *age* – the frequency of hypertension increases steadily with age, at least to age 50; (3) *sex* – hypertension is generally more common in females, perhaps due to its relation to toxemia of pregnancy, but the fulminating form, malignant hypertension, is more common in males; (4) *climate* – hypertension is more common in temperate than in tropical climates.

Secondary hypertension

In the remaining 10 percent of the cases of hypertension, some organic or functional disorder is believed to account for the elevation of blood pressure [44]. These include: (1) *increased intracranial pressure,* usually due to head trauma, brain tumor, or meningitis; (2) *spinal cord lesions,* such as bulbar poliomyelitis; (3) *diseases of the urinary tract,* including a wide variety of congenital and acquired lesions (polycystic kidneys, glomerulonephritis, pyelonephritis, obstruction of blood flow in one or both renal arteries, obstruction of one or both ureters); (4) *endocrine disturbances,* particularly lesions of the adrenal gland associated with increased secretion of aldosterone, and pituitary or adrenal gland lesions causing Cushing's syndrome; (5) *toxemia of pregnancy;* (6) *coarctation of the aorta.* If hypertension begins before age 30 or after age 50, it is often secondary rather than idiopathic.

Renal hypertension

Of the various disorders listed above, most consideration has been given to the *renal origin* of hypertension. As noted by Dustan et al. [45], renal lesions associated with hypertension may be perinephric, parenchymal, or arterial, and may be unilateral or bilateral. These workers propose that renal hypertension is due to a polypeptide which they have extracted from the kidney and have named *angiotensin.* Just how this vasopressor or humoral mechanism acts, and whether it may have significance in essential hypertension, is almost entirely unknown. Furthermore, the interrelationships of angiotensin, renin, aldosterone, and sodium chloride still require further elucidation.

Relationship to atherosclerosis

Although hypertension and atherosclerosis commonly occur in the same patient, it is generally believed that the two are independent. It is likely that hypertension accelerates and aggravates atherosclerosis, and it is certain that the combination of the two makes for a situation particularly hazardous to the patient.

3. Natural History of Hypertension

Early stages of essential hypertension

In the earliest stage of essential hypertension, the blood pressure elevation is usually *transitory.* In the female the onset frequently coincides with the nonconvulsive form of *toxemia of pregnancy.* In either sex the onset may be marked by a period of tension: nervousness, insomnia, palpitation, etc. This and other factors suggest that a *neurogenic mechanism,* acting through the autonomic nervous system, may cause spasm of the arterioles, initiating the disease. (Renal biopsies taken early in the course of hypertensive disease show no vascular or other lesions. Patients dying early in the disease from cerebral hemorrhage may show little or no pathologic evidence of arteriolar disease.) For a long period of time – nearly 20 years, on the average – the patient is able to live a normal life, although occipital headaches, dizziness, and insomnia are fairly common. Gradually the blood pressure becomes stabilized at a higher level, as the result of development of diffuse arteriolar sclerosis.

Complications

Whether the elevation of blood pressure is of idiopathic type, as above, or secondary to some known factor, the end result, if the elevation continues, is an extra burden upon the cardiovascular system generally, and a predisposition to certain complications. These complications of *hypertensive cardiovascular disease* are largely dependent upon three factors, one or more of which may be active in a particular case: (1) the extra burden of the high diastolic pressure upon the heart, resulting in dilatation and hypertrophy of the left ventricle and in *heart failure;* (2) the secondary development of sclerosis of the small renal arterioles, leading to reduced glomerular filtration, *nitrogenous retention,* papilledema, and proteinuria; and (3) the concurrent development of atherosclerosis, especially in the cerebral and coronary arteries, leading to *thrombotic occlusion* or *rupture with hemorrhage.* In a series of 500 patients with hypertensive cardiovascular disease followed by Perera [46] until their deaths, congestive failure developed one or more times in 50 percent of the cases, uremia in 18 percent, cerebrovascular accident in 12 percent, and myocardial infarction in 8 percent. Even after the development of one or more of these complications, most patients survived several years, except that papilledema and nitrogenous retention generally indicated the terminal phase of the disease.

Life expectancy

On the average, life is shortened in patients with hypertensive disease; the *average age at death is 52 years,* or about 15 years less than the general life expectancy. Perera's figures [46] do not reflect the beneficial results that have been observed to follow the use of combinations of *reserpine, hydrochlorothiazide,* and *hydralazine;* in a well-controlled prospective study in the Veterans Administration [47], the incidence of complications of hypertension was greatly reduced by this therapy. Significant adverse reactions occurred in only one of 73 patients treated. Females with the disease generally live longer than males, and whites longer than nonwhites. (It should be noted that the duration of life as given is a mathematical average. Individual patients with hypertension run a risk of sudden and unexpected death and hence averages mean little.)

Mode of death

Sudden death, chiefly cerebral or cardiac, occurred in about 43 percent of Perera's patients, *congestive heart failure* in 22 percent, *cerebrovascular accident* in 9 percent, *myocardial infarction* in 6 percent, renal failure and *uremia* in 6 percent, *rupture* of an arteriosclerotic aneurysm in 2 percent. Death was due to multiple factors or uncertain mechanisms in 12 percent.

4. *Malignant Hypertension*

Malignant hypertension, sometimes called the *accelerated phase of essential hypertension,* develops in about 7 percent of patients with hypertensive cardiovascular disease; in some instances the disease is apparently malignant from the beginning. Clinically the usual criterion for separating malignant from benign hypertension is the presence in malignant cases of measurable elevation of the optic disk and retinopathy as seen on *ophthalmoscopic examination.* In addition, the *blood pressure is usually higher* in these cases; *albuminuria, hematuria,* and *nitrogenous retention* are often noted; and the course of the disease is greatly accelerated. Most cases of malignant hypertension occur in males (approximately 5 males to 3 females). Thirty years ago, only 2 percent of patients with malignant hypertension survived 5 years; in 1962, 5-year survival was approximately 50 percent, whether treatment was by splanchnicectomy or antihypertensive drugs. It is unlikely that the groups are strictly comparable [48].

CORONARY ARTERY DISEASE AND MYOCARDIAL INFARCTION: ISCHEMIC HEART DISEASE

1. *Basic Data in Coronary Artery Disease*

Frequency

While atherosclerosis may affect any system of arteries in the body, its most common and most significant involvement is of the coronary arteries. *Coronary artery disease, or ischemic heart disease (IHD)* as it is coming to be called, accounts for more than *half a million deaths in the U.S. each year,* or *55 percent of all deaths from cardiovascular diseases.* Both morbidity and mortality from ischemic heart disease appear to be increasing; in males the increase in the last 20 years is sufficient to nullify all the lifesaving benefits of penicillin and other medical advances [49].

Causative factors:

Coronary artery disease, like atherosclerosis in general, is intimately related to *cholesterol metabolism, blood coagulation,* and *fibrinolysis;* perhaps cholesterol and the other lipoprotein fractions account for even the variations in coagulation and fibrinolysis. (Cholesterol is emphasized rather than the other fractions because more data are available on it; it may or may not be the most important fraction.) For a given population group, the *fat content of the diet in relation to total calories* may be the determining factor. The data from Capetown, South Africa, given in Table 18-3, show the picture clearly.

TABLE 18-3. Capetown Study of Ischemic Heart Disease in Middle-Aged Men*

Population group	Deaths per 100,000 from IHD	Blood cholesterol, mg. per 100 ml.	Animal fat in diet	
			Grams	% total calories
European	628	242	82	40
Cape Colored	274	195	60	25
Bantu	"Very low"	168	40	17

*Mean figures, as developed by population surveys, matched as to age within the age range of 40 to 59 years.

From Morris [49]. Reprinted (in part) by permission of the American Heart Association, Inc. For a full discussion, see also Morris, J. N., *Uses of Epidemiology.* Baltimore: Williams & Wilkins, 1970.

activity

Within a given population group, *degree of physical activity, smoking habits,* and *blood pressure* have causal significance. Thus in a large group of men age 25 to 64 in New York City [50], the least active men showed 64 percent more instances of myocardial infarction per year and more than twice as many deaths from myocardial infarction as did the most active group.

smoking

In the Framingham (Massachusetts) and the Albany (New York) studies [51], the rate of occurrence of myocardial infarction in men aged 40 to 49 was more than three times greater in cigarette smokers than in nonsmokers; men who had formerly smoked but had stopped smoking before the study began had approximately the same rate as nonsmokers. (It is possible that cigarette smoking acts by elevating cholesterol [52].)

blood pressure

In the Framingham study, individuals with a systolic blood pressure greater than 180 mm. of mercury had almost seven times as great a risk of IHD as did individuals with systolic blood pressure below 120 [53].

other factors

Obesity as an isolated factor was apparently not significant [53]. Prior to age

50 the incidence of IHD is many times greater in men than in women; thereafter the incidence is nearly equal in the two sexes.

2. Pathologic Changes in Coronary Occlusion

Mechanisms of occlusion

Occlusion of a coronary artery results from *thrombosis* in about two-thirds of the cases, but it may follow a *tear in the coronary intima adjacent to a plaque,* permitting blood to dissect the plaque upward by subintimal hemorrhage; presumably this is the mechanism by which direct trauma to the chest may cause occlusion. Occasionally a coronary artery is occluded as a result of *embolism,* as in bacterial endocarditis. When coronary occlusion is due to thrombosis, it usually occurs at a point of narrowing of the artery by atherosclerosis; rarely, an active arteritis rather than atherosclerosis accounts for the narrowing. Rupture of new capillaries in the plaque may lead to surface breaks on which platelets are deposited. Fibrin then forms on the platelet coagulum, and cellular elements of the blood are enmeshed to form the thrombus.

Location of lesions

The *anterior descending branch of the left coronary artery* is the vessel which usually shows the greatest evidence of atherosclerosis and has the highest frequency of thrombotic occlusion. Corresponding infarcts occur at the apex of the left ventricle, and especially in the apical portion of the interventricular septum. Occlusion of the *right coronary artery* or the *circumflex branch of the left coronary artery* usually causes infarction of the posterior or lateral wall of the left ventricle. Infarction of the right ventricle or of either atrium is extremely rare.

Pathogenesis of infarction: chemical changes

In the area of ischemia, *certain chemical changes precede the development of visible lesions:* a *decrease in muscle glycogen* and a *disappearance of the cardiac muscle enzymes, creatine phosphokinase* (CPK), *glutamic oxalacetic transaminase* (GOT), *lactic dehydrogenase* (LDH), and *hydroxybutyrate dehydrogenase* (HBD). As these enzymes disappear from the infarcted muscle, *values for them rise markedly in the serum* [54]. Serum CPK begins to rise within 3 hours and reaches its peak about 36 hours after onset of the attack, returning to normal about the third day. Serum GOT begins its rise a few hours later than CPK, peaks at about the same time, and remains elevated for about 4 days. Serum LDH and HBD rise more slowly, peak at about the fourth day, and remain elevated until about the 10th day after onset. While each of them may *give positives in conditions other than myocardial infarction* – CPK in skeletal muscle disease; GOT, LDH, and HBD in liver disease, hemolytic processes, and pancreatitis – these tests are very useful as aids in the diagnosis of myocardial infarction, especially if the electrocardiogram is equivocal or has a prior abnormality. Furthermore, the enzyme tests, and particularly CPK, are apt to be abnormal before ECG abnormalities appear.

morphologic changes

Morphologic changes follow these chemical changes: an hour or two after experimental occlusion [55], the *regular myofibrillar pattern is disrupted* by a foamy cytoplasmic change, contraction bands are prominent, fibers become separated by edema fluid. Beginning about the fourth hour after onset, the *cell cytoplasm undergoes striking changes* leading to protein coagulation, followed by nuclear changes of necrosis. Somewhat later, *leukocytes begin to invade* the infarct from the periphery. At this stage the infarct appears grossly as a yellowish area with hemorrhagic borders; definite changes in the electrocardiogram, due to alterations in the electric potential in the infarcted area, appear at about this time.

If the infarct extends to the endocardial or epicardial surface, *fibrin* will form on that surface. In the case of the endocardium, because of the presence of blood in the chamber, a *mural thrombus* will form over the area of infarction. In the case of the epicardium, fibrin on the surface may lead to the development of a *pericardial friction rub.* As a result of lytic action of the leukocytic enzymes, dead muscle fibers are broken up, beginning about 5 days after thrombosis; the debris is cleared, leaving the connective tissue framework of the area. Fibroblasts proliferate, collagen is laid down, and a *scar* is formed. Stretching of the scar is common, due to inelasticity, and an old infarct is usually marked by a thin, white area of outpouching of the ventricular wall. If this is extreme, the lesion is referred to as an *aneurysm of the heart.*

related lesions

Occasionally focal myocardial lesions resembling infarcts are found at autopsy in persons having no significant evidence of coronary artery disease. In some cases the lesions are true infarcts and have resulted from coronary embolism. In others they may be due to *potassium deficiency* or *sodium excess.* Such lesions are seen only in severe instances of electrolyte disturbance, as in patients who have been receiving diuretics over a long period of time, or who have been experiencing prolonged vomiting or diarrhea. Transaminase elevations and electrocardiographic alterations suggestive of infarction are sometimes associated with these lesions. There are focal areas of muscle fiber necrosis, marked off abruptly from unaffected fibers by zones of leukocytic infiltration.

3. Clinical Manifestations in Coronary Artery Disease

In coronary sclerosis

Narrowing of the lumen of a coronary artery results in *relative ischemia of the myocardium.* This is usually first revealed as a *limitation of cardiac reserve,* resulting in *dyspnea on exertion* and *angina on effort.* Occasionally ischemia may be sufficient to precipitate *cardiac failure.* In some instances of coronary sclerosis, myocardial infarction occurs without complete coronary occlusion; e.g., if sudden severe blood loss occurs, resulting in shock and reducing the oxygen-carrying capacity of the blood, myocardial infarction may result in that portion of the heart where the blood flow was already minimal from atherosclerosis. This is the concept of myocardial infarction from *relative coronary insufficiency.*

In coronary occlusion

Coronary occlusion is usually manifest by *sudden crushing substernal pain,* commonly *radiating down the left arm,* occasionally into the neck, shoulder, or even down the right arm. This is followed usually by an appreciable *fall in blood pressure,* sometimes to shock levels. *Dyspnea, cyanosis, sweating,* and *anxiety* are usually marked. Some hours later, as the affected area of myocardium becomes necrotic, *slight fever* is commonly noted, and with this there is usually moderate *leukocytosis* and *increase in the erythrocyte sedimentation rate.*

Complications

If the patient survives the *hypotensive phase* of the first few days, a second critical period is sometimes noted 5 to 12 days after the onset. At this time, corresponding to the phase of softening and lysis of the infarct, blood from the ventricular cavity may occasionally get between endocardial muscle fibers and cause *tearing of the heart wall* in the area of infarction. The result depends upon the location of the infarct, its size, and whether or not it affects the full thickness of the muscle wall. Thus rupture of the ventricle may occur, with the tear extending through the wall, resulting in *hemopericardium* and *cardiac tamponade.* More rarely the tear may be through the interventricular septum, producing an *intracardiac shunt,* or through a papillary muscle, leading to *mitral insufficiency* by loosening the "guy ropes" of the cusp; in such cases a sudden *violent disturbance of heart action* appears, often manifest by *cyanosis, increased venous pressure,* and the sudden appearance of *heart murmurs.*

4. End Results in Myocardial Infarction

Mortality

The period of greatest danger is the *first 24 hours* after onset of the attack: about 25 percent die during this period in the case of first attacks of myocardial infarction [56]. An additional 6 percent die during the first month, and another 9 percent by the end of the first year after the attack. Thus the *total mortality during the first year after a first myocardial infarction is about 40 percent. Advanced age* and *hypertension* are the two factors most commonly associated with mortality during this period; obesity has no significant effect.

Causes of death

Of those persons that die from acute myocardial infarction, 43 percent die from *myocardial failure* (left or right ventricle failure), 23 percent from *coronary failure* (recurrent pain suggesting extension of the infarct), 15 percent from *rupture of the heart,* 9 percent from *shock,* 3 percent from *pulmonary embolism,* 3 percent from *systemic embolism* from a mural thrombus, and 4 percent from miscellaneous causes [57]. Even if the patient recovers, he still has his coronary atherosclerosis and is therefore subject to *recurrent attacks.* With appropriate readjustment of diet and living habits, many patients live years after their first episode. *Heart failure,* due to combined factors, may come on at any time. *Sudden arrhythmias* (heart block, ventricular fibrillation) may also develop, causing *sudden death;* some cases of death during sleep, or while driving a car, or sudden collapse at home or office are undoubtedly due to arrhythmias.

CARDIOVASCULAR SYPHILIS

Frequency

The cardiovascular system is probably affected in about 20 percent of the cases of untreated syphilis; necessarily this figure is little better than a guess. Cardiovascular syphilis is usually a manifestation of *acquired syphilis,* rarely of congenital syphilis. In all its forms cardiovascular syphilis probably accounts for less than 3 percent of all cardiovascular deaths at the present time.

Myocarditis

Diffuse *syphilitic myocarditis* and *gumma* of the heart have been described but are extremely rare.

Syphilitic aortitis

All other forms of syphilis of the cardiovascular system have their beginnings in syphilitic aortitis. The interval between the appearance of the chancre and clinical evidence of syphilitic aortitis is usually *5 to 15 years,* but may rarely be as short as 6 months. The spirochete seems to have an affinity for the aorta, especially for the three limbs of the aortic arch – *ascending, transverse,* and *descending;* the abdominal aorta is rarely affected. *Grossly* the affected portion is somewhat dilated. Syphilitic fibrosis of the media, with destruction of muscularis and elastica, results in puckered stellate depressions of the intima, separated by wrinkled areas. (Fatty deposits, ulceration, and calcification are not characteristic, although atheromatous lesions may coincide with syphilitic ones.) Areas of medial thinning are often noted, and small knobby outpouchings may be seen. The aorta is greatly weakened. *Microscopically* the changes are noted chiefly in the media and adventitia. Typically the media shows scattered foci of necrosis and fibrous scarring; the adventitia and outer portion of media show perivascular infiltration by plasma cells and lymphocytes. Treponemas are rarely demonstrable. Uncomplicated syphilitic aortitis is usually *asymptomatic.* If cardiovascular symptoms or findings are present in a known syphilitic, one or more of the following complications should be suspected: aortic insufficiency, narrowing of coronary ostia, or aneurysm.

Aortic insufficiency

Insufficiency of the aortic valve results when the syphilitic fibrosis of the aortic media spreads to the commissures of the aortic valve, separating one cusp from another, and causing *thickening, shortening,* and *rolling of the cusp edges.* Ordinarily there is no narrowing of the orifice: the functional effect is almost a *pure insufficiency.* Dilatation of the aortic valve ring sometimes occurs as a result of the destructive changes in the aortic media; this adds to the regurgitation. Left ventricular dilatation and hypertrophy develop, and often become extreme. Later there is *left ventricular failure,* with pulmonary edema. Other heart valves are not affected by the treponemas.

Narrowing of coronary ostia

Coronary insufficiency is an important although uncommon complication of syphilitic aortitis. When the inflammatory fibrosis of the aortic wall happens to surround one or both coronary ostia, the scarring may narrow the lumen sufficiently to cause symptoms. *Sudden death* is common in such cases. Myocardial infarction is rarely seen as a result of syphilis.

Syphilitic aneurysms are discussed in the section following.

ANEURYSMS

1. General Features

Definitions and types

Any localized dilatation of the lumen of a blood vessel may be called an aneurysm; it is also known as a *true aneurysm.* A *false aneurysm* is a localized external widening of a vessel without dilatation of the lumen; it is obviously a result of a change in the vessel wall, usually a hematoma between its layers, hence often a result of trauma. A *dissecting aneurysm* is a special type of false aneurysm, not traumatic in origin, in which blood splits the layers of the artery apart and the false channel extends (dissects) for some distance along the course of the vessel. A *saccular aneurysm* is one having a small opening at its point of origin from the vessel, then bulging outward like a balloon; saccular aneurysms are usually a result of syphilitic aortitis. A *fusiform aneurysm* is one in which the vessel is more or less uniformly dilated for a distance, the bulge occurring in all directions instead of from one side as with the saccular type. All aneurysms are, of course, filled with either blood or thrombus.

Locations

Most aneurysms occur in the *aorta or its major branches;* less commonly, aneurysms affect *popliteal, splenic, renal,* and *intracranial* arteries. Rarely do they affect the pulmonary arterial bed or the venous system, except that one form of aneurysm connects an artery with a vein *(arteriovenous aneurysm).*

Causes

Aneurysms may result from any disease or condition which produces a *localized area of weakening in the vessel wall. Atherosclerosis, syphilis,* and *trauma* are the major causes; bacterial or other *infections of the vessel wall,* and *congenital defects,* are minor causes. All aneurysms are more common in males.

Manifestations

Aneurysms in the *thorax* usually cause pain, cough, or wheezing, by compressing adjacent structures. Aneurysms in the *abdomen* usually do not compress other structures particularly, hence pain is less often a symptom there than in the thorax; often the patient first notes a swelling, and the fact that it is pulsating. Sometimes the first symptoms of aneurysm are those resulting from *rupture of the aneurysm, with hemorrhage.* Symptoms and signs are often not sufficient to establish the diagnosis. *X-ray* is of great help, especially when combined with a *radiopaque dye* which fills the vessel and shows the area of dilatation.

Outcome

Aneurysms are naturally prone to rupture, since a weakened arterial wall is the reason for their existence in the first place. When rupture does occur, it may cause *exsanguinating hemorrhage,* or the *accumulation of blood may so compress vital structures as to cause death.* Thus a patient is apt to bleed to death if an aneurysm of the thoracic aorta ruptures into the esophagus, trachea, or pleural sac. A ruptured aneurysm of the abdominal aorta bleeds more slowly because it lies in the retroperitoneal space; such aneurysms may be cured by surgical excision and replacement by an aortic graft, especially if the renal arteries are not involved. When an aneurysm of an intracranial artery ruptures, it usually causes death by *increased intracranial tension* before blood loss is itself fatal. Small aneurysms, especially those of the abdominal aorta or its branches, may cause no trouble, being incidental findings at autopsy.

In the sections following, aneurysms are discussed in relation to their causes, since their differing manifestations are often determined by their causes.

2. Syphilitic Aneurysms

Manner of development

Syphilitic aneurysm, a common complication of syphilitic aortitis, occurs at a point *where the media of the vessel has been largely replaced by scar tissue* and hence greatly weakened. The blood pressure in the aorta forces the intima through the medial defect, and a saccular aneurysm balloons outward. At first the aneurysm wall is composed of thickened intima and adventitia. Later, as it enlarges and compresses adjacent tissues, the wall may come to include other structures, such as pleura, bone, lung. The intermittent *pulsing pressure* can erode the hardest structures such as vertebrae, ribs, or tracheal rings; elastic structures, like intervertebral disks and skin, tend to resist this force somewhat longer. Often a thrombus lines a part of the sac; sometimes this thrombus obscures the *expansile pulsation synchronous with cardiac systole,* which is the most distinctive clinical feature of aneurysm. This feature can be appreciated visually on *fluoroscopy,* or, if the aneurysm is just beneath the skin, can be detected with the hands. Some syphilitic aneurysms become as large as 30 cm. in diameter; most are 5 to 10 cm.

Occurrence

Syphilitic aneurysms occur chiefly in males between the ages of 40 and 60. They usually arise from either the ascending, transverse, or descending limbs of the aortic arch. A few arise from the innominate artery, but usually involve the aorta as well. They may bulge in any direction: forward, backward, right, or left.

Manifestations

Aneurysms arising from the ascending limb of the aortic arch are often called *aneurysms of symptoms,* because they tend to compress the trachea or anterior chest wall, producing pain, cough, and dyspnea. Those arising from the transverse portion of the arch have been called *aneurysms of signs,* because they compress the left bronchus (giving tracheal tug), the sympathetic nerve chain (giving unequal pupils), and the recurrent laryngeal nerve (giving laryngeal paralysis and hoarseness). Aneurysm in any position is apt to produce *pain,* which is dependent upon the stretching and erosive force of the aneurysm. Erosion of the vertebrae and spinal cord may produce *paralysis. Heart failure* is rarely a manifestation of syphilitic aneurysm; when it does occur, it is usually a result of one of the following: (1) an *arteriovenous shunt* due to erosion into some other vessel, such as the superior vena cava; (2) involvement of the aortic ring, producing dilatation and *aortic insufficiency;* (3) *dampening of the driving force* of systole; or (4) rupture into the pericardial sac, causing *cardiac tamponade.*

Outcome

Syphilitic aneurysm usually causes death by *exsanguinating hemorrhage.* Rupture may occur into the esophagus, trachea, pleura, or externally through the chest wall. Sometimes death is due to compression of the trachea or a bronchus, with the development of pneumonia or abscess. Rarely does a syphilitic aneurysm "heal" by its cavity becoming filled with thrombus.

3. Aneurysms Due to Atherosclerosis

In recent years, as syphilis has become less of a problem, *atherosclerosis has become the most frequent cause of aortic aneurysm.* In most instances the affected patients are males in the seventh or eighth decade. The *abdominal aorta,* generally below the renal arteries, is the most common site. The *iliac arteries* are the next most frequent sites of atherosclerotic aneurysm development. *Popliteal, splenic,* and *renal* arteries are occasionally involved. *Multiple aneurysms* due to atherosclerosis are common.

Pathogenesis

Atheromatous lesions tend to weaken the affected vessels and, when combined with loss of elastica in the media, result in aneurysmal dilatation. (See earlier section on Atherosclerosis.) Atherosclerotic aneurysms ordinarily do not exceed 3 to 10 cm. in transverse diameter. Arteriosclerotic aneurysms are usually spindle-shaped or *fusiform,* gradually widening out to full size and then tapering again to the normal size of the affected artery.

Clinical findings

An unruptured arteriosclerotic aneurysm of the abdominal aorta usually causes no symptoms, although the *mass* may sometimes be felt and be noted to *pulsate.* Sometimes there is pain, but pain usually signifies incipient *rupture.* When rupture occurs, it is usually into the *retroperitoneal* tissues, where a mass appears and enlarges over a period of a few hours. *Exsanguination* is the usual end result, but many patients are saved by surgical excision of the aneurysm and replacement with a graft or prosthesis. Arteriosclerotic aneurysms are common incidental findings in autopsies on elderly persons.

4. Congenital Aneurysms

Congenital aneurysms tend to affect *smaller arteries,* such as the cerebral, renal, and splenic arteries. They are usually saccular, 0.5 to 2.0 cm. in diameter, and tend to occur at points of bifurcation. Symptoms are rarely noted unless *rupture* occurs. *Cerebral aneurysms comprise a particularly important group;* they are considered in Chapter 26.

5. Traumatic Aneurysms

Of the aorta:

A few years ago most traumatic aneurysms were encountered in the *extremity arteries* and were a direct *result of penetrating wounds.* Since the early '60s, an increasing number of aneurysms of the thoracic aorta have come to be recognized as traumatic in origin, so that *trauma is now believed to be a more common cause of thoracic aneurysms than is syphilis.*

mechanism

Autopsies on individuals dying as a result of *airplane crashes* very commonly show, in addition to other injuries, *tears of the aorta at the site of the ligamentum arteriosum,* and *massive intrathoracic hemorrhage.* With sudden deceleration, the relatively mobile heart apparently jerks forward in the thorax, shearing the aorta transversely at its point of greatest fixation, namely where the descending portion of the arch begins, which is also a point of inherent weakness because of scar tissue corresponding to the obliterated ductus. Other forms of sudden violent deceleration due to trauma may also cause rupture of the aorta at this site: head-on automobile collisions at high speed, especially when the victim is thrown from the car; *pedestrians killed by speeding cars;* or *falls from high altitude* are the most likely mechanisms. In an autopsy study by Greendyke [58], 13 percent of all fatalities due to automotive accidents were a result of aortic rupture. In those who survive such accidents, *aneurysms may develop at this same site;* in some reported instances the aneurysms were *treated surgically,* and successfully, *8 to 20 years after the injury* that was believed to be responsible [59].

pathology

Aneurysms resulting from trauma of this type have a rather *characteristic gross appearance* [60]: the dilatation has an abrupt beginning and ending, due to the tear in the aortic wall that caused the aneurysm. The sac itself includes practically no media. In some instances a short dissection of the aortic wall occurs. Dense adhesions between the aneurysm and adjacent tissues are often noted.

manifestations

In most cases described as aneurysms (as contrasted to immediate traumatic rupture), the patients appear to have *recovered completely from the injuries* received several years previously. They may present for any of the usual symptoms of thoracic aneurysm: pain, hoarseness, hematemesis, or shock from hemorrhage.

outcome

In the hands of skilled thoracic surgeons, reconstruction of the aorta, perhaps with graft, is usually successful. Conceivably some cases of mild degree may heal spontaneously. Unquestionably aneurysms of this type are being seen at autopsy years later, with death resulting from rupture.

Of extremity arteries

Traumatic aneurysms of extremity arteries are usually a result of *penetrating wound* with *direct injury of an artery,* as by a bullet, knife, or bone fragment from a fracture. This may cause a *hematoma in the arterial wall* (false aneurysm). Presumably the affected vessel is nicked but not actually penetrated at the time of injury. Later the inner layers may bulge outward through the defect resulting from the nick. After a period of some months, rupture may occur into the tissues causing a hematoma. Sometimes both the artery and the vein are nicked at the same time. This may be followed later by the development of a communication (fistula) between the artery and vein, i.e., *traumatic arteriovenous aneurysm.*

6. Arteriovenous Aneurysms

Arteriovenous aneurysms, or *fistulas,* may be either *congenital* or *traumatic.* Their sacs provide communications between arteries and veins. They produce striking local manifestations *(murmurs, thrills),* and may in some instances cause *heart failure* if the shunt is large.

7. Mycotic Aneurysms

Mycotic aneurysms result when there is weakening of the arterial walls, usually by *bacterial action,* as with embolism during *bacterial endocarditis.* These aneurysms occur *at points of bifurcation,* and are often *multiple.* Mycotic aneurysms are also seen in some cases of *polyarteritis nodosa.* Mycotic aneurysms often terminate by *rupture.*

8. Dissecting Aneurysms

Definition

A dissecting aneurysm is a *spontaneous form of false aneurysm* in which there is a *splitting of the wall of the aorta,* usually at the juncture of the inner third and the outer two-thirds. Blood enters the split and extends it, resulting in an elongated hematoma in the wall. Rarely dissection may occur in the pulmonary artery or in smaller systemic arteries such as the renals.

Causes

The great majority of patients with dissecting aneurysm have a long history of *hypertension,* often of severe degree. Some patients with dissecting aneurysm have no hypertension, but show evidence of *Marfan's syndrome,* a congenital disorder of the mesenchymal tissues (see Chapter 28). Zones of *medial necrosis,* sometimes associated with small, slitlike cysts (medial cystic necrosis of Erdheim), are often found in aortas showing dissecting aneurysm and are believed by many to be causative. Syphilitic aortitis is not a cause, and probably would actually prevent dissection because of the scarring in the media. Arteriosclerosis is probably not a factor; aortas showing dissections are usually not particularly sclerotic, and, further, the intimal tear in dissecting aneurysm rarely occurs at an atheromatous lesion.

Pathogenesis

Assuming that a medial defect is the primary lesion in dissecting aneurysm, it is uncertain whether the blood gains access to the media from an intimal tear in the aorta or as a result of rupture of vasa vasorum in the wall. Intimal tears are not always found; when present they may conceivably represent either sites of breakthrough from the medial cleft into the lumen, or portals for entry of blood from the lumen into the media. *Intimal tears* are most commonly found either *just above the aortic valve,* where they are usually transverse, or adjacent to the aortic dimple corresponding to the *ligamentum arteriosum.* Both these locations are theoretically sites of stress. (Intimal tears are sometimes found at these sites in the absence of dissections.) After blood gets between the layers of the media, presumably in a plane of cleavage due to medial necrosis, it may dissect around the vessel, proximally and distally and along its branches.

Clinical features

Severe *chest pain,* usually substernal or in the back, and described as ripping or tearing, commonly marks the onset. The pain *extends with the dissection* – down along the spine, or to the legs. In patients with dissection of the ascending aorta, the murmur and other manifestations of *aortic insufficiency* may appear; this is a result of loosening of a commissure of the aortic valve so that one valve sags below the others. Other manifestations are usually due to *interruption of blood flow* in the aortic branches. Thus there may be signs of coronary occlusion due to dissection of a coronary artery when the aneurysm is in the ascending aorta, or signs of occlusion of the mesenteric, renal, iliac, spinal, or other arteries when the abdominal aorta is affected.

Outcome

The false or dissecting channel usually ruptures externally, often at some distance from the intimal tear. Death is often due to *hemopericardium* and cardiac tamponade when the aneurysm is proximal. In other cases death may be a result of *exsanguinating hemorrhage* into the pleural or abdominal cavity. Very rarely the dissection may cease, endothelium may line the false channel, and a "double-barreled" aorta may result.

COR PULMONALE

Definition

Cor pulmonale signifies *right ventricular strain.* As the term is generally used, it implies a chronic disorder, associated with *right ventricular hypertrophy. Acute cor pulmonale* is the term occasionally used for the sudden right ventricular strain that is a sequel to massive pulmonary embolism.

Forms:

The many causes of right ventricular strain can be divided into two groups on the basis of the mechanisms involved [61]: (1) those conditions in which the primary problem is *obstruction to pulmonary blood flow;* and (2) those conditions in which the primary problem is difficulty in ventilation *(dysventilation syndrome).* It is important to make the distinction because the treatment of the two groups is different in the early stages. Late in the course of development the distinction becomes less important because heart failure itself overshadows the causative mechanisms.

obstruction to pulmonary blood flow

Primary obstruction to pulmonary blood flow may be due to (1) *stenosis of the pulmonic valve;* (2) conditions which block blood flow in *major pulmonary arteries* (recurring pulmonary embolism, extrinsic compression), in *pulmonary arterioles* (idiopathic pulmonary hypertension; left-to-right shunts due to septal defects or persistent ductus arteriosus; pulmonary schistosomiasis), in *pulmonary veins* (extrinsic compression), in the *left atrium* (atrial myxoma, atrial thrombosis); or (3) *stenosis of the mitral valve orifice.* During early stages of their disease these patients' chief symptoms are those due to *low cardiac output:* easy fatigue, angina, or syncope. Cyanosis occurs only if shunts are present. On examination of the chest no expiratory wheezes are found, and pulmonary function studies in the early stages are not abnormal unless a shunt is present. *Cardiac catheterization* demonstrates marked *right ventricular hypertension.*

dysventilation syndrome

Primary difficulty in ventilation may result from *emphysema* (about 80 percent of the cases), *pulmonary fibrosis* (pneumoconiosis, sarcoid, radiation pneumonitis), *diffuse pleural fibrosis,* or *diseases restricting thoracic mobility* (kyphoscoliosis, ankylosing spondylitis, scleroderma, neurologic disorders, extreme obesity). Patients with these conditions show *cyanosis* and *dyspnea,* and examination reveals *thoracic deformity* and *expiratory wheezes.* Pulmonary function studies show severe disturbances: low $P_{A O_2}$, elevated $P_{A CO_2}$, and low pH. *Erythrocytosis* is commonly observed. Cardiac output is usually normal.

idiopathic pulmonary hypertension

Rarely *pulmonary hypertension* exists *without explanation,* i.e., without intrinsic lung disease and without demonstrable reason for interference with pulmonary blood flow. These cases occur usually in young women and seem comparable to essential hypertension in the systemic circulation.

Clinical features

In the final stages the manifestations of right ventricular strain occur in cases in both groups, no matter what the cause. These may include *dyspnea, cyanosis, increased venous pressure, painful enlargement of the liver, polycythemia, clubbing of the fingers,* and *accentuated pulmonic second sound.* Occasionally, especially in severe kyphoscoliosis, there may be heart murmurs, either systolic or diastolic. The electrocardiogram usually shows *right axis deviation* and sharply elevated P waves. The chest radiograph usually shows a *broadening of the heart shadow* due to hypertrophy and dilatation of the pulmonary conus. In some instances a neurologic disorder including papilledema and uncontrollable jerky movements of the extremities occurs, presumably due to the prolonged cerebral anoxia and continued high venous pressure; brain tumor or parkinsonism may be closely simulated [62].

Pathologic changes

The increased pulmonary arterial pressure causes *dilatation and hypertrophy of the right ventricle* – the characteristic autopsy evidence of cor pulmonale. Pulmonary arteries and arterioles may show hypertrophy of the muscular coat and atheroma of the intima; these changes are generally believed to be secondary to the increased pulmonary arterial pressure, comparable to the sclerosis of systemic arterioles in systemic hypertension.

METABOLIC HEART DISEASE

Cardiac manifestations may be noted with various diseases of metabolism. Since *correction of the cardiac dysfunction depends upon the success of treatment of the underlying metabolic disorder,* it is important that these cases be recognized. Several categories have been defined by Leiter [63].

Cardiac deposits of abnormal metabolic products

Abnormal deposits, resulting from metabolic disorders, may occur in the myocardium. *Amyloidosis of the heart* is rare, but may occur either as a part of primary or secondary amyloidosis or the heart may be the only organ affected (primary cardiac amyloidosis). This latter form occurs chiefly in males over the age of 70. The deposits may be focal and nodular, but more commonly are diffuse, separating individual muscle fibers, and involving endocardium and pericardium. Usually there is no obvious basis for the occurrence of the amyloid. *Glycogenosis of the heart* is also rare, presumably familial; it is seldom seen after 1 year of age. Heavy glycogen deposits may occur in skeletal muscle and in the tongue, as well as in the myocardial fibers. In *gargoylism,* a form of lipochondrodystrophy, a complex glycoprotein is deposited in the heart as well as in the liver, spleen, bones, and nervous system. Death is usually due to congestive heart failure at about 11 years of age. In the *muscular dystrophies* the myocardium is affected along with the skeletal muscles; strange vacuolative and degenerative changes occur in the fibers, and interstitial fibrosis may be noted. In the *malignant carcinoid* syndrome, fibrotic changes are noted in the pulmonic valve cusps and the endocardium of the right side of the heart; these changes are believed to be due to serotonin and perhaps catecholamines secreted by the tumor [64]. In *Marfan's disease* there is a congenital chemical abnormality of connective tissues involving the aorta and other large vessels; aneurysms may occur in affected vessels, usually in early adulthood.

Defects in cardiac metabolism

In other conditions the *metabolic machinery of the heart muscle* may be directly affected as a part of the systemic disturbance. Thus in *beriberi* it appears that myocardial energy production is affected as a result of the enzyme and vitamin deficiency. Most cases of beriberi heart disease in the Occident are associated with alcoholism. Characteristically the heart failure is of the high-output type. In *hyperthyroidism* there may also be high-output failure, presumably related to the heart's own increased metabolism. Cardiac arrhythmias are common in this condition. With *hypothyroidism,* low cardiac output is noted, sometimes with heart failure. Myxedema fluid may on rare occasions be noted in the myocardium at autopsy. In *hemosiderosis,* iron deposits occur in the myocardial fibers, and degenerative changes may be noted, resulting clinically in heart failure. *Cobalt* added to beer was apparently the agent accounting for the remarkable syndrome of heart failure that occurred in men drinking 30 or more pints of beer per day for many years [65] ; the metal was believed to cause the degenerative changes seen in the muscle fibers. In patients with *pheochromocytoma of the adrenal medulla,* the cause of death is commonly heart failure, believed to be a result of the focal myocarditis that occurs, apparently as a result of excessive secretion of catecholamines [66].

Circulatory overload

In another group of diseases *unusual arteriovenous shunts* occur in different parts of the body as a result of disease in those parts; the result may be heart failure from circulatory overload. Such effects have been described in *Paget's disease of bone,* in *cirrhosis of the liver,* and in *pregnancy;* in the last the shunts are apparently in the uterine wall and broad ligaments.

NEOPLASMS OF THE HEART

Primary

Primary neoplasms of the heart are extremely rare and are *usually benign. Rhabdomyoma* and *hamartoma* have been noted in the familial disorder, epiloia, in which cerebral, renal, and dermal lesions also occur. *Lipomas* occur occasionally in the interatrial septum; they apparently do not produce clinical manifestations. *Myxoma* is the most common primary neoplasm of the heart [67]. It is a soft mass, consisting of edematous connective tissue irregularly covered by thrombus, commonly attached to the endocardium by a pedicle, and hanging free into a cavity, usually the left atrium. It may block the mitral orifice, producing a murmur like that of mitral stenosis. Embolism from the surface thrombus is common. In a case of ours, an adult patient developed clubbing of the fingers within a few months. If suspected, the diagnosis could be made by angiocardiography; surgical removal should not be difficult.

Metastatic

Metastatic neoplasms of the heart are not uncommon; they were found in 20 percent of autopsies on patients dying with malignant neoplasms in the George Washington University Hospital [68]. The neoplasms commonly giving rise to cardiac metastases were those *primary* in the *breasts* and the *lungs,* and *lymphomas,* in that order as regards total numbers. Malignant *melanoma,* a much less common tumor than breast cancer, had cardiac metastases in every case of our series. Myocardium and pericardium are about equally affected, the endocardium less frequently. *Manifestations* of cardiac neoplasms are varied: if any findings are present, they are usually *arrhythmia* or signs of *cardiac failure,* in a patient dying with widespread metastases. Rarely cardiac or mediastinal metastasis may be manifest as heart failure appearing many years after removal of a primary neoplasm, in which case the correct diagnosis may be easily overlooked during life.

PERIPHERAL VASCULAR DISEASES

1. *Diseases of the Peripheral Arteries*

Segmental arterial disease

Atherosclerosis is the most important disorder of the peripheral arteries; the frequent association of atherosclerosis of the arteries of the legs and feet with *diabetes mellitus* should be emphasized. When *atherosclerosis of peripheral arteries is combined with thrombosis,* serious clinical symptoms may result; they have been described earlier in this chapter under the clinical features of atherosclerosis. Mönckeberg's *medial sclerosis* is common in the leg arteries, but produces little functional effect unless it is combined with the intimal lesions of atherosclerosis (see page 423).

Buerger's disease

The following disorders of the peripheral arteries, although relatively rare, must also be considered. *Thromboangiitis obliterans* (Buerger's disease) is a rare disorder of the vessels of the lower extremities, occurring chiefly in young adult males. Ischemia of the feet results, often leading to painful ulcers of the toes. There is an *inflammatory reaction* in the walls of *arteries and veins,* often associated with *venous thrombosis. Cigarette smoking* aggravates the disability. McKusick and his associates [69] have reviewed the aspects of this disease which mark it as a clinical and pathologic entity rather than a syndrome.

Reynaud's disease

Reynaud's disease is an angiospastic disorder affecting chiefly the fingers, often resulting in symmetric gangrene of the distal phalanges.

Endarteritis obliterans

Endarteritis obliterans is a term usually restricted to the physiologic closure of vessels, as of the ductus arteriosus, and the arteries of the uterus after the menopause.

Polyarteritis nodosa

Polyarteritis nodosa and the conditions allied to it (hypersensitivity angiitis, necrotizing angiitis, granulomatous arteritis) are inflammatory disorders affecting chiefly medium-sized arteries. They usually present as part of a hypersensitivity state (see Chapter 4), but sometimes are manifest by symptoms of arterial thrombosis.

Temporal arteritis

Temporal arteritis is probably a special form of granulomatous arteritis, but the reason for the peculiar affinity for the temporal artery is unknown.

Platelet thrombosis

Arteriolar and capillary *platelet thrombosis* may occur during the course of thrombotic thrombocytopenic purpura.

2. Diseases of the Veins

Circulatory role of veins

The veins have generally been considered to be a system of passive tubes having little function in the circulation. Guyton [70] has pointed out the inadequacy of this concept. The veins, by virtue of their plasticity, *serve as a storehouse* for blood, releasing it as required to maintain arterial blood volume. This is accomplished by a *pumping action,* activated by contraction of the skeletal muscles and by movements of the body, with the aid of the *venous valves.* The veins thus provide the heart with that amount of blood required for tissue needs, under the regulatory control of the *sympathetic nervous system.* Thus it seems likely that disorders of the venous valves may lead to disturbances of cardiac output, a concept that should receive more critical clinical appraisal than it has had to date.

Varicose veins:

In certain individuals, sometimes following a familial pattern, *peripheral veins are dilated, tortuous,* and *thick-walled,* bulging beneath the skin: *varicose veins.* The lower extremities are chiefly affected. The condition is particularly common in *women who have borne children* and in *people on their feet much of the time,* such as barbers and store clerks. Increased venous pressure, as from heart failure, or from direct compression of veins by the pregnant uterus or neoplasms, may lead to *incompetence of the valves* of the veins, aggravating venous stasis. *Sclerosis of the veins,* sometimes with calcium deposits, follows. *Edema* develops in severe cases. Skin circulation is sometimes impaired, and may lead to *chronic leg ulcers.* In most cases the condition is simply disfiguring, and there are no serious manifestations, but varicose veins are susceptible to *thrombosis,* and fatal pulmonary embolism occurs occasionally.

sites

The following are the important local sites of varicosities: (1) *saphenous veins,* which often become distended as a result of pregnancy, valvular incompetence, and thrombosis of the deeper veins of the leg; (2) *hemorrhoids,* either internal or external, often due to multiple pregnancies, pelvic tumors, or portal hypertension; (3) *varicocele,* sometimes painful, rarely disabling; (4) *prostatic* and *pelvic* varicosities, in which thrombi tend to become organized and calcified (phleboliths), causing confusion occasionally with ureteral calculi on x-ray; and (5) *esophageal varices* resulting from portal hypertension, as in cirrhosis of the liver. (This last is the only form of varicosity in which *massive hemorrhage* is apt to occur.)

Secondary thrombosis occurs commonly in the foregoing processes, but in the following conditions thrombosis is the chief, often the primary, process.

Phlebothrombosis

In phlebothrombosis, coagulation of the blood in the veins occurs *without antecedent inflammation.* Both *systemic and local factors* undoubtedly play a role. There is evidence that *dietary fats* influence the frequency of venous thrombosis in the population just as they influence the frequency of coronary artery thrombosis. The role of *"the pill"* in venous thrombosis and pulmonary embolism has attracted much attention. *Pancreatic neoplasms* predispose to venous thrombosis, presumably through some specific effect upon the coagulation mechanism. Local factors probably operate chiefly by inducing *venous stagnation.* Thus heart failure, compression of veins by neoplasms or by the pregnant uterus, and prolonged bed rest (as following surgery, fractures, or delivery) all cause local stasis of blood and predispose to thrombosis. When thrombosis occurs in the *veins of the calf* – perhaps the most common site for phlebothrombosis – it is usually associated with some increase in the circumference of the calf even if there is no visible edema, and often there is pain at the back of the knee or calf when the ankle is forcibly flexed (Homan's sign). The chief importance of phlebothrombosis is the *danger of pulmonary embolism.* If embolism does not occur, the thrombi may gradually become organized and converted into hyaline, fibrous branching cords, transforming the lumen of the vessel into a spongelike structure.

Thrombophlebitis

When thrombosis of a vein is secondary to *inflammation of the wall* of the vein, as in the leg veins following cellulitis or infected compound fractures, the process is called thrombophlebitis. *Pulmonary embolism is less likely in thrombophlebitis* than in phlebothrombosis, because the inflammatory reaction, if low-grade, tends to hold the thrombus more firmly in place. On the other hand, when virulent pyogenic organisms are present in the thrombus, partial *lysis of the thrombus* may occur, causing *embolism.* In such a case, the emboli may be septic, producing abscesses in the lung. This is often noted in cases of acute osteomyelitis due to staphylococci. Thrombophlebitis of the *portal vein* and of the large *venous sinuses of the cranium* may occur following serious infections of these drainage beds.

REFERENCES

1. *Cardiovascular Diseases in the U.S.: Facts and Figures.* New York: American Heart Association, 1965. (An excellent summary of statistical data from several sources, well presented.)
2. Schroeder, H. A. Municipal drinking water and cardiovascular death rates. *J.A.M.A.* 195:81, 1960.
3. Carroll, R. E. The relationship of cadmium in the air to cardiovascular disease death rates. *J.A.M.A.* 198:267, 1966.
4. Guyton, A. C. Regulation of cardiac output. *New Eng. J. Med.* 277:805, 1967.
5. Pittman, J. G., and Cohen, P. The pathogenesis of cardiac cachexia. *New Eng. J. Med.* 271:403, 453, 1964.
6. Braunwald, E., Ross, J., Jr., and Sonnenblick, E. H. *Mechanisms of Contraction of the Normal and Failing Heart.* Boston: Little, Brown, 1968. (Morphologic, biochemical, and hemodynamic aspects of cardiac function are stressed.)
7. Spann, J. F., Jr., Mason, D. T., and Zelis, R. F. Recent advances in the understanding of congestive heart failure. *Mod. Conc. Cardiovasc. Dis.* 33:73, 1970. (An excellent summary of current theory.)
8. Urquhart, J., and Davis, J. O. Role of the kidney and adrenal cortex in congestive heart failure. *Mod. Conc. Cardiovasc. Dis.* 32:781, 1963.
9. Rudolph, A. M., and Nadas, A. S. The pulmonary circulation and congenital heart disease. *New Eng. J. Med.* 267:968, 1022, 1962. (An excellent discussion of congenital heart disease and its physiologic effects.)
10. Jackson, B. T. The pathogenesis of congenital cardiac anomalies. *New Eng. J. Med.* 279:25, 80, 1968. (A wonderful article, giving satisfying answers to many questions, this is drawn on heavily in the section on congenital heart disease here.)
11. Warkany, J., Passarge, E., and Smith, L. B. Quoted by Jackson [10].
12. Emerit, I., de Grouchy, J., Vernant, P., and Corone, P. Quoted by Jackson [10].
13. Brown, G. C., and Evans, T. N. Serologic evidence of coxsackievirus etiology of congenital heart disease. *J.A.M.A.* 199:183, 1967.
14. Morton, W. E., and Huhn, L. A. Epidemiology of congenital heart disease. *J.A.M.A.* 195:1107, 1966.
15. MacMahon, B., McKeown, I., and Record, R. G. Incidence and life expectancy of children with congenital heart disease. *Brit. Heart J.* 15:121, 1953.
16. Wiland, O. K. Extracardiac anomalies in association with congenital heart disease. *Lab. Invest.* 5:380, 1956.
17. Noonan, J. A., Nadas, A. S., Rudolph, A. M., and Harris, G. B. C. Transposition of the great arteries: A correlation of clinical, physiologic and autopsy data. *New Eng. J. Med.* 263:592, 637, 684, 739, 1960.
18. Lev, M., Rimoldi, H. J. A., Eckner, F. A. O., Melhuish, B. P., Meng, L., and Paul, M. H. The Taussig-Bing heart: Qualitative and quantitative anatomy. *Arch. Path.* (Chicago) 81:24, 1966.
19. Peery, T. M. Brucellosis and heart disease. I. The shaky foundations of rheumatic heart disease. *Postgrad. Med.* 19:323, 1956. (The significance of "rheumatic stigmata" and of "a history of rheumatic fever" is questioned.)
20. Streptococci and rheumatic fever (Editorial). *Lancet* 1:485, 1967.
21. Murphy, G. E. The characteristic rheumatic lesions of striated and non-striated or smooth muscle cells of the heart. *Medicine* 42:73, 1963. (The

author presents convincing pictorial evidence that Aschoff bodies are essentially lesions of muscle cells.)

22. Kaplan, M. H., Bolande, R., and Blair, J. Presence of bound immunoglobulins and complement in the myocardium in acute rheumatic fever. *New Eng. J. Med.* 271:637, 1964.
23. Clawson, B. J. The Aschoff nodule. *Arch. Path.* 8:664, 1929. (A classic, often-quoted paper on the pathology of rheumatic fever.)
24. Bland, E. F., and Jones, T. D. Rheumatic fever and rheumatic heart disease: A 20-year report on 1000 patients followed since childhood. *Circulation* 4:836, 1951. (An extremely valuable study, but its applicability to the milder forms of rheumatic fever currently prevalent is subject to question.)
25. Peery, T. M. Brucellosis and heart disease. IV. The etiology of calcific aortic stenosis. *J.A.M.A.* 166:1123, 1958.
26. Angrist, A. A., and Oka, M. Pathogenesis of bacterial endocarditis. *J.A.M.A.* 183:249, 1963.
27. Lerner, P. I., and Weinstein, L. Infective endocarditis in the antibiotic era. *New Eng. J. Med.* 274:199, 259, 323, 388, 1966.
28. Mattingly, T. W. Changing concepts of myocardial diseases. *J.A.M.A.* 191:33, 1965.
29. Burch, G. E., Shih-Chien, S., Kang-Chu, C., Sohal, R. S., and Colcolough, H. L. Interstitial and coxsackievirus B myocarditis in infants and children. *J.A.M.A.* 203:1, 1968.
30. St. Geme, J. W., Noren, G. R., and Adams, P., Jr. Proposed embryopathic relation between mumps virus and primary endocardial fibroelastosis. *New Eng. J. Med.* 275:339, 1966.
31. Dalton, J. C., Pearson, R. J., Jr., and White, P. D. Constrictive pericarditis: A review and long-term follow-up of 78 cases. *Ann. Intern. Med.* 45:445, 1956.
32. Friedman, M. Plasma cholesterol concentration. *J.A.M.A.* 198:657, 1966.
33. Brown, D. F. Blood lipids and lipoproteins in atherogenesis. *Amer. J. Med.* 46:691, 1969. (This excellent article is part of a symposium on atherosclerosis featured in the same issue.)
34. Frederickson, D. S., Levy, R. I., and Lees, R. S. Fat transport in lipoproteins: An integrated approach to mechanisms and disorders. *New Eng. J. Med.* 276:94, 148, 215, 273, 1967. (A comprehensive review of lipoproteins, emphasizing the types of hyperlipoproteinemia and their clinical management.)
35. Getz, G. S., Vesselinovitch, D., and Wissler, R. W. A dynamic pathology of atherosclerosis. *Amer. J. Med.* 46:657, 1969.
36. Duguid, J. B. The role of connective tissues in arterial diseases. In Page, I. H. (Ed.), *Connective Tissue, Thrombosis and Atherosclerosis.* New York: Academic, 1959.
37. Astrup, T. Role of blood coagulation and fibrinolysis in the pathogenesis of arteriosclerosis. In Page, I. H. (Ed.), *Connective Tissue, Thrombosis and Atherosclerosis.* New York: Academic, 1959.
38. Friedman, M., and Byers, S. O. Experimental thrombo-atherosclerosis. *J. Clin. Invest.* 40:1139, 1961.
39. Conn, J. W., Cohen, E. L., Rovner, D. R., and Nesbit, R. M. Normokalemic primary aldosteronism: A detectable cause of curable essential hypertension. *J.A.M.A.* 193:200, 1965.
40. Laragh, J. H., Sealey, J. E., and Sommers, S. C. Patterns of adrenal secretion and urinary excretion of aldosterone. *Circ. Res.* 18(Suppl.):1, 1966. Plasma renin activity in normal and hypertensive subjects. *Circ. Res.* 19(Suppl.):1, 1966.

41. Schroeder, H. A. Cadmium as a factor in hypertension. *J. Chronic Dis.* 18:647, 1965.
42. Carroll, R. E. The relationship of cadmium in the air to cardiovascular disease death rates. *J.A.M.A.* 198:267, 1966.
43. Dahl, L. K. Salt intake and salt need. *New Eng. J. Med.* 258:1152, 1205, 1958.
44. Schroeder, H. A. Pathogenesis of hypertension. *Amer. J. Med.* 10:189, 1951. (The psychogenic, neurogenic, renal, and endocrine factors in the etiology of hypertension are brought together in a single concept.)
45. Dustan, H. P., Page, I. H., and Poutasse, E. F. Renal hypertension. *New Eng. J. Med.* 261:647, 1959.
46. Perera, G. A. Hypertensive vascular disease: Description and natural history. *J. Chronic Dis.* 1:33, 1955. (An exceptionally important study.)
47. Veterans Administration Cooperative Study Group on Antihypertensive Agents, E. D. Fries, Chairman. Effects of treatment on morbidity in hypertension. *J.A.M.A.* 202:1028, 1967. (An excellent study, of a type that the Veterans Administration is particularly well adapted to conduct.)
48. Kinsey, D., Whitelaw, G. P., Walther, R. J., Theophilus, C. A., and Smithwick, R. H. The long-term follow-up of malignant hypertension. *J.A.M.A.* 181:571, 1962.
49. Morris, J. N. Epidemiology and cardiovascular disease of middle age. *Mod. Conc. Cardiovasc. Dis.* 29:625, 1960.
50. Frank, C. W., Weinblatt, E., Shapiro, S., and Sager, R. V. Myocardial infarction in men: Role of physical activity and smoking in incidence and mortality. *J.A.M.A.* 198:1241, 1966.
51. Doyle, J. T., Dawber, T. R., Kannel, W. B., Kinch, S. H., and Kahn, H. A. The relationship of cigarette smoking to coronary heart disease. *J.A.M.A.* 190:886, 1964.
52. Kershbaum, A., and Bellet, S. Cigarette smoking and blood lipids. *J.A.M.A.* 187:32, 1964.
53. Dawber, T. R. Coronary heart disease: Morbidity in the Framingham study and analysis of factors at risk. *Bibl. Cardiol.* 13:9, 1963. (An important prospective study.)
54. Coodley, E. L. Enzymes in myocardial infarction. *Hosp. Practice* 2:66, 1967.
55. Sommers, H. M., and Jennings, R. B. Experimental acute myocardial infarction. *Lab. Invest.* 13:1491, 1964.
56. Pell, S., and D'Alonzo, C. A. Immediate mortality and five year survival of employed men with a first myocardial infarction. *New Eng. J. Med.* 270:915, 1964.
57. Edwards, J. E. Pathologic spectrum of occlusive coronary arterial disease. *Lab. Invest.* 5:475, 1956. (A survey of the wide range of manifestations of coronary atherosclerosis.)
58. Greendyke, R. M. Traumatic rupture of the aorta: Special reference to automobile accidents. *J.A.M.A.* 195:527, 1966.
59. Garamella, J. J. Schmidt, W. R., Jensen, N. K., and Lynch, M. F. Traumatic aneurysms of the thoracic aorta. *New Eng. J. Med.* 266:1341, 1962.
60. Groves, L. K. Traumatic aneurysm of the thoracic aorta. *New Eng. J. Med.* 270:220, 1964.
61. Neal, R. W., Nair, K. G., and Hecht, H. H. A pathophysiological classification of cor pulmonale. *Mod. Conc. Cardiovasc. Dis.* 37:107, 1968.
62. Austen, F. K., Carmichael, N. W., and Adams, R. D. The neurologic manifestations of chronic pulmonary insufficiency. *New Eng. J. Med.* 257:579, 1957.

63. Leiter, L. Metabolic heart diseases. *Mod. Conc. Cardiovasc. Dis.* 26:403, 1957.
64. Mengel, C. E. Carcinoid and the heart. *Mod. Conc. Cardiovasc. Dis.* 35:75, 1966.
65. Beer – With or Without Cobalt (Editorial). *Lancet* 2:928, 1967.
66. Van Vliet, P. D., Burchell, H. B., and Titus, J. L. Focal myocarditis associated with pheochromocytoma. *New Eng. J. Med.* 274:1102, 1966.
67. Pritchard, R. W. Tumors of the heart: Review of the subject and report of 150 cases. *Arch. Path.* 51:98, 1951. (A classic study.)
68. Cohen, G. U., Peery, T. M., and Evans, J. M. Neoplastic invasion of the heart and pericardium. *Ann. Intern. Med.* 42:1238, 1953.
69. McKusick, V. A., Harris, W. S., Ottesen, O. E., Goodman, R. M., Shelley, W. M., and Bloodwell, R. D. Buerger's disease: A distinct clinical and pathologic entity. *J.A.M.A.* 181:5, 1962.
70. Guyton, A. C. The venous system and its role in the circulation. *Mod. Conc. Cardiovasc. Dis.* 27:483, 1958.

19 THE RESPIRATORY SYSTEM

RESPIRATORY DISEASES: Incidence and mortality

Diseases of the respiratory system cause about 100,000 *deaths* annually in the United States, as compared to over 600,000 deaths attributed to diseases of the cardiovascular system. About 40 percent of all deaths in infants under 1 year are respiratory in nature, most being due to atelectasis of the lungs or pneumonia.

The *incidence* of respiratory diseases, especially infections, is, of course, much higher than the number of deaths therefrom. Upper respiratory infections, notably the common cold, are the most frequently occurring group of ills that human flesh is heir to.

In general the incidence and death rates of respiratory diseases are decreasing. This is particularly true of the infections. Public health measures, immunization, and modern forms of therapy have brought under control the formerly dreaded respiratory infections of childhood such as diphtheria, pertussis, and tuberculosis. Antibiotic therapy has greatly reduced the morbidity and death toll of the pneumonias. On the other hand, the incidence of *bronchogenic carcinoma* steadily rises. Today it is probably the most common type of cancer involving an internal organ, causing over 15 percent of all cancer deaths.

DISEASES OF THE UPPER RESPIRATORY SYSTEM

1. Upper Respiratory Infections

Upper respiratory infections (URI) due to *viruses* (the common cold, influenza, and adenovirus infections) are discussed in Chapter 7. *Bacterial diseases* involving the nasopharynx, oropharynx, larynx, and trachea, such as scarlet fever, septic sore throat, and diphtheria, are described in Chapter 5.

RHINITIS:

Rhinitis is an inflammation of the nasal cavity. It may be initiated by viruses or allergens. Allergic rhinitis is discussed in Chapter 4. The viral rhinitides are very frequently complicated by superimposed bacterial infections, the common organisms being streptococci, staphylococci, pneumococci, and *Hemophilus influenzae.* Bacterial infections may also develop during acute allergic rhinitis. An underlying factor in bacterial rhinitis is injury to the mucosal cilia caused by viruses, allergens, exposure to cold or dampness, excessive drying, or dust inhalation.

Clinical features

Clinically there is usually a fever with malaise and muscle aching. Breathing through the nose is difficult or impossible, because of the nasal mucosal swelling. The watery or mucoid nasal discharge becomes thick and mucopurulent when bacterial infection develops. Concomitant inflammation of the sinus, pharynx, and larynx is common.

Pathologic changes: acute rhinitis

In *acute rhinitis* the nasal mucosa is pinkish gray to angry red and moderately to severely swollen. The surfaces are covered with serous fluid or thin mucus early and with a mucopurulent discharge or frank pus later. Superficial ulceration may occur. Focal submucosal thickenings due to edema give rise to polypoid masses. The *nasal polyp* is pinkish gray and edematous, and it may attain a remarkably large size. *Microscopically* it is lined by pseudostratified columnar or stratified squamous epithelium. The stroma is loose, edematous, and infiltrated with eosinophils and mononuclear cells. Mucous retention cysts or false cysts due to pooling of serous fluid may be present. Choanal polyp arises in the nose or a maxillary sinus and hangs by a long pedicle in the nasopharynx. The persistence of these polyps leads to *chronic hypertrophic rhinitis.*

atrophic rhinitis

Atrophic rhinitis (rhinitis sicca, ozena) occurs following a prolonged suppurative infection. The nasal mucosa becomes shiny and dry. The epithelial surface is thin and shows focal squamous metaplasia. Collagenous scarring is found in the submucosa, and the mucous glands are atrophic.

Complications

Complications of rhinitis are uncommon but include septic cavernous sinus thrombophlebitis, osteomyelitis of adjacent bones, epidural, subdural, and/or brain abscess, and meningitis.

SINUSITIS:

Sinusitis is an inflammation of one or more accessory nasal sinuses and may be acute or chronic.

Acute sinusitis:

Acute sinusitis may be due to coagulase-positive and coagulase-negative staphylococci, streptococci, pneumococci, or gram-negative bacilli. Obstruction of the sinus orifice is a contributory etiologic factor. *Clinically* acute sinusitis is characterized by headache, pain and tenderness in the region of the affected sinus, disturbances in the sense of smell, purulent discharge from the affected sinus, and failure of transillumination of light through the sinus.

pathologic changes

The *sinus mucosa* is edematous and red, showing microscopically an acute inflammation. The edema may occlude the orifice, and a purulent exudate may collect within the sinus *(empyema of the sinus).*

complications

Complications include ulceration of the mucosa, cellulitis or abscess of the orbit, osteomyelitis of the adjacent bone, especially the maxilla from maxillary sinusitis, cavernous sinus thrombophlebitis from ethmoidal or sphenoidal sinusitis, and extradural, subdural, or brain abscess from frontal, ethmoidal, or sphenoidal sinusitis.

Chronic sinusitis:

Chronic sinusitis may be caused by the same bacteria as the acute form, which it usually follows. Chronic sinusitis, bronchiectasis, and dextrocardia or situs inversus viscerum make up *Kartagener's triad.*

pathologic changes

The *hypertrophic type* is characterized by sessile or pedunculated polyps projecting into the sinus. The *polyps* consist of loose myxomatous tissue covered by pseudostratified columnar or stratified squamous epithelium. The core is infiltrated with eosinophils and mononuclear cells. The *atrophic type* shows a thin submucosa with a few mucous glands. The accumulation of large amounts of mucus produces a mucocele of the sinus.

PHARYNGITIS:

Acute pharyngitis (sore throat) is common in upper respiratory infections. Septic sore throat and scarlet fever, due to beta-hemolytic streptococci, and diphtheria are discussed under Acute Bacterial Diseases in Chapter 5. Other types of pharyngitis are caused by alpha-hemolytic streptococci, staphylococci, pneumococci, and *Hemophilus influenzae.*

Pathologic changes

The *pharyngeal mucosa* is red, swollen, and velvety. A mucous, purulent or fibrinous exudate may cover it. *Microscopically* there is acute inflammation in the mucosa and submucosa, with hyperplasia of the submucosal lymph follicles.

Complications

Occasionally a pharyngitis may be severe enough to produce a *retropharyngeal* or *lateral pharyngeal abscess.* In these the suppuration extends between the pharyngeal wall and the cervical fascia. In *retropharyngeal abscess* a mass bulges in the midline. In *lateral pharyngeal abscess* the tonsil and tonsillar pillars bulge medially. The process may extend into the mediastinum and posterior triangle of the neck. Streptococci are the most common cause of these complications.

TONSILLITIS:

Chronic tonsillitis

Tonsillitis may be acute or chronic, the latter form being characterized by a persistent tonsillar enlargement to a diameter greater than 2 cm. due to lymphoid hyperplasia. Such enlargement, especially of the adenoids, may lead to chronic mouth breathing and the development of a high-arched palate and a characteristic dull, open-mouthed facies. In the later stages of chronic tonsillitis, fibrosis results in marked shrinkage of the glands.

Acute tonsillitis:

Acute tonsillitis is common in upper respiratory infections due to streptococci, staphylococci, pneumococci, and meningococci. The palatine tonsils are enlarged and edematous, with marked lymphoid hyperplasia (follicular tonsillitis). The crypts are filled with a purulent, patchy, white exudate. This exudate may inspissate and calcify, producing a *tonsillolith.*

complications

Complications include *peritonsillar abscess (quinsy)* (an extension of the tonsillar infection into the surrounding tissue, anterior pillars, uvula, and adjacent soft palate, the tonsils being pushed toward the midline), *lateral pharyngeal abscess,* and *retropharyngeal abscess.*

Tonsillar tuberculosis

Tuberculosis of the tonsils may occur as a primary infection, sometimes due to the bovine tubercle bacillus. The tonsils may contain large foci of caseation, and the mucosa may ulcerate. The anterior cervical lymph nodes are often involved in the tuberculous process. Tuberculous cervical lymphadenitis is known as *scrofula (king's evil).*

LARYNGITIS:

Acute laryngitis

Acute laryngitis may occur in upper respiratory infections, producing hoarseness clinically. Severe inflammation causes respiratory obstruction, which requires tracheotomy. Laryngitis may be caused by streptococci, pneumococci, or *Hemophilus influenzae.* Nonbacterial causes include steam and noxious gases such as chlorine. The *larynx* is red and edematous. *Microscopically* there is acute inflammation in the submucosa. Fibrin may be deposited on the mucosa.

Chronic laryngitis:

Chronic laryngitis is associated with excessive cigarette smoking [1], chronic alcoholism, or overuse of the vocal cords. Hoarseness and huskiness of the voice are typical. Tuberculosis and syphilis may also produce chronic laryngitis.

pathologic changes

The surface is opaque and covered with small papillary projections. The mucosa is acanthotic *(pachydermia laryngis)*, and lymphocytes are found in the submucosa.

Acute epiglottitis:

Acute epiglottitis (bacterial croup) [2], a dire medical emergency, is an acute inflammation which appears most commonly in children from about 1 to 5 years of age. The majority of cases are due to *Hemophilus influenzae* type B, other causative organisms being *Diplococcus pneumoniae*, beta-hemolytic streptococci, and *Staphylococcus aureus*. *Clinically* the infant or child rapidly develops sore throat, fever, respiratory distress, a "croupy" cough, drooling, leukocytosis, cyanosis, and even coma. Death due to respiratory obstruction may result unless a tracheotomy is performed.

clinical features

pathologic changes

The bulging *epiglottis* is bright cherry red and moderately to markedly swollen, sometimes to five to 10 times its normal size. The swelling produces laryngeal obstruction. *Microscopically* the epiglottic submucosa is intensely edematous, hyperemic, and infiltrated with neutrophils.

Acute laryngotracheitis:

Acute laryngotracheitis (croup) is an acute respiratory infection of infants and young children characterized clinically by a hoarse, ringing cough and difficulty in breathing. It is caused by streptococci, *Hemophilus influenzae*, and viruses such as those of influenza and adenoviruses.

pathologic changes

Grossly the mucosa of the epiglottis, larynx, and trachea is swollen and brilliant red. *Epiglottic edema* may be marked, producing extreme respiratory difficulty. The mucosa of the epiglottis, larynx, and trachea is covered by a thin *fibrinous membrane*. Large amounts of mucus are found in the trachea. The submucosa is infiltrated with neutrophils. The *anterior cervical lymph nodes* are often enlarged and show lymphoid hyperplasia.

Necrotizing tracheitis:

Necrotizing tracheitis [3] occurs below a tracheostomy stoma, beginning at the site of impingement of an inserted cannula. It is most common in patients with burns of the face and neck. The most frequent causative organisms are *Staphylococcus aureus, Pseudomonas aeruginosa*, and *Proteus* species.

pathologic changes

There is erosion of the tracheal mucosa sometimes extending down to the rings of cartilage. *Microscopically* an acute inflammatory reaction and necrosis are found. In some cases, especially those due to *Pseudomonas*, there is an acute vasculitis with bacterial invasion of arterial walls.

BRONCHITIS:

Acute bronchitis:

Acute bronchitis is usually due to extension downward of an upper respiratory infection. It may be due to streptococci, pneumococci, *Staphylococcus aureus*, or *Hemophilus influenzae*. A tracheitis is usually associated *(acute tracheobronchitis)*.

pathologic changes

The inflammation may be catarrhal or mucopurulent in nature. Abundant mucus is found in the bronchial lumen, and the bronchial wall is bright red grossly. There is a polymorphonuclear leukocytic or mononuclear infiltrate in the submucosa.

Chronic bronchitis: clinical features

Chronic bronchitis usually occurs in cigarette smokers, typically appearing after several years of smoking. It is characterized *clinically* by a chronic cough (smoker's hack), which is often productive of mucoid sputum; scattered rhonchi and wheezing; and, in many cases, signs of an associated pulmonary emphysema. *Bacteria* isolated from bronchial secretions in cases of chronic bronchitis include *Diplococcus pneumoniae, Staphylococcus aureus,* and *Hemophilus influenzae. Clinical flare-ups* appear to be caused by *viruses,* especially the respiratory syncytial virus, influenza virus, and adenoviruses, and the pleuropneumonia-like organism, *Mycoplasma pneumoniae* [4]. A majority of patients with chronic bronchitis show a positive test for anti-gamma globulin rheumatoid-like factors, indicating that there is an auto-immune response in this disease [5].

pathologic changes

Mucus is often found in the lumen of the bronchi, and the bronchial mucous glands are hyperplastic. The bronchial walls are somewhat thickened by fibrosis. In the submucosa there is an infiltration of lymphocytes and macrophages. There may be foci of squamous metaplasia of the bronchial epithelium, and the epithelial basement membrane is thickened. In a few cases the bronchial mucosa becomes very dry and thin (atrophic chronic bronchitis).

2. *Upper Respiratory Neoplasms*

NEOPLASMS OF THE NASAL CAVITY AND SINUS:

Neoplasms of the nasal cavity and paranasal sinus include *basal cell carcinoma* of the mucocutaneous junction, papilloma, epidermoid carcinoma and adenocarcinoma, and olfactory nerve tumors.

Papilloma

Squamous or transitional cell papilloma [6] is uncommon in the nasal cavity and occurs less often in a paranasal sinus. The neoplasm is more common in men than women and may reach a large size and obstruct the nasal fossa. It frequently recurs following surgical removal. *Grossly* the papilloma is firm and verrucous when it develops on the nasal septum *(septal papilloma). Microscopically* it consists of a papillary mass lined by squamous or transitional epithelium. Mitoses and dyskeratosis (the loss of cellular polarity and the presence of atypical cells) are frequent. An *inverted papilloma* is characterized by an inward growth of a squamous or transitional papilloma and usually arises from the middle meatus or middle or inferior turbinate. Malignant change to an epidermoid carcinoma with metastases is not uncommon. A few nasal or sinus papillomas are *adenomatous polyps* arising from submucosal mucous glands.

Carcinoma

Carcinoma of the nasal cavity and paranasal sinus [7] occurs most frequently in a maxillary antrum. Only about 25 percent arise in the nasal cavity. Most of the cases develop in the 40 to 70 year age group, and about 65 percent of the patients are men. The most common clinical signs are nasal obstruction, epistaxis, cheek swelling, and radiologic evidence of bone destruction. *Grossly* the neoplasms are papillary or fungating and frequently ulcerated. *Microscopically* about 80 percent are epidermoid carcinoma arising from the mucosa. The remainder are adenocarcinoma derived from submucosal mucous glands. Invasion of adjacent bone is common, but *metastases* to cervical lymph nodes are infrequent despite the usually advanced stage of these neoplasms by the time they are diagnosed.

Olfactory neuroepithelioma

Olfactory esthesioneuroepithelioma [8] arises high in the nasal fossa from neuroepithelial cells of the olfactory membrane. It is equally common in males and females. *Clinically* there are progressive nasal obstruction and epistaxis. The neoplasm almost always recurs after surgery. It is *highly radiosensitive. Grossly* it is polypoid, friable, and gray or grayish red. *Microscopically* there are two cell types, cylindrical cells arranged about a lumen *(rosettes)* and sheets and cords of undifferentiated neuroblasts with abundant cytoplasm and indistinct cell membranes. The cells forming rosettes are derived from the bipolar nerve cells of the olfactory organ. The neoplasm is highly vascular, and foci of necrosis are common. It *invades locally* into the paranasal sinus, hard palate, orbit, cranium, and brain. *Occasionally there are metastases* of undifferentiated cells to the lungs, lymph nodes, and bones.

Nasal glioma

Nasal glioma is developmental in origin and consists of a distorted mass of glial tissue within the nasal fossa.

NEOPLASMS OF THE NASOPHARYNX: Carcinoma

Carcinoma of the nasopharynx [9] makes up about 1 percent of all malignant neoplasms and is more common in men than women by 3:1. In the United States it usually occurs in the 50 to 70 age range; it is especially common in the Chinese. The *primary lesion* is often silent, becoming apparent due to bone erosion or cervical lymph node metastases. Exophytic neoplasms cause obstruction of the nose or eustachian tube. Hearing loss, epistaxis, cranial nerve involvement, and development of a cervical mass are common findings. *Cervical metastases* are present in about two-thirds of the cases at the time of diagnosis. Neoplasms which are limited to the nasopharynx are designated as *stage 1,* those with palpable cervical lymph nodes as *stage 2,* those with local invasion of the skull, orbit, and sinus and/or neurologic signs as *stage 3,* and those with distant metastases as *stage 4. Most* of these carcinomas *are radiosensitive,* and radiation is the treatment of choice. They may recur 10 or more years after apparent "cure." *Nasopharyngeal carcinoma arises most commonly on a lateral wall.* Some are exophytic, but most are infiltrative and ulcerated. *Microscopically about 85 percent are classified as epidermoid carcinomas, and of these about 80 percent are undifferentiated (grade III or IV).* Mucosal (clear cell), spindle cell, transitional cell, and mixed types of epidermoid carcinoma are recognized. Occasionally *mucinous adenocarcinoma* which is often papillary and very well differentiated, *adenoid cystic carcinoma,* and *mucoepidermoid carcinoma* occur in the nasopharynx. When the atypical epithelium in a nasopharyngeal carcinoma maintains its relationship to the underlying lymphoid tissue, the neoplasm is sometimes referred to as a *lymphoepithelioma.*

Angiofibroma:

Angiofibroma of the nasopharynx [10] usually occurs in adolescent boys and sometimes regresses spontaneously at about 25 years. It arises in the ventral periosteum or the fascia basalis, usually in the nasopharyngeal recess or at the base of the sphenoid bone. Occasionally it is multicentric in origin. The neoplasm tends to recur following excision. *Clinically* the early signs are nasal congestion and hemorrhage. The voice becomes flat. Later there are pain and a mucopurulent discharge. Exophthalmos occurs if the orbit is invaded, and with very large fibromas a "frog face" develops.

clinical features

pathologic changes

The *angiofibroma* may attain a large size and is usually pedunculated. The tumor is pinkish gray and spongy, and its surface may be ulcerated. Growth is expansive, and there is sometimes extension into the cranial cavity. *Microscopically* it consists of highly vascular and cellular fibrous tissue. Hemorrhages are common.

Sarcomas:

Sarcoma of the nasopharynx makes up about 35 percent of neoplasms of this region, in the United States. The types include plasmocytoma, malignant lymphomas, fibrosarcoma, and very rarely sarcoma botryoides. Fibrosarcoma has developed in an angiofibroma following x-radiation therapy [11]. About 75 percent of reported *extramedullary plasmocytomas* have occurred in the upper respiratory tract and oral cavity [12]. Those in the nasopharynx, nasal cavity, and maxillary sinus are more common in men than women and usually appear in the 50 to 60 year age group. Grossly the plasmocytoma is a red or gray, highly vascular, polypoid submucosal mass with a pink to yellowish gray cut surface. Microscopically it consists of sheets of tightly packed atypical plasmocytes. Some of these neoplasms develop in existing cases of multiple myeloma, and a significant number of solitary extramedullary plasmocytomas eventuate in plasma cell myeloma.

Plasmocytoma

NEOPLASMS OF THE LARYNX: Laryngeal papilloma

Papilloma of the larynx is the most common neoplasm in that organ. It has a nasty tendency to recur despite seemingly adequate surgical removal. Laryngeal papillomata occur most often in children, in whom they are usually multiple, rarely become malignant, and tend to regress spontaneously at puberty. Papillomata in children are possibly caused by a virus. In adults the lesion is common in singers (tenor's nodes) and has a tendency to become malignant. It is most common on the vocal cords and anterior commissure, which lies just behind the thyroid cartilage. The papilloma is squamous cell in type and has a verrucous appearance. The submucosa is edematous and is infiltrated with lymphocytes and macrophages.

Laryngeal carcinoma:

Carcinoma of the larynx [13] constitutes about 1 percent of all malignant neoplasms. It is more common in men than in women by about 10:1, and most cases appear at about age 60. Most cases of intrinsic carcinoma occur in cigarette smokers. The heavy drinking of whiskey is also predisposing, especially for extrinsic carcinoma [14] In many patients there is a preceding history of chronic inflammation, leukoplakia, or a papilloma of the larynx. *Hoarseness* is the earliest and most prominent symptom.

pathologic changes

About 95 percent of laryngeal carcinomas are epidermoid, with a few transitional cell, basal cell, or adenocarcinomas arising there. The lesion begins as a papillary neoplasm or as a flat, indurated mucosal patch. In time ulceration and destruction of adjacent structures occur.

intrinsic carcinoma

Intrinsic carcinoma of the larynx arises on a vocal fold (usually on the anterior third) or ventricular fold or in a ventricular pouch. Most of these carcinomas are grade I or II. *Metastases* in this type are late and go first to the deep cervical lymph nodes.

extrinsic carcinoma

Extrinsic carcinoma of the larynx arises from the epiglottis [15], an aryepiglottic fold, the pyriform sinus, or a vallecula epiglottica. Most of these carcinomas are grade III or IV. Metastases to the cervical lymph nodes occur early.

NEOPLASMS OF THE TRACHEA: Papilloma

Tracheal neoplasms are extraordinarily rare. Among the benign tumors is the *squamous papilloma* [16]. This neoplasm occurs about one-hundredth as frequently as laryngeal papilloma. It consists of a verrucous mass projecting into the tracheal lumen. *Microscopically* thick sheets of stratified squamous epithelium cover a slender fibrovascular stroma.

Carcinoma:

Tracheogenic carcinoma [17] constitutes less than 0.1 percent of fatal malignant neoplasms and about 50 percent of tracheal tumors in adults. Strangely there has been *no increase in incidence of carcinoma of the trachea* to parallel the marked rise in frequency of bronchogenic carcinoma, even though epithelial cellular atypia, basal cell hyperplasia, squamous metaplasia, and mucosal thickening have been noted in cigarette smokers and patients with pneumonia [18]. This phenomenon has not been completely explained. It has been hypothesized that the lower incidence of malignant change in the trachea is due to the greater velocity of cilial motility in the trachea, a moving mucous shield ("mucus raft") in the trachea, decreased viscosity and adhesiveness of the tracheal mucus, and/or the straightness and relatively large lumen of the tracheal tube. All these factors plus a vigorous cough reflex are thought to decrease the concentration of cigarette smoke condensate and other carcinogens in the tracheal mucosal cells. *Clinically* tracheal carcinoma is characterized early by a hacking, irritating cough occasionally productive of blood-streaked sputum and slight wheezing. Later dyspnea, hoarseness due to recurrent laryngeal nerve paralysis by extension of the neoplasm, wheezing, and a crowing stridor occur together with cervical lymphadenopathy.

pathologic changes

Grossly the neoplasm is an *elevated, ovoid mass* measuring up to 6 cm. in diameter. It may show extensive central necrosis and ulceration. *Microscopically* it is typically a *poorly differentiated epidermoid carcinoma. Metastases* occur late in the course. The cervical lymph nodes are involved first. In a few cases widespread metastases have occurred.

3. Miscellaneous Upper Respiratory Diseases

Acne rosacea

Acne rosacea involves the skin of the nose, cheek, and occasionally chin and forehead. It is more common in men than women, and is often associated with chronic alcoholism or occupational exposure to heat or cold. It begins in early adult life as *erythematous foci* which disappear periodically and then gradually become permanent. The involved skin is red and oily, and papules and pustules develop within it. The sebaceous gland ducts are plugged with inspissated sebum. *Microscopically* the *sebaceous glands* are enlarged and surrounded by lymphocytic infiltrates, and the dermal capillaries are telangiectatic.

Rhinophyma

Rhinophyma (Pfundnase) is the final stage of acne rosacea. There is a moderate to marked *nodular thickening of the skin of the nose,* especially of the alae nasae. *Microscopically* there are *hypertrophy and possibly hyperplasia of the sebaceous glands* as well as squamous metaplasia of the sebaceous glandular epithelium. The ducts are filled with cellular debris. Infestation with the mite *Demodex folliculorum* is common. A dermal lymphocytic infiltrate and telangiectasia are frequently seen.

Wegener's granulomatosis:

Wegener's granulomatosis [19] is rare and probably represents a profound hypersensitivity reaction. *Clinically* there are sinusitis, pulmonary disturbances, otitis, albuminuria, hematuria, and later uremia. Death often occurs within a year of the onset.

pathologic changes

In the paranasal sinus, nasal and oral cavities, larynx, and trachea there is ulceration. A *necrotizing granulomatous reaction* with many giant cells and foamy macrophages may be present in the submucosa. Necrotic granulomatous foci are also found in the lungs, spleen, liver, lymph nodes, and elsewhere. In the kidneys the characteristic lesion is a *focal necrotizing glomerulitis* resembling the "flea-bitten" kidney of subacute bacterial endocarditis. In many organs there is a focal necrotizing vasculitis involving arteries and veins. The *arterial lesions* are like those of periarteritis nodosa and often show healing by fibrosis.

Lethal granulomatosis

Lethal midline granulomatosis [20] is a rare, idiopathic, *necrotizing granulomatous inflammation* which progressively destroys the soft tissues and bones of the nose, paranasal sinus, soft palate, and pharynx. *Microscopically* there is a heavy inflammatory cellular infiltrate consisting predominantly of macrophages. Foreign-body giant cells may be present. There is extensive necrosis of the involved tissues. No or minor vascular lesions are found. Death results from the tissue destruction and secondary infection.

Hyperkeratosis of tonsil

Hyperkeratosis of the tonsil (mycosis leptothrica) occurs in young adults and is characterized by *white flaky patches on the tonsillar surfaces* which do not bleed on removal. *Microscopically* there are acanthosis and hyperkeratosis of the mucosa with keratin plugs within the crypts. Mycelia and colonies of *Leptothrix* species are present within the crypts. The tonsillar lymphoid tissue shows atrophy and fibrosis.

Pharyngeal bursitis

The pharyngeal bursa is a deep crypt in the adenoid tissue of the nasopharyngeal wall. It normally obliterates after puberty. *Pharyngeal bursitis (Thornwaldt's disease)* occurs in children and adolescents due to occlusion of the orifice by hyperplastic lymphoid tissue. The bursa becomes distended by accumulation of an inflammatory exudate, mucus, cellular debris, and cholesterol.

"Granulomas" of larynx

Postintubation "granulomas" of the larynx [21] occur in 1 in about 800 endotracheal anesthesias. The "granuloma" appears from 2 weeks to 7 months after the anesthetic procedure. The cause is thought to be the autonomic movements of the arytenoid cartilages against the endotracheal tube. It occurs much more commonly in women than men, and the majority of cases has been associated with thyroid surgery. Most "granulomas" occur on the posterior third of the vocal cords. They are not uncommonly bilateral. The lesions begin as ulcers, and bilateral lesions may oppose each other as "kissing ulcers." Granulation tissue grows in from the base and mounts up into a polypoid *pyogenic granuloma* consisting of capillaries, fibroblasts, and inflammatory cells. Later the mass becomes fibrous, and re-epithelialization covers the ulcer surface.

ASTHMA

ASTHMA:

Asthma may be due to bacterial or nonbacterial causes, about 2 percent of the cases being infectious in origin (bronchitic asthma). In both types hypersensitivity is the mechanism, in the former to bacterial protein and in the latter to a variety of organic and inorganic substances. The hypersensitivity leads to bronchial spasm, edema of the bronchial wall, and secretion of large amounts of viscid mucus. About 2 percent of Americans have bronchial asthma, and over 5000 deaths are attributed to it annually. *Clinically* it is characterized by paroxysmal episodes of dyspnea, in which there is great difficulty in expiration. Wheezing and rhonchi are heard. Deaths related to asthma may occur in *status asthmaticus* or may be due to cardiac and pulmonary complications, such as cor pulmonale, pulmonary emphysema, or pneumonia.

Pathologic changes

The *larger bronchi* contain large amounts of mucus, and the mucosa is edematous and injected. The walls of *medium-sized and small bronchi* are thickened, and their lumina are narrowed and filled with mucus. There are a thickening and hyalinization of the epithelial basement membrane in the medium-sized bronchi. The epithelium is thickened and may show ulceration or squamous metaplasia.

There is hypertrophy of the musculature of these bronchi. The submucosa shows moderate fibrosis and eosinophilic infiltration. Bronchial glands are often distended with mucus. In pronounced cases the *lungs* are emphysematous.

Sputum findings

The sputum contains twisted spirals of mucus from bronchioles (Curschmann's spirals), Laennec's pearls, Charcot-Leyden crystals which are derived from the nuclei of eosinophils [22], plugs of inspissated mucus, epithelial cells, macrophages, and eosinophils. *Curschmann's spirals* are irregularly wound, long, thin mucus threads. *Laennec's pearls* are tiny, bright, round or tear-shaped granules, and *Charcot-Leyden crystals* have the shape of two very broad-based, flat pyramids placed base to base.

Churg-Strauss syndrome

The *Churg-Strauss syndrome* [23] is asthma associated with disseminated necrotizing granulomatous vasculitis. *Clinically* there are severe asthma, mild fever, cutaneous and subcutaneous nodules, cutaneous purpura or an erythematous maculopapular or pustular rash, abdominal pain, bloody diarrhea, pericardial effusion, and eosinophilia. The onset usually occurs in adult life, and death typically ensues within 3 years of the onset. *Pathologically* there are widespread necrotizing granulomata about medium-sized arteries and veins. In a few cases the lesions are indistinguishable from those of polyarteritis nodosa. The lesion typically begins within the vessel wall or its supporting connective tissue. The *fully developed granuloma* shows a central zone of necrosis surrounded by epithelioid cells, which are often palisaded about the necrotic focus, and an outer zone of eosinophils and lymphocytes. The lesions are especially common in the lungs, myocardium, liver, and spleen.

DEVELOPMENTAL DEFECTS OF THE LUNGS

Malformations of the lungs severe enough to affect pulmonary function seriously are uncommon. *Developmental defects* include abnormalities in size, lobulation, position, and composition.

1. *Abnormalities in Size*

AGENESIS

Complete agenesis of the lungs occurs only in acephalic and acardiac monsters. *Bilateral primary aplasia or hypoplasia* is rare and is associated with severe malformations elsewhere. *Unilateral agenesis or aplasia* is also rare. When the right lung is absent, there may also be dextrocardia.

APLASIA

In *aplasia* there are only a few rudimentary bronchi without pulmonary or vascular structures.

HYPOPLASIA

Secondary hypoplasia may be due to any condition which decreases the thoracic space early in fetal life. The most severe secondary hypoplasias are associated with diaphragmatic hernia, especially in the lung ipsilateral with the diaphragmatic defect. Pulmonary hypoplasia may also be associated with idiopathic cardiac hypertrophy and polycystic kidneys which elevate the diaphragmatic leaves. Moderate hypoplasia is associated with bilateral renal agenesis. *Microscopically in severe hypoplasia* the bronchi are disproportionately increased in number, and the alveolar ducts and alveoli are less numerous and incompletely differentiated.

2. Abnormalities in Lobulation

Incomplete lobar separation is common, partial fusion of the right upper and middle lobes being the most frequent form. Rarely complete lack of lobar separation is found in one or both lungs. SEPARATION DEFECTS

The *azygos lobe* is an additional one found at either apex and has no clinical significance. AZYGOS LOBE

Sequestration is the formation of pulmonary tissue without communication with a bronchial tree. *Sequestered masses of pulmonary tissue may be intralobar, extralobar* (in a separate lobe still attached to the lung), *or completely separated from the lungs (accessory lung).* The extralobar and complete types occur almost exclusively on the left side, often in association with a defect of the left diaphragmatic leaf. Infection is common in intralobar sequestration. *Microscopically* the sequestered pulmonary tissue appears normal. SEQUESTRATION

3. Abnormalities in Position

Abnormal position of a lung is secondary to (1) diaphragmatic hernia with displacement of abdominal viscera into the thorax, (2) unilateral pneumothorax, or (3) pleural effusion. In *situs inversus* the positions of the right and left lungs are reversed. ABNORMAL POSITION

4. Abnormalities in Composition

Cystic disease of the lungs is the presence of one or more bronchogenic cysts. *Congenital polycystic lungs* may be associated with cysts of the liver, pancreas, and kidneys. Cysts may be present throughout both lungs or limited to part or all of one lobe. In size they may vary from microscopic to several centimeters in diameter. Cysts develop by sequestration of bronchial tissue or abnormal diverticulum formation during embryonic development of the tracheobronchial tree. Although they are *bronchogenic in origin,* many become separated from their bronchial communication. *Bronchogenic cysts* which appear in young adults represent a less severe form of defective bronchial development [24]. POLYCYSTIC LUNGS:

Congenital polycystic disease of the lungs is found most often in stillborn fetuses. Less severe forms are compatible with life and may remain asymptomatic until infection of a cyst occurs. Some patients complain of chest pain or discomfort, and some have a cough productive of thick mucoid sputum. Cysts which have no communication with a bronchus are filled with thick mucinous fluid; those with a bronchial communication may show air or fluid levels on chest x-ray films.

Grossly the cyst is round or ovoid and thin-walled. The inner lining is smooth and glistening and may show trabeculations. Most large cysts are subpleural. *Microscopically* the cysts are typically lined by a single layer of columnar epithelium. In large cysts the epithelium may have disappeared. Squamous metaplasia is sometimes found. In the cyst wall atrophic smooth muscle strands, foci of cartilage, and distorted mucous glands may be present. Pathologic changes

THE PNEUMONIAS

1. *Infectious Pneumonitides*

Pneumonia (pneumonitis) is an inflammation of the lungs characterized by consolidation; it is usually acute. Pneumonia ranks high as an immediate cause of death in the United States. However, most of these deaths are cases of bronchopneumonia secondary to some other disease process. Pneumonia may be a primary disease or secondary to some other process, such as chronic passive congestion of the lungs in which case it is known as *hypostatic pneumonia* and is often found in the dependent portions of the lungs. Pneumonia also is common in cases of debilitation. *Postoperative pneumonia* is due to aspiration, mucus-plug formation, and depression of the cough reflex by anesthesia. *Post-traumatic pneumonia* is due to compression of the respiratory cage. *Viral pneumonias* are discussed in Chapter 7.

Incidence

Pneumonia is more common in males than in females, and in infants and aged persons than in adults.

General pathologic changes

Agents causing pneumonia may reach the lungs either aerogenously or hematogenously *(embolic pneumonia)*, i.e., by inhalation or by septic pulmonary embolism. Aerogenous infection is by far the more common method. The *essential feature* of the pneumonias is inflammation of the lungs, with the accumulation of an exudate in the tissues and spaces of the respiratory tract. If the exudate is rich in fibrinogen, it will clot as fibrin and keep the tissues firm as long as the alveolar walls are intact. This feature often accounts for the *consolidation* which is typical of many pneumonias.

LOBAR PNEUMONIA:

Lobar pneumonia constitutes over 90 percent of all primary bacterial pneumonias, and about 95 percent of the cases of lobar pneumonia are due to the *pneumococcus, Diplococcus pneumoniae. D. pneumoniae* is a small, nonmotile, gram-positive coccus with one pointed or lance-shaped end. The organism usually occurs in pairs as a diplococcus. The pneumococcus is encapsulated and produces alpha hemolysis, a leukocidin, a necrotizing substance, and hyaluronidase. It is bile-soluble and ferments inulin. The capsule swells in type-specific antiserum (Neufeld quellung reaction). Many individuals are *carriers* of pneumococci, and other factors besides the presence of the organisms appear to be necessary for the development of clinical disease. Among these are exposure to cold or dampness. Pneumonia is more common in debilitated persons and chronic alcoholics than in healthy individuals. Lobar pneumonia occurs most often in the winter and early spring, and it is more frequent in men than in women by 3:1. Before the advent of antibiotic therapy the mortality in lobar pneumonia ranged as high as 30 percent, but today it is less than 5 percent. (Lobar pneumonia due to *Klebsiella pneumoniae* is discussed on page 101.)

Clinical features

Clinically lobar pneumonia is characterized by the sudden onset of shaking chills, fever, prostration, chest pain, cough, dyspnea, and rusty sputum. Pneumococci are found in the sputum. There is dullness on percussion over the affected lobe, with bronchial breath sounds and fine crackling and/or crepitant rales on auscultation. Leukocytosis is usually pronounced. On x-ray, infiltration of the pneumonic lobe is seen. The disease runs an acute febrile course which ends suddenly in untreated, nonfatal cases with a crisis on the ninth day, following which recovery is rapid. With the use of antibiotics the course is now run in about 3 days. *Walking (ambulatory) pneumonia* is an occasional cause of sudden death.

Patho-genesis

Pneumococci enter the affected lung through the respiratory tree and become entrapped in mucus in small bronchi and bronchioles. They proliferate in these tubes and spread to the alveoli, where they produce an acute inflammatory reaction. This process spreads rapidly through the lung until a natural barrier such as interlobar fissure is reached. Bacteremia is common in lobar pneumonia.

Pathologic changes:

Lobar pneumonia occurs in the right lung in about 50 percent of the cases, in the left lung in about 40 percent, and in both lungs *(double pneumonia)* in about 10 percent. Lobar pneumonia occurs more often in the lower lobes than in the upper lobes by about 9:1.

red hepa-tization

Red hepatization is the typical picture during the first 3 days of the disease. In this stage the affected lobe is red, consolidated, and heavy; it will sink in water. The parenchyma is friable. *Microscopically* the lung shows an intense hyperemia, the small vessels and alveolar capillaries being engorged. The *alveolar exudate* consists of large numbers of red cells and polymorphonuclear leukocytes. Large amounts of fibrin are found in the alveolar spaces.

gray hepa-tization

Gray hepatization is the characteristic stage from the fourth to the eighth day in the typical course of untreated lobar pneumonia. In this stage the involved lobe is often covered with fibrin. The cut surface is gray, dry, and granular. *Microscopically* the alveoli are uniformly filled throughout the lobe with a fibrinous network which connects through the pores of Kohn. Within the alveoli are many neutrophils and some erythrocytes. The alveolar walls are edematous and the capillaries hyperemic. The *alveolar walls are remarkably intact.* This is explained by the fact that, although suppuration occurs and proteolytic enzymes are released by the breakdown of neutrophils, there is sufficient space in the alveoli for the exudation of large amounts of plasma containing antienzymes which neutralize the proteolytic enzymes, preventing tissue destruction.

resolution

Resolution begins on about the third day in the portion of the lobe involved earliest and is present throughout the lobe on about the ninth day in the course of untreated lobar pneumonia. In this stage there is a decrease in the firmness of the involved lobe due to dissolution of the fibrin. *Microscopically* by this time the neutrophils are degenerated, macrophages and lymphocytes have appeared in the alveolar spaces, and removal of the exudate has begun. Typically the exudate is completely resorbed without tissue destruction in about 2 weeks, and the lobe is left just as it was before the start of the pneumonic process.

organiza-tion (carnifica-tion)

Although the usual outcome of lobar pneumonia is a complete resolution of the inflammatory process, in a few cases the involved lung becomes organized. In these cases the fibrin within the alveoli is invaded by fibroblasts, and the alveolar spaces are filled with a dense cellular fibrous tissue which grows along the fibrin network. The fibrin on the pleura may also be organized by the invasion of fibroblasts, with the formation of dense fibrous adhesions which obliterate the pleural space. *Grossly* areas of the lung which have undergone organization are firm and gray, with a somewhat fleshy appearance. The portions of the lung in which this *intra-alveolar fibrosis* occurs lose their capacity for aeration, and if the large foci are involved, respiratory difficulty will follow.

complications

Complications of lobar pneumonia include pleural effusion, which may be serous or serofibrinous; empyema (a large collection of pus in the pleural cavity); fibrinous or fibrinopurulent pericarditis; acute otitis media and mastoiditis; acute bacterial endocarditis; meningitis; arthritis; peritonitis (in children); herpes simplex; and shock due to peripheral vascular collapse.

BRONCHOPNEUMONIA:

Bronchopneumonia (lobular pneumonia) is usually secondary to chronic passive congestion of the lungs, aspiration, debilitation, or some disease of the respiratory tract such as pertussis, rubeola, scarlet fever, or influenza. Plugging of the bronchi with mucus appears to be an important factor in the pathogenesis. There is an extension of a purulent bronchitis into the adjacent alveoli. The most common *causes* of bronchopneumonia are coagulase-positive *Staphylococcus aureus* and gram-negative bacteria such as *Pseudomonas aeruginosa, Klebsiella-Aerobacter* group, *Escherichia coli,* and *Proteus* species. Streptococci and pneumococci also cause bronchopneumonia, as does *Salmonella typhi* rarely.

Pathologic changes

The pleural surface may be covered by a fibrinous exudate. On palpation of the *lungs,* shotty foci of increased resistance are felt. These foci vary in color from grayish yellow to dark red. The foci are patchy and mainly located around small bronchi and bronchioles. Drops of purulent material can be exuded from the center of these foci. *Abscess formation* is common in cases of bronchopneumonia due to staphylococci, especially in pyemia. The bronchial mucosa is red and swollen in the affected portions of the lungs. *Microscopically* the bronchial lumina are filled with neutrophils. Their walls are edematous, congested, and infiltrated by polymorphonuclear leukocytes. The alveoli surrounding the bronchi and bronchioles are filled with neutrophils, eosinophilic fluid, fibrin, and macrophages. The patches of bronchopneumonia may coalesce into large foci *(confluent bronchopneumonia).*

Complications

Bronchopneumonia, itself an often terminal complication of a debilitating disease, may be complicated by empyema or organization. In infants and children, *empyema* is a common complication of staphylococcal pneumonia. Other *complications of staphylococcal pneumonia* include *pneumatocele* (the development of an air-containing cavity in the lung) and *pyopneumothorax* (the presence of air and pus in the pleural cavity as the result of the development of a bronchopleural fistula).

INTERSTITIAL PNEUMONIA:

Interstitial pneumonia occurs in some cases of rubeola, pertussis, influenza, and other upper respiratory infections. The cause has been attributed to streptococcal toxins and to the viruses or bacteria of the various concomitant infections.

Pathologic changes

The affected portions of the lungs show foci of atelectasis. Numerous yellowish red foci, measuring up to 1 cm. in diameter, are found about small bronchi. The interlobular septa are prominent and edematous. *Microscopically* [25] the bronchial walls are edematous, hyperemic, and infiltrated by lymphocytes, plasmocytes, and macrophages, with only an occasional neutrophil. The bronchial epithelium may be desquamated. The *mononuclear infiltrate* extends into the interstitial tissue about the bronchus and into the interlobular septa. In a few alveoli there may be a mononuclear inflammatory reaction. The tracheobronchial *lymph nodes* are enlarged and soft. In some cases a diffuse interstitial *myocarditis* is associated with interstitial pneumonitis [26].

PRIMARY ATYPICAL PNEUMONIA:

Primary atypical pneumonia may be produced by *Coxiella burnetii* and a number of filtrable viruses such as those of influenza and psittacosis and adenoviruses. Most of the cases in which cold agglutinins are found are caused by *Mycoplasma pneumoniae* (Eaton agent), a pleuropneumonia-like organism [27].

Clinical features

Clinically primary atypical pneumonia occurs chiefly in young adults, especially military personnel in camps. It is characterized by coryza, fever, chills, headache, and cough, and typically lasts 2 to 3 weeks. In over half the cases due to *M. pneumoniae, cold hemagglutinins* appear during the second week of the disease. *Agglutinins for nonhemolytic Streptococcus MG* are demonstrable in about the same proportion of cases. This raises the possibility that *M. pneumoniae* is a stable L-form of *Streptococcus MG.* In about 25 percent of the cases a *positive serologic test for syphilis* is reported, and *eosinophilia* is found in the peripheral blood in about 20 percent of patients. An antibody reacting with lung tissue antigens has been found in the serum of about 70 percent of a series of patients with severe primary atypical pneumonia [28].

Pathologic changes

The *lungs* typically show patchy foci of dark red consolidation. The alveoli are infiltrated by macrophages, eosinophils, polymorphonuclear leukocytes, fibrin, and erythrocytes, and the alveolar walls are congested and edematous. There is a *marked tendency to organization* with the production of patchy fibrosis in the lung.

2. Noninfectious Pneumonitides

ASPIRATION PNEUMONIA:

Peptic-aspiration pneumonitis (Mendelson's syndrome) [29] is due to the *aspiration of gastric contents.* Vomiting is not a prerequisite to the entrance of gastric contents into the respiratory tree, for silent regurgitation may occur. *Aspiration is a constant menace in the anesthetized patient.* It occurs more commonly in obstetric patients and surgical emergencies than in routine surgical cases because of the lack of preparation in the former groups. The aspiration occasionally occurs during anesthesia but usually takes place postoperatively. Aspiration may be divided into two types, the *obstructive form,* in which solid material from the stomach gains access to the respiratory tree, and the *asthmatic form,* which is due to the aspiration of fluid. The obstructive type must be treated promptly by bronchoscopic removal because of the possibility of acute asphyxia from mechanical blockage of the tracheobronchial tree. The *aspiration of a significant amount of liquid vomitus* leads to the dramatic onset, 2 to 5 hours later, of cyanosis, dyspnea, tachycardia, and shock. There is evidence of severe bronchospasm with rales, wheezes, and rhonchi throughout both lungs. Bloody, frothy sputum is produced, and a chest film shows a soft, patchy mottling scattered throughout the lung fields.

Pathologic changes

Pathologically there is an *acute tracheobronchitis* with marked edema and injection of the tracheobronchial mucosa and the presence of pink, frothy edema fluid in the lumina. *Microscopically* there are a marked neutrophilic reaction, focal necrosis of the bronchial mucosa, and peribronchiolar hemorrhages. Free hydrochloric acid can be demonstrated in the bronchi. The asphyxia in these patients is due to respiratory obstruction caused by the edema fluid and inflammatory exudate in the bronchial tree, as well as the bronchial spasm. The serosanguineous fluid interferes with pulmonary ventilation and the diffusion of oxygen and carbon dioxide. Experimentally the *acute phase* of aspiration pneumonia consists of pulmonary edema, congestion, hemorrhage, a neutrophilic reaction, and sloughing of the bronchial mucosa [30]. With *aspirates free of gross particles, with a pH from 2.5 to 7,* and a volume less than 25 ml. in the rabbit, the reaction does not proceed beyond this acute phase. With *aspirates containing gross particles or with a pH below 2.5,* the inflammatory reaction continues. Highly acid aspirates provoke an extensive neutrophilic response. Gross particles stimulate a granulomatous foreign body reaction which may evolve over a period of 2 to 3 weeks. An *aspiration pneumonia will always result when the pH of the aspirate is less than 2.5.* Its *complications,* such as abscesses, bronchiectasis, and gangrene, are due to bronchial obstruction by the aspirated material and/or the inflammatory exudate. The enzymes in aspirated gastric contents are of little importance in the tissue reaction. *Aspiration of gastric contents occurs* not only in relation to anesthesia but *in debilitated patients* with serious medical disorders such as malignant neoplasms and cirrhosis of the liver, sometimes being the terminal event.

Milk-aspiration pneumonia

Milk-aspiration pneumonia [31] is a form of lipid pneumonia and is frequent in premature infants or those with central nervous system defects or esophageal obstruction. In adults it is most common in bedridden persons, the elderly, and the mentally ill. *Grossly* the milk can be identified in the tracheobronchial tree, and the lungs show *bronchopneumonia with hemorrhage and focal emphysema,* mainly dependently. Abscesses are sometimes present. *Microscopically* there is a mainly mononuclear reaction except in the early acute phase. The milk in the bronchi and alveoli stains pink, resembles fibrin, and may be plastered along the alveolar walls like hyaline membranes. The macrophages are foamy and finely vacuolated, and the milk lipids are sudanophilic. After several days the reaction becomes granulomatous with alveolar septal thickening and the appearance of epithelioid cells. Giant cells, which are sometimes bizarre and vacuolated, may be present. Fibrosis results, with long-standing granulomatous reactions. No differences are found in the reactions to cow's and human milk.

RHEUMATIC PNEUMONITIS:

Rheumatic pneumonitis has been described in some cases of rheumatic fever, but the lesions are not specific. Similar changes occur in uremic and viral pneumonitis. *(Uremic pneumonitis* is treated on page 568.) The pulmonary lesions occur during active rheumatic disease.

Pathologic changes

Grossly the lungs show no characteristic changes. They are dry and may show small pleural hemorrhages. *Microscopically* there is an interstitial infiltration of lymphocytes, plasmocytes, macrophages, and a few polymorphonuclear leukocytes. There is a scanty fibrinocellular intra-alveolar exudate, and the alveolar walls in the affected foci are covered with hyaline membranes. Later granulomatous foci consisting of fibroblasts and atypical histiocytes occur, but Aschoff bodies are not found in the lungs. Organization of the exudate following rheumatic pneumonitis leads to diffuse fibrosis of the lungs. Pulmonary hypertension and cor pulmonale result.

EOSINOPHILIC PNEUMONIA:

Eosinophilic pneumonia [32] is a part of *Löffler's syndrome.* This disease presents a usually mild clinical course with marked eosinophilia and transitory pulmonary lesions, but the lungs show an alarming x-ray picture. The disease appears to be *allergic* in nature and various cases have been thought to be due to infestation with *Ascaris lumbricoides,* as well as to hypersensitivity to pollens or bacteria.

Pathologic changes

Scattered focal areas of consolidation consist of fibrous tissue infiltrated with eosinophils. Some of the lesions are granulomatous with fibrinoid degeneration of collagen. Vascular lesions like those of periarteritis nodosa have also been found. In some cases the bronchi show the pathologic picture of asthma.

HEMORRHAGIC AND INTERSTITIAL PNEUMONITIS:

Hemorrhagic and interstitial pneumonitis with nephritis (Goodpasture's syndrome) [33] is characterized *clinically* by hemoptysis (which is often recurrent), hematuria, azotemia, and edema in patients with a hypersensitivity state such as glomerulonephritis or periarteritis nodosa.

Pathologic changes

The *lungs* are heavy, the combined weight often being over 2000 gm. There is an *acute necrotizing alveolitis* with hemorrhage. Into the areas of destruction there is a heavy infiltrate of neutrophils and a few eosinophils. Surrounding alveolar walls may show fibrous thickening, either dense and collagenous or loose and myxomatous. The lining cells are often cuboidal. The *kidneys* are usually heavy and show acute necrotizing or subacute glomerulonephritis (these are described in detail in Chapter 22). *Electron microscopy* has shown that alterations in the alveolar epithelial basement membrane are similar to those in the glomerular capillary membrane in acute glomerulonephritis [34]. The same antigen probably causes the changes in both the lungs and kidneys. Immunofluorescence has demonstrated gamma globulin and complement along alveolar septa [35]. In some cases of Goodpasture's syndrome the necrotizing angiitic lesions of periarteritis nodosa are found.

STEVENS-JOHNSON SYNDROME:

Mucosal respiratory (Stevens-Johnson) syndrome (erythema multiforme exudativum) is usually considered to be a *hypersensitivity reaction,* and some have classified it as a collagen disease.

Pathologic changes

Vesicles or bullae appear in the *buccal mucosa* rather suddenly. These quickly ulcerate, with the development of a membrane. Similar lesions appear in the *conjunctival* and *genital mucosa.* Erythematous or hemorrhagic lesions may appear in the *skin.* In the *lungs* there are foci of consolidation. The alveoli are filled with an edematous exudate containing lymphocytes and macrophages. The bronchial mucosa is sloughed in places, and the bronchial walls are infiltrated with mononuclear cells.

LIPID PNEUMONIA:

Lipid pneumonia is due to aspiration of oils in nose drops and laxatives or of cod liver oil. The latter type of aspiration is most common in children who have a cleft palate or who are debilitated. Occasional cases are due to aspiration of a foreign body containing oils, such as a peanut. The degree of pulmonary reaction depends on the free fatty acid content of the oil. In general, vegetable oils are less irritating than animal fats. The most common irritant in infants is cod liver oil and in adults, mineral oil.

Pathologic changes

Bland oils usually produce foci of consolidation about bronchi in the lower lobes. These foci are gray and spherical or pyramidal. The fat appears as large droplets. Large *vacuolated macrophages* containing the oil are found in the alveolar spaces. Lymphocytes and plasmocytes also infiltrate the alveoli. The presence of the oil is best identified by the fat stains. *Mineral oil* stains with scarlet red, but not with osmic acid. *Cod liver oil* becomes acid-fast on oxidation, and it can be identified in this way.

Secondary bronchopneumonia

In many cases a severe acute inflammation supervenes, due to secondary bacterial infection in the form of *bronchopneumonia.* Small and large, roughly spherical, firm yellow nodules may be found throughout both lungs in these cases. *Microscopically* the alveoli are distended with neutrophils, a little fibrin, and many vacuolated macrophages. The alveolar walls are thickened and lined by cuboidal cells. There is an interstitial fibrous tissue proliferation. The *regional lymph nodes* show numerous macrophages containing fat vacuoles.

SUPPURATIVE AND GRANULOMATOUS DISEASES OF THE LUNGS AND BRONCHI

1. Bronchiectasis

BRONCHIECTASIS: *Bronchiectasis* signifies a permanent *dilatation of the bronchi,* usually associated with suppuration. Two anatomic types are commonly described. *Saccular bronchiectasis* consists of rounded, cavity-like dilatations, and is commonly confined to a single segment or lobe of a lung. It is often found in children, and is usually purulent in nature. *Cylindrical bronchiectasis* shows a tubular dilation of the bronchi, and is typically found in adults. It often affects several lobes and may be bilateral. The left lung is affected slightly more often than the right, and the lower lobes are involved more often than the upper. Upper lobe bronchiectasis is probably a sequel of tuberculosis in most instances. When an upper lobe is involved, it is common for an adjacent segment of the middle or lower lobe to be affected also.

Causes

In most instances it seems that several causes act together to produce the bronchial dilatation. Some form of *bronchial obstruction* is often noted proximal to the dilatation. A foreign body in a bronchus is an especially important form of obstruction, but benign and malignant tumors of the bronchus or external compression, as from calcified tuberculous lymph nodes, may also contribute. *Infection* is usually combined with obstruction, each accentuating the other. As the bronchial mucosa becomes inflamed, obstruction by a foreign body becomes more complete, and as obstruction becomes more complete, the localized inflammatory effect is aggravated. Bronchial infection without obstruction may cause bronchiectasis in some cases, especially if there is actual ulceration of the mucosa and damage to the muscular and elastic coats of the bronchi. In *mucoviscidosis,* a childhood disorder in which there is chronic pancreatic disease, faulty absorption and digestion of fats and proteins, and defective absorption of fat-soluble vitamin A, bronchiectasis is a common feature. With *situs inversus* there is often chronic bronchiectasis, although the significance of this association is unknown.

Clinical features

When quantities of pus accumulate in the bronchi, this causes violent paroxysms of cough and expectoration, especially in the morning or on change in position. The sputum and other findings and the eventual outcome are generally the same as with lung abscess (see page 463). Massive, even fatal, hemoptysis sometimes occurs, usually from the varicosities which develop in the walls of the dilated bronchi.

Pathologic changes

Grossly the affected lobes are usually shrunken, atelectatic, and adherent to surrounding structures. Bronchi are dilated, thin-walled, and often distended with pus. Parenchymal tissue is collapsed and may be fibrotic. *Microscopically* the bronchial walls show a relative reduction in muscular and elastic elements. Ciliated bronchial epithelium is often replaced by squamous epithelium, promoting stagnation of secretions. Alveolar walls are thickened by fibrosis and chronic inflammation, and the air sacs in the affected areas are reduced in size and number. If the lungs are examined during a period of infection, the dilated bronchi may be empty. Increased vascularity of the affected lobes is almost always noted, due to the development of shunts between the bronchial and pulmonary arteries [36]. Probably as a result of increased pulmonary hypertension, sclerotic changes in the small arterioles are commonly noted.

2. Lung Abscess

LUNG ABSCESS:

A *lung abscess* is a localized area of tissue destruction and suppuration within the lung parenchyma. Bronchiectasis may convert to lung abscess if complicated by destruction of lung parenchyma. Before the introduction of antibiotics and the development of the specialty of anesthesiology, lung abscesses were much more common than they are today. Abscess is somewhat more frequent in the right lung than in the left, and in lower lobes than in upper ones.

Causes: infection

Infection is the basic cause of lung abscess, and the infectious agent can usually be demonstrated in the sputum and in tissue sections. Mixed bacterial infections are common, with anaerobic and saprophytic organisms predominating; occasionally fungi are responsible. In different cases one or more of the following factors permits the infection to gain a foothold.

aspiration

Aspiration of particles of wood, vegetable materials, tooth, dental prosthesis, blood, gastric contents, or septic material from the mouth or throat often precedes the development of lung abscess. Formerly aspiration was fairly common during the course of surgical anesthesia, and was often unrecognized because of the inhibition of the cough reflex. If there was aspiration of vomitus, the acid gastric juice with its digestive enzymes caused a rapidly progressive destruction of tissue; this was probably the mechanism for that special form of abscess known as *gangrene of the lung,* rarely seen today. Close attention to the airway during anesthesia minimizes the risk of aspiration.

septic embolism

Septic embolism, as following puerperal endometritis, osteomyelitis, or cavernous or lateral sinus thrombosis, usually produces multiple bilateral *septic infarcts* or abscesses. The authors' experience suggests that *lung abscess may also follow bland pulmonary embolism,* such as that occurring with heart disease; the ischemic or infarcted lung tissue tends to break down and form an abscess when secondarily infected from the bronchial tree, whereas normal lung tissue is able to resolve the exudate without tissue loss.

post-pneumonic abscess

It is distinctly unusual for lung abscess to follow directly after pneumococcal pneumonia, but it may follow *streptococcal* or *staphylococcal pneumonia,* especially when these pneumonias complicate heart failure and pulmonary embolism. When *empyema* complicates pneumonia, this may in turn lead to lung abscess by rupturing into the lung.

extension

An abscess near the diaphragmatic surface of the liver may rupture through the diaphragm, and if adhesions prevent its emptying into the pleural sac, it may rupture into the lung. Other forms of subdiaphragmatic or paravertebral abscesses may do the same thing.

abscess with carcinoma

Bronchogenic carcinoma should be suspected in adults when signs of abscess develop without apparent cause. Infected material retained behind the blockage in a bronchus leads to tissue destruction.

Clinical features

Cough and *expectoration* are the outstanding manifestations of lung abscess. The sputum is copious and often *foul-smelling,* and tends to separate into layers on standing. Chest pain, fever, and leukocytosis are the rule. There are impaired resonance and bubbling rales over the affected area, and sometimes signs of cavity are present. The chest radiograph shows an opaque area, often with a central radiolucent zone in which a fluid level is evident.

Pathologic changes

The *gross appearance* of lung abscess depends on the duration of the process and on the causative factors. In acute abscess, as following aspiration of vomitus and rapid bacterial invasion, a large segment of lung may be hemorrhagic and indurated and show a ragged cavity filled with sanguineopurulent material. *Most lung abscess is chronic.* The affected lung shows a shrunken lobe covered with dense adhesions; on section it shows an airless, fibrotic zone surrounding a cavity containing pus and communicating with a bronchus. *Microscopic features* are self-evident: a cavity lined with granulation tissue and filled with pus, surrounded by a zone of atelectatic and fibrotic lung tissue, heavily infiltrated with leukocytes. The causative agents can usually be demonstrated in sections stained appropriately.

Complications

Lung abscess, in contrast to abscesses in most other organs, *tends to become chronic* unless actively treated by antibiotics and/or excision. Lung abscess persists because the conditions which lead to its formation usually tend to persist; the foreign body cannot be coughed up, the necrotic tissue cannot regenerate, and infection is rarely completely eliminated. Usually the abscess *ruptures into a bronchus,* if there was no such communication at the beginning. *Rupture into the pleural sac* is also common, producing empyema, pneumothorax, and bronchopleural fistula. In some cases, with the establishment of adequate drainage via a bronchus, the infection may subside and the cavity may become lined with epithelium; this results in a sort of bronchiectasis localized to one bronchus. Often pleural adhesions, parenchymal fibrosis, and bronchial distortion with atelectasis bring about *chest deformity* and, in some cases, *cor pulmonale.*

Brain abscess may complicate any of the chronic suppurative lesions within the thorax: lung abscess, bronchiectasis, empyema, or suppurative pericarditis. The causative organisms apparently reach the brain via the vertebral plexus of veins. *Secondary amyloidosis,* involving the liver, spleen, kidneys, and adrenal glands, *may complicate chronic pulmonary suppuration.*

3. Pulmonary Tuberculosis

TUBERCULOSIS:

The cause, pathogenesis, and general features of tuberculosis have been discussed in Chapter 6.

Statistics

Pulmonary tuberculosis accounts for almost all deaths from tuberculosis generally, and for almost all disability from tuberculosis. In 1900 the death rate from tuberculosis in the United States was 194 per 100,000; by 1966 it had fallen to 3.6 per 100,000, one of the lowest rates in the world. In recent years a shift has also occurred in the age incidence of tuberculosis. In the 1930s tuberculosis was chiefly a disease of young adults, but now the majority of patients in tuberculous hospitals are above 40 years of age and many are above age 60. This change is believed to be a result of tuberculosis case-finding programs. Chest x-ray surveys have resulted in recognition of minimal lesions, before symptoms have appeared, and the isolation and treatment of these potential source cases have reduced the number of new cases in the younger age groups.

Avenues of infection

Since direct inhalation of contaminated air droplets or dust accounts for infection in most cases, it is natural that the respiratory tract is most commonly affected. In addition, the lungs are liable to infection by dissemination of bacilli from other sources via lymphatic-hematogeneous routes. The reaction of the host to first infection by the tubercle bacillus is different from reaction to reinfection. This is due largely to the influence of *acquired resistance* and *hypersensitivity* to the tubercle bacillus or its byproducts.

First-infection tuberculosis:

First-infection tuberculosis used to be chiefly a disease of children but at the present time an increasing proportion of such cases is seen in adults. The localization of lesions is apparently determined by chance distribution of inhaled particles. The Ghon lesion is typically subpleural in a lower lobe, the right more commonly than the left.

usual course

The *lesion of first-infection tuberculosis* shows a chronic proliferative and granulomatous reaction, followed by caseation, but usually no liquefaction. A comparable lesion, with granulomatous reaction and caseation, commonly develops in the regional lymph nodes. These lymph nodes plus the parenchymal lesion constitute the *primary complex*. In most instances these lesions *heal spontaneously*. A fibrous capsule forms, contracting the lesion. Calcium is deposited in the wall surrounding the granulomatous lesion. Bacilli may remain viable in the caseous center for years, walled off from the host.

course in fatal cases

If healing does not ensue, the disease is relatively *acute* and usually *continuous;* chronic tuberculosis is rarely a manifestation of first infection. With massive infection, bacilli spread from the hilar lymph nodes to the tracheobronchial, mediastinal, and cervical lymph nodes, and may gain entrance to the superior vena cava via the thoracic duct. In such cases *miliary tuberculosis* ensues, chiefly of the lungs, but often also of other organs, particularly the meninges. *Tuberculous meningitis* is a common mode of death in progressive first-infection tuberculosis. Sometimes the lymph node lesions extend and erode a bronchus or the pericardium, causing a rapidly fatal local spread of the infection.

Reinfection tuberculosis:

Reinfection tuberculosis is the common form of tuberculosis in adults; it is rare in children. Most cases of reinfection are presumed to come from a new *exogenous exposure* to bacilli, but an unknown number may come from endogenous reinfection. Localization of lesions is determined by unknown factors, apparently not related to chance distribution of inhaled particles. Lesions are primarily *apical* and often *bilateral.*

pathologic changes

The *lesions* in reinfection tuberculosis are less stable and more *exudative* than those in first-infection tuberculosis. Softening and *liquefaction* of the caseous areas occur, often resulting in hemoptysis, rupture into a bronchus, emptying of the liquefied material, and *cavity formation.* There is little tendency to involvement of lymph nodes. Prior to cavity formation, healing may occur by gradual resolution of the exudate, leaving little scar. After cavity formation, spontaneous healing is less likely and the bacilli grow more readily, presumably because of aerobic conditions. The granulomatous tissue in the cavity wall serves as a veritable factory for the production of tubercle bacilli.

significance of cavities

Patients with *open cavities,* i.e., ones communicating with a bronchus, are the chief sources of danger in tuberculosis, both to themselves and to others. Open cavities collect exudate containing viable tubercle bacilli. This exudate (the equivalent of sputum) may be aspirated to other parts of the same lung or to the opposite lung, and may be coughed into the mouth and swallowed. Wherever this exudate lodges, it inoculates unaffected tissue with tubercle bacilli, causing the spread of infection within the host. When the exudate is discharged from the body by cough, as a fine vapor spray, the contained tubercle bacilli may infect others directly, or indirectly via dust inhalation after drying. When the sputum (exudate) from a patient with an open cavity is stained appropriately, it is usually found to be teeming with acid-fast organisms, i.e., a "positive sputum."

mode of spread

Extension of the infection within the patient is chiefly by the spread of exudate along *natural passages,* as outlined above, with inoculation of other portions of the same or opposite lung, of bronchi, trachea, larynx, tonsils, and gastrointestinal tract. The pleura may be affected by *direct contiguity* with the parenchymal lesion, giving either a fibrinous *tuberculous pleuritis,* pleurisy with serous effusion, or a tuberculous empyema. Less commonly, spread is via *lymphatics* and *bloodstream,* giving *miliary tuberculosis.*

clinical forms

Minimal tuberculosis signifies a lesion of limited extent and without cavities; often it causes no symptoms and is discovered only as a result of a routine chest x-ray. *Tuberculous pneumonia,* or caseous pneumonic tuberculosis, is a rapidly fatal form of reinfection tuberculosis seen in heavily infected young adults, especially Negroes and American Indians. The areas of exudation become coalescent, as in lobar pneumonia, and scattered small cavities develop. Tremendous numbers of bacilli are found in the sputum. *Fibroid phthisis* is a very chronic form of tuberculosis, usually seen in elderly persons, especially in whites. Cavities are common, but fibrosis is marked and bronchi are distorted. Symptoms in these patients (shortness of breath, wheezing, cough) are often due more to mechanical factors than to tuberculosis itself, and may be mistakenly ascribed to heart disease. The sputum contains bacilli, but these patients are relatively well and usually ambulatory. Patients with this type of the disease are a great danger to others because they may not be recognized as having tuberculosis. Rarely in *endobronchial tuberculosis* a tuberculous ulcer of a bronchus may cause cough, expectoration, and hemoptysis without a parenchymal lesion being evident on x-ray. The sputum may be positive and parenchymal lesions may develop later. *Tuberculoma* signifies a dense, walled-off tuberculous lesion, probably the lesion of first infection in the adult. It is usually found accidentally in a patient without symptoms of tuberculosis. The lesion has a caseous center and a laminated fibrous wall, often with shell-like calcium deposits. Tubercle bacilli are often difficult to demonstrate. Lesions having an almost identical gross appearance have been described in histoplasmosis [37] and brucellosis [38]. Although tuberculous lesions of bones, kidneys, adrenal glands, and peritoneum are sometimes seen during the course of the reinfection type of pulmonary tuberculosis, it is rare for these lesions to assume clinical significance.

sequelae

Once cavities have formed in the lungs, spontaneous healing is rarely complete; even if the tubercle bacilli are eliminated by antibiotic therapy, the cavities remain as pockets for continued pyogenic infection. There may also be serious disability from distortion of the bronchi and vessels, thickening of the pleura, fixation of the mediastinum, and varying degrees of fibrosis of the lung parenchyma. *Emphysema, bronchiectasis,* and *kyphoscoliosis* are all common. The bronchial arteries often become greatly enlarged, and may communicate with branches of the pulmonary arteries. These *shunts,* which may also develop in bronchiectasis and chronic lung abscess, may cause increased blood flow in the pulmonary vascular bed. These various factors, singly and especially in combination, may *reduce pulmonary ventilation, promote anoxia,* and lead to *pulmonary hypertension* and *cor pulmonale.* These late effects of pulmonary tuberculosis have become more apparent in recent years as more patients have been cured of their tuberculous infection by antibiotic and surgical therapy.

mode of death

In untreated cases there is usually progressive involvement of more and more lung parenchyma, followed by *tuberculous laryngitis* and *tuberculous enteritis,* with toxemia, fever, and exhaustion. *Miliary tuberculosis* or *tuberculous meningitis* may occur, but are unusual complications of pulmonary tuberculosis in the adult. Rarely there may be *fatal hemoptysis,* as from a Rasmussen aneurysm of a pulmonary vessel in the wall of a cavity. Occasionally *spontaneous pneumothorax,* from rupture of a cavity or emphysematous bleb, may cause death.

relationship to other diseases

Silicosis predisposes to pulmonary tuberculosis, but it is less certain that other forms of pneumoconiosis have an effect. Tuberculosis is commonly encountered in the rejected homeless victims of *chronic alcoholism,* but this is thought to be related to poor housing and diet and other aspects of general immunity rather than to any specific factor. *Secondary amyloidosis* is sometimes a late complication of pulmonary tuberculosis. A study of a large number of cases of *pulmonary tuberculosis* showed that *bronchogenic carcinoma occurs about 20 times as frequently in patients with tuberculosis* as in the general population [39]. The incidence of the coexistence of tuberculosis and bronchogenic carcinoma increased with the age of the patient. The carcinoma developed in the tuberculous lobe in about two-thirds of the cases and in the same lung in over 80 percent. The incidence of coexistence in this series was 0.2 percent.

4. *Bronchopulmonary Mycoses*

All the diseases in this group tend to produce chronic lung abscess; the clinical picture is usually similar to that in tuberculosis. The specific organisms may be identified in smears or cultures of sputum or pus. Systemic dissemination of fungi is rarely observed except in seriously debilitated individuals. The morphologic features and characteristics of the different fungi have been discussed in Chapter 8.

CANDIDIASIS

Candida albicans may become pathogenic after suppression of the normal bacterial flora by prolonged *antibiotic therapy.* Fatal cases have also been described following treatment of *acute leukemia* with anti-folic acid compounds. The tissue reaction is a *chronic suppurative and granulomatous* one in which numerous branching and budding forms of the fungus are seen. Milder examples of the infection occur as a grayish white membrane on the mucosa of the trachea or bronchi, comparable to thrush in the mouth of debilitated infants.

ACTINOMYCOSIS

Actinomycosis of the lungs is less frequent than the abdominal and the cervicofacial forms, to either of which it may be a complication. A *chronic suppurative and granulomatous reaction* is noted in typical cases, and there is a strong tendency toward the formation of *sinus* in the chest wall. Sulfur granules, consisting of a meshwork of threadlike mycelia with peripherally arranged radial clubs, are usually evident in the sputum or in sections of the lung abscesses. The infection usually responds to proper antibiotic therapy.

NOCARDIOSIS

Nocardiosis produces a tissue reaction which resembles actinomycosis in the tendency to abscess and sinus formation and induration, but the tissue reaction is somewhat more acute with *Nocardia* than with *Actinomyces.*

CRYPTO-COCCOSIS

Cryptococcosis (torulosis) affects the brain and meninges more often than the lungs. In the lungs there may be relatively little inflammatory response, but in chronic cases a *granulomatous reaction* occurs. A sort of pseudocaseation is sometimes noted. Cryptococcosis of the lungs is rarely seen except as a *late complication in the lymphomas.*

BLASTO-MYCOSIS

Blastomycosis may be caused by either *Blastomyces dermatitidis* or *B. brasiliensis.* It produces an insidious abscess of the lungs which may be confused with tuberculosis or carcinoma.

HISTO-PLAS-MOSIS

In *histoplasmosis* of the lungs, *miliary lesions* having a tendency to heal and calcify are the form usually recognized. Many of the *laminated caseous nodules* of the lung parenchyma, previously believed to be tuberculomas, are due to *Histoplasma capsulatum* (histoplasmomas).

COCCIDI-OIDO-MYCOSIS

Coccidioidomycosis, a disease rather sharply limited to the San Joaquin Valley of California, may be manifest as a mild acute respiratory infection of short duration or (much less commonly) as a *chronic suppurative disease* of the lungs resembling tuberculosis. Abscesses may form, but more characteristically there is an inflammatory infiltration of the parenchyma. The various forms of *Coccidioides immitis* can be demonstrated in sputum and in lung sections.

ASPERGIL-LOSIS AND MUCOR-MYCOSIS

Aspergillosis and *mucormycosis* are rare forms of pulmonary mycosis. They may occur in diabetics and patients with aplastic anemia or cancer, especially lymphomas, as terminal infections. Each may cause a chronic suppurative and granulomatous pulmonary lesion, and the causative agent may be demonstrable in sputum or in lung sections.

FOREIGN BODIES IN THE RESPIRATORY PASSAGES

Foreign bodies in the respiratory passages are usually of an emergency nature, but may remain undetected and produce serious and irreversible pulmonary changes. Most respiratory foreign bodies are found in children [40]. *Sudden death* may result from lodgment of such a body in the larynx or from complete tracheal obstruction. In *nonfatal cases* the initial signs are choking, gagging, hoarseness, dyspnea with wheezing, coughing, and even cyanosis. The violent coughing spell may dislodge the foreign body. In about half the cases the foreign body is opaque and can be visualized by x-rays. Bronchoscopic removal can be accomplished in over 90 percent of the cases when performed early. Later swelling of the object or mucosal edema may make removal difficult. A *migratory foreign body in the trachea* may bob up and down with inspiration and expiration. As it strikes the rima of the glottis, an auditory slap is produced, and as it strikes the sides of the trachea, a palpatory thud may be felt. Foreign bodies more commonly enter the right bronchus than the left because of the more vertical course of the former. When a foreign body lodges in a bronchus, the reaction depends on the character of the object, the degree of obstruction it produces, and its location in the bronchial tree. *Complete bronchial obstruction* will lead to atelectasis distal to the obstruction. *Trapping of secretions and infection* may produce a chronic pneumonitis followed by *abscess formation. Incomplete bronchial obstruction* may cause emphysema and bronchiectasis. *Inhaled vegetable matter often evokes a violent tissue reaction.* In the case of the peanut this is due to the presence of arachidic acid. A dried bean is especially dangerous because it swells rapidly by the imbibition of tissue fluids. Occasionally the intrabronchial foreign body is endogenous, a calcified hilar lymph node eroding into it and acting as a foreign body *(broncholith)*. Modern therapy has reduced the *mortality* from inhaled foreign bodies to about 2 percent.

MIDDLE LOBE SYNDROME

Middle lobe syndrome [41] is due to an interference with the drainage of the right middle lobe bronchus, especially by enlarged tracheobronchial lymph nodes. There are intermittent fever, productive cough, hemoptysis, and right middle lobe pneumonitis. The changes are reversible early, but *bronchiectasis may result from prolonged obstruction.*

THE PNEUMOCONIOSES

Pneumoconiosis is a collective term for the pathologic changes caused by particulate matter which has been inhaled into the lungs. Most cases of pneumoconiosis are occupational in origin, occurring among miners and processors of certain harmful substances. In general, any dust with a concentration greater than 60 million particles per cubic foot containing 5 percent free silica under 10μ in diameter, or any dust containing 10 million particles per cubic foot with 35 percent free silica is dangerous.

ANTHRACOSIS:

Anthracosis is the deposition in the lungs of black coal pigment. *Occupational anthracosis* is an excessive accumulation of coal dust pigment in the lungs. The major pathologic changes are due to the accompanying silicosis, so that the condition is a modified silicosis (anthracosilicosis). *Nonoccupational anthracosis* occurs in urban dwellers, the degree depending on the impurity of the atmosphere. Small quantities of silica are also found in the lungs in persons living in dusty atmospheres. Clinical signs are usually absent.

Pathologic changes

Varying degrees of *black mottling* are found on and in the *lungs*, most conspicuously at the apices, anterior borders of the upper and lower lobes, and posterior borders of the upper lobes. The pigment may form a fine tracery over the pleural surfaces, the lines conforming to the interlobular septa. On *cut surface* the pigment is found in the interlobular septa and the adventitial tissue about the bronchi and great vessels. The *hilar and tracheobronchial lymph nodes* are slightly enlarged, firm, and uniformly black. *Microscopically* pigment is found free within the interstitial tissue and within macrophages.

Complications

Cavity formation occurs occasionally when anthracosis is very severe. The apical deposits of pigment may cause tissue necrosis and the formation of a cavity 2 to 4 cm. in diameter. *Rupture into a bronchus or vessel* may occur when tracheobronchial lymph nodes containing tremendous amounts of pigment soften or liquefy. The wall of an adherent bronchus or blood vessel may be eroded, with discharge of the black liquid into the lumen. Pigment entering the bloodstream is filtered out mainly by the liver and spleen. Small pigmented foci are found in the portal spaces in the liver and in the malpighian bodies in the spleen. Rarely a bronchus and vessel are eroded at the same time, resulting in a severe or even fatal hemoptysis. *Severe emphysema* may be produced in coal miners without fibrosis [42].

Relation to other lung diseases

Defects in resolution of pneumonic processes are found in persons with severe anthracosis, probably due to blockage of lymphatic drainage of the inflammatory exudate. Tuberculous lesions are often smaller and more localized in anthracotic than nonanthracotic lungs. This has been explained on the basis of blockage of lymphatics, preventing the spread of the process.

SILICOSIS:

Silicosis is a disease caused by the deposition of silica particles which have been inhaled into the lungs. It is an occupational disease in coal and gold miners, sandblasters, and metal grinders and polishers.

Pathogenesis

When a silica particle less than 2μ in diameter enters an alveolus, it is immediately phagocytized by a macrophage. The cell migrates toward the tracheobronchial lymph nodes via the lymphatics. The toxic ingested silica causes death of the cell, and the necrotic cytoplasm attracts a few polymorphonuclear leukocytes and macrophages. The latter become epithelioid cells, and later giant cells are formed. Fibroblastic proliferation leads to the formation of the silicotic nodule. Collagen is laid down within 60 to 90 days, and the epithelioid cells and most giant cells disappear. When silica is introduced into the lungs of rabbits, large amounts of phospholipid similar to that in the tubercle bacillus are released. This may account for the similarity of the silicotic nodule to the tubercle.

"Acute" silicosis

"Acute" silicosis produces death within 2 to 4 years. The *gross appearance* of the lung is less striking in the acute than in the chronic form. The lungs are voluminous and firm. The nodules average less than 0.5 mm. in diameter. They are numerous, especially just beneath the pleura. *Microscopically* they are similar to those of chronic silicosis.

Chronic silicosis:

In *chronic silicosis* a history of occupational exposure for 10 to 25 years is obtained. Progressive dyspnea and a chronic productive cough are the main *clinical signs.* Nodular densities with a reticular pattern are seen bilaterally on a chest film.

pathologic changes

A *chronic bronchitis* with edema, congestion, and mucus secretion in the bronchial walls is common. The *lungs* are voluminous, and dense fibrous adhesions obliterate most of the pleural cavities. Throughout the lungs numerous firm, spherical, grayish white nodules, 1 to 3 mm. in diameter, are found. The nodules consist of whorls of hyalinized fibrous tissue containing pigment granules. At the periphery a few lymphocytes are found, and occasional Langhans-type giant cells may be present. The *silicotic nodules* are discrete early, but they eventually coalesce, producing widespread fibrosis. The nodules often have a laminated, onion-skin appearance. *Silica* appears as radiant, anisotropic particles under polarized light. The lining of the intact alveoli may become cuboidal (fetalization of the alveolar lining). Emphysema is common about the nodules. The *tracheobronchial lymph nodes* contain nodules like those within the lungs. Occasionally nodules are found in the liver and spleen.

Relation to other lung diseases

The incidence of *organized pneumonia* is higher among persons with silicosis and other pneumoconioses than among the general population. This is believed to be due to the blockage of the lymphatic drainage of the inflammatory exudate. Many patients with silicosis (pure or modified) die of pulmonary tuberculosis *(silicotuberculosis); miner's phthisis* is a pneumoconiosis plus active pulmonary tuberculosis. The incidence of bronchogenic carcinoma is higher among persons with silicosis than among the general population.

Anthracosilicosis is common among anthracite and bituminous coal miners. The *pathologic picture* is that of silicosis plus dense deposits of black pigment. Anthraco-silicosis

Siderosilicosis occurs among miners of iron ores containing silica. The *lungs* are rusty red, the iron pigments being concentrated in small nodules. Grayish white *silicotic nodules* are also found. *Microscopically* there is diffuse fibrosis in addition to the whorled silicotic nodules. Within the fibrous tissue, large amounts of brown granular *iron pigment* are found. Pigment is also deposited in the thickened intima of medium-sized and small blood vessels. The *tracheobronchial lymph nodes* are red and fibrotic. *Tuberculosis* is commonly associated with siderosilicosis. Sidero-silicosis

ASBESTOSIS:

Asbestosis occurs among the workers who crush asbestos rock or card the asbestos and among workers who handle asbestos products such as insulation material. Both Canadian asbestos (chrysolite) and South African asbestos (crocidolite) contain about 50 percent silicon as hydrated silicates of calcium, magnesium, iron, and manganese.

Pathogenesis

Lesions are due to the inhaled silica dust plus the presence of asbestos fibers. The *asbestos body* is produced by the deposition of protein and iron pigment from the inflammatory exudate upon the surface of the asbestos fiber.

Pathologic changes

The *pleura* is thickened, and the pleural cavities may be obliterated by fibrous adhesions. The *lungs* are firm and nodular. On cut surface the nodules are grayish white or blue. In the upper lobes they tend to remain discrete, while in the lower lobes they are usually confluent. There is also a *diffuse fibrosis,* especially about bronchioles. Within the fibrous tissue are the characteristic *asbestos bodies,* which are golden yellow, segmented, and globular. They have the appearance of shishkebab. These bodies give a positive Prussian blue reaction. Foreign-body giant cells are occasionally found about the asbestos bodies. The *tracheobronchial lymph nodes* are enlarged and fibrotic. In the *trachea* and *bronchi,* chronic inflammation is common.

Relation to other lung diseases

The *incidence of bronchogenic carcinoma in cases of asbestosis* is about 14 percent as compared with an incidence of 7 percent in cases of silicosis and other pneumoconioses [43]. These incidences are much higher than that of bronchogenic carcinoma in the general population for comparable age groups. Bronchogenic carcinoma associated with asbestosis is especially common in female workers. The average interval between initial exposure to asbestos dust and the development of bronchogenic carcinoma is 16 to 18 years. In 80 percent of these cases the carcinoma is in a lower lobe, and epidermoid carcinoma is the most frequent type. *Mesothelioma of the pleura* and even of the *peritoneum* occurs significantly more commonly among workers with asbestos than do these rare neoplasms among the general population [44].

CALCIOSILICOSIS

Calciosilicosis is observed among workers in quartz, marble, granite, cement, and talc. The changes are mainly due to the silica, the calcium producing little effect on the lungs.

KAOLINOSIS

Kaolinosis is a pneumoconiosis due to the occupational inhalation of clay dust [45]. Kaolin is a clay derived from the disintegration of feldspar or mica. A clay is a dispersion of crystalline fragments of hydrated aluminum silicate in which most particles are smaller than 2μ. The *pulmonary deposits* are mainly in the upper lobes and are blue. Involvement may be patchy or diffuse. *Nodular fibrosis* with extensive whorls of collagen occur about the kaolin deposits. There is fibrous thickening of the alveolar walls, and an extensive obliterative endarteritis with thrombosis of pulmonary arteries occurs. Prominent emphysema is found in the lung parenchyma between nodules.

CARBORUNDUM PNEUMOCONIOSIS

Carborundum pneumoconiosis is caused by the inhaled dust of silicon carbide which, although it contains no free silica, produces a mild fibrosis of the lungs in occupational workers.

BERYLLIOSIS:

Beryllium pneumoconiosis (berylliosis) is produced by occupational exposure to the dust or fumes of the metal and its compounds. Beryllium metal and its oxide, fluoride, sulfate, and hydroxide, and lamp phosphor ($ZnMnBeSiO_2$) have been implicated as causes.

Pathologic changes

In the *acute lesions* the lungs are heavy and inelastic. The cut surface is a homogeneous pinkish or bluish gray. The alveoli are filled with fluid, lymphocytes, and plasmocytes. Multinucleated cells are common. Later the exudate organizes, leaving a central mass of eosinophilic debris. Fibrous tissue proliferation begins. In the *chronic phase* the lungs weigh up to 2000 gm., and small nodules up to 2 mm. in diameter are found throughout the lungs. *Microscopically* these nodules reveal a characteristic *granuloma* in which a peripheral layer of loose fibrous tissue surrounding a central mass of necrotic granular eosinophilic debris, similar to fibrinoid or caseation necrosis, is found. Sometimes a Langhans giant cell is present centrally. The granuloma is infiltrated by lymphocytes and macrophages. The intervening lung parenchyma is emphysematous. The alveolar walls may be thickened and infiltrated by mononuclear cells. Fibrosis is often extensive in the lungs. Similar granulomatous lesions may be present in the *tracheobronchial lymph nodes.* When beryllium is introduced into the *subcutaneous tissues,* a granuloma like that in the lungs develops.

BAUXITE PNEUMOCONIOSIS:

Bauxite pneumoconiosis [46] occurs in workers with alumina abrasives, due to the inhalation of fumes. It is not certain whether the lesions are due to aluminum particles or to the silica contained in the alumina ores (atypical form of silicosis). The involved lungs may contain up to 40 percent of alumina in their ash. *Clinically* dyspnea is extreme, and spontaneous pneumothorax is common. The course is rapidly downhill.

Pathologic changes

Grossly the lungs show numerous emphysematous bullae. *Microscopically* there is a diffuse interstitial fibrosis without nodule formation. The fibrous tissue is infiltrated by mononuclear cells. Bronchioles are dilated, some showing squamous metaplasia. Arterial walls are thickened. The tracheobronchial lymph nodes show fibrosis.

CADMIUM PNEUMONITIS

Cadmium pneumonitis is due to occupational inhalation of cadmium oxide fumes. The first phase of the reaction is a *stage of acute congestion and edema* similar to that due to noxious gases. This is followed within a few days by a *proliferative stage,* with hyperplasia of the alveolar and bronchiolar epithelium. The alveolar epithelium becomes cuboidal. Leukocytic infiltration is scanty. In the third stage there is *fibrosis,* mainly about the larger bronchi and blood vessels.

PHYTOPNEUMOCONIOSIS:

Phytopneumoconiosis is due to the inhalation of plant dusts. The important forms are bagassosis and farmer's lung.

Bagas-sosis:

Bagassosis is due to the prolonged inhalation of bagasse, the residue of sugar cane after the sugar has been removed. It occurs among workers in plants using bales of old, dehydrated bagasse, as in paper mills and wallboard manufacturing plants. Experimental studies show that inhaled *bagasse dust causes progressive thickening of the alveolar septa* with an infiltration by macrophages and the formation of foreign-body giant cells containing birefringent particles [47]. This reaction does not depend on hypersensitivity to bagasse or on the presence of contaminating saprophytic bacteria or fungi. However, the presence of such organisms is important in perpetuating the process and causing irreversible lung damage. *Clinically* there are cough, dyspnea, hemoptysis, night sweats, and fever. Chest x-ray films show tiny foci of pulmonary consolidation. The mortality rate in the acute phase is about 10 percent, but most patients recover completely 3 to 6 months after cessation of exposure to bagasse dust.

pathologic changes

There is *diffuse interstitial fibrosis* of the lungs. The fibrosis may be due not to the dust, but to fungi which are inhaled. Species of *Aspergillus* and *Rhizopus* and other fungi have been isolated from bagasse. *Byssinosis* is a similar condition due to the inhalation of cotton dust.

Farmer's lung

Farmer's lung [48] is due to the inhalation of the dust of moldy hay, oats, wheat, barley, tobacco, and corn fodder. It is possible that fungi such as *Candida albicans* play a causative role. In the *acute attack* there is a rapid onset of cough sometimes productive of blood-streaked sputum and dyspnea several hours after initial exposure to the dust. Repeated exposure over a period of months may lead to the *subacute phase* in which there are progressive dyspnea and cough with a sandstorm or miliary appearance in a chest film due to fine, nodular densities throughout the lung fields but with some concentration in the medial portions. The *chronic phase* follows repeated exposure for years and is characterized by severe pulmonary insufficiency due to fibrosis and emphysema. Some patients have a *marked eosinophilia* in the peripheral blood, indicating that the *pulmonary lesion may be due to hypersensitivity.* In the early stages lung biopsies show focal, noncaseating peribronchiolar granulomas with peripheral giant cells and an interstitial infiltration of macrophages and lymphocytes. Later extensive pulmonary fibrosis and emphysema are found.

ENDOGENOUS "PNEUMOCONIOSIS":

Endogenous "pneumoconiosis" [49] *is a pulmonary fibrosis due to alteration in the elastic tissue of the lung* as a primary degeneration or secondary to elastic injury. The condition occurs in adults but has a definite resemblance to *idiopathic pulmonary hemosiderosis* (essential brown induration of the lungs) of children.

Clinical features

Clinically the pulmonary signs and symptoms are gradually progressive with an average duration of about 7 years. There are dyspnea, hemoptysis, episodes of fever, cyanosis, polycythemia, and peripheral edema. The elastic changes do not appear to be secondary to cardiac disease or failure, although similar changes have been described in the lung in cases of mitral stenosis and severe left ventricular failure.

Pathologic changes

Grossly the lungs are heavy and show congestion, edema, emphysema, and a diffuse, fine fibrosis. *Microscopically* the vascular and interstitial elastic fibrils are strongly basophilic, thickened, and fragmented. The basophilia is due to the imbibition of iron compounds, and the fibers give a strongly positive reaction for iron. Larger vessels are dilated, but involved arterioles show luminal obliteration.

A marked foreign-body giant cell reaction occurs around the degenerated elastic fibers in vessel walls and interstitial tissue. There is a *diffuse fibrosis of alveolar walls and pulmonary septa.* Numerous siderophages (hemosiderin-laden macrophages) are present. Where these cells aggregate, the alveolar epithelial cells show cuboidal metaplasia. About 75 percent of these cases have developed *cor pulmonale.* This is often of marked degree, the right ventricular myocardium measuring over 1 cm. thick.

EMPHYSEMA OF THE LUNGS

EMPHYSEMA:

Emphysema of the lungs (pulmonary emphysema) is a condition in which the air spaces distal to the terminal bronchioles are enlarged due to overdistention or destruction of their walls. Today emphysema is the *most common chronic pulmonary disease,* estimates running as high as 10 million cases in the United States. The marked increase in incidence in recent years appears to be related to cigarette smoking [50] and exposure to air pollutants in urban areas. Pulmonary fibrosis and emphysema have been produced experimentally in dogs which have smoked cigarettes for over a year [51].

Pathogenesis

The *pathogenesis of pulmonary emphysema* is unsettled. The principal theories that have been proposed are that emphysema is due to air trapping resulting from expiratory bronchial obstruction; to inflammatory damage to respiratory bronchioles, alveolar ducts, and alveoli; or to ischemic damage to these structures secondary to vascular obstruction. According to the *obstructive concept* a chronic bronchiolitis produces obstruction of bronchioles by the accumulation of mucus and pus. Air enters the alveoli distal to the obstruction by collateral circulation through unobstructed bronchioles and pores of Kohn during inspiration. It becomes trapped, and when the pressure exceeds the elastic limit of the alveolar walls, they are ruptured. The *inflammatory concept* considers that loss of elastic tissue and weakening of muscle fibers is due to chronic bronchiolitis or the reaction to coal dust pigment. *Anthracotic pigment in the lungs,* long thought to be innocuous, is now suspected to be a causative factor by damaging the elastic tissue of the lungs. Degenerative changes in elastic fibers have been demonstrated at the sites of anthracotic pigment accumulation [52]. The *loss of elasticity in bronchioles and bronchi* due to pigment deposition, chronic bronchitis, or bronchial asthma may be an important factor in the expiratory difficulty experienced by emphysematous patients [53]. Such inelastic and atrophic bronchioles and bronchi may collapse on expiration and produce severe obstruction in that phase of ventilation. The rupture of alveoli behind bronchiolar and bronchial obstructions may be preceded by alveolar damage due to an *interstitial alveolitis* [54]. Such alveolar inflammation leads to destruction of the elastic tissue of the alveolar septa and obliteration of alveolar capillaries. The *vascular obliterative theory* is not widely accepted, and it is likely that the narrowing and even obliteration of small arteries and arterioles in and around areas of emphysema are an effect rather than a cause.

Associated diseases

Pulmonary diseases which frequently precede or are associated with emphysema are chronic bronchitis, bronchial asthma, mucoviscidosis, silicosis and other pneumoconioses, and tuberculosis.

Clinical features

Clinically in pulmonary emphysema the chest becomes barrel-shaped, due to an increase in the anteroposterior diameter. Respiratory movements are diminished, and expiration is difficult and prolonged. Wheezing is common. Hypercapnia (carbon dioxide retention) results from the diminished respiratory exchange and frequently produces respiratory acidosis. Dyspnea and cyanosis may develop, and there is often a chronic cough. Emphysematous lungs are hyperresonant on percussion. Rupture of an emphysematous bleb produces pneumothorax. The right ventricle becomes hypertrophied because of the increased pulmonary blood pressure (cor pulmonale), and a secondary polycythemia frequently develops. The *pathogenesis of increased pulmonary arterial pressure and cor pulmonale* in emphysema is not entirely clear. The development of precapillary anastomoses between the pulmonary and bronchial arterial circulations has been demonstrated. There also is an increase in the bronchopulmonary venous collateral circulation in emphysema. With the development of the incompetency of valves at the junctions of bronchopulmonary and azygos veins, a right-to-left flow develops. This may contribute to the systemic arterial oxygen desaturation and hypercapnia which is noted in the late stages of emphysema [55]. The frequency of *pulmonary atherosclerosis* in cases of chronic pulmonary emphysema may be due to episodes of pulmonary embolism with organization of the thrombotic material into atheromatous plaques [56]. The incidence of *pulmonary embolism* is significantly higher in patients with advanced emphysema than in control populations (45 percent as compared to 15 percent in one series) [57]. The emboli are large in the great majority of cases, and frequently are the direct cause of death. Pulmonary embolism does not occur more frequently in emphysema patients with right ventricular failure or polycythemia than in those without these complications.

Pathologic changes:

Emphysema may be diffuse or focal. In the diffuse type the lungs are voluminous and fill the entire pleural cavities. Large or small blebs may be found beneath the pleura, especially at the apices. The lungs have a soft, feathery feel. *Microscopically* the alveolar walls show knoblike thickenings, called *spurs,* on their ends. The walls are greatly stretched or ruptured, and the alveolar spaces much enlarged. The elastic tissue in the walls is diminished. Small arterioles are thickened, and the larger pulmonary artery branches show moderate atherosclerosis.

centrilobular emphysema

Pulmonary emphysema is divided pathologically into centrilobular, panlobular, and focal forms. *Centrilobular emphysema* [58] is the most common type and is much more prevalent in men than women. It is the form of emphysema to which cigarette smoking appears to be particularly related [59]. Centrilobular emphysema develops first in the upper lobes and begins centrally in secondary lobules of Miller in the region of respiratory bronchioles. Such bronchioles are frequently surrounded by black pigment cuffs in coal miners and city dwellers. This form of emphysema is constantly associated with bronchial, bronchiolar, and respiratory bronchiolar inflammation. Obstruction is uncommon until the process is extensive and involves the entire secondary lobule.

panlobular emphysema

Panlobular (panacinar destructive) emphysema [60] occurs more commonly in men than women. It generally develops in an older age group than the centrilobular form. Generalized panlobular emphysema is associated with kyphoscoliosis, endobronchial tuberculosis, silicosis, congenital absence of bronchial cartilage, and Marfan's syndrome. Partial obstruction or connective tissue deficiencies in bronchi and large bronchioles appear to be the main factors in its pathogenesis. The emphysema begins in the lower lobes and involves all parts of the secondary lobules simultaneously. The degree of involvement varies from mild to severe. In its most extreme form panlobular emphysema results in the so-called "cotton candy" or vanishing lung.

focal emphysema

Focal emphysema is localized to areas adjacent to foci of industrial or nonindustrial anthracosis and to tuberculous or other pulmonary scars. Large bullae or giant cysts may develop in relation to scars.

Special forms: compensatory emphysema

Compensatory emphysema is an overdistention of the alveoli of remaining lung following surgical removal of a lung, lobe, or portion of a lobe. Such overdistention does not ordinarily cause permanent damage to or disruption of alveolar walls, but in older patients destructive changes eventually occur in overdistended alveolar walls, and pulmonary functional capacity is decreased.

bronchiolar emphysema

Bronchiolar emphysema (cystic cirrhosis of the lungs) [61] is very rare. It is characterized *clinically* by progressive dyspnea and a chronic productive cough. *Grossly* the lungs are heavy and the pleural surfaces are bosselated (knobby). The *cut surfaces* are honeycombed by numerous small cysts with thick fibrotic walls. These are due to dilatation of small bronchioles. *Microscopically* the lung parenchyma is extensively replaced by dense fibrous tissue within which numerous varisized *bronchiolar cysts* are found. These are lined by columnar or cuboidal epithelium and show focal ulceration or squamous metaplasia. The cyst walls are made up of vascular fibrous tissue and contain numerous irregular bundles of hypertrophic smooth muscle which presumably arises from the bronchiolar walls. The heart shows moderate to marked right ventricular hypertrophy and dilatation.

infantile lobar emphysema

Infantile lobar emphysema [62] has been reported a number of times and is unexplained. The involved lobe (usually an upper lobe) is moderately to markedly emphysematous, and the other lobe (or lobes) is (are) atelectatic due to compression. Congenital fibrous dysplasia with overstretching of the inelastic fibrous alveoli, maldevelopment of bronchial cartilages, and congenital bronchial mucosal folds have been proposed as the cause.

interstitial emphysema

Interstitial emphysema is the accumulation of air in the tissue spaces of a lung. Acute or chronic inflammation of the involved lung is usually associated, especially when fibrosis is present. It may occur during the violent paroxysms of pertussis. Occasionally it appears in an apparently normal lung. The wall of a small bronchiole ruptures, and air dissects along its wall, then into the loose connective tissue of the septa out to the pleura or the hilum of the lung. It may rupture into the mediastinum *(mediastinal emphysema, Hamman's syndrome)* or appear subcutaneously in the neck or on the chest wall. The involved lung has a crackling feel. The air appears as beads within the fibrous tissue or as blebs beneath the pleura. An *acute* or *chronic mediastinitis* may follow due to the introduction of the cause of the pulmonary inflammation into the mediastinum.

ATELECTASIS

PRIMARY ATELECTASIS:

Atelectasis is a collapsed or airless state of all or a part of a lung. At birth both lungs are atelectatic *(primary atelectasis)*. With the onset of respiration, the alveoli expand. Once the alveoli are even partially expanded, the lung will float in water. This is a simple test which in most cases distinguishes whether the infant has breathed or not, an important medicolegal point. Factors which act to retard the initial expansion of the alveoli after birth are: (1) plugging of the bronchi by desquamated epithelium and other debris in amniotic fluid; (2) cohesion of the bronchial and alveolar walls; (3) an imperfectly developed or a damaged respiratory center; and (4) an imperfectly developed thoracic musculature.

Pathologic changes

The *totally atelectatic lung* is dark or bluish red and firm. In a *partially* atelectatic lung there are dark or bluish red foci, with the lighter pink, aerated portions projecting up above the depressed firm areas. In the atelectatic foci *microscopically* the alveolar walls are thick and flattened upon each other. The bronchiolar and bronchial walls are irregularly folded. In those cases due to bronchial plugging, curled squamous epithelial cells are found within the bronchi and expanded alveoli.

SECONDARY ATELECTASIS:

Secondary atelectasis includes any collapse of the alveoli after the primary expansion in neonatal life has taken place.

Compression atelectasis

Compression atelectasis is due to extrinsic pressure on all or part of a lung, driving the air out and producing collapse. It is complete when the pressure is great and uniform, as in a large pleural effusion, empyema, or pneumothorax. *Partial collapse* of a lung may be due to local pressure of a tumor mass, an enlarged heart, or an elevated diaphragm. The last may result from an acute dilatation of the stomach. Unless adhesions have formed on the pleura, the lung will reexpand when the cause of the collapse is removed.

Obstructive atelectasis

Obstructive atelectasis is due to complete blockage of a bronchus caused by a neoplastic mass, mucus, an inhaled foreign body, or a diphtheritic membrane. The air distal to the block is absorbed, leading to collapse of the involved portion of the lung. Except in the case of a foreign body, weakening of the respiratory movements due to debility or anesthesia is also a factor. Mucus secretions and tumors are the most common causes of bronchial obstruction.

Contraction atelectasis

Some cases of pulmonary atelectasis in which no bronchial plugging or external compression is found may be due to the contraction of smooth muscle fibers in the walls of alveolar ducts and in alveolar septa *(contraction atelectasis)* [63]. Such contraction is postulated as being due to increased neuromuscular reflex activity.

Acute massive collapse

Acute massive collapse of a lobe or an entire lung is due to bronchial obstruction plus respiratory weakness. It usually occurs a few hours following abdominal surgery. The patient suddenly develops extreme dyspnea, marked cyanosis, and prostration. There is no respiratory movement on the affected side. The heart is shifted to that side, and the leaf of the diaphragm on the affected side is high.

Physiologic changes

Focal atelectasis causes no physiologic alterations and no clinical signs or symptoms, except an area of dullness on percussion. *Massive atelectasis* alters the physiologic action of the lungs and heart. The blood volume flow through the lung is decreased, as well as the vital capacity and residual air, and the alveolar and blood carbon dioxide is increased. Dyspnea and cyanosis may be severe.

Pathologic changes

Atelectatic portions of a lung are firm, inelastic, airless, and sunken below the surface of the aerated portions. The color of the affected areas is steel blue or purple. If an entire lung is involved, it has the appearance of a squeezed sponge lying against the posterior chest wall and vertebral column. *Microscopically* the alveolar walls are pressed together so that the alveolar spaces are nearly obliterated. If the atelectasis is of prolonged duration, fibrosis may occur.

MISCELLANEOUS DISEASES OF THE LUNGS

1. Pulmonary Alveolar Proteinosis

PULMONARY ALVEOLAR PROTEINOSIS:

Pulmonary alveolar proteinosis [64] is a chronic lung disease of undetermined cause. It occurs more commonly in males than females by 2.5 to 1, and the reported cases have frequently developed in persons exposed occupationally to irritating fumes and dusts.

Clinical features

Clinically there are "creepingly progressive" dyspnea, cough productive of thick yellow sputum, chest pain, no or slight fever, and fatigability. Cyanosis may appear terminally, and clubbing of the fingers occurs in a few cases. Physical signs are slight. X-ray findings show a soft, feathery or nodular perihilar density with a radiating butterfly pattern.

Pathologic changes

Grossly in fatal cases the lungs may be enormously heavy (up to 3500 gm.). They are massively consolidated, and milky or thick yellow fluid oozes from the cut surface. The unconsolidated lung parenchyma is salmon-colored or dark red. *Microscopically* many alveoli are filled with eosinophilic, granular, and floccular proteinaceous material which is positive to PAS (periodic acid-Schiff) stain and is lipid-rich. This material appears to derive from the degeneration of sloughed-off alveolar septal cells. Acicular (needle-shaped), doubly refractile crystals and laminated bodies are found within the intra-alveolar material.

2. Hyaline Membrane Disease

HYALINE MEMBRANE DISEASE:

Hyaline membrane disease (respiratory distress syndrome) has been recognized as a common cause of death in newborn infants, especially premature children, those delivered by cesarean section, and those born of diabetic mothers. It causes about 25,000 deaths among infants yearly in the United States. In this disease the newborn infant respires normally for 8 to 24 hours. This is called the quiet or latent period. After that time respirations become labored and accelerated, and dyspnea and cyanosis appear. There are marked thoracic retractions as the infant struggles to breathe. Death usually occurs within 24 to 48 hours.

Cause

Left ventricular failure appears to be an etiologic factor because of the accumulation of edema fluid in the alveoli. The disorder occurs in about 90 percent of the cases of congenital cardiac anomalies which lead to pulmonary engorgement [65]. It is probable that thromboplastin in aspirated amniotic fluid induces clotting of fibrinogen leaked from the alveolar capillaries. In most newborn infants these fibrin clots are lysed by the action of fibrinolytic enzymes, and the *absence of a fibrinolytic enzyme system in the lungs* due to a genetic defect may be an important predisposing factor in hyaline membrane formation [66]. Lung plasminogen activator activity was absent in the lungs in a series of cases of hyaline membrane disease. The placenta has been found to contain high levels of an inhibitor of plasminogen activator, and placental infarction related to maternal diabetes mellitus or impending abortion may release this into the fetal circulation [67]. A new pathogenetic concept proposes that hyaline membranes result from the *absence of a powerful detergent-like agent* in the lungs [68]. This surface-acting agent is a lipoprotein containing dipalmitoyl lecithin. It is apparently produced in the mitochondria of alveolar epithelial cells. In its absence the surface tension at alveolar interfaces remains high, leading to the leakage of fluid from the capillaries and subsequent hyaline membrane formation.

Pathologic changes [69]

Grossly the lungs are reddish purple, usually show extensive *foci of atelectasis,* and may sink in water. The atelectasis is of the resorptive type, the lungs having previously been expanded. *Microscopically* the typical lesion is the presence of numerous eosinophilic, homogeneous, PAS-positive *membranes* lining the alveoli, alveolar ducts, and small bronchioles. It has been demonstrated by electron microscope that these membranes are basically *fibrin.* Desquamated epithelial cells and other debris are often found in the alveolar spaces. The blood vessels are markedly congested.

3. Acute Diffuse Interstitial Pulmonary Fibrosis

ACUTE DIFFUSE PULMONARY FIBROSIS:

In *acute diffuse interstitial pulmonary fibrosis (Hamman-Rich syndrome),* diffuse fibrosis develops within a month of the onset of symptoms. The disease is uncommon and occurs most often in middle-aged adults. The cause is unknown. Viruses, chemical agents, and repeated episodes of interstitial pneumonia have been blamed. Several cases have followed influenzal pneumonia. Hexamethonium and hydralazine have produced lesions identical with this disease. Dyspnea and cyanosis are prominent.

Pathologic changes [70]

Early there is an *acute pneumonitis,* with a large amount of fluid exudate and prominent hyaline membranes, but without much leukocytic infiltration. The alveolar lining becomes cuboidal. Later, fibroblasts, macrophages, and eosinophils appear. The fibroblasts invade the hyaline membranes, producing *intra-alveolar and interstitial fibrosis. Cor pulmonale* develops in chronic cases.

4. Alveolar Microlithiasis

ALVEOLAR MICROLITHIASIS:

Alveolar microlithiasis [71] is a rare chronic disorder which is often familial. It appears to be due to an inborn respiratory defect at the alveolar interfaces, probably in the carbonic anhydrase system. The pH increases, promoting the precipitation of calcium salts within the alveoli.

Clinical features

Clinically the diagnosis is usually made on a routine chest film, the disorder being asymptomatic until late in the course. The x-ray film shows startling, diffuse, fine calcific densities uniformly distributed in both lungs. Late in the disease, dyspnea, cyanosis, secondary polycythemia, clubbing of the fingers, and cor pulmonale develop.

Pathologic changes

Grossly the lungs are whitish, hard, and heavy (combined weights have reached 4000 gm.). They sometimes sink in water. The cut surface is extremely gritty, feeling like sandpaper. Apical emphysematous blebs are common. *Microscopically* numerous basophilic laminated concretions are found lying free in the alveolar spaces early in the disease. Later there is marked *intra-alveolar fibrosis* which encircles the concretions. Foreign-body giant cells are present. The masses consist mainly of calcium phosphate, with some calcium carbonate and magnesium carbonate. There is evidence of the presence of mucopolysaccharides. The heart may show right ventricular dilatation and hypertrophy. No other foci of calcification are found, and the bones are normal.

5. Alveolar Capillary Block

ALVEOLAR CAPILLARY BLOCK

Alveolar capillary block is caused by any pathologic process which alters the alveolar septa and thus reduces oxygen diffusion across the alveolar capillary membranes. *Alveolar capillary block affects oxygen diffusion more than that of carbon dioxide,* so that arterial oxygen unsaturation occurs with relatively little carbon dioxide retention. The block occurs in a variety of conditions such as hyaline membrane disease of the lungs; diffuse pulmonary fibrosis; fibrosis of the lungs due to tuberculosis, sarcoidosis, or pneumoconiosis; rheumatic pneumonitis; and pulmonary scleroderma.

6. Pulmonary Arteriosclerosis

PULMONARY ATHEROSCLEROSIS

Some degree of *atherosclerosis* is found *in the large pulmonary arteries* in most individuals over 50 years of age. This is usually but not always associated with systemic arterial atherosclerosis. In the pulmonary arteries, atheromatous plaques are typically situated at foci of high mechanical stress. The degree of atherosclerosis is *usually more severe in patients with pulmonary hypertension* than in normotensive individuals. It *occurs frequently in patients with congenital heart disease* in which there is a left-to-right shunt. *Pulmonary thromboembolism* is frequently found in cases of pulmonary sclerosis, and some authorities believe that organization of thrombi and emboli plays an important role in the development of atheromatous plaques. Pulmonary atherosclerosis per se is of limited clinical importance.

PULMONARY ARTERIOLOSCLEROSIS:

Much more serious is *sclerosis of the small pulmonary arteries and arterioles.* In the fetus the small pulmonary arteries and arterioles are thick-walled with small lumina. As the ductus arteriosus narrows and then becomes obliterated, a greatly increased amount of blood passes through the lungs. The pulmonary arterial and arteriolar lumina widen and the vessel walls become thin and seldom have a continuous muscle coat. Rarely the dilatation and thinning of small pulmonary arteries and arterioles does not occur after birth *(primary pulmonary arterial disease)* [72]. This leads to pulmonary hypertension in early life, with death due to right heart failure in infancy or childhood.

Primary arteriolosclerosis

Sclerosis of small pulmonary arteries and arterioles may be primary or secondary. Those cases for which no recognizable cause is found are classified as *primary.* Some of these are associated with *primary pulmonary hypertension,* which occurs most commonly in women between the ages of 20 and 40. It is characterized *clinically* by exertional dyspnea, episodes of precordial pain, syncopal (fainting) attacks, and dizziness and headaches on straining. On catheterization the mean *pulmonary arterial pressure* is elevated from a normal of 30/12 mm. of mercury to about 95/50. The mean *right atrial pressure* is raised to 9 mm. of mercury (normal -2 to +6), and the *right ventricular pressure* is elevated to 100/10 mm. of mercury (normal, 30/6). There is no systemic hypertension nor evidence of cardiac valvular disease. Electrocardiographic tracings show *right ventricular hypertrophy.* Chest films show prominence of the pulmonary arterial tree with a clear lung parenchyma. Sudden death occurs commonly in these patients. *Grossly* the lungs are not remarkable. *Microscopically* the significant changes are found in the small muscular arteries and arterioles which show concentric intimal fibroblastic proliferation and deposition of mucopolysaccharide with luminal narrowing or obliteration. The internal elastic lamina is split and fragmented. In the media, smooth muscle hypertrophy may be found. In some cases of primary pulmonary hypertension (as well as in some secondary cases), *plexiform (glomoid) structures* have been found in muscular pulmonary arteries [73, 74]. These have been attributed to a congenital vascular malformation, recanalization of thrombi or emboli, or reactive fibrosis resulting from increased pressure and flow or from gas bubble emboli. Just proximal to the structures, the artery is greatly narrowed by intimal thickening and becomes a tortuous *afferent channel.* The plexiform structure consists of a labyrinthine network of interconnected vascular channels measuring 4 to 18μ in diameter and is up to 800μ long. Distal to it the artery has a thin muscular coat and is otherwise normal. It ends in a normal arterial and capillary network. Such structures impart a high resistance to the pulmonary circulation, since according to *Poiseuille's law* the resistance to flow is inversely related to the fourth power of the radius of a vessel's lumen.

Secondary arteriolosclerosis

Secondary pulmonary vascular sclerosis is usually considered to be due to *increased pulmonary arterial pressure and/or flow.* However, at least some cases appear to be due to the *organization of multiple emboli or thrombi* in small pulmonary arteries and arterioles. Secondary pulmonary sclerosis occurs in cases of *congenital heart disease* with left-to-right shunt (interventricular and interatrial septal defects, persistent ductus arteriosus, and Eisenmenger's complex); *mitral stenosis,* in which the pulmonary vascular changes are often marked; *diffuse pulmonary fibrosis; emphysema of the lungs; multiple pulmonary emboli; kyphoscoliosis; and systemic hypertension. Chronic cor pulmonale* develops in most cases of secondary pulmonary sclerosis and hypertension. The right ventricular myocardium is hypertrophied; and the ventricle is frequently dilated. Death is often due to a right heart failure in these cases. A *secondary polycythemia* commonly develops as a compensatory phenomenon. Severe cases of pulmonary vascular sclerosis with marked dyspnea, polycythemia, and cyanosis (black cardiacs) are classified as *Ayerza's disease,* but the term is little used today.

NEOPLASMS OF THE BRONCHI AND LUNG

1. Benign Neoplasms

BRONCHIAL ADENOMA:

Adenoma constitutes about 10 percent of all bronchopulmonary neoplasms and is the most important benign tumor in this group. The incidence in men and women is about equal. The age period of greatest frequency is 20 to 40, 85 percent of bronchial adenomas occurring before age 50. Most adenomas occur in main-stem bronchi and are therefore visible on bronchoscopic examination. They are nearly equally divided between the right and left lung. Although the *carcinoid type of bronchial adenoma* rarely stains positively with silver (i.e., they are uncommonly argentaffin-positive) and mucin secretion occurs more commonly than in intestinal carcinoids, the bronchial neoplasm arises from Kultschitzky cells similar to those of the intestinal mucosa [75]. About 10 cases of *malignant carcinoid (Thorson-Biorck) syndrome* have been reported due to metastasizing bronchial adenomas [76]. This syndrome is related to the development of hepatic metastases and the elaboration of increased amounts of serotonin (5-hydroxytryptamine) and includes flushing and mottled cyanosis of the face, neck, and shoulders, asthma, diarrhea, and signs of right heart failure. Tricuspid and pulmonic valvular narrowing due to endocardial thickening is found. The *production of serotonin* by most carcinoid-type bronchial adenomas is indicated by the finding of increased blood serotonin and urinary 5-hydroxyindole acetic acid (5-HIAA) levels [77]. The origin of the *cylindromatous type* is probably from bronchial mucous glands.

Malignant carcinoid syndrome

Clinical features

Symptoms in cases of bronchial adenoma are primarily a result of bronchial obstruction, with stagnation of secretions and often with infection. There may be a history of *recurring pneumonia* affecting a particular lobe. Cough, intermittent and localized wheezing, and hemoptysis are commonly noted. If untreated, *bronchiectasis* may develop, giving copious sputum. The tumor itself is usually hidden in the mediastinal or cardiac shadows but the atelectasis resulting from local *bronchial obstruction* may be seen. Rarely the tumor may show as a rounded shadow (coin lesion) in the lung parenchyma near the hilum. *Bronchograms* reveal the tumor as a point of obstruction or as a filling defect.

Pathologic changes: carcinoid type — cylindromatous type — metastases

In most instances the tumor is round or oval, about 1 to 3 cm. in diameter, and projects as a tan *polyp* into the bronchial lumen. Some are firm, some soft; most tend to bleed easily. The mucosal covering is usually intact. About 85 percent of bronchial adenomas are of the *carcinoid type,* so named because of their resemblance to carcinoid tumors of the appendix. This type is composed of uniform cells with centrally placed, round or oval nuclei. The cells are arranged in clusters, sheets, or ribbons. Occasional acinar structures are present. Electron microscopy reveals that the neoplastic cells contain intracytoplasmic neurosecretory-type granules [78]. Foci of *bone* are found in about 15 percent of carcinoid adenomas [79]. The remaining 15 percent of bronchial adenomas are *cylindromatous,* i.e., the cells are arranged in a cylindrical pattern about small cores of hyaline material, resembling certain neoplasms of the salivary glands. As a class, *bronchial adenomas are borderline between benign and malignant neoplasms.* Although locally invasive, usually they do not recur after segmental resection or after lobectomy. If untreated, about 15 percent metastasize after a number of years, usually to the regional lymph nodes. Skeletal metastases with the carcinoid type are osteoblastic [80].

LEIOMYOMA

Rarely an encapsulated *leiomyoma* may arise from the smooth muscle of the bronchial wall and grow either inward into the lumen, as a polyp, or outward, pushing aside the lung parenchyma. These tumors cause hemoptysis and may be followed by bronchiectasis. *Leiomyosarcoma* develops very rarely in the lung.

CHONDROMA

Also uncommon is a benign encapsulated growth of cartilage, a *chondroma,* which arises from the bronchial wall, bulging either outward or into the lumen. It usually causes no symptoms and is a chance finding at autopsy.

HAMARTOMA

Somewhat more common than either the pure leiomyoma or the pure chondroma is a benign tumor composed of mixed connective tissue elements, sometimes mingled with an overgrowth of epithelium as well. When the tumor arises from well-differentiated cell elements normally found in the lungs, but in an abnormal, mixed-up pattern, the term *hamartoma* is commonly used. When different connective tissue elements are mingled but epithelium is lacking, the term *mesenchymoma* may be used.

2. *Bronchogenic Carcinoma*

BRONCHOGENIC CARCINOMA:

Lung cancer is almost synonymous with *bronchogenic carcinoma,* since the great majority of malignant tumors primary in the lower respiratory tract are epithelial in nature and arise from the *mucosa of the bronchial tree.*

Statistics

Bronchogenic carcinoma causes far more deaths than any other form of cancer in the male. In 1970 over 50,000 men died of lung cancer in the United States. Furthermore, it appears to be increasing in incidence more rapidly than any other cancer in the male; in 1930 the age-adjusted death rate from lung cancer among white males in the United States was 3.8 per 100,000, while in 1967 the figure was 40.6. The male to female ratio in bronchogenic carcinoma is about 5:1. This preponderance is chiefly in epidermoid carcinoma, adenocarcinoma being slightly more frequent in females. The peak incidence of bronchogenic carcinoma is in the 50 to 59 age group.

Causes: cigarette smoking

There is strong evidence that the increase in lung cancer is due to increased *cigarette smoking.* Among persons who smoke more than 40 cigarettes per day for a prolonged period, 12 percent die from bronchogenic carcinoma [81]. Controlled autopsy studies have demonstrated that *bronchial epithelial changes,* such as loss of cilia, increase in the number of cell rows, the presence of atypical cells, and carcinoma in situ, *are much more common in cigarette smokers than nonsmokers* [82]. The degree of such changes increases with the number of cigarettes smoked. The presence of numerous atypical cells in the bronchial epithelium is found more often in men than in women cigarette smokers and more frequently in cigarette than in cigar and pipe smokers. Bronchial basement membrane thickening, sometimes associated with squamous metaplasia, occurs in cigarette smokers; and alterations in bronchial elastic fibers resulting in some loss of elasticity are found in heavy smokers [83]. Controlled *experimental studies on rabbits* subjected to simulated cigarette smoking for several years revealed a significantly increased incidence of chronic rhinitis, bronchial epithelial changes (focal and generalized basal cell hyperplasia with and without atypical cells), and pulmonary emphysema [84]. *In dogs* in which main bronchi were treated with cigarette smoke condensate, epithelial hyperplasia, with and without atypical cells, and squamous metaplasia were significantly more common than in controls; and premalignant bronchial epithelial atypism, carcinoma in situ, and invasive carcinoma occurred only in condensate-treated dogs [85]. Alpha particle *radiation from* ^{210}*polonium,* a contaminant of tobacco, has been implicated in the genesis of bronchogenic carcinoma in cigarette smokers [86]. The report of the Advisory Committee to the Surgeon General of the U.S. Public Health Service states that "Cigarette smoking is causally related to lung cancer in men; the magnitude of the effect of cigarette smoking far outweighs all other factors. The data for women, though less extensive, point in the same direction" [87]. Diehards still argue against cigarette smoking's being a cause of lung cancer, as follows: Lung cancer has never been produced in experimental animals living in an air chamber loaded with cigarette smoke; its increase in incidence in women has not paralleled the increase in cigarette smoking; genetic factors may be involved; the observed association between smoking and lung cancer may be due to some outside common factor such as stress; and only 10 to 15 percent of heavy cigarette smokers develop lung cancer.

air pollution

Extensive studies have been undertaken to determine the *role of urban air pollution* in the causation of bronchogenic carcinoma. Known carcinogenic agents such as 3,4-benzpyrene, aliphatic hydrocarbon oxidation products, and chromium and nickel compounds are distributed widely in soot, gasoline, and diesel engine exhaust fumes and other air pollutants [88]. The benzene extract of gasoline engine exhaust condensate has about twice the carcinogenic activity of tobacco smoke condensate in producing skin neoplasms in mice [89]. Persons living in a large city have a 27 percent greater risk of developing lung carcinoma than those residing in rural areas, and urban cigarette smokers develop bronchogenic carcinoma more frequently than comparable smokers in rural areas. However, a study of Seventh-Day Adventists in smog-filled Los Angeles showed a significantly lower incidence of lung cancer in this nonsmoking group than in the general population [90].

other factors

In certain instances bronchogenic carcinoma appears to be an *occupational disease.* It has a very high frequency in cobalt, radium, and uranium miners and an increased frequency in workers in chromate, nickel, petroleum, and asbestos. Among hospitalized patients with *tuberculosis* there is an increased incidence of bronchogenic carcinoma.

Clinical features:

The neoplasm begins as a small mass in the mucosa of a bronchus, generally at the hilum, and is asymptomatic at first. Later, when it bulges into the lumen as a polypoid mass, it produces wheezing, hemoptysis, and cough. Bronchoscopic examination at this time may reveal the growth. Still later it may grow to surround the lumen and produce bronchial obstruction, atelectasis, and stagnation of secretions. *Chronic pneumonitis, bronchiectasis,* or *abscess formation* may follow, giving a febrile illness with much expectoration; about 25 percent of bronchogenic carcinomas form abscess cavities. The tumor extends to the pleura and to hilar and mediastinal lymph nodes. There is reduction of vital capacity due to parenchymal infiltration, bronchial obstruction, and pleural effusion. Dyspnea, cyanosis, and chest pain are terminal manifestations. Distant metastasis is common; the liver, bones, adrenal glands, kidneys, brain, heart, and mediastinum are often affected. The earliest lesions may show on x-ray as rounded parenchymal shadows *(coin lesions)* or may be hidden in the mediastinal shadows. Later the x-ray manifestations are more an indication of associated changes than of the primary tumor itself: *localized emphysema* (due to partial obstruction of the bronchus) or *atelectasis* (due to complete obstruction of the bronchus), *pleural effusion* (due either to pleural extension or lymphatic blockage), and *abscess* occur in different cases at different times. The lesions are slightly more frequent in the upper than in the lower lobes, but right and left lungs are about equally affected.

extra-pulmonary manifestations

A number of cases of *oat cell carcinoma* have developed *adrenocortical hyperplasia and manifestations of Cushing's syndrome* [91]. These cases have occurred mainly in men and have been characterized by increased ketosteroid and corticosteroid excretion, diabetes mellitus, and hypertension. The cause of the adrenocortical hyperplasia is adrenal corticotropin-like material which has been extracted from such neoplasms. In several cases of bronchogenic carcinoma without Cushing's syndrome, bilateral adrenal cortical hyperplasia has been found. This could be due to increased secretion of adrenal weight-maintaining corticotropin by the neoplastic cells or the anterior pituitary, or the nonspecific stress of a prolonged illness [92]. Chronic adrenal cortical insufficiency *(Addison's disease)* may be produced by bilateral adrenal destruction due to metastatic bronchogenic carcinoma [93]. Other extrapulmonary manifestations of bronchogenic carcinoma [94] include *hypercalcemia* unrelated to bony metastases and due to the secretion of a parathyroid hormone-like agent by the neoplastic cells [95], *increased antidiuretic hormone secretion* unrelated to pituitary metastases; *peripheral neuropathy* with degeneration of posterior root ganglion neurons and peripheral nerves; *muscle weakness* secondary to motor neuron degeneration or due to primary muscular degeneration *(carcinomatous myopathy); clubbing of the finger tips* in about 10 percent of the cases; *hypertrophic osteoarthropathy,* with which bronchogenic carcinoma is the most frequently associated condition; *migratory phlebothrombosis* in about 2.5 percent of cases; *terminal endocardiosis;* and *hypofibrinogenemia* due to tissue thromboplastin elaboration. Arginine vasopressin-like antidiuretic activity has been demonstrated in plasma and extracts of bronchogenic carcinoma from cases with inappropriate antidiuresis [96].

Pathologic changes:

There are *four histologic types* of lung cancer – epidermoid, anaplastic or oat cell, giant cell, and adenocarcinoma; each has its characteristic location and manner of growth, subject, of course, to considerable individual variation within the class. The first two, *epidermoid carcinoma* and *oat cell carcinoma,* are probably derived from the same parent cell, differing chiefly in the degree of cell differentiation. It is these two types which occur most frequently in men and which are presumably related to smoking.

epidermoid carcinoma

Epidermoid carcinoma arises from surface epithelium of main-stem bronchi or the next subdivision, and constitutes about 50 percent of all bronchogenic carcinomas. Microscopically this tumor is fairly well differentiated, but rarely shows keratin or pearly bodies. Sometimes there is pleomorphism with spindle and giant cells. This neoplasm grows more slowly than the anaplastic carcinoma, and spread is chiefly by *direct extension* to hilar lymph nodes, chest wall, and mediastinum. *Metastases* are present in about 35 percent of the cases at autopsy.

anaplastic carcinoma

Anaplastic epidermoid (oat cell) carcinoma arises from surface epithelium, especially of the main stem bronchi, and comprises about 35 percent of all bronchogenic carcinomas. *Microscopically* this neoplasm is composed of *small cells* resembling lymphocytes, with scanty cytoplasm and frequent mitoses. Its *spread* is chiefly *via lymphatics,* but distant hematogenous spread is common. Metastases are present in 90 percent of the cases at autopsy. *Metastases* in lymph nodes are found in 98 percent of the fatal cases, the liver in about 60 percent, one or both adrenal glands in 50 percent, bones and pancreas in about 40 percent, and the opposite lung and the brain in about 35 percent [97].

giant cell carcinoma

Giant cell carcinoma [98] is rare, constituting about 1 percent of bronchogenic carcinoma. It tends to develop peripherally and averages about 4 cm. in diameter. Microscopically the neoplasm consists largely of bizarre giant cells with one or more nuclei. The nucleus often has a horseshoe or ring configuration. Cytophagocytosis is often shown by the giant cells. There are also undifferentiated round cells and spindle cells. Tissue culture has established the epithelial nature of the cells of this neoplasm [99]. The course in giant cell carcinoma is rapid, death usually occurring within a year after detection.

adenocarcinoma

Adenocarcinoma presumably arises from the epithelial cells of the glands or ducts of the bronchial submucosa, lying below the covering epithelium. This tumor comprises about 10 percent of all lung carcinomas and affects both sexes about equally. It is generally located more peripherally in the bronchial tree than the other types. *Microscopically* it is composed of gland-forming, mucin-secreting epithelial cells. Its spread is chiefly by the bloodstream. *Metastases* are present in 86 percent of the cases at autopsy.

Special forms: bronchiolar carcinoma

Terminal bronchiolar carcinoma (pulmonary adenomatosis, alveolar cell carcinoma) [100] is a rare subvariety of adenocarcinoma of the lung. It arises in the epithelium of terminal bronchioles and grows slowly, rarely producing bronchial obstruction. *Grossly* this neoplasm resembles in some cases the uniform consolidation of lobar pneumonia; in other cases it is multicentric in origin, resembling a metastatic neoplasm. *Microscopically* groups of alveoli are lined with tall, clear *mucin-secreting cells.* The sputum is abundant and mucoid. Progressive extension reduces functioning lung tissue, causing dyspnea, clubbing of the fingers, and cyanosis. Metastasis occurs in 25 to 50 percent of the cases but is largely confined to the hilar nodes. Histologically the neoplasm resembles a viral disease in sheep known as *jaagsiekte.*

pulmonary scar carcinoma

Pulmonary scar carcinoma arises in fibrous scar resulting from chronic pneumonitis, an abscess, bronchiectasis, tuberculosis, infarction, siderosilicosis, or trauma [101]. Possibly its development results from the bronchiolar epithelial proliferation which has been noted about some of these lesions [102, 103]. Most of these neoplasms are *peripheral,* and the overlying pleura is puckered. A focus of dense fibrous scarring is found in or about the tumor, but it is not always certain whether such fibrosis preceded or developed secondarily with the neoplastic growth. *Such carcinomas appear to arise from bronchiolar epithelium,* but *histologically they may be adenocarcinoma, adenosquamous carcinoma, or epidermoid carcinoma.*

pulmonary sulcus tumor

The special manifestations of the superior *pulmonary sulcus tumor (Pancoast tumor)* are dependent upon location at or adjoining the thoracic inlet. While bronchogenic carcinoma is the usual neoplasm in this position, thyroid cancer and mediastinal neoplasms may produce similar effects. Infiltration of the brachial plexus gives pain and muscle atrophy in an arm; involvement of the cervical sympathetic chain causes *Horner's syndrome;* and compression of the superior vena cava results in edema of the face and upper extremities *(superior vena cava syndrome).*

carcinosarcoma

Carcinosarcoma of the lung [104] is very rare and usually grows as an intraluminal mass in a large bronchus. Microscopically the epithelial element has been epidermoid, mucinous, or anaplastic carcinoma. The connective tissue component is typically fibrosarcoma or chondrosarcoma.

PRIMARY LYMPHOMAS

While pulmonary involvement is found at autopsy in 25 percent of cases of disseminated lymphomas, *primary lymphoma* arising in a lung is uncommon [105]. Its origin is from peribronchial lymphoid tissue. About 65 percent of the cases are lymphosarcoma, 25 percent Hodgkin's disease, and 10 percent reticulum cell sarcoma. With the exception of some cases of Hodgkin's disease, the growth of these neoplasms is slow and spread is intra-alveolar, with late extension to the hilar lymph nodes.

3. *Metastatic Neoplasms to the Lungs and Pleura*

METASTATIC NEOPLASMS:

Metastatic neoplasms of the lungs and pleura are more common than primary neoplasms. Such metastases occur in about 25 percent of all fatal malignant neoplasms. In the authors' experience the most common neoplasms giving rise to pulmonary or pleural metastases, arranged in descending order of frequency, are carcinoma of the breast, gastrointestinal tract, female genital tract, and kidneys; melanocarcinoma; and male genital cancer. Neoplastic cells may reach the lung by direct extension, as through the diaphragm from the liver or stomach; by pulmonary arterial embolism, as in the case of osteogenic sarcoma; or by retrograde lymphatic extension from the mediastinal lymph nodes, as in Hodgkin's disease. Doubtless more than one path is used in many cases.

Clinical features

Clinical symptoms are sometimes minimal, even with widespread metastases. Pain, usually of pleuritic type, is probably the most frequent manifestation. Hemoptysis, cough, and dyspnea are also common signs. Often there is pleural fluid – serous, serofibrinous, or bloody – and the diagnosis of neoplasm can frequently be made by aspirating some of the fluid, centrifuging it, and studying the strained sediment for malignant cells.

Metastatic neoplasms in the lungs are typically multiple and bilateral. When they are in the parenchyma of the lungs, they are usually rounded. At the pleural surface they tend to be hemispheric or umbilicated. When spread is by lymphatic channels, the pleura often shows threadlike extensions of tumor, and the bronchi may show white thickening of the mucosa and submucosa. In such cases the hilar and mediastinal nodes are usually enlarged and replaced by neoplasm, and the parietal pleura often shows neoplasm extending along the intercostal vessels and nerves. Sometimes metastatic neoplasm is so diffusely spread throughout the lungs that it resembles pneumonia or fibrosis grossly.

Pathologic changes

DISEASES OF THE PLEURA

1. *Inflammations*

Acute pleuritis (pleurisy) commonly occurs in inflammation of the lungs due to pneumococci, staphylococci, streptococci, or the tubercle bacillus; lung abscess and gangrene; pulmonary infarct; bronchogenic carcinoma; and pericarditis. The exudate may be serous *(pleural effusion),* serofibrinous, fibrinous, or purulent *(empyema).* The last is usually associated with pneumococcal or streptococcal pneumonia and lung abscess. The pleura is covered with a thick purulent exudate filled with polymorphonuclear leukocytes. The pleural space may contain large amounts of thick purulent fluid.

Acute pleuritis

Chronic pleuritis leads to great thickening of the pleura by fibrosis. It is caused by the organization of a fibrinous exudate to produce numerous dense, fibrous pleural adhesions. These may obliterate the pleural space.

Chronic pleuritis

2. *Fluid Collections*

Hydrothorax (pleural effusion) is the presence of a fluid transudate in a pleural cavity. The fluid is straw-colored or clear, with a specific gravity below 1.018 and protein content below 4 gm. per 100 ml. The *causes* include pneumonia, congestive heart failure, renal edema, carcinoma of the lung, and fibroma of the ovary *(Meigs' syndrome).*

Pleural effusion:

Unilateral effusion is more common on the right side, possibly due to pressure of a dilated right auricular appendage on the right pulmonary veins. The amount of fluid varies from 100 to 2500 ml. Large effusions embarrass respiratory excursion. The fluid may contain blood *(sanguineous pleural effusion).*

pathologic changes

Hemothorax is the presence of blood in a pleural cavity due to rupture of an aortic aneurysm, tearing of an intercostal vessel by a fractured rib, or other trauma to the chest.

Hemothorax

Chylothorax is the presence of lymph (chyle) in a pleural cavity (usually the left) due to perforation or obstruction of the thoracic duct by trauma, malignant neoplasm, tuberculosis, or filariasis. Milky fluid is found in one or both pleural cavities; the amount varies from 50 to 500 ml.

Chylothorax

Chyliform fluids resemble chyle, being milky due to fine fat droplets or albuminous material (pseudochyle). Fat-laden fluids may be present in tuberculosis or bronchogenic carcinoma.

3. Pneumothorax

PNEUMOTHORAX:

Pneumothorax is the presence of air within the pleural cavity. It may be due to a penetrating wound of the chest wall; tearing of a lung by the jagged end of a fractured rib; rupture of a bleb on a lung; a bronchopleural fistula; or spontaneous rupture of a lung *(spontaneous pneumothorax).* Pneumothorax is used therapeutically, under controlled conditions, in the treatment of tuberculosis.

Spontaneous pneumothorax

Spontaneous pneumothorax [106] is most often due to rupture into the pleural space of one or more subpleural emphysematous bullae. Rarely a subpleural bronchogenic cyst may rupture. In a number of cases no demonstrable pulmonary or pleural abnormality can be found. Most cases occur in otherwise healthy young men, and most do not recur following reexpansion. *Clinically* there is a sudden onset of unilateral, often anterior pleuritic pain. The severity of dyspnea which follows depends upon the degree of pulmonary collapse. With extreme degrees of pneumothorax, especially when there is underlying pulmonary disease, cyanosis and shock may appear. On chest film a dark, homogeneous area without bronchovascular markings is found peripherally in the pleural space. The *mediastinum may be shifted* to the opposite side. *Complications* include sanguineous pleural effusion, failure of the collapsed lung to reexpand, empyema rarely, and mediastinal emphysema (pneumomediastinum).

Tension pneumothorax

Tension pneumothorax occurs under conditions in which air enters the pleural cavity during inspiration and cannot be pushed out during expiration, leading to a build-up of the pressure within the pleural cavity.

Open pneumothorax

Open (sucking) pneumothorax occurs when there is free passage of air into the pleural space from without due to an open wound of the chest wall. A hissing sound is heard as air enters and leaves the chest. The patient is cyanotic and dyspneic.

Pathologic changes

The pleural cavity is filled with air. The lung on the affected side is partially or totally collapsed and atelectatic, depending on the degree of the pneumothorax and the presence or absence of pleural adhesions. The mediastinum is pushed to the opposite side.

4. Primary Neoplasms

Primary neoplasms of the pleura are relatively rare. Fibroma, mesenchymoma, and fibrosarcoma may occur as local pleural nodules.

Mesothelioma

Mesothelioma [107] is the most important primary neoplasm of the pleura. It occurs as a localized or diffuse growth, affecting both the visceral and parietal layers, and often producing bloody pleural fluid within which atypical mesothelial cells can be identified [108]. The frequency of this neoplasm is unknown, because of varying criteria used by different authors; some so-called mesotheliomas are probably metastatic rather than primary neoplasms of the pleura. There is an increased incidence of mesotheliomas in persons with pulmonary asbestosis. *Microscopically* the tumor is composed chiefly of polyhedral or spindle cells, arranged usually in whorls or sheets and sometimes in a papillary form. *Metastases* to the mediastinal lymph nodes are common, but distant metastasis is rare.

TUMORS OF THE MEDIASTINUM

MEDIASTINAL TUMORS

Space-occupying lesions of the mediastinum include primary and metastatic neoplasms, cysts, and thyroid enlargements. About one-third of mediastinal tumors are neurogenous, 25 percent are cysts, 15 percent thymomas, 10 percent teratomas, and 5 percent lymphomas. Individual types of tumors are discussed elsewhere. The following is a list of mediastinal tumors (excluding metastatic neoplasms) arranged in order of relative frequency in various sites [109]: (1) *anterior mediastinum* – thymoma, teratomas (benign teratoma, teratocarcinoma, choriocarcinoma), goiter, parathyroid adenoma, lymphomas, lipoma, fibroma, lymphangioma, hemangioma; (2) *superior mediastinum* – goiter, bronchogenic cyst, parathyroid adenoma, lymphomas; (3) *middle mediastinum* – bronchogenic cyst, lymphomas, pericardial cyst, plasmocytoma; and (4) *posterior mediastinum* – neurilemmoma, neurofibroma, ganglioneuroma, fibrosarcoma, lymphomas, goiter, xanthofibroma, and gastroenteric cyst.

REFERENCES

1. Ryan, R. F., McDonald, J. R., and Devine, K. D. The pathologic effects of smoking on the larynx. *A.M.A. Arch. Path.* 60:472, 1955.
2. Vetto, R. R. Epiglottitis. *J.A.M.A.* 173:990, 1960.
3. Teplitz, C., Epstein, B. S., Rose, L. R., and Moncrief, J. A. Necrotizing tracheitis induced by tracheostomy tube. *Arch. Path.* (Chicago) 77:6, 1964.
4. Carilli, A. D., Gohd, R. S., and Gordon, W. A virologic study of chronic bronchitis. *New Eng. J. Med.* 270:123, 1964.
5. Bonomo, L., Gillardi, U., and Tursi, A. Anti-γ-globulin and antinuclear factors in chronic bronchitis. *Amer. J. Clin. Path.* 45:313, 1966.
6. Oberman, H. A. Papillomas of the nose and paranasal sinuses. *Amer. J. Clin. Path.* 42:245, 1964.
7. Frazell, E. L., and Lewis, J. S. Cancer of the nasal cavity and accessory sinuses. *Cancer* 16:1293, 1963.
8. Aldave, A., and Gallager, H. S. Olfactory esthesioneuroepithelioma. *A.M.A. Arch. Path.* 67:43, 1959.
9. Yeh, S. A histological classification of carcinomas of the nasopharynx with a critical review as to the existence of lymphoepitheliomas. *Cancer* 15:895, 1962.
10. Hubbard, E. M. Nasopharyngeal angiofibromas. *A.M.A. Arch. Path.* 65:192, 1958.
11. Batsakis, J. G., Klopp, C. T., and Newman, W. Fibrosarcoma arising in a "juvenile" nasopharyngeal angiofibroma following extensive radiation therapy. *Amer. Surg.* 21:786, 1955.
12. Webb, H. E., Harrison, E. G., Masson, J. K., and Re Mine, W. H. Solitary extramedullary myeloma (plasmacytoma) of the respiratory tract and oropharynx. *Cancer* 15:1142, 1962.
13. Sweeney, F. J., and Taylor, G. W. Carcinoma of the larynx. *Med. Ann. D.C.* 31:85, 1962.
14. Wynder, E. L., Bross, I. J., and Day, E. Epidemiological approach to the etiology of cancer of the larynx. *J.A.M.A.* 160:1384, 1956.
15. Shaw, H. J., and Epstein, S. S. Cancer of the epiglottis. *Cancer* 12:246, 1959.
16. Stein, A. A., and Volk, B. M. Papillomatosis of trachea and lung. *A.M.A. Arch. Path.* 68:468, 1959.

17. Ranke, E. J., Presley, S. S., and Holinger, P. H. Tracheogenic carcinoma. *J.A.M.A.* 182:519, 1962.
18. Ide, G., Suntzeff, V., and Cowdry, E. V. A comparison of the histopathology of tracheal and bronchial epithelium of smokers and nonsmokers. *Cancer* 12:473, 1959.
19. Godman, G. C., and Churg, J. Wegener's granulomatosis. *A.M.A. Arch. Path.* 58:533, 1954.
20. Sproul, E. E. Wegener's and lethal midline granulomatosis. *J.A.M.A.* 177:921, 1961.
21. Howland, W. S., and Lewis, J. S. Postintubation granulomas of the larynx. *Cancer* 9:1244, 1956.
22. Welsh, R. A. The genesis of the Charcot-Leyden crystal in the eosinophilic leukocyte of man. *Amer. J. Path.* 35:1091, 1959.
23. Abul-Haj, S. K., and Flanagan, P. Asthma associated with disseminated necrotizing granulomatous vasculitis, the Churg-Strauss syndrome. *Med. Ann. D.C.* 30:670, 1961.
24. Heller, E. L., Householder, J. H., and Benshoff, A. M. Bronchogenic cysts, a manifestation of congenital polycystic disease of the lungs. *Amer. J. Clin. Path.* 23:121, 1953.
25. Wolman, M., and Goldberg, M. G. The microscopical criteria of interstitial pneumonia. *A.M.A. Arch. Path.* 65:272, 1958.
26. Song, Y. S., and Sprung, D. H. Nonbacterial diffuse myocarditis associated with interstitial pneumonia. *A.M.A. Arch. Path.* 65:666, 1958.
27. Grayson, J. T., Alexander, E. R., Kenny, G. E., Clarke, E. R., Fremont, J. C., and MacColl, W. A. *Mycoplasma pneumoniae* infections. *J.A.M.A.* 191:369, 1965.
28. Thomas, L. Circulating autoantibodies and human disease, with a note on primary atypical pneumonia. *New Eng. J. Med.* 270:1157, 1964.
29. Dines, D. E., Baker, W. G., and Scantland, W. A. Aspiration pneumonitis – Mendelson's syndrome. *J.A.M.A.* 176:229, 1961.
30. Teabeaut, J. R. Aspiration of gastric contents: An experimental study. *Amer. J. Path.* 28:51, 1952.
31. Moran, T. J. Milk-aspiration pneumonia in human and animal subjects. *A.M.A. Arch. Path.* 55:286, 1953.
32. Christoforidis, A. J., and Molnar, W. Eosinophilic pneumonia. *J.A.M.A.* 173:157, 1960.
33. Parkin, T. W., Rusted, I. E., Burchell, H. B., and Edwards, J. E. Hemorrhagic and interstitial pneumonitis with nephritis. *Amer. J. Med.* 18:220, 1955.
34. Botting, A. J., Brown, A. L., Jr., and Divertie, M. B. The pulmonary lesion in a patient with Goodpasture's syndrome as studied with the electron microscope. *Amer. J. Clin. Path.* 42:387, 1964.
35. Koffler, D., Sandson, J., Carr, R., and Kunkel, H. G. Immunologic studies concerning the pulmonary lesions in Goodpasture's syndrome. *Amer. J. Path.* 54:293, 1969.
36. Liebow, A. A., Hales, M. R., and Lindskog, G. E. Enlargement of the bronchial arteries, and their anastomoses with the pulmonary arteries in bronchiectasis. *Amer. J. Path.* 25:211, 1949.
37. Zimmerman, L. E. Demonstration of histoplasma and coccidiodes in so-called tuberculomas of lung. *A.M.A. Arch. Intern. Med.* 94:690, 1954.
38. Weed, L. A., Dahlin, D. G., Pugh, D. G., and Ivins, J. C. *Brucella* in tissues removed at surgery. *Amer. J. Clin. Path.* 22:10, 1952.

39. Campbell, R. E., and Hughes, F. A., Jr. The development of bronchogenic carcinoma in patients with pulmonary tuberculosis. *J. Thorac. Cardiovasc. Surg.* 40:98, 1960.
40. Schwartz, E. Retained foreign bodies in the tracheobronchial tree of children. *J.A.M.A.* 175:242, 1961.
41. Effler, D. B., and Erwin, J. R. The middle-lobe syndrome: A review of the anatomic and clinical features. *Amer. Rev. Tuberc. Pulm. Dis.* 71:775, 1955.
42. Gross, P. Current concepts of pneumoconiosis. *J.A.M.A.* 172:546, 1960.
43. Telischi, M., and Rubenstone, A. I. Pulmonary asbestosis. *Arch. Path.* (Chicago) 72:234, 1961.
44. Selikoff, I. J., Churg, J., and Hammond, E. C. Relation between exposure to asbestos and mesothelioma. *New Eng. J. Med.* 272:560, 1965.
45. Lynch, K. M., and McIver, F. A. Pneumoconiosis from exposure to kaolin dust: Kaolinosis. *Amer. J. Path.* 30:1117, 1954.
46. Wyatt, J. P., and Riddell, A. C. R. The morphology of bauxite fume pneumoconiosis. *Amer. J. Path.* 25:447, 1949.
47. Smetana, H. F., Tandon, H. G., Viswanathan, R., Venkitasubramanian, T. A., Chandrasekhar, S., and Randhawa, H. S. Experimental bagasse disease of the lung. *Lab. Invest.* 11:868, 1962.
48. Jackson, D., and Yow, E. Pulmonary infiltration with eosinophilia: Report of two cases of farmer's lung. *New Eng. J. Med.* 264:1271, 1961.
49. Walford, R. L., and Kaplan, L. Pulmonary fibrosis and giant-cell reaction with altered elastic tissue: Endogenous "pneumoconiosis." *A.M.A. Arch. Path.* 63:75, 1957.
50. Mitchell, R. S., Vincent, T. N., and Filley, G. F. Cigarette smoking, chronic bronchitis, and emphysema. *J.A.M.A.* 188:12, 1964.
51. Auerbach, O., Hammond, E. C., Kirman, D., and Garfinkel, L. Emphysema produced in dogs by cigarette smoking. *J.A.M.A.* 199:241, 1967.
52. Wright, R. R. Elastic tissue of normal and emphysematous lungs. *Amer. J. Path.* 39:355, 1961.
53. Wright, R. R. Bronchial atrophy and collapse in chronic obstructive pulmonary emphysema. *Amer. J. Path.* 37:63, 1960.
54. Anderson, A. E., Jr., and Foraker, A. G. Pathogenic implications of alveolitis in pulmonary emphysema. *Arch. Path.* (Chicago) 72:520, 1961.
55. Liebow, A. A. The bronchopulmonary venous collateral circulation with special reference to emphysema. *Amer. J. Path.* 29:251, 1953.
56. Kernen, J. A., O'Neal, R. M., and Edwards, D. L. Pulmonary arteriosclerosis and thromboembolism in chronic pulmonary emphysema. *A.M.A. Arch. Path.* 65:471, 1958.
57. Ryan, S. F. Pulmonary embolism and thrombosis in chronic obstructive emphysema. *Amer. J. Path.* 43:767, 1963.
58. Wyatt, J. P., Fischer, V. W., and Sweet, H. Centrilobular emphysema. *Lab. Invest.* 10:159, 1961.
59. Anderson, A. E., Jr., Hernandez, J. A., Eckert, P., and Foraker, A. G. Emphysema in lung macrosections correlated with smoking habits. *Science* 144:1025, 1964.
60. Pratt, P. C., Hague, M. A., and Klugh, G. A. Correlation of postmortem function and structure in panlobular pulmonary emphysema. *Lab. Invest.* 11:177, 1962.
61. Ravines, H. T. Bronchiolar emphysema of the lungs. *A.M.A. Arch. Path.* 69:554, 1960.
62. Bolande, R. B., Schneider, A. F., and Boggs, J. D. Infantile lobar emphysema. *A.M.A. Arch. Path.* 61:289, 1956.

63. Corssen, G. Changing concepts of the mechanism of pulmonary atelectasis. A study of smooth muscle elements in the human lung. *J.A.M.A.* 183:314, 1963.
64. Rosen, S. H., Castleman, B., and Liebow, A. A. Pulmonary alveolar proteinosis. *New Eng. J. Med.* 258:1123, 1958.
65. Shanklin, D. R. Cardiovascular factors in development of pulmonary hyaline membrane. *A.M.A. Arch. Path.* 68:49, 1959.
66. Lieberman, J. A new concept of hyaline membrane disease. *New Eng. J. Med.* 260:619, 1959.
67. Lieberman, J. The nature of the fibrinolytic-enzyme defect in hyaline-membrane disease. *New Eng. J. Med.* 265:363, 1961.
68. Clements, J. A. Surface tension in the lungs. *Sci. Amer.* 207:121, 1962.
69. Gilmer, W. S., and Hand, A. M. Morphological studies of hyaline membranes in the newborn infant. *A.M.A. Arch. Path.* 59:207, 1955.
70. Pokorny, C., and Hellwig, C. A. Diffuse interstitial fibrosis of the lungs. *A.M.A. Arch. Path.* 59:382, 1955.
71. Sosman, M. C., Dodd, G. D., Jones, W. D., and Pillmore, G. U. The familial occurrence of pulmonary alveolar microlithiasis. *Amer. J. Roentgen.* 77:947, 1957.
72. Goodale, F., Jr., and Thomas, W. A. Primary pulmonary arterial disease. *A.M.A. Arch. Path.* 58:568, 1954.
73. Naeye, R. L., and Vennart, G. P. The structure and significance of pulmonary plexiform structures. *Amer. J. Path.* 36:593, 1960.
74. Moschcowitz, E., Rubin, E., and Strauss, L. Hypertension of the pulmonary circulation due to congenital glomoid obstruction of the pulmonary arteries. *Amer. J. Path.* 39:75, 1961.
75. Weiss, L., and Ingram, M. Adenomatoid bronchial tumors. *Cancer* 14:161, 1961.
76. Anlyan, W. G., Hargrove, M. D., Jr., Ruffin, J. M., Wallace, D. K., Weaver, W. T., and Kirshner, N. Metastasizing bronchial adenoma. *J.A.M.A.* 174:415, 1960.
77. Warner, R. R. P., Kirschner, P. A., and Warner, G. M. Serotonin production by bronchial adenomas without the carcinoid syndrome. *J.A.M.A.* 178:1175, 1961.
78. Bensch, K. G., Gordon, G. B., and Miller, L. R. Electron microscopic and biochemical studies on the bronchial carcinoid tumor. *Cancer* 18:592, 1965.
79. Kinney, F. J., and Kovarik, J. L. Bone formation in bronchial adenoma. *Amer. J. Clin. Path.* 44:52, 1965.
80. Jatlow, P., and Rice, J. Bronchial adenoma with hyperserotinemia, biventricular valvular lesions, and osteoblastic metastases. *Amer. J. Clin. Path.* 42:285, 1964.
81. Hammond, E. C., and Horn, D. Smoking and death rates – Report on forty-four months of follow-up of 187,783 men. II. Death rates by cause. *J.A.M.A.* 166:1294, 1958.
82. Auerbach, O., Stout, A. P., Hammond, E. C., and Garfinkel, L. Changes in bronchial epithelium in relation to cigarette smoking and in relation to lung cancer. *New Eng. J. Med.* 265:253, 1961.
83. Hayashi, Y., Cowdry, E. V., and Suntzeff, V. Microscopic properties of the basement membrane and elastic fibers of trachea and bronchus of smokers and nonsmokers. *Cancer* 14:1175, 1961.
84. Holland, R. H., Kozlowski, E. J., and Booker, L. The effect of cigarette smoke on the respiratory system of the rabbit. *Cancer* 16:612, 1963.

85. Rockey, E. E., Speer, F. D., Ahn, K. J., Thompson, S. A., and Hirose, T. The effect of cigarette smoke condensate on the bronchial mucosa of dogs. *Cancer* 15:1100, 1962.
86. Little, J. B., Radford, E. P., Jr., McCombs, H. L., and Hunt, V. R. Distribution of polonium^{210} in pulmonary tissues of cigarette smokers. *New Eng. J. Med.* 273:1343, 1965.
87. *Smoking and Health: Report of the Advisory Committee to the Surgeon General of the Public Health Service.* Washington: U.S. Government Printing Office, 1964, p. 196.
88. Kotin, P., and Falk, H. L. The role and action of environmental agents in the pathogenesis of lung cancer. I. Air pollutants. *Cancer* 12:147, 1959.
89. Wynder, E. L., and Hoffmann, D. A study of air pollution carcinogenesis. III. Carcinogenic activity of gasoline engine exhaust condensate. *Cancer* 15:103, 1962.
90. Wynder, E. L., Lemon, F. R., and Bross, I. J. Cancer and coronary artery disease among Seventh-Day Adventists. *Cancer* 12:1016, 1959.
91. Bornstein, P., Nolan, J. P., and Bernanke, D. Adrenocortical hyperfunction in association with anaplastic carcinoma of respiratory tract. *New Eng. J. Med.* 264:363, 1961.
92. Carnasos, G., and Ruebner, B. H. Adrenal width and metastasis in bronchogenic carcinoma. *Arch. Path.* (Chicago) 76:263, 1963.
93. Hill, G. J., and Wheeler, H. B. Adrenal insufficiency due to metastatic carcinoma of the lung. *Cancer* 18:1467, 1965.
94. Knowles, J. H., and Smith, L. H., Jr. Extrapulmonary manifestations of bronchogenic carcinoma. *New Eng. J. Med.* 262:505, 1960.
95. Turkington, R. W., Goldman, J. K., Ruffner, B. W., and Dobson, J. L. Bronchogenic carcinoma simulating hyperparathyroidism. *Cancer* 19:406, 1966.
96. Bower, B. F., Mason, D. M., and Forsham, P. H. Bronchogenic carcinoma with inappropriate antidiuretic activity in plasma and tumor. *New Eng. J. Med.* 271:934, 1964.
97. Watson, W. L., and Berg, J. W. Oat cell lung cancer. *Cancer* 15:759, 1962.
98. Hellstrom, H. R., and Fisher, E. R. Giant cell carcinoma of lung. *Cancer* 16:1080, 1963.
99. Ozzello, L., and Stout, A. P. The epithelial origin of giant cell carcinoma of the lung confirmed by tissue culture. *Cancer* 14:1052, 1961.
100. Laipply, T. C., Sherrick, J. C., and Cape, W. E. Bronchiolar (alveolar cell) tumors. *A.M.A. Arch. Path.* 59:35, 1955.
101. Strauss, F. H., Dordal, E., and Kappas, A. The problem of pulmonary scar tumors. *Arch. Path.* (Chicago) 76:115, 1963.
102. Berkheiser, S. W. Bronchiolar proliferation and metaplasia associated with bronchiectasis, pulmonary infarcts, and anthracosis. *Cancer* 12:499, 1959.
103. Berkheiser, S. W. Bronchiolar proliferation and metaplasia associated with thromboembolism. *Cancer* 16:205, 1963.
104. Prive, L., Tellem, M., Meranze, D. R., and Chodoff, R. D. Carcinosarcoma of the lung. *Arch. Path.* (Chicago) 72:119, 1961.
105. Sternberg, W. H., Sidransky, H., and Ochsner, S. Primary malignant lymphomas of the lung. *Cancer* 12:806, 1959.
106. Massaro, D., and Katz, S. Spontaneous pneumothorax. *Med. Ann. D.C.* 29:664, 1960.
107. Manguikian, B., and Prior, J. T. Mesotheliomas of the pleura. *Arch. Path.* (Chicago) 75:236, 1963.

108. Klempman, S. The exfoliative cytology of diffuse pleural mesothelioma. *Cancer* 15:691, 1962.
109. Schlumberger, H. G. Tumors of the mediastinum. Section V, Fascicle 18, in *Atlas of Tumor Pathology*. Washington: Armed Forces Institute of Pathology, 1951, p. 10.

GENERAL REFERENCES

Ash, J. E., Beck, M. R., and Wilkes, J. D. Tumors of the upper respiratory tract and ear. Section IV, Fascicles 12 and 13, in *Atlas of Tumor Pathology*. Washington: Armed Forces Institute of Pathology, 1964, pp. 11–213.

Liebow, A. A. Tumors of the lower respiratory tract. Section V, Fascicle 17, in *Atlas of Tumor Pathology*. Washington: Armed Forces Institute of Pathology, 1952.

Spencer, H. *Pathology of the Lung (Excluding Pulmonary Tuberculosis)* (2d ed.). London: Pergamon Press, 1968.

20 THE GASTROINTESTINAL TRACT

INTRODUCTION

Disorders of the gastrointestinal tract make up a large proportion of the illnesses which cause patients to consult their doctors. Less often do these disorders appear as causes of death.

"Food poisoning"

The digestive tract is particularly liable to transient disorders, often producing violent symptoms but subsiding spontaneously and leaving no ill effect. This feature is undoubtedly due in large part to the wide variety of ingested food and drink, variously derived, prepared, preserved, modified, and adulterated, according to whim and custom.

"Nervous indigestion"

Functional disorders

In addition, gastrointestinal complaints are often a result of emotional and psychogenic disorders, or of diseases which affect some other system of the body primarily. In such cases symptoms are probably related to disturbances of motility, or to chemical variations in digestive juices as a result of stimuli transmitted by the autonomic nervous system. For these reasons, serious functional digestive disorders (anorexia, nausea, vomiting, pain, diarrhea, hyperchlorhydria, achlorhydria, constipation) sometimes occur with little or no demonstrable organic change.

CONGENITAL ANOMALIES

Lips and mouth

Harelip (cheiloschisis) and *cleft palate* (anathoschisis) are due to failure of union of the nasal process with either or both of the lateral maxillary processes. Thus a fissure occurs on one side of the midline. There may be bilateral defects. Cleft palate rarely occurs except in association with the most severe cases of harelip. *Tonguetie* is an abnormal shortness of the membranous fold beneath the tip of the tongue, resulting in limited mobility of the tongue. *Macroglossia* is an unusually large tongue, preventing normal closure of the baby's mouth; this is sometimes seen in association with mongolism, but may also occur from unexplained edema, and be temporary. *Ranula* is a cyst occurring beneath the anterior portion of the tongue, and arising from a salivary gland. *Lingual thyroid* is occasionally seen as a bulging mass at the base of the tongue. *Congenital teratoma* may arise from the palate and fill the mouth (epignathus).

Neck

Congenital lesions of the neck are often cystic and may not be recognized until some time after birth. *Thyroglossal duct cyst* is located in the midline anteriorly, anywhere between the foramen cecum of the tongue and the thyroid gland; it is usually lined by columnar epithelium. *Branchial cyst* (fistula) is located laterally; it may be lined by ciliated, columnar, or squamous epithelium, and lymphoid tissue is usually abundant in the wall. *Cystic hygroma* is a rare, usually congenital, bulky tumor of the neck; it is composed of lymphatic vessels filled with lymph. *Congenital teratomas,* both cystic and solid, occur in the neck, frequently in association with the thyroid gland.

Esophagus

Atresia is probably the most common congenital defect of the esophagus, and is often associated with *tracheo-esophageal fistula.* There may be complete absence of esophageal lumen below the level of the bifurcation of the trachea; such cases have often been marked by polyhydramnios during the pregnancy (see Chapter 15). Tracheo-esophageal fistula is not compatible with life unless corrected in the first few days. *Congenitally short esophagus* may be encountered, associated with hiatus hernia of the stomach. In some instances *gastric mucosa* may occur in the esophagus and account for esophagitis or ulcer. Esophageal *diverticula* are sometimes congenital, and may cause stasis of food and inflammation of the wall of the pouch.

Stomach

Hypertrophic pyloric stenosis is said to occur principally in breast-fed male infants. The muscle of the pylorus is greatly thickened, often being palpable through the abdominal wall. This hypertrophy, plus spasm, prevents the normal emptying of the stomach contents into the duodenum. Reverse peristalsis sets in, sometimes marked by waves visible through the anterior abdominal wall. *Vomiting* after feeding is the usual manifestation. Some cases of infantile *colic* are due to pyloric stenosis.

Small intestine

The most extreme congenital abnormality of the intestine is *complete atresia.* In such a case the intestine usually ends as a blind pouch; the distal segment, which is, of course, blind proximally, may be normally patent throughout its length. When complete atresia occurs, it is most commonly located in the ileum. Incomplete obstruction, i.e., *congenital stenosis* of the small intestine, is most frequent in the duodenum. *Heterotopic pancreatic tissue* is often found in the submucosa of the duodenum, but has no known significance. *Diverticula* of the small intestine are probably of congenital origin in most cases. (Diverticula of the large intestine are much more common and are usually acquired.) *Meckel's diverticulum* is the most common congenital anomaly of the gastrointestinal tract, but rarely does it cause any symptoms. It is a remnant of the vitelline duct which connects the yolk sac of the embryo with the intestine. It may persist as a blind pouch projecting from the lower portion of the ileum, often connected with the umbilicus by a fibrous band. Rarely gastric mucosa may occur in Meckel's diverticulum and may cause peptic ulceration of the ileum just distal to the mouth of the diverticulum. As in any cul-de-sac, obstruction and inflammation may occur, and rarely perforation may follow. Occasionally, a Meckel's diverticulum may knot itself around a segment of intestine, causing intestinal obstruction.

Large intestine

Malrotation of the intestine may sometimes cause the cecum and appendix to be on the left side of the abdomen. *Defects of the mesentery* may be associated with malrotation or occur independently. These defects may result in herniation into abnormal peritoneal pouches, causing *intestinal obstruction* in early life, rarely in utero. The anus may be imperforate.

Meconium ileus is a rare congenital disorder in which meconium is extremely thick and ropy, causing obstruction, usually in the region of the ileum or cecum. It is believed to be a result of fibrocystic disease of the pancreas (mucoviscidosis) (see Chapter 21). Meconium ileus

DISEASES OF THE MOUTH AND RELATED STRUCTURES

1. *Diseases of the Mouth, Lip, Tongue, and Pharynx*

Gingivitis and *pyorrhea* are infections of the gums and about the teeth, due to various bacteria. (These diseases, and the various forms of *dental abscess,* fall in the field of dentistry rather than medicine.) *Canker sores* are ulcers of the buccal mucosa and tongue, particularly common in females; these sores are possibly of endocrine origin. *Mucous patches* are superficial ulcers of the buccal mucosa (usually multiple) due to syphilis. *Glossitis* may be a part of buccal inflammations generally, or may be a manifestation of pellagra (nicotinic acid deficiency), pernicious anemia (vitamin B_{12} deficiency), or sprue (unknown deficiency). *Syphilitic glossitis* shows fissures and irregular areas of leukoplakia; it is generally believed to be a precancerous lesion. *Leukoplakia* may occur in any part of the mouth, particularly in chronic alcoholics, and often in relation to jagged teeth or ill-fitting dentures; the lesion is believed to be precancerous. (For a discussion of tonsillitis and pharyngitis see Chapter 19.) Inflammations

A number of important neoplasms occur in the buccal cavity. Together they account for about 3.5 percent of all cancer deaths in the male, and about 1.4 percent of all cancer deaths in the female. The great majority of these neoplasms arise from the covering epithelium of the mucous membrane and are therefore *epidermoid carcinomas.* The *adenocarcinomas,* arising from the mucous glands of the mouth (the so-called minor salivary glands), do not occur nearly so frequently. Carcinoma:

Carcinoma of the lips is a common neoplasm of *elderly males,* and affects chiefly the *lower lip.* It is frequent in those exposed excessively to sunlight, and it seems to occur particularly in pipe smokers. The lesion begins as a crack with pearly thickening of its edges and a tendency to bleed. Later it progresses to form an indurated, crusted ulcer. The tumor extends through the full thickness of the lip, and to the cervical lymph nodes, but distant metastasis is rare and cure is common, either by surgery or irradiation. Microscopically it is an *epidermoid carcinoma,* generally of low grade (grade I or II – Broders). lip

Carcinoma of the floor of the mouth is an important neoplasm of the buccal mucosa, usually occurring between the mandible and tongue. *Alcoholics* and *smokers,* especially males, seem particularly susceptible, possibly due to vitamin deficiencies. *Metastases* in the *anterior cervical lymph nodes* may appear at a time when the primary lesion is barely noticeable as a small white mucosal patch or crack. It is an *epidermoid carcinoma,* usually about grade III (Broders). It metastasizes earlier and more widely than cancers of the lip and tongue, and cure is unusual. floor of mouth

Carcinoma of the tongue affects males chiefly. The *edges* of the tongue are most often affected. Irritation from *jagged teeth* or *rough dentures* or *syphilitic glossitis* may precede the development of cancer. There is induration and often ulceration of the mucosa. The tumor is an *epidermoid carcinoma* and may be of tongue any degree of malignancy. Metastasis is usually slow, involving the lymph nodes of the neck; rarely there may be rapid, widespread metastases. (Primary amyloidosis and scleroderma of the tongue, and the rare benign tumor, granular cell myoblastoma, may produce thickening and rigidity of the tongue and be confused with cancer.)

tonsils

Carcinomas of the tonsils may be of the more common *epidermoid type,* but are frequently anaplastic and intimately related to the tonsillar lymphoid tissue; such a tumor is sometimes called *lymphoepithelioma.* An identical tumor may occur in the mucosal lymphoid tissue of the nasopharynx or of the base of the tongue. The lymphoepithelioma is very sensitive to irradiation. *Lymphosarcoma* may occur as a primary neoplasm in these tissues, arising from the lymphatic elements of the tonsils or adenoids. Neoplasms of the tonsils spread early to the cervical lymph nodes, and may metastasize widely. Cure is unusual.

palate

Carcinomas of the palate are usually *adenocarcinomas,* and arise from the minor salivary glands; similar tumors may occur almost anywhere in the buccal mucosa, since these mucous glands are widely distributed. These neoplasms form a submucosal *nodule* which enlarges progressively and tends to *ulcerate.* A number of subvarieties of this tumor have been described (cylindromatous, mucoepidermoid), corresponding to the neoplasms of the major salivary glands (see the section following); the prognosis is generally worse for these neoplasms when they occur in the buccal mucosa than for the corresponding tumors in the major salivary glands, perhaps because they are not so readily excised.

2. *Diseases of the Major Salivary Glands*

Inflammations

The most common inflammatory lesion of the salivary glands, chiefly of the parotid gland, is *mumps* or epidemic parotitis. The salivary glands may be affected in *cytomegalic inclusion disease* of infants, usually believed to be of virus origin. (Both these diseases are considered in Chapter 7.) *Suppurative parotitis* is sometimes a terminal complication, as in chronic renal disease with uremia. It usually occurs as a result of poor oral hygiene in a comatose, debilitated patient. *Sarcoid* may, on occasion, involve the parotid gland; in such cases the uveal tract of the eye (iris, choroid, and ciliary body) and the lacrimal glands are also frequently affected (see Chapter 6). *Calculi* may form in the duct of any of the salivary glands (sialolithiasis), causing painful chronic or recurrent inflammation.

Neoplasms:

The most important disease processes affecting the major salivary glands in adults are *neoplasms.* The parotid gland is the site of origin of nearly 90 percent of the neoplasms of the salivary glands. Most of the remainder occur in the submaxillary gland; rarely is the sublingual gland affected. The same types of neoplasms occur also in the lacrimal glands [1]; indeed the lacrimal and salivary glands show a peculiar parallelism in many of their diseases.

mixed tumors

Mixed tumors comprise about 63 percent [2] of all salivary gland tumors. They are ordinarily considered benign, but there is recurrence in about 25 percent of the cases, often some years after surgery. They are rounded, firm masses, usually encapsulated, and often embedded in the gland. On section they have a mucoid appearance. Microscopically the tumor is *essentially epithelial,* but a peculiar change in the stroma is commonly noted, the stroma resembling *cartilage.* It is the presence of this cartilaginous material along with the epithelial elements which accounts for the name *mixed tumor.* In most instances the epithelium forms well-differentiated glands and appears completely benign, but occasionally the epithelium is atypical and distinctly malignant *(malignant mixed tumor),* while the stroma retains its mucoid or cartilaginous character. Malignant mixed tumors are prone to recurrence and to metastasis to the regional nodes.

muco-epidermoid tumors

Muco-epidermoid tumors make up about 11 percent of the neoplasms affecting the salivary glands. Grossly these tumors are poorly encapsulated. Microscopically mucus-secreting glandular epithelium and squamous epithelium are intermingled. Regional lymph node metastasis is the rule in this frankly malignant tumor.

Warthin's tumor

Papillary cystadenoma lymphomatosum (Warthin's tumor) is a benign neoplasm making up about 5 percent of all tumors occurring in the parotid gland; it is believed by some authors to arise from branchial cleft rests. Within a mass of lymphoid tissue embedded in the parotid gland are slitlike spaces lined with tall eosinophilic epithelium. Papillary projections into the cysts are common. There is no tendency toward recurrence or metastasis.

adeno-carcinoma

The remaining neoplasms of the major salivary glands include a number that can be grouped together simply as *adenocarcinomas;* they make up about 8 percent of the total, and include several neoplasms differing slightly in their histologic patterns (cylindromatous, adenoid cystic). They tend to metastasize to the cervical lymph nodes and later to distant sites.

tumor-like

Mikulicz's disease, also known as benign lymphoepithelial lesion [3], is a tumor-like process affecting chiefly middle-aged and elderly women. The disease is poorly understood and ill defined. Any of the salivary glands may be involved, and the lacrimal glands may also be affected. The glandular structure is largely replaced by lymphoid tissue in which islands of epithelial cells are noted. The clinical course of this disease is usually benign. (The term *Mikulicz's syndrome* is also used, generally to imply involvement of the salivary and lacrimal glands during the course of a systemic disease such as leukemia, lymphosarcoma, tuberculosis, or sarcoid. A *drying-up* of the salivary and lacrimal secretions and *painless swelling* of these glands are common features of the several diseases of the syndrome.)

3. Diseases of the Jaws

The jaws (i.e., the maxillae and mandible) are subject to the usual disease of bones (see Chapter 28). In addition, chiefly because of their relationship to the *teeth,* the jaws are subject to certain diseases not occurring in other bones.

Inflammations

Inflammations of the mandible or maxillae are usually a result of *dental infection.* Sometimes a soft red swelling occurs in the gum adjacent to a dental abscess; this *granuloma* may be confused with neoplasm. Theoretically *foci of infection* about the teeth may cause distant manifestations, as in the joints or prostate; however, this view is much less popular now than it was 35 years ago. Actinomycosis is an important cause of osteomyelitis of the jaws (see Chapter 8).

Cysts

Most of the cystic lesions of the jaws are related to the teeth or their accessory structures. The *radicular cyst* occurs in relation to the roots of the teeth and probably begins as an apical abscess, later becoming lined with epithelium from the surface. The *dentigerous cyst (follicular cyst)* arises from the epithelial sheath around an unerupted tooth. *Anterior median cysts* occur in the midline of the maxilla and are believed to arise from embryonic epithelial structures. All these cysts may appear as rarified areas in the maxilla or mandible on x-ray.

Neoplasms

The *adamantinoma (ameloblastoma)* is a neoplasm of low-grade malignancy, presumably derived from epithelium about the embryonic tooth (the "enamel organ"). The tumor is often cystic in part. Microscopically the picture is varied, but often resembles a basal cell carcinoma of skin. The *odontomas* are rare lesions which probably are not true neoplasms. They are usually extremely hard and arise directly from a tooth. (In some classifications odontoma is a broader term, including some solid epithelial tumors.) The *epulis* is a benign tumor of the gums or of the connective tissues about the teeth; the term usually refers to a giant cell tumor in this location. *Secondary carcinoma* is probably the most common malignant neoplasm of the jaws; it is usually a result of direct extension from carcinoma of the floor of the mouth or buccal mucosa. *Hemangioma-like* lesions of the gingiva occur commonly during *pregnancy* and recede thereafter. *Leukemic infiltration* of the gums causes soft red mucosal elevations which tend to bleed easily.

4. Diseases of the Neck

Inflammations

Inflammation of the neck, showing up primarily as an enlargement or *cellulitis,* is usually a result of tonsillitis and pharyngitis. *Ludwig's angina* (streptococcal) and *diphtheria* are the chief infections causing significant neck enlargement. *Retropharyngeal abscess,* due either to pyogenic infection or to *tuberculosis* of the cervical spine, is rarely encountered. Deep-seated *abscesses* of the neck usually are a result of suppuration in the cervical lymph nodes. They may be a complication of pyogenic infection of the teeth or tonsils. *Tuberculosis of the cervical lymph nodes* usually occurs in children and may closely simulate abscess.

Neoplasms

Neoplasms are among the most important diseases encountered in the tissues of the neck; the lymph node neoplasms are especially important. A neoplasm may be *primary* in the lymph nodes (Hodgkin's disease, lymphosarcoma), or *metastatic* from a primary site elsewhere (mouth, tongue, lung, breast). Neoplasms of the *thyroid gland,* benign and malignant, account for another important group of diseases which cause enlargement of the neck (see Chapter 27); *salivary gland tumors* are still another (see earlier section in this chapter). *Tumors of the carotid body* are rare neoplasms belonging to the group known as *paraganglioma.* They are benign, although their intimate relationship to the carotid artery may make removal difficult.

DISEASES OF THE ESOPHAGUS, STOMACH, AND DUODENUM

1. Diseases of the Esophagus

Acute esophagitis

Acute esophagitis may be due to: (1) ingestion of food which is too hot or of a corrosive chemical, such as a strong acid or alkali, mercuric chloride, or tincture of iodine; (2) a foreign body, such as a chicken or fish bone or a safety pin; (3) *Corynebacterium diphtheriae;* (4) streptococci, as in scarlet fever; or (5) continued vomiting from any cause. The mucosa is edematous and often ulcerated, and an acute inflammatory reaction is found. *Complications* include *hemorrhage* and *perforation.* Sharp foreign bodies are particularly dangerous; they may cause mediastinitis and may even perforate the aorta, causing fatal hemorrhage. Esophagitis with little inflammatory reaction is found fairly frequently at autopsy without there having been any evidence of esophageal symptoms during life. Some of these lesions may be agonal, related to relaxation of the cardiac sphincter. In debilitated patients, such lesions may be covered with a heavy fungus growth, usually *Candida albicans.*

Subacute and chronic esophagitis

Recurring inflammation of the esophagus is seen in those cases in which *food or gastric juice collects in the lower end of the esophagus;* cardiospasm or hiatus hernia may be the underlying cause of esophagitis. *Cardiospasm* occurs chiefly in young or middle-aged women, and is apparently due to a failure of the reflex mechanism by which the cardiac sphincter normally relaxes to permit passage of food from the esophagus into the stomach; the lumen of the esophagus becomes greatly dilated, as can be shown by barium swallow. In *hiatus hernia,* the cardiac sphincter of the stomach may be located above the level of the diaphragm, giving a pocket lined by gastric mucosa within the thorax. Since digestive juices are thought to play an important part in the inflammatory process which ensues, the condition is often known as *peptic esophagitis. Pain* is the chief symptom; it is often aggravated by change in position. Since the pain is often substernal, it may be confused with the pain caused by coronary artery disease. The wall of the lower end of the esophagus is greatly thickened and its mucosa edematous, hyperemic, and possibly ulcerated. In some instances of prolonged esophagitis with ulcer, stricture develops.

Stricture

Stenosis of the esophagus may be either congenital or acquired. The congenital form (see page 496) is often associated with tracheo-esophageal fistula. The acquired form occurs in middle-aged or elderly persons, and is usually a result of peptic esophagitis, as noted above. Another important form of acquired esophageal stricture is that which follows the *ingestion of a caustic chemical.* In children this is usually accidental; in adults it may be a suicide attempt. The common *agents* are lye (about 70 percent of the cases), Lysol, mercuric chloride, and strong acids. The common *sites* of stricture are the narrow portions of the esophagus: the level of the crossing of the left bronchus and the upper and lower ends. The acute ulcer produced by the chemical is filled in with abundant granulation tissue, which in turn is replaced in about 6 weeks by fibrous tissue. The latter contracts to form the stricture. The result is a gradually increasing *inability to swallow,* usually requiring surgery for relief.

Diverticulum

Two types of diverticula of the esophagus are described. The *pulsion diverticulum* usually occurs at the pharyngeal end of the esophagus, and shows a herniation of the inner layers of the wall between the muscle bands; a pouch is formed in which food collects, causing inflammation and discomfort. The *traction diverticulum* usually occurs at the level of the bifurcation of the trachea and shows a tentlike pocket, the apex of which is adherent to some old extrinsic locus of inflammation, as tuberculous tracheobronchial lymph nodes.

Plummer-Vinson syndrome

The *Plummer-Vinson syndrome,* consisting of dysphagia plus hypochromic microcytic anemia, is a disorder of middle-aged women, often accompanied by lesions of the lips and tongue suggesting a vitamin deficiency. The syndrome is sometimes complicated years later by epidermoid carcinoma of the upper end of the esophagus (postcricoid carcinoma).

NEO-
PLASMS:
Benign

Benign neoplasms of the esophagus are rare and include leiomyomas arising from the muscle coat, lipomas of the submucosa, and rarely, adenomas of the mucosa.

Carcinoma:

Carcinoma of the esophagus is much more common than benign neoplasms. It causes nearly 3 percent of all cancer deaths in males, compared to less than 1 percent in females. *Alcoholism* and *smoking* are contributory etiologic factors [4]. More than 60 percent of the patients with esophageal cancer are over age 50; when they are younger, there is usually some special factor such as a lifelong stricture following ingestion of lye in infancy [5]. *Clinically* there is gradually *increasing dysphagia,* first to solid foods and then to liquids. Emaciation is marked. *Pathologically* the most common site is at the level of crossing of the left bronchus; carcinoma is almost as common at the lower end and is least frequent at the upper end of the esophagus. Most cases of carcinoma at the upper end of the esophagus occur in females, especially those with the Plummer-Vinson syndrome. Carcinomas of the upper and midportion of the esophagus are usually epidermoid in type; those of the cardiac end are usually adenocarcinomas, arising from mucous glands in the submucosa.

natural
history

Carcinomas of the midportion of the esophagus begin as flat nodules in the mucosa and spread in the submucosa, slowly encircling the esophagus and narrowing the lumen. Terminally the neoplastic cells penetrate the walls of the esophagus and spread to adjacent structures in the mediastinum. Ulceration occurs in the advanced lesions and may permit bacterial infection to enter, causing mediastinitis. In other cases a fistula through the tumor area may form between the bronchus and the esophagus; in such cases death is usually a result of aspiration of food particles and pulmonary suppuration. Occasionally death is due to penetration of the neoplasm into the walls of the thoracic aorta, resulting in exsanguinating hemorrhage. Distant metastasis is unusual in carcinomas of the midesophagus. *Adenocarcinomas of the lower end* of the esophagus spread into the stomach wall as well as into the esophagus, and pursue a course much like that of gastric cancer; metastases occur to the lymph nodes of the lesser curvature of the stomach and to the liver. *Carcinomas of the upper end* of the esophagus behave like neoplasms of the oropharynx, spreading to the contiguous tissues and to the cervical lymph nodes, often involving the trachea terminally.

2. *Diseases of the Stomach and Duodenum*

GASTRI-
TIS:
Acute

Acute gastritis may be *irritative* (due to ingestion of alcohol, salicylates, iodides, or bromides), *corrosive* (due to strong acids and alkalis), *coagulative* (due to phenol or mercuric chloride), *phlegmonous* (primary streptococcal gastritis), or *hemorrhagic* (complicating acute infections or uremia). The mucosa is hyperemic, and ulcers, if present, are superficial.

Chronic

Chronic gastritis is a poorly defined condition. One form, *chronic atrophic gastritis,* is found in association with the achlorhydria of pernicious anemia or pellagra; the walls are thin, the rugae flattened, the mucous glands atrophic, and there is little inflammatory infiltrate. Atrophic gastritis appears to be a precursor lesion to gastric cancer in some cases of pernicious anemia. Another form, *chronic hypertrophic gastritis,* shows large rugae having a nodular mucosal pattern suggesting cobblestones, and microscopically an irregular infiltrate composed chiefly of lymphocytes and plasma cells. Usually this alteration of the gastric mucosa is associated with few symptoms, but in rare cases the enlargement of the rugae is extreme *(benign giant rugal hypertrophy,* or Menetrier's disease) and is a part of a disorder consisting of *benign neoplasms of several endocrine organs* (islet cells of the pancreas, parathyroid gland, pituitary gland, and adrenal cortex); hypoproteinemia is a feature of most cases in this group [6, 7].

ULCERS: Acute

Acute ulcers are more frequent in the stomach than duodenum. They occur in uremia, in association with burns *(Curling's ulcer)* and hypothalamic lesions, and, most commonly, agonally. Many of these lesions are apparently *stress ulcers* due to an increased secretion of hydrochloric acid and pepsin into the stomach following trauma or during surgery. Acute ulcers are usually small, often multiple, and occur in any part of the stomach. Usually they are silent, obscured by the symptoms of the underlying disease.

Chronic peptic ulcer:

Peptic ulcer is a chronic disease. It may occur in the *lower esophagus, stomach, duodenum, jejunum,* or adjacent to a *Meckel's diverticulum.* It is more common in men than women by about 3:1, and duodenal ulcer is especially frequent in men.

causes

The immediate cause of peptic ulcer is the *hypersecretion of acid gastric juice.* Evidence for this concept, as pointed out by Dragstedt [8], is: (1) peptic ulcers occur only in those portions of the gastrointestinal tract that come in contact with gastric juice; (2) neutralization or dilution of gastric juice has a healing effect; and (3) surgical procedures which reduce gastric secretion are also beneficial. In gastric ulcer the hypersecretion of gastric juice is said to be mediated by the liberation of the hormone, gastrin, from the stomach antrum due to food stasis there. In duodenal ulcers the hypersecretion of gastric juice is said to be mediated through the vagus nerves. Men 20 to 40 years of age with a personality type characterized by worry and nervous tension seem particularly prone to duodenal ulcer; presumably this is due to impulses initiated in the autonomic nervous system and transmitted by the vagi. Peptic ulcer is often precipitated by a period of overwork, incessant smoking, and irregular meals and sleep. In rare instances, recurring and intractable peptic ulceration, usually of the jejunum but also of the duodenum and stomach, is associated with benign islet cell tumors of the pancreas (Zollinger-Ellison syndrome) [6]. Rarely, too, peptic ulceration may be an important manifestation of hyperparathyroidism [9]. Patients under long-term steroid therapy, as for rheumatoid arthritis, are prone to develop gastric ulcer; the mechanism is not clear.

clinical features

Clinically the most prominent symptom is *intermittent epigastric pain* which comes on several hours after taking food and is *relieved by eating or by the ingestion of alkalis.* Confirmation of the clinical diagnosis is obtained by *gastric analysis* and by *radiography* of the upper gastrointestinal tract. In duodenal ulcer, large quantities of gastric juice are secreted at night, and the output of hydrochloric acid is high. Radiographic examination is usually done in order to prove the presence of an ulcer. Barium fills the ulcer, the lesion usually being revealed as a tiny bulge on the smooth contour of the barium-filled stomach or duodenum. In other instances the ulcer may be revealed as an area in which the peristaltic wave is distorted by spasm.

gross appearance

About 60 percent of all peptic ulcers occur in the duodenum, chiefly in the first part, the duodenal bulb. Most of the remaining 40 percent occur in the stomach, usually within 5 cm. of the pylorus and on or near the lesser curvature. Peptic ulcers rarely occur in the acid-producing portion of the stomach, i.e., the fundus. Similarly, when peptic ulcer occurs following gastrojejunostomy, it is on the jejunal side of the anastomotic line, and when it occurs in association with Meckel's diverticulum, it is in the adjacent intestinal mucosa, not in the acid-producing ectopic gastric mucosa of the diverticulum. Peptic ulcers are single in about 90 to 95 percent of the cases. Ulcers may be of any size, but most are 1 to 2.5 cm. in diameter. The edges are usually sharply punched out and the base usually consists of muscularis with a thin covering of scar tissue and exudate.

microscopic appearance

Microscopically the peptic ulcer shows four zones in its floor: (1) a surface inflammatory zone of fibrin and polymorphonuclear leukocytes; (2) a zone of necrotic granulation tissue; (3) a zone of viable granulation tissue; and (4) a zone of dense scar tissue. The margins of the ulcer show a variable degree of epithelial proliferation. The vessels about the ulcer show endarteritis obliterans.

course

The ulcer diathesis, based as it is upon personality conflict and autonomic stimuli, tends to persist for many years. Especially is this true of those patients whose ulcers are duodenal, in whom symptoms are often first noted in the late teens and return at intervals until the fifties, with or without some of the *complications* given below.

complications
(1) perforation

Perforation is the major complication of peptic ulcer, accounting for 65 per cent of deaths from ulcer. In some cases perforation seems to be precipitated by steroid or phenylbutazone therapy. When ulcers of the anterior surface of the stomach or duodenum perforate, the usual result is spillage of the gastric contents into the peritoneal sac. *Chemical peritonitis* ensues, followed by paralytic ileus and bacterial peritonitis, and death will result unless surgical treatment is prompt. When ulcers of the posterior surface of the stomach or duodenum perforate, the escaping gastric contents may be walled off from the peritoneal cavity by the pancreas or other structures in the retroperitoneal area. This prevents direct contamination of the peritoneal cavity, causing instead a localized *perinephric or subphrenic abscess.*

(2) hemorrhage

Hemorrhage is the other major complication, and tends to occur when the ulcer is so located that it involves an important blood vessel, such as the pancreaticoduodenal or the right or left gastric artery. In some instances it seems that hemorrhage is precipitated in cases of peptic ulcer by taking aspirin. The stomach or duodenum fills with blood, which rapidly is modified by gastric juice so that it becomes somewhat granular and dark brown. It may then be vomited (coffee-ground vomitus) or it may pass through the intestine and cause a tarry stool. Exsanguinating hemorrhage may occur and cause death; about 25 percent of deaths from peptic ulcer occur in this way.

(3) obstruction

Obstruction is the third important complication of peptic ulcer, and is seen chiefly in ulcers located at or near the pylorus. Scar formation in the ulcer base may block the lumen, resulting in gastric retention. Clinicians at the George Washington University Hospital have studied a patient with duodenal ulcer and pyloric obstruction who developed a most remarkable infiltration of the stomach wall by eosinophils, and who at the same time presented a pronounced eosinophilia of the peripheral blood [10]; this patient was known to be allergic to a large number of different foods, and it seems likely that retention of some allergenic food in the obstructed stomach called forth the eosinophilic response.

healing

The various factors which cause peptic ulcer tend to prevent healing; if these factors can be neutralized, the mucosa will grow over the defect, leaving only a slightly puckered, thin area marking the site of the ulcer. Therapy is directed at minimizing the neural stimuli by promoting tranquility in the environment; milk and alkalis are given to neutralize the acid of the gastric juice. In intractable cases not yielding to other forms of treatment, a large segment of the acid-secreting portion of the stomach may be removed surgically, or the vagus nerves may be severed on both sides to remove the neural stimuli to gastric secretion.

malignant change

It is difficult to say just how frequently carcinoma develops in benign peptic ulcer. Certainly it does not occur in duodenal ulcer; carcinoma of the duodenum in the usual area where ulcer occurs is extremely rare. In the stomach, benign ulcers are common and so are carcinomas. Furthermore, carcinomas of the stomach, like carcinomas of any other mucosal surface, are prone to ulcerate. Obviously ulceration in a carcinoma of the stomach is not proof that the carcinoma arose in a benign ulcer. On the other hand, if carcinoma is found only at one edge of an ulcerated lesion of the stomach, this suggests that ulcer preceded the neoplasm.

NEOPLASMS: Benign

Benign neoplasms of the stomach are uncommon and include *leiomyoma* (which forms a sometimes large submucous mass arising in the muscularis), *fibroma, lipoma, hemangioma,* and *adenoma.* Adenomas, usually in the form of multiple adenomatous polyps *(gastric polyposis),* are important because of a tendency for one or more to become malignant. However, less than 5 percent of gastric adenocarcinomas are believed to arise in preexisting polyps.

Gastric carcinoma:

Carcinoma of the stomach accounts for about 5 percent of all male cancer deaths and about 4 percent of all female cancer deaths. Most cases occur after age 40. The cause is essentially unknown, but certain *predisposing factors* are recognized. There is some tendency for gastric cancer to occur in families; this inheritance factor is emphasized by the observation that the occurrence of gastric cancer is significantly increased in persons of blood group A [11]. There is also a tendency for gastric cancer to occur in *certain ethnic groups;* the Japanese seem particularly susceptible, both in Japan and following migration to Hawaii and California [12]. The reason for this is not known. Gastric carcinoma is several times more frequent in *patients with pernicious anemia* than in the general population [13]. *Adenomatous polyps* of the gastric mucosa are generally believed to be precancerous.

clinical features

The presenting symptom in gastric cancer is usually *epigastric pain.* An earlier symptom is frequently *loss of appetite,* due presumably to infiltration of the stomach wall by cancer cells, interfering with hunger contractions. When the neoplasm is situated at or near the pylorus, obstruction is early, causing *fullness* and *discomfort after meals* and often vomiting. Ulceration may occur in any of the forms of cancer in any portion of the stomach, and is usually followed by melena, anemia, and hematemesis. Interference with nutrition may also cause anemia, often with evidence of vitamin deficiencies and sometimes with steatorrhea. Spread to the peritoneal surface is usually marked by the appearance of ascites, while spread to the liver and porta hepatis is often evidenced by jaundice.

sites

The most common location for gastric cancer is the *prepyloric region* (60 percent of the cases). The remainder of the cases are about evenly distributed from the cardiac orifice through the antrum.

gross forms

Three general forms of stomach cancer are recognized grossly and on radiographic examination.

1. The *fungating* growth bulges into the lumen of the stomach, and on the radiograph causes a filling defect in the barium shadow. This type may arise from an adenomatous polyp. This form of stomach cancer usually grows rather slowly; in spite of the fact that it often becomes large, it has the best prognosis of the three forms.

2. The *ulcerating* carcinoma has raised, indurated edges, and an ulcer crater for a base. It shows on x-ray as a slight projection from the barium shadow as the barium fills the ulcer niche. Ulcerocarcinoma can never be differentiated certainly from benign gastric ulcers, although the neoplastic ulcers tend to be somewhat larger.

3. The *infiltrating* carcinoma causes a marked thickening of the walls of the stomach and, on x-ray, a narrowing of the lumen and loss of mucosal folds.

Fairly frequently the gross characteristics may be combined in a single case. Thus an infiltrating or a fungating carcinoma may show areas of ulceration.

microscopic forms

The microscopic picture is quite varied. Most gastric carcinomas form recognizable *glands.* In some instances no glands are formed and the *cells infiltrate individually* as mucin-containing signet-ring cells *(mucinous carcinoma).* The fungating masses often consist of solid sheets of cells *(carcinoma simplex)* whose stroma shows a lymphocytic infiltrate; this microscopic picture has the best prognosis. In the infiltrating form there is a great *increase in the connective tissue* of the stomach wall; neoplastic cells may be quite scarce and difficult to identify, resembling lymphocytes or monocytes.

natural history

The courses of the different forms of gastric cancer sometimes follow a pattern, but more often they are unpredictable. The course and complications are as much related to the *site* of the growth as to the *type.*

Those neoplasms which begin as gastric polyps and those which begin in benign gastric ulcers may have a history of some months of pain, usually aggravated by food intake. The tumor cells spread superficially in the mucosa and then penetrate to the submucosa, invading veins and lymphatics, penetrating to the *serosal surface.* The veins of the stomach carry the tumor cells to the *liver* early, and liver metastasis may be very massive. The tumor cells spread by lymphatics to the *lymph nodes* along the greater or lesser curvature of the stomach, depending on the location of the neoplasm. Extension also occurs to contiguous tissues: pancreas, gastrohepatic ligament, and omentum. By this time the tumor mass in the stomach and adjacent lymph nodes is often large enough to be palpable as a *firm epigastric mass.* From the involved lymph nodes the tumor early invades the *thoracic duct,* spreading then to the mediastinal and left supraclavicular lymph nodes along the course of the duct. Hematogenous metastasis may then occur to the *lungs, bones,* and *other distant organs.*

In the case of the infiltrating type of gastric cancer, a different course is sometimes noted. The tumor cells, and the fibrous tissue reaction which they incite, may cause the stomach wall to become as much as *2 cm. thick,* with a corresponding narrowing of the lumen to about that of the small intestine. The tumor may spread from cardia to pylorus (almost never crossing to the duodenum), form *tiny nodules on the serosal surface* of the stomach, *seed the peritoneal cavity* extensively, and set up extensive metastases in the ovaries in females (Krukenberg tumor) or in the pelvic peritoneum in males. Ascites and intestinal obstruction may then occur, due to peritoneal metastases, without there being any metastases to lymph nodes or liver. This is, of course, somewhat unusual, but it has been seen by the authors in a number of instances of the linitis plastica, or "leather bottle stomach," type of gastric cancer.

outcome

The outlook for cure in gastric cancer at the present time is poor. Because symptoms are usually late, most patients are beyond the possibility of curative surgery when first seen. The 5-year survival rate for all cases is probably about 10 percent.

Other malignant stomach neoplasms

Sarcomas and other primary malignant neoplasms of the stomach are relatively rare. *Leiomyosarcoma* is probably the most common form, but the malignant lymphomas *(reticulum cell sarcoma, Hodgkin's disease, lymphosarcoma)* are also an important group. The clinical manifestations and course of these diseases are similar to those of carcinoma, the differentiation being largely of academic significance.

Carcinoma of the duodenum

Carcinoma of the duodenum is rare – so rare that it seems remarkable. Not only are primary neoplasms uncommon, but the duodenum is rarely invaded by extension from a carcinoma of the stomach. When duodenal carcinoma does occur, it is usually adenocarcinoma of the *duodenal papilla.* In this strategic location it may block the ampulla of Vater, causing obstruction jaundice and steatorrhea, and at the same time may cause melena as a result of ulceration of the duodenal mucosa about the ampulla.

FOREIGN BODIES

Foreign bodies that reach the stomach will usually pass through it without causing great trouble; it is those that lodge in the esophagus that are most dangerous. Coins, marbles, pins, and buttons are common objects swallowed, usually by children or the mentally deranged. *Bezoars* are conglomerations of organic material which sometimes become large enough to block the pylorus, producing discomfort and vomiting. Usually they are composed of hair, the *trichobezoar;* these occur chiefly in children, but sometimes in adults who have the strange habit of eating hair. Another form is the *phytobezoar,* composed of plant hulls and fibers; persimmon hulls are notorious in this regard. On radiographic examination the bezoars present a striking picture. In the barium-filled stomach they show as a filling defect; in the 6-hour film they are seen as a positive, sausage-like shadow because of the barium caught in the interstices of the mass.

PHYSIOLOGIC ALTERATIONS AFTER GASTRECTOMY

A variety of physiologic alterations may occur after partial or complete gastrectomy, less commonly after diffuse gastric disease. All do not occur in every patient, and it is not possible to predict which alterations, if any, will occur in which patients, or to avoid these complications by variations in surgical technique. The *dumping syndrome* is a particularly distressing picture, consisting of weakness, faintness, and collapse following eating; it is said to be the result of the rapid emptying of the gastric stump, releasing hypertonic solutions into the jejunum, where a reflex mechanism is excited [14]. In other patients a serious *nutritional defect* develops. There is limited food capacity, loss of appetite and weight, and often diarrhea [15]. Specific defects of fat absorption may also occur, suggesting sprue, with *steatorrhea, hypocalcemia,* and *osteomalacia,* the latter apparently due to inability to absorb vitamin D and calcium [16]. (Such cases must be differentiated from primary hyperparathyroidism causing peptic ulceration, for which gastrectomy may be done.) *Anemia* is also an important consequence of gastrectomy. There is first a microcytic anemia due presumably to blood loss, but after several years this may give way to macrocytic hyperchromic anemia similar to that seen with pernicious anemia [17], presumably due to loss of the intrinsic principle necessary for the manufacture of normal erythrocytes.

DISEASES OF THE INTESTINE

1. Diverticulosis and Diverticulitis

Definitions

A *diverticulum* of the intestine is an outpouching of the wall to form a sac whose mucosal lining is continuous with that of the intestine. (Note the difference between diverticulum and ulcer.) If multiple diverticula are present, as is common in the acquired form, the condition is spoken of as *diverticulosis.* If one or more diverticula become inflamed, the process is spoken of as *diverticulitis.*

Congenital diverticula

Congenital diverticula occur chiefly in the small intestine. *Meckel's diverticulum,* arising at about the midportion of the ileum, is the most important, but congenital diverticula may occur in the duodenum or jejunum as well, usually in the mesenteric border. Seldom do they cause symptoms.

Acquired diverticula

Acquired diverticula are much more frequent than the congenital, and are usually multiple. They are most *common in elderly persons,* especially those subject to constipation. In most instances acquired diverticula are about 1 cm. in diameter. They are most common *in the sigmoid portion of the colon,* where they bulge between the longitudinal muscle bands. Fecal matter collects in these pockets and often inspissates there, causing the patient periodic abdominal discomfort.

Complications

When a fecalith forms in a diverticulum, drainage from the pocket may be blocked, and pathogenic bacteria may penetrate the mucosa, giving rise to *diverticulitis;* this is the most common complication of diverticulosis. Symptoms may be identical to those occurring in appendicitis except that the pain is usually *on the left side,* corresponding to the location of the diverticula in the descending and sigmoid colon. In acute cases, perforation may occur, causing *peritonitis,* but usually diverticulitis is more chronic, causing much peridiverticular inflammation and fibrosis. This may lead to *chronic intestinal obstruction* and require surgical intervention. The affected segment of bowel is often very firm and bound down to surrounding tissue by the inflammatory process; the clinical and radiographic findings in such a case may be indistinguishable from obstruction due to carcinoma. Rarely a Meckel's diverticulum may cause intestinal obstruction, either by becoming turned inside out and blocking the lumen by intussusception, or by forming loops or bands that kink the bowel on itself. Other complications – melena and perforation – of Meckel's diverticulum are a result of peptic ulceration of the mucosa.

2. Regional Enteritis

Definition

Regional enteritis, also known as regional ileitis or Crohn's disease, is a chronic inflammatory disease, characterized pathologically by *hoselike thickening* of the distal portion of the small intestine.

Cause

Young adults are chiefly affected, the onset commonly being in the third decade. Males and females are equally susceptible. The cause of regional enteritis is unknown, although at one time or another the disease has been thought to be due to tuberculosis, protozoa, bacteria, viruses (especially that of lymphopathia venereum), sarcoidosis, allergy, or emotional disturbances.

Pathologic changes

In about 85 percent of the cases [18] the process is restricted to the small intestine; in 15 percent the colon is also involved. The *terminal ileum* is the segment usually affected, but jejunum and duodenum are sometimes involved. Usually only one segment of the bowel suffers, but "skip" areas and involvement of separate segments may be noted. The affected segments of intestine are sharply demarcated from healthy bowel, are thickened, gray-red, and stiff as a garden hose; the corresponding mesentery is edematous and thickened. *Localized obstruction of lymphatics seems to account best for these changes.* The mesenteric lymph nodes are often enlarged and soft. The lumen of the bowel becomes greatly reduced in size as the walls become thickened by edema. In acute cases an exudate consisting largely of macrophages and eosinophils appears in the tissue spaces. At this stage there is an acute inflammation of the small lymphatic vessels. Later ulceration and secondary infection occur and abscesses undermine the mucosa. In chronic cases there is a *granulomatous reaction* in all layers of the bowel and mesentery, affecting especially the lymph vessels (lacteals). Focal lesions develop in all layers of the bowel and in the mesentery; giant cells, epithelioid cells, eosinophils, monocytes, and lymphocytes may be seen microscopically. The lesions in the submucosa, mesentery, and lymph nodes may *resemble sarcoid* very closely. Lesions in other organ systems are rarely encountered, even in fatal cases, which are rare.

Clinical features

Mild *intermittent diarrhea* (2 to 5 stools daily), *abdominal pain,* and malaise, increasing over a period of several years, are usual. Perirectal abscesses and fistulas are common. In prolonged, severe cases there may be *anemia* and *deficiency states.* The stool is mushy, occasionally liquid, and contains mucus and occult blood. Barium meal reveals the extremely narrow, distorted lumen of the affected segment – the *string sign.* Spontaneous remissions of the disease may occur.

Complications

Acute perforation with peritonitis is rare, but *chronic walled-off perforation* is relatively common. The latter results in a *localized peritoneal abscess,* or a *fistula* to another segment of small or large intestine or to the urinary bladder. Sometimes intestinal obstruction develops, especially in long-continued cases with adhesions.

3. Antibiotic Enteritis

Definition

Antibiotic enteritis is an acute inflammation of the small intestine which develops in some patients receiving antibiotic therapy. It is rare today.

Cause

The *broad-spectrum antibiotics* such as chlortetracycline and oxytetracycline are the agents usually responsible for this disease, but penicillin, streptomycin, and other agents may at times incite the process. The route of administration of the drug is unimportant. Apparently the antibiotic eliminates the normal bacterial flora of the bowel, and antibiotic-resistant strains of bacteria invade in great numbers. In most instances an *antibiotic-resistant strain of staphylococcus* is the cause of the disease, and it can sometimes be recovered from the diarrheal stools in pure culture; in other cases mixed bacteria and occasionally fungi may be causative. Perhaps other factors, such as defective vitamin utilization in the absence of coliform bacteria, may be important. This iatrogenic disease may develop in medical or surgical patients, in or out of the hospital.

Pathologic changes

The intestinal tract may be inflamed throughout, but the changes are most pronounced in the *ileum.* The bowel is contracted and the lumen nearly empty. The mucosa and submucosa are congested, edematous, and hemorrhagic. Ulcerations are superficial and not numerous, and are usually capped with a fibrinous membrane. Ordinarily there are minimal changes in other organs; there is toxemia, but no bacteremia.

Clinical features

Fever and diarrhea are the chief symptoms, usually appearing about 3 to 8 days after starting antibiotic therapy. In severe cases the clinical picture may resemble Asiatic cholera, with shock, oliguria, and death in a few days. (Staphylococcal enteritis sometimes occurs as a food poisoning, without prior antibiotic therapy.)

4. Ulcerative Colitis

Definition

Ulcerative colitis is an inflammatory disease of the colon, of uncertain cause, characterized pathologically by ulceration of the mucosa and by varying degrees of scarring. (The term *ulcerative colitis* is usually not employed for the ulcerative diseases of the colon of specific cause, such as amebic colitis.)

Cause

A wide variety of etiologic factors and mechanisms have been proposed for ulcerative colitis, but none has been proved beyond question. The early idea that ulcerative colitis is a sequel of a specific bacterial *infection,* such as *Shigella dysenteriae,* has few followers now. *Allergy* has strong advocates, but the evidence is inconclusive; rheumatoid arthritis occurs in some patients with ulcerative colitis, but ordinary allergies, such as hay fever and asthma, are no more frequent in patients with ulcerative colitis than in the general population. *Excess of lytic enzymes* has been demonstrated in the feces of patients with ulcerative colitis, and it has been suggested [19] that these enzymes, secreted in excess by the intestinal mucosa, destroy the protective layer of mucus and act directly upon the mucosa to produce ulceration. The specific enzyme which has been suggested for this role is *lysozyme,* a bacteriolytic and mucolytic substance present in a number of body secretions. This theory seemed particularly attractive when first proposed, since it provided a mechanism by which *emotional disturbances* could aggravate the disease. A transitory rise in lysozyme content of the stool has been noted to occur even in normal persons during periods of frustration and anxiety. Later studies [20] seem to invalidate this theory, since they suggest that the increased lysozyme content of the stools in ulcerative colitis is due to the greatly increased number of leukocytes in the stool, and hence is the result rather than a cause of the ulcerations. The importance of emotional factors in the cause of the disease seems well established, however; perhaps they act through other disturbances of secretion, motility, or absorption to produce their effects. Most cases of ulcerative colitis have their onset between the ages of 20 and 40 years; both sexes are about equally susceptible.

Pathologic changes [18]

The *sigmoid* colon is most commonly affected. When the ascending segment of the colon is involved, the process is usually generalized throughout the colon. The ileum is also affected in some cases, especially those in which the process is most extensive. The serosa and mesentery are relatively uninvolved. In the earliest stages the mucosa shows scattered hemorrhages and marked hyperemia. Somewhat later the mucosa is irregularly ulcerated, leaving strips and islands of intact mucosa. If ulceration is shallow, there is a cobblestone effect; if deep, the patches of mucosa between the ulcers stand out prominently *(pseudopolyps).* Microscopically *crypt abscesses* are noted deep in the mucosa; these dissect in the submucosa and rupture onto the surface. In especially severe cases *acute inflammation of small arteries and veins* is noted. Inflammation, necrosis, regeneration, and fibrosis of the mucosa and submucosa are evident in different areas. In long-standing cases with extensive scarring, the length of the colon may be reduced by one-third.

Clinical features

In the rare fulminating case, diarrhea (5 to 20 stools per day) and rectal bleeding lead to anemia, electrolyte disturbances, nutritional deficiencies, and exhaustion, and to death within 6 months. Occasionally there is spontaneous recovery. More often there are *recurring episodes of diarrhea, abdominal pain, fever,* and *rectal bleeding* over a period of 20 or more years, often precipitated by emotional crisis, intercurrent infection, or dietary indiscretion. The stool is watery or purulent and contains blood and mucus, but little formed fecal matter. *Barium enema* reveals obliteration of the normal intestinal haustration, leaving a smooth narrow shadow which has been compared to a lead pipe.

Complications

Perforation with *peritonitis* is rare, but is the most common cause of death in fatal cases. Sometimes *hemorrhage* is massive, even to the point of exsanguination. Intussusception, perirectal abscesses, fistulae, and stricture may occur. *Carcinoma* of the colon develops in about 5 percent of the cases of long duration. In fatal cases the liver may show fatty degeneration, hepatitis, or rarely cirrhosis. Arthritis, thrombophlebitis, interstitial pancreatitis, and various skin manifestations may complicate the picture. Degenerative changes of the renal epithelium are found in some fatal cases, presumably as a result of potassium depletion [21], but usually there is no clinical manifestation of renal disease.

5. *Intestinal Tuberculosis*

Primary

Tuberculosis of the intestine may be primary, or it may be secondary to tuberculosis elsewhere in the body. The ingestion of a large number of bacilli is necessary for primary intestinal infection to occur. Primary intestinal tuberculosis is usually contracted from drinking milk from tuberculous cows and is usually due to the bovine strain of *M. tuberculosis.* The infection is rare at any age in the United States, but when it does occur it is usually in children. Most of the lesions are localized to the ileum. The mucosa and submucosa are greatly thickened over Peyer's patches and are often ulcerated; the regional lymph nodes are enlarged and caseous. Typical microscopic lesions of tuberculosis are found in the submucosa of the ileum and in the lymph nodes.

Secondary

Intestinal tuberculosis is much more common as a secondary infection following advanced pulmonary tuberculosis with cavitation than as a primary infection. The sputum containing viable bacilli is coughed up into the pharynx and then swallowed. In most instances the lesions are found in the ileocecal region. The ulcerations often correspond in location to the Peyer's patches of the ileum and the lymphatic follicles of the cecum. The mucosa is ulcerated, the ulcer edges being slightly undermined and the base granular and necrotic. Tubercles are often seen in the serosa overlying these areas of ulceration. The infection spreads along the lymphatic channels toward the mesentery, so that the ulcers encircle the lumen at right angles to the long axis. In some cases the mesenteric lymph nodes are also affected.

Clinical manifestations

Both the primary and the secondary intestinal lesions are manifest clinically by abdominal pain and tenderness, and by diarrhea. In the secondary form the symptoms of intestinal involvement are apt to be overshadowed by the pulmonary symptoms.

Outcome

The lesions of primary intestinal tuberculosis tend to heal, usually without significant scarring; calcified lymph nodes in the mesentery may be the only residue of the disease. The lesions of secondary intestinal tuberculosis rarely heal, since the pulmonary lesions in such cases are usually far advanced and cause the patient's death. Perforation of the ulcers is rare; when it does occur, bacterial peritonitis, either diffuse or localized (abscess), is the usual result rather than tuberculous peritonitis.

6. *Intestinal Actinomycosis*

Actinomycosis of the intestine is rare. When it does occur, it is usually the cecum and appendix that are affected. The intestine shows ulcers lined with granulation tissue in which colonies of *Actinomyces bovis* are seen, the so-called sulfur granules. Intercommunicating abscesses commonly develop, involving the abdominal wall and the liver, and sinuses may connect these with the skin surface. The illness is chronic and is marked by fever, sweats, and weight loss (see Chapter 8).

7. *Other Specific Intestinal Infections*

Other specific intestinal infections are acute systemic diseases in which the intestinal lesions are only a part, although sometimes the dominant part, of the total picture. These diseases – typhoid and paratyphoid fevers, bacillary dysentery, cholera, amebiasis, balantidiasis – have been considered in earlier chapters.

8. *Neoplasms*

SMALL INTESTINE:

Primary neoplasms of the small intestine are rare, compared to neoplasms of the colon. Since the fecal matter in the small intestine and cecum is liquid, tumors in these locations rarely cause obstruction unless they produce intussusception.

Carcinoid tumors

Carcinoid tumors, although rare, are probably the most common primary neoplasms of the small intestine. They may be evident grossly as one or more *yellow, submucosal nodules,* growing slowly and infiltrating locally. In about 20 percent of the cases carcinoid tumors metastasize, usually to the liver. When there are large masses of functioning carcinoid tumor (this usually means that metastases have occurred), there is an increase in *serotonin* in the blood, resulting in episodic crises of skin *flushing, nausea,* and *diarrhea,* i.e., *the clinical syndrome of the malignant carcinoid tumor* [22]. Peculiar fibrous tissue deposits (fibrostenosis) may occur in the pulmonary and tricuspid valves, leading to *cor pulmonale.* These deposits are believed to be derived from serotonin itself, probably combined with body protein. Microscopically the carcinoid tumor shows nests of polyhedral cells, resembling closely the islet cells of the pancreas, embedded in a fibrous stroma. The cells are usually argentophilic.

Adenocarcinoma of the small intestine is distinctly unusual. It may arise in the *duodenal papilla,* causing obstructive jaundice. The rare adenocarcinoma of the jejunum is sometimes familial and associated with pigmentation of the buccal mucosa (Jeghers' syndrome). Adeno-carci-noma

Hodgkin's disease, lymphosarcoma, and *reticulum cell sarcoma* may rarely arise in the lymphoid tissue of the small intestine. More often these tumors spread to the intestine from adjacent lymph nodes. Steatorrhea and severe nutritional disorders sometimes are seen in association with intestinal Hodgkin's disease. Lym-phoma

A number of different types of *benign neoplasms* may rarely occur in the small intestine: *angiomas* (also called *telangiectasias),* occasionally familial in their occurrence and causing recurrent hemorrhage; *lipomas; leiomyomas;* and *neurofibromas.* Benign tumors

Metastatic carcinomas are the most common of all the neoplasms of the small intestine. They may involve the intestinal wall by peritoneal implantation or direct extension, or by retrograde lymphatic permeation, as from skin melanomas or breast cancer. Metastatic tumors grow in the submucosa as multiple, rounded, button-like lesions and may either ulcerate, causing hemorrhage, or obstruct the lumen. Metastatic neoplasms

True *benign neoplasms* (lipomas, carcinoid tumors, leiomyomas) *are rare* in the colon. A benign lymphoma, the so-called rectal tonsil, is sometimes discovered on routine proctoscopy as part of a periodic health examination; it presents as a nonulcerated, submucosal nodule in the rectum; rarely does it cause symptoms. COLON: Benign neoplasms

Adenomatous polyps and *papillary adenomas* occupy an intermediate position between benign and malignant neoplasms; some consider them a form of in-situ carcinoma, others as a precancerous lesion. They are found in 8 to 10 percent of autopsies in adults, are more numerous in males, and are often multiple. Most colonic polyps are found in the *rectosigmoid portion* of the colon, but they may occur in any part. They are usually 0.1 to 5.0 cm. in diameter. Some have a broad base (sessile polyps), others have a long pedicle. *Microscopically* they show piling up of the epithelium, cell atypism, loss of cell polarity, and frequent mitotic figures. Those with a long pedicle are relatively harmless, but those with a broad base tend to show infiltration of the base (adenoma malignum), and may recur after snare excision. *Familial* (hereditary multiple) *polyposis* is a rare disorder apparently transmitted genetically as a dominant trait. It is usually encountered in children. Carcinoma of the colon very commonly develops in such cases. Polyps

Cancer of the colon (including rectum) is one of the most *common* forms of malignant neoplasm. It accounts for 1 cancer death in 8 in males, and is second only to cancer of the breast as a cause of cancer deaths in females. Of all cases of cancer of the colon, *65 percent occur in males* and 35 percent in females. Nearly three-fourths of all cancers of the colon occur in the *rectosigmoid* portion; this means that they can usually be seen on proctoscopic examination. In about 10 percent of the cases the neoplasm is in the cecum or ascending colon. The remainder occur in the transverse colon or in the hepatic or splenic flexures. Carcinoma:

Although there are some dissenters [23], most students of this disease believe that cancer of the colon usually arises in an adenomatous polyp. The distribution relation to polyps of polyps in the different portions of the colon corresponds closely to the distribution of colon cancers; patients with colon cancer often have adenomatous polyps as well; multiple cancers of the colon are common, as are multiple polyps; transition of polyps to cancer is occasionally noted clinically; unquestionably malignant cell changes are often found in otherwise benign adenomatous polyps.

gross pathologic changes; natural history

Externally carcinoma of the colon often shows hypertrophy and dilatation of the colon proximally, and some invagination of the bowel wall at the site of the tumor. Early lesions often show a *polypoid intraluminal growth;* later the tumor extends around the bowel in an *annular* (ring) fashion, narrowing the lumen. Ulceration is common and may be deep. Rarely the neoplasm is superficial and spreads without ulceration. In early cases the tumor is limited to the wall of the bowel (group A of Dukes' staging); later it extends into the serosal tissues (group B); finally regional lymph node and distant metastases occur (group C). It may spread across the serosa, seeding the dependent portions of the peritoneal cavity. Venous invasion and hematogenous metastasis are common, the spread being by the portal vein into the liver. Metastases to distant organs may also occur. In mucoid carcinomas the cut section of the tumor has a glistening, tapioca-like appearance. (When carcinoma of the colon develops in a case of long-standing ulcerative colitis, it is often of the mucoid variety.)

microscopic appearance

Microscopically the neoplasm is composed of glandular epithelium (adenocarcinoma), which in some cases is fairly well differentiated, in other cases quite anaplastic. Gland formation is usually evident and there is variable evidence of mucus secretion. In the mucoid or colloid forms of the neoplasm, mucin is formed in large quantities and dissects between the layers of the bowel wall. In such cases tumor cells may be relatively difficult to find in the large pools of mucus.

prognosis

Attempts have been made to correlate the prognosis in carcinoma of the colon with the degree of cell differentiation, but they have not been very successful. Prognosis seems more closely related to the gross extent of the neoplasm at the time of resection (i.e., Dukes' staging) and to the presence or absence of venous invasion than to the degree of cell differentiation. Careful search of the bowel sections is always made for evidence of invasion of the small veins by tumor cells; when such invasion is found, it usually means that metastasis has already occurred.

clinical features

The clinical symptoms vary with the location of the lesion. In most cases of rectosigmoid carcinoma a *change in bowel habits,* especially obstinate constipation, is the first symptom. Rarely there are no symptoms prior to onset of complete *obstruction.* Symptoms of *perforation* and *peritonitis* are sometimes the first manifestation. Blood in the stool is commonly noted. Neoplasms of the cecum and ascending colon may cause no symptoms until blood loss has produced anemia. A *palpable mass* is often evident, especially with tumors of the cecum.

Other neoplasms

Epidermoid carcinoma occurs as a primary tumor at the *anus,* but is rare. *Lymphomas* are rare as primary tumors of the colon. Involvement of the colon as a result of *extension from some adjacent organ* is quite common. Carcinoma of the *cervix* commonly spreads to the perirectal lymphatics and to the rectal submucosa; it may ulcerate, causing a rectovaginal fistula. The transverse colon is often involved in primary neoplasms of the *stomach* or *pancreas.* Any malignant neoplasm of the *mesenteric lymph nodes* may extend retrograde into the colon. The serosa of the colon is often affected by tumors seeding in the peritoneal cavity, as in papillary carcinomas of the *ovaries.*

DISEASES OF THE APPENDIX

1. Appendicitis

Cause

Acute appendicitis is by far the most common and most important disease of this vestigial organ, which serves no known purpose in man. Appendicitis is a disease chiefly of children and young adults (50 percent of the patients are under age 20), and males are more often affected than females. Dietary factors may be of some importance, but the chief factors in acute appendicitis are *obstruction of the appendiceal lumen* and *bacterial invasion of the appendiceal wall;* the bacteria normally present in the lumen do not ordinarily invade the wall except when the lumen is obstructed.

Pathogenesis

Mild acute appendicitis may occur during the course of systemic infections, such as streptococcal sore throat, measles, or rheumatic fever, particularly in children. In these cases appendicitis is presumably a part of a general enteritis, and tends to subside with the enteritis. In the great majority of the cases of severe appendicitis, obstruction of the lumen is the basic factor, as emphasized by Wangensteen [24]. Gas-forming bacteria normally present then multiply in the lumen, increasing intraluminal tension, blocking venous drainage, causing devitalization of appendiceal walls, and permitting bacterial penetration, with or without visible ulceration of the mucosa. Appendiceal obstruction is usually due to a *fecalith,* but seeds, worms, pins, and other objects are sometimes found. Serosal bands may kink the appendix. Scar tissue or anomalous muscle bundles may narrow the lumen proximally. Trauma or even violent exertion may rarely precipitate obstruction, apparently by forcing a fecalith into the lumen of the appendix.

Pathologic types:

The so-called pathologic types of appendicitis, as determined by gross and microscopic examination of the organ after its removal, probably represent only different degrees or stages of the inflammatory process as related to varying degrees of obstruction of the lumen.

catarrhal

In *catarrhal appendicitis,* the mildest form, the inflammation is largely confined to the mucosa. There is slight general enlargement of the appendix associated with minimal *hyperemia of the serosa, swelling of the mucosa* and *submucosa* due to lymphoid hyperplasia and leukocytic infiltration, and *excess mucus production* in the glands. When the appendix shows only these mild changes, there will usually be little or *no obstruction* of the lumen, or, if obstruction is present, the attack will have been of short duration at the time the appendix was removed by the surgeon.

suppurative

In *suppurative appendicitis,* the appendix is more swollen, often being *bulbous* at the tip; the serosa is irregularly *covered with fibrin,* the walls are diffusely infiltrated by leukocytes and are stretched thin by *pus in the lumen.* Mucosal ulceration is usually noted. The lumen is obstructed proximal to the dilatation in about 72 percent of the cases [24].

gangrenous

Gangrenous appendicitis shows the same features as suppurative appendicitis, plus one or more *focal areas of gangrene of the walls* due to interference with the blood supply. Often the obstructing *fecalith,* found in almost 100 percent of such cases, lies immediately beneath the locus of gangrene. Compression of the walls of the appendix leads to *venous stasis* and even *thrombosis;* putrefactive organisms invade the wall from the lumen, producing the characteristic *discoloration* and *softening* of the necrotic tissue. The omentum is often found wrapped around the appendix, isolating the infection from the peritoneal cavity. The mesoappendix is commonly indurated due to leukocytic infiltration.

Clinical features

Colicky, *periumbilical pain* is usually the first symptom of appendicitis and is a result of obstruction of the lumen. When inflammation extends to the peritoneal surface, the *pain is referred to the right lower quadrant* of the abdomen. Muscular *rigidity, tenderness,* and *rebound tenderness* are due to peritoneal inflammation. *Fever* and *leukocytosis* are evidence of systemic reaction to the infection. *Nausea* and *vomiting* are common, presumably a reflex phenomenon due to pain, perhaps also due to ileus.

Complications

Whenever there is obstruction of the lumen, *rupture* of the appendix is apt to occur, usually through an area of gangrene of the wall. Rupture may take the form of a small hole near the tip, or the appendix may actually be found in two pieces. The outcome depends upon whether or not the infection is walled off from the peritoneal cavity generally. If there have been previous episodes of acute inflammation, or if the process has developed slowly enough to permit the omentum to wrap around the appendix, peritoneal adhesions will form, limiting the infection to a localized peritoneal *abscess.* Less commonly subphrenic abscess occurs, usually as a delayed complication. With more fulminating attacks, especially in infants and small children, rupture may occur before effective adhesions have formed, and *generalized peritonitis* may result. *Peritonitis is the usual cause of death in fatal appendicitis.* Liver abscesses are a rare but important complication; they are a result of septic thrombosis of the portal vein (pylephlebitis) and its tributaries.

Sequelae

The healing of acute appendicitis may result in scar formation, and if this is at the proximal end, it may constrict the lumen, predisposing to subsequent obstruction by a fecalith. Thus *recurring attacks* of appendicitis are common. Peritoneal *adhesions* following acute appendicitis may cause acute or chronic intestinal obstruction; this is more common after appendiceal abscess.

Chronic appendicitis

Chronic appendicitis, i.e., a long-continued smoldering infection, is rare, and may be due to tuberculosis, actinomycosis, or enterobiasis. In most instances in which this diagnosis is given, the infection is recurrent rather than chronic.

2. Mucocele

Mucocele of the appendix is a result of proximal *obstruction without infection.* The glands continue to secrete, and the lumen becomes distended with mucus. If rupture ensues, mucus is spilled in the peritoneal cavity. There is no acute peritonitis, since no bacteria are present. Adhesions form about the pools of mucus, and chronic intestinal obstruction may result. If living epithelial cells are spilled into the cavity along with the mucus, they may continue to grow, as on tissue culture, and to secrete mucus. In such cases large pools of mucus, resembling frog spawn, may be pocketed in scattered portions of the peritoneal cavity, a condition known as *pseudomyxoma peritonei.* An identical picture is sometimes seen following the intraperitoneal rupture of a mucus-producing ovarian cyst (see Chapter 24).

3. Neoplasms

The *carcinoid* tumor is the most common neoplasm of the appendix; it is less frequently malignant than is the carcinoid of the small intestine. It may obstruct the appendix, resulting in appendicitis. *Neurinoma,* a benign neoplasm of the sheath of a peripheral nerve, is sometimes noted in the appendix, and apparently may cause abdominal pain. *Adenocarcinoma* is a very rare primary tumor of the appendix. *Metastatic tumors* may involve the appendix, usually secondary to involvement of the peritoneum or mesoappendix.

INTESTINAL OBSTRUCTION

1. Causes and Forms

In order to understand the causes and effects of intestinal obstruction, one must consider the intestinal contents as a liquid being forced through a tube under pressure, like water in a garden hose. Cessation of the flow may be a result of *kinking of the tube, blockage of the lumen,* or *failure of the driving force.* The first two are commonly spoken of as *organic obstruction,* the third as *paralytic.*

Kinking: hernia

Kinking of the intestine usually causes sudden and complete intestinal obstruction. It is most commonly due to trapping of a mobile loop, usually jejunum or ileum since their mesentery is longest, in a narrow, preformed pocket known as a *hernial sac.* Such pockets are usually *congenital* in origin, being defects left after imperfect closure of an embryonic opening; their common sites are the inguinal canal, femoral canal, umbilicus, and diaphragm. Some pockets are *acquired,* as when the peritoneum does not unite properly after laparotomy. The actual herniation usually occurs during some *strain* such as lifting, forcing a loop of intestine into the sac by the increase in intra-abdominal pressure. With prompt attention it is usually possible to return the viscus to the abdominal cavity, i.e., to reduce the hernia. If there is delay in reducing the hernia, edema of the intestine often develops as a result of *venous blockage,* the vessels being pinched shut in the narrow peritoneal ring at the neck of the sac. Edema, plus gas formation in the lumen of the intestine as a result of bacterial action, may make reduction of the hernia impossible after a few hours. This will lead to *gangrene of the bowel* unless prompt surgery relieves the strangulation. Hernia is thus a particularly dangerous as well as a common form of intestinal obstruction.

volvulus

Sometimes violent peristalsis will cause a *twisting of the intestine on its mesentery,* often at the site of a peritoneal adhesion. This condition, known as *volvulus,* occurs most frequently in elderly persons; it causes venous obstruction and gangrene of the strangulated segment of bowel if it is not corrected. Since volvulus most commonly affects the sigmoid portion of the colon, it is sometimes possible, if the condition is recognized promptly, to correct it without surgery by gently inserting the sigmoidoscope into the colon; the procedure has some hazard, however, both for the patient and the physician.

extrinsic masses

The intestine may be kinked upon itself as the result of *compression* by a mesenteric cyst, an aneurysm, a growing pregnancy in the presence of peritoneal adhesions, or a neoplasm external to the bowel.

Blockage of lumen: intrinsic masses

The *lumen of the intestine may be blocked as a result of tissue changes in the wall of the intestine, or by abnormal structures in the lumen.* Obstruction of this sort is usually *gradual in onset,* and only *slowly becomes complete. Neoplasms* of the intestine comprise the most important segment of this group. Most common is the annular or the polypoid form of *carcinoma of the rectosigmoid colon;* intrinsic tumors of the small intestine and cecum ordinarily do not block the lumen because the fecal stream is liquid in these areas.

strictures

Chronic inflammatory diseases of the intestine, such as *regional enteritis* and *lymphopathia venereum,* may cause strictures of the intestine. *Atresias* and *congenital strictures* of the intestine may also occur (see earlier section of this chapter).

foreign bodies

Rarely do foreign bodies cause blockage of the lumen; when they do, it is usually at a natural point of narrowing, such as at the *ileocecal valve.* Occasionally a large *gallstone* will get into the intestine, either passing down the biliary duct system or crossing from the gallbladder into the intestine through a fistula. Rarely a phytobezoar will block the intestine; more commonly it causes obstruction at the pylorus. Sometimes, especially in children, a large number of roundworms will become entangled to form a mass and obstruct the lumen.

viscid feces

Increased viscosity of the feces may sometimes cause obstruction, especially in elderly persons and newborn infants. Poor dietary habits, inadequate fluid intake, and lack of exercise make constipation a common difficulty in very elderly persons. Hard, dry fecal masses may distend the sigmoid colon *(fecal impaction);* instruments are sometimes required to remove them. In infants with pancreatic disease the meconium may be extremely viscid and sticky, causing chronic intestinal obstruction *(meconium ileus).*

intussusception

Rarely a *proximal segment of intestine becomes invaginated into a more distal segment* and blocks the lumen. This condition, known as *intussusception,* is most common in male *infants,* in whom it may occur without prior disease of the bowel; in adults intussusception is usually secondary, as to a polypoid tumor of the mucosa. Peristalsis moves the proximal segment (intussusceptum) along in the lumen until it becomes *strangulated* from venous blockage of the mesentery. A *palpable mass* is often noted, and *melena* may occur. The distal portion of the *ileum is usually invaginated into the cecum,* and strangulation of the mesentery usually occurs at the ileocecal valve. *Gangrene of the intussusceptum* occurs. In rare instances the gangrenous segment has been known to slough and to be passed per anum, with spontaneous anastomosis of the two ends; more commonly peritonitis results if surgical intervention is delayed. (Agonal intussusception is a condition that is easily distinguishable from the real thing. It is apparently a result of irregular segmental peristalsis as death approaches. The bowel is rarely invaginated for more than a few centimeters, and there is no strangulation or discoloration of the walls.)

Failure of the driving force:

Failure of peristalsis can cause intestinal obstruction just as effectively as can organic lesions. Such failure may be due to *anatomic defects in the neuromuscular mechanism* or to toxic or chemical injury, with *reflex blocking of the mechanism.*

congenital megacolon

In rare instances there may be a congenital *absence of the ganglion cells* in the distal segment of the colon [25]; some of these children have urinary tract difficulties as well. The peristaltic wave moves the fecal stream down to the distal portion of the colon but, lacking a neural pathway to transmit the stimulus further, there is no peristalsis in the distal segment, and no emptying of the bowel. As a result the bowel becomes greatly distended proximally (congenital megacolon or Hirschsprung's disease) and the abdomen becomes progressively larger and more tense. Surgical resection of this narrow, paralyzed distal segment, with anastomosis of the sigmoid colon to the anus, has resulted in a cure in most cases.

mesenteric embolism or thrombosis

Occlusion of a mesenteric artery, as by embolism or thrombosis, results in *infarction* of the mesentery and bowel wall. The necrotic intestinal wall is unable to transmit the peristaltic impulse, and gas and fluid distend the affected segment of bowel. *Melena* is commonly noted. If only a short length of intestine is affected, surgical resection and anastomosis may be effective, but since the condition is often a *complication of myocardial infarction and mural thrombosis,* or of *endocarditis,* a fatal outcome is more usual than recovery.

paralytic ileus

Paralytic ileus, also known as *adynamic ileus* and *inorganic obstruction,* may be due to gangrene of the bowel wall (as in mesenteric thrombosis) or to other factors blocking nerve impulses. *Injuries of the spinal cord, severe systemic infections* such as pneumonia, *metabolic disturbances* such as hypokalemia or water intoxication, *inflammation of the peritoneum,* and many other conditions may cause ileus. The "gas pains" which commonly follow manipulation of the viscera at surgery, or immobilization in a body cast, are a result of ileus. *Continued organic obstruction* of the intestine from any cause – incarcerated hernia, intussusception, volvulus, intrinsic neoplasm – is regularly followed by atony of the bowel proximal to the obstruction, i.e., by ileus. Thus *ileus may be either a cause or a result of intestinal obstruction.* The ileum is the segment of intestine most commonly affected in ileus. The bowel increases in diameter due to gaseous distention and fluid accumulation.

2. Effects

Pathologic changes

The tissue changes in intestinal obstruction are more distinctive in the gross than in the microscopic findings. Proximal to the obstruction, the intestine is *distended* with gas and (in the case of the small intestine) with fluid. Below the point of obstruction the lumen is empty, the bowel being very small. The walls proximally may be thick or thin, depending on the cause and duration of obstruction. With chronic partial obstruction there is often hypertrophy of the bowel wall proximally. The serosa is often dull from *fibrin* deposits. *Strangulation can be recognized by the discoloration of the bowel wall:* if of short duration, the serosa is merely dusky or cyanotic and will return to normal if the cause of strangulation is relieved; if the bowel is purplish black, edematous, and friable, the process is irreversible, and surgical resection of the involved segment is usually necessary.

Pathologic physiology: high obstruction

When intestinal obstruction is sudden in onset, complete, and high in the small intestine, and *especially if there is a closed loop* as in volvulus or strangulated hernia, there is much *vomiting,* with *loss of fluid and electrolytes.* This can be corrected only temporarily by intravenous replacement therapy, since these materials are promptly re-secreted into the upper small intestine. Reduction of plasma volume causes *hemoconcentration,* which is reflected by changes in hemoglobin, red cell count, and hematocrit. A histamine-like substance may be absorbed from the obstructed intestine, further *depressing the blood pressure. Oliguria* and *nitrogenous retention* follow. Loss of potassium results in *myocardial and renal damage.* Loss of chlorides results in alkalosis. A *profound toxemia and state of shock* develop in these cases.

low obstruction

When intestinal obstruction is gradual in onset, incomplete, and low in the colon, *vomiting is less,* and is *delayed in its onset;* fluid and electrolyte loss is also less. If the obstruction is unrelieved, paralytic ileus finally develops, the partial obstruction becomes complete, and toxic manifestations appear. Even when obstruction is low in the colon, if there is a closed loop, toxic absorption is great, and the clinical picture may closely resemble high obstruction. Intermittent, chronic, incomplete obstruction is often due to peritoneal adhesions.

strangulated bowel

With venous strangulation and gangrene the *bowel wall becomes devitalized* and normal intestinal *bacteria may penetrate to the peritoneal cavity,* resulting in *peritonitis.* Or the distended bowel may perforate, flooding the peritoneal cavity with feces. Gangrene may occur at any level; it is especially common with closed-loop obstructions because the mesentery is usually compressed in such cases, leading to edema, venous stasis, and thrombosis.

Clinical features

Cramplike pain indicative of violent peristalsis is the first symptom of obstruction. Auscultation of the abdomen reveals loud *rushing and tinkling noises. Abdominal distention,* which may be general or local, is a result of intestinal distention with gas and fluid. Feces and gas may be passed per anum until the segment below the obstruction is emptied. After this, there is *no evacuation of gas or feces* if the obstruction is complete. *Vomiting* is the result of reverse peristalsis, and the character of the vomitus is determined by the level and duration of obstruction, often being foul-smelling *(fecal vomiting).* If *dehydration* is unrelieved, the skin loses its elasticity and becomes drawn, the eyes appearing sunken. Finally the clinical picture of *shock* supervenes. A radiograph of the abdomen, taken in the upright position without contrast media (so-called flat plate) may reveal a stepladder pattern of *multiple fluid levels.* Excess amounts of gas are commonly noted; localization of gas helps to differentiate the various forms of obstruction. Death is the usual outcome if the obstruction is not relieved promptly, usually by surgery. *Death may be due to shock, aspiration of vomitus, or peritonitis.*

PERITONITIS

1. Types of Acute Diffuse Peritonitis

Acute diffuse peritonitis is usually of either chemical or bacterial origin. *Chemical peritonitis* may be a result of acute pancreatitis or of perforation of the gallbladder or stomach. Bile or gastric or pancreatic juice in the peritoneal cavity causes acute inflammation. Following the onset of ileus, bacteria may also appear in the exudate. *Bacterial peritonitis* is much more common. It is usually due to the ordinary intestinal bacteria. When there is massive hemorrhage in the intestinal mucosa and lumen, as in leukemia or thrombocytopenia, clostridia may sometimes penetrate the wall and cause peritonitis. Gas formation is common with other organisms as well.

2. Acute Bacterial Peritonitis

Causes: ruptured hollow viscus

Bacterial peritonitis usually results from *rupture* of, or *extension* of infection from, a diseased *hollow viscus* within the peritoneal cavity: appendix; gallbladder; intestinal diverticulum; perforated ulcer, as with typhoid fever, ulcerative colitis, and peptic ulcer; intestinal obstruction; gonorrheal salpingitis; and puerperal endometritis. The specific causative agent in many cases is the bacterium causing the primary disease, but often the peritonitis is due to mixed intestinal bacteria.

external injury

Less commonly bacterial peritonitis is a result of *penetrating injury,* as by a stab or gunshot wound or a surgical procedure. In such cases bacteria may be carried into the peritoneal cavity from the outside, or intestinal bacteria may be released into the peritoneal cavity by penetration of the bowel. Sometimes *crushing injuries* of the abdomen cause peritonitis without direct penetration of the peritoneal cavity from outside, as when *bone fragments* from a fractured pelvis penetrate the intestine, or when bowel wall is devitalized by contusion, permitting bacteria to penetrate the intestinal wall.

contiguous infection

Occasionally the peritoneal cavity is infected from a suppurative process in the *lung* or *pleura,* or from a retroperitoneal or subdiaphragmatic *abscess.*

blood-borne infection

Hematogenous infection of the peritoneum is uncommon. The *pneumococcus* is the usual organism; the streptococcus, staphylococcus, or gonococcus may occasionally be found. Peritonitis may be a result of bacterial infection of previously sterile fluid, as in the *ascites* of nephrosis or portal cirrhosis.

Pathologic changes

The peritoneal cavity contains a serous, fibrinous, purulent, or sanguineous *exudate,* depending upon the nature of the infection, the duration of the infection, and the circumstances generally. In infections due to intestinal bacteria, the exudate is generally *foul-smelling,* and gas may be noted. Often the omentum is drawn toward the area of perforation and aids the surgeon in finding the source of infection. *Fibrin* is almost constantly present, giving a granular appearance to the serosal surface and binding adjacent loops of intestine to each other loosely. Later fibrous adhesions may form, or they may indicate an older site of inflammation. The intestine becomes *distended* due to paralytic ileus.

Clinical features

Clinical manifestations are often complex, since they reflect the original disease process (e.g., appendicitis) as well as the complication (peritonitis), and since ileus is so regularly an added factor. *Fever* and *leukocytosis* give evidence of infection. At first there is *pain,* but later this may disappear. *Distension, nausea,* and *vomiting* are often marked and are due to ileus. Rarely is enough exudate present to give the physical signs of free fluid. Muscle *rigidity* is usually extreme; this is probably the most reliable physical sign. *Tenderness* and *rebound tenderness* are evident. A radiograph of the abdomen in the upright position often shows *gas under the diaphragm* and multiple fluid levels in the small intestine. (Note that *peritonitis may cause intestinal obstruction – ileus – and intestinal obstruction may cause peritonitis.)* Diffuse peritonitis is often fatal.

Sequelae

If the patient recovers from acute peritonitis, adhesions form as the exudate organizes; they may cause intermittent intestinal obstruction.

3. Peritoneal Abscesses

Localized peritonitis (peritoneal abscess) results when adhesions limit the spread of a peritoneal infection. The *location of an abscess generally indicates its origin.* Thus an abscess in the right lower quadrant is usually the result of appendicitis, but sometimes follows a perforated gallbladder or a ruptured duodenal ulcer; pelvic peritonitis in the female usually means infection of the female genitalia, as gonorrheal salpingitis or postabortal perimetritis, while in the male it usually means appendicitis; subphrenic abscess, either right or left, may follow perforated peptic ulcer, renal or liver abscess, ulcerative colitis, pancreatitis, perforated gallbladder, or ruptured appendix. Peritoneal abscesses tend to become chronic. They may be manifest by continuing pain, or as a mass in the abdominal cavity. The causative agents are usually the same as in acute diffuse bacterial peritonitis.

4. *Chronic Peritonitis*

Chronic peritonitis is distinctly unusual at the present time. Tuberculosis is the most important cause. The usual clinical problem is to differentiate the cases of chronic peritonitis from ascites due to portal hypertension. This can often be done by studying a sample of the peritoneal fluid to determine whether it is an exudate or a transudate (see page 57).

Tuberculous peritonitis

Tuberculous peritonitis is most common in females, presumably as a complication of tuberculous *salpingitis* (see Chapter 24). Occasionally it may be *hematogenous,* or it may be a complication of tuberculous *lymphadenitis* or spondylitis. Perforated tuberculous ulcer of the intestine does not ordinarily cause tuberculous peritonitis; why not? Peritoneal fluid may be blood-tinged. It shows the features of an exudate, although lymphocytes usually predominate; acid-fast organisms can be found if a careful search is made. The omentum may be rolled up and "caked" as a result of fibrin, forming a transverse upper abdominal mass which may be confused with the liver edge or with neoplasm. *Miliary tubercles* are usually easily recognized on the peritoneum. Tuberculous peritonitis is a terminal development in about 2 to 5 percent of cases of cirrhosis of the liver with ascites.

Foreign bodies

Foreign bodies may cause chronic inflammation and dense adhesions. *Talc* and *lycopodium,* formerly used on surgeon's gloves, cause chronic granulomas and adhesions. Occasionally *vegetable matter,* shot, wadding, etc., remaining after gunshot wounds or intestinal perforation, will cause chronic inflammation. *Gauze sponges,* instruments, etc. may rarely be left after surgery. *Lipiodol,* formerly used in x-ray studies to determine patency of the uterine tubes in cases of infertility, may cause chronic inflammation and adhesions, chiefly in the pelvis.

Miscellaneous

Chronic inflammation of the peritoneum, usually without bacterial infection, may also be a result of old or recurrent *hemorrhage* into the peritoneal cavity, as from neoplasms or endometriosis; *mucus* from ruptured mucocele of the appendix, or from ovarian and other cysts and tumors; *meconium* in infants with meconium ileus; and *lymph,* as from traumatic rupture of cisterna chyli.

REFERENCES

1. Reese, A. B. Tumors of the eye and adnexa. Section X, Fascicle 38, in *Atlas of Tumor Pathology.* Washington: Armed Forces Institute of Pathology, 1956.
2. Foote, F. W., and Frazell, E. L. Tumors of the major salivary glands. *Cancer* 6:1065, 1953. (A major landmark in the study of salivary gland tumors.)
3. Godwin, J. T. Benign lymphoepithelial lesion of the parotid gland; report of 11 cases. *Cancer* 5:1089, 1952.
4. Steiner, P. E. The etiology and histogenesis of carcinoma of the esophagus. *Cancer* 9:436, 1956. (A thoughtful and provocative study.)
5. Stout, A. P., and Lattes, R. Tumors of the esophagus. Section V, Fascicle 20, in *Atlas of Tumor Pathology.* Washington: Armed Forces Institute of Pathology, 1957.

6. Zubrod, C. G., Pieper, W., Hilbish, T. F., Smith, R., Dutcher, T., and Wermer, P. Acromegaly, jejunal ulcers and hypersecretion of gastric juice. *Ann. Intern. Med.* 49:1389, 1958.
7. Kenney, F. D., Dockerty, M. B., and Waugh, J. M. Giant hypertrophy of gastric mucosa: A clinical and pathological study. *Cancer* 7:671, 1954.
8. Dragstedt, L. R. Cause of peptic ulcer. *J.A.M.A.* 169:203, 1959. (A report of clinical and experimental studies by a well-known surgeon-physiologist.)
9. St. Goar, W. T. Gastro-intestinal symptoms as clue to diagnosis of primary hyperparathyroidism: Review of 45 cases. *Ann. Intern. Med.* 46:102, 1957.
10. McCune, W. S., Gusack, M., and Newman, W. Eosinophilic gastroduodenitis with pyloric obstruction. *Ann. Surg.* 142:150, 1955.
11. Aird, I., Bentall, H. H., and Fraser-Roberts, J. A. A relationship between carcinoma of the stomach and the ABO blood groups. *Brit. Med. J.* 1:799, 1953.
12. Quisenberry, W. B. The epidemiologic approach to the problem of gastric cancer. In *Third National Cancer Conference Proceedings.* Philadelphia: Lippincott, 1957, p. 721.
13. Zamcheck, N., Grable, E., Ley, A., and Norman, L. Occurrence of gastric cancer among patients with pernicious anemia at Boston City Hospital. *New Eng. J. Med.* 252:1103, 1955.
14. Machella, T. E. Mechanism of the postgastrectomy dumping syndrome. *Gastroenterology* 14:237, 1950.
15. Zollinger, R. M., and Ellison, E. H. Nutrition after gastric operations. *J.A.M.A.* 154:811, 1954.
16. Melick, R. A., and Benson, J. A., Jr. Osteomalacia following partial gastrectomy. *New Eng. J. Med.* 260:976, 1959.
17. Paulson, M., and Harvey, J. C. Hematological alterations after total gastrectomy. *J.A.M.A.* 156:1556, 1954.
18. Warren, S., and Sommers, S. C. Pathology of regional ileitis and ulcerative colitis. *J.A.M.A.* 154:189, 1954.
19. Grace, W. J., Seton, P. H., Wolf, S., and Wolff, H. G. Studies of the human colon. I. Variations in concentration of lysozyme with life situation and emotional state. *Amer. J. Med. Sci.* 217:241, 1949.
20. Kirsner, J. B., and Palmer, W. L. Ulcerative colitis: Considerations of its etiology and treatment. *J.A.M.A.* 155:341, 1954. (The psychosomatic aspects of ulcerative colitis are emphasized.)
21. Relman, A. S., and Schwartz, W. B. The nephropathy of potassium depletion. *New Eng. J. Med.* 255:195, 1956.
22. Mattingly, T. W. The functioning carcinoid tumor – a new clinical entity. *Med. Ann. D.C.* 25:239, 1956. (A very thorough study, based on both clinical and pathologic observations.)
23. Spratt, J. S., Jr., Ackerman, L. V., and Moyer, C. A. Relationship of polyps of the colon to colonic cancer. *Ann. Surg.* 148:682, 1958.
24. Wangensteen, O. H. The problem of the vermiform appendix. In Portis, S. A., *Diseases of the Digestive System* (3d ed.). Philadelphia: Lea & Febiger, 1953, pp. 746–769. (A good discussion of appendicitis by a distinguished surgeon, teacher, and investigator.)
25. Swenson, O. Hirschsprung's disease (aganglionic megacolon). *New Eng. J. Med.* 260:972, 1959. (Swenson reports here on the end results of his operation after 10 years.)

21 LIVER, BILIARY TRACT, AND PANCREAS

NON-NEOPLASTIC DISEASES OF THE LIVER

THE LIVER

The *liver* is a moderately firm, smooth, reddish brown, solid organ lying mainly in the right upper quadrant of the abdomen beneath the diaphragm. It normally weighs 1400 to 1600 gm. in males and 1200 to 1400 gm. in females. It has many functions, including the metabolism of proteins, carbohydrates, fats, and vitamin A, metabolism of bilirubin, and detoxification. The blood supply of the liver is from the hepatic artery and portal vein. It is drained by the hepatic veins through the central veins. The structural and functional integrity of the liver is dependent on the intake of a number of dietary factors. Protein is essential to hepatic structure and function; a protein deficiency will lead to fatty metamorphosis and atrophy of the parenchymal cells. Certain amino acids are especially important. Among these are methionine, which supplies methyl groups for choline formation, and cystine, which contains sulfur atoms needed for the detoxification functions of the liver. Extremely important in the liver is the maintenance of a balance between the lipogenic substances (fats, carbohydrates, and ethyl alcohol), which increase the amount of fat in the liver, and the lipotropic substances (protein, choline, betaine, and methionine), which remove fat from the organ. The exact mechanism of this lipotropic action is not understood, but it may operate by the formation of lipoproteins and phospholipids which can be transported from the liver. Choline is a precursor of the phospholipid, lecithin, and it may be essential for hepatic fat oxidation. Vitamins A, K, and B_{12} (which supplies methyl groups for transmethylation) are also of importance in hepatic function.

A number of disease processes involving the liver are discussed elsewhere: amyloidosis, page 80; typhoid fever, page 97; Weil's disease, page 105; viral hepatitis, page 157; amebic "abscess," page 181; parasitic diseases, Chapter 8; deficiency states, Chapter 12; and eclampsia, page 359.

1. Developmental Defects

Developmental defects of the liver are rare, except for those which are associated with malformations of the diaphragm or abdominal wall. *Agenesis* of the liver occurs only in acardiac-acephalic monsters. *Riedel's lobe* is a tonguelike, irregularly shaped projection from the anterior margin of the right lobe measuring up to 5 cm. long. Its neck is often narrow and may be thinned to a fibrous pedicle. The condition is more common in women than men and is seen infrequently today, so that it may be an acquired defect due to rib compression caused by tight lacing of a girdle. In *situs inversus viscerum* the liver is reversed in position but is otherwise normal. When the left leaf of the diaphragm is absent, the left lobe of the liver may lie in the left side of the thorax. A deep cleft is often found in the left lobe due to pressure against the free diaphragmatic margin. *Ectopia of the liver* may also result from defective development of the abdominal wall muscles or an umbilical hernia.

2. Fatty Metamorphosis

Fatty metamorphosis of the liver has been discussed in Chapter 1, and its relationship to hepatic cirrhosis is treated on page 528.

REYE'S DISEASE

Encephalopathy with fatty changes in the liver and kidneys (Reye's disease) [1] occurs in infants and children from 6 months to 8 years of age. The *cause* is unknown. *Clinically* after a few days of malaise the patient develops severe vomiting, convulsive seizures, irregular respiration, and stupor or coma. In about half the cases there are hematemesis and a palpable liver. The child lies with hands clenched, elbows flexed, and legs extended. *Laboratory data* include decreased blood and cerebrospinal fluid glucose levels, an elevated blood urea nitrogen, and ketonuria. The *mortality rate* is about 75 percent.

Grossly the liver is enlarged, firm, and yellow. *Microscopic examination* reveals severe fatty metamorphosis involving almost every hepatocyte. In some cases there is marked peripheral lobular necrosis with an infiltration of lymphocytes, macrophages, and neutrophils [2]. The kidneys are increased in size, and there is lipid deposition in the cytoplasm of proximal convoluted tubular epithelium. Most cases have had superficial gastric ulcers, and blood is present in the stomach. The brain is diffusely edematous.

3. Hepatic Necrosis

ZONAL NECROSIS

FOCAL NECROSIS

Hepatic necrosis may be zonal, focal, or diffuse. *Zonal necrosis* is central in chronic passive congestion, midzonal in yellow fever, and peripheral in eclampsia and phosphorus poisoning early. In *focal necrosis* small areas are affected without uniform distribution; it occurs in typhoid fever, bacillary dysentery, tularemia, and poliomyelitis.

DIFFUSE NECROSIS: Cause

Diffuse necrosis (toxic hepatitis) may be caused by drugs such as iproniazid, cincophen, and 6-mercaptopurine; chemicals such as phosphorus and carbon tetrachloride; bacteria *(Leptospira icterohaemorrhagiae);* the viruses of infectious hepatitis and homologous serum jaundice (viral hepatitis is discussed on page 157); and eclampsia, although peripheral zonal necrosis is more typical.

Clinical features

Clinically in mild cases there is slight jaundice, with nausea and vomiting. In severe cases the signs are fever, nausea and vomiting, jaundice, right upper quadrant pain, proteinuria, coma, and death.

Pathologic changes

The *pathologic changes* vary from slight damage to a massive, rapidly fatal necrosis. In *mild cases* there are diffuse foci of necrosis of parenchymal cells, with little inflammatory response. Later there is regeneration of liver cells. In *severe cases* the liver is small (it may be reduced to one-half its normal size), soft, mottled with red, yellow, and greenish areas, and wrinkled. *Microscopically* there is massive destruction of liver cells, leaving only a granular debris. The *supporting reticulum remains intact,* as is shown by silver stains. The venous sinuses are widely dilated and congested. There is little or no inflammatory response. In the kidneys, necrosis of the epithelium of the convoluted tubules occurs, and bilirubin casts are present.

SUBACUTE NECROSIS

Subacute necrosis with nodular hyperplasia is due to repeated attacks of necrosis. It may be caused by any of the toxins which produce diffuse necrosis. *Clinically* there are repeated episodes of jaundice, fever, nausea and vomiting, and epigastric and right upper quadrant pain. Scarring with fibrosis may lead to postnecrotic cirrhosis of the liver.

NEONATAL HEPATITIS

Neonatal hepatitis is characterized by the development of jaundice shortly after birth and a failure to thrive in the absence of erythroblastosis fetalis, congenital syphilis, mucoviscidosis, galactosemia, or defective development of the extrahepatic or intrahepatic bile duct system [3]. The condition is difficult to distinguish clinically from atresia of the bile ducts. The feces are pasty and clay-colored. Both direct and indirect bilirubin levels are elevated, and urinary urobilinogen is typically absent. The serum alkaline phosphatase level is elevated. *Grossly* in neonatal hepatitis the liver is enlarged and dark green with a finely granular surface. *Microscopically* most cases show numerous *giant parenchymal cells* measuring up to 400μ in diameter and containing up to 30 nuclei [4]. These cells contain a large amount of glycogen and hemosiderin. The hepatocytes often show a ductlike pattern with a bile thrombus in a central lumen. Hydropic and nuclear degeneration are common. Neutrophils, lymphocytes, and plasmocytes infiltrate the portal areas and liver parenchyma. Death usually occurs within a few weeks after birth.

The *cause* of neonatal hepatitis is uncertain. It has been attributed to intrauterine infection with hepatitis virus, but in some cases the changes of cytomegalic inclusion disease have been found. Neonatal hepatitis may also be produced by the virus of herpes simplex.

HYPERSENSITIVITY

Hepatitis due to hypersensitivity [5] has been described occasionally as part of a generalized allergic reaction, usually to drugs. The cholestatic hepatitis associated with chlorpromazine and other drugs is probably due to hypersensitivity. *Grossly* in hypersensitivity hepatitis the liver is somewhat enlarged. *Microscopically* the portal areas show a marked *eosinophilic infiltration.* The bile ductules may be filled with eosinophils. The inflammatory reaction disappears in about 2 weeks.

LUPOID HEPATITIS

Lupoid hepatitis is the designation for marked liver changes in cases of lupus erythematosus, the term *hepatic lupus* being confined to those with mild liver damage. Hepatomegaly is noted in about 35 percent of cases of lupus erythematosus. In *lupoid hepatitis* [6] there are focal or diffuse hepatocellular necrosis, regenerating hepatic lobules surrounded by fibrous bands, and lymphocytic infiltration. The liver changes and other manifestations of systemic lupus erythematosus are believed to be due to an auto-immune antigen-antibody reaction. In *hepatic lupus* there are fatty metamorphosis commonly, focal or central lobular necrosis, focal granulomas, and arteritis. *Not all authorities have accepted the concept of lupoid hepatitis.* In one series of cases of hepatitis and cirrhosis in young women with hyperglobulinemia and other clinical manifestations of "lupoid hepatitis," no histologic evidence of lupus erythematosus was found [7].

IMMUNOLOGIC ASPECTS

In *hepatic necrosis due to viral hepatitis and portal, postnecrotic, and biliary cirrhosis, gamma globulin* has been demonstrated immunocytochemically within mesenchymal cells, especially plasmocytes [8]. Intracellular gamma globulin is most constantly associated with *peripheral piecemeal necrosis* in cases of cirrhosis. Piecemeal necrosis is characterized by the death or disappearance of hepatocytes at the periphery of lobules or nodules, together with a striking infiltration of lymphocytes, plasmocytes, and macrophages, and bile ductule proliferation. The finding of gamma globulin in hepatic mesenchymal cells in hepatitis and cirrhosis supports the concept that *hepatic necrosis in these conditions is at least in part immunologic* due to antibody production against hepatocytic cytoplasmic components. The necrosis and fibrosis of cirrhosis may be due to an *autoimmune mechanism* based on the development of circulating antibodies against specific hepatic antigens such as hepatocytic cytoplasmic components, bile duct epithelium, or bile. *Circulating antibodies against bile ductular cells* are found in about 75 percent of patients with primary biliary cirrhosis, 65 percent with viral hepatitis, 45 percent with postnecrotic cirrhosis, 30 percent with posthepatic obstruction, 20 percent with portal (alcoholic) cirrhosis, and 10 percent of persons without apparent liver disease [9].

4. Cirrhosis

Cirrhosis is a progressive, chronic, diffuse inflammation of the liver, characterized by necrosis of many hepatocytes, regenerative proliferation of the surviving parenchymal cells, and fibrous scarring.

PORTAL CIRRHOSIS: Cause: role of ethyl alcohol

Portal (Laennec's, alcoholic, septal, fatty nutritional) cirrhosis is the most common form. *Ethyl alcohol* is an important causative factor. Up to 80 percent of the patients with portal cirrhosis give a history of chronic alcoholism, and 5 to 8 percent of chronic alcoholics develop cirrhosis. Ethyl alcohol is lipogenic in the liver because it supplies calories. *Alcohol also has direct and indirect toxic effects on the liver* which may play a role in the pathogenesis of portal cirrhosis [10]. The fatty metamorphosis of the liver associated with an excessive alcohol intake appears to be due mainly to the mobilization of free fatty acids in adipose tissue and their deposition in hepatocytes. Increased hepatocytic fatty acid synthesis and increased fatty acid esterification to triglycerides are other effects of alcohol on the liver which favor fat accumulation within hepatocytes. When alcohol is fed to normal subjects daily, it produces fatty metamorphosis within 2 days [11]. By 8 days hepatocytic mitochondria are large and distorted. Some giant mitochondria appear. Parallel stacks of rough endoplasmic reticulum almost disappear, and smooth endoplasmic reticulum is increased in amount.

role of diet

Fatty metamorphosis and sometimes cirrhosis occur in children in *kwashiorkor,* a nutritional disease due to a high-calorie, low-protein diet (see Chapter 12). Some cases of portal cirrhosis, especially in elderly persons, develop with no discernible evidence of excessive alcohol intake. In such patients the cirrhosis is apparently secondary to fatty metamorphosis of the liver induced by a high-carbohydrate, low-protein diet deficient in lipotropic factors.

Clinical features

Clinically portal cirrhosis is most common in men ranging in age from 45 to 65 years, and the overall male to female ratio is about 7:3. The disease is characterized by weight loss, vague epigastric pain, nausea, vomiting, diarrhea, ascites, a palpable nodular liver, jaundice, hemorrhagic tendencies, edema, palmar erythema, redness of the tongue, vascular spiders, enlargement of the breasts, and testicular atrophy. The jaundice is typically mild and intermittent. It may be marked early in the course in alcoholics with fatty metamorphosis of the liver, during episodes of decompensation in fullblown portal cirrhosis, and preterminally in patients with hepatic coma [12]. The *spider angiomata* (vascular spiders) in cirrhosis are practically limited to regions drained by the superior vena cava and are rare below the diaphragm. They blanch on pressure except for the central arteriole. *Dupuytren's contracture* of the palmar fascia develops in some cases of alcoholism and portal cirrhosis, but has also occurred in postnecrotic cirrhosis. *Atrophy of the hand muscles* is common in cirrhosis. *Finger clubbing* and flatness and paleness of the fingernails occur, and ridges may be seen in the nails.

Laboratory findings

The *laboratory findings* include anemia, leukopenia, thrombocytopenia, moderate elevations in the serum bilirubin level and icterus index, Bromsulphalein (BSP) retention, increased thymol turbidity and cephalin flocculation, decreased levels of serum albumin and cholesterol esters, increased serum globulin level, below normal prothrombin activity, and a moderately increased serum alkaline phosphatase level. The circulating level of aldosterone is increased in cirrhosis, while that of the glucocorticoids is diminished. Pituitary depression due to malnutrition probably causes the latter effect. The *serum and hepatic zinc levels are decreased,* the latter to about one-third of the normal level, and the urine zinc is increased [13]. There is also a deficiency of the zinc-containing metalloenzyme alcohol dehydrogenase in the liver.

Pathologic changes

Grossly the liver may be enlarged early, weighing up to 5000 gm. or more, due to fatty metamorphosis, but later it becomes atrophic and may be reduced to one-half its normal size. The consistency of the liver is firm, and it is difficult to cut. Its surface is coarsely nodular *(hobnail liver),* as is the cut surface. The nodules usually measure from 0.3 to 1.0 cm. in diameter. The color varies, being reddish brown, yellow, tawny brown, orange-brown, or green. *Microscopically* the earliest change is a periportal connective tissue proliferation. Later, groups of hepatic cells, usually several lobules, are surrounded by fibrous strands. The central veins disappear, and there is a severe disruption of the lobular architecture. Some degenerating hepatocytes contain a hyaline material which stains deeply with eosin *(Mallory body).* This material is in the form of droplets or fused masses in the cytoplasm. Electron microscopy shows large snakelike masses made up of tangles of small filaments [14]. The *alcoholic hyalin* histochemically is a lipoprotein complex [15]. Other hepatocytes contain fat vacuoles, and in some cases there is extensive fatty metamorphosis. Besides degeneration and necrosis of hepatocytes, foci of regenerating parenchymal cells are often seen. Early the connective tissue may be cellular, but later it loses this characteristic. The fibrosis is mainly multilobular in distribution, and the fibrous tissue is infiltrated by lymphocytes and other mononuclear cells. There is moderate bile ductule proliferation, but bile ductules appear more numerous than they actually are due to the loss of parenchymal cells.

Extrahepatic changes include testicular atrophy, especially in men under 50 years, hyperplasia of the male breasts, peptic ulcer of the stomach or duodenum in about 10 percent of the cases, atrophy of the adrenal cortex in some cases, and splenomegaly. In the *spleen* there is marked congestion of the red pulp with deposition of hemosiderin. Reticular fibrosis is commonly found in the spleen after prolonged congestion. Histochemical studies indicate that gamma globulin is produced in increased amounts by lymphocytes and plasmocytes in the splenic red pulp and medullary cords of the lymph nodes [16]. In about 25 percent of patients with portal or postnecrotic cirrhosis, splitting, fraying, or thickening is found in the glomerular basement membrane *(cirrhotic glomerulosclerosis).* Electron microscopic studies reveal basement membrane thickening, subendothelial and mesangial deposits, and fusion of the epithelial foot processes [17]. Immunofluorescence reveals gamma globulin within the basement membrane, but complement has not been demonstrated. Similar but less advanced renal changes have been found in cases of acute hepatic diseases, and the term *hepatic glomerulosclerosis* has been suggested for these renal alterations in liver disorders.

Pathogenesis

The hepatic changes in portal cirrhosis are initiated by the piecemeal necrosis in hepatocytes. Just how this process perpetuates itself is uncertain. The gradual progression of the necrosis may be due to the continued ingestion of ethyl alcohol and/or to prolonged nutritional deficiencies. The hepatic necrosis appears to be at least partly immunologic due to the development of circulating antibodies against hepatocytic cytoplasmic components. Another concept of the pathogenesis of portal cirrhosis [18] postulates that the swelling of hepatocytes resulting from injury produces obstruction of the flow of lymph and blood in the liver, mainly in the sinusoids. The sinusoidal and lymphatic endothelial cells proliferate and form new channels. The lumina of many of these new vessels become obliterated, and they are replaced by fibrous tissue. The proliferating vascular channels and the resulting fibrous scars surround more and more hepatocytes and cause their death by compression and ischemia. According to this concept the *obstruction of lymph and blood vessels* underlies the development of cirrhosis, and the *fibrous bands* which characterize cirrhosis result from the obliteration of new lymphatic and venous channels, the proliferation of bile ductules, and the condensation of the supporting reticulum of degenerated hepatocytes. Another study indicates that the *fibrosis* of portal cirrhosis results from proliferation of fibroblasts in the portal areas and around newly formed bile ductules as well as by the proliferation of reticulum fibrils in the tissue spaces around degenerating hepatocytes and the condensation of the reticulum network due to collapse following necrosis of hepatocytes [19].

Clinicopathologic correlation: portal hypertension

Portal hypertension causes the digestive symptoms (by means of congestion of the stomach and intestines), ascites, and splenomegaly. The portal hypertension is due to the compression of small venous radicles by fibrosis and by regenerating nodules of liver cells, and to an increase in the number and extent of arterioportal venous shunts. Injection-corrosion studies show enlargement of the hepatic arterial bed with reduction and distortion of the venous bed, especially of the hepatic veins [20]. Occasionally gross anastomoses between the portal vein and hepatic artery are found. The arteriovenous anastomoses lead to the transmission of arterial pressure to the portal venous system, the portal vein pressure rising from a normal of 60 to 100 mm. of water to up to 300 to 350 mm. In an attempt to overcome the obstruction, various *collateral channels* develop, and about 85 percent of the portal venous blood bypasses the liver through collaterals. The collateral channels include:

1. Dilatation of the anastomoses between the left coronary vein of the stomach and the esophageal veins which open into the azygos or intercostal veins. *Esophageal varices* may form, and rupture of such a varix is the most common cause of fatal hemorrhage in cirrhosis.

2. Dilatation of anastomoses between the branches of the inferior mesenteric vein and the superior hemorrhoidal vein. This leads to the development of *hemorrhoids* in patients with cirrhosis.

3. Dilatation of the epigastric veins of the anterior abdominal wall which communicate with the hilus of the liver through the round ligament. This leads to the formation of varicosities about the umbilicus – *caput medusae.*

4. Dilatation of the veins of Retzius originating in the intestinal wall, which form a trunk entering the inferior vena cava.

5. Dilatation of the veins of Sappey (accessory portal veins), which may drain into the paraumbilical veins.

6. Recanalization of the umbilical vein *(Cruveilhier-Baumgarten syndrome). (Cruveilhier-Baumgarten disease* is a congenitally patent umbilical vein with the shunting of blood from the portal into the epigastric vein, cirrhosis of the liver and congestive splenomegaly resulting.)

In relation to the *development of collaterals* secondary to portal hypertension, venous injection studies have demonstrated free anastomoses between periesophageal veins and mediastinal, pleuropericardial, and azygos veins in all cirrhotics, and anastomoses between mediastinal and bronchial veins in 40 percent [21]. *Portapulmonary venous shunts* bypassing the lungs are occasionally demonstrated and probably account for the decreased arterial oxygen saturation and finger clubbing in cirrhotics. Fine peripheral pulmonary arteries and arterioles are markedly dilated, and spider angiomata are sometimes found on the visceral pleura [22]. Peripheral pulmonary arteriovenous shunts have been demonstrated. *The collaterals in cirrhosis are not efficient.* Several surgical operations have been developed to provide collaterals (portacaval shunts, anastomosis of the splenic to the left renal vein, and omentopexy). In a series of elective *portasystemic venous shunt procedures* on patients with at least one prior episode of bleeding from esophageal varices [23], the portacaval shunt produced a greater drop in portal venous pressure than the splenorenal shunt. The side-to-side portacaval shunt was most successful in relieving ascites, but the splenorenal procedure was more effective in alleviating the pancytopenia resulting from hypersplenism. *Peptic ulceration* occurs in about 15 percent of the cases postoperatively. Experimentally this results from gastric hypersecretion of hydrochloric acid, which appears to be due to increased histamine synthesis in the stomach [24]. *Ammonia intoxication* with encephalopathy due to increased absorption of ammonia from the intestine and elevated levels in the peripheral blood develops in 20 percent. *Excessive deposits of iron* in the liver, pancreas, thyroid, heart, and kidneys have occurred in a few cases following portasystemic shunts, presumably due to an increased absorption of iron from the small intestine [25].

ascites

Ascites develops by transudation of fluid from the mesenteric veins and by lymphatic "weeping" from the liver. The transudation is due to the portal hypertension and to the hypoproteinemia which leads to a low serum osmotic pressure. Another etiologic factor is water retention, possibly due to the failure of the liver to inactivate the antidiuretic hormone of the posterior pituitary or to sodium retention caused by the failure of the liver to inactivate aldosterone. A rare and frequently fatal *complication* of massive ascites is *spontaneous perforation of the umbilicus.* Death in these patients may be due to peritonitis, hepatic and/or renal failure, or shock.

hypoproteinemia

Hypoproteinemia is due to the deficiency of protein metabolism by the damaged liver. The plasma colloidal osmotic pressure is lowered, and this contributes to the formation of edema and ascites. *Failure of estrogen inactivation* by conjugation in the damaged liver leads to enlargement of the breasts, testicular atrophy, pectoral and axillary alopecia, vascular spiders (central arterioles with radiating vessels), redness of the tongue, and palmar erythema. The urine estrogen level is high. **blood changes** *Anemia, leukopenia,* and *thrombocytopenia* are due to hypersplenism, with excessive destruction of blood elements and depression of the bone marrow. The hypersplenism is caused by chronic passive congestion of the spleen and may progress to a fullblown splenic anemia. A macrocytic anemia due to deficiency of hematopoietic factors occurs in some cases. The *hemorrhagic tendency* is due to a defect in the hepatic formation of prothrombin and coagulation factors V, VII, IX, and X. **jaundice** *Jaundice* is partly due to hepatocellular damage, but is mainly the result of intrahepatic bile stasis, so that pruritis is often noted.

death

Death in cirrhosis is due to cholemia (liver failure), ruptured esophageal varices with hemorrhage, bronchopneumonia, or the formation of a hepatocarcinoma.

Subacute portal cirrhosis:

Subacute portal cirrhosis (florid cirrhosis, binge drinker's liver) is a rapidly progressive variant of portal cirrhosis. It almost always occurs in alcoholics, and death usually follows a prolonged drinking bout.

clinical features

Clinically it is more common in men than in women (3:2) and is seen in the 40 to 50 age group. A poor dietary intake for months or years is noted. Weakness, weight loss, icterus, gastrointestinal bleeding, spider angiomata, splenomegaly, fever, and leukocytosis are common. Death is usually due to cholemia.

pathologic changes

Grossly the liver is brown, yellow, or green, with a smooth surface. It is generally enlarged, usually weighing about 2500 gm. *Microscopically* the picture varies. There is often pronounced regenerative activity alternating with foci of necrosis and fatty changes. In over 75 percent of the cases the liver contains large amounts of fat. Periportal fibrosis is usually marked and shows active fibroblastic proliferation. Neutrophils and some lymphocytes are found in the portal areas. The spleen is enlarged, averaging about 300 gm. in weight.

POSTHEPATITIC CIRRHOSIS

Posthepatitic cirrhosis (trabecular cirrhosis) [26] presumably results from an underlying smoldering inflammation of the liver, probably often resulting from subclinical viral hepatitis. *Pathologically it is intermediate between portal and postnecrotic cirrhosis. Grossly* the liver is normal or slightly decreased in size and reddish brown. There is a uniform distribution of nodules measuring 0.5 to 1.5 cm. in diameter surrounded by narrow fibrous strands. *Microscopically* the fibrous bands project out from the portal areas, surround 2 to 5 lobules, and measure 1 to 3 mm. wide. The fibrous tissue is infiltrated with lymphocytes, especially around bile ductules. The hepatocytes have a relatively normal lobular pattern, and fatty metamorphosis is absent to slight. The central veins are usually unaltered. It is questionable whether this entity represents a distinctive form of cirrhosis.

POSTNECROTIC CIRRHOSIS: Cause

Postnecrotic cirrhosis (toxic cirrhosis, coarse nodular cirrhosis) constitutes 10 to 15 percent of the cases of cirrhosis in the United States. It is caused by agents producing single or repeated attacks of diffuse hepatic necrosis, such as the viruses of infectious and serum hepatitis, chloroform, carbon tetrachloride, and cincophen. About half the patients give a history of excessive alcohol intake, so that ethanol may be an important causative factor in postnecrotic cirrhosis [27].

Clinical features

Clinically postnecrotic cirrhosis is similar to portal cirrhosis except that the signs of hepatic insufficiency are often more conspicuous than and precede those of portal hypertension. The course is usually more rapid than in portal cirrhosis. Distinct nodules may be palpated in the liver in the postnecrotic type. A distinctive laboratory feature is a marked elevation in the serum gamma globulin level, which may be over 4 gm. per 100 ml.

Pathologic changes

Pathologic changes in the liver are similar to those in portal cirrhosis. In the postnecrotic form typically the nodules are larger (usually above 2 cm. in diameter), vary strikingly in size, and are not uniformly distributed; there is little or no fatty metamorphosis; bile staining of the liver is a prominent feature; and the fibrosis is not entirely periportal in distribution. However, distinction between the postnecrotic and portal types is often impossible.

Pathogenesis

In *postnecrotic cirrhosis* [28] the internodular septa result from the condensation of collagen from portal areas and reticulum fibers in foci in which the hepatocytes have been completely destroyed. The collapse of the reticular framework is indicated by the parallel arrangement of argentophilic (silver-staining) fibers. There is little formation of new fibrous connective tissue by fibroblasts. Thus the *septa develop passively from the caving-in of preexistent stromal elements.* Bile ductule proliferation is more marked than in portal cirrhosis [29].

Wilson's disease:

Wilson's disease (hepatolenticular degeneration) is a familial degenerative disease of early life characterized pathologically by postnecrotic cirrhosis of the liver and by degenerative changes and glial proliferation in the lenticular nuclei of the basal ganglia. There is often a golden pigmentation at the corneal margins *(Kayser-Fleischer ring).*

cause

The *cause* is uncertain, but the disease appears to be inherited as a recessive trait and probably represents a primary defect in copper metabolism. There is an increased deposition of copper in the liver and brain; the hepatic accumulation of copper is the stimulus for the fibrosis. A *hepatic copper concentration* above 1000 mcg. per gram of dry weight is diagnostic of Wilson's disease. In most cases a *deficiency of ceruloplasmin* (a protein-copper complex) is found, the serum ceruloplasmin level being below 20 mg. per 100 ml. However, the concept that the deposition of copper in the liver and brain is related to the ceruloplasmin deficiency has been questioned [30]. Some patients with hepatolenticular degeneration have a normal serum ceruloplasmin, and a deficiency of ceruloplasmin may be present in heterozygotes for "Wilson's disease gene" who are free of the disease [31].

clinical features

Two clinical forms of hepatolenticular degeneration occur [32]. The *juvenile form (progressive lenticular degeneration)* has its onset between 7 and 15 years and is characterized by dystonia, with abnormal postures of the extremities when they are outstretched or during walking; a fixed facial expression; and rapid tremors of the fingers. In this type a breakdown of blood-brain barrier allows loosely bound plasma copper to accumulate in the brain parenchyma and produce cavitation there. The second clinical form, *pseudosclerosis,* appears between 20 and 35 years and is manifested by flapping wrist tremors, "wingbeating" of the shoulders, and dysarthria (difficulty in speech articulation). The dystonia of juvenile Wilson's disease may not be directly due to the deposition of metallic copper in the brain, but to a hepatic factor related to defective protein synthesis. In both forms there are clinical signs of hepatic cirrhosis.

pathologic changes

In the majority of cases of hepatolenticular degeneration the *gross and microscopic changes are most characteristic of postnecrotic cirrhosis* [33]. There is an irregular distribution of coarse nodules separated by fibrous septa together with regenerative foci. Fatty metamorphosis is more prominent than in other types of postnecrotic cirrhosis, and nuclear glycogen vacuolization of hepatocytes and enlargement of Kupffer cells are commonly found. Electron microscopy reveals that the excessive amounts of copper may be deposited in cytoplasmic lysosomes [34]. The distribution of copper in the hepatic lobules is markedly variable, lobules filled with copper being surrounded by copper-free ones. Copper may be finely or heavily distributed throughout the hepatocytic cytoplasm or concentrated about the nucleus. The Kupffer cells are free of copper. In the *Kayser-Fleischer ring,* copper is deposited in an abnormal matrix in Descemet's membrane in the cornea.

Plasma cell hepatitis

Plasma cell hepatitis [35] is described as a variant of postnecrotic cirrhosis. The *cause* is unknown, although many cases appear to be related to previous viral hepatitis. *Clinically* there are jaundice, hepatomegaly, splenomegaly, evidence of severe hepatocellular damage by liver function tests, and a markedly increased serum gamma globulin level. About half the patients have arthritis or joint pains and a skin rash. In contrast to other patients with postnecrotic cirrhosis these show *marked improvement on adrenocortical steroid therapy. Liver biopsies* show central lobular necrosis and periportal inflammation and fibrosis. The most striking feature is the *large number of plasmocytes in the infiltrate.*

PIGMENTARY CIRRHOSIS:

Pigmentary cirrhosis occurs in *hemochromatosis* in which there are excessive deposits of iron-containing pigments in the liver, pancreas, and skin (see also page 270). *Clinically* it is charactrized by bronzing of the skin and signs of diabetes mellitus and chronic liver disease.

Pathologic changes

Grossly the liver is usually enlarged, and is chestnut brown in color due to the enormous deposits of the iron-containing pigments, hemosiderin and hemofuscin. *Microscopically* there is marked fibrosis, which is mainly multilobular in distribution. Large deposits of these pigments are found in the hepatocytes and fibrous tissue.

CONGESTIVE CIRRHOSIS:

Congestive cirrhosis (cardiac cirrhosis) is a fibrosis and alteration in the liver architecture associated with severe and prolonged passive congestion, usually due to congestive heart failure. It is most commonly secondary to chronic constrictive pericarditis and rheumatic heart disease.

Pathologic changes [36]

Grossly the liver is normal or slightly decreased in size, firm in consistency, and dark reddish brown or purplish red in color. The surface is slightly nodular and the capsule is thickened. The cut surface is mottled with gray or yellowish gray foci separated by irregular brownish red zones. *Microscopically* the fibrosis is in the central and portal zones, with a scanty lymphocytic infiltration. There is a moderate alteration of the lobular architecture.

SYPHILITIC CIRRHOSIS

Hepatic fibrosis may develop in either congenital or acquired syphilis. In *congenital syphilis* the liver is enlarged early, but may be contracted later. The surface remains smooth. *Microscopically* there is a diffuse fine fibrosis which separates parenchymal cells and penetrates the lobules. Spirochetes are shown by Levaditi's stain. The picture may be complicated by the presence of gummata. In *acquired syphilis* the healing of large and small gummata of the liver leads to the formation of dense fibrous tissue which produces deep fissures. These separate the liver into large irregular "lobes" (*hepar lobatum,* sofa pillow liver). This lesion is rare today, and doubt has been cast on the spirochete as an etiologic factor in some cases. Arsenical therapy, formerly used in the treatment of syphilis, and the virus of homologous serum jaundice, injected during therapy, can produce hepatic necrosis with resultant fibrosis, and some cases of "syphilitic cirrhosis" have no doubt been caused by these agents. However, hepar lobatum occurred before arsenical therapy or injections were used, so some examples appear to be definitely syphilitic in origin.

SCHISTOSOMAL CIRRHOSIS

Schistosomal cirrhosis (Symmer's pipe stem cirrhosis) is due to liver infestation by the ova of *Schistosoma mansoni* and less frequently *S. japonicum* or *S. haematobium.* Fibrosis occurs in the liver, causing the formation of firm, pale gray nodules. The fibrosis is seen mainly about large portal vein radicles. The characteristic spined ova and the larvae are present. Eventually hepatocarcinoma develops in many cases. The late stages of schistosomal cirrhosis are clinically like those of portal cirrhosis. (Schistosomiasis is also discussed in Chapter 8.)

BILIARY CIRRHOSIS:

Biliary cirrhosis is rare, making up about 5 percent of the cases of cirrhosis in the United States. In most cases biliary cirrhosis is secondary to chronic obstruction in the biliary passages *(obstructive biliary cirrhosis).* The obstruction may be caused by a stone in the common or hepatic duct; carcinoma of a bile duct, ampulla of Vater, or head of the pancreas; metastatic carcinoma in the periductal lymph nodes; Hodgkin's disease or other lymphomas involving these nodes; or congenital atresia of the bile ducts. *Primary biliary cirrhosis* is uncommon and is related to prolonged intrahepatic cholestasis. The initial stage is a chronic necrotizing cholangitis and pericholangitis involving the septal and interlobular bile ducts and causing bile regurgitation [37]. Chronic cholangitis and pericholangitis with intrahepatic cholestasis occurs in a number of patients with *chronic ulcerative colitis* [38]. In some of these cases primary biliary cirrhosis develops, while others eventuate in portal or postnecrotic cirrhosis. A few cases of biliary cirrhosis are due to congenital hypoplasia of the bile ducts *(acholangic biliary cirrhosis).*

Clinical features

Clinically biliary cirrhosis is characterized by severe jaundice, pruritis, hepatomegaly, splenomegaly, and debility. There is usually no ascites until the patient is near death. The serum cholesterol is very high, sometimes reaching 2000 mg. per 100 ml. The serum alkaline phosphatase is usually markedly elevated, as is the direct-acting serum bilirubin level. Fat-soluble vitamin and lipid absorption from the intestine is defective because of the deficiency or absence of bile.

Pathologic changes

Grossly in biliary cirrhosis the liver is normal in size or moderately enlarged. It is often an intense green in color. The surface is smooth or very finely granular. The cut surfaces show dilated and tortuous bile ducts. *Microscopically* the fibrosis is mainly monolobular, encircling individual lobules. The earliest change is a periportal infiltration by lymphocytes and other mononuclear cells *(granulomatous stage).* Then highly cellular fibrous tissue appears in the periportal spaces *(fibroblastic stage).* Later the connective tissue loses its fibrous cellularity, but it remains infiltrated by chronic inflammatory cells. The bile ducts are dilated, and there is pronounced new duct formation. The bile canaliculi are distended with thick bile. Inspissated bile may be found between parenchymal cells and the walls of the sinusoids. The *spleen* is usually enlarged.

Fibroxanthomatous biliary cirrhosis

Fibroxanthomatous biliary cirrhosis is rare and occurs in the lipidoses and xanthomatoses. It is pericholangiolitic in type. There is chronic inflammation about tiny bile ducts in the portal areas, with duct obstruction and bile stasis. Lipid-laden xanthoma cells are present in the fibrous tissue.

5. Hepatic Infarcts

Hepatic infarcts are rare because the liver has a dual blood supply from the portal vein (75 percent) and the hepatic artery (25 percent) plus collaterals from the diaphragm; the liver cells are accustomed to relative anoxia; and the hepatic artery does not arise from the aorta, making embolism in it rare. Infarction may be due to embolism in or periarteritis nodosa of the hepatic artery, thrombosis of the portal vein, or laceration of the liver in a crushing injury *(traumatic infarction).* The hepatic infarct is *usually hemorrhagic,* but may be anemic.

NEOPLASMS AND CYSTS OF THE LIVER

Primary neoplasms of the liver are uncommon in the United States, although metastatic tumors to the liver are very frequent.

1. Benign Neoplasms

Hemangioma

Cavernous hemangioma is the most common benign hepatic neoplasm and is probably congenital. *Grossly* it is a circumscribed, spongy, dark red mass varying in size from a few millimeters to several centimeters. *Microscopically* the neoplasm consists of large, blood-filled, endothelially lined spaces separated by dense fibrous tissue. Occasionally a large surface hemangioma ruptures, causing intraperitoneal hemorrhage.

Adenoma

Adenoma [39] is a circumscribed, liver-colored or greenish mass consisting of well-differentiated hepatocytes and bile duct epithelium without lobular organization. The pure *bile duct adenoma* is usually cystic.

Hamartoma

Hamartoma of the liver consists of irregular masses of hepatocytes, strands and cords of bile duct epithelial cells sometimes forming ducts, large blood lakes, lymphatic vessels, and fibrous tissue. *Mesenchymal hamartoma* may occur in infancy. The tumor is reddish brown and contains cystic foci. Microscopically it consists almost entirely of collagenous fibrous tissue. A case of hamartoma with associated secondary polycythemia has been reported [40]. The polycythemia was considered to be due to the production or storage of erythropoietin, an erythropoietic-stimulating substance, by the neoplasm; the polycythemia underwent remission following surgical removal of the hamartoma.

2. Malignant Neoplasms

PRIMARY MALIGNANT NEOPLASMS:

Primary malignant neoplasms of the liver are almost always carcinomas, few sarcomas having been reported. Primary liver carcinomas are of four types: (1) *hepatocarcinoma (hepatoma),* derived from parenchymal liver cells; (2) *cholangiocarcinoma (cholangioma),* derived from bile duct epithelium or rarely from cholangiolar epithelium *(cholangiocellular carcinoma);* (3) mixed carcinoma *(hepatocholangiocarcinoma);* and (4) *undifferentiated carcinoma. Hepatoblastoma* is a rare embryonic neoplasm which usually occurs in children and contains malignant epithelial and mesenchymal elements.

Clinical features

Clinically a painful mass in the right upper quadrant of the abdomen, jaundice, ascites, lower extremity edema, and weight loss are common in primary liver carcinoma. There is a peculiar geographic distribution. In the United States and in Europe primary hepatic carcinoma is uncommon, in South African Bantus it constitutes about 35 percent of all malignant neoplasms, and in the Orient it is common. The age range is principally 45 to 60, but a few cases have occurred in infants and children. The male to female distribution in adults is about 4:1; in children, 2:1.

Causes

Hepatic cirrhosis is an associated finding in about 75 percent of hepatocarcinomas and 30 percent of cholangiocarcinomas [41]. About 8 percent of patients with cirrhosis develop primary liver carcinoma. It is probable that the carcinomas derive from regenerative nodules of parenchymal cells or proliferating bile ducts. *Diet* is doubtless an important factor in the geographic variations in incidence.

Hepatocarcinoma:

Hepatocarcinoma (hepatoma) is the most common type of primary liver carcinoma, constituting 70 to 80 percent of the cases. A number of cases of hepatocarcinoma have been associated with *marked hypoglycemia* [42], and a significant depression in blood sugar has been reported in about 30 percent of cases. The hypoglycemia is perhaps best explained by excessive use of glucose by and storage of glycogen in the neoplastic cells [43]. *Polycythemia,* sometimes of marked degree, is occasionally associated with hepatocarcinoma, possibly due to the elaboration of erythropoietin by the neoplastic cells. *Hypercalcemia* has rarely occurred in cases of hepatocarcinoma, presumably due to synthesis of a parathormone-like substance by the neoplastic cells [44]. In a few cases of hepatocarcinoma in children a *gonadotropin-like substance has been secreted* by the neoplastic cells and produced interstitial (Leydig) cell hyperplasia in the testes and sexual precocity [45].

pathologic changes

Grossly the liver is usually greatly enlarged, weighing over 3000 gm. The neoplasms show three forms: *multinodular* (about 90 percent of the cases), presenting varisized, circumscribed masses throughout the liver; *massive,* which is a large single mass; and *diffuse.* The neoplastic nodules are yellowish tan, often showing hemorrhagic or yellow necrotic foci. The liver usually shows an underlying portal cirrhosis. *Microscopically* there are trabeculae or sheets of large atypical parenchymal cells, with numerous multinucleated neoplastic giant cells. Abnormal lobules are often formed. The fine stroma is highly vascular, and clusters of neoplastic cells are often found within portal vein radicles. Some of the multinodular hepatocarcinomas appear to be multicentric in origin.

Cholangiocarcinoma:

Cholangiocarcinoma (cholangioma) constitutes less than 20 percent of primary liver carcinomas. The clinical course is usually more rapid than with hepatocarcinoma.

pathologic changes

Grossly the liver is enlarged and bile-stained. The neoplasm is usually multinodular. *Microscopically* there is typically a well-differentiated adenocarcinoma, showing numerous ductular structures lined by atypical bile duct epithelial cells.

Spread

Primary liver carcinoma tends to spread rapidly within the *liver,* forming multiple nodules, although some cases are thought to be multicentric in origin. The *portal vein* is frequently invaded, sometimes producing fatal intraperitoneal hemorrhage. In about 50 percent of the cases there are metastases to hepatic lymph nodes and the *lungs.*

Hemangioendothelial sarcoma

Hemangioendothelial sarcoma (angiosarcoma, Kupffer cell sarcoma) [46] occurs rarely in the liver. Multiple hemorrhagic, grayish pink nodules averaging about 3 cm. in diameter are found at autopsy. *Microscopically* these consist of many irregular vascular spaces lined by atypical endothelium which resembles Kupffer cells. Numerous phagocytic multinucleated tumor giant cells are present. Foci of necrosis are common. Vascular invasion is frequently seen, and metastases to the lungs occur.

META-STATIC NEO-PLASMS:

Metastatic neoplasms are extremely common, malignant cells reaching the liver via the portal vein, hepatic artery, and lymphatics. Liver metastases are found at autopsy in about 35 percent of all fatal malignant neoplasms and in 50 percent of carcinomas of areas drained by the portal vein, carcinomas of the breasts, and carcinomas of the stomach. *Metastatic carcinoma is rare in the liver of patients with portal cirrhosis* [47]. This is due to a decreased incidence of extrahepatic malignant neoplasms in patients with cirrhosis as well as to the altered vasculature of the cirrhotic liver.

Pathologic changes

The liver is enlarged, weighing as much as 10 kg., by multiple neoplastic nodules of varying size and shape. Large masses show foci of necrosis. Those on the surface have central depression *(umbilication)* due to necrosis. *Microscopically* most of the metastatic neoplasms are carcinomas. Rare cases of metastatic carcinomatous cirrhosis have been reported in women with scirrhous breast carcinomas.

3. Cysts

Congenital cysts

Congenital cysts (polycystic liver) [48] are uncommon and usually are associated with cysts in the kidneys. The hepatic cysts are multiple and tend to be small and subcapsular. They contain clear fluid and are lined by flat or columnar epithelium.

Hydro-hepatosis

Hydrohepatosis is a cystic dilatation of the intrahepatic bile ducts due to intermittent, incomplete, or slowly developing bile duct obstruction with bile retention. Eventually bile products are resorbed, leaving a watery fluid.

Peliosis hepatis

Peliosis hepatis is rare and consists of the presence of a large number of blood-filled cystic spaces in the liver [49]. Its pathogenesis is unknown. It may represent a congenital defect, ruptured sinusoids following hepatic inflammation, or the result of hepatocytic necrosis due to toxic damage or congestion. In *phlebectatic peliosis,* which occurs predominantly in men, the cysts appear to be formed by dilatation of the first part of central veins and are at least partly lined by endothelial cells. In *parenchymal peliosis* the cysts apparently result from severe congestion and focal necrosis. They are lined by hepatocytes.

HEPATIC FAILURE AND HEPATIC COMA

HEPATIC FAILURE

Hepatic failure (cholemia) ensues when such a large part of the hepatic parenchyma has been destroyed that the organ is unable to carry on its functions. It develops suddenly in acute hepatic necrosis, as in cases of fulminant viral hepatitis, and more slowly in chronic liver disease such as cirrhosis.

HEPATIC COMA: Causes

Hepatic coma results from the effects of hepatic failure on the brain. *The encephalopathy of hepatic failure* is due directly or indirectly to a *marked elevation in the serum ammonia level* [50]. The coma may result from an intracerebral depletion of alpha-ketoglutarate due to the presence of excessive amounts of ammonia. A significant decrease in the cerebral acetylcholine level is found during ammoniagenic coma. The *increased level of ammonia* results from the decreased ability of the liver to produce urea, increased absorption of ammonia from the intestine secondary to gastrointestinal hemorrhage and a high protein diet, or increased ammonia retention due to the administration of diuretics such as acetazolamide and chlorothiazide. The *bacterial production of ammonia in the intestine* can often be controlled by the use of nonabsorbable antibiotics such as neomycin and kanamycin. *Other factors* in the pathogenesis of hepatic coma may be an *elevation of blood methionine;* a *decrease in cerebral oxygen uptake; adrenocortical failure* secondary to adrenal atrophy (manifestations of hepatic failure such as hypotension, increased pigmentation, low serum sodium, high serum potassium, and oliguria are typical of adrenocortical failure); *abnormal degradation of testosterone* with production of the pyrogen etiocholanolone which may be responsible for the fever of hepatic failure; the frequently associated *oliguria and uremia due to renal failure; and arterial oxygen unsaturation.* The *hypotension* of liver failure other than that due to hemorrhage may be due to depletion of tissue norepinephrine stores [51].

Clinical features

Clinically hepatic coma is characterized by tachycardia, high fever, increased icterus, accentuated hemorrhagic phenomena (ecchymoses, coffee-ground vomitus, melena), foul-smelling diarrhea, drowsiness passing through stupor to deep coma, delirium, convulsions, "liver flap" (asterixis, a coarse flapping tremor of the upper extremities), *fetor hepaticus* (an aromatic sweet-sour odor in the breath and urine due to the presence of methyl mercaptan), and characteristic electroencephalographic changes. *Laboratory data* show a *marked increase in blood ammonia* (normal, 40 to 70 mcg. per 100 ml.); elevations in the blood and spinal fluid alpha-ketoglutarate, glutamine, and pyruvic acid levels; increased plasma and urine amino acids; and elevated spinal fluid protein level.

Pathologic changes

Grossly in hepatic encephalopathy the brain may be slightly or moderately swollen. *Microscopically* there are proliferation and enlargement of protoplasmic astrocytes throughout the gray matter, especially the lenticular nuclei, thalamus, and substantia nigra.

NON-NEOPLASTIC DISEASES OF THE GALLBLADDER AND BILE DUCTS

THE GALLBLADDER:

The *gallbladder* is a thin-walled, pear-shaped structure having a capacity of about 50 cc. Its functions are to store and concentrate hepatic bile and to deliver it periodically on demand. A fatty meal causes the release of the hormone cholecystokinin, which stimulates the gallbladder to contract.

Graham test

The functional capacity of the gallbladder can be studied in the individual patient by means of the Graham test; since indirectly it often shows evidence of gallbladder disease, it is a valuable clinical test. The radiopaque dye, tetraiodophenolphthalein, taken by mouth, is normally absorbed from the upper gastrointestinal tract and carried to the liver by the portal vein. In the liver it is excreted into the biliary system, passing to the gallbladder. Here the dye is concentrated by water absorption. The normal gallbladder filled with concentrated radiopaque material is readily visible in radiographs of the upper abdomen. If a fatty meal is then taken, the gallbladder is stimulated to empty itself; a subsequent radiograph shows disappearance of the shadow. Failure of the gallbladder to visualize with the Graham test is usually due either to obstruction of the cystic duct, so that hepatic bile cannot enter the gallbladder, or to inability of the gallbladder to concentrate the dye sufficiently (i.e., disease of the mucous membrane of the gallbladder). Gallstones can often be revealed as "negative shadows" in the gallbladder containing the dye.

Chemistry of bile

Gallbladder bile contains cholesterol, bile pigments, bile salts, calcium, mucus, and alkaline phosphatase in solution or suspension in water. Some of these are manufactured in the liver; others are excreted as threshold substances. Under various conditions these substances may come out of solution and form gallstones.

1. Developmental Defects

AGENESIS

HYPOPLASIA

Agenesis of the gallbladder [52] is relatively rare; the cystic duct is also usually absent, although occasionally a vestigial duct stump is found. Other congenital anomalies such as tracheo-esophageal fistula, cardiac defects, and polycystic kidneys are frequently associated with agenesis. Somewhat more common is *hypoplasia* of the gallbladder, in which the organ is small. Choledocholithiasis (the presence of one or more gallstones in a hepatic or common bile duct) occasionally occurs in cases of cholecystic agenesis or hypoplasia. Rarely *two gallbladders,* each with its own cystic duct, develop. *Reduplication of the cystic duct* with a single gallbladder also occurs.

SEPTATE GALLBLADDER

In *bilobate (divided) gallbladder* a longitudinal septum divides the organ into two relatively equal compartments. A transverse septum partially dividing the gallbladder near its distal end is common; it produces a *Phrygian or stocking-cap gallbladder* in which the fundus hangs downward. Such a septum at the middle results in an *hourglass or dumbbell gallbladder.* Rarely the organ is entirely embedded within the liver *(intrahepatic gallbladder). Congenital hydrops* of the gallbladder is usually associated with atresia of the cystic duct. The hydropic gallbladder may be very large and is filled with tenacious, whitish mucus.

CONGENITAL BILIARY ATRESIA

Congenital biliary atresia is the most important developmental defect of the biliary tree. It occurs in 1 in about 20,000 live births and is associated with other developmental anomalies in about 25 percent of the cases. *Clinically* the infant develops a progressively deepening jaundice within the first few days of life. Difficulty in fat and protein digestion becomes apparent early. Most of the patients die within 6 months.

Forms

Several *different forms* of biliary tree occlusion are found [53]. In about 65 percent of the cases there is *partial absence and/or atresia of the hepatic or common bile duct. Complete absence of the extrahepatic bile ducts* and *complete absence or atresia of the hepatic bile ducts* with a normal gallbladder and common duct each occurs in about 10 percent of the cases. In 7 percent there is *atresia of the intrahepatic portions of the large hepatic bile ducts* with normal extrahepatic ducts. In another 5 percent there is *atresia of the small intrahepatic ducts.* In 3 percent *localized stenosis of the common duct* is found. In 20 percent of the cases a dilated extrahepatic bile duct segment suitable for surgical anastomosis is found.

Pathologic changes

The liver in congenital biliary atresia [54] is large, green, and finely nodular. *Microscopically* there is bile ductule proliferation, and numerous *bile thrombi* are present in dilated bile canaliculi. The hepatocytes frequently have a ductlike arrangement and vary in size and shape. A moderate number of *giant hepatic cells* containing 10 to 30 nuclei are found. Many giant cells contain intracytoplasmic bile pigment particles. *Periportal fibrosis* is also present. Necrosis of hepatic cells and inflammatory reaction are usually slight and focal. The intrahepatic branches of the hepatic artery are enlarged, and their walls are thickened.

2. *Cholecystitis*

ACUTE CHOLECYSTITIS:

Cholecystitis is an inflammation of the gallbladder. Its *cause* is somewhat obscure, but, as with appendicitis, *bacterial infection* and *obstruction* both seem to play a part. The irritating nature of bile itself is also undoubtedly important. Obstruction of the cystic duct may result from edema of the gallbladder mucosa due to acute inflammation, displacement of the gallbladder and kinking of the duct due to impingement of enlarged lymph nodes or neoplasm, gallstones, and perhaps increased viscosity of the bile. Bacteria may reach the gallbladder via three routes: (1) ascending the lumen of the bile ducts from the intestine; (2) descending from the liver, either via the ducts or the lymphatics of the gallbladder and liver; or (3) by the bloodstream. Cholecystitis is usually due to organisms normally found in the intestine. Probably because of the higher incidence of cholelithiasis in diabetics (25 percent as compared to about 8 percent in nondiabetic patients), *cholecystitis is fairly frequent in cases of diabetes mellitus* [55].

Clinical features

It is generally believed that *acute cholecystitis without stones* is a mild affair. When signs and symptoms (pain in the right upper quadrant of the abdomen, vomiting, fever, and leukocytosis) are present, the inflammation is usually recurrent and stones are usually present.

Pathologic changes

The *acutely inflamed gallbladder* is enlarged and tense. Its wall is thickened due to edema and leukocytic infiltration, and the cystic duct may be closed by this same process. The serosa is covered with fibrin flecks, and the mucosa may be ulcerated. The lumen contains leukocytes and often cholesterol crystals. Stones may or may not be present.

Complications

When *acute cholecystitis* occurs *in the presence of stones,* the gallbladder wall may become so swollen that foci of *gangrene* develop where the stones compress the mucosa. *Rupture* of the gallbladder may then occur, causing *generalized peritonitis* with both chemical and bacterial features. In some cases inflammation extends along the bile ducts into the liver, causing *suppurative cholangitis.*

End results

It is uncertain whether the gallbladder, once inflamed, ever fully recovers. Perhaps crystals of bile salts or cholesterol become embedded in the inflamed mucosa, continuing the inflammatory process and predisposing to obstruction and stone formation. Certainly there is a *great tendency toward recurrent attacks of cholecystitis, and,* with recurring attacks, *for stones to form.*

Acute pneumocholecystitis

Acute pneumocholecystitis [56] is rare and is characterized by the presence of air within the lumen or wall of an acutely inflamed gallbladder. It is most frequently due to *Clostridium perfringens, Escherichia coli,* or staphylococci. Gangrene of the gallbladder is frequent. If significant amounts of pus are also present within the gallbladder, the condition is known as *pyopneumocholecystitis.*

CHRONIC CHOLECYSTITIS: Cause

Three factors – *obstruction, chemical action of bile,* and *bacterial invasion* – are important in *chronic cholecystitis.* The relationship of chronic cholecystitis and *gallstones* is poorly understood. Stones are found in nearly all cases of true chronic cholecystitis and also in most cases of recurrent acute inflammation.

Clinical features

Colicky pain in the right upper quadrant of the abdomen and belching and fullness after meals are the usual *signs and symptoms in chronic cholecystitis.* Often these symptoms are noted specifically to follow fatty meals. Presumably they are incited when the fatty food causes muscular contraction of the diseased gallbladder. Other signs, such as jaundice, chills, and fever, are due to complications.

Pathologic changes

In *chronic cholecystitis* the *gallbladder* is usually *smaller than normal* because of the contraction of scar tissue in its wall. There are adhesions between the gallbladder and the surrounding viscera. The mucosa loses its velvety appearance and becomes coarse and irregular. *Microscopically* the villous pattern of the mucosa is lost. This probably accounts for inability of the gallbladder to concentrate the dye in the Graham test, and hence for the failure of such a gallbladder to visualize. The lumen of the gallbladder is small and usually filled with faceted gallstones neatly packed against each other. The submucosa and muscularis are thickened due to fibrosis and lymphocytic infiltration.

Complications: cholangitis

In most instances the *complications* are dependent upon the presence of stones. A stone in the gallbladder may pass into the common bile duct and cause *obstructive jaundice.* If bacteria are present along with obstruction of the common duct, the infection may spread upward into the liver, giving *cholangitis.* In this condition the liver is deeply jaundiced, often appearing olive green. As the secretion of bile continues above the obstruction, the intrahepatic tributaries of the bile ducts become greatly distended, and when the liver is sectioned, dilute greenish bile mixed with pus runs from the many openings, as from a sponge. Occasionally protozoan parasites, chiefly *Giardia lamblia,* may cause cholangitis in the absence of gallstones and cholecystitis, but this is rare in the United States. *Clinically* cholangitis is usually manifest by recurring chills and fever in the presence of clinical and laboratory evidence of obstructive jaundice.

common duct stricture

Occasionally cholangitis may result in scarring and *stricture of the common bile duct;* in other cases stricture of the common bile duct may be a complication of the surgical procedure itself. Long-continued obstruction of the common bile duct, plus persisting infection, may cause *biliary cirrhosis.* Rarely the gallbladder may become densely adherent to the duodenum or transverse colon and may rupture, producing a *biliary fistula.* A large stone may pass from the gallbladder into the lumen of the intestine and may cause *intestinal obstruction.* Continued inflammation of the gallbladder over a period of many years, in the presence of stones, sometimes results in *carcinoma of the gallbladder.*

3. Hydrops

HYDROPS

Hydrops of the gallbladder is a rare type of chronic cholecystitis. It is usually associated with a gallstone in the cystic duct. Apparently the resulting blockage develops when the gallbladder is free of bile and uninfected. A clear, slightly viscid mucoid fluid collects in the gallbladder as a result of secretion by its lining cells. The wall becomes thin and smooth, the organ being greatly enlarged and often palpable. Later, infection may supervene and empyema may develop.

4. Cholelithiasis

CHOLELITHIASIS:

Cholelithiasis is the formation of calculi *(gallstones)* [57] in the gallbladder. Gallstones are found in about 10 percent of autopsies on patients dying after age 20, being more common in elderly persons. Stones are about three times as frequent in females as in males, and are especially frequent in women who have borne children, in diabetics, and in the obese.

Pathogenesis

The *pathogenesis* of gallstones is poorly understood. Two mechanisms are generally recognized: (1) As bile is concentrated perhaps as much as 10 times by absorption of water in the gallbladder, substances present in greater than normal concentration may crystallize, changes in the basic chemical composition of the bile also promoting crystallization. (2) Inflammation of the gallbladder may cause a nidus of dead tissue or fibrin to collect in the lumen, and crystalline material may aggregate on it, much as rock candy forms on a string in a supersaturated solution of sugar. Electron microscopic study of the gallbladder epithelium in cholecystitis reveals extrusion of cytoplasmic granules which might act as nuclei for calculus formation [58]. Additional factors such as stagnation of bile may also be involved.

Types of gallstone:

Almost all the chemical substances normally present in solution in bile may be found in gallstones. Stones composed of pure cholesterol or of pure bile pigment are often encountered in conditions in which the metabolism of these substances is at fault; they are spoken of as *metabolic gallstones.* Stones of a varied composition, either *combined* or *mixed,* usually have a protein matrix and are thought to result from inflammation of the gallbladder.

cholesterol stones

About 10 percent of all gallstones are composed of pure *cholesterol.* Such a stone is usually about 1 to 2 cm. in diameter, light in weight, and rounded. Often only one stone is present. It has a somewhat sandy, stonelike surface and on section shows a radial arrangement of glassy white crystals. It is usually said to be a "silent" stone, but many do cause symptoms. Normal bile contains a large amount of cholesterol (up to about 600 mg. per 100 ml.), and many of the conditions which predispose to gallstone formation (pregnancy, diabetes, obesity) are associated with an increase in blood cholesterol and presumably also with an increase in bile cholesterol. There is a suspicion, but no proof, that *cholesterolosis of the gallbladder* is concerned in the formation of cholesterol stones. In this condition the mucosal folds become loaded with cholesterol, often hanging into the lumen as tiny polyps. *Strawberry gallbladder* is another name for this condition, the tiny yellow deposits of cholesterol on the reddish mucosal surface suggesting the seeds on a ripe strawberry.

pigment stones

About 10 percent of all gallstones are composed solely of *bile pigment.* They are usually 2 to 5 mm. in diameter, multiple, faceted, dark green to black, and smooth; they crumble easily on pressure and are homogeneous and putty-like. This type of stone is commonly found in the gallbladder in long-standing cases of hemolytic anemia. The bile contains an excessive amount of pigment, and this may come out of solution as the bile is concentrated.

mixed and combined stones

Mixed and combined stones together make up about 80 percent of all gallstones. They contain both cholesterol and bile pigment, often in concentric layers of nearly pure substance, together with calcium carbonate and calcium bilirubinate. For a gallstone to give a *positive shadow on x-ray,* it must contain an appreciable amount of calcium. Other stones may show as *negative shadows* after the use of gallbladder dye, or they may be associated with a nonfunctioning gallbladder, i.e., one that does not concentrate the dye sufficiently to be radiopaque after the Graham test. Mixed and combined stones are multiple, usually have numerous flattened surfaces or facets, and vary from a few millimeters to 1.5 cm. in diameter. Their external surfaces are typically quite smooth. On section some show a central mass of pure cholesterol or pigment stone surrounded by concentric layers of chalklike but variegated material; this type is sometimes spoken of as a *combined stone.* It is likely that the central portion is formed as a result of some metabolic error, but that once formed it incites an inflammatory reaction in the gallbladder and becomes coated with other substances during the process. Other stones of varied chemical composition show on section a pattern that is variegated and laminated all the way to the central core. This type is often spoken of as a *mixed stone;* it is likely that it is formed as a sequel to gallbladder inflammation.

Effects of gallstones

Gallstones are irritating to the gallbladder mucosa, as any other solid foreign body in the gallbladder would be. Inflammation of the gallbladder usually results from the presence of stones, even if, in a particular case, the gallbladder plays no part in their formation. Thus chronic or recurrent cholecystitis usually accompanies cholelithiasis, and may be either cause or effect. The *clinical manifestations* of gallstones and the possible complications are the same as those of chronic cholecystitis. Cholelithiasis is found in almost all cases of gallbladder carcinoma, and probably plays a role in its development.

Choledocholithiasis

In 10 to 20 percent of patients undergoing surgery for cholelithiasis, one or more stones is found in the common bile duct *(choledocholithiasis).* Even despite choledocholithotomy (incision into a bile duct for removal of stones), *residual stones* remain in about 10 percent of patients. In most cases the stone is single and less than 1 cm. in diameter. It is frequently hidden in a hepatic duct. Gallstones may also reform in the common duct, but these are usually soft and mushy and do not become clinically apparent until several years after surgery.

Gallstone ileus

Gallstone ileus is a form of intestinal obstruction due to one or more gallstones which have entered the intestine, usually through a *cholecystoduodenal fistula.* About 80 percent of the cases occur in women. The *obstruction is most commonly in the ileum.* The obstructing gallstones range from 2.5 to 5 cm. in diameter. The overall mortality in gallstone ileus is about 15 percent.

NEOPLASMS AND CYST OF THE GALLBLADDER AND BILE DUCTS

1. Benign Neoplasms

Papilloma of gallbladder

Papilloma of the gallbladder is unusual and may occur singly or in groups. It is not prone to become malignant. Occasionally a papilloma breaks off and forms the center of a frambesiform (mulberry-shaped) mixed calculus. *Grossly* the papilloma is a cauliflowering or fronded projection on a stalk. *Microscopically* the delicate fibrous stalk is covered by a layer of columnar epithelium. The stroma may be infiltrated with macrophages filled with doubly refractile lipids.

Adenoma

Adenoma of the gallbladder is rare. It forms a slight, broad elevation under the mucosal surface and is composed of glandular spaces lined by cuboidal or columnar epithelium separated by scanty fibrous stroma. It is not a precursor of carcinoma. Cholecystic fibroadenoma occurs very rarely.

Adenomyoma

Adenomyoma of the gallbladder is the most frequent benign neoplasm of the organ. It is a hamartoma and always occurs in the fundus. *Grossly* it is a small, firm mass in the wall. *Microscopically* it shows acinar tubular structures lined by cuboidal or columnar epithelium, with a thin fibrous stroma between interlacing bundles of smooth muscle.

Papilloma of common duct

Papilloma of the common duct may be single or multiple and occurs most often at the ampulla of Vater. Jaundice due to common duct obstruction is the most common presenting sign, although chills and fever due to bile duct and liver infection herald the onset of some cases. *Microscopically* the papilloma may consist of numerous fronds covered by a single layer of columnar epithelial cells with a fibrovascular stroma or as numerous cystic spaces lined by flattened epithelial cells *(cystic papilloma).* Foci of atypical epithelial cells (carcinoma in situ) are found in some papillomas, and invasive *papillary bile duct adenocarcinoma* sometimes originates in a papilloma.

2. Malignant Neoplasms

CHOLECYSTIC CARCINOMA:

Carcinoma of the gallbladder [59] occurs about four times as often in women as in men and constitutes about 2 percent of all cancer deaths. *Cholelithiasis* is present in about 90 percent of the cases. It is possible that carcinogenic derivatives of cholic acid may be present in such stones, which are usually of the mixed pigment type. *Cholecystitis* and *cholesterolosis* do not appear to play any causative role per se. However, chronic cholecystitis is commonly associated with cholelithiasis in cases of carcinoma.

Clinical features

Clinically most cases occur in persons over 60 years of age. The picture is often vague, but right upper quadrant pain, weight loss, bloating and flatulence, anorexia, intolerance to fatty foods, and, with the development of hepatic or bile duct metastases, hepatomegaly and jaundice are often present.

Pathologic changes

The *common sites* of cholecystic carcinoma are the fundus and neck of the gallbladder. Some carcinomas are multicentric in origin. *Grossly* the neoplasm may infiltrate the wall locally or diffusely (most common form), stiffening and thickening it, or it may present as a large or small polypoid mass in the lumen. Ulceration may occur in the diffuse type. *Microscopically* over 90 percent of the neoplasms are columnar cell adenocarcinomas, presenting varying degrees of cell differentiation and a fibrous stroma. Mucin production may be abundant, and rarely signet-ring cells are found. Occasionally epidermoid carcinoma is found, and rarely *adenoacanthoma* (mixed adenocarcinoma and epidermoid carcinoma) occurs. The carcinoma may extend into the cystic and common ducts, producing regurgitative jaundice.

Metastases

Regional lymph nodes (cystic and hepatic) are involved early in about 70 percent of the cases. *Liver metastases* occur in about 60 percent. The lungs, peritoneum, and ovaries are other usual sites of metastases.

BILE DUCT CARCINOMA:

Carcinoma of the bile ducts is generally held to be rare, but it is possible that some "carcinomas of the head of the pancreas" actually originate in the common duct. Bile duct carcinoma is slightly more frequent in men than in women and is most common in the sixth and seventh decades. *Clinically* neoplasms in the hepatic or common duct produce obstruction and regurgitative jaundice.

Pathologic changes

The *incidence* in the three ducts varies in different series, but about 40 percent occur at the duct junction, 30 percent in the common duct, 25 percent in the hepatic duct, and less than 5 percent in the cystic duct. The neoplasm causes a local stiffening and thickening of the duct wall, with gradual occlusion of the lumen. *Microscopically* it is a columnar cell adenocarcinoma, usually scirrhous in type. The proximal ducts are dilated and eventually contain "white bile" (hydrohepatosis). Carcinoma of the cystic duct causes hydrops of the gallbladder.

Metastases

Metastases are less frequent than in gallbladder carcinoma, largely because the course is more rapid. *Regional lymph nodes* are involved in about 50 percent of the cases, and the *liver* and *peritoneum* in 20 percent; lung metastases are less common.

3. Cyst

CHOLEDOCHUS CYST:

Choledochus cyst [60] is a rare, idiopathic, congenital cystic dilatation of the common bile duct. About 75 percent of the cases occur in girls, the diagnosis usually being made before the patient is 10 years of age. *Clinically* there is an upper abdominal cystic mass with right upper quadrant pain and jaundice.

Pathologic changes

The *cyst* may measure up to 20 cm. in diameter and involves mainly the proximal portion of the common duct. Its wall is fibrous and may be 5 mm. thick. The cyst fluid is bile-tinged and blood-tinged.

NON-NEOPLASTIC DISEASES OF THE PANCREAS

1. Developmental Defects

Developmental defects of the pancreas are uncommon. Variations in the major excretory ducts are the most frequent form. Sometimes the duct of Wirsung enters the duodenum at a point separate from the entrance of the common bile duct. *Heterotopic pancreatic tissue* may be found in the wall of the stomach, small intestine, or occasionally a Meckel's diverticulum. Unencapsulated splenic tissue is sometimes included in the body of the pancreas. Less often the tail of the pancreas is fused to the spleen, and pancreatic tissue is found within the splenic parenchyma. *Pancreas divisum* is due to a failure of fusion of the dorsal and ventral pancreatic primordia. *Annular pancreas* encircles the duodenum and may produce intestinal obstruction.

2. Pancreatitis

PATHOGENESIS: Acute pancreatitis

The *pathogenesis* of both acute and chronic pancreatitis is still unsettled. There is fairly general agreement that *acute pancreatitis* is related to duct obstruction either within the pancreas, at the sphincter of Oddi, or in the duodenum, associated with increased enzyme activation or secretion within the pancreas. It has been suggested that increased intraductal pressures cause a *reversal of the exocrine-endocrine secretion ratio* so that a higher percentage of enzymes is secreted into the interstitial tissue fluid, thus exhausting their inhibitors and allowing activated lipases and proteases to produce chemical irritation [61]. These enzymes cause an *edematous pancreatitis* by increasing the endothelial permeability of small blood vessels. Serous or serosanguineous fluid collects between the lobules. In the absence of venous stasis, pancreatic necrosis does not ensue. Experimentally *partial venous outflow occlusion results in the conversion of the edema to necrotizing pancreatitis* [62]. Venous stasis evidently allows the enzymes and extravasated fluid to incubate together and produce a vasotoxic substance. This causes vascular necrosis and hemorrhage in the pancreas. The extensive destruction of elastic tissue in foci of pancreatic necrosis indicates that *elastase* (endopeptidase), released by activation of proelastase by trypsin, may play an important role in inducing the vascular injury [63].

Interstitial pancreatitis

Experimentally gradual or intermittent duct occlusion, combined with the stimulation of enzyme secretion, can initiate the development of *chronic interstitial pancreatitis* [64]. Incubated mixtures of trypsin and serum or plasma can initiate marked fibroplasia when introduced into the interstitial tissue of the pancreas. In *interstitial pancreatitis* [65] the inflammatory reaction, consisting of neutrophils and edema in the acute form and lymphocytes and plasmocytes in the more common chronic type, is confined to the interstitial tissue and there is little parenchymal necrosis. This type of pancreatic inflammation is significantly associated with alcoholism and is usually mild. In the healed form, dense fibrous bands or scars sparsely infiltrated with lymphocytes and plasmocytes are found in the pancreatic interstitium.

Relationship to hyperparathyroidism

Pancreatitis occurs in about 10 percent of cases of hyperparathyroidism due to hyperplasia, adenoma, or carcinoma [66]. The pancreatitis may be acute or chronic and sometimes follows parathyroid surgery. In some cases calculi resulting from the hypercalcemia of hyperparathyroidism develop in pancreatic ducts and lead to obstruction and inflammation. Focal thromboendarteritis and pancreatic necrosis have been produced experimentally by the administration of high doses of parathormone. It is also possible that excess ionic calcium may accelerate the calcium-dependent activation of trypsinogen to trypsin [67]. A clue to the diagnosis of hyperparathyroidism in relation to pancreatitis is the finding of an elevated or normal serum calcium level in acute pancreatitis. A few cases of pancreatitis have occurred in patients taking *chlorothiazide diuretics.*

ACUTE PANCREATITIS: Clinical features

Acute pancreatitis is a very serious disorder seen chiefly in males after age 40 and often associated with obesity and alcoholism. In about 50 percent of the cases gallstones are also present. The onset usually occurs after a heavy meal or overindulgence in alcohol. Apparently a heavy meal stimulates an increased flow of pancreatic juices and causes increased pressure in the ducts. There is extremely severe upper abdominal pain, usually radiating to the back and often simulating a ruptured viscus, myocardial infarction, or dissecting aneurysm. Distention and vomiting are a result of paralytic ileus. Hemoconcentration and shock develop. Death may occur during the first 24 to 48 hours from shock and dehydration. In about 50 to 75 percent of the cases there is a gradual recovery.

Pathologic physiology

With the *release of pancreatic enzymes into the interstitial tissue of the pancreas,* a series of related biochemical and physiologic changes occur. The enzymes amylase, lipase, and trypsin begin the digestion of the interstitial tissue. *Fat necrosis* develops in the pancreas and peripancreatic tissues, and often in the mesentery and omentum as well. These same enzymes are absorbed into the blood, where they may appear in very high levels for a few days (amylase and lipase are the substances usually studied clinically). Meanwhile, in the *foci of fat necrosis,* the neutral fat has been split into fatty acids and glycerol. The latter, being water-miscible, is carried away; the fatty acids unite with calcium from the blood to produce calcium soaps. The *level of the serum calcium is lowered* by this transfer to the tissues, in some cases in quantities sufficient to precipitate the clinical picture of tetany. Measurement of serum calcium may permit the diagnosis of pancreatitis to be made in patients whose blood lipase and amylase have returned to normal levels. The serum calcium level is also a prognostic guide, since severe depletion of calcium usually means very widespread fat necrosis. From the areas of fat necrosis, lipids may be absorbed in sufficient quantity to produce grossly evident lipemia, and even fat embolism in rare cases. *Alterations in the coagulability of the blood* also occur, but the mechanisms are obscure. In some instances there is a tendency toward thrombosis, perhaps related to trypsin activity; in others there is a tendency to hemorrhage. *Disturbances of carbohydrate and electrolyte metabolism* are common, the latter often being associated with signs of shock. Vomiting aggravates the electrolyte disturbance and the shock; in severe cases death occurs during this phase of the disease.

Pathologic changes

Locally the activity of the digestive enzymes results in widespread destruction of the pancreas. These is extensive hemorrhage into the gland *(acute hemorrhagic pancreatitis),* flecks of fat necrosis are widespread, and a serosanguineous exudate accumulates in the retroperitoneal tissues and peritoneal cavity. The chemical peritonitis leads to paralytic ileus. This may cause devitalization of the bowel wall and permit bacteria to pass to the peritoneal cavity, causing bacterial peritonitis. The necrotic foci in the pancreas are infiltrated with neutrophils, and the foci of fat necrosis show calcium deposition.

Complications

If the patient recovers, a *subphrenic abscess* may develop as the area of autolysis and inflammation is walled off. This may require surgical drainage. In some instances a *pancreatic pseudocyst* may form. Some fibrosis of the gland and adhesions about it are inevitable. These may lead to recurrence of acute pancreatitis *(chronic relapsing pancreatitis),* or it may even result in *diabetes mellitus,* usually in a rather mild form.

CHRONIC PANCREATITIS: Clinical features

Chronic pancreatitis presents most of the features of acute pancreatitis, but in a milder and recurrent form. Most patients give a history of a severe attack at the onset; in others there may be recurrent seizures of upper abdominal pain for a number of years, usually radiating to the back and requiring morphine for relief (in fact, drug addiction is common). Excessive eating and alcohol often precipitate the attacks. To these features are added those resulting from deficiency of pancreatic enzymes and hormones: diarrhea, later with bulky, fatty stools *(steatorrhea); weight loss;* and *diabetes mellitus.* Rarely are deficiency states as severe in chronic pancreatitis as in congenital fibrocystic disease, however.

Pathologic changes

Grossly the pancreas may be large or small; it is usually surrounded by adhesions. All or any part of the gland may be affected. Multiple small cysts and areas of fat necrosis are common. Calcium deposits may be noted in the parenchyma or as *calculi* in the pancreatic ducts, and demonstration of calcification on x-ray is a very helpful sign. On section the pancreas is fibrous and straplike, often feeling gritty to the touch. Its ducts are often dilated. The normal lobular architecture of the gland may be completely obscured.

3. Fibrocystic Disease

FIBROCYSTIC DISEASE:

Fibrocystic disease (cystic fibrosis) of the pancreas [68] is a congenital, recessively transmitted hereditary disease which is usually first recognized in infancy. About 95 percent of cases occur in Caucasians. Fibrocystic disease is not primarily pancreatic but a *disturbance in the function of many exocrine glands.*

The names *diffuse exocrinopathy* and *mucoviscidosis* have been proposed. The tracheobronchial mucous glands, pancreatic duct acini, biliary canaliculi, salivary gland secretory epithelium, and sweat glands may be involved. The basic defect in mucoviscidosis is not known. It may be a defect in glycoprotein synthesis or in the splitting of the kinins from their globulin precursor by kallikrein.

Clinical features

In about 10 percent of the cases there are signs of *intestinal obstruction* at birth, due to *meconium ileus.* The fecal matter, lacking all pancreatic secretions, is extremely viscid and sticky. This may at times lead to perforation of the bowel in utero, giving a sterile peritonitis *(meconium peritonitis).* In most cases the disease is recognized some months or years after birth, either because of obvious *nutritional deficiency* or because of recurring respiratory infections of unusual severity and persistence. The nutritional deficiency, as in chronic recurrent pancreatitis in the adult, involves all elements of the diet, but the utilization of lipids is the most notably affected; stools are bulky and greasy (steatorrhea) and vitamin deficiencies are commonly noted. The abdomen becomes distended (potbelly) from the bulky intestinal contents, and the extremities reveal muscle wasting. Osteoporosis and stunting of growth are common in those children that survive beyond infancy. Since the islet cells of the pancreas are not seriously affected, there is no diabetes, although carbohydrate absorption may be disturbed. Moderate to severe oral glucose intolerance has been found in about 40 percent of patients with cystic fibrosis [69]. The *sodium and chloride content of sweat is two to three times the normal level,* either a sweat chloride or a sweat sodium level above 60 milliequivalents per liter being diagnostic of mucoviscidosis in children. Children with this disease often taste salty when kissed, and salt may precipitate on their foreheads after exertion. In cases surviving infancy, the pulmonary changes overshadow those of the pancreas clinically. Usually pulmonary involvement accounts for death at an early age from bronchiectasis, recurrent pneumonia, and pulmonary insufficiency. Rarely do victims of this disease survive beyond their teens.

Pathologic changes

The pancreas is variable in size because of the cysts which are often present. The parenchyma is atrophic and fibrous. *Microscopically* the acinar tissue is almost completely absent, but islets of Langerhans usually remain. There is little beta-cell loss, but infiltration by fibrous tissue may cause an anatomic disorganization of islets. In the pancreas, atrophy of acinar cells is apparently secondary to the inspissation within ducts of mucus secreted by goblet cells. *Electron microscopic studies of the atrophic acinar cells* shows dilatation of ergastoplasm, a decrease in zymogen granules, mitochondrial spherulation, and microvillar atrophy [70]. In the liver there is cholangiolar proliferation behind inspissated mucus in intrahepatic biliary ducts. Biliary *cirrhosis* may result from the intrahepatic duct obstruction caused by inspissated mucus. Nutritional or postnecrotic cirrhosis develops occasionally. *Meconium ileus* occurs in about 10 percent of infants with cystic fibrosis. In children with severe degrees of pancreatic insufficiency, the feces become so bulky, inspissated, and putty-like as to cause *intestinal obstruction* mechanically or by intussusception. *Rectal prolapse* occurs in almost 25 percent of the childhood cases. *Bronchiectasis* results from bronchial obstruction by highly viscous mucus and superimposed infection. *Adult males* with fibrocystic disease show a *strikingly decreased fertility.* The vasa deferentia may be absent, and the epididymes are small and fibrotic [71]. The testes may be smaller than normal, and biopsies reveal decreased spermatogenesis with numerous abnormal spermatozoa.

4. Conditions Clinically Similar to Pancreatic Insufficiency

Several *malabsorption diseases* in which there is an inability to absorb fats result in a clinical picture closely resembling that in chronic pancreatic diseases, but show no gross or microscopic changes in the pancreas.

SPRUE:

Sprue (idiopathic steatorrhea, adult celiac disease) is a *complex deficiency state* which occurs chiefly in women and presents as a syndrome of malnutrition resulting from defective intestinal absorption. Sprue is a familial and inherited disorder in which the hydrolysis of certain polypeptides is impaired in the intestinal mucosa. Tryptophan metabolism is abnormal. Steatorrhea, weight loss, and multiple vitamin deficiencies with their effects are common. In addition, there is usually marked megaloblastic anemia due to insufficient absorption of vitamin B_{12}. *Tropical sprue* is a variant which occurs in the tropics in persons on a low-protein, vitamin-deficient diet. Sprue can usually be distinguished clinically from chronic pancreatic disease, since in the latter mild diabetes mellitus and x-ray evidence of calcification in the pancreas are common; these findings are lacking in sprue.

Pathologic changes

In sprue the *tongue* is bright red and sometimes ulcerated. Filiform papillae are enlarged. The small intestine appears normal grossly. In the *small intestine microscopically* there are blunting and atrophy of the villi and plasmocytic, lymphocytic, and eosinophilic infiltration of the lamina propria. *Electron microscopy* reveals a reduction in the size and number of microvilli, a marked decrease in pinocytotic vesicles in the cytoplasm of columnar cells, and absence of the terminal web of dense cytoplasm at the base of microvilli [72]. A *gluten-free diet* results in clinical improvement and gradual restoration of villi to a nearly normal mucosal pattern over several weeks [73]. In *tropical sprue* [74] the jejunal lesions are similar to those of idiopathic steatorrhea. Dissecting microscopic examination in cases of tropical sprue reveal swollen, packed, finger-like villi early, with flattening of the villi in late, atrophic cases. *Microscopically* there are shortening and swelling of the villi, with blunting of their tips. The number of epithelial cells is decreased. In the lamina propria there is a lymphocytic and plasmocytic infiltrate; in some cases numerous eosinophils are present.

CELIAC DISEASE:

Celiac disease is usually considered to be an *infantile and childhood type of sprue.* Clinically it shows most of the features of congenital fibrocystic disease of the pancreas, but the pancreas is normal on gross and microscopic examination. Celiac disease is usually not manifest for several months after birth, and recovery may occur.

Gluten-induced enteropathy

Celiac disease [75] is divided into a number of entities which produce the malabsorption syndrome. *Gluten-induced enteropathy* is due to a defect in small intestinal enzymatic activity accentuated by the ingestion of wheat gluten. The *gliadin fraction* of wheat gluten which contains large amounts of glutamine is the specific agent responsible for the onset of intestinal malabsorption. Most cases become apparent between the ages of 6 and 18 months. Intestinal biopsies in children with celiac disease show shortening or loss of microvilli on surface mucosal cells [76]. On electron microscopy all cytoplasmic organelles are seen to be affected. After a gluten-free diet, the intestine becomes normal. *Many cases of nontropical sprue (adult celiac disease) are also gluten-induced.* Episodes of *celiac crisis* may occur in infants due to active dehydration and electrolyte

Exudative enteropathy

depletion. In *exudative enteropathy* there is an excessive loss of serum proteins through the gastrointestinal mucosa from abnormally permeable lymphatic vessels. Malabsorption and steatorrhea are due to the lymphatic abnormalities. In *acanthocytosis (a-beta-lipoproteinemia),* which occurs most commonly in Jewish infants and children, there are a failure to thrive, steatorrhea, retinal changes, and ataxia. Somewhat crenated, cogwheel-shaped erythrocytes, which give the disorder its name, are found in the peripheral blood. *Laboratory findings* include increased fecal fat; decreased serum vitamin A, cholesterol, total lipid, and phospholipid levels; and absent serum beta-lipoprotein. The disorder is apparently an inborn metabolic defect transmitted as an autosomal recessive. The erythrocyte, ocular, and central nervous system abnormalities are due to defects in intestinal fat absorption and fat transport and to the inability of the patient to synthesize beta-lipoprotein.

Acanthocytosis

INTESTINAL LIPODYSTROPHY:

Intestinal lipodystrophy (Whipple's disease) is idiopathic. The histologic changes produced in the small intestine after varying periods of experimental chylostasis closely resemble those of intestinal lipodystrophy, thus indicating that mechanical lymphatic blockage is an important factor in its pathogenesis.

Clinical features

Clinically Whipple's disease is a *malabsorption syndrome,* there being almost complete failure to absorb lipids. The blood cholesterol may be as low as 50 mg. per 100 ml., thus providing chemical evidence of the failure of fat absorption. Chronic arthritis and fibrous pericarditis are found in some cases. The disease usually occurs in males at about age 50. Now that Whipple's disease can be diagnosed histologically during life by means of intestinal biopsy, mild to moderate forms are recognized, and the intestinal changes are sometimes reversible on adrenocorticosteroid therapy.

Pathologic changes

Grossly the mucosal folds of the *jejunum* and *ileum* show yellowish foci and dilated lacteals. *Microscopically* numerous *vacuolated macrophages containing glycoprotein* are present in the lamina propria. The glycoprotein is PAS (periodic acid-Schiff stain)-positive, and similar material may be found in reticulum cells within lymph nodes. Lipid is demonstrated intercellularly and within macrophages in the lamina propria. *Electron microscopy* has revealed that the microvilli of the small intestinal mucosal epithelial cells are normal in length and width and that these cells contain a normal number of cytoplasmic organelles. Electron-dense, sickle-shaped particles within macrophages have been variously interpreted as representing virus-like particles [77], bacteria [78], and the cristae mitochondriales of altered mitochondria [79]. The last interpretation would indicate that Whipple's disease represents a mitochondrial defect within macrophages or other reticuloendothelial cells. *Sickle-form, PAS-positive particles* have been found in macrophages in the myocardium, lungs, spleen, liver, pancreas, mesenteric and retroperitoneal soft tissues, lymph nodes, adrenal glands, and brain. The *mesenteric lymph nodes* may be yellow and contain much fat microscopically. The fat incites a granulomatous reaction, with macrophages and occasionally foreign-body giant cells.

JEJUNOCOLIC FISTULA

The deficiency syndrome seen in the malabsorption diseases is sometimes closely mimicked by the clinical picture resulting from a *fistula between the upper small intestine and the colon.* Such a fistula may occur spontaneously during the course of regional enteritis or may in some cases be a complication of abdominal surgery.

NEOPLASMS AND CYSTS OF THE PANCREAS

1. Benign Neoplasms

CYSTADENOMA

Cystadenoma of the pancreas [80] is an uncommon, slowly growing, encapsulated, spherical, cystic, coarsely lobulated mass measuring 2 to 8 cm. in diameter and occurring most often in the tail of the pancreas. The neoplasm is derived from duct epithelium and consists of cystic spaces lined by flat or cuboidal epithelium separated by dense fibrous bands. Papillary infoldings are sometimes found. The secretion is mucinous. Pancreatic cystadenoma occurs much more often in women than in men and is significantly associated with diabetes mellitus and other endocrine disturbances [81].

ISLET CELL ADENOMA

Islet cell adenoma is discussed on page 733.

2. Malignant Neoplasms

CARCINOMA:

Carcinoma of the pancreas causes about 3 percent of deaths from cancer. It is more frequent in men than in women by 2:1 and occurs usually in the sixth and seventh decades. The *cause* is entirely unknown, but diabetes mellitus may be a predisposing factor.

Clinical features

Clinically anemia is usually slight in pancreatic carcinoma. Glycosuria and hyperglycemia are present in about 20 percent of the cases. *Carcinoma of the head* of the pancreas causes progressive regurgitative jaundice by compression of the common duct, as well as epigastric pain, anorexia, and, late, weight loss and cachexia. The average survival period is 9 months. *Carcinoma of the body and tail* of the pancreas is manifested by back pain, digestive disturbances, ascites, hepatomegaly, and severe weight loss. A *migratory phlebothrombosis* is associated in about one-third of the cases *(Trousseau's syndrome).* A single thrombosis occurs in about 55 percent of the cases. Its cause is unknown, but it may be the release of trypsin, which is thromboplastic. While this thrombotic process is most often associated with carcinoma of the body or tail of the pancreas, it also occurs with carcinoma of the head of the pancreas and other visceral carcinomas [82].

Pathologic changes

About 75 percent of pancreatic carcinomas appear in the head, although some so diagnosed are neoplasms of the common duct. The gross and microscopic pictures are identical in the head, body, and tail. *Grossly* the neoplasm is a poorly defined, hard, nodular, light tan mass measuring 1 to 10 cm. in diameter within the pancreas. Multiple separate masses are not uncommon, and some carcinomas are multicentric in origin. *Microscopically* most of the neoplasms are *adenocarcinomas* derived from *duct epithelium,* showing irregular spaces lined by one or more layers of atypical cylindrical epithelium. Papillary formations are frequent. A dense fibrous stroma is often present. Less common is the *acinar cell carcinoma,* which is often pleomorphic, with a few clusters of cells resembling acini, sheets of poorly defined cells with large hyperchromatic nuclei, and bizarre multinucleated cells. *Fat necrosis* is common about the pancreas, metastases, and elsewhere, because of great amounts of lipase produced by acinar cell carcinomas. *Epidermoid* and *mucinous carcinomas* and *cystadenocarcinomas* occur rarely in the pancreas.

Metastases

Metastases are most common to the periaortic and mesenteric lymph nodes, *peritoneum* (especially from the body and tail), *liver* (in about 65 percent of the cases), and *lungs* (in 25 percent). Metastases are usually more widespread in carcinoma of the body and tail than of the head, because of the more rapid course in the latter.

ISLET CELL ADENOCARCINOMA

Islet cell adenocarcinoma is discussed on page 733.

3. Cysts

RETENTION CYSTS

Retention cysts result from duct obstruction by a gallstone or pancreatic stone, with cystic dilatation of a duct. The cysts are most frequently located in the distal body or tail, and sometimes reach a large size. They are lined by flat to tall columnar epithelium and have a dense fibrous wall. Most are unilocular, but they may be multilocular.

PSEUDOCYSTS

Pseudocysts are encapsulated collections of fluid in or around the pancreas caused by hemorrhage or suppuration. Peritoneum or adherent omentum forms the cyst wall. The cavity contains cloudy or brownish fluid.

OTHER CYSTS

Parasitic cysts are unusual and include echinococcal cysts and amebic "abscesses." *Angiocystic disease of the pancreas* occurs independently and in association with vascular cerebellar cysts of Lindau and retinal angiomatosis of von Hippel. *Congenital cysts* are associated with cystic disease elsewhere, especially polycystic kidneys, and *neoplastic cysts* include cystadenomas and dermoid cysts.

THROMBOSIS OF THE PORTAL, HEPATIC, AND SPLENIC VEINS

1. Portal Vein Thrombosis

PORTAL VEIN THROMBOSIS:

Thrombosis of the portal vein is associated with cirrhosis of the liver (most commonly), periportal lymphadenopathy, gastrointestinal infections, and carcinoma of the pancreas or liver. Stasis is the usual etiologic mechanism. Some cases are due to phlebosclerosis, often with calcification.

Pathologic changes

Complete, rapid occlusion of the portal vein may produce infarction and gangrene of the small intestine. *Gradual, chronic occlusion* produces ascites, splenic congestion, and esophageal varices. The portal vein may become a fibrous cord or undergo cavernomatous transformation (replacement by an angiomatous mass up to 8 cm. in diameter).

PYLEPHLEBITIS:

Septic thrombosis of the portal vein (pylephlebitis) occurs most commonly with acute appendicitis. It is also associated with chronic ulcerative colitis, diverticulitis, typhoid fever, and other gastrointestinal infections, as well as scarlet fever, pneumonia, bacterial endocarditis, endometritis, and other female genital tract infections. The most common causative organism is a streptococcus. Other frequent organisms found are *Klebsiella pneumoniae, Escherichia coli, Pseudomonas aeruginosa,* and *Proteus vulgaris.*

Pathologic changes

The intrahepatic branches of the portal vein are filled with a soft, yellowish gray, friable thrombus. This may extend down into the portal vein, and even into the mesenteric veins. The liver is riddled with abscesses *(portal pyemia)*, especially in the right lobe.

2. Hepatic Vein Thrombosis

HEPATIC VEIN THROMBOSIS:

Thrombosis of the hepatic veins (Budd-Chiari syndrome) is rare and idiopathic, occurring equally in males and females usually between 20 and 40 years of age. An underlying *endophlebitis* (narrowing due to intimal thickening) of the larger radicles of the hepatic veins and the main hepatic veins is found in most cases. About 30 percent of cases of hepatic vein thrombosis occur in other illnesses such as polycythemia, renal adenocarcinoma, ulcerative colitis, and trauma.

Clinical features

Clinically acute and chronic forms occur. In the *acute type* there is a sudden onset of abdominal pain, nausea, vomiting, and shock; later there are ascites, hepatomegaly and splenomegaly, delirium, coma, and death in 1 to 4 weeks. In the *chronic type* the onset of epigastric pain, ascites, and hepatomegaly is gradual. Jaundice is rare. Death occurs in about 6 months.

Pathologic changes [83]

The *acute type* is due to sudden thrombosis of veins previously narrowed by endophlebitis. In the *chronic type,* collaterals have developed through the umbilical veins and those of the gastrohepatic ligament. Thrombi in varying stages of organization are found in the hepatic veins and their tributaries. The vein walls show fibrous intimal thickening with luminal narrowing. The endophlebitis may involve the inferior vena cava, and thrombosis may occur there. *Grossly* the liver is enlarged, very firm, smooth, and intensely congested. On the cut surface dark red (hyperemic) areas alternate with irregular yellow (fatty) patches. *Microscopically* there is marked congestion with central zonal atrophy and necrosis.

3. Splenic Vein Thrombosis

SPLENIC VEIN THROMBOSIS

Thrombosis of the splenic vein is rare and is usually associated with portal hypertension or splenic infection. In the latter cases the thrombosis may be septic. Infarction of the spleen or splenic anemia may result from splenic vein thrombosis.

PORTAL HYPERTENSION

Portal hypertension is an increase in the portal venous pressure above the normal 60 to 100 mm. of water. It may be due to obstruction of the infrahepatic or intrahepatic portal venous system, impaired venous outflow from the liver, excessive arterial flow (splanchnic or hepatic) to the liver, or transmission of hepatic arterial pressure to the portal vein branches. The *cause* of portal hypertension may be *suprahepatic* (failure of the right side of the heart, tricuspid insufficiency, constrictive pericarditis, or thrombosis of the hepatic veins); *intrahepatic* (portal, postnecrotic, pigmentary, syphilitic, or schistosomal cirrhosis; biliary cirrhosis (late); primary hepatic carcinoma; or fatty metamorphosis); or *infrahepatic* (thrombosis of the portal vein or compression of the vein by an inflammatory or neoplastic mass). The *manifestations* of portal hypertension are described under Portal Cirrhosis earlier in this chapter.

NEOPLASMS AND CYSTS OF THE PERITONEUM, OMENTUM, AND MESENTERY

MESOTHELIOMA

Mesothelioma is the very rare primary neoplasm of the peritoneum. Its incidence is significantly increased among workers occupationally exposed to asbestos.

Grossly a gray or tan, granular, firm tumor spreads over the serosal surfaces. *Microscopically* epithelium-like tubular or papillary structures are found. Fibrous and fibrosarcomatous mesotheliomas also occur. In *malignant peritoneal mesothelioma* [84] clinically there is progressive abdominal discomfort, gastrointestinal disturbances, recurrent ascites, and marked weight loss. The neoplasm gradually overgrows extensive areas of visceral and parietal peritoneum. There is only superficial parenchymal invasion, and metastases are usually limited to regional lymph nodes.

METASTATIC NEOPLASMS

Metastases to the peritoneum are extremely common. Most are from carcinoma of the stomach, colon, or ovaries, less often of the gallbladder, pancreas, or uterus. Spread is transperitoneal (as by ascitic fluid), lymphatic, or even hematogenous. The peritoneum may become studded by firm, yellowish gray, shotlike masses (carcinomatosis). Ascites (often hemorrhagic) is common, and neoplastic cells are often found in the fluid.

CYSTS

Lymphatic cysts of the mesentery and omentum are probably congenital lymphangiomata appearing in childhood or young adulthood. They average 4 cm. in diameter, have an endothelial lining, and contain clear or milky fluid. *Echinococcal cysts* are fairly common in the mesentery, often forming large multiple masses.

TUMORS OF THE RETROPERITONEUM

NEOPLASMS

Retroperitoneal neoplasms are derived from the fibrous and adipose tissue of the posterior abdominal wall. They include *lipomas, liposarcomas, myxomas, myxosarcomas, and fibrosarcomas;* they often grow to an enormous size. In occasional cases of large retroperitoneal fibrosarcomata or other malignant mesodermal neoplasms, *hypoglycemia* has been produced. This is explained by increased glucose utilization by a large mass of neoplastic cells and by the secretion of tryptophan metabolites by these cells [85]. In one case the hypoglycemia disappeared following surgical removal of the neoplasm and reappeared when the tumor recurred.

RETROPERITONEAL FIBROSIS

Idiopathic retroperitoneal fibrosis is most likely inflammatory rather than neoplastic in origin [86]. The process is limited to the perirenal (Gerota's) fascia and has been considered a *perirenal fasciitis.* It has been attributed to low-grade infection, organization of hematomata, tuberculosis, syphilis, brucellosis, or an associated regional ileitis. Several cases have occurred in patients using methysergide maleate for migraine [87]. The fibrosis often regresses after cessation of the drug. Idiopathic retroperitoneal fibrosis occurs in men twice as often as women; over half the cases become apparent in the 40 to 60 age group. In 80 percent of the cases the process is bilateral and often symmetric. *Pathologically* it consists of a *fibrous mass or plaque* 2 to 6 cm. thick over the sacral promontory extending laterally about the ureters and upward as far as the lower pole of the kidney. The fibrous mass is sharply defined but unencapsulated. It closely envelops retroperitoneal structures but does not invade them. *Microscopically* there are varying amounts of adipose tissue and collagenous fibrous tissue sometimes arranged in whorls. There is a moderate infiltration with macrophages, lymphocytes, eosinophils, and neutrophils. *Compression of one or both ureters* is the major effect of retroperitoneal fibrosis, and varying degrees of hydronephrosis and renal failure secondary to ureteral obstruction are found.

NEOPLASMS OF THE ABDOMINAL WALL

DESMOID TUMOR

Fibroma (desmoid tumor) arises from the rectus sheath and tends to infiltrate the muscle. *Grossly* it is extremely hard, and its cut surface shows interlacing fibrous bands. *Microscopically* the incorporated myofibrils often form syncytial masses. About 80 percent of these tumors occur in parous women, and a history of trauma is usually obtained in other cases. Some desmoids recur repeatedly after removal. *Extra-abdominal desmoid tumors* [88] are occasionally found closely associated with skeletal muscle in a jaw (masseter muscle), shoulders, back (trapezius), thigh (quadriceps), and calf (gastrocnemius).

LIPOMA

Lipoma occurs fairly frequently in the subcutaneous fat of the abdominal wall.

REFERENCES

1. Dvorackova, I., Vortel, V., and Hroch, M. Encephalitic syndrome with fatty degeneration of viscera. *Arch. Path.* (Chicago) 81:240, 1966.
2. Case Records of the Massachusetts General Hospital. *New Eng. J. Med.* 276:47, 1967.
3. Ruebner, B. The pathology of neonatal hepatitis. *Amer. J. Path.* 36:151, 1960.
4. Smetana, H. F., and Johnson, F. B. Neonatal jaundice with giant cell transformation of the hepatic parenchyma. *Amer. J. Path.* 31:747, 1955.
5. Herrold, K. M., Rabson, A. S., and Smith, R. R. Involvement of the liver in generalized hypersensitivity reaction. *A.M.A. Arch. Path.* 66:306, 1958.
6. King, J. D. Lupoid hepatitis with advanced atrophic cirrhosis. *A.M.A. Arch. Path.* 68:669, 1959.
7. Jones, W. A., and Castleman, B. Liver disease in young women with hyperglobulinemia. *Amer. J. Path.* 40:315, 1962.
8. Paronetto, F., Rubin, E., and Popper, H. Local formation of γ-globulin in the diseased liver, and its relation to hepatic necrosis. *Lab. Invest.* 11:150, 1962.
9. Paronetto, F., Schaffner, F., Mutter, R. D., Kniffen, J. C., and Popper, H. Circulating antibodies to bile ductular cells in various liver diseases. *J.A.M.A.* 187:503, 1964.
10. Isselbacher, K. J., and Greenberger, N. J. Metabolic effects of alcohol on the liver. *New Eng. J. Med.* 270:351, 402, 1964.
11. Rubin, E., and Lieber, C. S. Alcohol-induced hepatic injury in nonalcoholic volunteers. *New Eng. J. Med.* 278:869, 1968.
12. Zieve, L. Jaundice in cirrhosis. *J.A.M.A.* 191:475, 1965.
13. Vallee, B. L., Wacker, W. E. C., Bartholomay, A. F., and Hoch, F. L. Zinc metabolism in hepatic dysfunction. *Ann. Intern. Med.* 50:1077, 1959.
14. Smuckler, E. A. The ultrastructure of human alcoholic hyalin. *Amer. J. Clin. Path.* 49:790, 1968.
15. Becker, B. J. P. The nature of alcoholic hyaline: A histochemical study. *Lab. Invest.* 10:527, 1961.
16. Glagov, S., Kent, G., and Popper, H. Relation of splenic and lymph node changes to hypergammaglobulinemia in cirrhosis. *A.M.A. Arch. Path.* 67:9, 1959.
17. Fisher, E. R., and Perez-Stable, E. Cirrhotic (hepatic) lobular glomerulonephritis. *Amer. J. Path.* 52:869, 1968.
18. MacDonald, R. A. Pathogenesis of nutritional cirrhosis. *Arch. Intern. Med.* (Chicago) 110:424, 1962.

19. Popper, H., Paronetto, F., Schaffner, F., and Perez, V. Studies on hepatic fibrosis. *Lab. Invest.* 10:265, 1961.
20. Hales, M. R., Allan, J. S., and Hall, E. M. Injection-corrosion studies of normal and cirrhotic livers. *Amer. J. Path.* 35:909, 1959.
21. Calabresi, P., and Abelmann, W. H. Porto-caval and porto-pulmonary anastomoses in Laennec's cirrhosis and in heart failure. *J. Clin. Invest.* 36:1257, 1957.
22. Berthelot, P., Walker, J. G., Sherlock, S., and Reid, L. Arterial changes in the lungs in cirrhosis of the liver – Lung spider nevi. *New Eng. J. Med.* 274:291, 1966.
23. McDermott, W. V., Palazzi, H., Nardi, G. L., and Mondet, A. Elective portal systemic shunt. *New Eng. J. Med.* 264:419, 1961.
24. Fischer, J. E., and Snyder, S. H. Histamine synthesis and gastric secretion after portacaval shunt. *Science* 150:1034, 1965.
25. Tisdale, W. A. Parenchymal siderosis in patients with cirrhosis after portasystemic-shunt surgery. *New Eng. J. Med.* 265:928, 1961.
26. Gall, E. A. Posthepatitic, postnecrotic, and nutritional cirrhosis. *Amer. J. Path.* 36:241, 1960.
27. Popper, H., Rubin, E., Krus, S., and Schaffner, F. Postnecrotic cirrhosis in alcoholics. *Gastroenterology* 39:669, 1960.
28. Smetana, H. Histogenesis of coarse nodular cirrhosis. *Lab. Invest.* 5:175, 1956.
29. Masuko, K., Rubin, E., and Popper, H. Proliferation of bile ducts in cirrhosis. *Arch. Path.* (Chicago) 78:421, 1964.
30. Simpson, J. F. Metabolic aspects of Wilson's disease. *Univ. Mich. Med. Bull.* 29:145, 1963.
31. Sternlieb, I., and Scheinberg, I. H. The diagnosis of Wilson's disease in asymptomatic patients. *J.A.M.A.* 183:747, 1963.
32. Denny-Brown, D. Hepatolenticular degeneration (Wilson's disease). Two different components. *New Eng. J. Med.* 270:1149, 1964.
33. Schaffner, F., Sternlieb, I., Barka, T., and Popper, H. Hepatocellular changes in Wilson's disease. *Amer. J. Path.* 41:315, 1962.
34. Goldfischer, S. The localization of copper in the pericanalicular granules (lysosomes) of liver in Wilson's disease (hepatolenticular degeneration). *Amer. J. Path.* 46:977, 1965.
35. Page, A. R., and Good, R. A. Plasma cell hepatitis. *Lab. Invest.* 11:351, 1962.
36. Neustein, H. B. Cardiac cirrhosis. *A.M.A. Arch. Path.* 61:512, 1956.
37. Rubin, E., Schaffner, F., and Popper, H. Primary biliary cirrhosis. Chronic nonsuppurative destructive cholangitis. *Amer. J. Path.* 46:387, 1965.
38. Stauffer, M. H., Sauer, W. G., Dearing, W. H., and Baggenstoss, A. H. The spectrum of cholestatic hepatic disease. In Symposium: Ulcerative colitis. *J.A.M.A.* 191:829, 1965.
39. Garancis, J. C., Tang, T., Panares, R., and Jurevics, I. Hepatic adenoma. *Cancer* 24:560, 1969.
40. Josephs, B. N., Robbins, G., and Levine, A. Polycythemia secondary to hamartoma of the liver. *J.A.M.A.* 179:867, 1962.
41. Patton, R. B., and Horn, R. C., Jr. Primary liver carcinoma. *Cancer* 17:757, 1964.
42. Lowbeer, L. Hypoglycemia-producing extrapancreatic neoplasms. *Amer. J. Clin. Path.* 35:233, 1961.
43. Landau, B. R., Wills, N., Craig, J. W., Leonards, J. R., and Moriwaki, T. The mechanism of hepatoma-induced hypoglycemia. *Cancer* 15:1188, 1962.
44. Keller, R. T., Goldschneider, I., and Lafferty, F. W. Hypercalcemia secondary to a primary hepatoma. *J.A.M.A.* 192:782, 1965.

45. Case Records of the Massachusetts General Hospital: Case 46451. *New Eng. J. Med.* 263:965, 1960.
46. Burston, J. Kupffer cell sarcoma. *Cancer* 11:798, 1958.
47. Ruebner, B. H., Green, R., Miyai, K., Caranosos, G., and Abbey, H. The rarity of intrahepatic metastasis in cirrhosis of the liver. *Amer. J. Path.* 39:739, 1961.
48. South, C., Jr., and Haug, W. A. Congenital polycystic disease of the liver. *A.M.A. Arch. Path.* 67:650, 1959.
49. Yanoff, M., and Rawson, A. J. Peliosis hepatis. *Arch. Path.* (Chicago) 77:159, 1964.
50. Chalmers, T. C. Pathogenesis and treatment of hepatic failure. *New Eng. J. Med.* 263:23, 77, 1960.
51. Mashford, M. L., Mahon, W. A., and Chalmers, T. C. Studies of the cardiovascular system in the hypotension of liver failure. *New Eng. J. Med.* 267:1071, 1962.
52. McIlrath, D. C., Re Mine, W. H., and Baggenstoss, A. Congenital absence of the gallbladder and cystic duct. *J.A.M.A.* 180:782, 1962.
53. Stowens, D. Congenital biliary atresia. *Amer. J. Gastroent.* 32:577, 1959.
54. Kasai, M., Yakovac, W. C., and Koop, C. E. Liver in congenital biliary atresia and neonatal hepatitis. *Arch. Path.* (Chicago) 74:152, 1962.
55. Mundth, E. D. Cholecystitis and diabetes mellitus. *New Eng. J. Med.* 267:642, 1962.
56. Zuidema, G. D., and Nardi, G. L. Acute pneumocholecystitis. *J.A.M.A.* 181:440, 1962.
57. Small, D. M. Gallstones. *New Eng. J. Med.* 279:588, 1968.
58. Chapman, G. B., Chiarodo, A. J., Coffey, R. J., and Wieneke, K. The fine structure of mucosal epithelial cells of a pathological human gall bladder. *Anat. Rec.* 154:579, 1966.
59. Thorbjarnarson, B., and Glenn, F. Carcinoma of the gallbladder. *Cancer* 12:1009, 1959.
60. Vlachos, J., Cassimos, C., and Trigonis, G. Choledochus cyst in a newborn. *A.M.A. Arch. Path.* 67:395, 1959.
61. Dreiling, D. A. The pathological physiology of pancreatic inflammation. *J.A.M.A.* 175:183, 1961.
62. Anderson, M. C. Venous stasis in the transition of edematous pancreatitis to necrosis. *J.A.M.A.* 183:534, 1963.
63. Geokas, M. C. Rinderknecht, H., Swanson, V., and Haverback, B. J. The role of elastase in acute hemorrhagic pancreatitis in men. *Lab. Invest.* 19:235, 1968.
64. Anderson, M. C., Wright, P. W., and Bergan, J. J. Chronic interstitial pancreatitis. A new concept of pathogenesis. *J.A.M.A.* 178:560, 1961.
65. Czernobilsky, B., and Mikat, K. W. The diagnostic significance of interstitial pancreatitis found at autopsy. *Amer. J. Clin. Path.* 41:33, 1964.
66. Mixter, C. G., Jr., Keynes, W. M., and Cope, O. Further experience with pancreatitis as a diagnostic clue to hyperparathyroidism. *New Eng. J. Med.* 266:265, 1962.
67. Turchi, J. J., Flandreau, R. H., Forte, A. L., French, G. N., and Ludwig, G. D. Hyperparathyroidism and pancreatitis. *J.A.M.A.* 180:799, 1962.
68. di Sant'Agnese, P. A., and Talamo, R. C. Pathogenesis and physiopathology of cystic fibrosis of the pancreas. *New Eng. J. Med.* 277:1287, 1344, 1399, 1967.
69. Handwerger, S., Roth, J., Gorden, P., di Sant'Agnese, P., Carpenter, D. F., and Peter, G. Glucose intolerance in cystic fibrosis. *New Eng. J. Med.* 281:451, 1969.

70. Porta, E. A., Stein, A. A., and Patterson, P. Ultrastructural changes of the pancreas and liver in cystic fibrosis. *Amer. J. Clin. Path.* 42:451, 1964.
71. Landing, B. H., Wells, T. R., and Wang, C. Abnormality of the epididymis and vas deferens in cystic fibrosis. *Arch. Path.* (Chicago) 88:569, 1969.
72. Ashworth, C. T., Chears, W. C., Jr., Sanders, E., and Pearce, M. B. Nontropical sprue. *Arch. Path.* (Chicago) 71:13, 1961.
73. Yardley, J. A., Bayless, T. M., Norton, J. H., and Hendrix, T. R. Celiac disease. A study of the jejunal epithelium before and after a gluten-free diet. *New Eng. J. Med.* 267:1173, 1962.
74. Swanson, V. L., and Thomassen, R. W. Pathology of the jejunal mucosa in tropical sprue. *Amer. J. Path.* 46:511, 1965.
75. di Sant'Agnese, P. A., and Jones, W. O. The celiac syndrome (malabsorption) in pediatrics. *J.A.M.A.* 180:308, 1962.
76. Biempica, L., Toccalino, H., and O'Donnell, J. C. Cytochemical and ultrastructural studies of the intestinal mucosa of children with celiac disease. *Amer. J. Path.* 52:795, 1968.
77. Cohen, A. S., Schimmel, E. M., Holt, P. R., and Isselbacher, K. J. Ultrastructural abnormalities in Whipple's disease. *Proc. Soc. Exp. Biol. Med.* 105:411, 1960.
78. Watson, J. H. L., and Haubrich, W. S. Bacilli bodies in the lumen and epithelium of the jejunum in Whipple's disease. *Lab. Invest.* 21:347, 1969.
79. Fisher, E. R. Whipple's disease: Pathogenetic consideration. *J.A.M.A.* 181:396, 1962.
80. Glenner, G., and Mallory, G. K. The cystadenoma and related nonfunctional tumors of the pancreas. *Cancer* 9:980, 1956.
81. Soloway, H. B. Constitutional abnormalities associated with pancreatic cystadenomas. *Cancer* 18:1297, 1965.
82. Durham, R. H. Thrombophlebitis migrans and visceral carcinoma. *A.M.A. Arch. Intern. Med.* 96:380, 1955.
83. Tseng, H. L. Thrombosis of hepatic veins. *A.M.A. Arch. Path.* 60:319, 1955.
84. Winslow, D. J., and Taylor, H. B. Malignant peritoneal mesotheliomas. *Cancer* 13:127, 1960.
85. Silverstein, M. N. Tumor hypoglycemia. *Cancer* 23:142, 1969.
86. Ormond, J. K. Idiopathic retroperitoneal fibrosis. *J.A.M.A.* 174:1561, 1960.
87. Elkind, A. H., Friedman, A. P., Bachman, A., Siegelman, S. S., and Sacks, O. W. Silent retroperitoneal fibrosis associated with methysergide therapy. *J.A.M.A.* 206:1041, 1968.
88. Gonatas, N. K. Extra-abdominal desmoid tumors. *Arch. Path.* (Chicago) 71:214, 1961.

GENERAL REFERENCES

Ackerman, L. V. Tumors of the retroperitoneum, mesentery, and peritoneum. Section VI, Fascicles 23 and 24, in *Atlas of Tumor Pathology*. Washington: Armed Forces Institute of Pathology, 1954.

Edmondson, H. A. Tumors of the liver and intrahepatic bile ducts. Section VII, Fascicle 25, in *Atlas of Tumor Pathology*. Washington: Armed Forces Institute of Pathology, 1958.

Frantz, V. K. Tumors of the pancreas. Section VII, Fascicles 27 and 28, in *Atlas of Tumor Pathology*. Washington: Armed Forces Institute of Pathology, 1959.

22 THE URINARY SYSTEM

NORMAL AND PATHOLOGIC PHYSIOLOGY OF THE KIDNEYS

The *functions of the kidneys* are the *formation of urine* and poorly understood *effects on the blood pressure and erythropoiesis.* Renal diseases may affect one or all of these functions.

Excretion of urine

The *excretory function* of urine formation plays an important role in maintaining the constant composition of body fluids; it is carried out by glomerular filtration, tubular reabsorption, and tubular secretion. Each of the 2.5 million nephrons in the kidneys acts as a functional unit in excretion. Composing each nephron is a glomerulus and a complex tubular system. Electron microscopy has vastly increased our knowledge of *fine glomerular structure.* The glomerular capillaries are lined by *endothelial cells* which show characteristic interruptions (pores or vesicles). Beneath the endothelium is a *basement membrane* about 3300 angstroms thick [1], which has a central dense, homogeneous layer (lamina densa) and pale outer zones (lamina rara interna and externa). The *lamina densa* [2] is a continuous membranous sheet lying between the capillary endothelium and mesangium and the epithelial cells of the glomerulus. Histochemically it appears to be a mucopolysaccharide or glycoprotein. The lamina densa is probably the *ultrafilter of the glomerulus* and normally blocks the passage of practically all serum proteins. The *epithelium* [3] consists of rather large cells (podocytes) which have abundant cytoplasm with numerous branches *(foot processes).* These insert on the basement membrane. Where it is present the *glomerular mesangium* lies between the capillary endothelial cells and the basement membrane. Composing it are *mesangial (stalk) cells,* which form a continuous latticework to which the endothelial cells are attached, and an intercellular *mesangial matrix* [4]. The latter consists of fine interlacing fibrils (sponge fibers of the stalk) which form a spongy network enmeshing the cytoplasm of mesangial cells. The *functions of the mesangium* have been variously considered to be glomerular support, collagen formation, contractility, and/or phagocytosis. A striking resemblance between mesangial cells and cells of the juxtaglomerular apparatus (JGA) in morphology and reactivity has been noted; it is possible that the stalk cells secrete renin as do those of the JGA [5].

Glomerular filtration

Glomerular filtration is a process for which the capillaries are well suited because their hydrostatic pressure is high (65 mm. of mercury). Pressures opposing filtration are the colloidal osmotic pressure of plasma proteins (25 mm. of mercury), the renal interstitial pressure (10 mm.), and the pressure necessary to drive fluid through the convoluted tubules (10 mm.), totaling 45 mm. Thus there is an *effective filtration pressure* of about 20 mm. of mercury. The glomerular filtrate is practically a protein-free ultrafiltrate of plasma. The normal renal plasma flow is 650 ml. per minute. About 120 ml. of filtrate is formed per minute (160 liters per day). The normal urine volume is 800 to 1600 ml. per day.

Tubular reabsorption:

Tubular reabsorption and secretion begins in the *proximal convoluted tubules,* where there is an isosmotic reabsorption of about 80 percent of filtrate water, all the glucose, and most of the sodium (about 85 percent), chloride, and ascorbic acid. The tubular epithelium transfers the resorbed material via the interstitial fluid into the peritubular capillaries. *Secretion* of creatinine and penicillin into the urine occurs from the proximal tubular epithelium. In the *descending limb of the loop of Henle* the filtrate has a low solute content. The flat epithelium acts as a selective dialyzing membrane, resorbing water. In the *ascending limb* the fluid is neutral in reaction, with a specific gravity of about 1.010. In the *distal convoluted tubule,* urine formation is completed by facultative reabsorption of water, sodium, chloride, phosphate, and sulfate ions, and secretion of ammonium and hydrogen ions. The secretion of these ions conserves base. Hydrogen ions are formed in the tubular cells by the action of carbonic anhydrase. Ammonia is released from amino acids and glutamine (by enzymatic action, as by amine oxidase) and combines with hydrogen ions to form ammonium ions. Both hydrogen and ammonium ions substitute for sodium ions in the urine, the latter being reabsorbed by the tubular epithelium as sodium bicarbonate and sodium chloride.

extrarenal controls

Extrarenal endocrine controls of tubular reabsorption are by the posterior pituitary-hypothalamic complex and the adrenal cortex. Secretion of the posterior pituitary *antidiuretic hormone* (ADH) is stimulated by a slight increase and depressed by an extremely slight decrease in plasma osmotic pressure. This hormone causes the distal tubular epithelium to reabsorb a hypotonic solution, so that the urine is hypertonic and of small volume. In the absence of ADH these cells reabsorb hypertonic fluid, the urine becoming dilute and of large volume *(diabetes insipidus). Adrenal cortical hormones* (aldosterone and to a lesser extent desoxycorticosterone) stimulate sodium resorption and prevent excessive potassium resorption.

1. Clinical Manifestations of Renal Disease

PROTEINURIA:

Proteinuria is the presence of excessive amounts of protein in the urine. Normally the glomerular capillary is very retentive of protein, and the small amounts which pass through the glomerular membranes are reabsorbed by the tubular epithelium. Proteinuria may have an origin that is either glomerular (due to a "leak" of an excessive amount of protein into the filtrate) or tubular (due to failure of reabsorption). The glomerular "leak" is by far the more common mechanism. In glomerular "leaks" the small albumin molecules predominate, although significant amounts of globulin pass into the filtrate. Certain large proteins such as hemoglobin may be of such a configuration and molecular weight as to pass through normal glomerular membranes and tubules.

Glomerular change

The only constant structural change in the glomerulus in proteinuria, as seen by electron microscopy, is a *transformation of the epithelial foot processes into broad cytoplasmic sheets* which abut onto the lamina rara externa of the basement membranes. This epithelial foot process fusion is secondary to basement membrane damage and appears to represent an attempt to halt the loss of protein through the glomerular filter. Increased metabolic activity of the epithelial cells is indicated by increased numbers of mitochondria and prominence of the Golgi apparatus. The foot process alteration can often be observed while the glomeruli appear normal by light microscopy. It is reversible and clears during remissions. In almost all conditions characterized by appreciable proteinuria, electron microscopy reveals *swelling or definite thickening of the glomerular basement membrane.* The increased permeability is evidently due to a disruption of the polymerized molecular structure of the basement membrane by the deposit of exogenous material such as antigen-antibody complexes. *Gamma globulins, complement, and fibrinogen* bound to glomerular capillary walls have been demonstrated in acute glomerulonephritis, membranous glomerulonephritis, and lupus erythematosus [6].

Orthostatic albuminuria

Orthostatic (postural) albuminuria is the urinary excretion of albumin only when the individual is erect. It may be due to circulatory changes in the kidneys caused by compression of the left renal vein between the superior mesenteric artery and the aorta, or reflex renal vasoconstriction initiated by a decreased amount of blood in the thoracic viscera. In cases of *fixed and reproducible orthostatic proteinuria,* renal biopsies reveal glomerular capillary wall thickening without basement membrane thickening, focal glomerular hypercellularity, and slight Bowman's capsular thickening in 45 percent of the cases [7]. Evidence of definite parenchymal renal disease is found in less than 10 percent of the cases. Electron microscopic studies of such renal biopsies [8] reveal focal glomerular capillary collapse, hypercellularity, and deposition of increased amounts of basement membrane material. There are also focal fusion of the epithelial foot processes and swelling of the cytoplasm of glomerular epithelial cells with intracytoplasmic vacuoles and accumulation of protein-like aggregates. These changes are probably the result of an increased uptake of protein-containing fluid which escapes through focal basement membrane defects that are not microscopically evident. The fine structure of many glomerular capillaries is completely normal.

Clinical aspects

Proteinuria is a prominent feature of acute, subacute, and membranous glomerulonephritis, amyloidosis, diabetic glomerulosclerosis, lupus erythematosus, and myeloma nephrosis. The effects of proteinuria are the physical loss of protein and tubular obstruction by inspissated casts.

CYLINDRURIA:

Cylindruria is the presence of *tubular casts* in the urine. They are found rarely in the absence of renal disease. Proteinuria must precede cast formation, which occurs in the distal tubules and collecting ducts where resorption of water and acidification of the urine favor coagulation of the protein. The actual precipitant is a nondialyzable, heat-resistant X-body, chemically related to chondroitin sulfate, which reaches its highest concentration in the distal tubules. Most casts are washed out by the increased fluid pressure from above, the tubules dilating about the coagula and casts appearing in the urine.

Tubular blockage

Tubular obstruction by casts is severe in hypoxic nephrosis (dense pigment casts blocking the distal convoluted tubules) and in severe globulinuria (as in some cases of acute glomerulonephritis and in myeloma nephrosis, or *globulinuric obstructive nephropathy).*

Classification

Casts are classified as *noncellular* (hyaline, finely and coarsely granular, waxy, fatty, and pigmented) or cellular (red, white, or epithelial cell casts). *Granular casts* contain lipid, especially cholesterol, granules and are common in membranous glomerulonephritis. The dense, short *pigment casts* contain bilirubin, hemoglobin, or myoglobin pigments. *Cellular casts* indicate exudation into the nephron. *Renal failure casts* are short and very broad, having been formed in the terminal collecting ducts of Bellini. Cast formation here means great slowing of the urinary flow has occurred due to loss of most of the nephrons draining into these ducts.

HEMATURIA: *Hematuria* is the presence of an abnormal number of erythrocytes in the urine. Normally up to 500,000 erythrocytes per 12 hours are passed. Centrifugation with microscopic examination of the sediment will distinguish hematuria from hemoglobinuria and myoglobinuria.

Causes *Renal causes* of hematuria include glomerular lesions (acute glomerulonephritis – gross hematuria; chronic glomerulonephritis – microscopic hematuria), tubular lesions (sulfonamide crystalluria, lithuria), vascular lesions (infarction, focal embolic glomerulonephritis, periarteritis nodosa, lupus erythematosus, and arteriolonephrosclerosis), interstitial lesions (pyelonephritis, tuberculosis), neoplastic lesions (adenocarcinoma, nephroblastoma, hemangioma), polycystic kidneys, and essential hematuria due to anomalous submucosal papillary venules. *Unilateral hematuria* occurs in pyelonephritis, tuberculosis, neoplasms, and essential hematuria. *Gross bilateral hematuria* indicates acute glomerulonephritis, arteriolonephronecrosis, or periarteritis nodosa. Blood is frequently found in the uncatheterized urine of women during menstruation.

PYURIA *Pyuria* is the presence of an abnormal number of leukocytes in the urine. Normally up to 1.9 million leukocytes may be found in a 12-hour specimen. Pyuria may be unilateral or bilateral and occurs in acute pyelonephritis, some cases of chronic pyelonephritis, and tuberculosis. A few white cells are normally found in the urine of uncatheterized females.

HYPOSTHENURIA: *Hyposthenuria* is a decreased capacity to form hypertonic urine. *Neurohumoral hyposthenuria* is due to inhibition or loss of the posterior pituitary-hypothalamic control of water balance. *Renal hyposthenuria* is due to a temporary or permanent loss of the ability of the distal tubular epithelium to perform the osmotic work required to concentrate or dilute the tubular fluid. In *arteriolonephrosclerosis* it is due to ischemia of the tubular cells. In *chronic glomerulonephritis* it is probably secondary to the arteriolar changes. A result of hyposthenuria is nocturia – the nocturnal formation of a large volume of urine with low specific gravity due to the mobilization of dependent edema fluid in congestive heart failure.

Effect An effect of hyposthenuria is an increase in the minimum urinary volume necessary for adequate excretion of metabolic wastes. A normal person can excrete 35 gm. of urinary solids daily in 500 ml. of urine with a specific gravity of 1.028. At specific gravity 1.010 a urinary volume of about 1500 ml. is needed. Failure to provide this volume leads to azotemia and uremia.

OLIGURIA: *Oliguria* is a failure of the kidneys to form urine in amounts sufficient to meet metabolic demands. The urine volume at which oliguria begins depends on the concentrating power of the kidneys, varying from 400 to 1500 ml. per day. *Anuria* is the failure of the kidneys to form urine. Since it may begin or terminate in oliguria, the two conditions are related and can be considered as one. The *causes of oliguria and anuria may be extrarenal* (dehydration, cardiac failure, shock, or painful stimuli), *renal,* or *obstructive.* The obstruction may be intrarenal (tubular blockage), pelvic, ureteral, vesical, or urethral. Complete anuria is uncommon and is usually associated with bilateral cortical necrosis.

Hyper-sthenuric oliguria

Hypersthenuric oliguria is characterized by an inadequate urine volume and a specific gravity greater than 1.023. It is caused by inadequate water intake or by a decrease in glomerular filtration without loss of tubular function, as by hypotension, decreased renal flow, or decreased filtration surface. The *cause* is usually extrarenal, but it does appear in acute glomerulonephritis.

Hypos-thenuric oliguria

Hyposthenuric oliguria is characterized by an inadequate urine volume and a specific gravity of about 1.010. It is due to a decrease or loss of tubular concentrating power, which may be caused by anoxia from shock, tubular damage by toxic agents, or loss of tubules. The *cause* is usually some type of renal parenchymal damage.

Reflex oliguria

Reflex anuria or oliguria due to painful stimulation is poorly understood. Corticomedullary vasomotor shunting via the vasa recta has been proposed, but it is not established. In some way cortical ischemia is the cause.

Mecha-nisms of oliguria

In most cases of oliguria or anuria, more than one mechanism plays a part. In *hypoxic nephrosis* the mechanisms are vasoconstrictive renal ischemia due to neurogenic shock, ischemic damage to tubules by redistribution of renal blood flow, and pigment deposition, due to a filtration of circulating pigment through glomeruli or passage of red cells through injured glomeruli. In *toxic nephrosis* the oliguria or anuria may be due to tubular blockage and/or reabsorption of fluid through the denuded tubular walls. In the *nephrotic syndrome* the cause of oliguria may be sodium retention, water being held to dilute the increased interstitial sodium.

RENAL EDEMA: Nephritic edema

Nephritic edema occurs in acute glomerulonephritis and eclampsia. The edematous skin is rubbery and nonpitting, and the edema is most marked in the eyelids and face. The protein content of the fluid is higher than in other edema fluids. Three mechanisms play a part: (1) decreased glomerular filtration due to glomerular damage and vasoconstriction, without tubular damage, producing a glomerulotubular imbalance which leads to hypersthenuric oliguria with retention of sodium and water; (2) loss of protein in the urine, which lowers the plasma colloidal osmotic pressure; and (3) generalized increased capillary permeability due to arteriolar constriction.

Nephrotic edema

Nephrotic edema occurs in subacute and membranous glomerulonephritis, amyloidosis, and diabetic glomerulosclerosis. It is due to hypoproteinemia, resulting from proteinuria in excess of the body's ability to replace the protein, and to sodium retention caused by the glomerulotubular imbalance. The accompanying lipemia appears to be due to resorption of lipids from the proteins in the tubular fluid; the accompanying frequent infections, such as erysipelas of edematous skin or pneumococcal peritonitis, to the loss of gamma globulin and complement in the urine.

DIURESIS:

Diuresis is an increase in the volume of urine. The process is usually initiated by the use of certain drugs known as *diuretics.* The three types of diuresis are: osmotic, filtration, and water.

Osmotic diuresis

Osmotic diuresis is achieved by increasing the amount of water and solutes reaching the distal portions of the nephrons. This can be done by raising the concentration of osmotically active substances in the glomerular filtrate (urea, glucose, hypertonic saline, mannitol); or by blocking proximal tubular reabsorption of glucose (by phlorizin), sodium and chloride ions (by organic mercurials and chlorothiazides), sodium and bicarbonate ions (by acetazolamide), or potassium ions (by furosemide and ethacrynic acid).

Filtration diuresis

Filtration diuresis is accomplished by elevating the glomerular filtration rate by increasing the cardiac output (as by digitalis in congestive heart failure), by raising the blood pressure (as by vasopressor agents), or by producing renal vasodilation (as by xanthine diuretics).

Water diuresis

Water diuresis is brought about by a reduction in water reabsorption in the distal tubules. It occurs in diabetes insipidus due to a deficiency of antidiuretic hormone and in renal diseases characterized by decreased distal tubular reabsorption (regenerative phase of tubular necrosis, as following certain poisonings, and nephrocalcinosis). Water diuresis may be induced by suppression of ADH secretion through forcing fluids and glucose injections.

EXTRARENAL AZOTEMIA

Extrarenal azotemia is a marked nitrogen retention not caused by kidney disease. It is due to congestive heart failure, hypotension, dehydration (as a result of severe diarrhea or of vomiting caused by intestinal obstruction), and massive gastrointestinal hemorrhage. Absorption of nitrogen compounds and reduction of the renal plasma flow cause the azotemia in gastrointestinal hemorrhage.

UREMIA:

Uremia is the complex terminal stage of organic or functional renal insufficiency. *Intrarenal causes* include vascular changes (sclerosis, necrosis, thrombosis), parenchymatous damage (glomerulonephritis, diabetic glomerulosclerosis, toxic and hypoxic nephrosis), interstitial injury (pyelonephritis, abscesses, tuberculosis), and damage to renal tissue as a whole (infarction, cortical necrosis). *Extrarenal causes* include severe blood loss or anemia, circulatory failure, marked sodium loss, and reflex anuria.

Mechanisms of renal failure

The *mechanisms of renal failure* are a decrease in glomerular filtration, tubular reabsorption and/or excretion, and, theoretically, loss of a detoxifying renal function. Loss of about 60 percent of *glomerular filtration* is followed by retention of nitrogenous metabolites, phenols, and electrolytes. *Decreased tubular reabsorption* results in loss of water and electrolytes, and an inability to form ammonium is the result of decreased tubular secretion. *Failure of detoxification and/or a failure to produce erythropoietin* may account for the hematopoietic depression in uremia.

Acute failure

In *acute renal failure* [9] due to shock, crush syndrome, burns, and hemoglobinuric and toxic nephrosis, the underlying pathologic change is *acute tubular necrosis.* Sudden renal insufficiency due to acute glomerulonephritis and bilateral cortical necrosis is classified as *acute parenchymal renal failure.* Acute renal failure is characterized *clinically* by a small urine volume with an initially high specific gravity.

Renal ischemia is considered the common denominator in the causation of acute renal failure. How the renal ischemia develops is poorly understood. Endotoxins of gram-negative bacteria cause peripheral vasoconstriction by intensifying the local effects of epinephrine. It is possible that *polysaccharides related chemically to bacterial endotoxins* may be liberated from necrotic tissue in crushing injuries and burns or from devitalized cells after prolonged shock. Such circulating substances may produce renal vasoconstriction and ischemia. In crushing injuries, burns, transfusion reactions, and paroxysmal hemoglobinurias associated with acute renal failure, *blood and muscle pigments* are released and frequently precipitate as tubular casts. Capillary blockage by such pigments may be a causative factor in the renal ischemia.

Most cases of acute renal failure are associated with *major surgery, obstetrical accidents, trauma, severe burns,* or *chemical poisoning.* Among surgical patients the highest incidence is in those undergoing aortic and open-heart operations. *About 80 percent of the cases of obstetrical renal failure are related to criminal abortion,* often with infection. *Antepartum and postpartum hemorrhage* is a major factor in over half the cases of obstetrical renal failure. The acute renal failure in *burn patients* is related to excessive fluid loss and hemoglobinuria. The latter is due to the hemolysis of 10 to 20 percent of circulating erythrocytes resulting from the high temperature at the burn site. Mercuric chloride, carbon tetrachloride, and ethylene glycol are the most common *chemical agents* producing acute renal failure. *Acute alcoholism* may also cause renal failure by producing a marked fluid and electrolyte depletion. Acute renal insufficiency occasionally results from the *hepatorenal syndrome,* as in the combined hepatic and renal failure of terminal cirrhosis. The kidney shutdown following *biliary tract surgery* may be due to the release of a vasodepressor substance by manipulation of the pancreas. Pathologically when renal failure is produced by a *nephrotoxin,* a large segment of the proximal convoluted tubule shows *epithelial cellular necrosis* which extends down to but does not include the basement membrane. In cases due to *renal ischemia* there is a complete disruption of tubular structure including the basement membranes *(tubulorrhexis). Many nephrons are uninvolved and carry on some renal function.*

The *oliguria or anuria* of renal failure is variously attributed to a more than 50 percent reduction in renal blood flow caused by ischemia, tubular collapse due to a predominance of increased interstitial pressure over the intratubular pressure, and tubular back-diffusion due to blockage by swollen epithelial cells and/or casts. The formation of *fibrin thrombi in glomerular capillaries* and the deposition of fibrinogen along basement membranes may contribute to the oliguria by causing reduced glomerular filtration [10]. During the phase of decreased urine volume the *elevation of serum potassium* is due to release of this ion from hemolyzed erythrocytes and depleted glycogen stores, as well as the development of metabolic acidosis. *Hyponatremia and hypochloremia* result from the accumulation of excess body water by the catabolism of protein and fat. The oliguric or anuric phase is followed after a number of days by the *diuretic phase,* in which tubular function returns and the urine volume increases by 50 to 100 percent daily.

Septicemia is an important cause of death during renal failure, the causative organism frequently being an antibiotic-resistant staphylococcus, gram-negative bacillus, or fungus. The *mortality rate among patients undergoing hemodialysis* for acute renal failure is about 50 percent.

Chronic failure

Chronic renal failure results from prolonged progressive kidney disease. The urine volume is usually large with low specific gravity until the terminal stage.

Thus the serum potassium is decreased or even depleted, although a terminal potassium intoxication may appear.

Clinical features

Clinically uremia is characterized by nausea and vomiting, *uremic frost* (urea crystals) on the face, neck, and chest, pericardial rub, dyspnea, irritability, twitching, convulsions, and coma. A "mousy" uriniferous odor is present. The *blood findings* include elevated nonprotein nitrogen (NPN), blood urea nitrogen (BUN), uric acid, creatinine, sulfate, phosphate, chloride, and ammonia levels. The calcium level falls due to phosphate retention. The *nervous hyperirritability, muscle twitching,* and *convulsions* are at least partly explained by the decreased blood calcium. *Vomiting, anorexia, apathy,* and *depression* may be due to free blood phenols. *Stomatitis* and *diarrhea* appear to be related to the blood urea elevation, possibly due to the action of oral or intestinal bacterial ureases on the urea in saliva and intestinal fluid to release ammonia. *Dyspnea* is related to the acidosis due to sodium loss or chloride retention.

Pathologic changes

The *lesions* are variable and unpredictable. Most patients show only a few of the many changes associated with uremia. The *brain* may show marked edema, and urea deposits occur in the cerebrum. A *fibrinous pericarditis* is common, sometimes with a serous effusion. Electrocardiographic evidence of *myocardial damage* due to hyperkalemia may be present, but no specific myocardial lesion is found. Tiny focal necroses or calcification of myocardial fibers may occur. *Calcium oxalate crystals* have been found in the myocardium in 10 percent and in the kidneys in 70 percent of cases of chronic renal disease with uremia [11]. Necrosis of myofibrils is seen adjacent to the crystal deposits. The finding of calcium oxalate crystals indicates that a *defect in glycine metabolism* may be present in uremia. *Fibrinous pleuritis* occasionally occurs in severe renal insufficiency. In *uremic pneumonitis,* butterfly-like densities radiate out from the pulmonary hila on x-ray. These densities are due to intra-alveolar hemorrhage and accumulation of protein-rich fluid. Hyaline membranes line numerous alveolar walls. In the *gastrointestinal tract* there may be a stomatitis and a necrotizing and ulcerative enterocolitis. The ulcers resemble those of bacillary dysentery. Massive hemorrhage may result from the ulcerations. In *uremic pancreatosis,* inspissation of secretions in dilated acini is often found, and an increased cytoplasmic eosinophilia in groups of acinar cells has been noted. The *multiple foci of necrosis* which occasionally occur in the spleen in uremia produce a *Fleckmilz (speckled spleen)* [12]. The necrotic foci are grayish and usually measure 3 to 4 mm. but may reach a large size. They are found centrally as well as peripherally in the spleen. Emboli are not found in relation to the necrotic foci. In the *vagina* there may be a hemorrhagic ulcerative colpitis. *Parotitis* (due to bacterial infection from the mouth), *hemorrhages* (due to thrombocytopenia), and *anemia* (due to failure of erythopoietin production and possibly to hemolysis caused by unknown toxic metabolites) are commonly associated with chronic renal failure. Urea may be demonstrated on the skin (uremic frost) and in the brain and pulmonary lesions by the xanthydrol reaction.

DEVELOPMENTAL DEFECTS OF THE KIDNEYS

1. Abnormalities in Number or Size

AGENESIS:

Agenesis of the kidney(s) may be unilateral or bilateral. It is due to lack of the metanephrogenic primordium, failure of the ureteral bud to develop from the wolffian duct, or failure of contact of the ureteral bud and the nephrogenic cord on one or both sides.

Bilateral agenesis

Bilateral agenesis is rare, is more common in male than female fetuses by 2.5:1, and is usually *associated with oligohydramnios.* Almost all fetuses with bilateral agenesis of the kidneys are stillborn. The ureters are commonly absent, and other developmental defects, particularly of the genital tract, are frequently present. A *characteristic facies* occurs with bilateral renal agenesis: a flat nose; wide-set eyes with prominent epicanthal folds; large, flabby, and low-set ("Dumbo") ears; and a receding chin. Rarely meningocerebral angiomatosis is associated with it.

Unilateral agenesis

Unilateral agenesis is somewhat more common on the left than on the right side and is more common in men than in women by about 2:1. The corresponding *ureter* is typically absent. Other developmental anomalies, especially of the genital tract, are often present. The single kidney is much heavier than normal, due to compensatory hypertrophy and hyperplasia. It is in the usual location in most cases, but is sometimes located in the pelvis.

HYPOPLASIA:

Hypoplasia (dysplasia) is the failure of complete development of one or both kidneys. The underdevelopment may affect only a portion of the renal parenchyma *(local hypoplasia).* Renal dysplasia occurs predominantly in females. It is difficult to distinguish the contracted kidney of chronic renal inflammation in early life from a hypoplastic kidney. The situation is further complicated because pyelonephritis (infection of the renal parenchyma) is common in renal dysplasia.

Cause

The *cause* is thought to be abnormal ureteral budding, so that the metanephrogenic mass is poorly organized. When the dysplasia is bilateral and marked, the fetus is usually stillborn. In less severe cases the individual survives for several months or even years. Hypertension usually develops in unilateral renal dysplasia.

Pathologic changes

Grossly the hypoplastic kidney is small (the upper limit of weight is set at 60 gm). Two forms occur: in one the organ is an adult kidney in miniature, having 3 to 5 lobes and calyces instead of the normal 12; in the other there may be one or more cysts grossly, and *microscopically* there are primitive glomeruli and tubules in a dense fibrous or fatty interstitium. Some tubules end blindly.

SUPERNUMERARY KIDNEY

Supernumerary kidney is extremely rare. The third kidney is probably due to the development of a second ureteral bud from the mesonephric duct on one side. It usually lies below the normal kidney and may be in the pelvis. The smaller supernumerary organ may be completely free of or loosely attached to the adjacent kidney. Their ureters usually fuse somewhere along their courses.

2. Abnormalities in Location or Shape

ECTOPIC KIDNEY

Ectopia of the kidney(s) is a congenital displacement of the organ(s). Ectopic kidneys typically lie horizontally in the iliac fossa, at the pelvic brim or in the pelvis. They are often altered in size and shape by the pressure of their abnormal neighbors. In *crossed ectopia* the displaced kidney usually lies caudally to the normal (fixed) kidney. The ureters typically enter the bladder in the normal position, the ureter of the ectopic kidney crossing the midline. Renal function may be normal in ectopic kidneys, but ureteral obstruction is more common than with normal kidneys.

FUSED KIDNEYS

Median fusion of the kidneys occurs in several variants, the most common of which is the *horseshoe kidney*. This fairly common anomaly is due to fusion of renal blastemas early in fetal development. In 90 percent of the cases the fusion is at the lower poles. Disorders due to urinary stasis, including renal calculi, occur more frequently in horseshoe than in normal kidneys, because in the former the ureters are often angulated. In most cases horseshoe kidneys are asymptomatic, but in some patients pressure of the isthmus on underlying nerves and vessels produce upper abdominal pain while standing or sitting (Rovsing syndrome). Other fusion types are the *L-shaped or sigmoid kidneys*.

FETAL LOBULATION

Persistence of fetal lobulation of the kidney is the most common anomaly of this organ. Deep grooves are seen on the external surface of the kidney, marking the renal lobes. It has no clinical significance.

3. Cystic Kidney

POLYCYSTIC KIDNEY: Clinical features

Polycystic kidney is an important renal anomaly; it may be unilateral or bilateral. *Clinically* there are two forms: the infantile and the adult. In the *infantile form,* cystic disease is usually apparent at birth. The cystic kidneys may interfere with delivery and lead to intrapartum death. They usually cause death from uremia in the first month of life. In the *adult form* the patient remains apparently well until the age of 40 to 50 years or older and then develops hypertension, proteinuria, and uremia. About 7 percent of one series of cases of polycystic kidney showed a relative polycythemia (normal hematocrit during severe uremia) [13]. Death occurs within 4 years of the onset of clinical signs in about 50 percent of the cases.

Pathologic changes: type 1

Extensive *microdissection studies* have demonstrated that there are *four types of polycystic kidney* [14]. *Type 1 is due to hyperplasia of the epithelium of the interstitial portions of the collecting tubules* [15]. The malformation appears to be transmitted homozygously as a recessive gene. It is invariably associated with cystic hyperplasia of intrahepatic bile ducts. This form is always bilateral and is incompatible with prolonged extra-uterine survival, although the cause of early death is not clear in these cases. *Grossly* the kidneys are symmetrically enlarged, often being the size of adult organs at birth. The external and cut surfaces are studded with cysts measuring 1 to 2 mm. in diameter in both the cortex and medulla. Because of the appearance of the sagittal section surface, the name *sponge kidney* is sometimes used. *Microscopically* cystic tubules are lined by cuboidal epithelium; they are elongated in the cortex and round or oval in the medulla. There is no increase in interstitial fibrous tissue. *Microdissection* reveals no tubular obstruction or discontinuity and shows that the dilated or cystic parts of tubules communicate openly with uninvolved portions and with the dilated renal calyces and pelvis. Cystic dilatation is most marked in the last generation of collecting tubules, which normally form the cortical rays. The enlargement is associated with hyperplasia of the epithelial cells, and the urine within the cysts is not under excessive pressure. The nephrons proximal to the collecting tubules appear relatively normal.

type 2

Type 2 is attributed to inhibition of activity in the ampullae, the zones of growth at the advancing ends of developing collecting tubules [16]. The malformation may involve both kidneys (death due to uremia occurs shortly after birth), one kidney, or, rarely, only part of one kidney. This form of polycystic kidney is often associated with developmental defects in other organs. *Grossly,* involved kidneys are usually larger, but may be smaller than normal. The cysts are thick-walled and spherical and form rounded elevations beneath the thickened capsule. *Microscopically* there is an almost complete absence of normal renal parenchyma between the cysts, which are lined by cuboidal cells and embedded in fibrous tissue. *Microdissection* reveals only 4 to 10 generations of collecting tubules instead of the normal 12 to 20. Almost all tubules terminate in small or large cysts. The cyst fluid is a secretion of the lining epithelial cells.

Type 3 is the form of bilateral polycystic kidneys found in patients who survive for more than a few weeks after birth *(polycystic kidneys of the adult)* [17]. This type occasionally is unilateral. It is *due to multiple abnormalities of renal development. Grossly* the kidneys are usually enlarged, their size depending on age and the degree of tubular involvement, and the amount of fluid collected within cysts. A pair may weigh up to 3500 gm. At birth the involvement is usually microcystic. In adults the cysts may be very large. They are filled with clear to straw-colored watery fluid or with dark brown or blue fluid due to hemorrhage. *Microscopically* varying numbers of normal or compressed, functional nephrons are present between cysts. When the latter arise from collecting tubules, they are surrounded by dense fibrous tissue; cysts from other tubular components are not invested by fibrous tissue and thus are thin-walled. *Microdissection* demonstrates an intermingling of normal nephrons and collecting tubules with cystic ones. Cysts develop in either the ampullary or interstitial portions of collecting tubules or in any part of nephrons. In the latter they arise most commonly in Bowman's space and the loop of Henle. Such cysts communicate with collecting tubules which open into the calyces. Cysts originating in collecting tubules are rarely connected to nephrons and are larger than those arising in nephrons. type 3

Type 4 is secondary to developmental urethral obstruction, usually by membranous folds at the level of the verumontanum [18]. Backpressure damages the ampullae of collecting tubules in both kidneys, disturbing their normal branching, and the distal portions of the nephrons. In the most severe cases the urinary bladder, ureters, and renal pelves are greatly distended, and cysts are found throughout the cortex. These arise in both collecting tubules and nephrons. Foci of extramedullary erythropoiesis and cartilage are present in the interstitial tissue. In the less severe cases the bladder wall is hypertrophic, the ureters are dilated and elongated, and the pelves are only slightly distended. Renal cysts are small and arise in the terminal (proximal) portions of collecting tubules, loops of Henle, and Bowman's spaces. Rarely obstruction at a ureterovesical or ureteropelvic junction causes unilateral renal cystic changes. type 4

Medullary sponge kidney [19], which may be considered a fifth type of polycystic kidney, is uncommon, usually bilateral, and characterized by many, usually small medullary cysts. These result from cystic dilatation of collecting tubules and may contain microcalculi. It is uncertain whether the condition is developmental or acquired. The condition may cause no clinical manifestations or may become manifest in the third through the fifth decade of life in the form of hematuria and flank pain. On pyelograms the cysts and their diverticula resemble a bunch of flowers or show a brushlike pattern. Medullary sponge kidneys are compatible with a normal life span unless they are complicated by pyelonephritis. Medullary sponge kidney

Solitary (simple) cyst of the kidney is rare in infants and children and common in adults. This indicates that it is probably acquired rather than developmental. The *cyst* is usually 5 to 10 cm. in diameter, thin-walled, and lined by a single layer SOLITARY CYST of flat or cuboidal epithelium. About 70 percent of these cysts occur at the lower pole. The cyst fluid is clear and may contain albumin and urea.

4. Other Abnormalities

HEREDITARY NEPHRITIS WITH NERVE DEAFNESS: *Hereditary nephritis with nerve deafness* [20] is most likely transmitted as an autosomal dominant with preferential association with the X chromosome during meiosis. *Clinically* hematuria is the most striking urinary finding, but proteinuria and pyuria may also occur. Urine cultures are negative. Male patients usually die of gradually progressive renal failure before they are 30. Females typically live much longer. The *deafness* is bilateral and pronounced. The main loss is for high-pitched sounds. In some affected families there is a high frequency of beta-hemolytic streptococcal otitis media. *Ocular anomalies* are sometimes present. They include spherophakia, lenticonus, cataracts, retinitis pigmentosa, and progressive myopia. The pathogenesis of the lesions in this syndrome is not known.

Pathologic changes: *Grossly* the kidneys are markedly atrophic. The cortices are thin, pale, and often streaked with yellow lines. *Microscopically* the glomeruli show increased cellularity, basement membrane thickening, and epithelial crescent formation. Lipid deposits are found in the epithelial cells of the glomerular tuft. The functioning tubules are dilated, but many others are atrophic. The tubular epithelial cells contain lipids. Tubular casts are common. The cortical interstitial tissue is fibrotic and infiltrated with lymphocytes, plasmocytes, and clusters of large cells with foamy, lipid-filled cytoplasm. These are degenerated and disorganized tubular epithelial cells.

PELVIC ANOMALIES: *Anomalies of the renal pelvis* include *double pelves* (which may indicate a double fused kidney) and *extrarenal pelvis,* in which the calyces and pelvis lie outside the renal parenchyma.

ARTERIAL ANOMALIES: Anomalous renal arteries include upper or lower polar arteries arising from the aorta or from the main renal artery, and multiple (2 to 4) renal arteries. *Lower polar arteries* occur in one in about 15 kidneys and may obstruct the ureter to produce hydronephrosis (dilatation of the pelvis and calyces with atrophy of the kidney due to backpressure).

DISEASES PRINCIPALLY AFFECTING THE GLOMERULI

1. Glomerulonephritis

DIFFUSE GLOMERULONEPHRITIS: *Diffuse glomerulonephritis* is a generalized inflammation of the glomerular tufts with secondary tubular, interstitial, and vascular changes. Its *cause* in most cases is *hypersensitivity to beta-hemolytic streptococci.* In about 90 percent of patients with *acute glomerulonephritis* there is an associated type 12 beta-hemolytic streptococcal infection, but occasional cases are associated with type 4, type 1, and Red Lake streptococci. Acute glomerulonephritis sometimes occurs following a streptococcal infection in which the organisms were promptly eradicated by antibiotic therapy. Usually the preceding infection is deep-seated. It may be in the form of scarlet fever or streptococcal pharyngitis, tonsillitis, mastoiditis, bronchopneumonia, osteomyelitis, or bacterial endocarditis. Occasionally acute glomerulonephritis follows staphylococcal, pneumococcal, meningococcal, gonococcal, *Hemophilus influenzae,* viral, or rickettsial infections. It occurs in about

40 percent of cases of anaphylactoid purpura, and it is associated with pulmonary hemorrhages and/or hemosiderosis in Goodpasture's syndrome (see page 461). A few cases have followed bee stings. *Antihuman kidney antibodies (AHK) are found in about 40 percent of cases of glomerulonephritis* [21]. Presumably the damage to renal tissue produced by streptococcal toxin causes the release into the circulation of a protein product which stimulates antibody production by the reticuloendothelial system. Such antibodies are not found in other forms of renal disease nor in normal controls.

Acute glomerulonephritis: clinical features

Acute glomerulonephritis typically follows the antecedent infection after an interval of 2 to 6 weeks. About 70 percent of the cases occur in the 5 to 20 age group, and the incidence in males is about twice that in females. There is no correlation between the occurrence of acute rheumatic carditis and acute glomerulonephritis. The *clinical manifestations* of acute glomerulonephritis include chills, moderate fever, headache, nausea and vomiting, pallor, edema of the eyelids, face, and external genitalia, hypertension, lumbar pain, and urgency and frequency of urination. The *urine* may be smoky or coffee-colored. There are hematuria, proteinuria, cylindruria, and oliguria, the daily urine volume averaging about 500 ml. Occasional cases of acute glomerulonephritis develop a *nephrotic syndrome* with marked proteinuria, hypoalbuminemia, hypercholesterolemia, and massive edema. Cardiac insufficiency of some degree develops in about 75 percent of cases. The *circulatory failure* in acute glomerulonephritis, evidenced by dyspnea, pulmonary congestion and edema, cardiac enlargement, increased venous pressure, and peripheral edema, is due to fluid retention resulting from decreased renal excretion of sodium and water. This is caused by a *severe reduction in the glomerular filtration rate.* Since tubular function is much less severely impaired than glomerular function, a more complete reabsorption of sodium and water occurs. The antistreptolysin and antistreptokinase titers are often elevated in acute glomerulonephritis. This stage usually lasts a few weeks. Over 80 percent of the patients recover fully, and recurrent attacks are rare following complete healing of the initial one. About 2 percent die during the acute phase due to cardiac and/or renal failure. The remaining cases go into the subacute or chronic stages of glomerulonephritis directly or after a latent period of months or years.

pathologic changes

Grossly the kidneys are large, swollen, red, and smooth, with tense capsules which strip easily. Their surfaces may be dotted by punctate hemorrhages. On cut surfaces the cortices are bulging, thickened, and usually deep red, although they may be pale. Corticomedullary differentiation is sharp, the pyramids being extremely congested. *Microscopically* most of the glomeruli in both kidneys are enlarged. There is usually marked endothelial proliferation, with less epithelial hyperplasia *(acute proliferative glomerulonephritis).* The capillary endothelial swelling and overgrowth narrows or closes the lumina, and capillary thrombi occur. Occasionally a patchy fibrinoid necrosis of the capillary walls is found *(acute necrotizing glomerulonephritis).* Polymorphonuclear leukocytes, sometimes in large numbers *(acute exudative glomerulonephritis),* may be present intravascularly and extravascularly. Many erythrocytes may be found in Bowman's spaces *(acute hemorrhagic glomerulonephritis).* Fibrin is present in the exudate.

Immunofluorescence reveals the presence of *gamma globulin* and *complement* along the glomerular basement membranes in most cases of acute glomerulonephritis, and fibrinogen derivatives are found mainly within proliferating endothelial and mesangial cells. Fluorescein-labeled immunoglobulin G (Ig G) from the serum of patients with acute glomerulonephritis (and from many normal persons) stains the glomerular basement membrane and mesangium in biopsies from cases of early acute poststreptococcal glomerulonephritis [22]. Previous absorption of the Ig G fraction on the plasma membrane of beta-hemolytic streptococci abolishes this staining. No other bacteria have this effect, and staining does not occur in other renal diseases. In one study, fluorescein-labeled antiserum to type 12 *streptococcal antigen* was found within glomeruli, and ferritin-labeled antiserum to gamma globulin and streptococcal antigen was localized in the glomerular basement membranes and proliferating endothelial and mesangial cells in cases of acute glomerulonephritis [23].

By *electron microscopy* there is focal widening of the glomerular basement membranes with occasional protuberances *(humps)* up to 2.5μ in diameter [24]. The humps may represent antigen-antibody complexes and are almost pathognomonic of poststreptococcal glomerulonephritis. They are on the epithelial side of the basement membrane, and two or more epithelial foot processes are fused over the larger humps. Otherwise the foot processes are generally discrete. The epithelial cells show cytoplasmic vacuolization. The glomerular capillary lumens are narrowed and even occluded due to the increase in number and size of the endothelial and mesangial cells. Cytoplasmic swelling and vacuolization are seen in the endothelial cells. Strands of basement membrane-like material *(hyaline fibers)* are found between endothelial cells. Sequential renal biopsies in a case of acute glomerulonephritis [25] reveal that *resolution of the glomerular changes* is in progress within a month after the onset. At this time, repair of glomerular basement membrane defects on the epithelial side is under way. At about 10 weeks endothelial cells are engaged in basement membrane repair. After about 18 months glomeruli appear normal except for focal basement membrane defects and collapsed capillary loops and persistence of increased numbers of mesengial cells. The tubules show lipid vacuolization and hyaline droplet formation in the epithelial cells and dilatation of the proximal tubules. Hyaline or cellular casts fill many lumina. In the necrotizing and hemorrhagic forms, degenerating red cell casts are found in the distal tubules. Under electron microscopy the *epithelial cells of the proximal and distal convoluted tubules* show thickened and flattened microvilli, and their cytoplasm contains many vesicles and channels [26]. Flocculation and later homogenization of granular material in large vesicles lead to the formation of *hyaline droplets.* Lipid droplets unrelated to the swollen mitochondria are found basally in the cells. The interstitial tissue of the kidneys is edematous and may be infiltrated by polymorphonuclear leukocytes.

Subacute glomerulonephritis: clinical features

Subacute glomerulonephritis may follow the acute form directly or after months or years. Many patients give no history of a preceding acute phase. *Clinically* a nephrotic syndrome, with massive proteinuria, severe edema, hypercholesterolemia, anemia, and mild hypertension, is characteristic. This stage lasts for several months to a year and may progress into the chronic phase of glomerulonephritis. Death is usually from uremia or infection, most often pneumonia.

pathologic changes

Grossly the kidneys are large, pale, and soft. The capsules are slightly adherent. On cut surface the cortices are wide and pallid. *Microscopically* there is widespread glomerular involvement, *epithelial crescents* being very numerous. They develop within 2 to 4 weeks of onset and are formed by the proliferation of Bowman's capsular epithelium, or possibly by an ingrowth of proliferating proximal tubular epithelium. The epithelial cells become spindled and appear morphologically like fibroblasts. The crescent may become honeycombed and take on an *adenomatoid appearance. Adhesions* frequently form between the glomerular tuft and capsule, and they may obliterate the capsular space. Phase and electron microscopy show *capillary basement membrane* thickening in most cases. In about 20 percent of the cases, especially those showing the nephrotic syndrome clinically, *membranous transformation* occurs, a hyaline layer forming between the basement membrane and the epithelial layer [27]. This may be due to the trapping of protein. Loss of the foot-process pattern and vacuolization of the epithelium occur. The *tubular epithelium* shows hyaline droplet formation and vacuolization. Tubular casts are common.

Chronic glomerulonephritis: clinical features

Chronic glomerulonephritis is the slowly progressive end phase of diffuse glomerulonephritis. It may follow the acute stage directly or appear after the subacute stage. Acute flare-ups may punctuate the chronic phase. *Clinically hypertension* increases steadily with progression of the disease. Renal findings include a loss of the ability to concentrate urine, the development of a *fixed specific gravity* near 1.010, *slight proteinuria,* and elevation of the blood urea and nonprotein nitrogen levels. *Anemia* (usually normocytic but occasionally macrocytic) may be pronounced late. This stage may last for years, often terminating in uremia and death.

pathologic changes

Grossly the kidneys are shriveled and firm, with tightly bound capsules which decorticate on stripping. The external surfaces are irregularly granular and pitted. On cut surface the cortices are narrowed, varying between 1 to 6 mm. in width. *Microscopically* many glomeruli are partially or completely hyalinized *(chronic sclerosing glomerulonephritis).* In well-established cases 40 to 90 percent of the glomeruli are hyalinized. The glomerular obsolescence is due to capillary collapse with loss of circulation [28]. The capillary collapse is caused by intercapillary fibrosis, capillary wall thickening, epithelial crescent formation, and/or afferent arteriolosclerosis. Electron microscopy reveals that obsolescent glomeruli contain a collapsed remnant of capillary basement membrane and mesangial matrix and endothelial nuclei enmeshed in masses of material resembling basement membrane [29]. Many *tubules* are small or are replaced by *interstitial fibrous tissue.* The latter is infiltrated by lymphocytes. A few small groups of dilated tubules are present. Most of these drain functioning hypertrophied glomeruli. Middle-sized and small *arteries* show intimal and medial hyaline thickening. The degree of the vascular changes correlates with the severity of hypertension and clinical course.

ACUTE MEMBRANOUS GLOMERULONEPHRITIS: Pathologic changes

Acute membranous glomerulonephritis occurs in preeclampsia and eclampsia, as the initial stage of chronic membranous glomerulonephritis, and possibly in syphilitic nephrosis. The changes are usually reversible in the toxemias of pregnancy and in syphilis.

Grossly the kidneys are swollen, and hemorrhages beneath the capsules and in the parenchyma may be seen. *Microscopically* there is a velvety fibrinoid swelling of the glomerular capillary walls. The capillaries are ischemic and may contain fibrin thrombi. In *preeclampsia and eclampsia,* electron microscopy reveals marked endothelial cytoplasmic swelling, causing almost complete luminal occlusion. Fibrinoid material is deposited between the endothelium and basement membrane and between endothelial cells. There are no basement membrane changes and only focal and limited epithelial foot-process alterations are seen by electron microscopy despite the severe proteinuria [30]. After delivery, endothelial swelling subsides, and the fibrinoid is removed by endothelial cells. In some cases the endothelial swelling persists post partum in renal biopsies for up to 2 years. During preeclampsia or eclampsia, various degenerative changes, ranging from cloudy swelling to necrosis, are found in the proximal convoluted tubular epithelium. Proteinaceous material and debris are present in the tubular lumina.

CHRONIC MEMBRANOUS GLOMERULONEPHRITIS: Clinical features

Chronic membranous glomerulonephritis (idiopathic nephrotic syndrome, lipid nephrosis) is of unknown cause. It usually occurs in children or young adults and may be a variant of subacute glomerulonephritis with a profound nephrotic component. However, a previous history of infection is usually vague or absent. *Clinically* the condition is characterized by anasarca, massive proteinuria, waxy pallor, decreased plasma proteins, and marked hypercholesterolemia. Renal function is good. The course is irregular with frequent remissions. Most patients with lipid nephrosis recover completely, especially with adrenocorticosteroid therapy. However, some cases progress to renal insufficiency. Death is usually due to intercurrent infection.

Pathologic changes

The kidneys are slightly to moderately enlarged, soft, and a pale, mottled, yellowish red. The capsule of each kidney strips easily, revealing a smooth surface which bulges slightly. The cortex is slightly widened and streaked with yellow. *Microscopically* the glomeruli in chronic membranous glomerulonephritis show slight but definite thickening of the capillary basement membrane and even some proliferation of endothelial cells. The thickening is seen best with the PAS (periodic acid-Schiff) stain. Glomerular endothelial cells may be swollen due to intracytoplasmic lipids. By means of *electron microscopy* two forms can be differentiated [31]. The *foot-process type,* which occurs mainly in early childhood, is characterized by endothelial and mesangial cell swelling; focal, flocculated subendothelial precipitates; only slight, localized basement membrane thickening; and extensive fusion of the epithelial cell foot processes. Early the *membranous type,* found principally in adults, shows occasional projections like the teeth of a comb on the epithelial side of the basement membrane, dense subepithelial protein deposits, and epithelial cell foot process fusion. The basement membrane eventually becomes quite thickened and homogeneous, and the foot processes are diffusely fused. The relationship between the two types is uncertain. By light microscopy in some cases the glomerular lesions consist of the presence of four to eight spherical hyaline masses of fairly uniform size in each glomerulus *(lobular glomerulonephritis).* In membranous glomerulonephritis the tubules are dilated, and the epithelium, especially in the proximal convoluted tubules, shows degenerative changes such as cloudy swelling and hydropic degeneration. In the cells lining the proximal convoluted tubules are found numerous vacuoles containing both *isotropic* and *anisotropic fat,* the latter forming a typical *Maltese cross in polarized light.* The fat is from lipoproteins which are reabsorbed from the protein-rich glomerular filtrate. Similar doubly refractile fat globules are found within the eosinophilic debris in the lumina. This leads to the presence of fat in the urinary sediment.

The *membranous change* (thickening of the capillary basement membrane) is similar to the glomerular wire-loop lesion of lupus erythematosus, and the *lobular change* is like the glomerular lesion of diabetic glomerulosclerosis. However, in chronic membranous or lobular glomerulonephritis the lesions are more widespread than in the other diseases, almost every glomerulus being involved in a uniform manner.

Focal glomerulonephritis has been discussed under Subacute Bacterial Endocarditis in Chapter 18.

2. Other Glomerular Lesions

DIABETIC GLOMERULOSCLEROSIS:

Diabetic (intercapillary) glomerulosclerosis (Kimmelstiel-Wilson disease) is one of the most distinctive renal lesions in diabetes mellitus. It is found in about 15 percent of autopsies of diabetic patients. The *cause* is unknown. The lesion is *not* pathognomonic of diabetes mellitus, since it occurs occasionally in acute pancreatitis, portal cirrhosis and fatty metamorphosis of the liver, and glomerulonephritis [32]. Similar lesions have been produced in rabbits by cortisone administration. Glomerulosclerosis is not related to insulin therapy. One etiologic concept is that the lesions result from fat embolism in the glomerular capillaries with a consequent exudation of fibrin. The lesions are similar to the small capillary aneurysms which develop in diabetic retinopathy.

Clinical features

Clinically the disease occurs chiefly after age 40 and is somewhat more common in females than in males. There are marked proteinuria (it is one of the most common causes of the *nephrotic syndrome* in adults), hypoproteinemia, edema, hypertension, and retinopathy. Lipids and fatty casts appear in the urine. Uremia develops terminally.

Pathologic changes

Grossly the kidneys are usually slightly larger than normal and are not distinctive. *Microscopically* in the *nodular type* there are round, focal *hyaline masses,* ranging from 20 to 120μ in diameter, scattered through the glomeruli. These masses stain as mucopolysaccharides. In the *diffuse type* there is a generalized thickening of the glomerular basement membranes. Hyaline deposition begins in the primary bifurcation of afferent arterioles and extends to affect the more peripheral capillary loops. Eventually the entire glomerulus may be completely converted to hyalin. Electron microscopic studies in *diffuse diabetic glomerulosclerosis* show that in the early stages the basement membrane is two to three times the normal thickness and in the late stages, up to 10 times the normal thickness [33]. In the *nodular type* of glomerulosclerosis there is widening of the mesangium (intercapillary space) due to the conspicuous deposits of hyaline or basement membrane-like material. In more advanced cases the capillary basement membrane becomes involved and may be thickened to three to five times the normal width. *The diffuse and nodular forms of diabetic glomerulosclerosis frequently occur together.*

Other diabetic lesions

Other *renal lesions in diabetes mellitus* include reduction in the number of juxtaglomerular cells [34], necrotizing papillitis, and both fatty degeneration of and the accumulation of glycogen in the convoluted tubular epithelium. In the rare *Armanni-Ebstein diabetic nephropathy,* glycogen vacuoles are found in the epithelium of the terminal straight segment of the proximal convoluted tubules [35]. The lesion is considered to be pathognomonic of diabetes. *Arteriolonephrosclerosis* is common in diabetics in association with hypertension. Distinctive of diabetes is a hyaline thickening of the efferent as well as the afferent arterioles. *Atherosclerosis of the renal and intrarenal arteries* is also common and usually begins at an earlier age than in nondiabetics. *Acute and chronic pyelonephritis* occur fairly frequently in diabetics.

AMYLOID GLOMERULOSIS:

Amyloid glomerulosis (amyloid nephrosis) occurs in secondary amyloidosis (discussed on page 80). *Clinically* the symptoms are marked proteinuria and edema. Hypertension and uremia are unusual.

Pathologic changes

The kidneys are large, pale, firm, and waxy. In protracted cases they may become contracted and granular. *Microscopically* the eosinophilic *amyloid* is deposited in the glomeruli, the walls of the arterioles, and around the collecting tubules. By electron microscopy the amyloid is seen to be deposited subendothelially at first. Later it is apparently deposited in the capillary basement membrane, which becomes irregularly and focally thickened up to 20 times normal. Ultrastructurally the amyloid consists of fibrils averaging about 100 angstroms in diameter [36]. The epithelial cells show intracytoplasmic vacuoles and replacement of the foot processes by broad cytoplasmic sheets, as in other disorders characterized by marked proteinuria. Eventually the glomeruli are converted to amyloid masses. When this occurs the corresponding tubules atrophy and are replaced by fibrous tissue. Earlier the tubular epithelium may show fatty vacuoles, and eosinophilic "colloid" casts may be found in their lumina.

RENAL LESIONS IN LUPUS ERYTHEMATOSUS:

Glomerular lesions in disseminated lupus erythematosus (see page 78) are inconstant. Classically there is a *nephrotic syndrome* with proteinuria and massive edema. The *urine is telescopic* in that it shows all elements found in other renal diseases – erythrocytes; leukocytes; hyaline, cellular, granular, and fatty casts; and lipid bodies. Hypertension and uremia are rare. The condition appears in women from age 18 to 35 chiefly.

Pathologic changes

Grossly the kidneys are usually slightly enlarged. *Microscopically* there is an endothelial proliferation in the glomerular capillaries. The most distinctive lesion is a patchy hyaline thickening of the basement membrane of the glomerular capillaries, giving a wire-loop appearance when the glomerular tuft is cut in cross section. With electron microscopy the most characteristic change is shown as a variable thickening of the basement membrane up to six times normal. Fibrinoid accumulates subendothelially. The *wire-loop lesion* is an extension of these processes, the loop being composed of a greatly thickened portion of a basement membrane adjacent to a broad subendothelial fibrinoid deposit. Immunofluorescence has shown that the fibrinoid material contains gamma globulins, complement, and fibrinogen [37]. Organized extracellular deposits have been found by electron microscopy in the glomerular mesangium, between the basement membrane and endothelial cells, within the basement membrane, and subepithelially [38]. The deposits show parallel curved bands or cross striations.

DISEASES PRINCIPALLY AFFECTING THE RENAL TUBULES

NEPHROSIS

The term *nephrosis* is used by pathologists to designate degenerative *renal lesions which are manifested mainly in the tubules,* especially the sensitive *convoluted tubules.* Unfortunately confusion has arisen because of the *clinical use* of the terms *nephrosis* and *nephrotic syndrome* for any renal disease characterized by proteinuria, massive edema, and hypercholesterolemia, in the absence of hematuria and marked hypertension and nitrogen retention.

1. Acute Nephrosis (Acute Tubular Necrosis)

TOXIC NEPHROSIS: Causes

Toxic nephrosis may be caused by exogenous (chemical and infectious) or endogenous (metabolic) toxins. Among the chemical agents which cause toxic nephrosis are mercuric chloride, potassium dichromate, uranium nitrate, chloroform, carbon tetrachloride, dioxane, ethylene glycol, and diethylene glycol. *Bacterial toxins* may produce tubular degeneration. *Metabolic agents* which produce nephrosis include the substances active in eclampsia and in jaundice (probably an abnormal aminoaciduria as well as the effects of shock). *Cholemic nephrosis* is discussed under Jaundice on page 277.

Clinical features

Clinically oliguria or anuria, nitrogen retention, and acute renal failure occur. The oliguria or anuria may be due to tubular blockage and/or reabsorption of the glomerular filtrate. After a week, if the patient survives, diuresis with a dilute urine ensues.

Pathologic changes

The kidneys are *markedly swollen.* The renal capsule is tense, stripping easily to reveal a smooth pale red or yellow surface; the flabby kidney bulges when its capsule is removed. The pale cortex is thickened and sharply demarcated from the dark medulla. Yellow streaks may course through the medulla. *Microscopically* the changes are most profound in the proximal convoluted tubules, the epithelium of which may show cloudy swelling, hydropic degeneration, fatty metamorphosis, necrosis, and/or calcification. The necrosis extends down to but does not include the basement membrane. In the *acute nephrosis due to chloroform and carbon tetrachloride,* severe fatty degeneration occurs in the tubular epithelial cells. In *ethylene glycol poisoning,* wheat sheaf- or fan-shaped calcium oxalate crystals are found within the tubules. Severe hydropic degeneration is produced by diethylene glycol and dioxane. The tubular lumina are narrowed by the epithelial swelling and are filled with desquamated cells and other debris. The glomeruli may show degenerative changes, and eosinophilic debris may collect in the glomerular spaces. After a week, if the patient survives, the tubules are relined by a low columnar epithelium. Later a normal epithelium returns.

OSMOTIC NEPHROSIS

Osmotic nephrosis is produced by the intravenous injection of *hypertonic sucrose.* Similar lesions have been produced by the injection of 30 percent acacia intravenously. A hypertonic concentration of sucrose in the tubular epithelium probably causes the imbibition of water into the cells, producing a sievelike trelliswork of vacuoles in the cytoplasm *(hydropic degeneration).* Electron microscopy reveals that vacuole formation is due to progressive enlargement of cytoplasmic lysosomes [39].

HYPOKALEMIC NEPHROSIS

Hypokalemic (kaliopenic) nephrosis or *nephropathy* is due to a low serum potassium level. It has been found in some cases of chronic intestinal disease, such as regional enteritis, ulcerative colitis, chronic diverticulitis, and carcinoma of the colon, in which there is a severe potassium loss by vomiting or diarrhea. The degree of renal dysfunction is usually not severe. *Microscopically* the convoluted tubular epithelial cells are ballooned out to fill the entire lumen by large clear vacuoles. These vacuoles do not contain protein, lipids, or glycogen. The nuclei are pushed basally. *Electron microscopy* reveals that the round or ovoid intracytoplasmic vacuoles are bound by a single osmiophilic membrane and that most vacuoles are empty [40]. The tubular basement membranes are thickened, and some smaller vacuoles appear to form extracellularly beneath separated basement membranes (subbasilar vacuolation) [41]. These extracellular fluid collections may be due to the hypernatremia which occurs in potassium deficiency.

HYPOXIC NEPHROSIS:

Hypoxic nephrosis (lower nephron nephrosis) may occur in shock, burns, crush syndrome, heat stroke, hemolytic transfusion reactions, and blackwater fever (malaria), and postoperatively. No constant factor is present in all these conditions, although hemoglobin casts are present in some types. *Shock* with decreased renal cortical blood flow is most likely the basic cause. Spasm of the renal arterioles may be a factor. Similar changes can be produced by shunting the blood directly from the arcuate arteries to the renal medulla, with consequent hypoxia of the renal cortex. Bilateral cortical necrosis may represent an extreme degree of hypoxic nephrosis.

Clinical features

Clinically oliguria or anuria, associated with azotemia, edema, and hypertension or hypotension, is common. The *renal insufficiency* is probably due to blockage of the tubules by pigment casts and the swelling of the epithelial cells, and vasoconstrictive renal ischemia due to shock.

Pathologic changes

The kidneys are enlarged, flabby, and pale. They bulge when their capsules are stripped. The cortex is widened and moist. The medulla is dark and shows increased striations. *Microscopically* the picture varies somewhat with the cause, but typically within 24 hours lipid vacuoles and other degenerative changes appear in the epithelium of the ascending limb of the loops of Henle. After 24 to 36 hours *hemoglobin or myoglobin casts* appear mainly in the distal convoluted and collecting tubules; however, they may occur in any part of the tubular system, so that the nephrosis is not strictly lower nephron in type. By the third to fifth day there is necrosis as well as beginning regeneration of the tubular epithelium. After the fifth day tubules may rupture, small granulomatous foci appearing about them. Interstitial edema and lymphocytic infiltration are found.

Myoglobinuric nephrosis

Myoglobinuric nephrosis, a form of hypoxic nephrosis, occurs in its most severe form following crushing injury to muscle (crush syndrome). However, milder forms occur in cases of primary idiopathic myoglobinuria, which is paroxysmal and sometimes related to acute alcoholism, electric shock therapy, high-voltage electric injury, and muscular dystrophy. Transient, usually *mild myoglobinuria may occur following muscular exertion,* as in the *squat jump syndrome* in which swelling of the quadriceps muscles follows this form of calisthenics [42]. Patients with the squat jump syndrome exhibit transient proteinuria, hematuria, myoglobinuria, and hemoglobinuria. *Renal biopsies* show myoglobin and hemoglobin casts in the renal tubules and slight degenerative changes in the tubular epithelial cells. The quadriceps muscles show interstitial edema and focal hemorrhages.

2. Chronic Nephrosis

MYELOMA NEPHROSIS:

Myeloma nephrosis occurs in some cases of multiple myeloma, a malignant plasmocytic neoplasm of the flat bones (see page 381). *Bence Jones protein* (a peculiar protein – molecular weight 37,000 – which precipitates at 50 to 60°C. and redissolves at about 80°C.) appears in the urine in over 50 percent of the cases. In these cases there is commonly severe renal damage due to precipitation of the protein in the tubules.

Pathologic changes

Grossly the kidneys are slightly or markedly reduced in size. The external surface is smooth, and the cut surface pale and waxy. *Microscopically* many *distal convoluted tubules* are blocked by highly eosinophilic Bence Jones protein casts. These usually show fragmented centers, and may show foci of calcification and protein crystals. The adjacent tubular epithelium shows a syncytium interpreted as a multinucleated *foreign-body* giant cell *reaction.* Proximally in the affected tubules the epithelium shows degenerative changes. *Electron microscopy* studies on renal biopsies in patients with plasma cell myeloma reveal doubling of the thickness of the glomerular basement membrane and focal blunting and fusion of the epithelial cell foot processes [43]. These are the glomerular changes found in other nephropathies with significant proteinuria.

Other renal lesions associated with multiple myeloma include metastatic calcification in the glomeruli from destructive bone lesions, occasional plasma cell infiltration (myelosarcoma) in the interstitial tissue, and amyloid deposits in the glomeruli from prolonged myeloma.

MELANURIC NEPHROSIS

Melanuric nephrosis occasionally occurs in relation to a melanocarcinoma (see page 788). *Clinically* there is a nephrotic picture with terminal oliguria and uremia. *Grossly* the kidneys are grayish or brownish black, the medulla being slightly darker than the cortex. *Microscopically* brown and black granules of melanin are found in the Bowman's capsules, cytoplasm of tubular cells, and interstitial tissue.

DISEASES PRINCIPALLY AFFECTING THE RENAL BLOOD VESSELS

The *renal blood supply* is very abundant, being designed to provide the free flow of blood through the glomerular capillaries at a relatively high pressure which is essential for glomerular filtration as well as for tissue nourishment. Any lesion which interferes with adequate blood flow at an adequate pressure decreases the competency of renal function. A peculiarity of the renal vascular tree is the presence of *two sets of capillaries:* the *glomerular* from the afferent arterioles (the pressure is relatively high), and the *peritubular* from the efferent arterioles (the pressure is relatively low, and the blood supply depends on the flow through the glomerular capillaries). Sclerosis of renal and intrarenal arteries and arterioles is extremely important because of the association of these changes with hypertension.

ATHEROSCLEROSIS

Atherosclerosis of the renal arteries is associated with hypertension only when the arteries are occluded sufficiently to cause renal ischemia. The plaques usually occur near the aortic opening.

FIBROMUSCULAR DYSPLASIA

Fibromuscular dysplasia of the renal arteries [44] occurs much more often in women than in men. Its cause is unknown. Most of the affected women are multiparous. The majority of patients are under 40 when hypertension is diagnosed. The blood pressure ranges from 160 to 220/110 to 120 mm. of mercury. The right renal artery usually is more severely affected than the left. The arterial lumen is narrowed by encroachment of the wall. In *fibromuscular dysplasia of the media* there is alternate thickening and thinning of the arterial wall. The medial thickening is due to fibrous hyperplasia and muscular hypertrophy. The elastic tissue is deficient. In some cases there is only marked fibrosis of the outer media. In *fibromuscular dysplasia involving the adventitia* the artery is surrounded by excessive fibrous tissue containing some muscle bundles.

ARTERIAL NEPHROSCLEROSIS:

Arterial nephrosclerosis (atherosclerotic nephrosclerosis, *senile arteriosclerotic kidney)* is rarely associated with marked hypertension or impairment of renal function.

Pathologic changes

Large and medium-sized intrarenal arteries are involved by atherosclerosis. *Grossly* the kidneys show a patchy distribution of irregular depressed areas, similar to healed infarcts, on their surfaces. The kidneys are slightly reduced in size. *Microscopically* there are wedge-shaped foci of fibrosis in the involved areas due to the fanlike distribution of the arteries. There is a loss of most of the glomeruli and tubules in the affected areas. Lymphocytes and plasma cells infiltrate the surrounding areas.

ARTERIOLONEPHROSCLEROSIS:

Arteriolonephrosclerosis is the most constant pathologic finding in benign essential hypertension. However, renal biopsies early in hypertensive patients fail to show the lesion. Therefore the arterionephrosclerosis evidently results from, rather than causes, the hypertension. While the *role of the kidneys in* initiating *hypertension* is incompletely understood, there is growing evidence that increased production of the proteolytic enzyme, *renin,* is a major factor. *Renin appears to be secreted by cells of the juxtaglomerular body of Goormaghtigh.* The juxtaglomerular apparatus is a baroreceptor. A drop in afferent arteriolar pressure of as little as 5 mm. of mercury causes renin secretion by juxtaglomerular cells. An increased number of cells, especially of active, large, clear cells, has been found in the juxtaglomerular bodies in cases of essential hypertension, unilateral renal arterial occlusion with hypertension, acute, subacute, and chronic glomerulonephritis, and pheochromocytoma [45].

Renin acts on angiotensinogen (hypertensinogen, renin substrate), a circulating hepatogenous globulin, to split off the decapeptide, angiotensin-1. In the pulmonary circulation this is converted to the octapeptide, angiotensin-2 (angiotonin, hypertensin), the most powerful known vasoconstrictor agent. It also stimulates adrenal cortical cells to secrete aldosterone, which in turn leads to sodium retention. Angiotensin-2 has a very short half-life. It is inactivated by several enzymes known as *angiotensinases.*

According to the concept of *renoprival hypertension,* hypertension results from loss of the capacity of the renal parenchyma to destroy pressor amines through its monoamine oxidase system. Another factor in the production of renoprival hypertension is an absence or deficiency of renomedullary prostaglandin (medullin), an antihypertensive agent [46]. Thus disease processes which temporarily or permanently damage the renal parenchyma extensively, such as glomerulonephritis, chronic pyelonephritis, and metastatic carcinoma, could produce hypertension by these mechanisms.

The clinical features of benign essential hypertension are discussed on page 424.

Pathologic changes

Grossly in arteriolonephrosclerosis the kidneys are normal in size early, but later become moderately and even markedly atrophic. The capsule strips with difficulty, fragments of cortical tissue being torn off *(decortication).* The external surface is finely granular and slightly pale. Tiny retention cysts are often present in the cortex. On cut surface the cortex is moderately to severely narrowed. The small vessels are prominent and do not retract. It is often impossible to distinguish this condition from chronic glomerulonephritis or chronic pyelonephritis, but the surface granularity does tend to be finer in arteriolonephrosclerosis. *Microscopically* the essential lesion is a sclerosis of the small arteries and arterioles which is most marked in the afferent arterioles just proximal to the glomerular tuft. The small arteries and arterioles show hyaline changes characterized by a sharply defined, smooth, eosinophilic thickening of the intima. The hyaline deposits may be derived from the incorporation of thrombi into the arteriolar walls [47]. The lumina are narrowed or even obliterated. Electron microscopic observations in cases of arteriolonephrosclerosis demonstrate that *hyaline material is deposited entirely or mainly within the intima of involved arterioles* [48]. The *hyalin* is made up of compact fine granules and appears to arise by excessive filtration of plasma proteins into the intima of arterioles. The closure of the arteries and arterioles produces changes in the glomeruli supplied by them. These alterations include thickening of the basement membrane, hyalinization of the tuft, and marked thickening of the connective tissue of Bowman's capsule, which fuses with the hyalinized tuft and obliterates the capsular space. The *glomerular changes* in arteriolonephrosclerosis begin with a wrinkling of the capillary basement membrane, followed by its thickening and collapse [49]. Bowman's space becomes filled with hyalin. The *ischemic glomerulus* becomes a knot composed of wrinkled capillary basement membrane compressed by the hyaline material. Some glomeruli may be resorbed and disappear completely. As glomeruli become sclerosed, the corresponding tubules atrophy. Uninvolved surrounding tubules may appear normal or be dilated. In *essential hypertension* the arterioles of the spleen, pancreas, adrenal capsules, liver, retinae, and brain may show changes similar to those in renal arterioles in a lesser or greater degree. Edema of the brain is common, and the retina may show edema and hemorrhages. The myocardium is hypertrophic.

MALIGNANT NEPHROSCLEROSIS:

Malignant nephrosclerosis is associated with *malignant hypertension* (discussed on page 426). It constitutes about 7 percent of cases of hypertension. In some cases of *malignant hypertension,* malignant nephrosclerosis is superimposed on a preexisting benign arteriolosclerosis *(accelerated hypertension).* The kidneys show a mixture of the changes of the two processes. Some cases of glomerulonephritis and pyelonephritis terminate in malignant nephrosclerosis.

Pathologic changes

Grossly the kidneys are normal in size or slightly enlarged, and their surfaces are smooth. Occasionally sufficient time elapses before death for contraction and granularity to develop. The surfaces are covered with hemorrhages which are typically large and blotchy, but may be petechial. *Microscopically* two types of changes occur in the arterioles: cellular hyperplasia (hyperplastic arteriolosclerosis), the more common type; and arteriolonephronecrosis (arteriolar necrosis, necrotizing arteriolitis). In *cellular hyperplasia* the walls of small arteries and arterioles are thickened by concentric fibroblastic proliferation, giving an onion-skin appearance. Collagen may be laid down. The thickening may occur in the intima (endarteritis) or in the media. *Arteriolonephronecrosis* is most typical in the afferent arterioles. Their walls have a smudged appearance due to fibrinoid degeneration and they stain deeply with eosin. Aneurysmal dilatation may occur. Hemorrhage is common into the necrotic wall. Both types of changes are often present in the same kidney, and *immunofluorescence reveals the presence of gamma globulin, fibrinogen, and complement* (beta 1C globulin) *in the walls of arterioles and glomeruli showing fibrinoid necrosis* [50]. The finding of complement indicates that an immune reaction plays a role in the pathogenesis of the lesions of malignant nephrosclerosis.

Changes in the renal parenchyma associated with malignant hypertension are tubular degeneration with hyperplasia of the epithelium and focal degenerative glomerulitis. The latter is characterized by fusion and necrosis of the capillary loops; capillary thrombosis; swelling, fatty, hyaline, or necrotic degeneration of the tuft epithelium; and formation of fibrinous adhesions between glomerular loops and the lining of Bowman's capsule. There is a patchy fibrinoid necrosis of the tuft with hemorrhage into the capsular space. Characteristic arteriolar changes may also occur in the adrenal glands, pancreas, retinae, and brain. In almost all patients with malignant nephrosclerosis *treated with antihypertensive drugs* [51], the acute lesions, such as thrombosis and arteriolar and glomerular necrosis, show improvement or healing. In the medium-sized and large renal arteries an intimal fibrous hyperplasia with narrowing of the lumina occurs. This lesion leads to progressive renal ischemia and death.

RENAL LESIONS IN PERIARTERITIS NODOSA

The kidneys are among the most commonly involved organs in periarteritis nodosa (discussed on page 78). Similar renal lesions may be produced by sulfonamide hypersensitivity. The *gross and microscopic lesions* may closely resemble those in the kidneys in malignant hypertension. Usually there are numerous small foci of infarction or necrosis of parenchymal tissue, with acute fibrinoid necrosis of small arteries. The involved vessels show thrombosis and marked polymorphonuclear leukocytic infiltration in and about their walls.

RENAL LESIONS IN SYSTEMIC SCLERODERMA

The kidneys may be involved in *generalized scleroderma (progressive systemic sclerosis)* [52]. The scleroderma kidney is *grossly* slightly enlarged with a smooth external surface except for small foci of infarction. The surface may be dotted with petechiae. The cortex is pale and is well demarcated from the congested medulla. *Microscopically* focal glomerular changes are found. These include localized or diffuse basement membrane thickening, with a wire-loop lesion like that seen in lupus erythematosus in a few cases; fibrinoid deposits in the capillary lumina; and hyaline-droplet formation within tuft epithelial cells. The tubular epithelium shows degenerative changes. In the interlobular arteries the most constant lesion occurs: there is moderate to marked luminal narrowing due to intimal deposits of mucopolysaccharide material. The arterial changes produce small cortical infarcts. In the afferent arterioles there are fibrinoid deposits and thromboses.

INFARCTION:

Clinical features

Infarction of the kidney is fairly common and is often associated with mitral or aortic bacterial endocarditis, atrial fibrillation with left intra-auricular thrombosis, and myocardial infarction with mural thrombosis. Symptoms and signs are sharp back pain, costovertebral angle tenderness, nausea and vomiting, hematuria, and, rarely, anuria and uremia.

Pathologic changes

Early the infarct is hemorrhagic, the central necrotic area being surrounded by a zone of congestion. Soon it becomes pale with an adjacent zone of congestion and acute inflammation. *Later* there is pitting of the surface and a wedge-shaped focus of fibrosis with loss of parenchymal tissue. The subcapsular zone is often spared because of the capsular arteries. An embolus is usually found in a branch of the renal artery. Occasionally thrombosis in a renal vein tributary produces a hemorrhagic infarct.

ATHEROEMBOLIC RENAL DISEASE:

Clinical features

Atheroembolic renal disease [53] results from obstruction of small renal arteries by atheromatous material dislodged from the aortic wall. It occurs in patients with severe atherosclerosis either spontaneously or following trauma or aortic surgery. *Clinically* sudden massive atheroembolism, usually seen after surgery, is characterized by oliguria or anuria and uremia. With lesser degrees of atheroembolism, hypertension is common.

Pathologic changes

Grossly the kidneys are usually smaller than normal and have a granular external surface with wedge-shaped scars. Recent infarcts are sometimes present. Atheroemboli occlude arcuate, intralobular, and smaller arteries. *Microemboli* show cleftlike spaces, from which cholesterol has been dissolved out, surrounded by amorphous eosinophilic material. Foreign-body giant cells are found in older lesions.

CORTICAL NECROSIS:

Bilateral cortical necrosis of the kidneys is an unusual condition occasionally associated with toxemias of pregnancy, scarlet fever, pneumonia, diphtheria, and dysentery. Similar lesions result from poisoning by dioxane and diethylene glycol. Bilateral cortical necrosis also occurs in the generalized Shwartzman reaction.

Clinical features

Clinically there is pain or tenderness in the epigastrium or loins, with oliguria or anuria at the onset. Death usually occurs in 4 to 12 days.

Cause

The necrosis is generally held to be *ischemic in origin* due to widespread organic or functional occlusion of the interlobular arteries and arterioles. The mechanism of obstruction – intense vasoconstriction, vasoparalysis, thrombosis, or necrosis of arterial walls – varies.

Pathologic changes

Grossly the kidneys are swollen and soft. The capsule strips easily, revealing a smooth surface with irregular, patchy, reddish yellow mottling. The cut surface bulges, and the cortex is largely replaced by opaque yellowish necrotic foci. These irregular foci may be outlined by a red zone of congestion beneath the capsule and in surrounding cortical and medullary areas. *Microscopically* there is widespread coagulation necrosis of the cortex, the necrotic foci being bordered by a hemorrhagic or hyperemic zone, with a polymorphonuclear leukocytic infiltration. A ghostlike pattern of the destroyed parenchymal tissue may remain. Arterioles and small arteries may show luminal occlusion by fibrin thrombi, and even necrosis of their walls.

RENAL VEIN THROMBOSIS:

Thrombosis of the renal vein or of the inferior vena cava above the level of these veins *may cause the nephrotic syndrome* [54]. Its pathogenesis is incompletely understood but is apparently related to the increased intrarenal venous pressure, especially in the peritubular capillaries. The massive proteinuria is due to increased protein filtration through the glomeruli plus decreased tubular reabsorption of protein.

Pathologic changes

Grossly the kidneys are swollen and dark red or purplish due to venous congestion. *The capsular veins are dilated and tortuous. Microscopically* the most striking lesion is *diffuse thickening of glomerular basement membranes,* which may develop within 2 weeks of the onset of the thromboses. Electron microscopy reveals that the thickening is due to irregular aggregations of material between the basement membrane and the epithelial foot processes. The *glomerular epithelial cells* show fusion and broadening of their foot processes, and numerous vacuoles are seen within their cytoplasm. The proximal *tubular epithelial cells* undergo vacuolar cytoplasmic degeneration. Many tubules are dilated, and distal tubules often contain proteinaceous casts. The *renal veins* are partially or completely occluded by old or recent thrombi. Older thrombi are partially recanalized.

DISEASES PRINCIPALLY AFFECTING THE RENAL INTERSTITIAL TISSUE

ACUTE DIFFUSE INTERSTITIAL NEPHRITIS:

This inflammatory renal lesion occurs during various bacterial, rickettsial, and viral infections, including scarlet fever, diphtheria, typhoid fever, typhus, and smallpox, as well as during sulfonamide therapy. It appears to be due to toxic products of the organisms and hypersensitivity to the drug. *Clinically* there is a sudden onset of oliguria or even anuria with azotemia. The cause of the renal shutdown is presumably the pressure of the rapidly accumulating interstitial cellular infiltrate on intrarenal vessels. Severe cases almost always prove fatal.

Pathologic changes

Grossly the kidneys are swollen (up to twice their normal size) and soft. The external surfaces are smooth and have a mottled purplish red to yellowish brown color, with petechiae. The cut surface shows a thick, moist cortex and a deep red medulla. *Microscopically* there is a diffuse infiltration of the cortical interstitial tissue with plasmocytes, macrophages, eosinophils, and a few neutrophils. The glomeruli are not involved. The *tubular epithelium* may show degenerative changes, and degenerated neutrophils are found in the distal tubules.

1. Infections of the Kidneys

PYELO-NEPHRITIS:

Pyelonephritis is the term which denotes an infection of the kidney and renal pelvis. It differs from the other major inflammatory lesion of the kidney – glomerulonephritis – in that in pyelonephritis the causative organisms actually infect the organ. However, in some cases of chronic pyelonephritis it is difficult or impossible to isolate the organism from the urine or even the kidney. In pyelonephritis the *infecting organisms may reach the kidneys either hematogenously or urogenously,* the latter via the ureteral lumen or periureteral lymphatics as an ascending infection. Some type of obstruction to the normal outflow of urine is usually present, especially in the ascending types. The normal kidney can often excrete bacteria entering it if no blockage is present. However, an asymptomatic bacteriuria may lead to the development of acute or chronic pyelonephritis, probably due to a patent ureterovesical valve in the absence of obstruction [55].

Incidence of urinary infections

There is a uniformly *higher incidence of urinary tract infection in females than males* due to the shortness of the female urethra and ureteral kinking and compression during pregnancy. The *prevalence* of urinary tract infections as evidenced by significant bacteriuria (the presence of over 100,000 bacteria per milliliter of urine in at least two clean catch specimens) among school children is 1 percent in girls and 0.04 percent in boys [56]. Only 3 percent of the children with bacteriuria have definite clinical evidence of urinary tract infection. In about 85 percent of the cases in one series the *infecting organism* was of the *Escherichia coli* group [57]. The incidence of significant bacteriuria in pregnant women is about 5 percent. Bacteriuria is more frequent in multiparous women and in Negro women. The *most common causative organisms* are *Escherichia coli, Aerobacter aerogenes, Proteus* species, and coagulase-negative staphylococci. Acute pyelonephritis develops in about 2 percent of women during pregnancy. Its incidence is 10 times higher in women with untreated, persistent bacteriuria than in those without bacteriuria early in pregnancy.

Causes

The *sources of infection in hematogenous pyelonephritis* include dental infections, sinusitis, otitis media, tonsillitis, furunculosis, lung abscess, bronchiectasis, appendicitis, diverticulitis, prostatitis, cervicitis, and septicemia. The *causes* of the urinary obstruction underlying *ascending infection of the kidney*(s) include congenital anomalies, renal calculi (stones), ureteral stricture or kinking, prostatic hyperplasia (by bladder neck and urethral compression), and urethral stricture. The *causative organisms* in pyelonephritis are most commonly *Staphylococcus aureus* (especially in hematogenous infections), *Escherichia coli* (the most common organism in ascending infections with acid urine), *Aerobacter aerogenes, Proteus vulgaris,* and streptococci, including *S. faecalis,* which is commonly found in alkaline urine. Two or more organisms are found in about 25 percent of the cases.

Clinical features

Clinically, acute pyelonephritis is characterized by chills, fever, pain in one or both flanks, tenderness on fist percussion over the affected kidney(s) (Murphy punch), leukocytosis, dysuria, and neutrophils, some erythrocytes, bacteria, and "pus" casts in the urine. Urine culture demonstrates the causative organism. *Chronic pyelonephritis* is protean in its manifestations and is often diagnosed only at autopsy. It may follow acute pyelonephritis or may develop insidiously. In up to two-thirds of the cases *hypertension* develops. There may be protracted low-grade fever and slight flank pain with signs of renal failure such as hyposthenuria. Neutrophils, erythrocytes, and bacteria in small numbers are usually found in the urine. *Glitter cells* (granular motility cells) are large neutrophils found in the urine showing Brownian movement of the cytoplasmic granules. With the Sternheimer-Malbin supravital stain (crystal violet and safranine), the glitter cells are colorless or light blue as compared to the orange-purple staining of other neutrophils. *The presence of glitter cells in the urine is highly suggestive of the diagnosis of pyelonephritis.*

Acute suppurative pyelonephritis:

Acute suppurative pyelonephritis (pyemic kidneys) is *hematogenous* and is usually due to *Staphylococcus aureus* as part of a pyemia. It is commonly secondary to acute osteomyelitis and wound infections.

pathologic changes

Both kidneys are involved. *Grossly* they are enlarged and hyperemic, and numerous yellow, discrete *abscesses* are found in the cortices. The formation of a single large abscess is known as a *carbuncle of the kidney. Microscopically* the abscesses contain degenerated neutrophils and necrotic tissue debris.

Acute obstructive pyelonephritis:

Acute (obstructive) pyelonephritis may be unilateral or bilateral, depending on the site of the obstruction. Mild cases, erroneously called *pyelitis* (inflammation of the renal pelvis), are common in infant girls due to congenital anomalies such as dysplasia, and in pregnant women due to ureteral kinking or compression by the enlarging uterus.

pathologic changes

Grossly the kidney (or kidneys) is (are) enlarged and hyperemic. Yellow abscesses of various sizes are found in the medulla. These radiate up into the cortex. The *pelvic mucosa* is red and edematous, and the calyces and pelvis contain pus. The ureter(s) is (are) dilated due to obstruction. *Microscopically* the interstitial tissue of the kidney(s) is infiltrated with polymorphonuclear leukocytes, and some neutrophils are found in the tubules. The abscesses are filled with degenerated neutrophils. The calyces and pelvis contain pus, and their mucosa may be ulcerated. The submucosa is hyperemic and infiltrated with neutrophils. Occasionally acute pyelonephritis is complicated by a large *perinephric or subphrenic abscess.* Removal of the cause of the obstruction usually is followed by subsidence of the infection with only moderate residual renal damage.

Necrotizing papillitis:

About two-thirds of the cases of *necrotizing renal papillitis (papillitis necroticans)* occur in diabetics, and the lesion is found in about 3 percent of diabetics at autopsy. The papillitis is usually associated with a severe ascending acute pyelonephritis. The *cause* of the papillary necrosis appears to be ischemia due to compression of the medullary arterial supply by a sudden increase in intrapelvic pressure plus the pressure of the interstitial exudate on the papillary capillaries. Necrotizing renal papillitis has occasionally occurred in patients taking excessive amounts of acetophenetidin [58]. The prognosis in these patients is better than the grave outlook in diabetics with papillary necrosis.

pathologic changes

Grossly there are yellow or white, friable foci of necrosis sharply limited to the papillae. One or more papilla(e) may be affected unilaterally or bilaterally. Usually there is widespread involvement. *Microscopically* the *papillae* appear infarcted and show a dense polymorphonuclear leukocytic infiltrate. A papilla may slough off into the pelvis. The arteries show no lesions that might produce infarction.

Chronic pyelonephritis:

Chronic pyelonephritis is now recognized as the cause of atrophic, contracted kidneys somewhat less commonly than arteriolonephrosclerosis and more often than chronic glomerulonephritis. It is not always possible to distinguish these lesions even microscopically in the scarred and contracted kidneys. Cases of chronic pyelonephritis often show progressive renal failure (usually with hypertension) and slight proteinuria, pyuria, and hematuria. Bacteria are seldom found in the renal parenchyma in these cases. It is possible that bacterial variants or protoplasts which are not discernible microscopically or by usual culture methods are present in cases of chronic pyelonephritis in which the kidneys are apparently sterile [59]. Bacterial antigen from *Escherichia coli* has been detected in renal tissue in cases of chronic pyelonephritis in which no bacteria can be found [60].

pathologic changes

Grossly the kidneys (the lesion is usually bilateral) are small, often weighing less than 100 gm. each. Points which tend to differentiate the contracted kidneys of chronic pyelonephritis from those of arteriolonephrosclerosis and chronic glomerulonephritis grossly are the presence of wide U-shaped depressions on the external surfaces, the presence of dilated calyces and pelves indicating urinary obstruction, and grayish white scarring of the pelvic and calycine submucosa. *Microscopically* there are clusters of hyalinized glomeruli adjacent to foci of dilated tubules containing eosinophilic "colloid" casts *(thyroidization of the kidney),* periglomerular fibrosis, interstitial fibrosis with a moderate to marked interstitial infiltration with lymphocytes, plasmocytes, and macrophages, and hyaline thickening of the walls of arterioles and small arteries. The latter change accounts for or is the result of the development of hypertension in the majority of cases of chronic pyelonephritis.

Megalocytic interstitial nephritis

Megalocytic interstitial nephritis [61] is rare and is usually associated with lower urinary tract infection. It occurs more commonly in females than males. The *cause* is not clear, but the condition is frequently related to infection with gram-negative bacteria, especially *Escherichia coli. Grossly* the kidneys show varisized gray or grayish yellow foci, mainly in the cortex. These foci consist of clusters of large polyhedral cells 12 to 20μ in diameter. Their cytoplasm is acidophilic and granular. It is negative with fat stains, but positive with the periodic acid-Schiff (PAS) stain. The nucleus is located peripherally. These cells probably originate from proximal convoluted tubular lining cells. The presence of Michaelis-Gutmann calcospherites in some of the polyhedral cells indicate that megalocytic nephritis is a renal form of malakoplakia.

Xanthogranulomatous pyelonephritis

Xanthogranulomatous pyelonephritis [62] is a rare form of chronic pyelonephritis. Urinary obstruction usually precedes its development. Both clinically and pathologically xanthogranulomatous pyelonephritis may closely mimic renal adenocarcinoma. *Grossly* the kidney is enlarged and is widely replaced by poorly circumscribed, bright yellow nodules interspersed with firm, grayish white tissue. The perirenal fat may be involved. *Microscopically* the nodules consist of sheets and clusters of macrophages with finely vacuolated, sudanophilic cytoplasm (foam cells). A few multinucleated giant cells are present, and the foci are infiltrated with lymphocytes, plasmocytes, and a few neutrophils.

RENAL TUBERCULOSIS: Clinical features

Renal tuberculosis usually begins in one kidney by hematogenous spread from a pulmonary lesion. Destructive renal tuberculosis occurs in less than 5 percent of cases of lung tuberculosis. Typically one kidney is involved first, with later spread to the other. *Clinically* there are persistent pyuria and hematuria from one or both kidneys. Acid-fast *Mycobacterium tuberculosis* may be found in the urine by concentration, culture, or guinea pig inoculation.

Pathologic changes

The *earliest gross lesion* in the kidney is in the medulla, especially in a papilla. Caseous foci develop and enlarge in the medulla and cortex. The entire kidney may be destroyed. *Microscopically* the caseous parenchymal foci show the typical tuberculous granuloma. The infection spreads to the ureter, where fibrosis may produce ureteral stricture and urinary obstruction. A *tuberculous cystitis* may develop, with tiny tubercles appearing about the ureteral orifices at first. Later the entire wall may become involved by the tuberculous process, with mucosal ulceration. Tuberculous cystitis is also, but less often, due to hematogenous spread directly to the bladder and to spread from tuberculous prostatitis or seminal vesiculitis. The ureteral and vesical lesions tend to heal if a singly infected kidney is removed surgically. The second kidney may be involved by an ascending infection from the bladder along the periureteral lymphatics or by independent hematogenous infection.

Glomerular alterations have been found in occasional cases of *pulmonary tuberculosis,* some of whom also have renal tuberculosis [63]. The glomeruli show endothelial hyperplasia, patchy or diffuse basement membrane thickening, and a slight neutrophilic infiltration. The findings were similar to those of acute glomerulonephritis or lupus nephritis and are sometimes termed tuberculous nephritis. They represent a hypersensitivity reaction in the kidneys.

NEOPLASMS OF THE KIDNEYS

1. Benign Neoplasms

Benign neoplasms of the kidneys include adenomas, fibromas, leiomyomas, lipomas, hamartomas, hemangiomas, and papillomas of the renal pelvis.

ADENOMA

Adenoma of the kidney occurs asymptomatically as a yellowish gray, encapsulated cortical nodule measuring a few millimeters to 3 cm. in diameter. The neoplasm usually arises from tubular epithelium *(tubular adenoma)* and consists microscopically of cystic tubular structures which sometimes show a papillary pattern. The cells often have an abundant clear cytoplasm like those of adenocarcinoma of the kidney. Some adenomas apparently become malignant, especially those composed of solid sheets of clear cells. A few adenomas have glomerulus-like intracystic projections *(glomerulomas).*

FIBROMA

LEIOMYOMA

Fibroma of the kidney occurs as a small (0.3 to 1 cm.) white nodule in the medulla. *Leiomyoma* of the kidney is a tiny subcapsular nodule and probably derives from smooth muscle of the capsule.

HAMARTOMA

Hamartoma of the kidney appears as a gray or yellow round nodule about 1 cm. in diameter, usually in the medulla. It consists of varying amounts of fibrous tissue, fat, smooth muscle, blood vessels, and tubular epithelium. This tumor is probably a developmental anomaly rather than a true neoplasm and may occur as part of *epiloia,* a congenital hamartial disorder. The *angiomyolipoma* is a common form of renal hamartoma. It may occur with or without other stigmata of epiloia and may be asymptomatic or be manifested by flank pain, hematuria, and/or a palpable mass. *Grossly* the angiomyolipoma is round and yellow or gray and appears encapsulated, averaging 9 cm. in diameter. *Microscopically* it consists of varying amounts of mature adipose tissue, smooth muscle, fibrous tissue, and often tortuous blood vessels mainly of an arterial type.

HEMANGIOMA

Hemangioma of the kidney is rare, but may cause moderate or severe hematuria. It is usually cavernous.

PELVIC PAPILLOMA

Papilloma of the renal pelvis is uncommon and is transitional cell in type. It is more common in men than women by over 2 to 1. *Clinically,* painless hematuria, pyuria, and signs of associated renal calculus formation are common. The papilloma grows into the pelvic lumen as a pinkish, fernlike mass. Because the 5-year survival rate following surgery is only about 50 percent, most pelvic papillomas are considered as low-grade carcinomas.

2. Malignant Neoplasms

ADENOCARCINOMA:

Adenocarcinoma of the kidney *(hypernephroma,* tubular carcinoma, *Grawitz's tumor)* constitutes about 85 percent of malignant renal neoplasms. It makes up about 2 percent of all cancer, occurs in men twice as often as in women, and develops after age 40 in 90 percent of the cases. The name *hypernephroma* stems from the old concept that this neoplasm arose from adrenal cortical inclusions in the kidney. The present concept is that it *arises from renal tubular epithelium* and is probably related to the renal adenoma.

Clinical features

Clinically the prominent features are painless hematuria, a mass in the flank, and fever due to necrosis. On a pyelogram, displacement of calyces is seen. In about 2 percent of cases of adenocarcinoma of the kidney there is an *associated erythrocythemia.* Elevated red cell counts have been especially common in renal adenocarcinoma in which the renal vein is grossly invaded and occluded by the neoplasm. The erythrocythemia may be due to *increased elaboration of erythropoietin,* an erythropoiesis-stimulating substance which is believed to be normally produced in the kidneys. A case of adenocarcinoma of the kidney with an associated *leukemoid reaction,* as defined by a leukocyte count over 50,000 per cubic millimeter and/or 2 percent blast forms in the peripheral blood, has been reported [64]. A similar case in which the leukocyte count was as high as 98,250 was seen at the George Washington University Hospital. In that patient the bone marrow showed marked granulocytic hyperplasia. The alkaline phosphatase reaction of the neutrophils was positive, indicating that they were mature and that this was a leukemoid reaction rather than leukemia.

A usually markedly *elevated urinary lactic dehydrogenase (LDH) activity* has been found in cases of carcinoma of the kidney and urinary bladder [65]. The elevation is present in both renal adenocarcinoma and papillary carcinoma of the renal pelvis and does not occur with benign neoplasms or cysts. The *urinary alkaline phosphatase activity* is elevated in renal adenocarcinoma but not in localized urinary bladder carcinoma. Increased urinary LDH and alkaline phosphatase activities also occur in acute and subacute glomerulonephritis, acute tubular necrosis, recent renal infarction, and some cases of pyelonephritis.

Pathologic changes

Grossly the neoplasm is typically a large, roughly spherical, partially encapsulated, golden yellow mass. The cut surface shows extensive foci of necrosis and hemorrhage. The neoplasm occurs most commonly at the upper pole and compresses the adjacent renal parenchyma. *Microscopically* the tumor is most frequently composed of clusters of *large cells with a clear cytoplasm.* The cells have a high lipid content, which gives the neoplasm its yellow color. Less often a tubular or papillary pattern is present; in such neoplasms the cells are spindle in type, resembling a sarcoma.

Metastases

Metastases are usually the result of invasion of the renal vein. Sometimes the neoplasm grows into the inferior vena cava, and even into the right atrium. *Metastases to the lungs* are discrete, spherical, *"cannonball"* masses. Other common metastases are to *bones* and the *liver.*

NEPHROBLASTOMA:

Nephroblastoma (Wilms' tumor, adenosarcoma or embryoma of the kidney) is an apparently congenital malignant neoplasm. It is rare, making up about 5 percent of renal cancer. Boys and girls are equally affected. The average age at which it is detected is 2 to 3 years. *It is believed to originate from cells of the metanephrogenic blastema.* A significant association of nephroblastoma with congenital defects such as aniridia (absence of the iris), hemihypertrophy (overdevelopment of the extremities and/or other parts on one side of the body), hypospadias, cryptorchidism, and horseshoe kidneys is found [66]. The relationship of Wilms' tumor with several anomalies of the urogenital tract suggests that development of this congenital neoplasm is enhanced by influences which induce such developmental defects. A small papova-like virus has been isolated from a tissue culture in a case of nephroblastoma [67].

Clinical features

Clinically the neoplasm is usually detected as an asymptomatic mass. There may be fever due to necrosis or hemorrhage in the tumor. Calycine distortion is seen on pyelogram. The neoplasm is highly radiosensitive, at least temporarily.

Pathologic changes

Grossly the nephroblastoma is grayish white, soft, and encephaloid. It begins in the renal cortex and eventually replaces almost the entire kidney. *Microscopically* there are sheets of closely packed, atypical spindle cells within which are embedded well-formed tubular or rosette-like structures. Glomeruloid structures are present. Electron microscopy shows these to consist of epithelial cells without capillaries or mesangial cells [68]. Rarely smooth or striated muscle or cartilage may be present. Sometimes the neoplasm occurs bilaterally.

Metastases

Metastases are both hematogenous and lymphogenous. They are common in the lungs, liver, brain, omentum, and regional lymph nodes.

CARCINOSARCOMA

Carcinosarcoma of the kidney (adult Wilms' tumor) [69] is rare and occurs more commonly in men than women. *Clinically* it is indistinguishable from renal adenocarcinoma. Flank pain, hematuria, and a palpable mass are found. The left kidney is involved slightly more often than the right one. *Grossly* the neoplasm is a large, white or tan, partly necrotic mass. *Microscopically* foci of clear or granular cell adenocarcinoma in a sheetlike or tubular pattern are found associated with sarcomatous elements. The latter may be fibrosarcoma, leiomyosarcoma, rhabdomyosarcoma, chondrosarcoma, and/or osteogenic sarcoma. *Metastases* consist of one or more sarcomatous elements and are most common in the lungs. Almost all patients die within a year after diagnosis.

PELVIC CARCINOMA:

Carcinoma of the renal pelvis occurs much less frequently than neoplasms of the kidney parenchyma, constituting about 10 percent of kidney cancer. It may be associated with leukoplakia of the pelvic mucosa or with renal calculi. *Clinically* hematuria appears early.

Pathologic changes

Grossly the neoplasm is usually papillary. *Microscopically* it is usually *transitional cell in type.* Less commonly, epidermoid carcinoma occurs and is often flat. Very rarely mucinous cystadenocarcinoma of the renal pelvis has been described. Pelvic carcinoma may block urinary outflow and produce hydronephrosis.

SYSTEMIC SYNDROMES SECONDARY TO RENAL INSUFFICIENCY

RENAL RICKETS

Renal rickets (renal dwarfism or infantilism, osteonephropathy) results from chronic kidney disease in infancy and/or early childhood. *Underlying renal lesions* include bilateral hypoplasia, polycystic kidneys, chronic pyelonephritis, chronic glomerulonephritis, and hydronephrosis. *Renal insufficiency* initiates a cycle of phosphate retention, calcium loss (hypercalciuria) resulting in hypocalcemia, acidosis, and nitrogen retention. A *secondary hyperparathyroidism* develops, depleting the bones of calcium and producing osteitis fibrosa cystica. *Clinically* the child is dwarfed and shows rachitic stigmata (bossing of the skull, rosary, leg bowing), which are refractory to vitamin D therapy. Sexual development is sometimes retarded.

DE TONI-FANCONI SYNDROME

De Toni-Fanconi syndrome (diabetes insipidus with aminoaciduria) is familial. There is a defect in tubular reabsorption. The entire proximal tubule is short, and the first portion is narrow and has a swan-neck appearance. In most of the childhood cases the underlying defect is a disordered cystine metabolism, and cystinosis develops [70]. Cystine crystals are deposited in the renal tubular epithelium, cornea, and bone marrow. Bony changes are like those of renal rickets, with osteomalacia in the occasional adult case. The *biochemical findings* include decreased serum inorganic phosphorus with a normal serum calcium level, hyperchloremia, normal serum nonprotein nitrogen, proteinuria, glycosuria, hyperaminoaciduria, especially cystinuria (with normal amino acid blood level), lactic and beta-hydroxybutyric aciduria, hyperphosphaturia, and, typically, an alkaline urine reaction. An acquired de Toni-Fanconi-like syndrome has occurred in patients taking degraded tetracyclines (see page 250).

CALCULUS FORMATION IN THE URINARY SYSTEM

UROLITHIASIS:

Urolithiasis is the formation of a calculus or calculi (stones) within the urinary tract. They most often begin in the renal calyces and pelvis, sometimes later being passed into the ureter or bladder; some calculi develop in the lower urinary tract. Urolithiasis is especially frequent in Egypt, Syria, and India, due to diet, and in the United Arab Republic, due to the high incidence of vesical schistosomiasis. In the United States it almost always occurs after the age of 30 and becomes common in persons over 50 because of the high incidence of urinary obstruction and infection. Men have a somewhat higher incidence of renal calculi than women.

Cause

The most important primary etiologic factor is a *supersaturation of the urine with crystalline material.* Most commonly this is in the form of calcium salts, the hypercalciuria being idiopathic or due to primary or secondary hyperparathyroidism (this accounts for less than 5 percent of renal calculi), extensive bone demineralization (as in multiple myeloma, metastases to bone, or sarcoidosis), hypervitaminosis D, or an excessive intake of milk and alkalis (as in peptic ulcer therapy). Other crystalline materials include acetylated sulfonamide drugs, especially sulfapyridine, and uric acid in cases of gout. Calculi develop in these patients particularly when there is prolonged recumbent bed rest with osteoporosis, or when there is dehydration due to inadequate fluid intake, fever, or hot weather. Stones due to supersaturation are typically bilateral and multiple in the kidneys and tend to recur. Infection commonly occurs proximal to the calculi because of urinary obstruction.

The most important secondary cause of urolithiasis is *urinary tract infection.* Crystalline material may encrust on a necrotic focus on the calycine, pelvic, or vesical mucosa. Calculi are therefore common in cases of chronic pyelonephritis and cystitis, and such stones may develop anywhere in the urinary tract and be unilateral or bilateral. *Obstruction* per se is probably not as important etiologically as the associated infection. Vesical calculi are often present in cases of urethral obstruction. The presence of an *indwelling* (Foley) *catheter or a foreign body in the bladder* commonly leads to stone formation. *Vitamin A deficiency* may predispose to urolithiasis by producing squamous metaplasia of the upper urinary tract mucosa.

Clinical features

Clinically a calycine or pelvic stone may remain silent for some time. Some grow to a very large size, filling the calyces and pelvis; or a calculus may pass into the ureter, and suddenly there are excruciating flank pain radiating into the groin, and hematuria. The stone may pass into the bladder, or it may become impacted in the ureter, usually at the ureteropelvic junction or at the bend in the ureter just lateral and posterior to the bladder. With time, signs of urinary obstruction and infection, such as pyuria, dysuria, and frequency, develop. Calculi which reach the bladder may grow to a large size, or they may enter the urethra and cause obstruction or be passed in the urine. Stones containing calcium are usually radiopaque. Radiolucent calculi are outlined as negative shadows by the use of radiopaque materials in the urinary tract. *Complications* of urolithiasis include pyelonephritis, hydronephrosis or pyonephrosis, and rarely rupture of the renal pelvis or bladder or carcinoma of the pelvis or bladder.

Pathologic changes

Nephrolithiasis (the formation of a calculus or calculi within the renal calyces and/or pelvis) should be distinguished from the deposition of granular crystalline material in the tubules, as in metastatic calcification *(nephrocalcinosis),* urates in gout, and acetylated sulfonamide compounds. *Renal stones* usually begin adjacent to the tip of a papilla. Some arise on the pelvic mucosa. As more and more crystalline material is laid down on the nidus, the stone becomes larger and larger. While it is still small, a calculus may break off and enter the ureter, or one or more may grow to an enormous size to fill the contours of the calyces and pelvis as a *staghorn (coralline) calculus.*

Chemical composition

The *chemical composition* of most urinary calculi is mixed. During their formation the urine usually undergoes episodes of infection and of changes in reaction, concentration, and composition. The stones are frequently laminated, with a different chemical composition in the various layers. However, certain crystalline materials usually predominate in a stone to make it characteristic. *Calcium oxalate stones* make up about one-third of all urinary calculi. In pure form they are due to hypercalciuria alone and occur in acid urine. They are dark brown, oval, extremely hard and rough-surfaced, and usually measure less than 1 cm. in diameter. These calculi are fairly common among vegetarians due to the calcium oxalate in many green vegetables, such as spinach. Hyperoxaluria is not a factor in the formation of most oxalate stones. However, in rare cases of *oxalosis* the formation of oxalate renal calculi is secondary to hyperoxaluria. In these cases there is an apparent defect in oxalate metabolism, either a failure to degrade oxalic acid or an overproduction of it from precursors such as glycine. Oxalate crystals are deposited widely in the tissues in oxalosis. Roughly 40 percent of urinary calculi consist of *calcium oxalate combined with calcium phosphate and calcium carbonate.* This stone occurs mainly in alkaline urine and is due to hypercalciuria with secondary urinary tract infection. About 20 percent of calculi are *magnesium and ammonium phosphate stones,* which are often combined with CaC_2O_4, $Ca_3(PO_4)_2$, and $CaCO_3$. These usually form in alkaline urine and in association with infection. They often encrust a foreign body or neoplasm in the urinary bladder. Phosphate stones are white, soft, smooth, and friable, and conform to the outlines of the spaces they occupy. They may become very large as staghorn calculi in the kidneys or as a pear-shaped stone in the bladder. Because of their calcium content, phosphate stones are usually radiopaque. *Uric acid stones* make up about 5 percent of calculi, are brown, moderately hard and smooth, and tend to form in acid urine. *Acetylated sulfonamide* (especially sulfapyridine) *stones* are very rare today and are small. *Xanthine* and *cystine stones* are rare and are related to metabolic disorders involving these compounds.

OBSTRUCTION OF THE URINARY SYSTEM

Tubular obstruction

Obstruction of the urinary tract may occur anywhere from the renal tubules to the urethral meatus. *Tubular obstruction* may be caused by luminal blockage due to necrotic epithelial debris (as in mercury poisoning) or pigment casts (as in hypoxic nephrosis). The obstruction is usually widespread and bilateral and produces oliguria or anuria. However, tubular compression by edema, ischemia of the kidneys due to shock, and excessive tubular reabsorption of water are contributing factors in the reduction of urine formation. This type of urinary obstruction is acute, the patient dying or recovering in a few days with little residual renal damage.

Pelvic and ureteral obstruction

Pelvic obstruction is usually partial and is caused by a large renal calculus or pelvic neoplasm. *Ureteral obstruction* may be due to (1) intraluminal blockage – from calculus, primary neoplasm; (2) external pressure – from lower polar renal artery; chronic periureteral inflammation; periureteral fibrosis; secondary neoplasm, especially carcinoma of the cervix by extension to one or both ureters; ligature mistakenly applied about a ureter during surgery; pressure of the enlarging uterus during pregnancy; congenital or acquired stricture; or (3) kinking – from pregnancy, ptosis (downward displacement of a kidney), congenital abnormality. Pelvic and ureteral obstruction are usually chronic and partial and may be constant or intermittent. Most cases are unilateral, although in certain types of renal calculi, pregnancy and ureteral involvement by cervical cancer often cause bilateral obstruction which is more severe on one side than the other.

Vesical and bladder neck obstruction

Vesical obstruction is caused by a large calculus and by primary or secondary neoplasm, especially in the trigone. Except for a neoplasm about a single ureteral orifice, obstruction in the bladder affects both ureters and kidneys. *Bladder neck obstruction* [71] is an important cause of urinary blockage in children. A few cases are associated with lumbosacral meningomyelocele. In most cases the *causative factor is obscure.* Bladder neck obstruction usually becomes manifest between the ages of 2 and 5 years. The child develops a urinary tract infection with fever, abdominal pain, flank pain, painful urination, and anemia. There may be difficulty in starting the urinary stream, and it may be thin. *Infection is the major sign* in 75 percent of the cases, *Escherichia coli* being the most common organism. Cinecystography enables visualization of the bladder neck narrowing or spasm of a thickened detrusor muscle. The *intraluminal bladder pressure* is increased, voiding pressures reaching two and one-half times normal. *Pathologically* the obstructing mass of soft tissues at the bladder neck consists of submucosal fibrous tissue showing chronic inflammation. The detrusor muscle is hypertrophied. With prolonged bladder neck obstruction, generalized bladder hypertrophy, hydroureters, and hydronephrosis will develop.

Urethral obstruction

Urethral obstruction is caused by compression due to hyperplasia or carcinoma of the prostate, which also constricts the bladder neck; gonorrheal stricture; urethral neoplasms; and congenital anomalies. Blockage of the urethra produces marked hypertrophy of the bladder, sometimes with the development of diverticula, and bilateral urinary obstruction.

Neurogenic obstruction

Besides mechanical blockage, urinary obstruction may be caused by a *neurogenic defect.* This is due to spinal cord lesions which interfere with the pathways for voluntary control of the bladder, so that it empties only by the automatic emptying reflex ("cord bladder"). Such lesions include spina bifida (a congenital vertebral and spinal cord defect), tabes dorsalis (a tertiary syphilitic lesion of the posterior columns of the spinal cord), multiple sclerosis, spinal cord compression due to neoplasm, and spinal cord damage due to trauma. Paraplegia (paralysis of the lower extremities) is often present. Hypertrophy of the bladder and bilateral hydronephrosis result. Lesions of the sacral plexus or cauda equina may destroy the emptying reflex, and the bladder then evacuates only by overflow.

HYDRONEPHROSIS:

Hydronephrosis is a progressive enlargement of a kidney with parenchymal atrophy and dilatation of the calyces and pelvis. It is almost always due to urinary obstruction, but in congenital idiopathic hydronephrosis no organic obstruction is found. Hydronephrosis may be unilateral or bilateral, depending on the site(s) of obstruction. Hydronephrosis is due to backpressure on the renal pelvis, calyces, and parenchyma caused by the urinary stoppage. The passage of a stone into a ureter with sudden complete obstruction may cause a rapid rise in the intrapelvic pressure above the glomerular filtration pressure. Urine formation may thus be suppressed in the kidney, so that hydronephrosis is very slight in the resulting atrophic organ. However, sudden obstruction can also lead to a progressive hydronephrosis [72]. With prolonged partial obstruction the degree of hydronephrosis may become extreme, such cases being unilateral in practically all instances because death due to renal failure occurs in bilateral hydronephrosis before severe dilatation can develop. However, bilateral congenital hydronephrosis may result in kidneys massive enough to interfere with labor. In utero nitrogenous wastes are excreted via the placenta, but the infant dies in uremia shortly after birth.

Clinical features

Clinically in hydronephrosis there is flank pain, and there may be a palpable mass. When infection develops, fever, chills, pyuria, and leukocytosis appear. When hydronephrosis is bilateral, signs of progressive renal failure terminating in uremia are present. Retrograde pyelography demonstrates the presence of hydronephrosis. Intravenous pyelography usually shows nonfunction in the affected kidney.

Pathologic changes

Grossly the hydronephrotic kidney is enlarged, the degree of increase in size depending on the duration of the lesion and type of obstruction. The changes begin in the pelvis, which becomes dilated and filled with urine. The chemical composition of the pelvic fluid is altered by pyelovenous backflow. Later the renal cortex becomes gradually thinned and atrophic. *Microscopically* the tubules and Bowman's spaces are dilated, and the tubular epithelium is flattened. Later the tubules atrophy and are replaced by fibrous tissue. The kidney becomes a cystic bag of fluid in severe cases of hydronephrosis. *Infection* is very common in the hydronephrotic kidney. It may be parenchymal (pyelonephritis), pelvic (pyonephrosis), or both. *Pyonephrosis* is an infected hydronephrosis with frank pus in the dilated calyces and pelvis. The kidney may be converted into a bag of pus. The pelvic mucosa is shaggy. The portion of the ureter proximal to an obstruction becomes dilated and filled with urine *(hydroureter).* If it is infected and contains pus, it is a *pyoureter.*

pyo-nephrosis

DEVELOPMENTAL DEFECTS OF THE URETERS AND URINARY BLADDER

1. Ureteral Anomalies

Ureteral anomalies are fairly frequent, but many are asymptomatic. Some types, however, are apt to cause complications and become of clinical importance.

Bifid ureter

Bifid (Y-shaped) ureter is the most common anomaly and is associated with double renal pelves. The ureteral segments usually unite somewhere along their courses and enter the bladder through a single orifice. Rarely the ureter is completely duplicated or even triplicated. In the rare *caudal bifid* (inverted-Y) *ureter* the tube begins singly and divides below to enter the bladder through two orifices.

Agenesis

Agenesis or hypoplasia of a ureter is always associated with agenesis of the ipsilateral kidney, since the ureteral bud acts as an organizer for the metanephrogenic mass.

Ectopia

Ectopia of a ureter is usually related to displacement or malformation of the corresponding kidney or to aberrant blood vessels. A ureter may lie behind the inferior vena cava *(retrocaval ureter).* Obstruction due to kinking or pressure is common. *Ectopic terminations* of a ureter may occur in the form of an opening into the prostatic urethra, seminal vesicle, or vas deferens in the male, into the urethra, vagina, uterus, or uterine tube in the female, and into the rectum or abnormal locations in the urinary bladder in either sex.

Luminal anomalies

Anomalies of the ureteral lumen include congenital stricture, kinks and twists, diverticula rarely, and megaloureter (a neurogenic, usually bilateral congenital dilatation). Obstruction is common in cases of ureteral stricture, kinking, or twisting.

2. Vesical Anomalies

Exstrophy

Exstrophy (ectropion) of the urinary bladder is rare and develops in the male fetus seven times as often as in the female. Due to an absence of the anterior surface of the bladder and the overlying abdominal wall, the posterior vesical wall is everted and protruded anteriorly. The symphysis pubis is typically absent also, and other pelvic anomalies are frequent. In males complete exstrophy is usually associated with hypoplasia of the penis with epispadias, the floor of the urethra and the bladder neck being exposed, and cryptorchidism (incomplete descent of the testes). In girls with complete bladder exstrophy the clitoris is cleft and the labia minora widely separated, exposing the vagina. Epispadias is typically present. The *cause* of exstrophy is probably a failure of union of the urogenital cleft. About half these patients die before the age of 10 years due to urinary tract obstruction and infection. Very rarely exstrophy may consist of a *superior or inferior vesical fissure* with only a slight defect in the anterior abdominal wall and a small protrusion of the everted superior or inferior portion of the bladder [73].

Diverticula

Developmental diverticulum of the urinary bladder is due to a focal failure of development of the muscularis, with outpouching of the mucosa through the congenital defect. It is rare. *Acquired diverticula* are more common than the developmental type and are produced by urethral obstruction. Occasionally they are congenital, but such diverticula are most frequent in men over 50 because of prostatic hyperplasia. *Vesical diverticula* are saccular pouches 1 to 10 cm. in size and are lined by a thin transitional epithelium. They are of clinical importance because urinary stasis and infection are common within them.

Others

Other anomalies of the urinary bladder are rare and include agenesis, duplication, hourglass configuration, and vesicovaginal or vesicorectal fistula (due to failure of development of the urorectal septum into the cloaca).

3. *Urachal Anomalies*

Anomalies of the urachus, which is normally a fibrous cord produced by the involution of the allantoic duct, are due to patency of part or all of the structure. *Umbilico-uracho-vesical fistula* occurs when both ends remain open; the bladder is undescended. In *umbilico-urachal fistula,* only the upper end is patent. *Urachal cyst* develops when the urachus is patent and both ends are closed. The cyst is filled with fluid and may attain a huge size. Rupture at the umbilicus or into the peritoneal cavity may occur.

INFECTIONS OF THE URETERS AND URINARY BLADDER

ACUTE URETERITIS

Acute ureteritis may result from a descending infection from an acute pyelonephritis, an ascending spread from an acute cystitis or, less commonly, a direct hematogenous infection of a ureter. In the first two types, organisms may reach the tube via its lumen or via the periureteral lymphatics. Urinary obstruction is commonly present, and the ureter is often dilated *(hydro-ureter).* Its mucosa may be ulcerated, and the lumen contains purulent material. *Microscopically* the edematous wall is heavily infiltrated with neutrophils.

URETERITIS CYSTICA

Ureteritis cystica is probably due to chronic infection and is commonly associated with similar lesions in the renal pelvis *(pyelitis cystica)* and urinary bladder. It may be unilateral or bilateral and usually occurs in persons over age 50. It is characterized by the presence in the submucosa of *cysts* up to 2 cm. in diameter. These are most common at the upper end of the ureter and are lined with several layers of transitional epithelium or a single layer of flat to columnar epithelium (in the larger cysts). They are formed by a central degeneration of the cell nests of von Brunn and contain a watery or mucinous fluid.

CYSTITIS:

Cystitis is an inflammation of the urinary bladder. It is usually secondary to infection in adjacent organs or to instrumentation of the bladder, as with a catheter or cystoscope. A study of the *effects of an indwelling catheter* in the urinary bladder on the development of cystitis has shown that bacteriuria develops in 7 percent of normal volunteers in whom the catheter is left in place for 18 to 24 hours, in 20 percent when it is present for 36 hours, and in 45 percent when it remains in place for up to 72 hours [74]. The incidence of cystitis during or following the use of an indwelling catheter is much higher in patients with bladder abnormalities or disease.

Acute cystitis:

Acute cystitis may be due to a descending infection from an acute pyelonephritis or an ascending infection from the urethra. The latter type is more common in females, because of the shortness of the urethra. Mild cases are not infrequent following the onset of sexual intercourse in women ("honeymoon cystitis"). The common *causative organisms* in acute cystitis include *Escherichia coli, Proteus vulgaris,* and *Streptococcus faecalis.*

clinical features

Clinically there is urinary frequency with burning and pain on micturition. The *urine* contains pus, erythrocytes, bacteria, and albumin (from the breakdown of neutrophils, red cells, and desquamated epithelium).

pathologic changes

Grossly the bladder wall is edematous. The *mucosa* is often ulcerated and hemorrhagic. *Microscopically* there is an acute inflammatory reaction in the submucosa.

special forms

Special types of acute cystitis include *gangrenous cystitis, phlegmonous cystitis, emphysematous cystitis* (which usually occurs in diabetics and is characterized by gas-filled mucosal vesicles up to 1 cm. in diameter), and *bullous cystitis* (which like the preceding type is often due to gas-forming clostridia).

Chronic cystitis:

Chronic cystitis usually follows one or more attacks of acute inflammation, but in some patients no history of an acute episode is found. It is caused by the same organisms as acute cystitis and is common in urinary obstruction due to prostatic hyperplasia or urethral stricture. The persistence of residual urine after voiding, as in cystocele, bladder diverticulum, or prostatic enlargement, is particularly predisposing to chronic cystitis.

clinical features

Clinically there is dysuria, and small amounts of pus and blood are found in the urine.

pathologic changes

Grossly the bladder wall is thickened and trabeculated, crisscross fibrous cords being seen beneath the mucosa. *Microscopically* the submucosa shows fibrous thickening and is infiltrated by lymphocytes, plasmocytes, and macrophages. The infiltrate may extend into the hypertrophied muscularis.

special forms

Special forms of chronic cystitis include the following:

1. *Cystitis cystica.* Degeneration of submucosa cell nests of von Brunn produces mucous cysts lined by transitional, cuboidal, or columnar epithelium. The cysts measure 0.1 to 3 cm. in diameter.

2. *Encrusted cystitis.* Ammonium salts are precipitated on the mucosa in alkaline urine, the condition usually occurring in postpartum women.

3. *Follicular cystitis.* In this condition small nodules of lymphocytes form in the submucosa, especially at the trigone.

4. *Interstitial cystitis* (Hunner's ulcer). This infection almost always occurs in women, is of unknown cause, and shows one or more shallow ulcers with marked underlying submucosal fibrosis.

5. *Malakoplakia.* This occurs predominantly in women over 30 and appears as multiple well-circumscribed, soft, yellowish mucosal plaques, 0.1 to 5 cm. in

diameter, with depressed centers. Microscopically it shows a granulomatous submucosal reaction containing calcospherites *(Michaelis-Gutmann bodies).*

6. *Leukoplakia.* This is a premalignant white mucosal plaque.

7. *Schistosomal cystitis (bilharziasis).* This infection is due to *S. haematobium* and rarely *S. mansoni.*

URETERAL INJURIES

Ureteral injuries, some of which lead to urinary obstruction, occur in about 0.5 percent of major pelvic operations [75]. *Such injuries occur in women about four times as commonly as in men.* Ureteral injuries are bilateral in about 15 percent of the cases, affect the left ureter only in about 55 percent, and the right ureter only in about 30 percent. Ureteral injury results from accidental clamping with a hemostat, complete or partial ligation by suture, complete or partial transsection, excision of a segment, or excessive stripping of the adventitia with resultant ischemia from loss of blood supply. A ureter may also be injured by a bullet or stab wound or as a result of severe flank trauma.

NEOPLASMS OF THE URETERS, URINARY BLADDER, AND URETHRA

1. Ureteral Neoplasms

Neoplasms of the ureters are unusual. Because of the narrow lumen, urinary obstruction occurs very commonly with ureteral neoplasm. Benign neoplasms are rare and include *transitional cell papilloma.* Transitional cell carcinoma may be papillary, infiltrating, or ulcerative. *Papillary carcinoma* is more common in men than in women by 2:1 and usually occurs in the lower third of the ureter. Hematuria is frequent early and may be gross. Metastases may be early and widespread.

2. Vesical Neoplasms

BENIGN NEOPLASMS

Benign neoplasms of the urinary bladder are uncommon and include fibromas, myxomas, leiomyomas, rhabdomyomas, hemangiomas, and neurofibromas. Because of their marked tendency to recur after seemingly adequate excision, the histologically benign *transitional cell papillomas* are often considered to be grade I carcinomas. Only those neoplasms with a transitional cell mucosa indistinguishable from normal and with a fine fibrovascular stroma should be considered benign papillomas [76].

MALIGNANT NEOPLASMS:

Malignant neoplasms of the urinary bladder are epithelial in origin in over 95 percent of the cases. The bladder gives rise to about 1 percent of all carcinomas. Most occur after age 50, especially between 55 and 70, and bladder carcinoma occurs about three times as frequently in men as in women.

Papillary carcinoma:

Papillary transitional cell carcinoma is by far the most common type of epithelial cancer occurring in the bladder. *Clinically* hematuria, dysuria, and infection are common. Cystoscopically a papillary mass is seen on the bladder wall.

causes

There is a *significantly high incidence of bladder carcinoma in workers exposed to aniline dyes, benzene, and alpha- and beta-naphthylamine, in patients with schistosomiasis of the bladder, and among heavy cigarette smokers.* In naphthylamine workers there is a 15 to 20 year lag before the development of carcinoma. The actual carcinogen may be 2-amino-1-naphthol. Free aminophenols may also play a carcinogenic role. Released by enzymes, they have been found in the urine of patients with bladder cancer. Another potent vesical carcinogen is *p*-diphenylamine. The development of frank carcinoma secondary to exposure to this chemical (and probably to other carcinogens) is preceded by mucosal dyskeratosis and carcinoma in situ [77]. Papillary transitional cell carcinoma has been produced in rats by feeding them high doses of a mixture of sodium cyclamate and sodium saccharin and by cyclohexylamine, a metabolite of cyclamates [78].

pathologic changes

Grossly the neoplasm usually is a pink, delicately fronded, soft papillary mass growing from the bladder mucosa. The more highly malignant ones are firm and verrucous, or flat and ulcerated. About half these neoplasms arise in the trigone; other common sites are on the lateral walls or about the ureteral orifices. *Microscopically* the papillary folds have a thin fibrous core and are lined by several to many layers of transitional cells. These vary histologically from only slightly atypical cells (grade I) to anaplastic types (grade IV), but most are well differentiated. Foci of squamous metaplasia frequently develop. According to the *Jewett and Strong classification,* stage 0 is carcinoma in situ; stage A, infiltration into subepithelial tissue; stages B1 and B2, infiltration into muscularis; stage C, infiltration into perivesical fat; and stage D, infiltration into adjacent organs and lymph nodes.

Epidermoid carcinoma

Epidermoid carcinoma of the urinary bladder is less common than the transitional cell type. It is sometimes associated with leukoplakia of the mucosa and, more often, with prolonged cystitis caused by the ova of *Schistosoma haematobium.* Invasive epidermoid carcinoma may be preceded by *carcinoma in situ* by 1 to 5 years [79]. *Clinically* epidermoid carcinoma is like transitional cell carcinoma. *Grossly* the neoplasm is flat, slightly raised, and ulcerated. It infiltrates the bladder wall. *Microscopically* most are fairly well differentiated, with foci of pearl formation. Some show an extensive reactive fibrosis.

Adenocarcinoma

Adenocarcinoma of the urinary bladder is very rare and apparently arises from cloacal or urachal rests or from the periurethral glands in the bladder neck. *Grossly* it is slightly elevated and ulcerated with rolled edges. *Microscopically* it is sometimes mucinous.

Metastases

Metastases from urinary bladder carcinomas usually occur late in the course. The neoplasms invade the bladder wall and spread to adjacent structures (ureters, prostate, vagina, rectum) and the pelvic lymph nodes. Hematogenous spread also occurs. *Complications* include ureteral obstruction and vesicorectal and vesicovaginal fistulae.

Sarcoma

Sarcoma of the urinary bladder is extremely rare and usually appears in young children or the aged. The types include leiomyosarcoma, rhabdomyosarcoma, and lymphosarcoma.

3. Urethral Neoplasms

Tumors of the urethra are rare; most common is the *urethral caruncle* which occurs only in the female urethra and represents a focal urethral prolapse with secondary infection rather than true neoplasia. It is exquisitely painful. The caruncle may be papillomatous, telangiectatic, or granulomatous. Transitional cell or squamous carcinoma may arise in a caruncle. *Benign neoplasms* of the urethra include squamous papillomas, adenomas (from periurethral glands), and fibromas. *Malignant neoplasms* are rare and include epidermoid carcinoma (the more common type) and adenocarcinoma, which in the female arises from Skene's glands. In the female, urethral carcinoma may be causally related to chronic irritation or infection; it coexists with a caruncle fairly frequently [80]. The carcinoma grows as a papillary or fungating mass which may protrude through the urethral orifice.

REFERENCES

1. Jørgensen, F., and Bentzon, M. W. The ultrastructure of the normal human glomerulus. Thickness of glomerular basement membrane. *Lab. Invest.* 18:42, 1968.
2. Kurtz, S. M. The fine structure of the lamina densa. *Lab. Invest.* 10:1189, 1961.
3. Jørgensen, F. Electron microscopic studies of normal visceral epithelial cells. *Lab. Invest.* 17:225, 1967.
4. Suzuki, Y., Churg, J., Grishman, E., Mautner, W., and Dachs, S. The mesangium of the renal glomerulus. *Amer. J. Path.* 43:555, 1963.
5. Dunihue, F. W., and Boldosser, W. G. Observations on the similarity of mesangial to juxtaglomerular cells. *Lab. Invest.* 12:1228, 1963.
6. Hadley, W. K., and Rosenau, W. Study of human renal disease by immunofluorescent methods. *Arch. Path.* (Chicago) 83:342, 1967.
7. Robinson, R. R., Glover, S. N., Phillippi, P. J., Lecocq, F. R., and Langelier, P. R. Fixed and reproducible orthostatic proteinuria. I. Light microscopic studies of the kidney. *Amer. J. Path.* 39:291, 1961.
8. Robinson, R. R., Ashworth, C. T., Glover, S. N., Phillippi, P. J., Lecocq, F. R., and Langelier, P. R. Fixed and reproducible orthostatic proteinuria. II. Electron microscopy of renal biopsy specimens from five cases. *Amer. J. Path.* 39:405, 1961.
9. Franklin, S. S., and Merrill, J. P. Acute renal failure. *New Eng. J. Med.* 262:711, 761, 1960.
10. Koffler, D., and Paronetto, F. Fibrinogen deposition in acute renal failure. *Amer. J. Path.* 49:383, 1966.
11. Bennett, B., and Rosenblum, C. Identification of calcium oxalate crystals in the myocardium in patients with uremia. *Lab. Invest.* 10:947, 1961.
12. Rabson, S. M., and Richter, M. N. Multiple necrosis of the spleen. "Fleckmilz" of Feitis. *Amer. J. Clin. Path.* 37:597, 1962.
13. Friend, D. G., Hoskins, R. G., and Kirkin, M. W. Relative erythrocythemia (polycythemia) and polycystic kidney disease, with uremia. *New Eng. J. Med.* 264:17, 1961.
14. Osanthanondh, V., and Potter, E. L. Pathogenesis of polycystic kidneys. Survey of results of microdissection. *Arch. Path.* (Chicago) 77:510, 1964.
15. Ibid. Pathogenesis of polycystic kidneys. Type 1 due to hyperplasia of interstitial portions of collecting tubules. *Arch. Path.* (Chicago) 77:466, 1964.
16. Ibid. Pathogenesis of polycystic kidneys. Type 2 due to inhibition of ampullary activity. *Arch. Path.* (Chicago) 77:474, 1964.
17. Ibid. Pathogenesis of polycystic kidneys. Type 3 due to multiple abnormalities of development. *Arch. Path.* (Chicago) 77:485, 1964.
18. Ibid. Pathogenesis of polycystic kidneys. Type 4 due to urethral obstruction. *Arch. Path.* (Chicago) 77:502, 1964.

19. Abeshouse, B. S., and Abeshouse, G. A. Sponge kidney. Review of literature and report of five cases. *J. Urol.* 84:252, 1960.
20. Krickstein, H. I., Gloor, F. J., and Balogh, K. Renal pathology in hereditary nephritis with nerve deafness. *Arch. Path.* (Chicago) 82:506, 1966.
21. Kramer, N. C., Watt, M. F., Howe, J. H., and Parrish, A. E. Circulating anti-human kidney antibodies in human renal disease. *Amer. J. Med.* 30:39, 1961.
22. Treser, G., Semar, M., McVicar, M., Franklin, M., Ty, A., Sagel, I., and Lange, K. Antigenic streptococcal components in acute glomerulonephritis. *Science* 163:676, 1969.
23. Seegal, B. C., Andres, G. A., Hsu, K. C., and Zabriskie, J. B. Studies on pathogenesis of acute and progressive glomerulonephritis in man by immuno-fluorescein and immunoferritin techniques. *Fed. Proc.* 24:100, 1965.
24. Herdson, P. B., Jennings, R. B., and Earle, D. P. Glomerular fine structure in poststreptococcal acute glomerulonephritis. *Arch. Path.* (Chicago) 81:117, 1966.
25. Strunk, S. W., Hammond, W. S., and Benditt, E. P. The resolution of acute glomerulonephritis. An electron microscopic study of four sequential biopsies. *Lab. Invest.* 13:401, 1964.
26. Flume, J. B., Ashworth, C. T., and James, J. A. An electron microscopic study of tubular lesions in human kidney biopsy specimens. *Amer. J. Path.* 43:1067, 1963.
27. Churg, J., and Grishman, E. Subacute glomerulonephritis. *Amer. J. Path.* 35:25, 1959.
28. Grishman, E., and Churg, J. Chronic glomerulonephritis. *Amer. J. Path.* 36:607, 1960.
29. Nagle, R. B., Kohnen, P. W., Bulger, R. E., Striker, G. E., and Benditt, E. P. Ultrastructure of human renal obsolescent glomeruli. *Lab. Invest.* 21:519, 1969.
30. Mautner, W., Churg, J., Grishman, E., and Dachs, S. Preeclamptic nephropathy. *Lab. Invest.* 11:518, 1962.
31. Churg, J., Grishman, E., Goldstein, M. H., Yunis, S. L., and Porush, J. G. Idiopathic nephrotic syndrome in adults. *New Eng. J. Med.* 272:165, 1965.
32. Raphael, S. S., and Lynch, M. J. G. Kimmelstiel-Wilson glomerulonephropathy: Its occurrence in diseases other than diabetes mellitus. *A.M.A. Arch. Path.* 65:420, 1958.
33. Kimmelstiel, P., Kim, O. J., and Beres, J. Studies on renal biopsy specimens, with the aid of the electron microscope. I. Glomeruli in diabetes. *Amer. J. Clin. Path.* 38:270, 1962.
34. Schindler, A. M., and Sommers, S. C. Diabetic sclerosis of the renal juxtaglomerular apparatus. *Lab. Invest.* 15:877, 1966.
35. Ritchie, S., and Waugh, D. The pathology of Armanni-Ebstein diabetic nephropathy. *Amer. J. Path.* 33:1035, 1957.
36. Shirahama, T., and Cohen, A. S. Fine structure of the glomerulus in human and experimental renal amyloidosis. *Amer. J. Path.* 51:869, 1967.
37. Paranetto, F., and Koffler, D. Immunofluorescent localization of immunoglobulins, complement, and fibrinogen in human diseases. I. Systemic lupus erythematosus. *J. Clin. Invest.* 44:1657, 1965.
38. Grishman, E., Porush, J. C., Rosen, S. M., and Churg, J. Lupus nephritis with organized deposits in the kidneys. *Lab. Invest.* 16:717, 1967.
39. Trump, B. F., and Janigan, D. T. The pathogenesis of cytologic vacuolization in sucrose nephrosis. *Lab. Invest.* 11:395, 1962.
40. Muehrcke, R. C., and Rosen, S. Hypokalemic nephropathy in rat and man. A light and electron microscopic study. *Lab. Invest.* 13:1359, 1964.

41. Biava, C. G., Dyrda, I., Genest, J., and Bencosme, S. A. Kaliopenic nephropathy. A correlated light and electron microscopic study. *Lab. Invest.* 12:443, 1963.
42. Howenstine, J. A. Exertion-induced myoglobinuria and hemoglobinuria. *J.A.M.A.* 173:493, 1960.
43. Fisher, E. R., Perez-Stable, E., and Zawadzki, Z. A. Ultrastructural renal changes in multiple myeloma with comments relative to the mechanism of proteinuria. *Lab. Invest.* 13:1561, 1964.
44. Crocker, D. W. Fibromuscular dysplasias of renal artery. *Arch. Path.* (Chicago) 85:602, 1968.
45. Turgeon, C., and Sommers, S. C. Juxtaglomerular cell counts and human hypertension. *Amer. J. Path.* 38:227, 1961.
46. Lee, J. B. Antihypertensive activity of the kidney – The renomedullary prostaglandins. *New Eng. J. Med.* 277:1073, 1967.
47. Still, W. J. S., and Hill, K. R. The pathogenesis of hyaline arteriolar sclerosis. *A.M.A. Arch. Path.* 68:42, 1959.
48. Biava, C. G., Dyrda, I., Genest, J., and Bencosme, S. A. Renal hyaline arteriosclerosis. An electron microscope study. *Amer. J. Path.* 44:349, 1964.
49. McManus, J. F. A., and Lupton, C. H., Jr. Ischemic obsolescence of renal glomeruli. *Lab. Invest.* 9:413, 1960.
50. Paronetto, F. Immunocytochemical observations on the vascular necrosis and renal glomerular lesions of malignant nephrosclerosis. *Amer. J. Path.* 46:901, 1965.
51. McCormack, L. J., Beland, J. E., Schneckcloth, R. E., and Corcoran, A. C. Effects of antihypertensive drugs on the evolution of the renal lesions in malignant nephrosclerosis. *Amer. J. Path.* 34:1011, 1958.
52. Fisher, E. R., and Rodnan, G. P. Pathologic observations concerning the kidney in progressive systemic sclerosis. *A.M.A. Arch. Path.* 65:29, 1958.
53. Kassirer, J. P. Atheroembolic renal disease. *New Eng. J. Med.* 280:812, 1969.
54. Panner, B. Nephrotic syndrome in renal vein thrombosis. *Arch. Path.* (Chicago) 76:303, 1963.
55. Kass, E. H. Bacteriuria and the pathogenesis of pyelonephritis. *Lab. Invest.* 9:110, 1960.
56. Kunin, C. M., Zacha, E., and Paquin, A. J., Jr. Urinary-tract infections in schoolchildren. I. Prevalence of bacteriuria and associated urologic findings. *New Eng. J. Med.* 266:1287, 1962.
57. Kunin, C. M., and Halmagyi, N. E. Urinary-tract infections in schoolchildren. II. Characterization of invading organisms. *New Eng. J. Med.* 266:1297, 1962.
58. Moolten, S. E., and Smith, I. B. Fatal nephritis in chronic Phenacetin poisoning. *Amer. J. Med.* 28:127, 1960.
59. Kalmanson, G. M., and Guze, L. B. Role of protoplasts in pathogenesis of pyelonephritis. *J.A.M.A.* 190:1107, 1964.
60. Aoki, S., Imamura, S., Aoki, M., and McCabe, W. R. "Abacterial" and bacterial pyelonephritis. *New Eng. J. Med.* 281:1375, 1969.
61. Ravel, R. Megalocytic interstitial nephritis. *Amer. J. Clin. Path.* 47:781, 1967.
62. Rios-Dalenz, J. L., and Peacock, R. C. Xanthogranulomatous pyelonephritis. *Cancer* 19:289, 1966.
63. Berman, L. B., Antonovych, T. T., and Duke, J. Glomerular abnormalities in tuberculosis. *A.M.A. Arch. Path.* 69:278, 1960.
64. Reiss, O. Leukemoid reaction due to hypernephroma. *J.A.M.A.* 180:1126, 1962.

65. Amador, E., Zimmerman, T. S., and Wacker, W. E. C. Urinary alkaline phosphatase activity. I. Elevated urinary LDH and alkaline phosphatase activities for the diagnosis of renal adenocarcinoma. *J.A.M.A.* 185:769, 1963.
66. Miller, R. W., Fraumeni, J. F., Jr., and Manning, M. D. Association of Wilms' tumor with aniridia, hemihypertrophy and other congenital malformations. *New Eng. J. Med.* 270:922, 1964.
67. Smith, J. W., Pinkel, D., and Dabrowski, S. Detection of a small virus in a cultivated human Wilms' tumor. *Cancer* 24:527, 1969.
68. Balsaver, A. M., Gibley, C. W., Jr., and Tessmer, C. F. Ultrastructural studies in Wilms' tumor. *Cancer* 22:417, 1968.
69. Newman, D., and Vellios, F. Adult carcinosarcoma (adult Wilms' tumor) of the kidney. *Amer. J. Clin. Path.* 42:45, 1964.
70. Madani, M., and Berman, L. B. The Fanconi syndrome with cystinosis. *Med. Ann. D.C.* 30:729, 1961.
71. Gross, R. E., Randolph, J., and Wise, H. M., Jr. Surgical correction of bladder-neck obstruction in children. *New Eng. J. Med.* 268:5, 1963.
72. Sheehan, H. L., and Davis, J. C. Experimental hydronephrosis. *A.M.A. Arch. Path.* 68:185, 1959.
73. Higgins, C. C. Exstrophy of the bladder. *J.A.M.A.* 171:1922, 1959.
74. Cox, C. E., and Hinman, F., Jr. Incidence of bacteriuria with indwelling catheter in normal bladders. *J.A.M.A.* 178:919, 1961.
75. Higgins, C. C. Ureteral injuries. *J.A.M.A.* 182:225, 1962.
76. Mostofi, F. K. Pathological aspects and spread of carcinoma of the bladder. *J.A.M.A.* 206:1762, 1968.
77. Melamed, M. R., Koss, L. G., Ricci, A., and Whitmore, W. F. Cytohistological observations on developing carcinoma of the urinary bladder in man. *Cancer* 13:67, 1960.
78. Price, J. M., Biava, C. G., Oser, B. L., Vogin, E. E., Steinfeld, J., and Ley, H. L. Bladder tumors in rats fed cyclohexylamine or high doses of a mixture of cyclamate and saccharin. *Science* 167:1131, 1970.
79. Melamed, M. R., Voutsa, N. G., and Grabstald, H. Natural history and clinical behavior of in situ carcinoma of the urinary bladder. *Cancer* 17:1533, 1964.
80. Monaco, A. P., Murphy, G. B., and Dowling, W. Primary cancer of the female urethra. *Cancer* 11:1215, 1958.

GENERAL REFERENCES

Allen, A. C. *The Kidney: Medical and Surgical Diseases* (2d ed.). New York: Grune & Stratton, 1962.

Corcoran, A. C., and Weller, J. M. In Sodeman, W. A. (Ed.), *Pathologic Physiology* (4th ed.). Philadelphia: Saunders, 1967, pp. 713–748.

Heptinstall, R. H. *Pathology of the Kidney.* Boston: Little, Brown, 1966.

Lucké, B., and Schlumberger, H. G. Tumors of the kidney, renal pelvis and ureter. Section VIII, Fascicle 30, in *Atlas of Tumor Pathology.* Washington: Armed Forces Institute of Pathology, 1957.

Mostofi, F. K., and Smith, D. E. (Eds.). *The Kidney.* Baltimore: Williams & Wilkins, 1966.

Potter, E. L. *Pathology of the Fetus and the Newborn* (2d ed.). Chicago: Year Book, 1961, pp. 421–449.

23 THE MALE GENITAL SYSTEM

GENITAL SYSTEM DISEASES IN GENERAL

The two important groups of genital system diseases are the venereal infections and the carcinomas of various genital organs.

Venereal diseases

The venereal infections have much higher morbidity than mortality rates. In 1968, about 19,000 cases of primary and secondary syphilis were reported in the United States, yet only about 2400 deaths are attributed to syphilis and its sequelae. Comparable figures for gonorrhea are 465,000 cases and 10 deaths, and for chancroid, lymphogranuloma venereum, and granuloma inguinale together, 1500 and 5. It is estimated, however, that in some areas there are 2 to 3 cases of syphilis and 5 to 10 of gonorrhea for each case reported. Because the causative organisms of these diseases are transmitted by a means which even the most eager-beaver public health officer would have little hope of controlling, the incidence of venereal disease will probably continue to be high. However, except in the case of gonorrhea, public health and police measures have produced a decline in the number of cases in the past 25 years; early adequate treatment has also greatly decreased the complications and late manifestations of these infections.

Genital cancer

Genital cancer is an important cause of death, especially in the female. Annually there are about 42,000 deaths in the United States due to malignant neoplasms of genital organs. Of these, about 24,000 are in females (about 15 percent of cancer deaths in women) and 18,000 in males (about 10 percent of cancer deaths in men). Among men the prostate gland is the most common site of genital cancer. Prostatic carcinoma causes about 17,000 deaths yearly (about 6000 deaths are attributed to "benign" hyperplasia of the prostate gland). Malignant neoplasms of the testes cause less than 1000 deaths each year, but most of these are in young men, whereas prostatic cancer occurs principally in men past 60.

Public attitude

Perhaps the most significant development in relation to genital system diseases in the past 25 years has been the change in the attitude of the public toward them. Much of the shame and degradation formerly attached to them (especially to venereal infections) has been erased. From a medical standpoint this means that patients seek treatment earlier and develop fewer psychologic scars than before this more enlightened outlook appeared. In 1881 Henrik Ibsen's dramatic study of congenital syphilis was regarded as a horrible and scandalous affront to decency; productions of *Ghosts* today raise hardly a single prudish eyebrow.

VENEREAL INFECTIONS IN THE MALE

1. Syphilis (Lues)

The general features of syphilis, the most important of the venereal diseases, are discussed on page 133.

Genital lesions

Typically 3 weeks after exposure the *chancre* (haircut sore) develops at the site of inoculation on the penis or, less often, on the scrotum. *Penile lesions* are usually on the glans near the frenum or inner prepuce, rarely on the shaft. The chancre is usually single, but may be multiple. It begins as a macule, which soon progresses to a painless indurated papule 0.5 to 2 cm. in diameter. The surface becomes superficially eroded, so that the characteristic chancre is an elevated, hard, circumscribed, superficially ulcerated, button-like, copper-colored lesion. A thin layer of adherent fibrin covers the smooth surface. The causative organisms, *Treponema pallidum,* can be demonstrated by dark-field examination of serum exuded from the chancre. Microscopically the mucosa or epidermis is ulcerated, and polymorphonuclear leukocytes are found near the surface. At the ulcer edges the rete pegs are elongated. The subepithelial tissue is heavily infiltrated with lymphocytes, plasmocytes, and macrophages. About the ulcer there is a zone of perivascular plasmocytic infiltration, and capillary proliferation and fibrosis are found. Silver stains outline numerous spirochetes. Even without therapy the inflammation subsides, and the chancre heals in 4 to 6 weeks, usually without a scar. *Secondary genital syphilids* include *mucous patches* (focal superficial ulcers) on the penis, containing many organisms, and *condylomata lata* (flat, verrucous lesions showing epidermal or mucosal hyperplasia with elongation of rete pegs and subepithelial perivascular lymphocytic and plasmocytic infiltration).

The *testes* are invaded in almost every case of syphilis, acquired or congenital. Often the spirochetes are present without causing demonstrable lesions. *Syphilitic orchitis* may occur in the acquired or congenital form. In contrast with genital tuberculosis, the testis is involved before the epididymis in acquired syphilitic orchitis. Two types are known: (1) diffuse interstitial syphilitic orchitis, and (2) gummata of the testis. *Diffuse interstitial syphilitic orchitis* is the more common form. The testis is often small, woody hard, and traversed by dense white fibrous bands. The tunica albuginea testis is thickened. *Microscopically* there is diffuse fibrosis in the late stages. Earlier there is a heavy inflammatory infiltrate with lymphocytes, plasmocytes, and multinucleated giant cells; spirochetes are found at this stage. Testicular atrophy is produced. *Gumma formation* in the testis may be single or multiple, and produces enlargement of the organ. The *epididymis* and *prostate* gland are occasionally involved in syphilis.

2. Gonorrhea (Blennorrhea)

Cause

Neisseria gonorrhoeae, a gram-negative, intracellular diplococcus which produces endotoxins, causes *gonorrhea (clap).* The organism is *spread* by sexual contact and, in young girls, by fomites such as towels or bed sheets. It can be found easily within neutrophils in the purulent urethral discharge from men, but is often difficult to detect in material from infected females. With the use of a conjugate of fluorescein isothiocyanate and globulin fractions of gonococcal K-antigen immune serum, gonococci can be visualized easily within a few minutes by *ultraviolet microscopy* in smears of male and female urethral exudate as well as in cervical and vaginal discharges [1]. A thick, purulent urethral discharge like that of gonorrhea is occasionally caused by *Neisseria meningitidis, N. catarrhalis, N. flava, Mima polymorpha,* and *M. polymorpha* var. *oxidans* [2].

Pathologic changes

From 2 to 5 days following infection during coitus an acute inflammation appears in the *mucosa of the anterior urethra* in males. There is a purulent exudate from the urethral orifice *(the drip).* After 2 to 4 weeks the inflammation subsides, even without treatment in uncomplicated cases. In the urethra the infection is limited to the intact mucosa and periurethral glands. *Endotoxins excite the purulent exudate.* A transient *gonococcemia* occurs in most cases.

Hematogenous complications

Hematogenous complications include:

1. *Septic arthritis.* This occurs twice as often in men as in women and may appear during the acute phase or months later. Usually it follows the onset by 1 to 3 weeks. In 80 percent of cases the arthritis is *polyarticular,* involving the knees, ankles, wrists, shoulders, and finger and toe joints. The *affected joint* is swollen, red, and tender. The joint fluid is purulent or serous, containing numerous polymorphonuclear leukocytes. Purulent involvement of a joint may lead to destruction of the articular cartilage and synovial membrane, causing *ankylosis* (fibrous fixation of the joint). Gonococci may be recovered from the joint fluid during the active phase. *Keratoderma blennorrhagica* may be associated with the arthritis; it occurs in 1 in about 5000 cases of gonorrhea and is 15 times as common in men as in women. There are vesicular lesions, which later show marked hyperkeratosis, on the feet, legs, trunk, arms, and face. Before chemotherapy 2 to 5 percent of cases of gonorrhea developed arthritis.

2. *Acute bacterial endocarditis, rarely.* About 85 percent of the lesions occur on previously normal valves. In about 70 percent of the cases the aortic valve is attacked, in 10 percent the pulmonic valve, and in 12 percent the tricuspid valve. Gonococci are therefore a frequent cause of *endocarditis of the right side of the heart.* The valvular vegetations are large and ulcerative, causing marked destruction of the valves. In one-third of the cases vegetations occur on the atrial endocardium and chordae tendineae. The endocarditis usually appears 1 to 3 weeks after the onset of urethritis.

3. *Pyemia.*

Genitourinary complications in males

Genitourinary complications of gonorrhea in men are frequent in inadequately treated patients. They include:

1. Acute balanitis.

2. Acute balanoposthitis.

3. Periurethral abscess.

4. Acute posterior urethritis (verumontanitis).

5. Acute cowperitis (inflammation of Cowper's glands).

6. *Urethral stricture.* This complication is rather common and may produce urinary obstruction. Fibrous bands develop and finally block the urethral lumen, sometimes years after the gonorrheal infection.

7. *Acute prostatitis,* infection here leading to abscess formation and chronicity.

8. Acute seminal vesiculitis.

9. *Acute epididymitis (strain).* This may produce sterility when it is bilateral. The infection appears 2 to 3 months after the urethritis. Early the globus minor is involved, but soon the entire organ is invaded, the epididymis becoming edematous and enlarged. Multiple tiny abscesses are found. Later there is marked fibrosis, with obliteration of seminiferous tubules. The process is usually unilateral.

10. Orchitis. Infection of the testis is uncommon, being produced by extension from the epididymis.

11. Acute cystitis.

12. Chronic urethritis with a thin mucopurulent discharge *(gleet).*

All these complications result from direct extension from the urethral infection.

Kerato-conjunctivitis:

Gonococcal keratoconjunctivitis usually occurs in children, although it may complicate gonorrhea in adults. It is most common in newborn infants *(ophthalmia neonatorum),* infection occurring during passage through the birth canal. *Ophthalmia neonatorum* formerly caused over 25 percent of blindness in children, but the prophylactic use of silver nitrate drops in the eyes or of antibiotics at birth has reduced this incidence greatly.

pathologic changes

There is a severe acute inflammation of the conjunctiva with ulceration of the cornea. This heals by fibrous scar formation, resulting in a *corneal opacity* which may produce blindness.

3. Chancroid

Cause

Hemophilus ducreyi, a gram-negative, short, nonmotile bacillus occurring in pairs and chains causes *chancroid* (soft chancre). The organism may exist as a harmless saprophyte in the vagina. *Transmission* is by sexual contact, the organism invading the skin through a small wound. Phimosis is commonly associated with chancroid. The *incubation period* is 3 to 10 days.

Pathologic changes

In men the lesions occur most commonly on the preputial orifice, the internal preputial surface, the frenum, and the fossa navicularis. The earliest lesion is a macule, which quickly becomes a papule, a vesicle, and then a pustule, which ruptures to produce a sharply defined *ulcer* with ragged, undermined edges. The ulcer base is covered by a grayish exudate. *Microscopically* the *epidermis* shows acanthosis and numerous small abscesses filled with polymorphonuclear leukocytes at the ulcer edges. The *dermis* is edematous, hyperemic, and infiltrated with neutrophils and some plasmocytes at the ulcer edges. The *inguinal lymph nodes* are enlarged and show central suppuration in over 50 percent of the cases. In a few cases the nodes become matted and ulcerate through the overlying skin. *Mixed chancre* is mixed infection due to syphilis and chancroid.

4. Lymphogranuloma Venereum

Cause

The cause of *lymphogranuloma (lymphopathia) venereum* (lymphogranuloma inguinale) is a chlamydia of the Chlamydiaceae group *(Miyagawanella* genus). The *Frei test* uses a yolk sac emulsion containing the chlamydia. An allergic, tuberculin-like reaction occurs at the site of inoculation of this emulsion in persons who have or have had the disease. A *complement-fixation* test is also used for diagnosis. *Transmission* is by sexual contact, especially in conditions of uncleanliness. The incubation period varies from 3 to 21 days.

Pathologic changes:

The *primary lesion* is a small, indurated vesicular nodule on the prepuce. This usually ulcerates. *Microscopically* the ulcer base shows a necrotic zone infiltrated with neutrophils. The underlying dermis is infiltrated with plasmocytes and macrophages. The epithelium at the ulcer edge shows hyperplasia and elongation of the rete pegs. The epithelium is edematous, and the cells undergo hydropic degeneration. The primary lesion is transient and disappears after a few days. Within 2 to 8 weeks inguinal, iliac, and sometimes femoral lymph nodes enlarge to form *buboes.* (The combination of the primary lesion and the enlarged nodes is the *primary-bubo complex.*) In about one-third of the cases the lymphadenitis is bilateral. The overlying skin becomes tense and violet. It may ulcerate or develop numerous sinus tracts from the lymph nodes. *Grossly* the lymph nodes are enlarged, conglomerated, and purplish pink. The abscesses are yellow and stellate. *Microscopically* the involved lymph nodes show lymphocytic and reticuloendothelial hyperplasia. Plasmocytes infiltrate the nodes, and macrophages accumulate in definite foci. As these foci enlarge, their centers become necrotic and neutrophils collect, disintegrating to form an abscess. Several abscesses run together to form the typical *stellate abscesses.* At the abscess margins the macrophages are palisaded and occasional giant cells are present. Later the abscesses are replaced by fibrous tissue.

chronic lesions

Chronic lesions may follow apparent recovery by weeks to years and are due to reactivation of the virus. They include *penile elephantiasis* (which leads to phimosis and balanoposthitis), *bubonuli* (nodule formation along the penis), and *anorectal stricture.* In the male anorectal infection follows rectal coitus in homosexuals. Early there is a *proctitis* with a mucopurulent discharge, shallow ulcers of the mucosa, and the formation of polypoid masses on the mucosa. *Rectal stricture* follows the proctitis and is usually within 6 cm. of the anus. The rectal wall is thick, fibrous, and rigid, and the lumen is greatly narrowed so that cigarette-shaped stools are formed. *Sinuses and fistulae* are common about the rectum. Cauliflowering growths may encircle the anus *(lymphorrhoids). Anal carcinoma* is significantly associated with chronic lymphogranuloma.

5. Granuloma Inguinale

Cause

Calymmatobacterium (Donovania) granulomatis, the *Donovan body,* a gram-negative, leishmania-like body with a definite capsule, causes *granuloma inguinale* (granuloma venereum, pudenda tropicum). The organisms are found intracytoplasmally in macrophages in the lesions. These bodies show a polar or bipolar condensation of chromatin. They stain purplish with hematoxylin and eosin and brown or black with silver stains, having a *safety pin* appearance.

Transmission

Granuloma inguinale is mildly contagious and is probably *spread* by sexual contact, being frequently associated with filth and neglect. In distribution the disease is universal, being most prevalent in tropical and subtropical areas. In the United States granuloma inguinale is much more common among Negroes than whites. The *incubation period* is 35 to 40 days.

Pathologic changes:

Ulcers occur most often on the *external genitalia and inguinal region,* the latter being infected secondarily by direct extension, auto-inoculation, and via lymphatics. The perineum, inner aspects of the thighs, anus, lower abdominal wall, and rectum may become involved. In about 5 percent of the cases *extragenital lesions* appear on the mucosa of the lips, mouth, pharynx, larynx, and esophagus by auto-inoculation from genital lesions. The lesions begin as papules, which become vesicles and then pustules or nodules 1 to 4 cm. in diameter. These ulcerate, the *ulcers* growing peripherally and sometimes becoming quite extensive. The ulcer base is composed of beef-red, velvety granulation tissue, and the margins are rolled. Ulcers may coalesce, and lymphatic extension may produce *satellite ulcers.* Lymphatic blockage may produce *elephantiasis. Secondary infection* of the ulcers, especially by fusospirochetes (Vincent's organisms), is common. *Inguinal ulcers* develop from a soft, subcutaneous fluctuant mass *(pseudobubo). Microscopically* in the early papule or nodule the epithelium is hyperplastic with elongation of the rete pegs. In the dermis or submucosa there is an infiltrate of polymorphonuclear leukocytes and of pathognomonic macrophages *(granuloma cells),* the latter being large cells (25 to 90μ in diameter) which contain 1 to 10 intracytoplasmic cysts filled with Donovan bodies. Their nuclei are pushed peripherally and are often pyknotic. With ulceration numerous plasmocytes appear within a luxuriant growth of granulation tissue in the ulcer base. There is a scarcity of lymphocytes in the lesions. The ulcers of granuloma inguinale may heal, leaving an atrophic depigmented scar. Nodular, hypertrophic, ulcerovegetative, and cicatricial lesions also occur.

lymph node involvement

In the unusual cases of involvement of *inguinal lymph nodes* these are slightly enlarged, firm, and grayish white. *Microscopically* the lymphocytes are widely replaced by plasmocytes, polymorphonuclear leukocytes, parasite-laden macrophages, and fibroblasts.

TUBERCULOSIS OF THE MALE GENITALIA

The *prostate gland* is frequently involved by tuberculosis, the infection being hematogenous. Tubercles form, enlarge, and finally convert most of the gland into a fibrocaseous mass. The *seminal vesicles* may become involved by extension from the prostate gland or by the hematogenous route. Thick fibrous walls surround the seminal vesicles which are filled by caseous material. The *epididymis* is a common site of genital tuberculosis and becomes infected hematogenously or by extension from the prostate gland and seminal vesicles. *Tuberculous epididymitis* is usually unilateral. The earliest lesions are discrete or massed yellow caseous foci in the globus minor. Eventually the entire epididymis becomes involved. The *testis* is rarely affected by tuberculosis without a preceding infection of the epididymis, and involvement of the testicular parenchyma is usually not marked. When *tuberculous orchitis* is extensive, the testis may become bound to the scrotum, with the formation of sinus tracts through the scrotal skin. The *tunica vaginalis testis* may be involved by extension from the epididymis, a serofibrinous or purulent exudate appearing. The tunica often acts as a barrier to extension into the testis.

DISEASES OF THE PENIS

1. Congenital Anomalies

Congenital anomalies include agenesis, hypoplasia, hyperplasia, and duplication (diphallus). *Agenesis* is usually associated with absence of all the genitalia except the testes and with imperforate anus. The anomaly is common in sympodial monsters (sirenomelus), in which the lower extremities are fused.

CONGENITAL ANOMALIES:

Ectopic locations of the urethral meatus are the most frequent malformation of the male genitalia. They are due to incomplete or abnormal fusion of the urethral folds along the inferior wall of the genital tubercle. Urinary tract infections are common in infants with such anomalies. *Hypospadias* is characterized by an abnormal urethral opening on the ventral surface of the penis. When the opening is at the penosacral junction, there is complete *hypospadias.* In this type the penis is hypoplastic and may be mistaken for a clitoris. If cryptorchidism is also present, determination of sex by external examination may be impossible. *Epispadias* is the presence of an abnormal urethral opening on the dorsum of the penis; this is less common than hypospadias. Occasionally a dorsal meatus may be present along with a normal one.

Ectopias of urethral meatus: hypospadias

epispadias

Congenital obstruction of the male urethra may be due to atresia of the meatus or to the development of two valvelike mucosal folds in the region of the verumontanum (colliculus seminalis), the male homologue of the hymen. Obstruction to urinary outflow results in vesical dilatation and hypertrophy, hydro-ureters, and bilateral hydronephrosis.

Urethral obstruction

2. Other Non-neoplastic Diseases

Phimosis is the inability to draw the prepuce back over the glans penis due to a congenitally narrow preputial orifice or to scarring of the foreskin following inflammation or trauma. Smegma accumulates beneath the prepuce, and bacterial infections are common. *Paraphimosis* is the inability to push the forcibly retracted prepuce forward over the glans. Constriction of the venous return by the tight foreskin produces a painful swelling of the glans penis. Urethral constriction causes acute urinary retention.

PHIMOSIS AND PARAPHIMOSIS

Priapitis is an inflammation of the penis. The pathologic changes due to venereal infections have been discussed.

PRIAPITIS:

Balanoposthitis is an infection of the glans and prepuce. It may be caused by staphylococci, streptococci, colon organisms, and *N. gonorrhoeae;* the condition is common with phimosis or redundant prepuce and in individuals with poor bathing habits. Most of these infections are purulent in nature, and ulceration of the glans mucosa may occur. Gangrene of the glans penis *(gangrenous balanitis)* may develop due to Vincent's organisms (fusospirochetosis) or streptococci. The glans may slough off. Chronic infections produce scarring with resultant phimosis.

Balanoposthitis

Herpes progenitalis is probably viral in origin. It is characterized by the formation of vesicles on the glans mucosa and preputial skin.

Herpes

Peyronie's disease (*fibrous cavernositis,* plastic induration of the penis) is characterized by the formation of indurated plaques, nodules, or cords along the

PEYRONIE'S DISEASE

dorsum of the penis, usually in men 50 to 70 years of age. Erections are painful and curved. The cause is unknown. There is proliferation of the fibrous tissue of Buck's fascia and the sheaths of the corpora cavernosa. Later cartilage or bone may develop by metaplasia.

PRIAPISM

Priapism is the existence of a prolonged penile erection not accompanied by sexual desire. It may be caused by cerebral or spinal cord injury or compression, and by thrombosis of the veins of the corpora cavernosa following sexual overactivity; it is seen in patients with leukemia (about 25 percent of cases of priapism occur in leukemia) and with sickle cell anemia. It may develop during transurethral prostatectomy. The onset is sudden and painful, and urination is difficult or impossible.

3. Neoplasms

BENIGN NEOPLASMS

Benign neoplasms include papillomas, which are fairly common, and lipomas, fibromas, and angiomas, which are rare. However, many of the papillomas are condylomata acuminata (venereal warts) which are probably viral in origin. The *condyloma acuminatum* is a raspberry-like or cauliflower-like verracous mass, usually on the coronal sulcus. The lesions of condyloma acuminatum may be multiple or confluent. *Microscopically* the epidermis shows acanthosis, and there is a lymphocytic infiltration in the dermis.

ERYTHROPLASIA

Erythroplasia of Queyrat is a premalignant lesion which usually occurs on the glans penis, but may involve the coronal sulcus or prepuce. *Grossly* the lesion is shiny, sharply defined, slightly elevated, and pinkish red. The surface is slightly eroded and velvety. Induration is present, and there is fixation to the underlying dermis. *Microscopically* the epidermis shows small erosions, acanthosis, and elongation of the rete pegs. The underlying dermis is edematous, hyperemic, and infiltrated by mononuclear cells, especially plasmocytes.

MALIGNANT NEOPLASMS: Epidermoid carcinoma:

Epidermoid carcinoma [3] is the most common malignant neoplasm of the penis. The ultimate *cause* is unknown, but *retained smegma,* which may be carcinogenic, and irritation by phimosis, chronic infection, or trauma are important causative factors. The importance of circumcision in preventing carcinoma of the penis is demonstrated by its extreme rarity in Jewish men and by its distribution in India and Pakistan, where its incidence is 10 percent of all skin cancer among uncircumcised Hindus, while the disease is almost unknown among Moslems, who practice the ritual. About 20 percent of patients with carcinoma of the penis have or have had venereal disease.

frequency

In the United States penile carcinoma constitutes less than 2 percent of skin cancer, being about three times more common in Negroes than white men; the highest incidence is between ages 45 and 60. In China it makes up about 20 percent of all skin cancer, and in Europe 5 percent.

pathologic changes

The most *common sites* of the neoplasms are on the glans penis, coronal sulcus, and prepuce. *Grossly* the neoplasm is papillary or flat, and ulcerative. Growth is slow. *Microscopically* most are grade I or II epidermoid carcinoma. In almost 50 percent of the cases there is *spread* to the inguinal lymph nodes. Visceral metastases are rare.

metastases

Other malignant neoplasms

Adenocarcinoma of the penis is extremely rare. The neoplasm may arise from the glands of Littré or Cowper or from the lacunae of Morgagni. Mucinous adenocarcinoma may derive from Cowper's glands. *Melanocarcinoma* may occur on the skin of the penis or on the mucosa of the glans penis or urethral meatus [4]. *Sarcoma* is exceedingly rare; fibrosarcoma, Kaposi's sarcoma, and angiosarcoma have been reported. *Metastatic carcinoma* is uncommon and is most frequently from primary neoplasms in the urinary bladder, rectum, and prostate gland [5].

DISEASES OF THE PROSTATE GLAND

1. Non-neoplastic Diseases

ACUTE PROSTATITIS

Acute prostatitis is usually due to extension of an infection of the prostatic urethra or urinary bladder and occasionally to hematogenous infection. It commonly follows urethral instrumentation, such as catheterization or cystoscopy. The causative organisms include *Staphylococcus aureus,* streptococci, *Neisseria gonorrhoeae,* and *Escherichia coli. Grossly* the prostate gland is swollen and soft. *Microscopically* acini are filled with neutrophils. Small or large abscesses often develop.

CHRONIC PROSTATITIS

Chronic prostatitis may follow the acute form. The prostatic stroma is infiltrated with lymphocytes, plasmocytes, macrophages, and some neutrophils. Occasionally a *granulomatous prostatitis,* with a foreign-body giant cell reaction, develops due to the presence of necrotic prostatic tissue or inspissated secretions.

HYPERPLASIA:

Hyperplasia (benign hypertrophy) is very common in men over age 50 and is almost universal to some degree in octagenarians. The *cause* is the development of a *relative hyperestrinism* following the male climacteric. The estrogenic hormone is produced mainly by the adrenal cortex. In the prostate gland the central mass responds to estrogenic stimulation, while the external portions are dependent on the remaining testosterone.

Clinical features

Clinically in a relatively small number of cases of prostatic hyperplasia, *partial or complete urinary obstruction* due to compression of the prostatic urethra and bladder neck develops. With urinary blockage there are dysuria, frequency of urination, dribbling, and difficulty in starting and stopping the urinary stream. Digital rectal examination reveals a nodular or uniform enlargement of the prostate. The presence of residual urine in the bladder leads to the development of cystitis. Prolonged urinary obstruction produces hydronephrosis and signs of renal failure.

Pathologic changes

Grossly the prostate gland is enlarged from two to 10 times its normal size, sometimes weighing over 200 gm. The hyperplasia is almost limited to the ambisexual *lateral and middle lobes.* These may be smooth or nodular, and they are encapsulated, firm, and rubbery. A milky fluid exudes from the light tan cut surface. *Microscopically* there is a hyperplasia of both the glandular and stromal elements. The increase may be principally in the acinar cells *(adenomatous hyperplasia)* or in the stromal cells *(fibromuscular hyperplasia).* Many glands are dilated and filled with eosinophilic corpora amylacea. They are lined with a single layer of columnar or cuboidal cells usually, and papillary projections into the glandular lumina are fairly common. In the *stroma* a lymphocytic infiltrate is often found. Electron microscopy reveals that the tall columnar cells are the actively proliferating ones and that low columnar and cuboidal cells are degenerating [6]. Each acinus is completely surrounded by a basement membrane.

CALCULI

Calculi of the prostate gland occur fairly often in men over 50. *Endogenous calculi* appear in cases of prostatitis, hyperplasia, and carcinoma. Stones develop about corpora amylacea or cell debris with the inspissation of secretions in obstructed acini. The calculi consist mainly of calcium phosphate and calcium carbonate and vary from 1 mm. to several centimeters in diameter. They are white to brown and usually multiple. *Exogenous calculi* are of urinary origin.

VASCULAR LESIONS

Vascular lesions of the prostate gland include infarction, which is caused by arteriosclerotic or thrombotic arterial occlusion, periarteritis nodosa, embolism in bacterial endocarditis, vascular damage due to trauma (urethral instrumentation, massage), and *thrombosis of the periprostatic venous plexus* in bedridden patients. In areas about a prostatic infarct the glandular epithelium may undergo squamous metaplasia. Pulmonary embolism may result from the phlebothrombosis.

2. *Neoplasms*

BENIGN NEOPLASMS

Benign neoplasms of the prostate gland are rare. The most common is the *leiomyoma,* which is derived from the smooth muscle of the stroma. It is firm, rubbery, and yellowish white, with a whorled cut surface. *Microscopically* there are interlacing bundles of smooth myofibrils with little fibrous tissue. The leiomyoma may attain a large size. Frequently hyperplastic nodules are mistakenly called adenomas, fibroadenomas, fibromas, or leiomyomas.

MALIGNANT NEOPLASMS: Adenocarcinoma:

Adenocarcinoma of the prostate gland causes about 10 percent of cancer deaths in men. It seldom occurs in men under 50, but it is found in about 40 percent of those over 80, mostly as latent (microscopic) carcinoma. Carcinoma was found in almost 10 percent of the prostates examined in a large autopsy series [7]. The *cause* is unknown, but it may be related to the atrophy of the posterior lobe which occurs with the gradual drop in the androgen level after the age of 40. Carcinoma is not causally related to prostatic hyperplasia.

clinical features

Clinically prostatic carcinoma usually is characterized by urinary obstruction and infection. The enlargement, usually in the posterior lobe, is palpable on rectal examination. In many cases metastases have occurred by the time of diagnosis, and some cases are discovered because of bone pain or pathologic fractures. By cytologic techniques malignant cells may be identified in prostatic smears following massage. The serum level of *acid phosphatase,* which is formed largely by prostatic epithelial cells, is elevated in about 85 percent of the cases with metastases, and in 50 percent the level is above 10 King-Armstrong units. The acid phosphatase level is raised by androgen administration and lowered by orchiectomy or estrogen therapy. When bony metastases are present, the *alkaline phosphatase* level is also elevated in about 85 percent of cases.

pathologic changes

About 75 percent of prostatic carcinomas arise in the *posterior lobe,* 15 percent in the anterior lobe, and 10 percent in the lateral lobes. Over 90 percent develop in the subcapsular regions. Occasionally multicentric neoplasms occur. *Grossly* the lesion is grayish white with yellow spots; it is hard and is indistinctly demarcated from the surrounding tissue. *Microscopically* there are small, fairly well differentiated glandular structures lined by atypical epithelium. The glands lie back to back with little or no intervening stroma. Adjacent non-neoplastic glands are atrophic. The stroma may be densely fibrous. *Perineural lymphatic invasion* is common. In the later stages invasion of the bladder base and periureteral lymphatic spread produces hydro-ureter and hydronephrosis unilaterally or bilaterally. Transitional carcinoma or mixed transitional and adenocarcinoma of the prostate gland is uncommon and probably originates in the epithelium of its ducts into the prostatic urethra [8].

Metastases are frequent, developing in about half the cases within a year of the clinical onset. Iliac, periaortic, and sacral *lymph nodes* are involved in about 75 percent of the fatal cases; *osseous metastases* are present in up to 70 percent, the pelvic bones and sacrum almost always being involved in such cases. Less often the lumbar vertebrae, femora, thoracic vertebrae, and ribs are affected. Involvement of bones occurs via perineural lymphatics, the vertebral venous plexus of Batson, and the systemic circulation. The bony metastases are *osteoblastic* and show typical foci of increased opacity on x-ray. metastases

Effects of estrogen therapy and orchiectomy on the carcinoma, more pronounced with the former, include a marked reduction in nuclear size, loss of mitotic activity, and pyknosis. The cytoplasm of affected cells becomes vacuolated and bursts. Estrogen effects are highly variable [9]. In some cases there is no morphologic indication of degenerative changes in any neoplastic cells. Even in tumors showing marked estrogen effects, a few unaffected malignant cells can usually be found. *Prolonged estrogen administration* produces hyperplasia and squamous metaplasia of the prostatic urethral and utricular epithelium, aspermatogenesis and tubular basement membrane thickening in the testis, gynecomastia (hyperplasia of the duct epithelium and stroma of the male breasts), and, rarely, carcinoma of the breast. effects of therapy

Sarcoma of the prostate gland is rare. About 30 percent of the cases occur in boys under age 10, with a rapidly downhill course. Urinary and rectal obstruction develop. The neoplasm may attain a large size, often surrounding the bladder neck and invading adjacent tissues. It is grossly soft and fleshy with foci of hemorrhage and necrosis. *Microscopically* fibrosarcoma, rhabdomyosarcoma, and leiomyosarcoma are the usual types. *Metastases* are most commonly to regional lymph nodes, bones, and lungs. Sarcoma

DISEASES OF THE SEMINAL VESICLES, SPERMATIC CORDS, AND EPIDIDYMIDES

1. Diseases of the Seminal Vesicles

Diseases of the seminal vesicles include *seminal vesiculitis,* which may be gonorrheal, tuberculous, or nonspecific. *Abscesses* may develop in the pyogenic infections. Calcification of part or all of a gland may follow tuberculosis. *Calculi* occur in dilated alveoli following ejaculatory duct obstruction. *Neoplasms* are rare and include cystadenoma and adenocarcinoma, derived from the columnar alveolar epithelium, and leiomyoma, from the smooth muscular stroma.

2. Diseases of the Spermatic Cords

Diseases of the spermatic cords include:

1. *Congenital anomalies* – agenesis, atresia, duplication of the vas deferens.

2. *Inflammations.* Those of the entire cord are called *funiculitis* and those of the vas deferens, *vasitis* or *deferentitis.* Infections occur by extension from the epididymis, urethra, or seminal vesicles, and include gonorrhea and tuberculosis. In *filarial funiculitis* there are lymphangiectasis and interstitial fibrosis, calcified filariae being encased in whorls of hyalinized fibrous tissue.

3. *Torsion.* This is due to twisting, often during exertion, and results in compression of the veins of the pampiniform plexus, which produces congestion, hemorrhage, and sometimes infarction of the ipsilateral testis, usually an undescended one. In most cases there is an underlying excessive mobility secondary to an abnormal persistence of the processus vaginalis testis.

4. *Varicocele.* This is a dilatation, elongation, and tortuosity of the veins of the pampiniform plexus, which may be secondary to pressure on the spermatic vein or its tributaries or primary (idiopathic and *usually on the left side*).

5. *Neoplasms.* These include lipomas (the most common type), fibromas, leiomyomas, hemangiomas and lymphangiomas, neurilemmomas, adenomatoid tumors, teratomas, and rare fibrosarcomas, leiomyosarcomas, and rhabdomyosarcomas.

3. Diseases of the Epididymides

Diseases of the epididymides include *acute epididymitis,* which is usually gonorrheal in type and may be followed by fibrosis and obliteration of the coils of the ductus epididymis; *tuberculous epididymitis; spermatocele,* in which there is cystic dilatation due to duct obstruction and which is filled with milky fluid and dead and viable spermatozoa; and *neoplasms,* which are rare, usually occur in the globus minor, and are twice as frequent on the left side as on the right. The *adenomatoid tumor* is the most common type of neoplasm; it is benign and arises from Müllerian mesenchymal vestiges, producing epithelial structures by metaplasia [10], or from mesothelium. It also occurs in women, usually along the uterine tubes. Most of these tumors appear between 20 and 40 years of age. The neoplasm is firm, spherical, white, and homogeneous, and measures 1 to 5 cm. *grossly. Microscopically* it consists of small glandlike structures lined by cuboidal or low columnar epithelium-like cells and solid cords of cells with abundant eosinophilic cytoplasm in a fine fibromuscular stroma. *Other neoplasms* include leiomyomas, fibromas, lipomas, angiomas, papillary cystadenomas, and very rare adenocarcinomas derived from the ciliated columnar duct epithelium.

DISEASES OF THE TESTES

Testicular disorders include the following:

1. *Congenital anomalies.* Rarely agenesis of one or both testes or fusion (synorchism) occurs. *Testicular dysgenesis* and *cryptorchidism* (incomplete descent of one or both testes) are discussed below. In ectopia a testis is located abnormally due to a deviation from the normal pathway of descent, common ectopic locations being the femoral canal, perineum, or subcutaneously in the penis.

2. *Inflammations.* Except for syphilis, these are usually an extension from an epididymitis. (Gonorrheal orchitis is discussed on page 608, syphilitic orchitis

on page 606, tuberculous orchitis on page 610, and mumps orchitis on page 153.

3. *Infarction.* This results from venous and occasionally arterial obstruction caused by torsion of the spermatic cord, the testis becoming greatly enlarged, soft, dark red due to hemorrhage, and necrotic.

4. *Atrophy.* This may be due to arteriosclerosis in elderly males, chronic orchitis, severe malnutrition or cachexia, hypopituitarism, hyperestrinism in cirrhosis of the liver, prolonged estrogen administration, x-ray radiation, cryptorchidism in adults, and blockage of the ductus epididymis or vas deferens.

5. *Neoplasms.* These are discussed below.

1. Testicular Dysgenesis

About two-thirds of the cases of *testicular or seminiferous tubular dysgenesis (Klinefelter's syndrome)* are due to development of only the medullary portion of the embryonic gonad so that an imperfect male reproductive system forms in a genetic female [11]. Patients with Klinefelter's syndrome often have *47 chromosomes* (instead of the usual 46) in their body cells due to the *presence of three sex chromosomes (XXY).* A few cases of testicular dysgenesis have been associated with mongolism (Down's syndrome) [12]; these have 48 chromosomes. In some cases of Klinefelter's syndrome, XXY/XY mosaicism has been found [13]. This is probably due to nondisjunction of the X chromosome during meiosis, followed by loss of one X chromosome in some cells early in ontogenesis. Cases with XY (normal male), XXXY, XXXXY, XXYY, and XXXYY chromosomal patterns have also been reported. Many cases show *female sex chromatin* in their body cells.

In Klinefelter's syndrome the *testes* are small (less than 3.5 cm. in long diameter in young adults) and show hyalinization and basement membrane thickening in the seminiferous tubules with absence of spermatogenesis. Scattered clusters of *interstitial cells* are found. These Leydig cells are large and have a foamy cytoplasm. The *gynecomastia* is characterized mainly by an overgrowth of periductal fibroblasts. The *breast hyperplasia may be related to the loss of inhibin* normally produced by seminiferous tubular cells, so that the effect of androgens on the mammary glands is unopposed. Patients with Klinefelter's syndrome are usually low normal or subnormal mentally and are subject to syncopal attacks. They are usually impotent and frequently complain of headaches, dizziness, hot flashes, and palpitations.

2. Cryptorchidism

Cryptorchidism is diagnosed in 0.4 percent of boys and 0.04 percent in men. In this condition the involved testis may have stopped in its downward descent anywhere along its path from the coelomic cavity to the inguinal canal. The *cause* is not always apparent, but in some cases a short spermatic cord, tight inguinal canal, incompletely developed gubernaculum testis, inflammatory adhesions, or a gonadotropic hormone deficiency may play a causative role. The lesion may be unilateral or bilateral, occurring more frequently on the right side than the left when it is unilateral. Until puberty the undescended testis remains normal, but *after puberty* a *gradually progressive atrophy* with hyaline thickening of the tubular basement membranes, loss of germinal tissue, and interstitial fibrosis occurs. Thus bilateral cryptorchidism in the adolescent or the young adult produces sterility. The undescended testis is roughly 10 times as likely to develop a neoplasm as is the normal scrotal testis.

3. Neoplasms

Neoplasms of the testes cause less than 1 percent of cancer deaths in men, but they are of definite importance because their highest incidence is in the 25 to 34 age group. They are less common in nonwhites than in whites, and they occur with equal frequency in the two testes. Testicular neoplasms are much more common in undescended or ectopic testes than in scrotal testes. *About 95 percent arise from germ (sex) cells of the testes.* The remainder originate in nongerminal elements, such as the interstitial cells and fibrous or vascular stroma. Because of the primitive nature of their cells of origin, the germinal neoplasms, except for the seminoma, are highly malignant. Similar germinal neoplasms occasionally appear in the anterior mediastinum [14]. It is uncertain whether such tumors arise from misplaced multipotential germ cells or represent atypical thymomas.

Clinical features

Clinically a palpable mass develops in a testis. It is painful in embryonal carcinomas, teratomas, and choriocarcinomas. The *Aschheim-Zondek test* is positive in about 15 percent of seminomas and 25 to 30 percent of embryonal carcinomas, teratomas, and choriocarcinomas. In choriocarcinomas, chorionic gonadotropin is produced by the neoplasm, and in the other types it is postulated that testicular destruction leads to an excessive formation of gonadotropin by the anterior pituitary. Studies of the *nuclear sex of the cells in germinal neoplasms* show that about 25 percent of embryonal carcinomas and teratomas are of female nuclear sex [15]. None of the seminomas examined has shown female sex chromatin. These findings indicate that *embryonal carcinomas and teratomas* arise from haploid germ cells by autofertilization and that *seminomas* originate from germ cells before reduction division.

GERMINAL NEOPLASMS: Seminoma:

Seminoma is the least malignant germinal neoplasm of the testes and in its pure form constitutes about 40 percent of such tumors. It occurs most often in the fourth decade of life and is the homologue of the dysgerminoma of the ovaries. Seminoma-like neoplasms also occur in the mediastinum, retroperitoneal region [16], and pineal gland without evidence of testicular origin. The seminoma is not closely related to the other germinal testicular neoplasms, but foci of seminoma are often found in the same testis as one or more of the other neoplasms, often as satellite nodules. In fact, only about 60 percent of germinal testicular neoplasms are purely of one type.

pathologic changes

Grossly the affected testis is partly or completely replaced by a firm, resilient, gray or tan mass with a glistening, bulging cut surface. Foci of coagulation necrosis are common. *Microscopically* the seminoma consists of sheets of polyhedral cells which uniformly measure about 20μ in diameter. Their clear cytoplasm is rich in glycogen. The nuclei are large with prominent nucleoli. Intratubular growth is found in about 25 percent of seminomas. Fibrous trabeculae lobulate the neoplasm, and the *fibrous stroma is typically infiltrated with lymphocytes.* The stroma sometimes shows a granulomatous reaction with the formation of sarcoid-like foci.

metastases

Metastases are most commonly to the periaortic and iliac lymph nodes, liver, and lungs. The left kidney and adrenal gland are much more frequently involved than the right because the lymphatics from the left testis drain to nodes about the left renal vein.

prognosis

The *prognosis* is fair, the 5-year survival rate being about 90 percent. *Seminomas are highly sensitive to radiation.* Those without a lymphoid stroma tend to be more highly malignant than seminomas infiltrated with lymphocytes. When the Aschheim-Zondek test is positive and the interstitial cells of the testis are hyperplastic, the prognosis is relatively poor.

Spermatocytic seminoma

Spermatocytic seminoma [17] is rare and is either a variant of the classic seminoma or a distinct neoplasm. It occurs only in the testes, where it is never associated with a teratoma. The average age of patients with spermatocytic seminoma is 50 years. The *prognosis* is less favorable with this neoplasm than with classic seminoma. *Grossly* spermatocytic seminoma is grayish tan to reddish brown and sometimes hemorrhagic or cystic. *Microscopically* it consists of sheets of polyhedral cells varying from 10 to 20μ in diameter. The smaller cells resemble spermatogonia, and larger forms are like primary spermatocytes. Intratubular growth is frequently seen. The cell sheets are separated by pools of acidophilic fluid representing liquefactive necrosis and fibrous trabeculae. The stroma is not infiltrated by lymphocytes.

Teratoma:

Teratoma in the testis is much more often highly malignant than its ovarian counterpart; the benign cystic teratoma (dermoid cyst), which is the most common form in the ovary, rarely occurs in the male gonad. Testicular teratoma arises from totipotential cells and constitutes about 10 percent of the germinal series. Another 20 percent of these neoplasms consist of a combination of teratoma with embryonal carcinoma and/or choriocarcinoma. Satellite nodules of seminoma may be associated with teratoma in any form. Teratoma is intermediate between the seminoma and embryonal carcinoma in grade of malignancy, the 5-year survival rate being about 70 percent.

pathologic changes

Grossly teratoma typically replaces all the testis, producing a nodularity in the capsule. The cut surface is variegated, showing numerous varisized cystic spaces filled with gelatinous materials, foci of cartilage, bone spicules, and zones of necrosis and hemorrhage. *Microscopically* there is a disorderly panoply of various fetal and adult tissue types from all three germ layers. Organoid differentiation is sometimes discovered. Squamous epithelium (ectoderm), gastrointestinal and respiratory epithelium (entoderm), and cartilage and smooth muscle (mesoderm) are found most frequently.

metastases

Metastases are very commonly found in the periaortic and iliac lymph nodes, liver, and lungs.

Embryonal carcinoma:

Embryonal carcinoma (trophocarcinoma) makes up about 30 percent of germinal neoplasms of the testes. It arises from totipotential germ cells. The *prognosis* is poor in patients with this highly malignant neoplasm, the 5-year survival rate being about 35 percent.

pathologic changes

Grossly the tumor is firm and grayish white with foci of hemorrhagic necrosis. It partly or completely replaces the testis and invades the capsule and surrounding structures. *Microscopically* the *totally undifferentiated type* consists of large, pleomorphic primitive cells in sheets. Numerous mitotic figures are found. A dense fibrous stroma is sometimes present. In the *slightly differentiated type* some of the pleomorphic cells are organized into structures resembling primitive epithelium *(testicular adenocarcinoma).* Some embryonal carcinomas contain *syncytial trophoblastic elements* and/or *embryoid bodies* (which superficially resemble 1- to 2-week embryos). Foci of seminoma are fairly frequently associated with embryonal carcinoma. Usually temporary *spontaneous regression* is common in embryonal carcinomas due to massive necrosis within the neoplasms.

metastases

Metastases are most common in the periaortic and iliac lymph nodes, lungs, liver, and bones.

Chorio-carcinoma:

Choriocarcinoma is rare, making up about 1 percent of germinal neoplasms. It arises from the totipotential germ cells and, like its placental counterpart, is extremely malignant. There have been no 5-year survivals; about 85 percent of the patients die within 2 years after the diagnosis is established.

pathologic changes

Grossly the choriocarcinoma is typically small and replaces only a portion of the affected testis. The neoplasm shows widespread necrosis and hemorrhage with a little viable tissue peripherally. Occasionally metastatic choriocarcinoma, which may be widespread, is detected, only a pigmented scar resulting from spontaneous regression of the primary neoplasm due to infarction being found in a testis. Such scars often contain hematoxylin-staining bodies representing nuclear debris from necrotic neoplastic cells [18]. *Microscopically* there are *cytotrophoblasts* (large uniform cells with a clear cytoplasm and a distinct cell membrane) and *syncytial trophoblasts* (large multinucleated cell masses with a vacuolated cytoplasm). *Chorionic villus-like structures* are present.

metastases

Metastases reach the periaortic and iliac lymph nodes, lungs, and liver in almost every case. Neither the metastases nor the primary neoplasm responds to irradiation.

NONGERMINAL NEOPLASMS:

Nongerminal neoplasms are rare. They are almost always histologically benign and include the interstitial cell tumor, androblastoma, Sertoli cell adenoma, fibroma, neurofibroma, angioma, adenomatoid tumor, and adenocarcinoma of the rete testis. It has been suggested that the androblastoma, Sertoli cell adenoma, and so-called granulosa and theca cell tumors of the testes be grouped together as *specialized gonadal stromal neoplasms* [19]. All are derived from cells of the supporting network for the germinal cells of the testes.

Interstitial cell tumor:

Interstitial cell tumor is *derived from the Leydig cells* and about 85 percent are benign. It is very rare, but cases have occurred in boys. Because the neoplasm often secretes excessive amounts of androgens, *precocious puberty* occurs in boys with this tumor. In about 10 percent of cases of interstitial cell tumor, *gynecomastia* is observed. This paradoxical feminine characteristic may be due to mammary stimulation by large amounts of circulating androgens or to a compensatory rise in estrogens.

pathologic changes

Grossly the interstitial cell tumor is 1 to 10 cm. in diameter, firm, well demarcated from the surrounding testicular tissue, spheroidal, and lobulated. On cut surface it is yellow or brown, homogeneous, and bulgy. *Microscopically* there are sheets of uniform polygonal cells with cytoplasmic lipid vacuoles, pigment granules and rod-shaped *Reinke crystalloids.*

Androblastoma:

Androblastoma (testicular adenoma) is the homologue of the ovarian arrhenoblastoma and arises from immature male gonadal cells. This extremely rare neoplasm is benign, occurs in boys and men, and *occasionally is feminizing,* producing gynecomastia. This is explained by the production of estrogen by Sertoli type cells in the neoplasm.

pathologic changes

Grossly the *mixed or diffuse androblastoma* is usually fairly large (up to 10 cm.), encapsulated, spheroidal, lobulated, and firm, with a yellow parenchyma traversed by grayish white fibrous septa. *Testicular adenoma* occurs as one or more tiny (1 to 5 mm.), spheroidal, yellow nodules within the testis. *Microscopically* three histologic types representing gradations in cell differentiation are recognized. The least differentiated is the *diffuse stromal androblastoma* in which there are small, densely packed spindle or round cells with hyperchromatic nuclei and sparse cytoplasm, resembling the adult ovarian stromal cells. In the *tubular androblastoma* (tubular adenoma) the structure is close to that of the fetal testis, with uniform, interlaced tubular structures lined by cuboidal *Sertoli type cells. Mixed androblastoma* is intermediate in differentiation, showing both stromal and tubular elements. The stroma contains foci of *Leydig-type cells.*

Sertoli cell adenoma

Sertoli cell adenoma, which is well known as a feminizing tumor in dogs, is somewhat controversial in man. Teilum [20] considers estrogen-producing androblastomas as Sertoli cell tumors. In cases of testicular feminization, in which persons with the outward appearance of females are found to have undescended testes and male nuclear sex chromatin in their body cells, Sertoli cell adenomas have been described [21]. These tumors have no discernible endocrine effect. *Grossly* they are discrete, sometimes encapsulated, firm, and light tan, and they may measure up to 25 cm. in greatest diameter. *Microscopically* they consist of tubular structures filled with Sertoli cells. These have a clear cytoplasm and small, darkly staining nuclei. No germ cells are present, but a few interstitial cells are found between the tubules. Both within the tumor and in the adjacent compressed testicular tissue, the tubules have the appearance of the infantile testis.

METASTATIC NEOPLASMS

Metastatic neoplasms [22] are rare, being most often from primary neoplasms in the lungs (bronchogenic carcinoma) and prostate gland. Foci of neoplasm are typically in the interstitial tissue and are surrounded by relatively normal seminiferous tubules.

DISEASES OF THE SCROTUM

Diseases of the scrotum include the following:

1. *Congenital anomalies.* Bifid scrotum with a separate pouch for each testis, cleft scrotum resembling labia majora in pseudohermaphroditism, or rudimentary development in cryptorchidism may occur.

2. *Skin lesions.* These include scabies, pediculosis, syphilids, and, commonly, epidermal inclusion cysts which may be multiple and may calcify (calcifying epithelioma).

3. *Gangrene.* This may result from trauma, gangrenous balanitis, chancroid, or clostridial infection.

4. *Elephantiasis.* This is caused by infestation of the draining lymphatics with *Wuchereria bancrofti.*

5. *Hydrocele.* This is a serous fluid accumulation (100 to 500 ml.) in the sac of the tunica vaginalis testis, the cyst being single or multiloculated.

6. *Hematocele.* This is the presence of blood in the sac of the tunica vaginalis and is usually due to trauma.

7. *Hematoma* within the scrotal wall due to crushing injury or in a hemorrhagic diathesis.

8. *Neoplasms. Epidermoid carcinoma of the scrotal skin* is the most important and the most frequent neoplasm of the scrotum. It was formerly common among chimney sweeps, and still has a high incidence among mule spinners (cotton mill workers) and petroleum and paraffin workers because of the impregnation of their trousers with carcinogenic hydrocarbon compounds. Scrotal cancer usually occurs in men over 50. *Grossly* a verrucous focus appears first; then it fungates and ulcerates. *Microscopically* it is usually fairly well differentiated squamous carcinoma. *Metastases* occur late to the inguinal lymph nodes. The 5-year survival rate is 50 to 70 percent. *Other scrotal neoplasms* include junctional nevus, fibroma, leiomyoma, lipoma, and rhabdomyosarcoma.

REFERENCES

1. Simpson, W. G., and Brown, W. J. Current status of the diagnosis and management of gonorrhea. *J.A.M.A.* 182:63, 1962.
2. Graber, C. D., Scott, R. C., Dunkelberg, W. E., and Dirks, K. R. Isolation of *Neisseria catarrhalis* from three patients with urethritis and a clinical syndrome resembling gonorrhea. *Amer. J. Clin. Path.* 39:360, 1963.
3. Staubitz, W. J., Lent, M. H., and Oberkircher, O. J. Carcinoma of the penis. *Cancer* 8:371, 1955.
4. Reid, J. D. Melanocarcinoma of the penis. *Cancer* 10:359, 1957.
5. Paquin, A. J., Jr., and Roland, S. I. Secondary carcinoma of the penis. *Cancer* 9:626, 1956.
6. Mao, P., Nakao, K., Raif, B., and Geller, J. Human benign prostatic hyperplasia. *Arch. Path.* (Chicago) 79:270, 1965.
7. Halpert, B., Sheehan, E. E., Schmalhorst, W. R., and Scott, R., Jr. Carcinoma of the prostate. A survey of 5000 autopsies. *Cancer* 16:737, 1963.
8. Ende, N., Woods, L. P., and Shelley, H. S. Carcinoma originating in ducts surrounding the prostatic urethra. *Amer. J. Clin. Path.* 40:183, 1963.
9. Franks, L. M. Estrogen-treated prostatic cancer. The variation in responsiveness of tumor cells. *Cancer* 13:490, 1960.
10. Jackson, J. R. The histogenesis of the "adenomatoid" tumor of the genital tract. *Cancer* 11:337, 1958.
11. Henry, W. L., Anderson, M. B., and Hall, A. S. Klinefelter's syndrome. *Med. Ann. D.C.* 28:141, 1959.
12. Lanman, J. T., Sklarin, B. S., Cooper, H. L., and Hirschhorn, K. Klinefelter's syndrome in a ten-month-old mongolian idiot. *New Eng. J. Med.* 263:887, 1960.
13. Lubs, H. A., Jr. Testicular size in Klinefelter's syndrome in men over fifty. *New Eng. J. Med.* 267:326, 1962.

14. Oberman, H. A., and Libcke, J. H. Malignant germinal neoplasms of the mediastinum. *Cancer* 17:498, 1964.
15. Theiss, E. A., Ashley, D. J. B., and Mostofi, F. K. Nuclear sex of testicular tumors and some related ovarian and extragonadal neoplasms. *Cancer* 13:323, 1960.
16. Abell, M. R., Fayos, J. V., and Lampe, I. Retroperitoneal germinomas (seminomas) without evidence of testicular involvement. *Cancer* 18:273, 1965.
17. Scully, R. E. Spermatocytic seminoma of the testis. *Cancer* 14:788, 1961.
18. Azzopardi, J. G., Mostofi, F. K., and Theiss, E. A. Lesions of testes observed in certain patients with widespread choriocarcinoma and related tumors. *Amer. J. Path.* 38:207, 1961.
19. Mostofi, F. K., Theiss, E. A., and Ashley, D. J. B. Tumors of specialized gonadal stroma in human male patients. *Cancer* 12:944, 1959.
20. Teilum, G. Classification of testicular and ovarian androblastoma and Sertoli cell tumors. *Cancer* 11:769, 1958.
21. Neubecker, R. D., and Theiss, E. A. Sertoli cell adenomas in patients with testicular feminization. *Amer. J. Clin. Path.* 38:52, 1962.
22. Price, E. B., Jr., and Mostofi, F. K. Secondary carcinoma of the testis. *Cancer* 10:592, 1957.

GENERAL REFERENCE

Dixon, F. J., Jr., and Moore, R. A. Tumors of the male sex organs. Section VIII, Fascicles 31b and 32, in *Atlas of Tumor Pathology*. Washington: Armed Forces Institute of Pathology, 1952.

24 THE FEMALE GENITAL SYSTEM

GENERAL CONSIDERATIONS – PHYSIOLOGY

The *chief function of the female genital system is reproduction.* In addition, the ovaries elaborate hormones under the influence of the pituitary and other endocrine glands, and these hormones contribute to the *femininity* and *general well-being* of the female.

Birth to puberty

At birth the ovaries are flat ovoid structures about 1.5 by 0.5 by 0.2 cm., and the uterus, consisting chiefly of cervix, is about 3 by 2 by 1 cm. The uterus enlarges progressively from birth to puberty, with the fundus undergoing the most evident changes. The endometrium becomes thickened and soft. The ovaries enlarge irregularly as the follicles mature; at the time of puberty each ovary is about 4 by 3 by 2 cm., and shows numerous "cysts" 1 to 1.5 cm. in diameter on its surface.

Cyclic changes

From the menarche (age 12 to 15) to the menopause (age 40 to 55), the uterus and ovaries are continually changing. Whenever the uterus is not pregnant, it is preparing for pregnancy. Under the influence of the *ovarian follicular hormone,* the endometrium thickens in preparation for the possible implantation of the embryo *(follicular or proliferative phase* of the endometrial cycle). When the follicle ruptures and the ovum starts its journey toward the uterus, the ovarian follicle is converted to the *corpus luteum* and its hormone, progesterone, continues the preparation of the endometrium for pregnancy. The glands of the endometrium become tortuous and their lining cells develop secretory vacuoles; the stroma becomes looser and more vascular *(lutein or secretory phase* of the endometrial cycle). If the ovum is not fertilized within a few days, the corpus luteum regresses, the crest of the hormone wave recedes, and the endometrium is shed (*menstrual phase* of the cycle). Only a thin layer of ragged tissue is left from which a fresh, new membrane must regenerate before the next ovum is ready. The cycle is repeated about every 28 days, except when interrupted by pregnancy.

Pregnancy changes

If the ovum is fertilized, the cycle is replaced by a period of continuous growth. The corpus luteum becomes larger, often being cystic at the center. The lutein phase in the endometrium persists and the stroma becomes progressively more vascular and cellular: the *decidual reaction* of pregnancy. The covering (trophoblastic) cells of the embryo anchor themselves in the soft, spongy, vascular decidua. As the embryo grows, the placenta becomes differentiated, and its cells add their hormone *(chorionic gonadotropin,* "pregnancy hormone") to the pool of hormones. The uterine vessels become greatly enlarged to provide the vascular bed for the placental circulation and for the maternal-fetal interchange of nutrients, waste products, oxygen, growth factors, and the like. The *entire uterus undergoes rapid and progressive growth* as the myometrial fibers increase in length and mass. As the uterus enlarges, it rises out of the pelvis, becomes a palpable abdominal organ, globular and soft, until at term it extends well above the umbilicus.

Post-partum changes

This growth process in the uterus is rapidly reversed, once the baby and placenta are born. After the sudden withdrawal of the placental hormones, the muscle fibers of the myometrium shrink back to normal, the uterine vessels become sclerotic, and the endometrium is shed. With the onset of lactation, the pituitary hormones suppress gonadal activity and the uterus experiences a rest for several months; normally the menstrual cycle is not resumed immediately. The stretched and bruised cervix and vulva gradually recover but are never quite the same after childbirth; the previously smooth contour of the cervix with its central dimple is converted into shallow fissures and scars radiating from the external os.

Menopausal changes

After the menopause and the associated loss of the hormone stimulus, the uterus normally shrinks somewhat. Usually it retains its normal position, but sometimes, because of weakening of the supporting ligaments, it tends to slip into a position of partial prolapse. When this occurs in parous women, the bladder and urethra may be distorted and displaced (cystocele); often the rectum is also affected (rectocele). Because of advances in obstetric practice, these relatively minor *sequelae of childbirth* are less frequent than they once were, and the more serious complications such as rectovaginal and vesicovaginal fistula are rarely seen.

Endocrine disturbances:

It is not surprising that the uterus and ovaries, subject as they are to puberty changes, intense cyclic stimulation, and menopausal influences, should at times fail in these normal responses. Such failure may be manifest by *precocious or delayed puberty, infertility* with or without suppression of the menses *(amenorrhea),* or *menstrual abnormalities at or near the menopause.*

pubertal abnormalities

Precocious uterine development, with periodic bleeding, is sometimes seen in association with neoplasms or hyperplasia of the *adrenal cortex,* or with estrogen-producing neoplasms, chiefly *granulosa cell tumors of the ovary* (see later section of this chapter). Delayed development may be due to *hypothyroidism* or to poorly understood deficiencies of other endocrine organs.

infertility and amenorrhea

Infertility may be due to many factors. In the female it may be due to *failure of ovulation, blockage of the oviducts,* or *faulty development of the endometrium.* Ovulation may be suppressed because of chronic systemic disease, some abnormality of pituitary function, or organic disease of the ovaries. When ovulation does not occur normally, the output of estrogen and progesterone by the ovaries is usually diminished. Lacking the ovarian stimulus to regeneration, the *endometrium becomes atrophic,* showing sparse glands, compact stroma, and thinning of the entire layer, comparable to the changes occurring normally at the menopause; *amenorrhea* is the usual result.

menopausal abnormalities

When a woman approaches the menopause, ovulation normally becomes somewhat irregular, some cycles being *anovulatory.* Usually *menstruation becomes scant,* and occasional periods are missed until finally there is complete cessation of the menses. Less commonly menstrual bleeding may be increased at the menopause. All such cases should be promptly and carefully investigated, since cancer may also cause bleeding at this age, and early recognition of genital cancer is essential if treatment is to be effective. *Functional uterine bleeding* at the menopause is apparently due to hyperestrinism without a balancing amount of progesterone. There is *irregular spotting* between periods or after the regular periods have stopped. Curettage yields thick, firm endometrium which is often polypoid. Microscopic examination shows greatly dilated *cystic endometrial glands* ("Swiss cheese" endometrium), corresponding to an exaggerated proliferative phase of the menstrual cycle. Curettage usually cures such cases.

CONGENITAL ABNORMALITIES

In spite of the complexity of the embryologic development of the female genital tract, *significant anomalies are quite unusual.* In the most extreme of these cases, both the internal and the external genitalia may be affected, often as a result of abnormalities of the fetal endocrine system. More commonly the defect involves one portion of the tract more or less exclusively.

ABNORMALITIES OF VULVA AND VAGINA

Quite rarely the external genitalia may be so abnormal that it is difficult to recognize the infant's sex – *hermaphroditism* or *pseudohermaphroditism* [1]. This may be due to abnormalities of development of the fetal gonads or adrenal glands, or rarely to abnormalities of the maternal endocrine system. The common congenital lesions of the external genitalia are *imperforate hymen* or *abnormalities of the vagina* (absence, atresia, or duplication). Obvious abnormalities are usually noted at birth, but some are not noted until the time of expected menstruation or even later.

ABNORMALITIES OF UTERUS AND CERVIX

Most congenital anomalies of the uterus and cervix are a result of imperfect fusion of the Müllerian ducts. The result may be *septate uterus* (the uterine cavity being divided into two parts by a septum extending downward from the fundus), a *bicornuate uterus* (a distinct portion of the uterine mass projecting laterally on each side), or *double uterus* (uterus didelphys), in which the entire uterus and cervix are duplicated more or less equally, corresponding to the normal pattern in certain lower animals, with or without a *double vagina.* In most instances the uterine deformity is not recognized until pregnancy occurs, when pelvic examination reveals the abnormality. Pregnancy may develop and proceed normally, but complications (abortions, difficult presentations, dystocia, retention of placenta, etc.) occur with much greater frequency than in normal cases.

ABNORMALITIES OF UTERINE TUBES AND OVARIES

Anomalies of the tubes and ovaries are quite uncommon. In rare cases there is failure of formation or development *(agenesis)* of the ovaries, either due to a primary ovarian defect or secondary to a lack of hormone stimulus from the pituitary gland. In either case there is usually a failure of development of the uterus, external genitalia, and breasts due to inadequate hormone stimulus. The infantile uterus, with amenorrhea and infertility, may persist throughout life.

VENEREAL INFECTIONS IN THE FEMALE

The general features of venereal diseases have been discussed in the preceding chapter. It remains only to consider the specific lesions in the female.

SYPHILIS

Rarely is the primary lesion of syphilis in the female evident to the patient on self-examination, and hence it *usually goes undetected.* This lesion (chancre) may develop on the mucosal surfaces of the labia minora, on the fourchette, adjacent to the clitoris, at the urethral meatus, or in any portion of the vagina or external surface of the cervix. The gross features of the chancre in the female are identical with those in the male. Secondary genital syphilids include *mucous patches* and *condylomata lata* on the vulva and in the vagina. These lesions often enlarge appreciably during pregnancy.

GONORRHEA: Initial stages

The initial stages of gonococcal infection in the female usually consist of acute inflammation of the *urethral meatus* and of the mucous glands in the genital area: the *periurethral* (Skene's) *glands, vulvovaginal* (Bartholin's) *glands,* and the *cervical glands.* There are usually a purulent exudate in the vagina and marked edema and reddening of the mucosa, with pouting of the external os of the cervix. Infection of Bartholin's glands may go on to abscess formation (Bartholin abscess), or the infection may subside, to be followed by stricture of the ducts and, at a later date, cyst formation (Bartholin cyst). In most cases the infection apparently subsides spontaneously or as a result of therapy.

Salpingitis and tubo-ovarian abscess

Salpingitis (inflammation of the uterine tube) is the most important genital complication of acute gonococcal infection in the female. The organisms are believed to traverse the uterine cavity, producing little or no effect upon the endometrium, but inciting an acute inflammation of the mucosa of both uterine tubes. At first the tubes are swollen and hyperemic, and the lateral ends leak a small amount of exudate into the peritoneal cavity, causing *pelvic peritonitis.* Later the fimbriae are agglutinated by fibrin deposits, the tubes become closed at both ends, and a purulent exudate accumulates in the lumen, giving the "pus tube," or *pyosalpinx.* If salpingitis develops at about the time of ovulation, the gonococcus may infect the open lesion on the surface of the ovary, the fimbriae of the tube surrounding the follicle so that tube and ovary become involved together, causing *salpingo-oophoritis (tubo-ovarian abscess).* During the acute phase of the tubal infection, the patient is acutely ill, with fever, vomiting, and bilateral lower abdominal pain. Pelvic examination usually reveals an extremely tender mass on each side of the uterus. Symptoms subside slowly over a few days as the organisms die out in the tubal sacs.

Sequelae

With time the exudate slowly changes character until it becomes serous *(hydrosalpinx).* Often there are several acute exacerbations of the tubal infection, eventually followed by *dense pelvic adhesions.* The adhesions may cause periodic attacks of *partial intestinal obstruction.* Frequently they interfere with follicle development and ovulation, resulting in *painful, irregular menstrual periods,* and *infertility.* In those patients in whom ovulation continues, the tubal disease will often interfere with the migration of the fertilized ovum, resulting in *ectopic pregnancy.*

Extragenital complications

Systemic complications may also occur with gonococcal infections. These include *septic arthritis, bacterial endocarditis,* and *gonorrheal ophthalmia;* they have been discussed in the preceding chapter.

CHANCROID

In women the *painful ulcerative lesions* of chancroid may occur on any portion of the external genitalia; the infection may spread to the *inguinal lymph nodes,* causing suppuration (abscesses) there, as in the male. Involvement of the uterus and adnexa uteri apparently does not occur.

LYMPHOGRANULOMA VENEREUM

The primary lesion of lymphogranuloma in the female is seen as a *small ulcerated lesion on the vulva,* followed by *inguinal adenitis,* with or without suppuration (bubo). In the female, *rectal stricture* is an important sequela of *lymphopathia* of the vulva. Its occurrence is usually ascribed to the fact that the lymphatics of the lower portion of the vulva tend to drain into the lymph nodes of the deep pelvis, which also receive the lymphatics from the rectum. The inflammatory reaction in *lymphopathia* is a *chronic suppurative and granulomatous* one somewhat akin to that in tuberculosis.

GRANULOMA INGUINALE

Granuloma inguinale is characterized by *chronic granulating ulcers* of the vulva, groin, and perineum. These ulcers heal slowly and are associated with much scarring. The lesions have been described in Chapter 23.

TUBERCULOSIS OF THE FEMALE GENITALIA

Salpingitis

When tuberculosis affects the female genital tract, it is the uterine tubes that are most commonly involved. In most instances the tubes are affected during the course of hematogenous dissemination from a primary site in the thorax. Tubercles appear first in the mucosa as *granulomatous and caseous foci,* later spreading to involve the entire wall. The infection often extends along the lumen of the tubes, so that bacilli may be disseminated throughout the *peritoneal cavity.* Clinically there often are no symptoms directly referable to the tubes. The abdomen is usually tense and shows *signs of free fluid.* The patient is usually chronically ill. If operation is done, the nature of the condition can usually be recognized grossly: tiny yellowish gray tubercles cover the peritoneal surface, and are especially evident over the serosa and fimbriae of the tubes.

Endometritis

Tuberculous endometritis results by extension from tubal infection and, rarely, from direct hematogenous spread. Small tubercles appear in the stroma, caseation being absent or slight. The condition is usually diagnosed on the basis of histologic examination of curettings. In some patients, indication for curettage has been vaginal bleeding; in others, infertility.

DISEASES OF THE VULVA AND VAGINA

1. Acute Nonvenereal Inflammation

The vulva and vagina may be affected by a wide variety of bacterial, fungus, and protozoan diseases. *Bacterial infections* are usually related to uncleanliness and scratching, or to widespread skin infections, as furunculosis.

Thrush

Fungus infections, often due to *Candida albicans* which causes thrush, tend to occur in diabetic women receiving antibiotic therapy for some infection; there is usually a thick, cheesy exudate containing spores and hyphae.

Trichomonas vaginitis

Trichomonas vaginalis, a protozoan parasite, is a common cause of *vaginitis* and *cervicitis,* manifest by a copious purulent vaginal discharge. The organism is a flagellate, readily recognized by its rapid motion in carefully handled moist preparations of the vaginal exudate.

Skin diseases

The vulva may also be affected in a variety of skin diseases such as *lichen planus, psoriasis,* and *contact dermatitis;* clinically these diseases are usually manifest by itching and burning.

2. *Changes With Aging*

Kraurosis vulvae

With aging the vulvar and vaginal tissues tend to shrink and atrophy. In the usual form, kraurosis vulvae, there is *degeneration of the fibrous and elastic tissue of the dermis* of the vulva and *thinning of the epidermis* with reduction in hair follicles and sebaceous glands. Grossly the skin of the vulva becomes thin, dry, and shiny. These changes are usually greatly accentuated if x-ray therapy has been employed over the vulva. The vagina may share in these atrophic changes, so that the introitus is narrowed (senile vaginitis) and intercourse is painful (dyspareunia).

Leukoplakia

In other aging women there are irregular *white areas* of induration in the skin and mucosa of the vulva, often *with scaling and fissuring. Microscopically* there is a thickening of the keratinized layer of the epidermis; often a marked prolongation of the rete pegs into the dermis may be seen. Many lymphocytes and monocytes are evident in the connective tissues of the superficial dermis. It is uncertain whether leukoplakial vulvitis is a later stage of kraurosis or a separate process of different cause. Patients showing leukoplakia must be studied closely, since there is a strong *tendency for epidermoid carcinoma* to develop in these lesions.

3. *Neoplasms of the Vulva*

Benign neoplasms

The usual *benign* skin neoplasms *(squamous papilloma, nevus, lipoma, neurofibroma,* and *hemangioma)* occur occasionally in the vulva. The *condylomata,* either flat or papillary, are apparently inflammatory hyperplasias, and not true neoplasms. The *hidradenoma* is a neoplasm of the vulva which rarely occurs on other skin surfaces. It originates from the epithelium of the apocrine sweat glands and grows as a discrete nodule, about 1 cm. in diameter, usually on the labia majora. Microscopically it is a cystic structure, usually filled with a papillary growth covered with columnar epithelium.

Malignant neoplasms: epidermoid carcinoma

The most common *malignant* neoplasm of the vulva is the *epidermoid carcinoma.* It is largely a disease of elderly women. In about half the cases some chronic inflammatory lesion, chiefly leukoplakial vulvitis, precedes the development of vulvar carcinoma. The first stage of vulvar cancer is sometimes noted as carcinoma in situ; when it occurs in skin surfaces, it is commonly known as *Bowen's disease.* Vulvar cancer usually begins as a small nodule on the labia, gradually enlarging and often ulcerating. It may *infiltrate extensively* in the external genitalia and *spread to the inguinal lymph nodes;* more distant metastasis is somewhat unusual. *Microscopically* the changes are characteristic of *invasive squamous cell cancer,* usually of medium-grade malignancy. In a number of cases of vulvar or perineal cancer studied in the George Washington University Hospital [2], carcinoma of the cervix also developed, either simultaneously or some time later. This phenomenon has been considered by Newman to be an example of multicentric field cancerization.

melanoma

Melanoma is the second most important malignant neoplasm of the female external genitalia. In some instances it arises in *preexisting nevi,* in others it appears to develop directly from the *heavily pigmented skin* of the area. The labia majora are the most common site, but the tumor may arise in the labia minora, clitoris, vestibule of the vagina, and also in the perineal and perianal skin. These lesions usually cannot be seen by the patient and may be first manifest by itching or occasionally hemorrhage after the neoplasm is well established.

Metastases occur early in the inguinal lymph nodes and by the bloodstream. The microscopic features of the neoplasm are like those of skin melanomas generally (see Chapter 29).

Paget's disease

Rarely a lesion comparable to *Paget's disease* of the nipple is seen in the vulva, often in association with a deeper adenocarcinoma of the vulva arising presumably from the apocrine sweat glands. The microscopic features are identical with those of the breast lesion (see Chapter 25).

4. Neoplasms and Cysts of the Vagina

Neoplasms

Primary neoplasms of the vagina are rare, but secondary neoplasms are quite common, usually a result of direct extension from carcinoma of the cervix. *Epidermoid carcinoma* is the most frequent primary malignant tumor of the vagina. It begins as a flat nodule in the mucosa of any portion, extends into the deeper tissues, and metastasizes to the regional lymph nodes. *Sarcoma botryoides* is a very rare embryonal sarcoma occurring chiefly in infants and young girls. It arises either from the vaginal surface of the cervix or from the vagina proper, bulging into the vagina in the form of multiple edematous grapelike masses.

Cysts

Cysts of the vagina are somewhat more common. Most large cysts – 2 cm. or more in diameter – are believed to derive from incomplete closure of *Gartner's duct* from embryonic life. They usually lie anterolaterally in the wall of the vagina, or in the vulva or broad ligament. Microscopically the Gartner's duct cysts are usually lined with a single layer of columnar epithelium. Small epidermal *inclusion cysts* may occur in any portion of the vaginal wall.

DISEASES OF THE CERVIX UTERI

1. Inflammatory Processes

Chronic cervicitis

Infections constitute an important segment of the diseases of the cervix. These may be acute and of specific origin, due to *Neisseria gonorrhoeae* or a streptococcus, but *chronic nonspecific cervicitis is much more common.* Sometimes chronic cervicitis is a sequel of acute cervicitis of pyogenic origin; more commonly it seems to be a result of laceration and low-grade infection following childbirth. The patient usually complains of a thin, mucoid *vaginal discharge,* often accentuated after the menstrual period, and sometimes of a low backache. Speculum examination reveals a *fissured, asymmetrical* cervix, with irregular areas of superficial mucosal erosion alternating with white hyaline patches of leukoplakia. Small *submucosal cysts* (Nabothian cysts) are common, due to distention of the mucous glands following blockage of their ducts. *Cervical polyps* are frequently seen in association with chronic cervicitis; they have no special tendency to become neoplastic.

Cervicitis and cancer

Chronic cervicitis may be clinically indistinguishable from cervical cancer. Vaginal smears and *cervical biopsy* are usually done before treating a case of cervicitis. *Schiller's test* may also be used. In this test a weak iodine solution is painted over the cervical mucosa; the areas of intact epithelium stain brown because of their glycogen content, while eroded areas remain pink and unstained. This procedure was thought at one time to be useful for the recognition of cancer of the cervix, but the test is not specific for cancer. It will, however, help to delineate areas from which biopsy should be taken. Of greater value is the examination of vaginal smears stained by the Papanicolaou technique. *This procedure should be a part of the periodic health examination in all women,* since *it serves to detect cervical cancer before symptoms have occurred, at a time when the disease is curable.* Atypical cells can be detected by this screening method. Since atypical cells may sometimes occur in healing erosions, *biopsy* is necessary for confirmation.

2. Carcinoma

Importance

The *most important disease of the uterine cervix is cancer;* carcinoma of the cervix is second in frequency only to breast cancer among the neoplasms causing cancer deaths in females in the United States. The *common cell type is epidermoid carcinoma;* this is meant when the term *cervical cancer* is used without qualification.

EPIDERMOID CARCINOMA: Cause

Cervical cancer is rare in nulliparas, occurring chiefly in women who have had many pregnancies, and especially in those having pregnancies early in life. It is especially common in low income groups. The neoplasm is extremely rare in virgins and in the marital partners of males circumcised in infancy. Type 2 herpes virus may be related to the development of cervical carcinoma [3]. An increased incidence of both in situ and invasive carcinoma is found in women with genital herpes.

Natural history: stage 0

Cervical cancer usually begins at or near the squamocolumnar junction of the external orifice of the cervix; occasionally it arises within the cervical canal. At first (stage 0) the neoplastic changes are confined to the surface epithelium and consist of *loss of the regular cell layers* and *replacement of normal cells* by cells having large nuclei and nucleoli, with scant cytoplasm, and showing frequent mitotic figures. During this stage or phase of development *(carcinoma in situ, intra-epithelial* or *preinvasive carcinoma)* there are *usually no symptoms,* although there may be slight intermenstrual spotting. A superficial erosion may be evident on speculum examination, but grossly there is no tumor or other distinctive features. *This stage can be diagnosed only by biopsy,* although it may be suspected on the basis of cytologic examination of vaginal secretions. During this stage the tumor is generally curable by hysterectomy, and perhaps even by lesser procedures.

stage I

After a long period of surface growth, apparently lasting 8 to 10 years, the malignant cells penetrate the basement membrane and infiltrate the submucosa, forming a *flat, nodular,* often *ulcerated* lesion which has a *granular base* and *bleeds* easily on manipulation. At this stage the patient may note some *intermenstrual* (or postmenopausal) *bleeding* and there may be some vaginal *discharge* – warning signs of cancer! Speculum examination by the physician may reveal a suspicious lesion, but during stage I – when the process is confined to the cervix (usually to one lip and at the external orifice) – the appearance is usually indistinguishable from benign ulcerative lesions grossly. Hysterectomy will usually effect a cure during stage I.

stage II

After stage I the spread of the neoplasm is relatively rapid. The cells infiltrate between the muscle bundles of the cervix to reach the *parametrium,* and within the mucosa to involve the *entire surface of the cervix and the upper portion of the vagina. Bleeding, discharge,* and *pain* are usually evident at this stage. On speculum examination the lesion is seen to involve *most of the vaginal portion of the cervix;* the surface of the neoplasm is usually *granular and bulging,* and is irregularly *ulcerated.* This stage can usually be recognized clinically if the speculum examination is combined with vaginal-abdominal examination; on the latter the *parametrial tissues are indurated* as a result of the extension of the neoplasm.

stage III

In stage III the ulcerating, fungating lesion extends downward to involve the *lower third of the vagina,* and laterally in the parametrium to reach the *pelvic walls.* On bimanual examination, all the tissues of the pelvis are indurated and fixed – the *frozen pelvis* of advanced cervical cancer. General symptoms such as *weakness* and *weight loss* are generally added to the local symptoms during this stage. Obviously surgical treatment is less likely to be successful at this stage than in the preceding ones.

stage IV

The final phase, stage IV, is reached when the neoplastic cells have extended locally to involve the *bladder and rectum,* have penetrated lymphatic channels to reach the *pelvic lymph nodes,* or have set up *metastases in distant organs. Vesicovaginal or rectovaginal fistula* may develop during this phase. Especially important is the tendency to infiltrate the lymphatics surrounding the lower portion of the ureters, resulting in *blockage of the urinary tract* and *hydronephrosis: urinary tract infection and uremia are the usual terminal events in cervical cancer.* Edema of one or both extremities is also common as a result of neoplastic invasion of pelvic lymphatics and veins.

Clinical application of staging

The stages of cervical cancer are more than mileposts in the course of the disease; they are the *chief basis for prognosis and therapy.* If the diagnosis of cervical cancer is made during stage 0 or stage I, and if proper therapy (radiation or surgery) is begun promptly, cure will be obtained in well over half the cases. If the disease has progressed to stage III or IV before therapy is started, the chance of cure is small; even when such patients are cured of cancer, most remain invalids because of the necessary extent of surgery or because of the side effects of irradiation. At present most patients with cervical cancer in stage 0 or stage I in the George Washington University Hospital are treated by surgery, and most patients with stage III or IV are treated by irradiation. The management of stage II is somewhat variable. The stage is not only a guide to prognosis and therapy in the individual patient, it also permits the *evaluation of new methods of treatment and the comparison of new and old methods.* For all these reasons the clinical gynecologist evaluates each case of cervical cancer carefully before beginning treatment, and records his estimate of the stage.

CERVICAL STUMP CANCER

The modern gynecologist insists that if there is indication for the surgical removal of the uterus, the entire organ, including the cervix, should be taken unless there is a specific contraindication of doing so. It was once considered good practice to leave the cervix behind when hysterectomy was done for leiomyomas, for the technical reason that the cervix provided better closure of the vaginal vault and better support for the other pelvic organs than could be obtained after its removal. It was found, however, that *carcinoma* occurred in the *cervical stump* more often than would have been expected under ordinary circumstances. It was the usual type of cervical cancer – epidermoid carcinoma. Why did it happen? It is generally believed that many of these patients had cancer of the cervix from the start, but because leiomyomas of the fundus were also present, attention was directed at the large abnormality to explain genital bleeding, the physician overlooking what may have been a minimal or in situ malignant neoplasm. Later, then, the cervical carcinoma became apparent in the cervical stump. (The authors have, on several occasions, found unsuspected cervical cancer in a uterus removed for leiomyomas.)

ADENOCARCINOMA

The *adenocarcinoma* of the cervix, arising from cervical glands, is much rarer than epidermoid carcinoma. Because of its location *within the cervical canal* it may cause uterine bleeding for some time before the growth is evident on speculum examination of the cervix. Cervical curettage is the usual method of diagnosis. The course of adenocarcinoma of the cervix is similar to that of epidermoid carcinoma. Local extension to the lower urinary tract is usual during the terminal phase.

3. Other Neoplasms

There are no other common neoplasms of the cervix. *Leiomyomas* and *leiomyosarcomas* of the uterus may occur at the cervical os, but they are essentially neoplasms of the fundus of the uterus rather than the cervix. *Cervical polyps* may cause genital bleeding and be confused with carcinoma, but generally they are of inflammatory rather than neoplastic origin. *Sarcoma botryoides* is a very rare tumor of the cervix and vagina, occurring principally in young children.

DISEASES OF THE FUNDUS UTERI

1. Inflammatory Processes

Infection of the uterus is relatively uncommon except as a complication of pregnancy. Rarely following spontaneous abortion or delivery at term, but commonly following *criminal abortions,* streptococcal and mixed bacterial infections of the uterus occur. Under such circumstances bacteria may be introduced into the pregnant uterus on a pencil, piece of wire, or dirty surgical instrument by an unskilled person, lacerating the tissues as the object is introduced blindly. The bacteria multiply in the endometrium, penetrate the uterine walls and vascular sinuses, and cause *pyometria, peritonitis, pyemia,* and *septic infarcts* of the lungs. A comparable situation occurs very rarely following long difficult labor at term. Clinically a foul-smelling bloody discharge (lochia) and chills, fever, and other systemic symptoms are usually noted.

2. Benign Neoplasms

LEIOMYOMA:

The *most common of all neoplasms in the female* is the *leiomyoma (fibromyoma, fibroid, myoma) of the uterus.* It is the benign neoplasm which arises from the smooth muscle cells of the myometrium. This neoplasm first appears during active sex life, grows during pregnancy, and regresses after the menopause. This tumor is especially common in Negroes. It is generally believed to be related to hyperestrinism; comparable tumors have been produced in animals by giving them excess estrogen.

Site

Leiomyomas are *often multiple.* They may occur in any part of the uterus, but are most frequent in the body of the uterus. All begin as *interstitial* or *intramural* tumors, and many remain so. As they grow, some, especially the largest tumors, bulge from the peritoneal surface and become *subserous.* Others project into the uterine cavity as rounded polypoid *submucous* growths. Some cause a symmetric enlargement of the uterus and *may be confused with pregnancy.* Occasionally a submucous leiomyoma may be extruded from the cervix (aborting fibroid) and cause eversion of the uterus.

Gross appearance

Leiomyomas are *well-encapsulated, white nodules,* having a watered-silk appearance on cut section. They may compress their blood supply, causing infarction (red degeneration), especially during pregnancy. After the menopause or after infarction, they may undergo cystic or hyaline changes, often followed by dystrophic calcification.

Microscopic appearance

The usual microscopic appearance is that of *bundles of normal-appearing smooth muscle fibers* running in all directions. The normal pattern of the myometrium is reproduced exactly; in fact, it may be impossible to recognize the neoplasm microscopically unless its capsule is shown in the section. Variable amounts of fibrous tissue may intertwine with the muscle fibers, especially in older women.

Clinical features

These neoplasms, when they occur in younger women, may *interfere with placental implantation,* causing infertility, abortions, or fetal death; they may also cause fetal malposition or may obstruct the passage of the fetus through the birth canal. In older women this neoplasm commonly causes *menorrhagia, metrorrhagia,* and *pressure symptoms* such as back pain, need for frequent urination, and a feeling of fullness in the rectum. Usually symptoms begin before the menopause; after the menopause these neoplasms usually cease to grow.

Malignant changes

In the great majority of cases, leiomyomas *remain benign* throughout their course. Perhaps as many as 2 percent become malignant in later life. (See Leiomyosarcoma, page 636.)

ADENOMYOMA

Adenomyoma of the uterus, also known as *endometriosis interna* or *uterine endometriosis,* is a benign tumor, occurring chiefly in the anterior or posterior uterine wall. *Clinically* it is manifest by dysmenorrhea, bleeding, and uterine enlargement. *Grossly* it is not encapsulated, and may be easily overlooked; sometimes it is recognized only because the uterine wall shows a local area of thickening. *Microscopically* there are deep nests of endometrial stroma and glands, separated by uterine muscle. Adenomyosis of the uterus is often associated with parametrial or ovarian endometriosis and is similarly under ovarian hormone influence. (See Endometriosis, page 641.)

3. Adenocarcinoma of the Endometrium

The *most common malignant neoplasm of the fundus* or body of the uterus, and the second most common malignant neoplasm of the uterus as a whole, is the *adenocarcinoma of the endometrium,* also known as *adenocarcinoma of the uterus, endometrial carcinoma, carcinoma of the body of the uterus,* and *fundus* or *corpus cancer.* The patient with endometrial carcinoma is generally first seen at about age 55 to 60, and her usual symptom is irregular vaginal bleeding. Nulliparas are commonly affected. Obese women and women who have hypertension and diabetes mellitus are especially prone to endometrial cancer. The neoplasm is generally believed due to *hyperestrinism;* sometimes it develops during the course of prolonged estrogen therapy.

Natural history

The cell alteration occurs first in a group of endometrial glands, the cells of which become enlarged, their nuclei being large and hyperchromatic, their cytoplasm clear and pale. As these cells multiply, they bud into the gland spaces and exfoliate into the endometrial cavity; routine vaginal smears taken at this time may show the atypical cells. Later the neoplastic cells penetrate their basement membranes and invade the endometrial stroma, forming small new glands lined with atypical epithelium. In time a thickening of the endometrium develops in this area, often bulging into the uterine cavity as a polyp. The polyp is soft, friable, and vascular; if the patient presents herself at the time of the first irregular bleeding, the neoplastic process may be confined to this polypoid mass, readily curable by hysterectomy. If either the patient or the physician temporizes, the neoplastic cells will spread to other portions of the endometrium and will invade the myometrium along lymphatic channels and tissue spaces. Even at this stage, cure is possible, because *endometrial carcinoma grows relatively slowly* – much more slowly on the average than epidermoid carcinoma of the cervix. In its late stages the neoplastic cells will penetrate to the serosa and seed over the pelvic peritoneum to the pelvic and retroperitoneal lymph nodes, and to the submucosa of the urinary bladder, rectum, and ureters. Vesicovaginal or rectovaginal fistula, urinary tract obstruction and infection, uremia, and peritonitis are the terminal findings in progressive cases.

"Atypical" hyperplasia of endometrium

Occasionally in younger women seen because of excessive menstrual bleeding (menorrhagia), curettage yields abundant soft polypoid tissue, and microscopic examination shows the glands lined by a regular row of large pale cells whose nuclei are somewhat hyperchromatic but lack the more definite features of cancer. Some of the glands may show papillary masses budding into their lumina. This is *"atypical" ("adenomatous") hyperplasia,* shown by Hertig and Sommers [4] to be *precancerous* or even carcinoma in situ. Bleeding is apt to recur in this type of case, the epithelium becoming progressively more atypical, until finally frank invasive endometrial cancer is evident.

4. *Other Malignant Neoplasms*

LEIOMYOSARCOMA

Leiomyosarcoma, the malignant neoplasm arising *from smooth muscle cells,* is the second most frequent cancer of the fundus of the uterus. It is usually thought to arise in a benign leiomyoma, but undoubtedly this neoplasm may also develop directly from the normal myometrium. It is a rather rapidly growing tumor, softer and more brainlike than its benign counterpart, and is prone to hemorrhage and necrosis. Beginning usually as an intramural or submucous uterine nodule in a woman near the menopause, it may cause *abnormal uterine bleeding* as an early symptom. Vaginal examination usually reveals one or more palpable masses in the uterus. Depending on the patient's age, desire for children, etc., the uterus may or may not be removed. If removed at this stage, it is usually with the diagnosis of fibroids; often the first suspicion of the presence of a leiomyosarcoma is the pathologist's report after removal of a uterus believed to contain benign leiomyomas. Under these circumstances, the patient is usually cured. If surgery is postponed, the patient will note a relatively rapid progression of symptoms: enlarging mass, increasing uterine hemorrhage, back pain, and weight loss. When this exaggeration of symptoms occurs *after the menopause,* one should suspect that the tumor is malignant. This tumor, if untreated, tends to invade veins and metastasize to distant organs (lungs, liver) as well as to spread locally to the peritoneum and contiguous organs.

OTHERS

Other malignant tumors of the uterus are relatively rare. The *mixed mesodermal tumor* of the uterus, also known as *carcinosarcoma,* has increased in frequency in recent years, according to the authors' experience. This neoplasm is composed of epithelial and connective tissue elements, either or both of which may be malignant. Cartilage, striated muscle, and other connective tissues may be represented. In some instances this tumor has developed years after radium or x-ray irradiation for benign conditions [5]. The *endometrial sarcoma* is a rare, spindle cell neoplasm thought to arise from the stromal cells of the endometrium. *Choriocarcinoma,* the rare, highly malignant neoplasm arising from the fetal trophoblast and invading the uterus, has already been considered (see Chapter 15).

DISEASES OF THE OVARIES

1. Normal Cyclic Changes

Since the normal cyclic variations in the ovaries are often confused with pathologic lesions, it is very important to review the normal anatomy of the ovaries. The adult ovaries are ovoid, about 4 cm. in maximum diameter, and during the reproductive period of life *their surfaces are covered with bulging "cysts,"* the largest generally about 1.5 cm. in diameter. *If an ovary has no "cysts" during the period of active sex life, it is distinctly abnormal.* Normal follicles contain a clear watery fluid and have a thin pale lining. The normal corpus luteum is golden yellow and soft, and usually has a cystic cavity filled with fibrin or clotted blood; with regression the corpus luteum becomes smaller, loses its yellow color, and eventually is represented by a firm white scar, the corpus albicans. If an ovary is seen shortly after the time of ovulation, an open defect, containing fibrin or blood clot, will mark the site of the recently ruptured follicle. After the menopause these normal "cysts" gradually become smaller and disappear and the ovaries become progressively smaller and more sclerotic.

2. Oophoritis

Gonococcal oophoritis

Inflammation of the ovaries is relatively uncommon. The *gonococcus* may infect the open lesion on the surface of an ovary which follows follicle rupture, the infection reaching the ovary via an infected uterine tube. Adhesions form between the fimbriae of the tube and the ovary, and the two structures fuse into a retort-shaped mass filled with pus – the *tubo-ovarian abscess* (see page 628).

Other forms

Rarely other pyogenic bacteria may infect the ovaries during the course of *puerperal sepsis.* Nonpyogenic oophoritis is quite rare, but occurs sometimes during the course of mumps.

3. Simple Cysts

"Simple" cysts of the ovary are those related to the normal cyclic changes; most other cysts are actually cystic neoplasms. The dividing line between *normal* follicles and corpora lutea on the one hand and *cystic* follicles and corpora on the other is not sharply drawn; the cysts are usually larger than the normal structures.

Follicle cysts

Follicular cysts are usually multiple and are located just beneath the ovarian capsule. Perhaps an abnormal thickness of the capsule prevents normal rupture of the follicles, which continue to enlarge until their lining cells become atrophic. Rarely hyperestrinism may result, giving the *Stein-Leventhal syndrome:* menstrual irregularity, variable masculinization, and infertility. More commonly there are no symptoms.

Lutein cysts

Lutein cysts represent changes in the corpus luteum. Perhaps incomplete luteinization of the cells lining the follicle, or excessive hemorrhage into the follicle, prevents the normal fading of the corpus luteum to the corpus albicans. No definite symptoms are attributed to lutein cysts.

4. Cystic Neoplasms

PSEUDOMUCINOUS CYSTADENOMA

The *multilocular or pseudomucinous cystadenomas of the ovary* are generally believed to arise as the result of one-sided development of an ovarian teratoma. *Grossly* they are usually unilateral, multilocular, thin-walled, and translucent. On section they contain *viscid mucoid fluid,* usually clear or whitish, collected in many separate cysts having common walls. They may become very large: the record is 328 pounds [6]! *Microscopically* the cysts are lined with a single layer of tall columnar epithelial cells having basal nuclei and mucin droplets in their cytoplasm. Clinically such a cyst is usually evident as a *slowly growing mass,* crowding other structures. Rarely it may rupture, causing pseudomyxoma peritonei. Occasionally it may become twisted on its pedicle, causing venous strangulation and symptoms of an acute abdominal emergency. In about 5 percent of the cases the lining cells take on malignant characteristics (see Cystadenocarcinoma, below).

PAPILLARY CYSTADENOMA: Pathologic changes

The *papillary or serous cystadenoma* probably arises by invagination of the covering epithelium of the ovary, but some believe this tumor begins in the uterine tube and involves the ovary secondarily. *Grossly* this tumor may be unilocular or multilocular, is frequently bilateral, and is usually 5 to 15 cm. in size. It contains *watery (serous) fluid* and the lining shows numerous soft, granular *papillary projections. Microscopically* these cysts are lined with cuboidal, sometimes ciliated, epithelium, and the papillae are similarly covered. The lining cells contain no mucin. Small calcified deposits (psammoma bodies) may occur in the papillae.

Clinical features

Clinically the papillary cystadenoma is usually first evident as a simple *mass,* compressing adjacent structures. Later the papillae tend to penetrate the cyst wall and project from the serosal surface. They may then *implant* over the peritoneal surface, causing widespread involvement of the *pelvic peritoneum* with *adhesions* and *ascites.* The cyst fluid often contains viable tumor cells; for this reason the gynecologist is very careful not to spill the contents of the cyst during the course of its removal. This neoplasm must be regarded as *potentially malignant* from the beginning. The common form of ovarian cancer, the cystadenocarcinoma, usually develops from this neoplastic cyst.

CYSTADENOCARCINOMA

Cystadenocarcinoma of the ovary is the *most common form of ovarian cancer;* it accounts for nearly 5 percent of all female cancer deaths in the United States. In most instances it *arises from the papillary cystadenoma.* This neoplasm is characterized by extensive *spread throughout the pelvis,* so that tubes, ovaries, uterus, and intestines are densely matted. At this stage any attempt at surgical removal is hopeless. Recurrent ascites and chronic intestinal obstruction lead to a state of profound cachexia. Distant metastasis may or may not occur. *Papillae,* covered with neoplastic epithelium, are the hallmark of this neoplasm;

they can be found free in the peritoneal fluid, and in the metastases in lungs or lymph nodes.

TERATOMAS:

The *teratoid tumor* of the ovaries may be *either solid or cystic.* The most common form is cystic and consists largely of dermal elements, hence the common name, *dermoid cyst of the ovary.*

Origin

There are many theories as to the origin of this cystic neoplasm; the two most popular are: (1) that these tumors are distorted fetuses, either included twins or formed as parthenogenetic offspring of the bearer's own ova, and (2) that they represent "areas of tissue which during early embryonic development escaped from the action of the primary organizer," as suggested by Willis [7].

Pathologic changes

The common dermoid cyst contains fatty material which tends to solidify at room temperature; this material is believed to be the *secretion of the sebaceous glands* in the wall of the cyst. The cyst wall usually shows a small mass bulging into the cavity, covered with skinlike epithelium from which hair arises and projects into the cavity. Near this bulging dermal mass the cyst often shows a thickening of the wall; teeth, cartilage, and bone can frequently be identified in this tissue. *Microscopically* a number of *other well-differentiated but totally unorganized tissues* can be made out, such as respiratory tract epithelium, thyroid tissue, gastric mucosa, salivary glands, dermal glands, neural tissue, and retina.

Clinical features

Usually these neoplasms are first recognized during *young adult life* (20 to 35 years) but sometimes they are evident in infancy. Symptoms are usually a result of *pressure* from the slowly expanding mass; at times dermoid cysts interfere with pregnancy or labor. The *cystic teratomas are seldom malignant; solid teratomas may be quite malignant,* as either a mixed malignant neoplasm or malignant in some one tissue, usually epidermoid carcinoma. Sometimes choriocarcinoma develops, but this is less common in the ovarian than in the testicular teratomas.

5. Solid Neoplasms

The two important *benign solid neoplasms of the ovaries* are the fibroma and the Brenner tumor; most other solid ovarian neoplasms are malignant, or at least potentially so.

FIBROMA

The *fibroma* is a common solid tumor of an ovary, often resembling a leiomyoma in gross appearance. Usually it is only a few centimeters in size, but sometimes it grows to be quite large. Occasionally, for unknown reasons, ascites and hydrothorax occur in association with a fibroma of an ovary *(Meigs' syndrome).* More commonly the fibroma is an incidental finding in an ovary removed for some other reason.

BRENNER TUMOR

The *Brenner tumor* is a firm, yellow neoplasm, thought to be derived from Walthard inclusions in the ovarian cortex. *Microscopically* it shows epithelial cell rests, sometimes solid, sometimes glandular, embedded in dense fibrous tissue. It has no endocrine effects and is almost uniformly benign.

PRIMARY CARCINOMA

Most ovarian carcinomas are cystic, but a few are solid and composed of sheets of undifferentiated cells, the so-called *medullary carcinomas* of the ovary. Others form well-defined glands which lie in a fibrous stroma; such neoplasms, perhaps derived from endometrial implants or from embryonal cell rests, are generally termed simply *adenocarcinomas.* They spread locally to the pelvic organs, and metastasize by lymphatic and hematogenous routes. Solid tumors containing cells of more than one type have already been considered under Teratomas (see page 639).

SECONDARY CARCINOMA

Secondary neoplasms of the ovaries are quite common, and are often bilateral. Whenever a patient shows bilateral, solid ovarian masses, the possibility that they are metastatic neoplasms should be considered. The primary growth is usually located in the *stomach, colon,* or *uterus.* A special form, known as the *Krukenberg tumor* of the ovary, is metastatic from the stomach, or rarely the colon, and shows a particular microscopic feature: individual signet-ring cells containing mucin droplets, which do not form glands, but which infiltrate the ovarian stroma. In these cases the primary gastric neoplasm may be silent, i.e., without symptoms, and the patient may present herself because of lower abdominal complaints.

HORMONE PRODUCING NEOPLASMS:

There remain for brief consideration a number of rare solid ovarian neoplasms which manifest themselves not only as *pelvic masses,* but also because they secrete certain *hormones.* These remarkable tumors are generally believed to arise from the primitive gonad, before it has definitely differentiated as an ovary. Although relatively slow in their growth, they should be considered as malignant neoplasms, since they may recur and metastasize.

Feminizing tumors

The *granulosa cell tumor* is the most important feminizing tumor. It is usually unilateral, and is solid and yellow on cross section; microscopically variable, it may show rosettes of small granular cells having ova-like structures (Call-Exner bodies), or it may have a cylindromatous pattern. If it appears *in childhood,* it may cause endometrial hyperplasia and bleeding, a form of *precocious puberty.* When this tumor appears during active sex life, no endocrine effects may be noted. If it develops *after the menopause,* it may cause endometrial hyperplasia and *irregular uterine bleeding.* Most of these tumors grow very slowly but perhaps 25 percent recur and metastasize (in one of the authors' patients the tumor recurred and caused death some 20 years after resection). After removal, the abnormal endocrine manifestations tend to disappear. The *theca cell tumor* is a rare neoplasm composed of lipid-containing cells resembling fibrous connective tissue. It is believed to arise from the theca interna of the follicle. These tumors usually occur after the menopause and produce a feminizing effect.

Masculinizing tumors

Masculinizing ovarian neoplasms are even rarer than feminizing ones. The *arrhenoblastoma* is the most common tumor in the group. It may arise either in an ovary or in the broad ligament adjacent to it. Grossly it is solid and yellow, and is unilateral. Microscopically it may show structures like seminiferous tubules of the testis, or other cell patterns. The *adrenal adenoma* of the ovary, sometimes known as masculinovoblastoma, is a very rare masculinizing tumor, sometimes occurring in the broad ligament. Its cells resemble those of the adrenal cortex. *Virilizing hilus cell tumor* (Berger's tumor) is an extremely rare tumor derived from cells in the hilus of the ovary comparable to Leydig cells of the testis. All these neoplasms, occurring in the female, produce *defeminizing* symptoms at first (amenorrhea, infertility, atrophy of the breasts, deepening of the voice); later, evidence of *masculinization* is noted, such as growth of a beard, male pattern of pubic hair distribution, prominence of the Adam's apple, and enlargement of the clitoris. Removal of the tumor may or may not cause disappearance of these symptoms. (Similar masculinizing effects are sometimes encountered in females having *adrenal cortical hyperplasia or adenoma,* or certain disorders of the pituitary. One of the authors' cases, long considered to be an instance of masculinization secondary to an arrhenoblastoma, has on restudy proved to be a case of hermaphroditism. In this case the arrhenoblastoma, with its structures resembling seminiferous tubules, was in fact a testis containing atrophic seminiferous tubules; the true nature of the case was revealed when a testis having a good tunica albuginea was removed from the opposite broad ligament some years later!)

Neutralizing tumor?

The *dysgerminoma* is a rare tumor having no definite endocrine effects, but it is found fairly often in females whose external genitalia have certain features resembling the male, i.e., in pseudohermaphrodites. The appearance of the genitalia does not change when the tumor is removed, however. It is often bilateral. Fairly often it is first discovered during pregnancy; it is said to be the most common ovarian tumor to appear during pregnancy. Microscopically the dysgerminoma shows an alveolated pattern of large vesicular cells and scattered lymphoid elements, resembling the seminoma of the testis rather closely. It is a relatively low-grade malignant tumor, recurring in about one-third of the cases.

DISEASES OF THE UTERINE TUBES

The only common diseases of the uterine tubes are *salpingitis* (usually gonorrheal, sometimes tuberculous) and *tubal pregnancy.* These have been considered previously. Nonvenereal inflammation of tubes due to streptococcus or other pyogenic organisms may occur post partum, usually as a complication of puerperal endometritis. Occasionally a chronic form of salpingitis is seen following the use of lipiodol to test tubal patency. The oily droplets remain in the tube and incite a chronic granulomatous reaction (*lipoid granuloma* of the tube). A residual effect after any form of salpingitis is often *tubal stenosis,* causing either infertility or abnormal implantation of the embryo.

Salpingitis isthmica nodosa, a condition in which the uterine end of the tube is irregularly nodular and firm and contains nests of epithelial cells, is of uncertain origin; it may be the end result of an inflammatory process, or it may be adenomyosis of the interstitial portion of the tube.

Hydatid cysts of Morgagni occur at the fimbriated ends of the tubes as grapelike structures, about 1 cm. in diameter, on a short stem. They are apparently unimportant congenital anomalies, arising from the mesonephros or Wolffian body.

Malignant tumors of the uterine tubes (carcinoma, sarcoma, choriocarcinoma in ectopic pregnancy) are extremely rare, according to most observers.

ENDOMETRIOSIS

Definition; sites of predilection

Endometriosis can be defined as the presence of endometrial tissue – glands and stroma – in any abnormal location. The most common site is the *pelvic peritoneum,* including the serosal surfaces of the pelvic organs: *ovaries, uterosacral ligaments, broad ligaments,* uterine tubes, uterus, rectum and sigmoid, and rectovaginal spetum. Endometriosis of any of these structures is sometimes referred to as *endometriosis externa,* in contrast to endometriosis of the myometrium, which is called *endometriosis interna.* Occasionally endometrial tissue is found in the inguinal canal, the umbilicus, appendix, vaginal wall, and surgical scars.

Theories of origin

The *retrograde menstruation* theory of Sampson seems to explain satisfactorily most instances of endometriosis: viable bits of shed endometrium are believed to be transported out of the uterine tubes and implanted on the peritoneal surfaces. Endometriosis in the scar of the abdominal wall following cesarean section seems most easily explained as mechanical *transplantation.* Under other circumstances, as in the myometrium and round ligament, *displaced embryonic cells* or *metaplasia* may account for the abnormal location of the endometrial tissues. None of these theories seems to explain a curious fact about endometriosis, noted by many observers, i.e., its greater frequency in high than in low income groups. On private gynecologic services, endometriosis is probably the most common disease for which oophorectomy is performed.

Dependency upon ovarian function

The aberrant endometrial tissue of endometriosis is under the control of the ovarian hormones. Like the normal endometrium of the uterus, the misplaced endometrium undergoes cyclic proliferation, luteinization, hemorrhage, and shedding, and develops a decidual reaction during the course of uterine pregnancy. Endometriosis is not recognized before puberty, and retrogresses with the cessation of ovarian function, either at the time of the natural menopause or as a result of oophorectomy.

Pathologic changes: endometriosis externa

Grossly endometriosis externa is usually evident as multiple, reddish brown or purple cystic nodules a few millimeters in diameter; these nodules are found on the surface of the ovaries, over the posterior surface of the uterus, or in the cul-de-sac. In the ovaries the cysts often become somewhat larger, even several centimeters in diameter, and are filled with a thick, reddish brown, pasty material (*"chocolate cysts"). Microscopically* the cystic lesions are lined, at least in part, with recognizable endometrial tissue containing both glands and stroma. As a result of recurring "menstruation" into the cysts, an inflammatory reaction develops in the cyst wall; old blood pigment collects in phagocytes, and, with time, dense fibrous adhesions and hyaline scar tissue form. Sometimes the endometrial tissue dies out in old lesions, and the diagnosis, suspected on the basis of the hemosiderin pigment, cannot then be proved beyond a doubt.

endometriosis interna

In the myometrium the endometrial tissue is interlaced with smooth muscle fibers so as to form solid areas of thickening of the uterine wall adjoining the uterine cavity. These deep-lying nests of endometrium are continuous with the endometrium lining the uterine cavity; hence they do not become cystic with recurring hemorrhage.

Clinical features

The usual symptom in endometriosis is *pain at or preceding menstruation,* i.e., *dysmenorrhea.* Pain is believed to be due to increased tension within the tissues as the endometrium thickens under ovarian hormone stimulation, and then bleeds at the time of menstruation. The discomfort is often referred to the back, and may be aggravated by defecation. In other cases the symptoms are those of partial *intestinal obstruction;* this may be due to adhesions between the intestine and the pelvic peritoneum or to an actual mass of endometrial tissue (endometrioma) in the intestinal wall, distorting and blocking the lumen. Patients with endometriosis sometimes present themselves because of *infertility;* presumably this is due to adhesions about the tubes and ovaries interfering with the rupture of the follicle or the migration of the ova.

Related conditions

Stromal endometriosis is similar to ordinary endometriosis in all features except that the growth is composed exclusively of *endometrial stroma, without glands.* It usually presents as an endometrial polyp with microscopic invasion of the myometrium. This condition is much rarer than the usual form of endometriosis. One type of *ovarian adenocarcinoma* is believed by some to arise in ovarian endometriosis, since it closely resembles a common form of endometrial cancer, and is unlike other ovarian neoplasms.

REFERENCES

1. Gold, J. J. Hermaphroditism and pseudohermaphroditism. In Saphir, O. (Ed.), *A Text in Systemic Pathology.* New York: Grune & Stratton, 1958. (An elaborate treatment of this facet of congenital anomalies of the genitalia.)
2. Newman, W., and Cromer, J. K. The multicentric origin of carcinomas of the female anogenital tract. *Surg. Gynec. Obstet.* 108:273, 1959.
3. Naib, Z. M., Nahmias, A. J., Josey, W. E., and Kramer, J. H. Genital herpetic infection: Association with cervical dysplasia and carcinoma. *Cancer* 23:940, 1969.
4. Hertig, A. T., and Sommers, S. C. Genesis of endometrial carcinoma: Study of prior biopsies. *Cancer* 2:946, 1949.
5. Hill, R. P., and Miller, F. N., Jr. Combined mesenchymal sarcoma and carcinoma (carcinosarcoma) of the uterus. *Cancer* 4:803, 1951.
6. Novak, E. R., and Woodruff, J. D. *Gynecologic and Obstetric Pathology* (6th ed.). Philadelphia: Saunders, 1967.
7. Willis, R. A. Teratomas. Section III, Fascicle 9, in *Atlas of Tumor Pathology.* Washington: Armed Forces Institute of Pathology, 1951.

25 THE MAMMARY GLANDS

STRUCTURE AND PHYSIOLOGY

The mammary glands undergo extensive structural changes depending on the age and sex of the individual and on the functional condition of the sexual apparatus. They resemble the sweat gland in structure and development and are *essentially modified apocrine sweat glands.* In males the mammary glands involute after birth. In females they continue to develop, reaching final development only at the end of pregnancy. After lactation they undergo partial involution. The glands become markedly atrophic after the menopause.

Resting mammary glands

Each *resting mammary gland* consists of 15 to 25 closely adjoining, irregular *lobes,* which radiate from the *mammary papilla (nipple).* The lobes are separated by layers of dense interlobar connective tissue and much adipose tissue. Each lobe has an excretory *lactiferous duct* which opens independently at the nipple. Each duct has a dilatation (sinus lactiferus) beneath the areola. It then becomes constricted again and curves toward its opening at the surface. The lobes are subdivided into *lobules* by layers of connective tissue rich in lobular masses of adipose tissue. This interlobular fibrous tissue is dense, while the intralobular connective tissue is more cellular, contains fewer collagenous fibers, and has practically no fat. This looseness of the fibrous tissue about the ducts allows for distensibility. The walls of the secretory portions of the breast *(terminal ductules and alveoli)* consist of a basement membrane, a layer of myo-epithelial cells with a contractile fibrillar cytoplasm, and a layer of low columnar cells. Electron microscopy reveals that the myo-epithelial layer is discontinuous [1]. Columnar cells reach the basement membrane where myo-epithelial cells are absent. Microvilli are present on the luminal surface of epithelial cells as well as between cells. In the virginal breast few if any alveolar buds are present, the ducts terminating in dilatations. In the distal direction the small alveolar ducts gradually unite into larger and larger ducts, finally forming the lactiferous duct. The small alveolar ducts close to the nipple enter the lactiferous duct directly. Each lobe is thus an independent compound alveolar gland. The duct epithelium is columnar from the finest alveolar ducts to the sinus lactiferus, where it becomes cuboidal. Distal to that it is stratified squamous in type. Over the nipple and areola the epidermis is deeply pigmented, especially after pregnancy. This pigmentation is under the influence of estrogens. Smooth muscle is found circularly about the nipple and along the lactiferous ducts. The *areolar glands of Montgomery* are special accessory mammary glands, intermediate in structure between the true mammary gland and the sweat gland.

Mammary glands during gestation

From the time of implantation of the ovum, progressive changes take place in the mammary glands. In the *first half of pregnancy* there is rapid multiplication of the epithelium at the ends of the secretory ducts. Lumenless ducts form with pocket-like evaginations, the alveoli. In the *second half of pregnancy* the multiplication of epithelial cells decreases in intensity, the ductules develop lumens, and the glandular cells begin to produce a secretion. At the *end of pregnancy,* colostrum appears.

Estrogens stimulate the ductular proliferation and an increase in the intralobular and interlobular fibrous tissue. *Progesterone,* acting following the estrogens and in company with them, produces lobular and alveolar development.

Mammary glands during lactation

The secretory epithelial cells of the alveoli fluctuate from tall columnar to cuboidal to flat, according to their functional activity. Their cytoplasm contains rod-shaped or granular mitochondria and large fat globules. *Milk secretion* is apocrine in type, the inner portion of the cell being pinched off and forming part of the secretion. The epithelium of the alveolar ducts is cuboidal or low columnar. Elongated, spindle-shaped myo-epithelial cells are also present along the ducts. Milk secretion is stimulated by the anterior pituitary hormone, *prolactin.* The ejection of milk requires: sucking, oxytocin secretion, and perialveolar and periductal myo-epithelial cellular contraction.

Post-lactational regression

The glands do not return to their original state following lactation. Many of the alveoli which have formed do not disappear, and secreted material may be retained for a long period.

Post-menopausal involution

In old age the epithelium of the secretory portions of the glands atrophies, and the glands return to the prepubertal condition. The interstitial fibrous tissue becomes less cellular, the number of collagenous fibers decreases, and the whole mass becomes homogeneous, even being partly hyalinized.

Blood supply

The *arterial supply* of each mammary gland is from the perforating branches of the internal mammary artery, the thoracic branches of the axillary artery, and the intercostal arteries. *Venous drainage* is through the internal mammary, axillary, and intercostal veins. These drain into the vertebral veins and may carry malignant cells from the breast to the vertebrae and brain.

Lymphatic drainage

The *breast lymphatics* begin in the connective tissue surrounding the alveolar ducts and alveoli and collect along the larger ducts in the subpapillary lymphatic network *(subareolar plexus).* They drain into the ipsilateral *axillary lymph nodes* (mainly from the lateral portion of the breast), the *infraclavicular lymph nodes* (mainly from the upper portion), and the *internal mammary (sternal) lymph nodes* (mainly from the medial portion)."

DEVELOPMENTAL ANOMALIES

Amastia

Polymastia

Amastia is the congenital absence (agenesis) of one or both breasts. It is often bilateral; the right gland is usually absent when amastia is unilateral. *Polymastia* is the presence of more than two breasts and is the most common anomaly of the organ. Extra mammary glands occur anywhere on the milk lines extending from the axilla to the groin. Accessory (supernumerary) breasts may not have nipples. These masses enlarge during lactation, and if nipples are present, they may even secrete milk.

Athelia is the absence of a nipple. It is a rare anomaly and may be associated either with amastia or with an otherwise normal breast. *Polythelia* is the presence of accessory nipples, and is rare. It may be associated with polymastia, with an otherwise normal breast, or alone along a milk line. The accessory nipple is often near the areola. Polythelia is more common in males than females.

Athelia

Polythelia

Developmental inversion of the nipples is a fairly common defect. It is probably due to failure of the ducts to elongate normally, so that there is tension on the nipples. Large and/or pendulous breasts are especially prone to have inverted nipples. The condition may interfere with nursing, or may be confused with acquired nipple inversion in breast carcinoma, especially when only one nipple is involved.

Nipple inversion

INFLAMMATIONS

Eczema of the nipple usually results from uncleanliness or from prolonged nursing. The affected nipple is red, painful, and weeping. It may be confused grossly with Paget's disease of the breast. *Microscopically* there is hyperkeratosis with vesiculation in the epidermis. The underlying dermis is infiltrated by lymphocytes.

NIPPLE ECZEMA

Acute mastitis is practically limited to the period of lactation, especially during the first few weeks and in the primiparous. The *causative agent* (usually *Staphylococcus aureus,* less commonly streptococci) invades the breast through fissures in the nipple, making its way via lymphatics or along ducts. *Clinically* the affected breast is exquisitely tender, painful, swollen, red, and hot. The changes may be diffuse or local. With the appearance of suppuration, localization occurs.

ACUTE MASTITIS:

Breast abscesses may be subareolar, parenchymal, stromal, or retromammary. The appearance is that of an acute abscess (or acute inflammation if an abscess is not formed). The *axillary lymph nodes* are frequently swollen and show edema and reactive hyperplasia microscopically. Acute mastitis may pass into subacute or chronic stages, with their typical cell responses and other features.

Pathologic changes

Chronic mastitis is usually a granuloma, except for the occasional chronic peripheral mastitis which follows an acute infection. In this lesion infiltration by lymphocytes and fibrosis are typical. *Tuberculous mastitis* is uncommon and usually occurs in young women secondary to tuberculosis of the lungs or of the cervical lymph nodes. The microscopic picture is typical of tuberculosis. *Syphilis* is rare in the breast and may appear as a chancre of the nipple (primary syphilis), as mucous patches and other secondary syphilids, or as a gumma (tertiary syphilis). The chancre may be confused with Paget's disease of the breast.

CHRONIC MASTITIS: Tuberculous mastitis

Syphilis

Gangrene of the mammary gland is rare and occurs in cases of diabetes mellitus, thrombophlebitis of mammary veins, and infections with gas-producing clostridia, as well as following plastic surgical procedures. Several cases have been reported following the administration of anticoagulant drugs such as bishydroxycoumarin and phenylindanedione [2]. In such cases trauma leads to hemorrhage into the breast with subsequent gangrene.

GANGRENE

Galactocele (milk cyst) develops in young women during lactation and is probably due to duct obstruction. This cyst, which may become quite large,

GALACTOCELE

contains milk or inspissated material. The surrounding stroma is infiltrated by lymphocytes.

STAGNATION MASTITIS

Stagnation mastitis (caked breast) is a nonsuppurative, mildly inflammatory condition due to a local engorgement of one or more lobules of the breast with milk during early lactation. One or more painful lumps are formed in the breast or breasts. Moderate engorgement of lactating breasts in women taking chlorpromazine has been observed.

COMEDOMASTITIS

Duct ectasia (comedomastitis) is a dilatation of the ducts at or after the menopause, especially in parous women. The dilated ducts are palpable and are filled with a putty-like material which can be extruded from the nipple. A mass 4 to 5 cm. in diameter may be formed; on palpation it feels like a bag of worms. The dilated ducts are filled with amorphous debris containing neutral fat and lipid-laden macrophages. The epithelium is desquamated. Lymphocytes and macrophages infiltrate the surrounding stroma *(periductal mastitis).*

PLASMA CELL MASTITIS:

Plasma cell mastitis is the severely inflammatory end stage of duct ectasia. It is rare today, and occurs most commonly in multiparous women above the age of 40. It is initiated by stasis and inspissation of secretions, and the lesion is a reaction to the escape of lipid-containing material into the periductal tissues. *Clinically* there is induration of the breast associated with lump formation, distortion of the breast contour, and retraction of the nipple. The breast may be painful and tender. Sometimes there is a purulent, serous, or sanguineous discharge from the nipple.

Pathologic changes

Grossly there is a firm, almost lardlike, whitish or yellowish mass which extensively involves the breast. It typically measures 3 to 5 cm. in diameter and is quite firm. The *cut surface* is level and is mottled with distorted and dilated ducts, expressible secretions, and foci of necrosis. *Microscopically* the dilated ducts are filled with lipid-containing amorphous debris, colostrum cells (vacuolated macrophages), and desquamated epithelial cells. There is a *heavy periductal infiltrate* made up of plasmocytes, lymphocytes, lipid-laden macrophages (foam cells), eosinophils, and neutrophils. Lipid crystals are embedded in the dense periductal fibrous tissue. Marked fibrosis is seen in older lesions. The *axillary lymph nodes* may show a reactive hyperplasia. Plasma cell mastitis may be confused with carcinoma of the breast grossly and on frozen section.

FAT NECROSIS:

Fat necrosis is a quiet degeneration of the adipose tissue of the breast, which may be due to trauma, suppurative disease, carcinoma, ischemia induced by pressure, or biopsy surgery. The necrosis with saponification may appear up to a year after the exciting cause. *Clinically* there is a hard, somewhat fixed lump in the breast which may be present for months or years.

Pathologic changes

Grossly the lesion is well defined, firm, solid, chalky, and lardlike early. Later, with necrosis and hemorrhage, the color may change to light yellow, orange, brown, or brownish red. With saponification the fat becomes a yellow oily liquid. Cyst formation, hemorrhage, calcification, and fibrosis are common in older lesions. *Microscopically* early there are opaque fat cells, and the adipose tissue is infiltrated by polymorphonuclear leukocytes, plasmocytes, lymphocytes, and macrophages. Epithelioid, foam, and giant cells may be found. Later there is necrosis, with cholesterol crystals, fibrosis, and calcification.

MAMMARY PHLEBITIS

The rare *subcutaneous mammary phlebitis* (Mondor's disease) [3] is characterized by the development of a painful, tender superficial cord beneath the skin in the lateral or inframammary region. Its cause is unknown. About 75 percent of the cases occur in women. *Microscopically* there is thrombosis of medium-sized subcutaneous veins with later fibrous thickening of the vein wall. The phlebitis clears spontaneously in a few weeks. Seldom is there a coexisting breast lesion.

ENDOCRINE DISTURBANCES

HYPERPLASIA IN FEMALES

Hyperplasia in females before puberty is usually bilateral. Many cases are unexplained, but some are due to estrogen-producing tumors, such as a granulosa cell tumor of an ovary. The breast changes are usually reversible after removal of the neoplasm. *Hyperplasia at or near puberty (virginal hypertrophy)* is due to an inherent abnormal sensitivity to estrogenic hormones. One or both breasts may be affected. The involved breast becomes pendulous, and there is an increase in lobule formation and fibrous tissue. This condition is sometimes associated with a follicular cyst of an ovary or with a fibroadenoma of the breast. The changes are irreversible.

HYPERPLASIA IN MALES:

Hyperplasia in males (gynecomastia) [4] may occur at any period, but is especially frequent in boyhood and old age; the highest incidence is between 10 and 19 years. A study of gynecomastia in *adolescent boys* [5] found that mammary hyperplasia in the form of a firm, discoid subareolar nodule is present in almost 40 percent of boys from 10 to 16 years of age, with a peak incidence at 14. In about 25 percent of the cases gynecomastia is unilateral. The condition usually disappears within 1 to 2 years. Adolescent gynecomastia is probably related to either relatively or absolutely elevated estrogen levels at the time of the onset of puberty. At any age gynecomastia may occur with estrogen or stilbestrol therapy, or it may be associated with estrogen-producing neoplasms and other tumors of the testes, with a decrease in androgen production (as in severe dietary deficiencies), or with failure of estrogen detoxification (as in cirrhosis of the liver). Gynecomastia appears in Klinefelter's syndrome as an overgrowth of periductal fibroblasts. Injury has been implicated as a causative agent, but is probably not one. Trauma may stimulate a rapid increase in growth in gynecomastia, however.

Pathologic changes

In men gynecomastia is usually unilateral, except when associated with testicular or adrenal neoplasms. The mammary hyperplasia is typically most marked in the subareolar region. Secretions may accumulate in the ducts and may be extruded from the nipple. In gynecomastia there is fibrous tissue proliferation together with variable degrees of duct multiplication, branching, and elongation. The stroma is infiltrated by lymphocytes. In about 25 percent of cases of gynecomastia secondary to prolonged estrogen therapy, acini are formed in small lobules [6]. These structures are not seen in gynecomastia due to other causes.

MAMMARY DYSPLASIA: Cause

Mammary dysplasia is a degeneration characterized by many gradations and variations in the amount of epithelial hyperplasia, fibrosis, and cyst formation. It is due to an *ovarian hormonal imbalance* – a progesterone deficiency with relative or absolute hyperestrinism – acting on a susceptible breast for a long period of time.

Clinical features

Clinically the condition is found especially in the last decade of reproductive life. However, it may develop then and show symptoms only after the menopause. The peak incidence is between 40 and 45 years. Most patients are unmarried. The condition is usually bilateral and is associated with premenstrual breast pain and tenderness and with irregular menses. The breasts are lumpy, especially in the upper and outer quadrants. The lesions may subside spontaneously or during pregnancy or lactation. Many of the changes of mammary dysplasia are found in a significant number of clinically normal breasts, so subclinical cases occur frequently.

Relationship to carcinoma

The *relationship of mammary dysplasia to breast carcinoma* is controversial. Foote and Stewart [7] did not feel that the changes of mammary dysplasia are premalignant although they found a direct transition between such lesions and malignant foci in occasional cases. Warren [8] found breast carcinoma to be 4.5 times more common in a large group of women with mammary dysplasia, irrespective of age, than in the general female population. In a study of over 800 cases of breast carcinoma at the George Washington University Hospital, coexistent lesions of fibrocystic mastopathy were present in 62 percent [9]. Grossly evident cysts were found in 27 percent of these cases. By comparison, the changes of fibrocystic mastopathy were seen at autopsy in one or both breasts of 53 percent of women with no history of breast disease, and gross cysts were noted in 19 percent of this group [10]. While the significance of the higher incidence of fibrocystic disease in breasts with carcinoma than in noncarcinomatous breasts is not entirely certain, the preponderance of evidence appears to indicate a relationship between this form of mammary dysplasia and breast cancer.

Pathologic changes:

Two variants of mammary dysplasia are recognized: fibrous and fibrocystic mastopathy. The former is less common and not important clinically. In any one patient one form usually predominates, but all gradations and transitions are found.

fibrous mastopathy

Fibrous mastopathy (mazoplasia) shows a lesser degree of changes in the breast in mammary dysplasia than the fibrocystic form. *Grossly* there is a fairly well-localized palpable mass, usually in the upper and outer quadrant of one breast. It is firm and difficult to cut. The cut surface is nonencapsulated, white or pearly gray, and dotted with minute pink foci of parenchyma. *Microscopically* there is an increase in the interlobular fibrous tissue, which becomes rather collagenous. The scattered ducts are slightly dilated to form microcysts. Their epithelium may be normal, multilayered, or flat. Fibrous mastopathy may eventuate in a marked fibrosis of the affected part of the breast, with duct obliteration [11].

fibrocystic mastopathy

Fibrocystic mastopathy (chronic cystic mastitis) may be local, with a single large cyst, or diffuse. When it is bilaterally diffuse, the condition is known as *Schimmelbusch's disease. Grossly* there are smooth, rounded, tense, movable masses, usually 3 to 4 cm. in diameter. The cut surface of one of the masses shows many cysts varying greatly in size (0.1 to 3 cm. usually). Some contain clear fluid and are translucent. Others are hemorrhagic and appear bluish through the cyst wall *(blue dome cyst)*. The fluid within the cysts is under great pressure. These cysts are formed from ducts which have not undergone involution following hyperplasia. Secretions increase the size of the cysts. *Microscopically* the lobules are irregular and small. Ducts are dilated and filled with an amorphous granular material. The larger cysts have flattened or absent epithelium with a dense surrounding stroma. The most typical feature is the presence in some cysts of a single layer of tall, plump, "gasoline pump" epithelial cells with a strongly eosinophilic cytoplasm and palely staining basilar nuclei. These cells represent *apocrine metaplasia.* By electron microscopy the apocrine cells are shown to be filled with cytoplasmic organelles [12]. The increase in mitochondria may account for the eosinophilia. Some cysts show papillary proliferation of the epithelium, and in some cases there may be a diffuse papillomatosis in the dilated ducts and cysts. *Duct papillomatosis* is the lesion of fibrocystic mastopathy most frequently associated with carcinomatous change. Trabeculae consisting of epithelial stalks may bridge the smaller cysts. *Epithelial hyperplasia* may almost completely fill some cysts. The stroma about the lobules and ducts is infiltrated by lymphocytes and plasmocytes.

ADENOSIS:

Adenosis (lobular hyperplasia) is often associated with mammary dysplasia, but may exist independently. It occurs most often in the 30 to 40 year age group and is characterized by varying degrees of epithelial hyperplasia and duct and/or alveolar proliferation. At times the hyperplasia may be alarming and be confused with carcinoma. The condition is usually bilateral, but is not infrequently unilateral. The *cause* is probably a hormonal imbalance with relative or absolute hyperestrinism.

Pathologic changes

Grossly the breast is usually small with a characteristic granular feel at the periphery. The lesion cuts with difficulty, revealing a poorly defined, pearly gray cut surface dotted with pinkish tan foci measuring 0.1 to 0.5 cm. in diameter. *Microscopically* the tiny foci consist of small collections either of hyperplastic terminal ductules *(blunt duct adenosis)* or of alveoli. Some ducts are dilated, and the hyperplastic epithelium may be piled up within the proliferating ducts, sometimes spilling out of them. Often there is a joint proliferation of ducts and intralobular fibrous tissue in numerous small lobules *(fibroadenomatosis).*

Sclerosing adenosis

Sclerosing adenosis is a variant in which there are separation and disorganization of lobules by extensive intralobular fibrosis and epithelial and especially myo-epithelial cell proliferation. The tightly packed and distorted acini have tiny central lumina, and each acinus is surrounded by a basement membrane. By electron microscopy the proliferation is shown to be almost entirely by myoepithelial cells [13]. Collagen fibers are laid down by these cells. In *florid sclerosing adenosis* the involved lobules have a wild appearance with hyperchromatic spindle and epithelial cells, so that it may be mistaken for carcinoma on frozen section.

NEOPLASMS

A sharp distinction between the epithelial and fibrous hyperplasia of mammary dysplasia and true neoplasia of these tissues cannot always be made. Duct papillomas are localized epithelial overgrowths into a dilated duct which may be related to papillomatosis. In the same way the epithelial and fibrous tissue overgrowth in a fibroadenoma may be related to dysplasia, although it appears to be a true neoplasm.

1. Benign Neoplasms

INTRADUCTAL PAPILLOMA:

Intraductal papilloma usually appears in parous women between 25 and 35 years of age. In over 50 percent of the cases there is spontaneous or induced *bleeding from the nipple.* The tumor may be palpable.

Pathologic changes

The neoplasm is commonly multiple and appears in the larger ducts as pedunculated, raspberry-like masses attached to the walls of dilated ducts or cysts, usually within the boundary of the areola. Those less than 1 cm. in diameter are pale and glistening, whereas larger ones are pink. A cloudy, sanguineous fluid may fill the duct or cyst. *Microscopically* there is a delicate branching villous pattern of narrow, vascularized connective tissue stalks covered by a single layer of epithelium. The height of the epithelium depends on the age of the lesion and on the tension within the duct or cyst. Tumors with almost no stroma which form many glandlike spaces lined with a single layer of flattened epithelium within the duct or cyst are *papillary cystadenomas.* A very small percentage of duct papillomata evidently develop into papillary adenocarcinoma.

FIBROADENOMA:

Fibroadenoma is a very common, slowly growing, estrogen-induced, fibroepithelial neoplasm, usually occurring in nulliparous women between 25 and 35 years of age. It is more frequent in Negro than in white women. There is often a history of irregular menses, dysmenorrhea, and premenstrual tension. Growth is rapid during pregnancy and lactation and usually ceases at the menopause. Often there is an increase in the size of the tumor during menstruation. Florid proliferation may occur in fibroadenomas in patients taking oral contraceptives [14]. Electron microscopy indicates the fibroadenoma develops by proliferation of stromal cells, and the duct epithelial growth is secondary [15]. Rarely carcinoma, especially lobular carcinoma in situ, develops in the epithelium of a fibroadenoma [16].

Pathologic changes

The neoplasm is usually single, but is unilaterally multiple in about 2 percent of the cases and bilateral in about 5 percent. The skin over the tumor is unchanged, and the tumor is movable under the skin. *Grossly* the tumor feels rubbery and is smooth or lobulated, sharply outlined, encapsulated, and 0.5 to 3.5 cm. in diameter. The color is pearly gray or pink. The cut surface is delicately fissured (the ducts), and feels moist or sticky. Old tumors may show hyalinization or calcification. *Microscopically* two types are described, but since both are usually found in each neoplasm there is little advantage in differentiating them. In the *intracanalicular fibroadenoma* the connective tissue is greatly proliferated and shows myxomatous degeneration in many cases. Polypoid masses of fibrous tissue, covered by flattened or cuboidal epithelium, grow into the parenchymal channels. Huge formations of this kind (over 10 cm. in diameter) are called *cystosarcoma phyllodes* [17]. These may become malignant and recur or metastasize *(malignant cystosarcoma phyllodes, adenofibrosarcoma)* in rare cases. The *pericanalicular fibroadenoma* is characterized by hyperplastic lobules distorted by dense fibrous tissue growth in sweeping encircling bands. The ducts are lined by one or two layers of cuboidal or columnar cells. All gradations in the relationship between the amounts of fibrous and epithelial tissues are found in fibroadenomata. Pure fibroma and pure adenoma are also rarely observed in the breast.

CYSTOSARCOMA PHYLLODES

ADENOMA:

Adenoma [18] is rare in its pure form. It occurs in young women and is often associated with pregnancy or lactation. Many pathologists do not classify the adenoma as a separate entity, considering the tumor to be a type of fibroadenoma or a hyperplasia of pregnancy or lactation. Rarely carcinoma may develop in an adenoma.

Pathologic changes

Grossly the tumor is usually single and is movable and firm on palpation. It is tan and varies from 1 to 10 cm. in diameter. *Microscopically* there is a remarkable epithelial proliferation in the form of regular, closely packed glands. The epithelium varies from cuboidal to tall secretory cells. In some tumors the glands resemble the small compact ones of the fetal breast *(fetal adenoma).*

OTHER BENIGN NEOPLASMS

Other benign neoplasms are rare and include fibroma, leiomyoma, lipoma (which must be distinguished from fat replacement in an atrophic breast), mixed tumor, hemangioma (capillary or cavernous), lymphangioma, granular cell myoblastoma, chondroma, and osteoma. (The last two must be distinguished from cartilaginous or osteoid degeneration in a neoplasm or inflammatory or degenerative lesion of the breast.)

2. Malignant Neoplasms

Malignant neoplasms of the mammary glands constitute about 10 percent of all cancer. The ratio of benign to malignant neoplasms in the breast is about 6:4, and over 99 percent of malignant neoplasms of the breast are carcinomas.

CARCINOMA:

Carcinoma of the breast occurs in one in about 17 women in the United States during a normal life span. About 67,000 new cases are diagnosed each year. Despite advances in surgical and medical therapy the mortality rate from breast carcinoma has remained uniform for over 30 years. It causes 20 percent of all cancer deaths in females and 0.2 percent of all cancer deaths in males. About 30,000 women die annually of mammary carcinoma in the United States. *Most breast carcinomas are discovered shortly before, during, or just after the menopause.* There is a bimodal *age distribution,* with the highest incidence (almost 20 percent of the cases) in the 45 to 49 year old age group and a smaller peak in the 55 to 59 year age group. Over 50 percent of patients with breast carcinoma are in the 40 to 59 year age group. In general, the older the patient, the more likely a single lump in the breast is a carcinoma.

Cause

The *cause* is not completely known, but it appears to be related to imbalances in the periodic hyperplasias and involutions in the breast under hormonal influences. *Estrogen stimulation* for prolonged periods seems to predispose to carcinoma in the breast. There is evidence that marked epithelial hyperplasia, especially in the form of intraductal papillomatosis, in *fibrocystic mastopathy* is related to the development of carcinoma [19]. Another bit of evidence incriminating the estrogens is that among women with breast carcinoma there is a greater than expected incidence of endometrial carcinoma. Stromal hyperplasia of the ovaries, a stigma of hyperestrinism, has been found in about 85 percent of postmenopausal women with breast carcinoma (as compared with 35 percent in controls). Not all breast carcinomas are estrogen-dependent, however. Breast carcinoma is significantly more common among unmarried than married women and among nulliparous or oligoparous than multiparous women [20]. Among parous women, breast carcinoma is somewhat more common in those who have not nursed their babies or who have done so only for short periods. *Hereditary factors* appear more prominently in breast carcinoma than in most other types of cancer, the occurrence in mothers and daughters and in sisters being frequently noted. A factor analogous to the virus-like Bittner milk factor in mice conceivably could play a role in this transmission. An RNA-containing virus closely resembling the Bittner factor has been isolated from the milk of mothers with breast carcinoma and has been found in mammary cancer cells [21].

Pathologic changes

Carcinoma may occur in either female breast, in accessory breast tissue, and in the male breast. The ratio of the incidence of carcinoma in the left breast to that in the right is 110:100. Simultaneous *bilateral carcinoma* [22] occurs in about 0.5 percent and successive bilateral cancer in about 3 percent of cases of breast carcinoma. It is often difficult to exclude the possibility of metastasis from one mammary gland to the other. The average interval between successive carcinomas is 8 years. *Carcinomas appear most commonly in the upper and outer quadrant of the breast* (about 50 percent of the cases), because more breast tissue is present in this portion than elsewhere. Roughly 15 percent of the cases occur in each of three regions – subareolar region, upper and inner quadrant, and lower and outer quadrant – and about 5 percent in the lower and inner quadrant. Lesions near the breast peripheries tend to metastasize to regional lymph nodes earlier than those in the center, while carcinomas in the inner quadrants develop mediastinal metastases more frequently than those in the outer quadrants. *Lymphatic spread within the breast* is first vertically downward to the retromammary fascia, after which it becomes centrifugal. About 99 percent *of breast carcinomas are derived from duct or alveolar epithelium (adenocarcinoma);* however, very few show a typical glandular pattern. The infiltrating duct carcinoma with fibrosis (scirrhous type) is the most common form. Carcinomas of the large lactiferous ducts are usually papillary in type. In the intermediate (lobar) ducts, duct cell and comedocarcinomas are commonly found. *Most carcinomas arise from the lobular duct epithelium.* Only occasionally do they derive from the alveolar epithelium. In any region the carcinomas may be infiltrating or noninfiltrating. The *average rate of growth* is estimated as 1 cm. per 3 months.

Metastases

Metastases in breast carcinomas are chiefly via lymphatic routes, especially to the axillary lymph nodes, but hematogenous spread is not uncommon. *About 60 percent of cases* of breast carcinoma have *axillary metastases at operation.* The occurrence of axillary metastases increases with the size of the breast lesion. Metastases also occur in the internal mammary, infraclavicular, supraclavicular, lower cervical, intercostal, and mediastinal lymph nodes. Involvement of epigastric nodes leads to spread to the mediastinal and abdominal lymph nodes. Extension across to the *opposite breast* is not uncommon. The *skin over the breast* may be involved via the periductal lymphatics, the lymphatics of Cooper's ligaments, or direct extension. Obliteration of the deep lymphatics by tumor cell clusters may cause edema of the skin, the swollen skin anchored down intermittently by hair follicles resembling pig skin or an orange peel *(peau d'orange).* Diffuse lymphatic edema produces a shieldlike effect in the skin *(cancer en cuirasse). Visceral metastases* in breast carcinoma go to the lungs and pleura (in about 60 percent of autopsied cases), the liver, bones, adrenal glands, and brain, in order of frequency. The stomach is involved in about 10 percent of autopsied cases of breast carcinoma. In about 50 percent of premenopausal women with widespread metastases, grossly evident or microscopic metastases are present in the ovaries. *Metastases to the bones* tend to be osteoclastic, the ribs, vertebrae, pelvis, and femora being most commonly involved. Spread to the vertebrae and brain is often via drainage from the intercostal into the vertebral veins.

Prognosis

The *prognosis* in breast carcinoma is generally worsened with increasing duration of symptoms, increasing size of the lesion [23], and the presence of axillary metastases. The overall *5-year survival rate* is about 40 percent. With radical mastectomy the 5-year survival rate is about 50 percent, the 5-year clinical cure rate being 40 percent. The prognosis is poorer in women under 40, when estrogenic activity is intense. In young women, especially during pregnancy, breast carcinoma is likely to be highly anaplastic and rapidly growing; this is probably related to the increased vascularity within the breast. In about 75 percent of persons who survive 5 years with breast carcinoma, a peripheral plasmocytic infiltrate is found, as compared with 25 percent of controls, indicating that this inflammatory reaction represents a form of host resistance to the neoplasm [24]. Early diagnosis is of the utmost importance in the control of breast cancer, and the *examination of exfoliated cells in nipple smears* is now used to diagnose asymptomatic cases of mammary carcinoma.

Classification

Classification of mammary carcinoma is confused, none of the many proposed classifications being completely satisfactory. A classification widely used in *surgical pathology* is that of the Memorial Hospital for Cancer and Allied Diseases in New York:

- I. Paget's disease of the nipple
- II. Carcinoma of mammary ducts
  - A. Noninfiltrating
    - 1. Papillary carcinoma
    - 2. Comedocarcinoma
  - B. Infiltrating
    - 1. Papillary carcinoma
    - 2. Comedocarcinoma
    - 3. Carcinoma with fibrosis
    - 4. Medullary carcinoma with lymphoid infiltration
    - 5. Colloid carcinoma
- III. Carcinoma of lobules
  - A. Noninfiltrating
  - B. Infiltrating
- IV. Relatively rare carcinoma
  - A. So-called "sweat gland carcinoma"
  - B. Intracystic carcinoma
  - C. Adenoid cystic carcinoma
  - D. Squamous cell carcinoma
  - E. Spindle cell carcinoma
  - F. Carcinoma with osseous and cartilaginous metaplasia

The following *simple classification* (cross-referenced to the Memorial Hospital system) will be used here:

- I. Papillary adenocarcinoma (MH II., A.1., B.1.)
- II. Intraductal carcinoma
  - A. Paget's disease of the breast (MH I.)
- III. Comedocarcinoma (MH II., A.2., B.2.)
- IV. Epidermoid carcinoma (MH IV., D.)
- V. Infiltrating duct carcinoma with fibrosis (MH II., B.3.)
- VI. Medullary carcinoma (MH II., B.4.)
- VII. Mucinous carcinoma (MH II., B.5.)
- VIII. Apocrine carcinoma (MH IV., A.)
- IX. Acute inflammatory carcinoma.
- X. Lobular carcinoma (MH III., A., B.)

Papillary adenocarcinoma:

Papillary adenocarcinoma constitutes less than 5 percent of mammary carcinoma and usually arises de novo in a large lactiferous duct, but occasionally it originates in a preexisting duct papilloma. *Clinically* there is commonly a bloody or serous discharge from the nipple. A large, bulky subareolar nodule is felt; this may be fluctuant due to hemorrhage or cyst formation. The axillary lymph nodes are involved late, and the 5-year clinical cure rate is about 75 percent.

pathologic changes

Grossly the neoplasm may be hemorrhagic or cystic, and it grows as a single intraductal soft mass or is found in several neighboring dilated ducts. *Microscopically* there is a papillary pattern in which epithelium varies from a single layer to large sheets of columnar cells showing moderate hyperchromaticism, lack of polarity, and frequent mitoses. In some cases there is no invasion of the stalk at the base, the papillary tumor being confined to the duct (noninfiltrating). If there is spread beyond the confines of the duct, the carcinoma is infiltrating. Frequently intraductal carcinoma showing a cribriform (sievelike) pattern is found in ducts adjacent to a papillary carcinoma [25].

Intraductal carcinoma:

Intraductal (duct cell) carcinoma is characterized *clinically* by bleeding or discharge from the nipple. It may or may not be palpable centrally.

pathologic changes

Grossly the involved ducts are filled with grayish tan neoplasm from which small tumor cell masses can be expressed. *Microscopically* the ducts are filled with a profuse, sometimes papillary growth of large atypical epithelial cells. There may be a central clear area or a small focus of necrosis. Focal disruption, thinning, or absence of the duct basement membrane is found in practically all cases of apparently noninfiltrating intraductal carcinoma [26]. A few cases have shown axillary or widespread metastases despite lack of evidence of stromal invasion. Obvious periductal infiltration may be present.

Paget's disease:

Paget's disease of the breast is a chronic eczematoid thelitis (inflammation of the nipple) associated with an intraductal carcinoma. It constitutes about 2 percent of all breast carcinoma. At operation about 50 percent of these cases have axillary metastases. The patients usually range from 40 to 60 years old. *Clinically* Paget's disease typically begins with burning, itching, or soreness of the nipple, which later becomes enlarged and red. Fissuring and weeping or oozing then occur. Sometimes the nipple changes are preceded by the finding by palpation of a central lump in the breast.

pathologic changes

Grossly beneath the nipple area the ducts are often dilated, thickened, and filled with a grumous paste. Obvious infiltration beyond the duct may be noted. *Microscopically* there are many vacuolated, large pale cells with hyperchromatic nuclei and frequent mitotic figures *(Paget cells)* in the rete pegs of the epidermis. These cells frequently contain mucin, and melanin granules may be found in their cytoplasm. The epidermis shows a "motheaten" appearance and is compressed. The dermis is edematous, hyperemic, and infiltrated by plasma cells and lymphocytes. The Paget cells almost always represent *intra-epidermal invasion by direct extension or by metastasis from the duct carcinoma.* In a few cases the epidermal neoplasm may be primary, producing intraductal carcinoma by descent into the breast, or it may exist independent of the duct carcinoma [27]. The associated intraductal carcinoma is typical and sometimes lies deep within the breast.

extra-mammary Paget's disease

Extramammary Paget's disease occurs, especially over an underlying sweat gland carcinoma, similar epidermal changes being found. It is more common in women than in men. The principal *sites* are the axilla and anogenital region (vulva, perineum, perianal region, penis, scrotum) [28].

Comedo-carcinoma:

Comedocarcinoma is a slowly growing variant of intraductal carcinoma. It constitutes less than 5 percent of breast carcinoma. *Clinically* this tumor occurs especially after the menopause. It is centrally located. There is a cloudy discharge from the nipple, and toothpaste-like ribbons can be extruded from the nipple. The course may extend over several years.

pathologic changes

Grossly the neoplasm is usually circumscribed and yellowish gray, averaging 5 cm. in diameter. Yellowish gray, pasty material may be expressed in ribbons from dilated ducts within the mass. *Microscopically* the ducts are filled with darkly staining, atypical epithelial cells and contain a central granular, amorphous, and eosinophilic *necrotic area*. The larger the mass of cells, the greater is the necrosis. The tumor may be confined to the ducts or may be infiltrating.

Epidermoid carcinoma

Epidermoid carcinoma in a duct originates in a focus of metaplastic epithelium. It is rare, constituting less than 1 percent of breast carcinoma, but it metastasizes early and widely. Foci of epidermoid metaplasia may be found in several types of adenocarcinoma of the breast.

Infiltrating duct carcinoma:

Infiltrating duct carcinoma with fibrosis (scirrhous carcinoma) is the most common type of carcinoma in the breast, constituting about 75 percent of all mammary carcinoma. Almost 70 percent of the patients have axillary metastases at operation. It usually arises in lobular ducts. *Clinically* the only early sign is the discovery of a small, rather fixed mass in the breast, most commonly in the upper and outer quadrant. It is best palpated by the palm of the hand. Late signs are retraction of the nipple, dimpling of the skin over the tumor, and the presence of an axillary mass.

pathologic changes

Grossly the scirrhous carcinoma averages 2 to 3 cm. in diameter and is very hard, fixed to the surrounding breast tissue, and tan with yellow streaks due to necrosis. It cuts with the grittiness of unripe fruit. The cut surface is concave and retracts below the level of the cut. Small cysts may be present in and about the tumor. *Microscopically* there is marked fibrosis with minute, angular, cleft-like spaces containing closely packed epithelial cells in thin columns or threads. The cells are often in single file. The epithelial cells in scirrhous carcinoma are small with deeply staining nuclei and little cytoplasm. Periductal and perivascular infiltration and invasion of fat are very common.

Medullary carcinoma:

Medullary (encephaloid, *circumscribed) carcinoma* makes up less than 5 percent of mammary carcinoma. *Clinically* there is usually a deeply seated, mid-zonal, circumscribed, slightly movable mass. These neoplasms are distinctly less infiltrating than scirrhous carcinomas of comparable size. They may fungate and reach a huge size without axillary metastases developing. There is often little or no skin attachment or dimpling over these neoplasms. The *prognosis* is much better than that in scirrhous carcinoma.

pathologic changes

Grossly the neoplasm is soft and bulky, often measuring more than 5 cm. in diameter. It is partly cystic or hemorrhagic, opaque, and grayish tan. *Microscopically* it is very cellular, with large oval or polygonal cells having a slightly basophilic cytoplasm and a vesicular nucleus. The scanty stroma is often *infiltrated by lymphocytes (medullary carcinoma with lymphoid stroma).*

Mucinous carcinoma:

Mucinous (colloid) carcinoma includes those breast carcinomas in which there is marked mucin secretion. Foci of mucin formation are not uncommon in breast carcinoma, but pure mucinous carcinoma is unusual, constituting about 2 percent of mammary cancer. The *prognosis* is more favorable than in most other forms of breast cancer, axillary metastases being found in only about 45 percent of the cases at operation [29].

pathologic changes

Grossly the tumor is fairly well outlined and unencapsulated. It is a moderately firm, spherical mass with a translucent, moist, gelatinous or slimy surface marked by a delicately interlacing pattern of more solid opaque tissue. When the tumor is cut, strings of mucin cling to the knife. *Microscopically* there is a multilocular cystlike formation, the spaces containing a light grayish blue-staining, amorphous material. At the periphery small clusters of deeply staining epithelial cells are found. Columns and nests of *signet-ring cells* are also found.

Apocrine carcinoma

Apocrine carcinoma [30] makes up about 1 percent of breast carcinoma. It represents apocrine anaplasia in the breast and sometimes appears to arise in areas of apocrine metaplasia. Almost all the tumors measure over 2 cm. in diameter, and about half are over 5 cm. It develops as either an intraductal carcinoma or an infiltrating carcinoma with moderate reactive fibrosis. The characteristic feature is the presence of large atypical epithelial cells with eosinophilic cytoplasm and a small nucleus. These cells are heaped up and partly fill the spaces they line; they may show a papillary growth.

Adenoid cystic carcinoma

Adenoid cystic carcinoma [31] is rare in the breast. The tumor presents as a sometimes tender mass. *Grossly* it measures 1 to 5 cm. in diameter and may be cystic. *Microscopically* there are clusters of small cuboidal cells with little cytoplasm. These cells are arranged about tiny cystic spaces in a cylindromatous pattern. The spaces contain a mucinous material. Perineural lymphatic infiltration is frequent. However, metastases are uncommon, and the prognosis is much better in mammary adenoid cystic carcinoma than in this type of neoplasm in other sites.

Inflammatory carcinoma:

Inflammatory carcinoma (carcinomatous mastitis, erysipeloid carcinoma) usually occurs in obese, pendulous breasts in young women, especially during lactation. It is rare, and about 75 percent of the patients have axillary metastases at operation. The condition may easily be confused with an acute mastitis. *Clinically* the onset is sudden with a rapidly developing reddish purple discoloration and induration of the breast. The nipple is encrusted and retracted.

pathologic changes

The *skin* is edematous and thick. There is a large, poorly defined, centrally located, reddish gray mass. *Microscopically* the tumor is usually a poorly differentiated adenocarcinoma with much lymphatic permeation. Clusters of neoplastic cells are found throughout the breast substance.

Lobular carcinoma

Lobular carcinoma [32] is found in about 5 percent of breast cancer and is the only type of carcinoma that does not occur in the male breast. It arises from the alveolar epithelium. Occasionally it is noninfiltrating (in situ lobular carcinoma) [33], well-demarcated clusters of alveoli being lined by atypical epithelial cells. Their cytoplasm is sometimes vacuolated *(Pagetoid change).* The gland lumina may be filled with neoplastic cells. In situ lobular carcinoma is bilateral in almost 25 percent of the cases. When alveolar carcinoma is infiltrating, it is sometimes difficult to distinguish from lobular duct carcinoma. However, a characteristic feature of the former is a circular arrangement of infiltrating cells about small ducts, producing the effect of a bull's eye in a target.

Male mammary carcinoma:

Carcinoma of the male mammary gland [34] is rare, being 100 times less common than carcinoma of the female breast. In general, it occurs in an older age group than in the female. A history of preceding trauma is obtained in 25 percent of the cases, and gynecomastia is associated in a few of the cases. A few cases have occurred in men who had received prolonged estrogen therapy. There is a high incidence of breast cancer in men with Klinefelter's syndrome. At operation about 50 percent have axillary node metastases. The *prognosis* is poor, the 5-year survival rate being 30 percent. Infiltration, fixation, and ulceration of the overlying skin are common, due to the small size of the male breast.

pathologic changes

Grossly the neoplasm is usually diffusely infiltrating and attached to the skin and pectoral fascia. It is opaque and gray, with a few small cysts and foci of hemorrhage or necrosis. *Microscopically* about 75 percent of these neoplasms are infiltrating duct carcinomas, but the tumor may be of any type except lobular carcinoma. Paget's disease of the nipple is rare in men.

Effects of therapy: surgery

The *treatment* of mammary carcinoma [35] is mainly *surgical.* When a definite mass is palpated in a breast, the standard procedure is to remove it surgically, in toto if feasible. A *frozen section diagnosis* is obtained within a few minutes. If the lesion is benign, no further surgery is necessary. However, if the pathologist's diagnosis is carcinoma, a *radical mastectomy* is then performed. This procedure, advocated by William Halsted in 1882, includes the removal of the entire breast and overlying skin, a subcutaneous dissection of the adjacent skin flaps, excision of the pectoralis major and minor muscles, and dissection of the axilla. The rationale of the operation is to remove the entire primary neoplasm as well as its routes for early extension and metastasis. Sacrifice of the pectoral muscles is necessary because of the possibility of direct retromammary spread into them and the existence in about 35 percent of women of the *interpectoral nodes of Rotter* which drain portions of the breast. Some surgeons modify the operation to include dissection of the *internal mammary chain of lymph nodes,* especially when the carcinoma is in the inner half of the breast, and/or the *supraclavicular nodes.* This has increased the 5-year clinical cure rate by about 10 percent. *Complications* of the Halsted procedure include breakdown of the skin flaps, necessitating skin grafting; cellulitis of the operative wound site; and edema of the ipsilateral upper extremity, most often due to removal of the deep lymphatic channels during surgery. Other factors include infection; angulation or spasm of the axillary vein, interfering with venous and lymphatic return from the arm; lymphatic obliteration by fibrosis caused by postoperative radiation; and obesity [36]. Rarely a *lymphangiosarcoma* develops in a markedly edematous arm *(Stewart-Treves syndrome). Simple mastectomy* (removal of the breast only) is sometimes performed in very elderly women, in obviously incurable breast cancer, or in cases of in situ lobular carcinoma.

radiation therapy

X-radiation and, less commonly, *radium radiation* are sometimes used either preoperatively or postoperatively. The usual tumor dose is 5000 to 7000 r. Radiation produces nuclear pyknosis and cytoplasmic vacuolization in neoplastic cells. Some cells usually remain viable and often are bizarre, large, and multinucleated. The stroma becomes densely collagenous and focally calcified. *Postoperative radiation* is sometimes aimed at the internal mammary, mediastinal, and supraclavicular lymph nodes when these have not been removed. X-radiation is effective in slowing growth and alleviating pain in bone metastases. The *disadvantages* of radiation therapy are the development of radiation dermatitis and, rarely, burns; the production of radiation fibrosis in the underlying lung; and the increased incidence of edema of the arm with postoperative radiation.

oophorectomy and adrenalectomy

Hormonal therapy [37] is used in many forms for breast carcinoma, but is almost always secondary to mammary surgery and radiation. The hormones are by no means curative, but are used as an adjunct to surgery, to slow the progress of the disease by suppressing or opposing hormonal stimulation of malignant cells, and/or to relieve pain. The failure of some breast carcinomas to respond to hormone suppression or administration is due to the fact that not all such neoplasms are hormone-dependent. In premenopausal women *castration by x-radiation or bilateral oophorectomy* is carried out fairly frequently because the growth of some mammary carcinomas is stimulated by estrogens. The interval before the recurrence of carcinoma following radical mastectomy and the 5-year survival rate are significantly increased by prophylactic oophorectomy [38]. *Bilateral adrenalectomy* [39] is used after oophorectomy in cases of disseminated carcinoma in premenopausal or postmenopausal women to remove the final source of estrogen production. Regression of the size of metastases in bones, viscera, and soft tissues or large primary tumors occurs in about 35 percent of the cases. In bone metastases, recalcification of previously osteolytic lesions is found. Survival for up to 3 years has been achieved in women with hormone-dependent carcinoma. *Combined bilateral oophorectomy and adrenalectomy* in patients with metastatic breast carcinoma have resulted in objective regression of metastases in about 40 percent of the cases, with subjective improvement in up to 60 percent [40].

steroid therapy

Prednisolone and cortisone have been administered to suppress adrenal function in the treatment of widely metastatic breast carcinoma. Their most effective use has been in cases with cerebral metastases, hypercalcemia due to bone destruction, and lymphedema. About 20 percent of disseminated breast carcinoma show temporary tumor regression on prednisolone. Pain decrease and subjective improvement occur in many patients without tumor regression. With *prednisone* about 50 percent of cases show objective improvement such as recalcification in osteolytic bony metastases [41]. In patients treated with *adrenal corticosteroids* an *increase in the frequency of metastases* to the stomach and duodenum, spleen, myocardium, lungs, liver, brain, and the opposite breast has been found [42]. This increase in metastatic lesions is explained by means of the effects of adrenal steroids on the "soil" of various organs in regard to the growth of malignant cells. Adrenal steroids are known to have inhibiting effects on the gastric and duodenal epithelium, the spleen, and the Kupffer cells. The generalized reduction of the immune response of the reticuloendothelial system during steroid therapy may be another factor in the increased incidence of metastases in patients on such therapy. The *average survival time* in patients treated with adrenal steroids is the same as in patients with breast carcinoma who receive no steroids (about 4.5 years from the time of onset).

hypophysectomy

Hypophysectomy or *pituitary irradiation* with radioactive yttrium (^{90}Y) is occasionally carried out in disseminated breast cancer because of experimental evidence that prolactin (mammotropin) from the eosinophilic cells has a growth-stimulating effect on the mammary glands independent of milk secretion [43]. Removal or destruction of the anterior pituitary also leads to decreased adrenal estrogen production. The degree of adrenal cortical atrophy is greater following hypophysectomy than after corticosteroid therapy. Temporary remissions have been produced in about half the cases treated by hypophysectomy. *Pituitary necrosis* is produced by the insertion of pellets of radioactive yttrium [44]. The radiation zone undergoes complete necrosis and is surrounded by a fibrous capsule which contains clusters of pituitary cells. The posterior pituitary is usually entirely destroyed.

androgen and estrogen therapy

Bilateral orchiectomy has been used palliatively in cases of carcinoma of the male breast. The mechanism is obscure, but does not appear to be androgen depletion. Soft tissue masses are affected more than bone metastases, and over 90 percent of the patients so treated are benefited. *Androgens* have been extensively used in postmenopausal women with advanced breast cancer, testosterone propionate being the most widely employed compound. The remission rate with androgens has been about 20 percent in both premenopausal and postmenopausal cases [45]. Both soft tissue masses (primary or metastatic) and bone metastases may respond. Paradoxically *estrogens* have given encouraging palliative results in postmenopausal women. The mechanism is obscure. Regressions are achieved in 35 percent of treated cases [45]. Soft tissue metastases are especially affected by estrogen therapy. The administration of massive amounts of estrogens in premenopausal women with metastatic breast carcinoma produces definite regression of the neoplasm for 6 to 21 months in about 15 percent of patients [46]. A decrease in serum and urine calcium levels is found in about 30 percent of the cases, indicating a metabolic response to therapy. The rationale of the large doses of estrogen is to produce anterior pituitary inhibition. However, there is evidence of growth stimulation in about 10 percent of cases so treated. Another complication of estrogen therapy in metastatic breast carcinoma is the development of *intractable hypercalcemia* in about 5 percent of the cases [47]. This occurs in patients with osteolytic metastases and is characterized by lethargy, weakness, marked hypercalcemia, renal insufficiency, and coma. Death occurs despite cessation of estrogen therapy and forced hydration. Both estrogens and androgens can cause exacerbation in some breast carcinomas and must be used with caution. It also must be remembered that annoying or serious side effects are common with hormone therapy.

chemotherapy

The *chemotherapy* of breast carcinoma includes the use of *nitrogen mustard* and various derivatives such as *sulfur mustard, triethylene phosphoramide* (TEPA), and *triethylene thiophosphoramide* (thio-TEPA, TSPA) intravenously. Critical studies indicate that about 50 percent of the cases undergo a marked regression in the size of primary or metastatic neoplasm except in bone. Part of the decrease in size is due to necrosis. The *cellular changes* with TSPA [48] include squamous metaplasia, cytoplasmic vacuolization, multinucleation, and the development of large bizarre cells within the neoplasm. In some areas malignant cells completely disappear; elsewhere they appear perfectly intact. Some remissions last over a year with repeated courses of these drugs. A serious side effect is a clinically significant *bone marrow depression* in about 40 percent of the cases, with the production of agranulocytosis and thrombocytopenia in a number of them.

SARCOMA

Sarcoma [49] makes up less than 1 percent of breast tumors. The most common type is the *malignant cystosarcoma phyllodes* (adenofibrosarcoma), which constitutes almost half of all mammary sarcomas. In this name, *-sarcoma* refers to the fleshy appearance rather than to malignancy, so that the qualifying adjective *malignant* must be used to separate this neoplasm from the benign cystosarcoma phyllodes. The malignant type usually consists of a fibrosarcomatous stroma containing a few distorted ducts. It metastasizes to the regional lymph nodes and lungs. *Primary sarcoma* may be fibrosarcoma, liposarcoma, angiosarcoma [50], lymphosarcoma [51], reticulum cell sarcoma [52], Hodgkin's disease, or extramedullary plasmocytoma. *Stromal sarcoma* [53] frequently shows a mixture of malignant fibrous, myxoid, and adipose tissues. Mammary sarcoma may appear at any age, and there is a definite history of trauma in 10 percent of the cases. These tumors tend to recur after surgical excision, but in general the prognosis is good, with a 5-year survival rate of about 60 percent. Less than 5 percent develop axillary metastases, hematogenous spread being the rule. Sarcoma may grow to a large size, being soft and homogeneous and resembling fish flesh. Foci of necrosis or hemorrhage are common.

REFERENCES

1. Tannenbaum, M., Weiss, M., and Marx, A. J. Ultrastructure of the human mammary ductule. *Cancer* 23:958, 1969.
2. Kipen, C. S. Gangrene of the breast – a complication of anticoagulant therapy. *New Eng. J. Med.* 265:638, 1961.
3. Hogan, G. F. Mondor's disease. *Arch. Intern. Med.* (Chicago) 113:881, 1964.
4. Treves, N. Gynecomastia. *Cancer* 11:1083, 1958.
5. Nydick, M., Bustos, J., Dale, J. H., Jr., and Rawson, R. W. Gynecomastia in adolescent boys. *J.A.M.A.* 178:449, 1961.
6. Schwartz, I. S., and Wilens, S. L. The formation of acinar tissue in gynecomastia. *Amer. J. Path.* 43:797, 1963.
7. Foote, F. W., and Stewart, F. W. Comparative studies of cancerous versus noncancerous breasts. *Ann. Surg.* 121:6, 197, 1945.
8. Warren, S. Relation of "chronic mastitis" to carcinoma of the breast. *Surg. Gynec. Obstet.* 71:257, 1940.
9. Miller, F. N., Jr., Dornfeld, L., and Horowitz, M. I. The relationship of fibrocystic mastopathy and breast carcinoma. Unpublished data, 1962.
10. Frantz, V. K., Pickren, J. W., Melcher, G. W., and Auchincloss, H., Jr. Incidence of chronic cystic disease in so-called normal breasts: Study based on 225 postmortem examinations. *Cancer* 4:762, 1951.
11. Vassar, P. S., and Culling, C. F. A. Fibrosis of the breast. *A.M.A. Arch. Path.* 67:128, 1959.
12. Murad, T. M., and von Hamm, E. The ultrastructure of fibrocystic disease of the breast. *Cancer* 22:587, 1968.
13. Murad, T. M., and von Hamm, E. Ultrastructure of myoepithelial cells in human mammary gland tumors. *Cancer* 21:1137, 1968.
14. Goldenberg, V. E., Wiegenstein, L., and Mottet, N. K. Florid breast fibroadenomas in patients taking hormonal oral contraceptives. *Amer. J. Clin. Path.* 49:52, 1968.
15. Murad, T. M., Greider, M. H., and Scarpelli, D. G. The ultrastructure of human mammary fibroadenoma. *Amer. J. Path.* 51:663, 1967.
16. Goldman, R. L., and Friedman, N. B. Carcinoma of the breast arising in fibroadenomas, with emphasis on lobular carcinoma. *Cancer* 23:544, 1969.
17. Obermans, H. A. Cystosarcoma phyllodes. *Cancer* 18:697, 1965.
18. Hill, R. P., and Miller, F. N., Jr. Adenomas of the breast. *Cancer* 7:318, 1954.
19. Kern, W. H., and Brooks, R. N. Atypical epithelial hyperplasia associated with breast cancer and fibrocystic disease. *Cancer* 24:668, 1969.
20. Wynder, E. L., Bross, I. J., and Hirayama, T. A study of the epidemiology of cancer of the breast. *Cancer* 13:559, 1960.
21. Todaro, G. J., Zeve, V., and Aaronson, S. Virus in cell culture derived from human tumour patients. *Nature* (London) 226:1047, 1970.
22. Farrow, J. H. Bilateral breast cancer. *Cancer* 9:1182, 1956.
23. Fisher, B., Slack, N. H., and Bross, I. D. J. Cancer of the breast: Size of neoplasm and prognosis. *Cancer* 24:1071, 1969.

24. Berg, J. W. Inflammation and prognosis in breast cancer. *Cancer* 12:714, 1959.
25. Kraus, F. T., and Neubecker, R. D. The differential diagnosis of papillary tumors of the breast. *Cancer* 15:444, 1962.
26. Ozello, L. The behavior of basement membranes in intraductal carcinoma of the breast. *Amer. J. Path.* 35:887, 1959.
27. Toker, C. Some observations on Paget's disease of the nipple. *Cancer* 14:653, 1961.
28. Helwig, E. B., and Graham, J. H. Anogenital (extramammary) Paget's disease. *Cancer* 16:387, 1963.
29. Melamed, M. R., Robbins, G. F., and Foote, F. W., Jr. Prognostic significance of gelatinous mammary carcinoma. *Cancer* 14:699, 1961.
30. Frable, W. J., and Kay, S. Carcinoma of the breast. Histologic and clinical features of apocrine tumors. *Cancer* 21:756, 1968.
31. Cavanzo, F. J., and Taylor, H. B. Adenoid cystic carcinoma of the breast. *Cancer* 24:740, 1969.
32. Warner, N. E. Lobular carcinoma of the breast. *Cancer* 23:840, 1969.
33. Newman, W. In situ lobular carcinoma of the breast. Report of 26 women with 32 cancers. *Ann. Surg.* 157:591, 1963.
34. Norris, H. J., and Taylor, H. B. Carcinoma of the male breast. *Cancer* 23:1428, 1969.
35. Moore, F. D., Woodrow, S. I., Aliapoulios, M. A., and Wilson, R. E. *Carcinoma of the Breast.* Boston: Little, Brown, 1968.
36. Treves, N. An evaluation of the etiological factors of lymphedema following radical mastectomy. *Cancer* 10:444, 1957.
37. Kennedy, B. J. Hormone therapy for advanced breast cancer. *Cancer* 18:1551, 1965.
38. Treves, N., and Finkbeiner, J. A. An evaluation of therapeutic surgical castration in the treatment of metastatic, recurrent, and primary inoperable mammary carcinoma in women. *Cancer* 11:421, 1958.
39. Harris, H. S., Jr., and Spratt, J. S., Jr. Bilateral adrenalectomy in metastatic mammary cancer. *Cancer* 23:145, 1969.
40. Nelsen, T. S., and Dragstedt, L. R. Adrenalectomy and oöphorectomy for breast cancer. *J.A.M.A.* 175:379, 1961.
41. Lemon, H. M. Prednisone therapy of advanced mammary cancer. *Cancer* 12:93, 1959.
42. Sherlock, P., and Hartmann, W. H. Adrenal steroids and the pattern of metastases of breast cancer. *J.A.M.A.* 181:313, 1962.
43. Furth, J., and Clifton, K. H. Experimental pituitary tumors and the role of pituitary hormones in tumorigenesis of the breast and thyroid. *Cancer* 10:842, 1957.
44. Kelley, W. A., Evans, J. P., Harper, P. V., and Humphreys, E. N. The effect upon the hypophysis of radioactive yttrium. *Surg. Gynec. Obstet.* 106:600, 1958.
45. Report to the Council on Drugs of the A.M.A. Androgens and estrogens in the treatment of disseminated mammary carcinoma. *J.A.M.A.* 172:1271, 1960.
46. Kennedy, B. J. Massive estrogen administration in premenopausal women with metastatic breast cancer. *Cancer* 15:641, 1962.
47. Kleinfeld, G. Acute fatal hypercalcemia: A complication in estrogen therapy of metastatic breast cancer. *J.A.M.A.* 181:1137, 1962.
48. Moore, G. E., and Pickren, J. W. Response of breast cancer to triethylene thiophosphoramide. *A.M.A. Arch. Path.* 65:98, 1958.

49. Oberman, H. A. Sarcomas of the breast. *Cancer* 18:1233, 1965.
50. Gulesserian, H. P., and Lawton, R. L. Angiosarcoma of the breast. *Cancer* 24:1021, 1969.
51. De Cosse, J. J., Berg, J. W., Fracchia, A. A., and Farrow, J. H. Primary lymphosarcoma of the breast. *Cancer* 15:1264, 1962.
52. Lawler, M. R., Jr., and Richie, R. E. Reticulum cell sarcoma of the breast. *Cancer* 20:1438, 1967.
53. Berg, J. W., De Cosse, J. J., Fracchia, A. A., and Farrow, J. Stromal sarcomas of the breast. A unified approach to connective tissue sarcomas other than cystosarcoma phyllodes. *Cancer* 15:418, 1962.

GENERAL REFERENCES

Haagensen, C. D. *Diseases of the Breast.* Philadelphia: Saunders, 1956. (A thoughtful treatise on mammary lesions, with a clinical emphasis.)

McDivitt, R. W., Stewart, F. W., and Berg, J. W. Tumors of the breast. Second Series, Fascicle 2, in *Atlas of Tumor Pathology.* Washington: Armed Forces Institute of Pathology, 1967. (A review of breast neoplasm, richly illustrated, based on long experience.)

26 THE NERVOUS SYSTEM

HISTOGENESIS OF THE NERVOUS SYSTEM AND ASSOCIATED TISSUES

The basis of the entire nervous system is the *neural plate,* a thickened band of *ectoderm* lying along the middorsal line of the early embryo. This plate folds into a *neural groove* bounded on each side by neural folds. These fuse and the structure becomes the *neural tube,* which gives rise to a *neural* (ganglionic) *crest* on each side. The cranial and spinal ganglia develop from the neural crests. Within the neural tube the epithelium differentiates in two directions; toward ependymo-epithelium and toward medulloblasts. According to the Kernohans' schema [1], *ependymo-epithelium* differentiates into ependymal cells (including those of the choroid plexuses), oligodendroglia, pinealocytes, and posterior pituicytes. *Medulloblasts* give rise to the spongioblast-astroblast-astrocyte and neuroblast-neurocyte (neuron) series and contribute to the formation of pheochromocytes of the adrenal medulla and other chromaffin cells. The microglia and the epineurium, perineurium, and endoneurium are derived from *mesoderm,* and the leptomeninges and pachymeninges are products of the neuroskeletal intertissue. From the notochord the nuclei pulposi of the intervertebral disks arise.

Vertebrae

The *vertebrae* develop from paired somitic sclerotomes lying segmentally along the notochord. Growth occurs in three directions: (1) medially to surround the notochord and form the vertebral bodies, (2) dorsally to form the neural (vertebral) arch, and (3) in the thoracic region, ventrolaterally to form the ribs. *Failure of fusion* of the paired structures forming the neural arch dorsally leads to *rachischisis (cleft spine) or spina bifida.*

Cranium

The *skull* derives from the desmocranium, a dense mesenchymal mass enveloping the cranial end of the notochord. This expands medially, laterally, and cephalad to form the brain case. Failure of fusion of the skull in the midline is *cranioschisis.* Failure of development of the skull is *acrania; hemicrania* is the failure of development of one-half of the cranium. Asymmetric development leads to *plagiocephaly* (twisted skull).

THE CEREBROSPINAL FLUID

The *cerebrospinal fluid* is normally produced by the epithelial cells of the choroid plexus, especially in the lateral ventricles, either by secretion or dialysis.

Under pathologic conditions it may be produced by the lining cells of all parts of the ventricles and arachnoid spaces. *Circulation* is a continuous, leisurely process of mixing and diffusion brought about by alterations in pressure within the fluid caused by brain pulsations, respiratory movements, and shifts in body position. Flow is from the lateral ventricles to the third ventricle via the foramina of Monro, then to the fourth ventricle through the aqueduct of Sylvius. The fluid then flows via the foramina of Luschka and the foramen of Magendie into the cisterna magna. From this distribution center the fluid reaches the other cisterns and the subarachnoid space. It is reabsorbed into the bloodstream by the Pacchionian granulations and into the lymph stream via the Virchow-Robin perivascular spaces and nerve sheaths.

Circulation

Characteristics and composition

Normally cerebrospinal fluid is a clear, colorless liquid with a specific gravity of 1.005 to 1.009 under a pressure of 70 to 170 mm. of water. It contains up to 5 lymphocytes per cubic millimeter, 15 to 45 mg. per 100 ml. of protein, 45 to 80 mg. per 100 ml. of glucose, and 119 to 128 milliequivalents per liter of chloride. Cerebrospinal fluid may be removed by means of a lumbar or cisternal tap for examination. Its pressure may be measured by a manometer. The *Queckenstedt test* is performed to determine the presence or absence of a spinal subarachnoid block to cerebrospinal fluid flow. In the test the jugular veins are compressed, raising the intracranial venous pressure. If the circulation is unimpeded, the spinal fluid pressure will be elevated 150 to 300 mm., returning to its original level within 10 seconds after the release of jugular pressure. The test should not be carried out when there is evidence of increased intracranial pressure. In fact, a spinal tap must be performed cautiously when the intracranial pressure is increased, because of the possibility of causing herniation of the medulla oblongata into the foramen magnum.

Abnormalities in pressure

Increased pressure of the cerebrospinal fluid is found in meningeal inflammations (meningitides), encephalitis, poliomyelitis, subarachnoid hemorrhage, and space-occupying intracranial lesions (subdural hematoma; epidural, subdural, or brain abscess; cerebral hemorrhage; and brain tumor). Pressures above 500 mm. are common, but rarely do they exceed 1000 mm. *Decreased pressure* occurs in some individuals normally; it also is seen in shock, dehydration, and subarachnoid block, and following intravenous injections of hypertonic fluids.

Alterations in gross appearance

Turbidity of the cerebrospinal fluid most commonly develops in cases of meningitis, the fluid becoming hazy when there are more than 500 cells per cubic millimeter. Frankly purulent fluid indicates a septic meningitis. *Clotting* results from the presence of fibrinogen in the fluid and occurs typically in septic and tuberculous meningitis. The fluid may coagulate solid, or a fine web or pellicle may form. *Grossly, bloody fluid* may be caused by tearing a vessel during the spinal tap *(traumatic tap),* but such bleeding usually appears in only the first tube of fluid withdrawn, and the supernatant fluid is not yellowish as it is in true hemorrhage into the subarachnoid space. Blood in the cerebrospinal fluid that is not the result of trauma from the spinal tap indicates a subarachnoid hemorrhage or rupture of an intracerebral hemorrhage into a ventricle or the subarachnoid space. *Xanthochromic* (yellow) *fluid* is caused by the release of blood pigments from degenerated erythrocytes. It develops a few days after bleeding into the subarachnoid space. Crenated (shrunken) erythrocytes are often present. Pigments may enter the subarachnoid space from without under conditions of abnormal permeability, so that xanthochromia may appear in cases of epidural and subdural hemorrhage. Yellowing of the cerebrospinal fluid is usually accompanied by an increase in protein and cells. Marked xanthochromia, pleocytosis, a greatly elevated protein level, and rapid coagulation of the fluid constitute *Froin's loculation syndrome,* which develops in the fluid below an obstruction of the spinal canal.

Pleocytosis is the presence of an abnormal number of cells in the cerebrospinal fluid. The highest counts (1000 to 10,000 neutrophils per cubic millimeter) are found in the septic meningitides. Moderate increases (10 to 250 lymphocytes per cubic millimeter) occur in poliomyelitis, encephalitis, tuberculous and fungus meningitis, lymphocytic choriomeningitis, and neurosyphilis. Slight rises in the cell count are sometimes seen in multiple sclerosis and brain tumors.

Pleocytosis

The *protein* level is elevated in most organic central nervous system diseases, because of development of abnormal permeability to serum proteins by the cells which produce cerebrospinal fluid. Severe increases occur in septic meningitis, in subarachnoid hemorrhage, and in pockets of fluid behind obstructions. The *glucose* level is often precipitously reduced in the acute bacterial meningitides. The level is moderately decreased in patients with widespread leptomeningeal neoplastic metastases. In patients with increased intracranial pressure, the glucose level is normal or slightly increased. The cerebrospinal fluid *chloride* level is definitely reduced in septic and tuberculous meningitis; it remains normal in localized inflammations (such as subdural, epidural, or brain abscess), poliomyelitis, encephalitis, lymphocytic choriomeningitis, and neurosyphilis.

Changes in chemical composition

By means of the manometric, gross, microscopic, chemical, microbiologic, and serologic examination of a small volume of cerebrospinal fluid, the diagnosis of many central nervous system diseases can be established. Thus lumbar puncture is one of the most valuable techniques available for the differentiation of neurologic disorders.

DEVELOPMENTAL DEFECTS OF THE CRANIUM, VERTEBRAE, AND NERVOUS SYSTEM

Oxycephaly (*acrocephaly,* turret skull) is due to a symmetric premature closure of the coronal sutures. The skull is tower-shaped. Exophthalmos occurs, and the facial expression is adenoidal. Syndactyly of the hands, polydactyly of the feet, and cardiac anomalies are sometimes associated with oxycephaly. *Craniofacial dysostosis* (Crouzon's disease) is hereditary and is characterized by oxycephaly, a beak-shaped nose, hypoplasia of the maxilla, exophthalmos, external strabismus, a short upper lip, and a protruding lower lip.

OXYCEPHALY

Scaphocephaly is caused by premature closure of the sagittal suture. The head is long and narrow, and the forehead and occiput bulge.

SCAPHOCEPHALY

Platybasia is a malformation of the base of the skull in which the posterior fossa is flattened and the space between the sella turcica and the foramen magnum is lengthened. The atlas may be fused to the base of the skull. Because of these defects, the medulla must course backward to reach the foramen magnum and may be bent sharply over the odontoid process of the axis. Increased intracranial pressure and exophthalmos are common. *Acquired platybasia* may develop in the course of osteitis deformans involving the skull.

PLATYBASIA

ARNOLD-CHIARI DEFECT

Arnold-Chiari malformation consists of fusion of the atlas and occipital bones, posterior displacement of the odontoid process of the axis, and a funnel-shaped posterior fossa. Herniation of the cerebellar tonsils and medulla into the defect is frequent, resulting in obstruction to the flow of cerebrospinal fluid. Hydrocephalus commonly results. Congenital stenosis of the aqueduct of Sylvius and spina bifida with meningomyelocele are often associated with Arnold-Chiari malformation. In about one-half the cases of Arnold-Chiari malformation, *vernicomyelia* (the presence of amniotic fluid squamae, lanugo hairs, and mucus in the spinal subarachnoid space and central canal) has been found [2]. The occurrence of vernicomyelia indicates that the "meningomyelocele" in the Arnold-Chiari defect is a degenerated neural plate.

KLIPPEL-FEIL SYNDROME

Klippel-Feil syndrome is characterized by a reduction in the number of cervical vertebrae and fusion of the bodies of two or more cervical vertebrae. *Clinically* the neck is short, the shoulders appearing to be high. The condition is neither hereditary nor familial, and males and females are affected equally. Neurologic disorders such as syringomyelia, Friedreich's ataxia, and mental deficiency are often associated. Typically the *cervical vertebrae* are a solid mass of bone. Spina bifida is frequently associated with the syndrome, and diplomyelia is sometimes present. Fusion and deformity of the ribs are common.

INIENCEPHALY

Iniencephaly is a rare, lethal malformation in which there are a defect in the squamous portion of the occipital bone, enlargement of the foramen magnum, and absence of the laminae and spinous processes of the cervical and thoracic vertebrae. The cervical and sometimes other vertebrae are reduced in number and are fused and deformed. There is hyperextension of the neck, the face pointing upward. The brain may be normally developed, but it and much of the short, malformed spinal cord occupy a single cavity. Ventricular dilatation may lead to cerebral cortical narrowing. Concomitant visceral defects are common.

HYPERTELORISM

Hypertelorism results from overdevelopment of the lesser wings of the sphenoid bone with underdevelopment of the greater wings. The cribriform plate is broader and the nasal aperture wider than normal. The head is broad and flat, with a prominent forehead, upturned (retroussé) nose, and eyes wide apart.

ANENCEPHALY:

Anencephaly is the failure of development of the forebrain and, in some cases, of the rest of the brain and the spinal cord (amyelia). The defect is incompatible with life. It is generally considered to occur predominantly in female fetuses, but about 75 percent of the authors' cases have been in males. Its *cause* is unknown, but injection studies of the major cephalic arteries and veins in cases of anencephaly have shown major vascular anomalies in 30 percent of the cases and poorly filling networks of branching and anastomosing sinusoids within the grossly defective brain tissue in the remainder of cases [3]. It is proposed that the cerebral abnormalities in anencephaly occur during the first 6 to 8 weeks of fetal development because of a failure of integration of the primordial cerebral vasculature into the systemic circulation. The presence of foci of hematopoiesis about the defective vessels in cases of anencephaly indicate definite cerebral anoxia. *Maternal polyhydramnios* is often present.

Pathologic changes

The *cerebral hemispheres* are soft, reddish purple, amorphous masses measuring a few centimeters in thickness and lying on the base of the skull. *Microscopically* the masses consist of dilated and congested vascular channels and small disorganized foci of cerebral tissue. The cranial vault is absent. The eyes bulge due to shortening of the anterior cranial fossa. *Club foot* (talipes) is almost always present. The *adrenal glands* are small and show marked cortical atrophy, apparently due to the absence of pituitary stimulation. The adrenal cortical atrophy occurs between the fifth and seventh month of gestation [4]. Multiple congenital defects are sometimes present in cases of anencephaly.

OTHER BRAIN ANOMALIES

Microcephaly is an anomaly in which the brain, especially the cerebrum, does not reach normal size. It has occurred in a number of fetuses exposed in utero to atomic bomb radiation. *Microgyria* is a failure in development of the cerebral convolutions, so that they remain smaller than normal. The sulci are excessively wide and deep. *Pachygyria* is the development of thick cerebral gyri due to inadequate formation of the sulci. The brain surface is abnormally smooth *(lissencephaly)*. *Porencephaly* is the failure of development of a superficial portion of a hemisphere, the defect being filled by fluid. The space or spaces communicate with the ventricular system. Porencephaly may also be traumatic in origin. *Arhinencephaly* is the failure of development of the olfactory bulb and tracts, corpus callosum, and interhemispheric fissure, one large ventricular cavity being found. Arhinecephaly has been found in a case of trisomy 13-15, and it is thought that other cases of this defect are associated with this abnormal chromosomal pattern [5]. Cases of arhinencephaly frequently also show harelip, cleft palate, microcephaly, microphthalmia (abnormally small eyes), and polydactyly or syndactyly, defects also found in cases of trisomy 13-15. *Cyclopia* (the development of a single central eye due to failure of cleavage of the optic cup) also occurs in association with arhinencephaly. *Agenesis of the corpus callosum* may appear as an isolated defect.

ENCEPHALOCELE

Encephalocele is the protrusion of a portion or all of the brain through a defect in the calvarium.

SPINAL CORD ANOMALIES

Amyelia is failure of the spinal cord to develop. It is often associated with anencephaly. *Diplomyelia* (diastematomyelia) is the development of two separate spinal cords, each containing only one anterior and posterior horn. A cystic cavity or fissure separates the two cords. *Myelocele* is an exposure of the spinal cord due to a defect in development of the dorsal arch.

SPINA BIFIDA

Spina bifida is a common defect, occurring once in every 1000 births. There is a failure of development of the dorsal arches of one or more vertebrae, usually in the lumbosacral region. Spina bifida is often associated with hydrocephalus and talipes. In *spina bifida occulta* there is no protrusion, the skin over the defect being wrinkled and covered with a patch of hair resembling a tail, or there may be a subcutaneous lipoma. A *tight filum terminale* may be associated with spina bifida occulta [6]. With it there are gait disturbances with limping and frequent stumbling and ankle sprains in early childhood. Later weakness and atrophy of the leg muscles and high-arched feet develop. Leg and back pains and limited flexion of the back are common. Frequently urinary bladder disturbances are associated with a tight filum terminale. If there is protrusion, a sac is formed *(spina bifida aperta)*. Its contents may be of three types: (1) *meningocele,* a leptomeningeal protrusion through a bony and dural defect in the skull or vertebral column (the latter is usually sacral); (2) *meningomyelocele,* a protrusion of both leptomeninges and cord through a bony and dural defect in the vertebrae; or (3) *syringomyelocele,* a rare defect in which the central canal of the spinal cord in myelocele is greatly distended with cerebrospinal fluid with resultant pressure atrophy of the spinal cord. Spina bifida aperta is present alone or in combination in 45 percent of central nervous system developmental defects. When a child has spina bifida aperta, its siblings have the defect six times as often as the expected rate in the general population.

PILONIDAL SINUS

Pilonidal sinus is variously explained as a persistence of the neurenteric canal in the coccygeal region, an epidermal inclusion, or a failure of fusion of the skin of the two halves of the body in this region. Many cases are acquired due to trauma (*"jeep seat"* or *rough-riding syndrome*). A similar lesion occurs occupationally in barbers, hairs being driven into the interdigital skin. The pilonidal sinus is lined by skin with numerous hairs and sweat and sebaceous glands. The sinus opens onto the skin over the coccyx. Not infrequently the sinus tract becomes infected, and a foreign body reaction to the included hairs often develops. In some persons the opening onto the skin is absent, a depression (postanal dimple) being found over the coccyx. There may be a *pilonidal tract* or *pilonidal cyst* under the skin in these persons.

AMAUROTIC IDIOCY:

Amaurotic familial idiocy is a hereditary degenerative disease which most often occurs in Jewish infants, but seldom in the firstborn. It is transmitted as a recessive. The condition may be a variant of Niemann-Pick's disease.

Pathologic changes

The *brain* is hard and small. The cells and fibers of the cerebral cortex, anterior and posterior horns of the spinal cord, and posterior root ganglia show widespread degeneration. The *degenerated cells of the brain and retina* are swollen and filled with lipids. These are gangliosides and contain neuraminic acid. There is diffuse gliosis in the central nervous system.

Clinical features

Clinically the most common form is *Tay-Sachs disease* which is congenital but becomes manifest at 3 to 4 months. *Bielschowsky-Jansky disease* begins at 3 to 4 years, *Spielmeyer-Vogt disease* at 7 to 12 years, and *Kuf's disease* in adulthood. Early signs of amaurotic idiocy are listlessness, hyperacusis (increased sensitivity to sound), blindness, and muscle weakness. A *cherry-red macular spot* is pathognomonic. Later the flaccid paralysis becomes spastic and convulsions develop. There is severe mental deterioration. In Tay-Sachs disease death occurs at about 2 to 3 years.

MONGOLISM

Down's syndrome (mongolism) is a gross congenital defect of unknown cause which develops during the eighth week of gestation. The infant has a low mentality, dry skin, a small head, slanting eyes, white flecks in the irises, fat cheeks and back of the neck, protruding tongue, short thumbs, bent fifth fingers, square palms, and markedly hypotonic musculature. Cardiac anomalies are common, especially persistent atrioventricular ostium *("mongol heart")*. The *brain* is small with defective gyri, the number of cerebral cortical neurons being greatly reduced. Most patients with Down's syndrome have *47 chromosomes in their body cells* due to an additional short, acrocentric chromosome (one in which the centrosome is located toward one tip) on chromosome 21 (trisomy 21) [7]; these children are usually the offspring of older mothers. In about 15 percent of cases of mongolism, 46 chromosomes are found, with reciprocal translocation of a small autosome on chromosome 15; the mothers of this group are usually young. A parent and one or more siblings without mongolism may be carriers of the translocation and have 45 somatic chromosomes [8]. Acute or subacute leukemia occurs in patients with mongolism over three times as often as the predicted rate *(mongoloid-leukemic syndrome)*.

TUBEROUS SCLEROSIS:

Tuberous sclerosis (Bourneville's disease) is a type of central nervous system sclerosis. Most cases are familial, and the defect appears to be transmitted as a mendelian dominant in such cases. Boys are affected about twice as often as girls. The tuberous sclerosis complex [9] is probably hamartial in nature and consists of, besides the central nervous system lesions, sebaceous adenomas of the face, rhabdomyoma of the heart, hamartoma of the kidney, and phacoma of the retina. This combination is known as *epiloia. Shagreen skin,* in which there are close-set papules resembling untanned leather, is present in some cases. Epilepsy and mental deficiency are characteristic in tuberous sclerosis.

Pathologic changes

There are numerous firm, whitish, opaque, spheroid nodules up to 3 cm. in diameter in the gray cortex, brain stem, cerebellum, and spinal cord. *Microscopically* these are made up of dense glial tissue and giant glial and ganglion cells. The *retinal phacoma,* which is pathognomonic of tuberous sclerosis, consists of a small gray or white focus on or near the optic disk. *Microscopically* there is a hamartial proliferation of glial cells with a few giant ganglion cells.

CEREBRAL PALSY:

Cerebral palsy is a generic term for a group of neurologic disorders caused by lesions occurring in the pyramidal or extrapyramidal tracts in the brain during embryonic, fetal, or early infantile life. About 15 percent of cases of cerebral palsy are postneonatally acquired due to lesions developing after the first 2 weeks of life [10]. *Clinically* 40 to 60 percent of the cases are characterized by *spasticity* of one or more extremities (due to pyramidal tract involvement), 20 to 40 percent show *athetoid movements* (due to extrapyramidal tract involvement), and less than 20 percent show *ataxic movements* (due to cerebellar damage). *Convulsions* may occur due to involvement of the motor cortex. *Mental retardation* is severe in about 30 percent of the cases.

Cause

The *cause* is not always clear, nor is it the same in all cases. Etiologically cerebral palsy may be divided into three types [11]:

1. *Developmental.* The lesions may be hereditary or induced. Pathogenetically there is an arrest of growth and differentiation, resulting in hypogenesis or dysgenesis of the motor cortex on one or both sides. There are patches of microgyria. Malformation of the brain has been found in about 30 percent of cases of cerebral palsy.

2. *Encephaloclastic due to systemic causes.* The causes include anoxia neonatorum which may produce focal necrosis in the motor cortex or internal capsule(s); prematurity, in which hemorrhage or necrosis may occur in these areas; and erythroblastosis fetalis with kernicterus.

3. *Encephaloclastic due to local causes.* Such causes include mechanical birth injuries which produce meningeal hemorrhage or cerebral laceration, hydrocephalus with damage to the motor cortex by compression, and, rarely, cerebral arterial thrombosis or embolism with infarction of the motor cortex or an internal capsule.

Postinfectious encephalitis, meningitis, and head injuries, with or without skull fracture or subdural hematoma, are important causal factors in *postneonatally acquired cerebral palsy.*

Spastic diplegia

Congenital spastic diplegia (Little's disease) is a type of cerebral palsy in which the lower extremities are spastic with increased deep reflexes and positive Babinskis. When the child begins to walk, the gait is "cross-legged" in type. The *cause* is usually agenesis of the motor neurons of the part of the motor cortex controlling the lower extremities and occasionally the upper extremities.

AMYOTONIA CONGENITA

Amyotonia (myatonia) congenita (Oppenheim's disease) is evident shortly after birth. The *pathologic change* is a paucity of anterior horn neurons in the spinal cord. The muscles, lacking a complete nerve supply, are atonic and profoundly weak.

DEVELOPMENTAL NEOPLASMS:

Sacrococcygeal tumors are developmental in origin and are teratomas. Most are benign, containing well-differentiated adult tissues, but they may be highly malignant, containing primitive tissues. Many are cystic, some being dermoid cysts. The neoplasms are usually apparent at birth or during infancy. They commonly develop posterior to the sacrum.

Chordoma:

Chordoma is rare and arises from notochordal rests. The *most common sites* are the sacrococcygeal (70 percent) and basisphenoid (20 percent) regions.

pathologic changes

Grossly chordoma is a soft, sticky, expansive mass which tends to invade or incorporate adjacent bone. The neoplasm may grow about and constrict the rectum. *Microscopically* there are cords and clusters of cells in a dense myxomatous stroma. The typical cell is a large, vacuolated *physaliferous* (bubble-bearing) *cell.* Electron microscopy also reveals intercellular vacuolated spaces [12]. About 15 percent of these neoplasms are histologically highly malignant, and a few metastasize to the lungs. All tend to recur after surgical removal because of their inaccessible locations.

EPILEPSY

EPILEPSY:

Epilepsy is a symptomatic paroxysmal cerebral dysrhythmia in which sudden, excessive, and unruly motor neuronal discharges occur. Alkalosis such as that due to hyperventilation, hypoxia, hypoglycemia, and water-logging tend to precipitate epileptic convulsions. *Musicogenic epilepsy* is a rare form of reflex epilepsy in which seizures are triggered by various forms of music. *Photogenic epilepsy,* in which seizures are set off by strong light, is probably the most common reflex form of the disease. Epilepsy may be idiopathic, post-traumatic, or postinfectious, the first type being by far the most common. There are about 800,000 cases of epilepsy in the United States. Most cases develop before the age of 21 years, and males and females are involved with about equal frequency.

Clinical features

Clinically epilepsy is characterized by *periodic grand mal convulsions* (generalized clonic convulsions with biting of the tongue and unconsciousness) or episodes of *petit mal* (loss of consciousness). The convulsions are preceded by an *aura* in about 50 percent of the cases and followed by depression or occasionally by an epileptic furor. During the *tonic phase* of a grand mal convulsion the patient is apneic and becomes cyanotic with venous engorgement. With the accumulation of carbon dioxide the *clonic convulsions* begin. Inspired air mixes with saliva to form the foam present at the lips. During a *grand mal convulsion,* spikelike high-amplitude waves (100 to 200 microvolts) at a rate of 15 to 40 per second are found on electroencephalogram as compared to the normal 20 to 60 microvolt waves at 8 to 12 per second. In *petit mal attacks* a sharp spike followed by slow, dome-shaped, high-amplitude waves (100 to 250 microvolts) at a rate of about 3 per second is found. *Status epilepticus,* in which prolonged and repeated convulsions occur sometimes for hours, develops in about 10 percent of epileptics.

Pathologic changes

In the *post-traumatic or postinfectious group,* foci of gliosis are sometimes found in the motor cortex. An arachnoiditis, with thickening and opacity of the overlying pia-arachnoid, may be present. In the *idiopathic group* no specific pathologic changes are recognized. Evidence of old or recent *injury to the tongue* due to biting during convulsions is very often present.

HYDROCEPHALUS

HYDRO-CEPH-ALUS:

Hydrocephalus (water on the brain) is a condition in which excessive amounts of cerebrospinal fluid collect within (and sometimes outside of) the ventricles, greatly dilating these cavities and compressing the surrounding cerebral tissue, causing atrophy. The greatest degrees of hydrocephalus occur in infants in whom the head is still capable of enlargement. In infants the enlargement of the head may be enormous, the cranial bones being widely separated.

Causes

Obstruction to the flow of cerebrospinal fluid may occur at any of three points: (1) in the aqueduct of Sylvius, (2) in the roof of the fourth ventricle, and (3) around the midbrain where it passes through the narrow opening in the tentorium. The first two cause *internal hydrocephalus;* the last, *communicating hydrocephalus,* in which the ventricles are open to the basal cisterns and spinal canal.

Hydrocephalus in children

Hydrocephalus of infants and children may be due to obstruction either in the roof of the fourth ventricle or in the aqueduct of Sylvius, probably due to adhesions resulting from a mild meningitis (arachnoiditis). In other cases a thin gossamer membrane may occlude the aqueduct due to a congenital defect. A congenital septum or membrane may occlude the fourth ventricular outlets (Dandy-Walker syndrome). Such obstructions may also result from inflammations. Rarely the *Arnold-Chiari malformation,* in which the brain stem is displaced through the foramen magnum thereby plugging it and preventing reabsorption of cerebrospinal fluid, may be the cause. *Meningitis,* especially tuberculous meningitis, may lead to hydrocephalus. In *tuberculous meningitis* the plastic exudate on the roof of the fourth ventricle may block the foramina of Luschka and Magendie. *Syphilitic meningitis* may similarly cause hydrocephalus. A few cases are due to an overproduction of cerebrospinal fluid by *choroidal papillomas* in the ventricles. Finally, there are many cases of hydrocephalus which are *idiopathic.*

Neoplasms

Intracranial neoplasms may cause hydrocephalus in three ways: (1) by direct compression of the pathways of the cerebrospinal fluid, as by a glioma of the midbrain; (2) by forcing the brain stem into the opening of the tentorium, as by a supratentorial tumor; or (3) by pressing the cerebral hemispheres upward against the skull, obliterating the cortical subarachnoid spaces and thus interfering with reabsorption. All degrees of dilatation of the ventricles and atrophy of the brain substance may be found, depending on the location and degree of the obstruction.

HYDRO-MYELIA

Hydromyelia is a dilatation of the central canal of the spinal cord. It may or may not be associated with hydrocephalus.

INFLAMMATIONS OF THE NERVOUS SYSTEM AND RELATED STRUCTURES

Infections of the nervous system may be due to a wide variety of agents, such as viruses, pyogenic organisms, tubercle bacilli, and fungi. As a rule, viruses involve the substance of the brain or spinal cord predominantly, while most other agents involve the meninges primarily. The *cerebrospinal fluid* often reflects the nature of the infectious process affecting these structures.

1. Meningitis

Strictly speaking, *meningitis* signifies inflammation of the meninges without regard to whether one or another of the three membranes is affected. In *leptomeningitis,* a more specific term for the usual form of meningeal infection, the pia mater and the arachnoid are affected, and the exudate accumulates between these two membranes, i.e., in the subarachnoid space surrounding the brain and cord. *Pachymeningitis* means inflammation of the dura mater, the membrane that is intimately related to the skull itself. When the term *meningitis* is used without specification, leptomeningitis is implied.

Routes of infection

Infectious agents may reach the meninges by any of three routes: (1) by the *bloodstream* and choroid plexus during bacteremia (the usual avenue in the case of leptomeningitis), (2) by *direct continuity* (such as from an area of osteomyelitis of the skull or spine or from mastoiditis), or (3) by *penetrating wounds* (such as fractures or gunshot wounds).

PYOGENIC MENINGITIS:

When the spinal fluid is visibly cloudy or creamy, the predominating cell is the polymorphonuclear leukocyte and the infection is usually due to one of the *pyogenic bacteria.* Ordinarily the organism can be demonstrated in the fluid by smear or culture. It is extremely important that the causative agent be identified promptly and its antibiotic sensitivity determined so that therapy can be fully effective. *Diplococcus pneumoniae, Hemophilus influenzae,* and *Neisseria meningitidis* cause the majority of cases of pyogenic meningitis. Less often the causative organism is a streptococcus, *Staphylococcus aureus, Escherichia coli, Pseudomonas aeruginosa, Proteus mirabilis, Klebsiella pneumoniae,* and *Listerella monocytogenes.*

Meningococcal meningitis:

Meningococcal meningitis is caused by *Neisseria meningitidis (N. intracellularis)* and is the only type of meningitis having any tendency to be *epidemic;* even this type may occur sporadically. The disease is not highly infectious as a rule. A "carrier epidemic" often precedes the appearance of a case epidemic. Epidemics usually occur in winter, and especially in closed groups such as military barracks or boarding schools. Epidemics of meningococcal meningitis have often occurred along with those of influenza. Children are especially susceptible. The *incubation period* is 1 to 10 days.

pathogenesis

The organisms apparently enter the bloodstream through the nasopharynx. *Bacteremia* leads to involvement of the choroid plexus which is followed by meningeal inflammation. In fulminating infections death may occur before meningitis develops; in such cases the *meningococcemia* is overwhelming, and there may be a shocklike state with purpura and adrenal hemorrhages *(Waterhouse-Friderichsen syndrome)*. Rarely a chronic form of meningococcal meningitis is seen, lasting several months with recurring bacteremia and meningitis.

pathologic changes

In fulminating cases with peripheral vascular collapse, *bilateral adrenal necrosis and hemorrhage* may be the only visceral lesions. In the usual case *meningitis* is the only grossly demonstrable lesion. The meninges show hyperemia, and a *serous to purulent exudate collects in the subarachnoid space,* especially in the posterior fossa. Creamy material may fill the entire subarachnoid space. The exudate consists of *neutrophils and fibrin.* The blood vessels of the pia-arachnoid are dilated and engorged. There is no involvement of the brain proper. Rarely meningococcal endocarditis, pericarditis, or septic arthritis may occur.

clinical features

In *fulminating meningococcemia* there is an abrupt onset of shaking chills, severe headache, and prostration. Cases with *adrenal hemorrhages* are characterized by shock and an extensive purpuric rash involving the skin and mucous membrane. The hemorrhages are due to endothelial damage and vascular necrosis caused by meningococci, which can be identified in the lesions. Death is due to peripheral vascular collapse and acute adrenal insufficiency. When there is little or no adrenal damage, a petechial rash and an *encephalitic picture* with rapidly developing, deep coma appear. In patients with *meningococcal meningitis,* as in other types of pyogenic meningitis, the increased intracranial pressure causes severe headache, nausea, vomiting (which may be projectile), and sometimes generalized or localized convulsions. Signs of meningeal irritation are neck stiffness, hyperextension of the head or even opisthotonos, hyperesthesia, hyperirritability, and increased deep tendon reflexes. Kernig's sign (inability to extend the leg completely on the flexed thigh) and Brudzinski's signs (flexion of the opposite leg when one is passively flexed and flexion of both legs when the neck is flexed by an examiner) are positive. In some cases of meningitis, signs of a meningococcemia, such as a hemorrhagic rash and shock, are present.

cerebrospinal fluid changes

The *cerebrospinal fluid* is under *increased pressure* and is usually *cloudy;* the *cell count* ranges from several hundred to thousands of cells per cubic millimeter *(mostly neutrophils). Gram-negative diplococci* are seen both intracellularly and extracellularly. The protein level is high, and glucose is absent. Meningococci are very fastidious in their requirements, tending to disappear from a culture after 24 to 48 hours unless subcultured.

outcome

When seen in epidemic form, the severity of the disease is relatively constant for that epidemic, so that in some epidemics the cases are mild and in others, severe. This difference seems to be a matter of *variable virulence of the organism.* With modern therapy most patients survive without residual damage to brain or meninges. In the fulminating cases death may occur in a few hours from acute adrenal insufficiency.

Pneumococcal meningitis

Pneumococcal meningitis is caused by *Diplococcus pneumoniae.* The organisms reach the meninges via the bloodstream and choroid plexus, usually as a complication of pneumococcal pneumonia, but sometimes from otitis media or endocarditis. Occasionally no other focus is found (primary pneumococcal meningitis). The mortality rate is about 20 percent.

Streptococcal meningitis

Streptococcal meningitis is usually secondary to infection of the middle ear or paranasal sinuses, but may develop during other streptococcal infections.

Staphylococcal meningitis

Staphylococcal meningitis is relatively rare, but occurs during the course of a bacteremia, as from pyelonephritis in diabetics, furunculosis in malnourished infants, or endocarditis due to *Staphylococcus aureus.*

Influenzal meningitis

Influenzal meningitis is due to *Hemophilis influenzae* and is important to infants and the elderly, but is rare otherwise. It often occurs without apparent pulmonary or other localization.

The *clinical, pathologic, and spinal fluid findings* in pneumococcal, streptococcal, staphylococcal, and influenzal meningitis are like those in meningococcal meningitis. Differentiation is made by identification of the causative organism in the cerebrospinal fluid.

Listeria meningitis

Listeria meningitis [13] is caused by *Listeria monocytogenes,* a motile, gram-positive, microaerophilic bacillus which produces beta hemolysis on blood agar. Almost all cases occur in the newborn and in young infants, and intra-uterine infection can occur. The organisms also enter the body in milk or meat. *Clinically* there are fever, anorexia, irritability, vomiting, and convulsions. Nuchal rigidity is uncommon in the newborn, but the fontanelle is typically tense or bulging. The *mortality rate* in untreated cases is 70 to 80 percent. In surviving infants, hydrocephalus commonly develops. Pathologically there is a *purulent meningitis* with neutrophilic infiltration of the pia-arachnoid and subarachnoid space. While meningitis is the most common form of listeriosis, occasionally a hematogenously *disseminated miliary granulomatosis* with small nodules in the abdominal and thoracic viscera, nervous system, and skin occurs, often as a result of intra-uterine infection.

Neonatal meningitis

Neonatal meningitis (meningitis of newborn infants) [14] is presumed to have resulted from in utero or birth canal infection when it becomes manifest within the first 48 hours of life. Cases which develop later are secondary to pneumonitis, gastroenteritis, pyoderma (a purulent skin infection), or otitis media in the infant. In almost all cases the organisms reach the meninges hematogenously and blood cultures are positive. *Escherichia coli* is the causative organism in about 35 percent of the cases. Paracolon organisms, hemolytic streptococci, and staphylococci are other important causal agents. Neonatal meningitis is more common in premature than full term infants due to the increased permeability of the gastrointestinal mucosa and the blood-spinal fluid barrier in prematures, as well as their immature immunologic and phagocytic responses. Neonatal meningitis is often difficult to diagnose because of the vagueness of its signs. Bulging of the fontanelle and nuchal rigidity are frequently absent. The *mortality rate* in neonatal meningitis is about 65 percent.

SEROUS MENINGITIS

Occasionally meningitis occurs without bacterial invasion of the subarachnoid space. Following simple lumbar puncture, intrathecal medication, fracture of the skull, or deep-seated brain lesions, the cell count and protein content of the spinal fluid may rise, although rarely to the levels found in pyogenic meningitis. Spinal fluid glucose is usually not appreciably lowered. These cases are known as *serous meningitis.* Symptoms are usually relatively mild, and the course is favorable.

LYMPHOCYTIC MENINGITIS:

In certain types of meningitis the spinal fluid cell count is only moderately increased (100 to 1000 per cubic millimeter), the fluid is either clear or barely opalescent, and lymphocytes are the dominant cell. Generally speaking, the clinical symptoms in such cases are slower in appearing and less violent in their manifestations than in septic meningitis.

TUBERCULOUS MENINGITIS:

Tuberculous meningitis is usually part of generalized *miliary tuberculosis,* especially in infants and small children. The blood-borne bacilli lodge in the choroid plexus, tubercles are formed, and the bacilli are seeded over the meninges by the cerebrospinal fluid. In some instances bacilli may reach the brain from the lungs via Batson's veins. Sometimes *tuberculomas* form in brain or meninges, and from these meningitis may occur some time after the hematogenous dissemination. Rarely tuberculous meningitis may complicate tuberculous spondylitis (Pott's disease).

Pathologic changes

Miliary tubercles are seen as minute yellowish gray dots in the *arachnoid membrane,* chiefly at the base of the brain about the cerebellum, pons, or midbrain. In addition, a general clouding of the meninges may be noted, often with adhesions, producing mild hydrocephalus. *Microscopically* typical miliary tubercles are seen in the meninges, choroid plexus, and ependymal lining of the ventricles. *Tuberculous arteritis* is commonly noted. A caseous, sometimes semiliquid nodule *(tuberculoma)* 0.5 to 2 cm. in diameter may be found in any part of the brain, spinal cord, choroid plexus, or meninges. Multiple tuberculomas are common. A tuberculoma may sometimes resemble a brain tumor clinically.

Cerebrospinal fluid changes

The *cerebrospinal fluid pressure* is increased, and the fluid is clear to slightly cloudy; the *cell count* is usually 50 to 500 per cubic millimeter with lymphocytes predominating. The protein content is increased, the glucose level is diminished, and the chlorides are low in relation to blood chlorides. A pellicle usually forms in the spinal fluid sample on standing. Acid-fast bacilli are present, but a long search is often needed to find them.

Outcome

A few years ago recovery from tuberculous meningitis was unknown, hence no sequelae were recognized. With antibiotic therapy occasional recoveries now occur, but in such patients mental deterioration is common.

TORULAR MENINGITIS

Torular meningitis, due to the yeast *Cryptococcus neoformans,* is a *chronic granulomatous meningitis,* often indistinguishable from tuberculous meningitis during life. Most cases currently seen occur as terminal infections in patients with Hodgkin's disease and multiple myeloma. The organisms enter the body by inhalation into the lungs in most instances, reaching the brain via the bloodstream. They have a large spherical nucleus surrounded by a doubly contoured refractile capsule and may sometimes be seen in the spinal fluid. The characteristic *pathologic changes* are cysts, 1 to 2 mm. in diameter, in the gray matter of the cerebral cortex and in the basal ganglia. These contain great numbers of the organisms. The meningitis is largely basal, the exudate consisting of macrophages and lymphocytes. *Spinal fluid findings* are identical with those in tuberculous meningitis except for the causative agent. The disease is almost uniformly fatal.

VIRAL CHORIOMENINGITIS

Benign lymphocytic choriomeningitis is a slightly contagious form of *viral meningitis* and is sometimes confused with tuberculous meningitis or with nonparalytic poliomyelitis. A virus specific for this disease has been recovered from the blood and spinal fluid, but some cases of aseptic meningitis are caused by Coxsackie, ECHO, and herpes simplex viruses. Since the condition is rarely fatal, the *pathologic changes* are almost unknown. Presumably there is a minimal lymphocytic exudate in the subarachnoid space. The *spinal fluid* is clear and under slightly increased pressure. The cell count is usually 20 to 600 per cubic millimeter, the cells being all lymphocytes. No organisms are found on smear or culture. Since facilities rarely permit demonstration of the virus in clinical practice, the diagnosis is usually made by exclusion of other causes. The spinal fluid protein content is slightly increased, but the chloride and glucose levels are normal. *Recovery* is usually rapid and complete, and there are no sequelae.

MISCELLANEOUS INFECTIONS

Various diseases affecting the brain and spinal cord primarily may involve the meninges secondarily and show a lymphocytic response in the spinal fluid. These include central nervous system syphilis, poliomyelitis, viral encephalitis, toxoplasmosis, and coccidioidomycosis. Rarely can the causative organism be demonstrated in the spinal fluid in the diseases belonging to this group. Some of these diseases can be distinguished by serologic tests, others by prolonged clinical observation. These diseases are often referred to as types of *meningoencephalitis.*

2. Abscesses of the Dura Mater

EPIDURAL ABSCESS:

Epidural abscess usually affects that portion of the dura mater which lines the cranial cavity, but this infection may also occur in the spinal canal as a result of trauma or bone disease. Pus forms between the bone and the dura mater, usually several weeks after infection of the overlying bone has occurred. The primary lesion is usually mastoiditis, frontal sinusitis, scalp abscess, gunshot wound, or compound fracture of the skull.

Pathologic changes

The *dura mater* is elevated from the bone by a collection of pus, which may contain fragments of bone or foreign bodies. The causative agent (staphylococci, streptococci, or other bacteria) can usually be demonstrated in the exudate. On x-ray, bone proliferation can sometimes be noted at the edges of the abscess, with rarefaction at the base. There is often a flattening of the underlying brain cortex as a result of compression. Occasionally the space between the dura mater and the arachnoid membrane becomes involved consequent to the extradural abscess; such an abscess, localized by adhesions from the rest of the subdural space, is known as a *subdural abscess.* It is less frequent than extradural abscess but is due to the same causes.

Subdural abscess

Clinical features

In most cases extradural and subdural abscesses are chronic, and symptoms are usually those of brain compression (headache, vomiting, convulsions), as in brain tumor. Surgical drainage usually results in relief of the symptoms.

3. Brain Abscess

BRAIN ABSCESS:

A *brain abscess* is a localized area of suppuration within the substance of the brain. It is usually either cerebral or cerebellar in location. *Clinical manifestations* are local, depending on size and location, and general (fever and chills). In some instances there are no symptoms until the abscess becomes large or ruptures into a ventricle or the pia-arachnoid.

Pathogenesis

The causative organisms may be introduced by trauma, or by extension from an infection in some adjacent structure, such as the ethmoid or frontal sinuses, mastoid air cells, orbits (abscess), or cavernous sinus (septic thrombosis). At first an extradural abscess may form, later a subdural one, and finally a brain abscess. In other instances the abscess may be metastatic, a result of septic embolism during the course of endocarditis, pyemia, or especially pyogenic infections of the thorax (lung abscess, empyema, bronchiectasis, or pericarditis). Streptococci, staphylococci, and pneumococci are the most common infecting organisms.

Pathologic changes

The *brain* is asymmetric in appearance, the affected portion being swollen and the surface markings somewhat obliterated by compression. The *meninges* are usually adherent at the most superficial portion of the abscess. On section a rounded or ragged cavity is found; it is often lined with a fibrous membrane and filled with creamy pus. Abscesses developing by direct extension are usually solitary; abscesses resulting from septic embolism are often multiple.

Outcome

If not drained, brain abscesses tend to rupture into the subarachnoid space or ventricular system, in either case causing a purulent bacterial meningitis. This is sometimes recurrent and is usually fatal. Prior to this development the spinal fluid may be nearly normal; although the protein level is generally elevated, the spinal fluid pressure and cell count are only slightly raised, and bacteria are not demonstrable on smear or culture.

4. *Septic Thrombophlebitis of Intracranial Venous Sinuses*

By virtue of their location and their tributaries, two sets of venous sinuses in the dura mater of the cranium are susceptible to infection – the cavernous sinuses and the lateral sinuses. When either is infected, there is a general picture of severe sepsis, often with evidence of septic emboli to the lungs. These conditions have become rare in recent years as a result of the effective antibiotic treatment of mastoiditis and cranial osteomyelitis.

CAVERNOUS SINUSITIS

The *cavernous sinuses* are paired, one being located on each side of the sella turcica; the two sinuses anastomose freely. They receive blood from the orbits and face. Infection may reach these sinuses from a furuncle on the nose or upper lip via the small veins of the face. Septic thrombosis blocks the venous tributaries first from one and then from both orbits. The deep tissues and conjunctivae become edematous, the eyes bulge and become discolored, resembling "black eyes" from trauma; there is great pain in the eyes. Bacteria within the thrombi cause fibrinolysis in the clot, and septic emboli are carried to the lungs. Meningitis is a common complication.

LATERAL SINUSITIS

The *lateral sinuses* lie just deep to the mastoid air cells and may be infected secondarily to mastoiditis. The involved bone may be eroded by the infection. An extradural abscess may form, followed by direct involvement and thrombosis of one of the lateral sinuses. Sometimes no local manifestation is evident, and the condition is first revealed by evidence of pulmonary embolism. If lateral sinus thrombosis is suspected, a lumbar puncture should be performed together with the Queckenstedt test; this will disclose complete obstruction if it is present and also will indicate the side affected. Meningitis is an important complication of lateral sinus thrombosis.

5. *Viral Infections of the Brain and Spinal Cord*

GENERAL FEATURES

Certain viruses have a special affinity for the central nervous system and hence are known as *neurotropic viruses;* the diseases due to these neurotropic viruses are considered in this section. Most other viruses (measles, mumps, chickenpox, smallpox) do not ordinarily affect the central nervous system but may on occasion do so, especially during convalescence. Certain neurotropic viruses invade the nervous system during the course of *viremia.* Others apparently enter the body through the skin or intestinal mucosa, and then spread proximally via the *peripheral nerves* to the central nervous system. In some instances (as in herpes simplex) it appears that the virus may remain dormant in the nervous system for long periods, later becoming activated. Most neurotropic viruses have a *specific localization* of effect and can be recognized by this feature plus the character of the tissue response. Foci of necrosis, lymphocytic infiltration, and later demyelinization occur in most cases, and inclusion bodies may be seen in nerve cells in some instances. The cellular exudate accumulates in the subarachnoid space and in its perivascular extensions – the Virchow-Robin spaces.

ENCEPHALITIS:

Encephalitis connotes an inflammation of the brain. In the United States encephalitis is usually due to viral infections and is uncommon. Occasionally *bacterial encephalitis* may occur terminally in a septicemia or be caused by emboli from an endocarditis or lung abscess. Small neutrophilic infiltrates are scattered through the brain. Encephalitis may be caused by a number of infectious agents including rickettsiae, plasmodia, *Toxoplasma gondii,* trypanosomes, and *Trichinella spiralis.* These infections are discussed in Chapters 7 and 8.

Type A encephalitis:

Encephalitis lethargica (type A or von Economo's encephalitis, sleeping sickness) is probably caused by a filtrable virus. The disease appeared epidemically from 1916 to 1926. Today, if it occurs at all, there are only sporadic cases.

pathologic changes

Grossly there is marked congestion of the meninges and brain, especially of the brain stem. Small hemorrhages occur on the floor of the fourth ventricle. *Microscopically* the interstitial lesions consist of intense vascular dilatation, with perivascular cuffing by lymphocytes and plasmocytes in the adventitia and in the Virchow-Robin spaces. This pathologic change is absent in the fulminating cases. The most severe lesions occur in the midbrain, especially in the periaqueductal region and substantia nigra; the diencephalon, basal ganglia, pons, and medulla are frequently involved. Neuronal degenerative changes occur in varying degrees, especially in the ganglion cells of the substantia nigra (with loss of pigmentation), the periaqueductal and periventricular gray matter, and the nuclei of the oculomotor nerves. The cerebrum, cerebellum, and spinal cord are occasionally affected.

clinical features

The onset may be sudden or gradual; the disease is characterized by somnolence (due to lesions about the hypothalamus) or by a hyperkinetic state (due to involvement of the basal ganglia). In the latter there are purposeless movements, muscle spasms, and hiccoughing. Oculomotor palsies, such as ptosis and strabismus, and dysphagia are common. A reverse Argyll Robertson pupil, which reacts to light but not to accommodation, is sometimes found. *Postencephalitic parkinsonism* is due to damage of the substantia nigra. There are muscle rigidity, tremors, masking of the face, and a mincing gait. Personality changes with behavior problems may appear in the chronic phase of encephalitis. *Mortality* has been about 25 percent in epidemics.

St. Louis encephalitis

St. Louis encephalitis is caused by a small filtrable virus and is transmitted by mosquitoes, such as *Culex tarsalis, C. quinquefasciatus,* and *C. pipiens.* The virus is closely related to that of Japanese B encephalitis and Russian tick-borne encephalitis. The *pathologic changes* [15] are like those of type A encephalitis except that the brain is more extensively involved, with prominent lesions in the midbrain, pons, medulla, and cerebellum; the spinal cord is more frequently affected; and the meningitis is more marked. *Clinically* the symptoms are high fever, headache, vertigo, signs of meningeal irritation, tremors, ataxias, and sometimes lethargy and spastic paralyses. Most patients are over 50 years of age, and the mortality rate varies from 10 to 30 percent. The *cerebrospinal fluid changes* include increased pressure and protein levels, a normal glucose level, and a moderate pleocytosis with lymphocytes predominating. Postencephalitic parkinsonism is rare.

Japanese B encephalitis

Japanese B encephalitis is similar to the St. Louis type and involves the cerebrum, basal ganglia, midbrain (especially the substantia nigra and red nuclei), cerebellum, and spinal cord. The cerebellar Purkinje cells are often destroyed. The mortality rate is about 35 percent.

Equine encephalomyelitis

Equine encephalomyelitis is an epizootic viral infection of horses, but may occur in human beings, especially children. Transmission is probably by mosquitoes. Eastern and western forms occur, the former being more severe clinically and pathologically, with a mortality rate of about 65 percent. There is an acute disseminated inflammation throughout the cerebral cortex, basal ganglia, pons, medulla, and spinal cord, with intense congestion, perivascular cuffing by neutrophils, an acute arteritis, and neuronal degeneration. In the cerebrospinal fluid the cell count is high, and 60 to 90 percent of the cells are polymorphonuclear leukocytes.

Disseminated encephalomyelitis:

Acute disseminated encephalomyelitis (toxic or degenerative encephalitis) is a group of poorly understood, frequently fatal disorders related to encephalitis on the one hand and to multiple sclerosis on the other. Some authorities consider the group to be a single basic virus disease, such as herpes simplex, activated by any one of several agents. Others consider each member of the group to be due to a separate virus, or even to be nonviral and due to hypersensitivity. All cases show *foci of demyelinization* (particularly about the veins in the white matter of the brain or spinal cord), *nuclear changes* in ganglion cells of the cortex, and *glial proliferation.* The lymphocytic inflammatory response is variable; in some cases it is intense, in others minimal.

postvaccinal encephalomyelitis

Postvaccinal encephalomyelitis is one of the best-studied members of this group. Symptoms (headache, fever, drowsiness, coma, and paralyses) develop about 10 days after vaccination against smallpox or rabies. In the cases following smallpox vaccination the involvement is mainly encephalitic, and with the antirabies vaccine it is principally myelitic. This complication of smallpox vaccination is extremely rare, but its mortality rate is 25 to 50 percent. Postvaccinal encephalomyelitis is reported in from 1:500 to 1:8500 in various series of cases treated prophylactically with the *Semple rabies vaccine* prepared in rabbit brain. So far no case of encephalomyelitis has been produced by *vaccine prepared on duck embryos* [16]. Reactions to duck embryo vaccine have included lymphadenopathy and urticaria due to egg hypersensitivity in a few cases.

demyelinating encephalomyelitis

Demyelinating encephalomyelitis occurs rarely following the administration of *tetanus antitoxin* [17]. It is a hypersensitivity reaction and is characterized pathologically by dotting of the cerebral subcortical white matter with deep brown perivascular foci of demyelinization averaging 1 mm. in diameter.

postinfectious encephalomyelitis

Postinfectious encephalomyelitis may follow measles, mumps, chickenpox, and sometimes other virus diseases. Often the patient has recovered from the preceding disease before signs of nervous system involvement appear. Most patients have a complete recovery from postinfectious encephalomyelitis.

POLIO-MYELITIS: **Cause**

Acute anterior poliomyelitis (infantile paralysis, Heine-Medin's disease) is an acute inflammation of the spinal cord and brain stem, involving mainly the anterior horns of the lumbar segments of the spinal cord. It is caused by a very small *neurotropic filtrable enterovirus* which can be recovered from the pharynx of a patient or carrier, from feces of acutely ill and convalescent patients, and from the intestinal wall and mesenteric lymph nodes at autopsy; it is also found in sewage. There are *three serologic types of poliovirus:* type 1 (Brunhilde), type 2 (Lansing), and type 3 (Leon); there is no cross immunity between strains. The virus is of low virulence, and most infected individuals show no symptoms, even though they develop strain immunity. Poliomyelitis is both endemic and epidemic. Its incidence is seasonal, principally June through September. It occurs mainly in children, although in some epidemics the incidence is as high as 20 percent in adults. It rarely occurs before the age of 1 year.

Modes of infection [18]

The method of *transmission* of the virus is mainly by ingestion. In most cases of clinical poliomyelitis the virus reaches the lower intestinal tract and multiplies in the mucosal epithelial cells. From there it evidently travels along nerve fibrils to the regional sympathetic or sensory ganglia, where it again multiplies. The corresponding segment of the central nervous system is then invaded. Virus from the intestinal mucosa may also reach the bloodstream via Peyer's patches, the mesenteric lymph nodes, and the thoracic duct. However, most of this virus is quickly removed from the blood by reticuloendothelial cells, so that significant viremia does not ordinarily occur except with virus strains capable of proliferating in non-neural tissues. In cases of *bulbar poliomyelitis* the virus evidently penetrates the oropharyngeal mucosa, especially in the tonsillar region and often following tonsillitis or tonsillectomy, and reaches the cranial nerve nuclei of the medulla and brain stem.

Pathologic changes

Grossly the *spinal cord* and *brain stem* are markedly edematous and bulge when the meninges are opened. Petechiae and minute necrotic foci are found on the cut surface. The meninges are congested. *Microscopically* profound changes may extend from the sacral spinal cord to the basal ganglia and even higher. The *lumbar segments* of the spinal cord are most frequently involved, then the cervical enlargement and brain stem. The medulla is affected in most fatal cases. Lesions involve both the gray and white matter, but are more intense in the former, especially in the anterior horns of the spinal cord. They sporadically appear in the posterior horn neurons. In about 50 percent of fatal cases the *meninges* are infiltrated by lymphocytes, macrophages, and a few neutrophils. The meningeal and parenchymal vessels are greatly congested, and hemorrhages are frequent. Both large and small vessels are cuffed by lymphocytes, with a few plasmocytes. These cells are mainly in the Virchow-Robin spaces. The interstitial lesions consist of collections of lymphocytes and polymorphonuclear leukocytes, with an enormous proliferation of microglia, as shown by silver stains. The neurons show degenerative changes in all cases. The most pronounced changes occur in the *ganglion cells of the anterior horn.* These show acute swelling, loss of Nissl granules, nuclear chromatolysis, fragmentation, and complete disappearance. Dead cells are surrounded and digested by phagocytic microglia and neutrophils *(neuronophagia).* Cell death may occur rapidly and is due to a direct action of the virus. Internuncial cells are damaged in about 25 percent of the cases. In the *brain stem,* even in fatal cases, cell damage is not marked. Later the involved spinal cord shows atrophy, the affected side being shrunken. The destroyed cells are replaced by astrocytic proliferation. Cavities may form in the areas of softening within the anterior horns. The involved *muscles* show atrophy, fatty replacement, and fibrosis. The lesions in other organs are nonspecific and include cloudy swelling of the liver and kidneys, focal necrosis in the liver, and lymphoid hyperplasia. Focal cellular infiltrates may occur in the myocardium.

Clinical features

Clinically acute anterior poliomyelitis characteristically shows a *prodromal period* of 1 to 3 days with fever, headache, sore throat, stiff neck, nausea and vomiting, and irritability. In many respects the onset is like that of the common cold. The prodromal stage is followed by the *paralytic stage;* however, paralysis never develops in many patients. Paralysis is flaccid in type and reaches its maximum extent rapidly. It is asymmetric and often unilateral, muscle involvement depending on the particular motor neurons affected. There is a definite correlation between the degree of muscle weakness and the amount of anterior horn neuron damage [19]. Up to 20 percent of these neurons in a segment can be destroyed without apparent muscle weakness. When 40 percent are damaged, there is almost complete paralysis of the muscles controlled by the affected neurons. In the *bulbar type* of poliomyelitis, cranial nerve signs and respiratory difficulties occur. Cerebral and cerebellar involvement is uncommon. There may be pain due to involvement of the posterior root ganglia, but it is usually not severe. The rigidity which occasionally occurs is meningeal in origin.

Cerebrospinal fluid changes

The *cerebrospinal fluid* is clear or has a faint ground-glass appearance. The pressure and protein level are moderately elevated. Glucose and chloride levels are often normal. Early there are usually 100 to 200 cells per cubic millimeter, with about half polymorphonuclear leukocytes and half lymphocytes. After about 24 hours the number of cells falls, and the cells are all lymphocytes.

Outcome

The overall mortality rate is variable in different epidemics but is usually about 5 percent. In the bulbar form of the disease the death rate is much higher. Some degree of recovery from paralysis occurs in most patients, and recovery is complete in many.

Conditions related to poliomyelitis:

Paralytic poliomyelitis-like disease has also been produced by Coxsackie virus types A7, A9, B3, B4, and B5 and ECHO virus types 2, 4, 6, and 9 [20]. Mild paralytic disease has been attributed to the mumps virus. Cases caused by *Coxsackie and ECHO viruses* are rarely as severe as those produced by polioviruses, although occasional deaths in infants have been caused by the former. Coxsackie virus type B5 can produce encephalitis as well as poliomyelitis-like disease in adults [21].

Landry's paralysis

Landry's ascending paralysis is an acute, even fulminant disorder in which first the legs, then the arms, and finally the intercostal muscles and diaphragm are paralyzed. It is probably due to a filtrable virus and may be a fulminating type of poliomyelitis. Death occurs in 3 to 4 days. The *pathologic changes* are remarkably slight. There is degeneration of the cells of the anterior horns and breaking up of the medullary sheaths of their fibers. Perivascular cuffing is not found.

Guillain-Barré syndrome

The cause of the *Guillain-Barré syndrome (acute idiopathic polyneuritis)* is uncertain but is probably viral. It is occasionally associated with herpes zoster and chickenpox. In one case related to chickenpox there was also an ascending (Landry's) paralysis [22]. Some cases of Guillain-Barré syndrome are associated with infectious mononucleosis. *Pathologically* in acute idiopathic polyneuritis the involved nerve fibers are swollen, and there are lymphocytic infiltrates in the posterior nerve roots and ganglia. Rarely the spinal cord and brain stem are involved. *Clinically* there is a usually transient paralysis. A more or less distinctive feature is the *albumino-cytologic dissociation* wherein the spinal fluid protein level is elevated although the cell count may be normal (similar findings may be obtained late in the course of poliomyelitis). Although the patient is critically ill for a while, there is usually complete recovery. Rarely death may occur from bulbar paralysis.

RABIES:

Rabies (hydrophobia) [23] is a uniformly fatal viral disease which affects certain lower animals (dog, cat, fox, wolf, bat, and others) and sometimes man. The rabies virus occurs as *street virus,* which is isolated from naturally infected animals, and *fixed virus,* which has been attenuated by passage through experimental animals. Only street virus strains form Negri bodies. By electron microscopy rabies virus resembles the rubeola virus structurally, consisting of granular filamentous elements enclosed in a membrane. The virus is present in the salivary glands of infected animals and hence may contaminate bites, scratches, or wounds. From the wound the virus travels to the central nervous system along the axis cylinders. The *incubation period* depends on the length of the nerve that the virus must traverse before reaching the brain. Bites about the face have an incubation period of several weeks; bites of the foot, a year or more. Obviously there can be no delay in prophylactic therapy in the case of face wounds.

Pathologic changes

Pathologic changes in the brain consist of perivascular collections of lymphocytes and *inclusion bodies (Negri bodies)* in the cytoplasm of ganglion cells, especially in the hippocampus major, medulla oblongata, and Purkinje cells of the cerebellum. Negri bodies are round or oval, and acidophilic. In only about 40 percent of cases of rabies in humans are Negri bodies identified in the brain. A case of rabies with an associated *diffuse interstitial myocarditis* has been reported [24]. The edematous interstitial tissue was infiltrated with neutrophils, macrophages, plasmocytes, and "immature Aschoff myocytes." Focal myofibrillar degeneration was also noted.

Clinical features

Clinical manifestations of rabies are neuromuscular irritability, convulsions, choking (which is due to pharyngeal spasm and causes the characteristic fear of strangling while attempting to drink water or other fluids), and vomiting. The outcome is death. Diagnostic oversight is easily possible in patients bitten more than a year before the onset of symptoms.

HERPES SIMPLEX

Herpes simplex is a viral disease believed to be activated from a dormant state in association with febrile diseases such as pneumonia. It causes blister-like lesions of the lip and nose ("fever blisters") and occasionally corneal ulcers. *Acidophilic intranuclear inclusions (Lipschütz bodies)* are found in the surface lesions and in ganglion cells of corresponding parts of the brain and spinal cord. Rarely a severe and highly fatal *encephalitis* is caused by the herpes simplex virus in infants, children, and young adults. In such cases the brain is mushy and shows extensive cortical and subcortical necrosis. The lesions are most marked in the cerebrum, with less involvement of the basal ganglia, brain stem, and cerebellum. *Microscopically,* besides widespread destruction of neural tissue, there are intranuclear inclusion bodies in remaining cortical neurons and in oligodendrocytes. Neuronophagia, perivascular cuffing, and vascular necrosis are seen adjacent to necrotic foci. Herpes simplex is also discussed on page 151.

HERPES ZOSTER:

Herpes zoster (shingles) is a generally nonrecurring viral disease in which clusters of blister-like lesions appear in the skin or mucous membranes. These superficial *lesions follow the course of a sensory nerve,* either cranial or peripheral. The *virus* is identical with that of chickenpox. The individual skin lesions are quite comparable, and herpes zoster may appear among the contacts of a patient with chickenpox.

Pathologic changes

The *sensory nerve* corresponding to the surface lesions shows a true neuritis. It is swollen and pale, and there is active inflammation. Corresponding cells in the *posterior ganglia* show cytoplasmic inclusion bodies. There may be Wallerian degeneration of the sensory columns in the spinal cord. The cells of various visceral organs may also show inclusion bodies.

Clinical features

Skin lesions are usually unilateral and, like the peripheral nerves, tend not to cross the midline of the body. A generalized form of herpes zoster resembling chickenpox is also seen occasionally, usually as a terminal event in leukemia, lymphoma, or multiple myeloma. The lesions are very *painful,* and the pain may persist for years after the skin lesions heal, especially in elderly persons.

6. Syphilis of the Central Nervous System (Neurosyphilis)

Public health measures for the prevention and control of syphilis in its communicable phases have been so effective that neurosyphilis has become relatively uncommon. It is still important, however, and occurs in extremely variable pathologic and clinical patterns. The involvement may be mainly interstitial (meningovascular syphilis and gummata) or parenchymal (paresis and tabes dorsalis).

MENINGO-ENCEPHALITIS:

Syphilitic meningoencephalitis (meningovascular syphilis) is primarily a meningitis and arteritis, affecting both the brain and the spinal cord. It may appear within months, more often years, after the primary infection.

Pathologic changes

Grossly both the *dura and pia-arachnoid* are usually involved. The exudate may be slight and milky or thick and gelatinous, and it may cover the entire cerebral hemispheres or only the base of the brain. Over the spinal cord it may involve the meninges patchily. *Microscopically* the exudate resembles that of tuberculous meningitis, with lymphocytes and plasmocytes. There may be gummatous foci. The inflammation spreads into the underlying cerebral or cord tissue, and the degree of encephalitis or myelitis may be severe. The small blood vessels are cuffed with lymphocytes and plasmocytes. In the arteries there is lymphocytic infiltration of the adventitia with some plasma cells. The intima thickens, narrowing or closing the lumen *(Heubner's endarteritis). Thrombosis* may occur in the involved arteries. A gummatous arteritis rarely occurs.

Clinical features

The *clinical picture* depends on the type and extent of the lesions. The *acute form* is similar to other types of acute meningitis, with nuchal rigidity, headache, and positive Kernig and Brudzinski signs. In the more *chronic type* thrombosis of branches of the middle cerebral artery may produce hemiplegia in a young individual. Involvement of cranial nerves by the exudate or gummata produces typical signs: optic nerve involvement causes optic neuritis and blindness; oculomotor nerve involvement causes ptosis; and trochlear and abducens nerve involvement causes strabismus and diplopia.

Cerebrospinal fluid changes

Typically the complement-fixation and agglutination tests for syphilis are strongly positive. The colloidal gold curve is elevated in the first or second zone. The pleocytosis ranges from 10 to 500 lymphocytes per cubic millimeter, and an elevation in the protein level is found. Fluid changes are most marked when the involvement is mainly meningeal; the cerebrospinal fluid may be almost normal when the lesions are chiefly vascular.

GUMMA

Gumma of the central nervous system is rare today. It usually develops in the meninges and involves the brain or spinal cord only superficially. The compressed nervous tissue shows gliosis and neuronal degeneration. A gumma acts as a space-occupying lesion, and the clinical picture depends on its size and location.

PARESIS:

General paresis (general paralysis of the insane, dementia paralytica) is a parenchymatous type of neurosyphilis in which the cerebrum is mainly involved. It is a late manifestation of syphilis, appearing 10 to 15 years after the primary infection, and it occurs in males about three times as often as in females. *Juvenile paresis,* resulting from congenital syphilis, usually becomes apparent at about the age of 10 years.

Pathologic changes

The *brain* is often atrophic, weighing 150 to 200 gm. less than normal; in such cases the gyri are narrowed and the sulci widened. The *pia mater* may be thickened, opaque, and adherent over the frontal lobes, so that there is decortication of brain substance on stripping. The *ventricles* are dilated, and their walls, especially the floor of the fourth ventricle, are granular and frosted *(granular ependymitis). Microscopically* the *meninges* are infiltrated by chronic inflammatory cells. In the *cerebral cortex* the architecture is destroyed, and the ganglion cells show severe degenerative changes, such as nuclear chromatolysis or pyknosis, and even cell disappearance. Few cells remain intact in the frontal and parietal lobes. Association fibers and the pyramidal tracts may degenerate secondarily. All blood vessels are surrounded by lymphocytes and plasmocytes in the adventitia and Virchow-Robin spaces. Heavy deposits of iron pigments are found about blood vessels extracellularly and within microglial cells. The latter are often elongated *(rod cells).* There is a peppering of the interstitial tissue with lymphocytes and plasmocytes, and teeming hordes of spirochetes can be demonstrated with silver stains in active cases. Neuroglial proliferation is marked, especially in the superficial portions of the cortex. Brushlike glial processes project into the pia mater and become adherent to it. Small subependymal mounds of neuroglia cause the granularity of the ventricular walls. The optic and other cranial nerves may show degenerative changes. In the *spinal cord* there may be secondary degeneration of the pyramidal tracts of the lateral columns. If the posterior columns are also involved, the condition is known as *taboparesis.*

Clinical features

Clinically the mental disorder varies from slight memory loss to megalomania and a mood of marked euphoria. The speech is often thick and slurred. Tremors are common due to degeneration of cells of the corpus striatum, and convulsions may occur. Generalized muscle weakness (paresis) is characteristic. A typical feature is *Argyll Robertson pupils,* which are miotic and react in accommodation but not to light.

Cerebrospinal fluid changes

The *cerebrospinal fluid* shows a positive complement-fixation test in about 95 percent of the cases. The cell count is usually 30 to 100 per cubic millimeter, being chiefly lymphocytes. The paretic colloidal gold curve is strongly first-zonal (typically 5555543200).

TABES DORSALIS:

Tabes dorsalis (locomotor ataxia) is a parenchymatous type of neurosyphilis principally involving the spinal cord. It is a late manifestation of syphilis, appearing 10 to 15 years after the primary lesion. It is much more common in males than females.

Grossly the pia mater is thickened over the affected portions of the spinal cord and may be adherent. The surface of the *posterior columns* is flattened and may even be concave. On cut surface these columns have a gray, translucent appearance, standing out from the adjacent white matter. The lumbar segments of the spinal cord are mainly involved, but changes may appear in the cervical segments. The *posterior nerve roots* are shrunken and gray. *Microscopically* there is a degeneration and disappearance of fibers of the lower afferent neurons (exogenous fibers) of the posterior columns. Since the column of Goll (fasciculus gracilis) consists of fibers from the lumbar and sacral regions, it is more often involved than the column of Burdach (fasciculus cuneatus). Both the medullary sheaths and the axis cylinders of these fibers disappear, and degenerated fibers remain unstained with Weigert's myelin stain. There is a marked neuroglial proliferation. The walls of small blood vessels may be thickened. The *posterior nerve roots* show changes similar to those in the columns. Secondary degeneration occurs in the posterior root ganglia. Degeneration of the second (optic), third (oculomotor), and seventh (facial) cranial nerves is common. Pathologic changes

Clinically an early sign is the feeling of walking on a rug. There may be lightning sensations down the legs due to irritation of the posterior nerve roots. Later, loss of the sensations of pain, position, vibration, and deep sensation occurs. Except for pain, these sensations normally pass upward in the posterior columns of the spinal cord and are explained on the basis of posterior column degeneration. Since pain sensations pass upward in the supposedly uninvolved spinothalamic tracts, the essential lesion in tabes dorsalis may be that in the posterior nerve roots. Other findings are incoordination with a positive Romberg sign, loss of deep reflexes, especially in the lower extremities, Argyll Robertson pupils, and cranial nerve changes. The cranial nerve changes include blindness (due to optic atrophy), ptosis, diplopia, and facial anesthesia. There may also be visceral crises, which are probably meningeal in origin, and trophic disturbances, which are secondary to the anesthesia and/or position sense loss. Among these are Charcot's joints and perforating ulcers of the feet. Clinical features

In the *cerebrospinal fluid* the complement-fixation test for syphilis is positive in over 70 percent of the cases. In active cases there are usually 10 to 15 lymphocytes per cubic millimeter, with increases during tabetic crises. The tabetic colloidal gold curve is typically positive in the midzone (something like 0012442100). Cerebrospinal fluid changes

7. *Myelitis*

Myelitis is an inflammation of the spinal cord. A diffuse myelitis may occur in conjunction with inflammation of the brain (encephalitis) to give the condition known as *encephalomyelitis;* or certain groups of cells in the spinal cord may be selectively involved, as is the case with the anterior horn cells in *anterior poliomyelitis.*

Transverse myelitis is localized and may affect both the sensory and motor fibers in the spinal cord, and also the nerve roots and ganglion cells at the particular level of involvement. It may be due to bacterial infections or trauma. TRANSVERSE MYELITIS:

The *bacterial causes* of transverse myelitis are chiefly those conditions affecting the vertebrae (such as tuberculosis and brucellosis), causing extradural abscess with secondary involvement of the spinal cord. The substance of the spinal cord may sometimes be involved directly, as in gumma or septic infarcts. *Mechanical* Causes *injury* to the spinal cord may be due to herniation of a nucleus pulposus, vertebral fracture or dislocation, severance of blood vessels to the spinal cord, or gunshot wounds. Mine injuries are particularly likely to involve the spine. The rare and poorly understood transverse myelitis following *spinal anesthesia* may or may not be traumatic.

Pathologic changes

Tissue changes depend upon the cause and mechanism of involvement. The dura mater is apt to be thickened, and in instances of bone disease it may be elevated from the underlying bone by necrotic tissue, pus, or tumor. The spinal cord may be swollen and edematous in acute trauma or compressed and flattened from chronic vertebral deformities. *Microscopically* there is swelling of myelin sheaths at the early stage, with later disappearance of myelin. Macrophages, lymphocytes, and swollen microglial cells (gitter cells) are common; less often neutrophils are seen. Neuronophagia is sometimes evident.

Clinical features

In extreme cases there is complete anesthesia and loss of all voluntary motor activity below the level of cord involvement. The paralysis may be upper motor neuron type (spastic) at certain levels, and lower motor neuron type (flaccid) at other, generally higher, levels. Reflex arcs may or may not be interrupted. There is usually loss of control of bowel and bladder function, either retention or incontinence being the result.

Outcome

If the spinal cord is involved from without, is not badly damaged, and is surgically decompressed promptly, there may be full or partial restoration of function. If spinal cord necrosis, disruption, or degeneration has occurred, there can be no regeneration of neurons. The end result is usually permanent *paraplegia*, confining the patient to a wheelchair for life. Along with paralysis, there is usually some degree of anesthesia and other sensory impairment below the level of spinal cord injury. *Urinary tract infection* is very common in these patients, and death is sometimes the result of secondary amyloid disease due to a persistent pyelonephritis [25].

8. *Neuritis*

The term *neuritis* is commonly used by nonmedical persons to signify any painful condition of the back or extremities in which the bones and joints do not seem to be affected. Even physicians tend to use the term rather loosely for a variety of disorders of unknown cause. *Neuralgia* is a better term for some of the disorders listed here, in that this term is appropriately noncommittal as to the cause of the affliction.

Causes

Disorders of the peripheral nerves may be caused by a number of factors, including the following: *vitamin B (thiamine) deficiency*, as in beriberi or Wernicke's disease (thiamine deficiency in alcoholics); *chemical poisoning* (lead, arsenic, jamaica ginger, or "jake paralysis" due to orthotricresyl phosphate, methyl alcohol, lathyrism); *bacterial toxins* (diphtheria); *virus infections* (herpes zoster); *metabolic disorders* (diabetes mellitus); *mechanical injury* (nerve compression by neoplasm, aneurysm, herniated nucleus pulposus, a crutch, bone fragments, or cast applied for immobilization of fracture); and *unknown causes* (facial nerve paralysis or Bell's palsy, trigeminal neuralgia or tic douloureux).

Pathologic changes

The *tissue changes* vary extremely according to the causes and nature of the process. Early there may be swelling and hyperemia of the nerve, with later myelin degeneration, proliferation of Schwann's sheath, and disappearance of neurons. Secondary changes occur in corresponding nerve nuclei, and *Wallerian degeneration* may extend long distances in the central nervous system. A patchy segmental demyelinization of Gombault develops in the polyneuropathy due to arsenic (motor and sensory nerves) or lead (motor nerves). In neuritis *trophic changes* may occur in skin, muscles, and organs of special sense. Localization may be to cranial or peripheral nerves, or both. Multiple peripheral nerves are often involved and in different portions of their course, hence the terms *polyneuritis, radiculitis, plexitis,* and *peripheral neuritis.*

Clinical features

Depending on the type and location of the nerve affected, and the degree and duration of nerve involvement, there may be paralysis, anesthesia, pain, hyperesthesia, muscle atrophy, blindness, deafness, anosmia, dysphagia, or Horner's syndrome. Foot drop and wrist drop are two common paralytic manifestations, especially noted in neuritis due to chemical poisoning, as by lead or arsenic.

Serum neuritis

Serum neuritis occurs occasionally following administration of tetanus antitoxin due to the horse serum in it [26]. The nerves of the brachial plexus are frequently involved. *Clinically* there is intense pain in the muscles supplied by the affected nerves early, and within a few hours a progressive flaccid paralysis ensues. The pain is replaced by numbness and paresthesias. Complete recovery occurs within 6 months in 80 percent of the cases. Occasionally death results from respiratory muscular paralysis. The *pathologic changes are little known,* but the *peripheral neuritis* is thought to be due to perineural edema and perivascular infiltrations about involved neurons and nerve fibers.

DEGENERATIVE DISEASES OF THE NERVOUS SYSTEM

Degenerative diseases of the central nervous system are those disorders in which there is degeneration of the parenchyma independent of hemorrhage, vascular occlusion, marked edema or inflammation, or neoplastic invasion. They may be due to deficiencies, heredofamilial factors, or senescence, but most are idiopathic.

MULTIPLE SCLEROSIS:

Multiple sclerosis (disseminated sclerosis) is a chronic disease of the nervous system characterized by curious remissions and relapses and by the presence of numerous areas of demyelinization scattered patchily throughout the white and gray matter of the brain and spinal cord. The *cause* is unknown. Among the proposed causes are filtrable viruses, spirochetes, hypersensitivity, a circulating lipolytic enzyme, and small venous thromboses with resultant infarction in the spinal cord and brain. The lesions are frequently found about veins. However, the thrombi may be secondary, due to thromboplastic substances released by degenerated myelin.

Pathologic changes

Grossly the lesions are firm, well-defined, gray, translucent plaques, 0.1 to 6 cm. in diameter, scattered asymmetrically throughout the central nervous system. They are especially numerous in the pons, medulla, and cerebellar peduncles, and are common in the optic nerve and chiasm as well as at the margins of the lateral, third, and fourth ventricles. In the spinal cord they are frequent in the lateral columns (pyramidal tracts), and they are not uncommon in the posterior columns. The *lesions are found more frequently in the white than in the gray matter* of the central nervous system. *Microscopically* there are demyelinization, chronic inflammation, and gliosis. Early the medullary sheaths break up into myelin droplets, and the vessels are cuffed by lymphocytes, plasmocytes, and Gitterzellen filled with lipid material. Later the vessels are surrounded by many neuroglial masses. Some axis cylinders degenerate, and some even disappear; others are remarkably intact. The lost nerve fibers are replaced by a dense glial network. The patches of degeneration remain isolated, with little secondary degeneration above and below.

Clinical features

There are between 100,000 and 250,000 cases of multiple sclerosis in the United States. It occurs more commonly in women than men by a ratio of 3:2 [27], and most cases have their onset between the ages of 20 and 40. The lesions are usually more widespread than the severity of the clinical picture would suggest. There is a bizarre variety of symptoms and signs depending on the location of the lesions. The remissions which frequently occur are apparently possible because of the intact state of many of the axis cylinders within the plaques. The most characteristic finding is *Charcot's triad* (nystagmus, intention tremors, and scanning speech, in which there are often long pauses between syllables) due to lesions in the cerebellar peduncles. Spastic paraplegia, increased deep reflexes, and positive Babinski signs are due to involvement of the pyramidal tracts. Temporary blindness or dimness of vision is frequent, being caused by lesions in the optic nerve or chiasm. The patients often show a remarkable euphoria. About 50 percent of the patients develop a *paretic-type colloidal gold curve* in the cerebrospinal fluid. The cerebrospinal fluid level of gamma globulin is significantly increased in about 70 percent of typical cases of multiple sclerosis and in about 55 percent of patients with unremitting disease or initial attacks [28]. The cases in which the gamma globulin is increased often also show pleocytosis and abnormal colloidal gold curves.

IDIOPATHIC DISSEMINATED ENCEPHALOMYELITIS:

Idiopathic acute disseminated encephalomyelitis (acute multiple sclerosis) is clinically and pathologically like the postinfectious form (see page 681) which may follow rubeola, varicella, variola, or vaccinia, but in the idiopathic cases the cause is inapparent.

Pathologic changes

In those dying very early in the course of the disease there may be no gross changes. As the foci of demyelinization coalesce, however, poorly defined, round, oval, or irregular yellow to yellowish gray patches are scattered through the white matter of the central nervous system. These vary from less than 1 mm. to several centimeters in diameter, and occasionally involve the gray matter. *Microscopically* the characteristic lesions are pericapillary or perivenous foci of demyelinization with a slight to absent inflammatory reaction and slight to moderate perivascular astrocytosis.

Clinical features

Clinically young adults are usually affected, and the onset is acute with headache, vomiting, and sometimes fever. The neurologic signs are varied according to the areas of involvement. They include mental changes, hemiplegia, paraplegia, ataxia, nystagmus, optic neuritis, paresthesias, and sensory losses. The cerebrospinal fluid may show an elevated protein level and a mild lymphocytic pleocytosis. Recovery is usually remarkably complete in 2 to 3 weeks, because most axis cylinders have survived; but relapses or later involvement of new areas of the central nervous system are not uncommon. When optic neuritis dominates the clinical picture, the condition is called *ophthalmoneuromyelitis* (Devic's disease).

DIFFUSE CEREBRAL SCLEROSIS:

Diffuse cerebral sclerosis is the generic term for a group of rare, often familial diseases characterized by widespread demyelinization of subcortical white matter with slight damage in the cerebral cortex, basal ganglia, and brain stem.

Sudanophilic cerebral sclerosis

Sudanophilic cerebral sclerosis (Schilder's disease) is a rare condition of children and young adults of *unknown cause.* It strongly resembles multiple sclerosis, but is usually more steadily progressive than that disorder. There are gelatinous, gray, translucent foci of demyelinization in the white matter of the cerebrum. *Microscopically* the demyelinization is accompanied by destruction of axis cylinders, perivascular cuffing, and gliosis. There is a marked secondary degeneration of fibers. Fat stains reveal all stages of myelin degeneration. Lipids are found mainly within microglial cells and swollen astrocytes. *Clinically* the onset is acute, and the course is rapidly progressive. Blindness, deafness, sensory loss, spastic paraplegia, and convulsions are common.

Pelizaeus-Merzbacher's disease

Pelizaeus-Merzbacher's disease has a strong familial tendency, begins in infancy or early childhood, and progresses slowly. The patients usually live 2 to 3 decades. Diffuse demyelinization occurs in the cerebral and cerebellar white matter and brain stem. Occasionally preserved myelin islands are found. *Clinically* there are incoordination, athetosis, spasticity, visual loss, and mental deficiency.

Krabbe's disease

Krabbe's disease is a familial diffuse sclerosis appearing in infancy. There is a complete destruction of the myelin sheaths and axons throughout the cerebral white matter. The cerebellum, basal ganglia, and spinal cord may also be involved. In foci of recent demyelinization, clusters of large mononuclear *epithelioid cells* and multinucleated *globoid cells* with basophilic cytoplasm are found about or near blood vessels.

Metachromatic leukodystrophy

Metachromatic leukodystrophy (metachromatic diffuse sclerosis or leukoencephalopathy) is part of a generalized metabolic disorder in which sulfatides accumulate in the central nervous system white matter, peripheral nerves, liver, gallbladder, pancreas, and renal tubular epithelium [29]. *Sulfatides* are lipids which contain the base sphinogosine and stain atypically with cationic aniline dyes such as cresyl violet and toluidine blue. Metachromatic pink-staining material is found in the fluffy portion of the urinary sediment. In the central nervous system white matter the ratio of sulfatides to cerebrosides is reversed. *Grossly* the white matter appears slightly grayer than normal. *Microscopically* there is diffuse but often incomplete demyelinization of the cerebral white matter, corticospinal tract, and white matter of the lateral cerebellar lobes. *Metachromatic substance* is found in oligodendrocytes, large astrocytes, Betz motor neurons, and neurons of the globus pallidus, thalamus, dentate nucleus, anterior horns, and retina. *Clinically* the disease usually becomes manifest in the second or third year of life by difficulty in walking due to spasticity and/or ataxia.

AMYOTROPHIC LATERAL SCLEROSIS:

Amyotrophic lateral sclerosis (Charcot's disease) is a chronic, progressive disease of *unknown cause* in which there is degeneration of both the upper and lower motor neurons. It is more common in males by 4:1 and usually appears in the fourth and fifth decades. The disease is common among natives of Guam, the Mariana Islands, and New Guinea.

Pathologic changes

A marked loss of anterior horn cells leads to atrophy of the anterior horns. Many cells disappear, and the remaining ones show all degrees of degeneration, including shrinkage, vacuolar degeneration, and chromatolysis. The *pyramidal tracts* degenerate, and there is a corresponding involvement of the *Betz cells of the motor cortex.* The *motor nuclei of the pons and medulla* degenerate late in the course. In the affected muscles there is marked atrophy, with replacement fibrosis.

Clinical features

Clinically the earliest signs are usually weakness, wasting, and fine tremors in the thenar, hypothenar, and interossei muscles of the hands; then the arms and shoulders become involved. Spastic paraplegia, with increased deep reflexes and positive Babinski signs, may appear due to the upper motor neuron lesions. Death due to bulbar paralysis usually occurs within 3 years of the onset.

Progressive spinal muscular atrophy

Progressive spinal muscular atrophy is a form of amyotrophic lateral sclerosis in which no clinical evidence of upper motor neuron lesions appears. Fibrillary tremors are prominent in this type and the disease may have a protracted course. *Microscopically* degeneration of both the spinal anterior horn neurons and the lateral columns is found. The *Aran-Duchenne type* usually appears between the ages of 30 and 40 years and is more common in men than women. The hands are usually involved first, then the entire upper extremities. Finally the lower extremities are affected. The course may be protracted. The *Werdnig-Hoffmann type* is familial and appears in infancy. It may be rapidly fatal because of involvement of the respiratory muscles, and death usually occurs by the fifth year of life. The *Charcot-Marie-Tooth type* [30] is familial and usually appears between the ages of 6 to 10 years. There is a symmetric degeneration of the lower motor neurons of the peroneal nerves, and fibrosis of these nerves may be found. Pes cavus (high arch), hammer toes, and peroneal muscle atrophy insidiously develop.

Progressive bulbar palsy

Progressive bulbar palsy (Duchenne's paralysis) may occur as a purely bulbar disease or as the final stage of amyotrophic lateral sclerosis. There is degeneration of the motor nuclei of the pons and medulla (cranial nerves VII, X, XI, and XII). *Clinically* this is a *glossolabiopharyngeal paralysis.* It begins with difficulty in articulation. The tongue wastes and shows fibrillary tremors. Difficulty in swallowing develops near the end of the course.

FRIEDREICH'S ATAXIA:

Friedreich's ataxia (hereditary spinal ataxia) is a rare familial abiotrophy (premature degeneration) of several tracts of the central nervous system in young individuals; its *cause is unknown.*

Pathologic changes

The *spinal cord* is atrophic. Translucent patches of degeneration occur in the *posterior and lateral columns* of the spinal cord. Clarke's column (nucleus dorsalis) is also involved. There is a degeneration of the myelin sheaths and axons with secondary gliosis.

Clinical features

Clinically Friedreich's ataxia is the spinal form of cerebellar ataxia. The cerebellar signs, due to involvement of the direct spinocerebellar tract, include "cerebellar reel," nystagmus, scanning speech, and a positive Romberg sign. The posterior column lesions produce loss of deep reflexes and position sense. Pyramidal tract degeneration leads to muscle weakness and positive Babinski signs. Pes cavus, hammer toes, and scoliosis are characteristic findings.

MARIE'S ATAXIA

Marie's ataxia (hereditary cerebellar ataxia) has an onset later than that of Friedreich's ataxia, to which it is related. There is atrophy of the cerebellar cortex, dentate nucleus, and olivary nuclei, with a variable degree of degeneration of the spinocerebellar tracts. Optic atrophy may also occur.

LOUIS-BAR SYNDROME

The *Louis-Bar syndrome* is characterized by progressive cerebellar ataxia and oculocutaneous telangiectasia [31]. A familial tendency and frequent pulmonary infections are sometimes found. There is *diffuse cerebellar cortical degeneration* affecting the Purkinje, granular, and basket cells, with little involvement of the cerebellar white matter. The disease becomes manifest in the first few years of life with nystagmus, dysarthria (imperfect articulation in speech), progressive cerebellar ataxia (failure of muscular coordination), choreo-athetosis, decreased or absent tendon reflexes, loss of facial expression, and drooling.

COMBINED DEGENERATION OF THE CORD: Cause

Subacute combined degeneration of the spinal cord (combined sclerosis) occurs in 30 to 50 percent of cases of *untreated pernicious anemia,* and rarely may precede the appearance of a hyperchromic, macrocytic anemia in the peripheral blood by several years. It is due to failure of vitamin B_{12} absorption because of a lack of the intrinsic factor. Subacute combined degeneration occurs rarely in other conditions, such as carcinoma of the stomach, diabetes mellitus, pellagra, sprue, and ergot poisoning.

Pathologic changes

Translucent patches of degeneration are found in symmetric arrangement in the *posterior columns,* crossed and direct pyramidal tracts of the *lateral columns,* and *cerebellar tracts.* The lesions are most marked in the midthoracic region, with secondary degeneration in the cervical segments in the ascending fibers, and in the descending fibers in the lumbar segments. The patches become porous and appear loosely meshed. *Microscopically* the lesions consist of the fusion of many tiny patches. Demyelinization is present, with complete destruction of the medullary sheaths. Later the axis cylinders disappear. Little gliosis occurs in the patches of degeneration.

Clinical features

Clinically the earliest signs are paresthesias – numbness and tingling (due to radicular irritation) in the fingertips ("pins-and-needles" sensation). Later, loss of vibratory and position sense and ataxia appear. Some patients show a spastic paraplegia with increased deep reflexes and positive Babinski signs. Finally there is a flaccid paralysis with complete sensory loss. Parenteral liver or vitamin B_{12} therapy arrests the degeneration and promotes astrocytosis. Folic acid is not effective.

SYRINGOMYELIA:

Syringomyelia is a rare, idiopathic disease which usually becomes manifest in young individuals. It is often associated with spina bifida and other congenital anomalies.

Pathologic changes

The underlying lesion is a *gliosis in the gray commissure and the base of the posterior horns,* usually in the lower cervical and upper thoracic segments. This glial tissue becomes softened and liquefied, so that a *tubular cavity (syrinx)* is formed *in the center of the spinal cord.* This cavity is separate from the central canal of the spinal cord, and it may extend the length of the cord and even into the brain stem *(syringobulbia).* The cavity is often lined by glial tissue.

Clinical features

Clinically the most characteristic sign is the *dissociated anesthesia* (loss of sensibility to pain and temperature, with preservation of touch) in the involved areas due to the crossing of the fibers for pain and temperature in the affected gray commissure. Touch fibers ascend in the ipsilateral posterior columns. There is spasticity of the legs due to pressure on the pyramidal tracts. Early there may be an *anesthesia dolorosa* (painful anesthesia) due to irritation of pain fibers. A muscular atrophy of the lower motor neuron type occurs in the upper extremities. Burns on the hands and legs are common because of the anesthesia.

Various trophic changes, such as ulcers and Charcot joints, are probably due to multiple traumata. The development of painless whitlows is called *Morvan's disease.*

PARALYSIS AGITANS: *Paralysis agitans (Parkinson's disease, parkinsonism,* shaking palsy) is the result of degenerative changes in the basal ganglia which may be caused by arteriosclerosis and carbon monoxide and manganese poisoning. Most cases are idiopathic, but are probably due to senile atrophy. Such cases appear most often in men in the sixth and seventh decades. *Parkinson's syndrome* occurs in about 15 percent of patients taking *tranquilizers of the phenothiazine group* for over 3 months, and some form of extrapyramidal reaction occurs in almost 40 percent [32]. Such drugs include chlorpromazine, triflupromazine, prochlorperazine, trifluoperazine, fluphenazine, and perphenazine. In the phenothiazine drugs a side chain containing an amine is essential and a halogen in the parent nucleus is important in causing parkinsonism [33]. Phenothiazines containing fluorine most commonly produce this syndrome. The symptoms disappear following withdrawal of the drug.

Pathologic changes

Pathologically in idiopathic and arteriosclerotic Parkinson's disease, tiny golden-yellow *lacunae* (foci of softening) are found in the striate body (caudate and lenticular nuclei). Many of these are perivascular, but they are thought to be metabolic rather than vascular in origin [34]. *Lewy bodies* (intracytoplasmic masses with a dark central zone and clearer periphery) are common in the neurons of the basal ganglia and brain stem.

Clinical features

Clinically the classic picture shows cogwheel muscle rigidity, rest tremors with the typical pill-rolling movements, masked facies, drooling, and a flexed attitude of the body. The patient has a mincing festination (hastening) gait. The signs are due to interruption of the extrapyramidal tracts. Pollakiuria (frequent micturition) is common due to hypertonicity of the detrusor muscle.

Postencephalitic parkinsonism

Postencephalitic parkinsonism is similar clinically to paralysis agitans, but is due to degenerative lesions in the substantia nigra and usually occurs in young individuals. Round intracytoplasmic inclusions *(Lewy bodies)* may be found in the nigral neurons. Oculogyric crises and personality changes are common.

Hepatolenticular degeneration (Wilson's disease) is discussed under Diseases of the Liver on page 533.

HUNTINGTON'S CHOREA

Huntington's chorea is a rare heredofamilial disease transmitted as a mendelian dominant. Males and females are affected about equally. The disease becomes manifest in middle life and is characterized clinically by involuntary choreiform movements and tremors, with mental deterioration. The *choreiform movements* are probably due to loss of controlling influences from the neostriatum (putamen and caudate nucleus). Atrophy of the cerebral cortical neurons and degeneration and disappearance of the cells of the putamen and caudate nucleus occur.

SYDENHAM'S CHOREA

Sydenham's chorea (St. Vitus' dance) is a manifestation of rheumatic fever which usually occurs in girls under 20. It has occurred in a few cases of disseminated lupus erythematosus and rarely in patients with Schönlein-Henoch (anaphylactoid) purpura. *Clinically* it is characterized by sudden irregular involuntary movements. In fatal cases, marked hyperemia, perivascular cuffing by lymphocytes, and slight degeneration of neurons are found in the *cerebral cortex and basal ganglia,* especially in the neostriatum.

MYASTHENIA GRAVIS: Cause

Myasthenia gravis is a chronic disease characterized by weakness of voluntary muscles, usually beginning in the muscles of the eyes and jaws. It commonly appears between 20 and 35 years and is typified by remissions and relapses. The cause is insufficient formation or too rapid destruction of acetylcholine at the myoneural junction. A serum muscle-coating globulin, presumed to be an *auto-antibody against skeletal muscle,* is present in about 25 percent of cases of myasthenia gravis [35]. Thyroglobulin antibodies are found in about 35 percent, and there are serum antinuclear factors in about 15 percent of patients with myasthenia gravis. These findings plus the occurrence of passive transfer during pregnancy and the pathologic finding of lymphorrhages in involved muscles support the concept that myasthenia gravis is an *auto-immune disease,* although the evidence is not conclusive. Concomitant chronic thyroiditis, in some cases a full-blown lymphocytic (Hashimoto's) thyroiditis, is found in about 20 percent of patients with myasthenia gravis [36], additional evidence of the auto-immune nature. In about 5 percent of patients with myasthenia gravis there is an associated hyperthyroidism [37]. Muscle weakness tends to be profound in cases with hyperthyroidism as well as those with hypothyroidism.

Pathologic changes

In the affected muscles there is a *lymphorrhage,* with focal collections of lymphocytes about the capillaries of the interstitial tissue. The muscle fibers appear to be normal. In about 50 percent of the cases there is *hyperplasia or a neoplasm in the thymus.*

CEREBRAL ATROPHY:

Cerebral atrophy is very common in persons over 60 *(senile atrophy).* In this condition there is a decrease in the number of neurons, with gliosis and arteriosclerotic changes. *Premature senile atrophy* occurs in persons under 60. It may be localized to certain gyri which become shrunken, especially in the frontal lobes *(Pick's convolutional atrophy),* or it may occur as a widespread atrophy of the gyri of all lobes but especially the frontal lobes *(Alzheimer's presenile dementia).* A psychosis is commonly associated with the latter. In Alzheimer's disease as well as in senile dementia, *senile plaques* are found in the cerebral cortex. These consist mainly of enlarged matted, twisted, and interwoven unmyelinated axonal processes with a few myelinated axons and rare glial cells [38]. These plaques contain amyloid-like fibrillar material and are positive with silver stain and with periodic acid-Schiff stain. *Ulegyria (lobar sclerosis)* is an infantile cortical atrophy involving one or more lobes in one or, asymmetrically, both cerebral hemispheres. There is a progressive loss of neurons with subsequent gliosis.

(Margin notes: Pick's atrophy; Alzheimer's disease; Ulegyria)

VASCULAR DISORDERS OF THE NERVOUS SYSTEM

1. Aneurysms of Cerebral Arteries

"CONGENITAL" ANEURYSM:

"Congenital" aneurysm (berry or miliary *aneurysm)* occurs usually on the circle of Willis, especially the anterior communicating artery, the middle or anterior cerebral arteries, or the basilar artery, usually at or near a point of bifurcation, where the media is defective normally.

Pathologic changes

"Congenital" aneurysms are multiple in about 20 percent of the cases [39]. In distribution, about 15 percent of these aneurysms are on the anterior communicating, 5 percent on each anterior cerebral, 15 percent on each middle cerebral, 10 percent on each internal carotid, 15 percent on the basilar, and 5 percent on each vertebral artery [40]. They are saccular in form and vary from 0.1 to

3 cm. in diameter. The wall of the aneurysm is composed of a greatly thickened intima, with complete absence of the media and internal elastic lamina. An atheroma is almost always present in the intima. With rupture or leakage of the aneurysm, *subarachnoid hemorrhage* develops. Bright red blood floods the subarachnoid space. *Rupture* is found in about 75 percent of cases of cerebral arterial aneurysm. Following rupture, *intracerebral hemorrhage* occurs in about 25 percent of cases, and *intracerebral and intraventricular hemorrhage* is present in another 40 percent. The common sites of intracerebral hemorrhage are the island of Reil and the temporal and frontal lobes. Hemorrhage into the *subdural space* occurs in almost 20 percent of cases.

Clinical features

Clinically before rupture an aneurysm in the anterior group of arteries may become large enough to compress the olfactory nerve (producing anosmia) and/or the optic nerve (causing unilateral hemianopia). Sometimes an aneurysm presses on the tuber cinereum, giving the signs usually associated with a pituitary neoplasm. An aneurysm of the posterior group of arteries is usually asymptomatic before rupture, but it may compress the ninth, tenth, and eleventh cranial nerves and cause clinical signs. *Leakage or rupture* of the aneurysm produces subarachnoid hemorrhage, often in young individuals. Marked dizziness and violent headache suddenly develop. If the hemorrhage is severe, coma follows quickly. The neck is rigid on flexion, the Kernig and Brudzinski signs are positive, Babinski reflexes are often positive, and the deep tendon reflexes are hyperactive. The cerebrospinal fluid is under greatly increased pressure and is grossly bloody.

ARTERIOSCLEROTIC ANEURYSM

Arteriosclerotic aneurysm occurs in persons over 50 at the site of an atheroma. It may occur in any of the cerebral arteries, but is especially common in the vertebral-basilar and internal carotid-middle cerebral axes. The aneurysm is fusiform in shape.

ARTERIOVENOUS ANEURYSM

Arteriovenous aneurysm occasionally develops in cerebral vessels due to a congenital defect in the capillary bed. A complex tortuous network of vessels makes up the aneurysm. Convulsions and/or motor and speech disturbances may occur, depending on the location of the aneurysm.

MYCOTIC ANEURYSM

Mycotic aneurysm is caused by septic embolism, usually to a middle or anterior cerebral artery. An acute arteritis leads to weakening of the arterial wall and aneurysm formation. Most emboli arise in vegetations of bacterial endocarditis.

2. Cerebrovascular Accidents

Cerebrovascular accidents include all lesions resulting from damage to blood vessels which produces infarction or hemorrhage in or about the brain or spinal cord. The major types are cerebral infarction and cerebral hemorrhage. Subarachnoid hemorrhage may be spontaneous, especially in patients with hypertension, but is usually due to rupture of or leakage from an aneurysm.

INFARCTION: Causes: arteriosclerosis and thrombosis

Cerebral infarction results from the occlusion of a cerebral artery due to thrombosis or embolism. *Thrombosis,* the more common cause, may occur in a cerebral artery damaged by arteriosclerosis, periarteritis nodosa, thromboangiitis obliterans, or syphilitic arteritis. *Cerebral arteriosclerosis* is the most frequent cause of thrombosis, common sites of occlusion being the middle cerebral, posterior cerebral, and basilar arteries. *Atherosclerosis* occurs in the large arteries at the base of the brain. *Medial fibrosis* with reduplication of the internal elastic lamina appears in the small arteries. *Intimal hyalinization* is the major change in arterioles. Cerebral arteriosclerosis often does not correlate with sclerotic changes elsewhere in the body and has no constant relationship to hypertension. Atherosclerotic plaques in cerebral arteries contain appreciably less calcium than comparable ones in coronary arteries. This "defective calcification" may explain the greater tendency of sclerotic cerebral arteries to rupture [41]. *Carotid artery occlusion* has been recognized in recent years as an important cause of cerebral infarction [42]. Such occlusion is usually due to generalized or segmental atherosclerosis with or without superimposed thrombosis in one or both internal carotid arteries. Atherosclerosis is typically more severe at the bifurcation of the common carotid artery, especially on the left because that common carotid artery comes directly off the aorta. Some cases of carotid artery occlusion are produced by extrinsic compression or kinking of the artery. Complete occlusion of an internal carotid artery results in infarction of the ipsilateral cerebral hemisphere if collateral circulation is insufficient.

"subclavian steal" syndrome

The *"subclavian steal" syndrome* is a form of cerebrovascular insufficiency secondary to atherosclerotic obstruction of the proximal segment of the left subclavian artery [43]. A reversal of blood flow through the ipsilateral vertebral artery to supply collateral circulation for the upper extremity results in a deficiency in the posterior cerebral circulation. Occasionally venous thrombosis produces cerebral infarction. In the cerebrum, *venous infarcts* are usually limited to the gray cortex.

embolism

Embolism in cerebral arteries most often originates from a thrombus in the left side of the heart, in a pulmonary vein, or in other veins by paradoxical embolism. Air and fat embolisms also occur. *Atheromatous plaques* dislodged from the intima of the aorta or a carotid artery by erosion or surgical manipulation may lodge as emboli in cerebral arteries [44]. Rarely a calcific segment of a stenotic mitral valve may break away during commissurotomy and become a cerebral embolus. Embolism is most frequent in branches of the middle cerebral artery, probably because it is a direct continuation of the internal carotid artery. It may produce sudden death without infarction.

angiography

Carotid angiography, in which a radiopaque dye is injected to outline the cerebral arterial system on x-ray films, occasionally results in cerebral infarction [45]. Small foci of hemorrhagic necrosis are seen in such cases. Sometimes an acute arteritis is found in nearby vessels, probably due to a direct toxic effect of organic iodides in the dyes employed in angiography.

vasospasm

In the numerous cases of cerebral infarction in which no organic occlusion can be found, sustained vasospasm may be the cause. However, partial or complete arteriosclerotic and/or thrombotic occlusion of supply arteries can be found upon careful search in small infarcts [46].

Pathologic changes

If the patient survives at least several hours, *cerebral infarction* always follows cerebral arterial occlusion because cerebral arteries are functionally end arteries. The infarct early shows slight softening *(encephalomalacia)* and a transient infiltration by polymorphonuclear leukocytes. After 2 to 3 days the focus is yellow, soft, and semiliquid, with an edematous or hemorrhagic border. *Microscopically* there is degeneration of neurons, axis cylinders, and glial cells, with liquefaction of the lipid material of the myelin. Later the necrotic material is removed by round phagocytic, ameboid *microglial cells* which are abundant and develop a foamy or vacuolated cytoplasm *(Gitterzellen).* *Large infarcts* have cystic centers filled with yellowish fluid *(apoplectic cyst)* and surrounded by glial tissue. *Smaller infarcts* heal by the formation of a dense neuroglial scar if the patient survives.

HEMORRHAGE: Cause

Cerebral hemorrhage varies from tiny petechiae to massive hematomata. *Small hemorrhages* result from poisons such as carbon monoxide, bacterial toxins, or purpuric conditions, such as leukemia. *Large hemorrhages (apoplexy)* result from vascular disease, especially atherosclerosis, with or without hypertension. The *most common site of rupture* is a lenticulostriate branch of a middle cerebral artery, with hemorrhage into the basal ganglia and internal capsule. Pontine and cerebellar hemorrhages are less common. The mechanism of hemorrhage is unknown. A previous small infarct may be a necessary precursor. In cases of increased intracranial pressure, midline midbrain and pontine hemorrhages *(Duret hemorrhages)* are common. They are probably due to venous compression where the brain stem is jammed into the incisura of the tentorium cerebelli.

Pathologic changes

In *large hemorrhages* the brain bulges on the affected side with flattening of the gyri. The hemorrhage dissects through the brain tissue and may rupture into a ventricle, causing gross blood to appear in the spinal fluid. A *ventricular cast* may be formed by clotted blood. Rupture onto the surface of the brain produces subarachnoid hemorrhage. *Pontine hemorrhages* are often "splinter" or "crow's feet" in type. In the hemorrhagic area there is complete disintegration of brain tissue. In time the clot softens, and the brain tissue liquefies, producing a cyst filled with milky or yellow fluid. Blood pigments in the adjacent yellowed tissue betray the origin of the cyst.

Clinical features in cerebrovascular accidents

Clinically the picture depends on the size and location of the infarct or hemorrhage. Usually *coma* is present in large lesions, often appearing quite suddenly. Death may be rapid in intraventricular or medullary hemorrhage. Extreme hyperpyrexia and miosis are common in *pontine hemorrhage.* Nystagmus and deviation of the eyes toward the side of the lesion are typical in *cerebellar hemorrhage.* The most common sign is a contralateral spastic hemiplegia (flaccid early) with a positive Babinski sign due to *infarction or hemorrhage in the internal capsule.*

NEOPLASMS OF THE NERVOUS SYSTEM

Neoplasms may occur in the central and peripheral nervous systems and their coverings. *Most neoplasms of the nervous system are derived from the supporting structures;* only occasionally do they arise from nerve elements. About 10 percent of nervous system diseases are neoplastic, and males are affected more commonly than females.

Malignancy

The *malignancy* of a central nervous system neoplasm depends on its rapidity of growth and its location relative to vital centers. In the cerebrospinal axis are found some of the most slowly growing neoplasms as well as some of the most malignant in the body. *Metastasis outside the central nervous system is extremely rare in primary neoplasms;* this is true even of those derived from nonspecific supporting tissues, such as blood vessels. Spread within the central nervous system is usually via the subarachnoid space, but such spread is commonly localized.

Clinical features

Clinically central nervous system neoplasms cause a great variety of signs and symptoms depending on their location and size. Intracranial neoplasms act as space-occupying lesions in a tightly enclosed cavity. They may be simulated by other space-occupying masses such as brain abscess or tuberculoma. The *effects of intracranial neoplasms* include:

1. *Circulatory changes.* Vascular shifts may be apparent on cerebral arteriograms.

2. *Compression, distortion, and displacement of other structures.* This may be discerned as a displacement of the calcified pineal gland to the opposite side on skull films, or of the ventricular system on pneumoencephalogram or ventriculogram.

3. *Increased intracranial pressure.* This produces papilledema (choked disks) and in some cases herniation of a cingulate gyrus beneath the falx cerebri, an uncus through the incisura of the tentorium cerebelli, or the cerebellar tonsils into the foramen magnum, compressing the medulla.

4. *Interference with cerebrospinal fluid flow.* This produces internal or communicating *hydrocephalus,* ventricular dilatation being found on pneumoencephalogram or ventriculogram.

General symptoms and signs of intracranial neoplasms are headache, which is typically constant and aggravated by posture changes and is caused by stretching of the dura mater and distortion of blood vessels; vomiting, which may be projectile; apathy; dullness; blurring of vision; bradycardia; generalized convulsions; and a slight leukocytosis – all are due to increased intracranial pressure. *Localizing signs* may develop early or late in the course. Neoplasms growing in silent areas of the brain may reach a large size before becoming detectable.

Pseudotumor cerebri

Pseudotumor cerebri is a syndrome simulating a brain tumor, with increased intracranial pressure manifested by headache and papilledema. In prolonged and severe cases blindness results from optic nerve atrophy. The syndrome occurs most commonly in overweight adolescent or young adult females, who often have menstrual irregularities. There are probably multiple causes, among them hypervitaminosis A and prolonged adrenal corticosteroid therapy [47]. The signs and symptoms clear after withdrawal of the vitamin or steroids. Pseudotumor cerebri occasionally develops in patients with Addison's disease. *Cerebral biopsies* in cases of the syndrome show only edema of the brain.

1. Primary Intramedullary Neurogenic Neoplasms

GLIOMAS:

Gliomas are derived from the supporting cells of the central nervous system and constitute about 50 percent of all brain neoplasms and 25 percent of all spinal cord neoplasms.

Ependymoma group:

The *ependymoma* group constitutes about 5 percent of intracranial gliomas and 50 percent of intraspinal gliomas. Roughly 70 percent of tumors of the filum terminale and conus medullaris are of this type. The *origin* of ependymomas is from ependymal lining cells of the ventricles and central canal and the secretory epithelium of the choroid plexus. Deeply intramedullary ependymomas derive from ependymal cells remaining after fusion of primitive ventricular walls in the brain. They are most common in the fourth ventricle (especially from the roof), thoracic cord, and cauda equina where they are extramedullary and may reach a huge size. These last arise from ependymal cell clusters in either the conus medullaris or the filum terminale. The *average age* of occurrence is 25 years, and the *duration* of the disease is usually from 1½ to 4 years.

paraphyseal cyst

choroidal papilloma

papillary ependymoma

epithelial ependymoma

cellular ependymoma

ependymoblastoma

The ependymoma group contains several variants. The *paraphyseal* (colloid) *cyst* is a slowly growing, histologically benign cyst of the third ventricle; it represents a persistence of the rudimentary paraphysis. The pedunculated cyst is lined by cuboidal choroid-like epithelium which is occasionally ciliated. The cyst fluid is mucinous. Such cysts cause sudden excruciating headaches which are relieved by a change of position. The *choroidal papilloma* projects as a papillary mass into one or more ventricles. The epithelial lining is tall columnar with intracytoplasmic mucin droplets. The mass may cause hydrocephalus by overproduction of cerebrospinal fluid in the lateral ventricles or by blockage of the cerebrospinal fluid flow in the fourth ventricle. *Papillary ependymoma* is similar, but does not derive from the choroid plexus. The lining cells are cuboidal and contain no mucin droplets. The fibrous stroma often undergoes myxomatous change. *Epithelial ependymoma* is characterized by the formation of numerous structures resembling central canals (rosettes) within the neoplasm. Blepharoplasts (intracytoplasmic pieces of cilia) are found within some tumor cells. *Cellular ependymoma* consists of sheets of ependymal cells with occasional pseudorosettes radiating about a central eosinophilic body. Rarely extracranial metastases have been found. *Ependymoblastoma* is highly malignant and rapidly growing. It is very cellular, mitoses and giant cells being common.

In general, intramedullary ependymomas are gray, soft, and circumscribed with a narrow zone of demarcation from the surrounding brain or spinal cord. Cerebral ependymomas are commonly cystic. From 10 to 20 percent of ependymomas show calcification grossly, and more show microscopic foci.

Oligodendroglioma:

Oligodendroglioma arises from oligodendrocytes, usually in the cerebral white matter of the frontal lobes. It constitutes about 5 percent of all central nervous system neoplasms. The *average age* of occurrence is 35 years, and the average *duration* of the disease is 5 years.

pathologic changes

Grossly the oligodendroglioma is usually fairly well demarcated, large, slowly growing, cystic, and grayish pink. Foci of necrosis and calcification are common. Occasionally the neoplasm breaks through the cerebral cortex and mushrooms out into the subarachnoid space *(meningeal gliomatosis)*. *Microscopically* there are broad sheets of large cells with darkly staining round nuclei surrounded by clear halos of cytoplasm. The cell membranes are well defined. *Oligodendroglioblastoma* is a malignant histologic variant. However, the prognosis is poor in all oligodendrogliomas.

Astrocytoma group:

The *astrocytoma group* originates from astrocytes or astroblasts of the neuroglia of the brain and, less commonly, of the spinal cord.

astrocytoma

Astrocytoma (astrocytoma, grade I) is the most common of all gliomas, constituting about 15 percent of intracranial neoplasms. It usually occurs in the cerebrum in adults (especially in the temporal lobes) and the cerebellum in children. The *average age* of occurrence is 30 years, and the *duration* of the disease is usually several years. *Grossly* there is a gray, poorly defined mass which often shows foci of necrosis, hemorrhage, cyst formation, and microscopic calcification. *Cerebellar astrocytomas* are very commonly cystic and often contain only a mural nodule of neoplastic tissue. Compression and narrowing of the fourth ventricle may produce internal hydrocephalus. *Microscopically* there are three types: (1) the *fibrillar or pilocytic astrocytoma,* consisting of well-differentiated astrocytes with a dense fibrillar stroma; (2) the *gemistocytic astrocytoma,* which consists of greatly swollen astrocytes with hyalin-like cytoplasm, eccentric nuclei, and short fibrillar processes; and (3) the uncommon *protoplasmic astrocytoma* in which atypical astrocytes with swollen cytoplasm are set in a cobweb-like acidophilic matrix interspersed with foci of microcystic degeneration. In all types the edges of the neoplasm blend with the surrounding tissue.

astroblastoma

Astroblastoma (astrocytoma, grade II) occurs in the cerebrum in about 65 percent of the cases and in the cerebellum in 15 percent. It constitutes less than 5 percent of intracranial neoplasms. The *average age* of occurrence is 35 years, and the *duration* of the disease is about 2 years. *Grossly* this is an expansive, unencapsulated, gray mass with foci of hemorrhage, necrosis, and cyst formation. *Microscopically* it consists of immature astrocytic cells arranged radially about the blood vessels to which they are attached by sucker feet.

spongioblastoma

Spongioblastoma polare (astrocytoma, grades I to IV, depending on the degree of anaplasia) usually occurs in the cerebrum in adults and the pons in children. It comprises about 5 percent of gliomas, and the *average age* of occurrence is 15 years. *Grossly* this is a slowly growing, poorly delineated, soft mass. *Microscopically* there are interlacing bundles of fibrils. The typical cell is a spindle-shaped astrocyte with either a single polar process or bipolar processes. Any degree of anaplasia from well differentiated (grade I) to bizarre (grade IV) may be found. *The spongioblastoma is probably a histologic variant rather than a distinct entity.*

glioblastoma multiforme:

Glioblastoma multiforme (astrocytoma, grades III and IV) is the most malignant of all brain neoplasms. It constitutes about 10 percent of intracranial neoplasms. Males are more frequently affected by 3:2. *About 90 percent occur in the cerebrum,* and about 10 percent are multicentric in origin. Of cerebral glioblastomas about 25 percent arise in the frontal lobes, 25 percent in the temporal lobes, 20 percent in the parietal lobes, and 5 percent in the occipital lobes, the rest involving more than one lobe [48]. The majority of cases occur in the 45 to 55 year age group, and the survival period after diagnosis is usually less than a year. *Grossly* this neoplasm is an irregular, partly hemorrhagic and necrotic, yellow, brown, or reddish gray expansile mass, often measuring up to 5 cm. in diameter. Infiltration across the corpus callosum into the opposite hemisphere is common *(butterfly tumor).* Rarely a diffuse glioblastomatous transformation of the cerebrum and brain stem occurs *(gliomatosis cerebri)* [49]. Glioblastomas spread by peripheral invasion and less frequently by meningeal invasion, implants seeding along the subarachnoid space. Meningeal gliomatosis may occur. *Microscopically* the picture is pleomorphic, with spongioblasts, gemistocytic astrocytes, multinucleated giant cells with bizarre mitotic figures, and a marked increase in vascular elements with endothelial proliferation in the capillary walls. In fact, the degree of *endothelial hyperplasia* closely parallels the degree of anaplasia throughout the astrocytoma series [50].

rare metastases

Very rarely a glioblastoma multiforme has developed extracranial metastases. Metastases of glial elements to the lungs and cervical lymph nodes have been recorded. The extreme rarity of extracranial metastases may be due to the inability of the component cells to invade blood vessel walls in the brain [51]. The rare metastases usually result after repeated surgery which enables the neoplastic cells to invade extracranial soft tissue and its vessels. Another factor in explaining the paucity of distant metastases is that the neoplasm consists of neuroglial tissue which is bathed in the cerebrospinal fluid, and this fluid is not present outside the central nervous system.

Medulloblastoma:

Medulloblastoma (granuloblastoma, glioblastoma isomorphe) is a highly malignant neoplasm of children. It *originates* either from medulloblasts or from residua of the external granular (Obersteiner's) layer of the cerebellum. Medulloblastoma occurs in the posterior vermis and, less often, in the hemispheres of the cerebellum. Its frequency is about 10 percent of all gliomas, and it is more common in boys by 2:1. The *average age* of occurrence is 12 years, and the *duration* of the disease is about 18 months. *Clinically* headache, vomiting, and a staggering gait are common.

pathologic changes

Grossly the neoplasm is often circumscribed. It usually grows into the fourth ventricle, producing internal hydrocephalus. It is pinkish gray and soft. *Microscopically* the typical cell is small and oat- or carrot-shaped with a hyperchromatic nucleus. Clusters of these cells often form *pseudorosettes.* The medulloblastoma may spread via the cerebrospinal fluid, forming secondary nodules in the brain and spinal cord. Very rarely *metastases outside the nervous system* occur, especially in lymph nodes and bones [52].

NEURONAL NEOPLASMS:

Neoplasms arising from parenchymal neural cells are uncommon within the central nervous system.

Neurocytoma

Neurocytoma (neuroastrocytoma) is a very rare, slowly growing, poorly delineated neoplasm composed of mature neurocytes in a glial stroma. The *neuroblastoma* is also rare within the central nervous system. It consists of primitive neural cells and resembles the medulloblastoma microscopically.

Pinealoma

Pinealoma (pinealocytoma) is a rare neoplasm which occurs most commonly in males between 15 and 25 years. *Grossly* it expands anteriorly into the third ventricle or posteriorly over the midbrain. *Microscopically* there is a mosaic of large cells and small, darkly staining cells resembling lymphocytes. The pattern is similar to that of the seminoma of the testis.

Gliomas (ependymoma, astrocytoma) *and teratomas* also occur in the pineal region. *Pineal teratoma* is sometimes associated with precocious puberty.

Retinoblastoma

Retinoblastoma is discussed under Diseases of the Eyes on page 818.

2. Primary Extramedullary Neurogenic Neoplasms

SUPPORTING CELL NEOPLASMS:

Primary extramedullary neurogenic neoplasms arise from supporting cells or from neural elements of the peripheral nervous system. The origin of some of these tumors is disputed. *Neoplasms arising from supporting cells* are quite common peripherally.

Neurilemmoma:

Neurilemmoma (neurinoma, schwannoma) is a fairly common peripheral nerve tumor. It is almost always benign, and its *origin* is probably from cells of the sheath of Schwann. Neurilemmoma develops along nerve roots (this is the most common neoplasm of the spinal canal) and large peripheral nerves. Almost one-half of neurogenous mediastinal neoplasms and about 15 percent of all mediastinal tumors are neurilemmomas [53].

pathologic changes

Grossly it is a round or ovoid, encapsulated, firm, yellow mass 1 to 10 cm. in diameter. Growth is along the surface of the nerve. The center of the tumor may be cystic or gelatinous. *Microscopically* it shows interlacing streams of spindle cells showing *palisading of the nuclei.* A small amount of intercellular collagen is found. In Antoni type A neurilemmomas, whorled and fanlike *Verocay bodies* are common. These tumors are rich in nuclei which often lie parallel to the fibrils. Antoni type B is characterized by large numbers of fibrillary processes and microcystic degeneration.

Acoustic neurinoma

Acoustic neurinoma is a histologically benign expansive neoplasm of the vestibular branch of the *eighth cranial nerve.* It is considered to be a neurilemmoma, which it resembles grossly and microscopically, although it is disputed whether the sheath of Schwann exists along this nerve. The neoplasm *occupies the cerebellopontine angle.* Rarely the fifth (trigeminal) or seventh (facial) nerve is the primary site of a neurinoma. *Clinically* the symptoms are ipsilateral tinnitus (ringing, buzzing, roaring), progressive deafness, dizziness, and nystagmus.

Neurofibroma:

Neurofibroma is a benign neoplasm occurring subcutaneously or along peripheral nerves. Its *origin* is probably from the cells of the sheath of Schwann.

pathologic changes

Grossly the neurofibroma is gray, firm, and spherical or ovoid. The neoplasm grows in the depth of the nerve, and nerve fibers may be seen coursing through it. *Microscopically* there are interlacing strands of long spindle cells. A moderate amount of intercellular collagen is present, and included nerve fibers may be found. In *storiform neurofibromas* the spindle cells are arranged like matting or a pinwheel [54]. Occasional cells contain melanin.

Neurofibromatosis

Multiple neurofibromatosis (von Recklinghausen's disease) is a rare familial entity in which there are hundreds of subcutaneous, often pedunculated neurofibromas, as well as associated lesions in the central nervous system and peripheral nerves (meningiomas, plexiform neuromas). The disease is transmitted as a mendelian dominant and begins in childhood. Small and large foci of brown pigmentation (café au lait spots), nevi, melanocarcinomas, and lipomas are often present. In about 10 percent of the cases a neurofibrosarcoma or soft tissue sarcoma develops [55].

Neurofibrosarcoma:

Neurofibrosarcoma (neurogenic sarcoma) is usually less malignant than the fibrosarcoma. Its origin is probably from cells of the sheath of Schwann. It develops along peripheral nerve trunks and in the retroperitoneal region paravertebrally.

pathologic changes

Neurofibrosarcoma is slowly invasive and eventually metastasizes. *Microscopically* there are three types: sclerosing (dense fibrous stroma with few atypical spindle cells), spindle cell (bundles of interlacing spindle cells), and anaplastic. The neoplasm tends to recur after surgical removal.

NEURAL CELL NEOPLASMS:

Neoplasms arising from peripheral neural cells and their processes are not common except for the nevus-melanocarcinoma group (discussed under The Skin on page 787). Carcinoid tumors are considered with gastrointestinal neoplasms on page 512.

Ganglioneuroma

Ganglioneuroma is a benign neoplasm arising from migrant undifferentiated nerve cells. These tumors are found paravertebrally most commonly, often being located in the posterior mediastinum. About 30 percent of neurogenous mediastinal neoplasms are ganglioneuromas. These neoplasms also occur retroperitoneally [56] and in the adrenal glands, gastrointestinal tract, and mesentery. *Grossly* they are firm, spheroid or ovoid, and usually large masses with grayish white or yellowish cut surfaces. *Microscopically* the presence of *large ganglion cells in a fibrous stroma* (probably of Schwann sheath origin) is typical. Foci of calcification are frequently found.

Ganglio-neuro-blastoma

Ganglioneuroblastoma is intermediate between ganglioneuroma and neuroblastoma in histologic appearance and degree of malignancy. It usually appears before the age of 6 years and occurs in the retroperitoneal region, posterior mediastinum, and adrenal medulla. *Grossly* the neoplasm resembles the ganglioneuroma, but the ganglioneuroblastoma is softer and has a tendency to undergo necrosis and hemorrhage. Calcific foci are frequently present. *Microscopically* it consists of both mature and immature ganglion cells and small, darkly staining neuroblasts. The latter cells are malignant and may spread by direct invasion of adjacent structures or by distant metastases, which occur in about 40 percent of the cases. The distribution of *metastases* is similar to that of neuroblastoma. Some cases of ganglioneuroblastoma, as well as of ganglioneuroma and neuroblastoma, have been associated with *hypertension and diarrhea,* evidently due to epinephrine and norepinephrine secretion by neoplastic cells. Bioassay reveals significant amounts of catecholamines in all three of this group of neoplasms [57].

Neuro-blastoma:

Neuroblastoma [58] is a highly malignant neoplasm which occurs in infants and young children. Its *origin* is from migrant neural blast cells in the adrenal medulla, paraganglia, and sympathetic ganglia. When the tumor arises from sympathetic blast cells, it may be called a *sympathicoblastoma.* In about 40 percent of cases the neuroblastoma develops in the adrenal medulla, and in about 35 percent, retroperitoneally. This neoplasm is usually radiosensitive. The mortality rate of patients with neuroblastoma is about 70 percent within a year after diagnosis. *Occasionally a neuroblastoma or sympathicoblastoma has matured to a ganglioneuroma* through the intermediate stage of a ganglioneuroblastoma [59]. Extremely rarely neuroblastomas undergo spontaneous regression.

pathologic changes

Grossly it is soft, white or yellow, and hemorrhagic; fibrous septa lobulate the mass. *Microscopically* the typical cell is small and has a large nucleus and scanty cytoplasm with short processes. *Rosette formations* are scattered through the section.

metastases

Two clinical types have been described: (1) the *Pepper type,* said to be more commonly from neuroblastomas of the right adrenal gland, with extensive metastases to the liver (which is involved in about 65 percent of neuroblastomas) and mesenteric lymph nodes, and (2) the *Hutchinson type,* with large metastases to the skull and periorbital tissues and said to be more often from neuroblastomas of the left adrenal gland. The lungs, gastrointestinal tract, and other bones are frequent sites of metastases.

Pheochromo-cytoma

Pheochromocytoma of the adrenal medulla is discussed on page 720.

Carotid body tumor:

Carotid body tumor (chemodectoma of the carotid body) [60] arises in the glomus caroticum at the bifurcation of the common carotid artery. These bodies are chemoreceptors sensitive to changes in the blood pH and carbon dioxide and oxygen tensions, and they regulate respiraton. The carotid body has generally been thought to be a nonchromaffin paraganglion; but definite argentaffin cells closely resembling Kultschitzky cells have been identified in the normal carotid body and its chemodectoma [61]. Such cells may secrete serotonin, and a functional carotid body-like tumor with argentaffin cells elaborating levarterenol has been described [62].

pathologic changes

The neoplasm is firmly adherent to the bifurcation of the artery, making resection difficult. It measures up to 5 cm. in diameter and is encapsulated. The cut surface is homogeneous and pinkish gray (or reddish brown from hemorrhage). *Microscopically* the neoplasm reproduces the normal carotid body, with *nests (Zellballen) of chief cells* in a highly vascular stroma. The chief cells have an epithelioid appearance. The carotid body tumor is almost always benign histologically. However, local recurrence following excision and lymph node or distant metastases occasionally occur. Comparable neoplasms are found in the glomus jugulare near the middle ear (see page 825), in the glomus intravagale (vagal body) [63], and in the aortic body [64]. Multiple tiny nodules centered about pulmonary venules with the histologic appearance of chemodectomas have occasionally been found in the lungs [65].

clinical features

Clinically the tumor occurs most commonly in the 20 to 40 age group, and is found equally in both sexes. It may appear in several members of a family and may be bilateral. The carotid body tumor grows as a painless, nontender, slowly enlarging, firm, oval mass at the angle of the jaw ("potato tumor"). It is movable from side to side and decreases in size on carotid artery compression.

Neuromas

Neuromas develop from peripheral nerve fibrils. The *myelinic neuroma* is a rare, massive retroperitoneal neoplasm showing a whorled pattern of nerve fibers with a large amount of associated myelin. *Plexiform neuroma* occurs along peripheral nerves as a tangled, spaghetti-like mass of large, well-differentiated nerve filaments. Occasionally a small neuroma is found in an obliterated appendix. *Traumatic neuroma* usually occurs at an amputation site *(amputation neuroma)* and consists of a bundle of neurofibrils and proliferated Schwann sheath cells.

3. Meningiomas

MENINGIOMAS:

Meningiomas constitute about 20 percent of intracranial and 25 percent of intraspinal neoplasms. The tumors occur most commonly in middle-aged adults. Their *origin* is from "cap cells" (meningocytes) on the outer surface of the pia-arachnoid. These cells are derived from the neural crest, so that meningiomas are neuroectodermal in origin. Electron microscopic studies indicate that almost all meningiomas are derived from a pluripotential meningothelial cell with both epithelial and mesenchymal propensities [66]. *Common locations* are parasagittal, over the free convexity of the brain, in the sphenoidal ridge, in the olfactory groove, and in the cerebellopontine angle.

Pathologic changes

Grossly the meningioma is nodular, encapsulated, gray, and firm, varying in size from microscopic to huge and weighing up to 200 gm. *Microscopically* [67] there are two main types: (1) the *meningotheliomatous meningioma* (the most common type), which shows whorled nests of large cells with indistinct cell boundaries and an interlacing stroma of elongated cells, and (2) the *fibroblastic meningioma,* which has interlacing strands of collagen and reticulin fibers with palisaded nuclei and nests of meningothelial cells. The *psammoma (psammomatous meningioma)* is a variant of the meningotheliomatous type in which there are many hyalinized or calcified laminated psammoma bodies. These bodies result from degeneration of nests of meningothelial cells, and a few are found in most meningiomas. A rare type is the *angioblastic meningioma* which is extremely vascular. *Metaplasia* appears to occur in some meningiomas; osteoblastic, chondroblastic, and lipomatous types have been described. Rarely a meningeal melanoblastoma develops from pial melanoblasts. *Most meningiomas are histologically benign,* causing their effects by compression of the underlying brain or spinal cord. Occasionally a histologically malignant meningioma *(meningiosarcoma)* occurs, usually of the fibrosarcoma type. This appears to arise from the arachnoid and stromal elements. Extracranial metastases are rare and are most common in the lungs and pleura [68].

4. Vascular Neoplasms

Neoplasms arising from neural blood vessels are not uncommon and occur in a variety of forms.

TELANGIECTASIS

Telangiectasis is a vascular malformatión and usually develops in the midbrain. Focally the capillaries are dilated and tortuous.

LINDAU'S DISEASE

Lindau's disease [69] is a rare congenital defect in which there are multiple hemangioendotheliomas of the retina, cerebellum, medulla oblongata, spinal cord, and liver; polycystic disease of the pancreas, liver, and kidneys; and focal hyperplasia of the adrenal cortex. Occasionally, an adenoma or adenocarcinoma of the kidney or a pheochromocytoma is associated.

VON HIPPEL'S DISEASE

Von Hippel's disease is an angiomatosis of the retinal blood vessels. About 20 percent of these patients have other lesions of Lindau's disease.

STURGE-WEBER-DIMITRI'S DISEASE

Sturge-Weber-Dimitri's disease [70] is an association of hemangiomas (often with calcification and iron pigment deposition) in the meninges over one cerebral hemisphere with a port-wine hemangioma over the distribution of the trigeminal nerve on the same side or bilaterally.

ANGIOMAS

Isolated *hemangioma* is rare within the central nervous system, but it occurs somewhat more frequently in the meninges. *Hemangioendothelioma (hemangioblastoma)* is a histologically benign vascular neoplasm which occurs in the cerebellum as a cystic mass with a mural neoplastic nodule. *Microscopically* it is highly cellular, with marked proliferation of endothelial cells, and contains foam cells. It may occur alone or with other stigmata of Lindau's disease. *Hemangiosarcoma* occurs rarely and has been known to metastasize widely outside the central nervous system.

5. Mesodermal Supporting Tissue Neoplasms

SARCOMAS: Fibrosarcoma

Primary sarcomas are rare in the central nervous system and meninges. *Fibrosarcoma* probably arises from fibroblasts in the adventitia of blood vessels. Some cases have developed a number of years after x-radiation therapy of the brain [71]. *Giant cell fibrosarcoma* [72] is a variant in which a few or many huge, bizarre, usually multinucleated giant cells are found together with abundant reticulin fibers in the less anaplastic sarcomatous foci. These unusual neoplasms are firm with foci of cystic degeneration, and occur most often in the temporal lobes. *Reticuloendothelial neoplasms* of the brain [73] make up about 15 percent of primary sarcomas there. They usually occur as a single tumor in the cerebrum. The average age of the patients is about 45 years, and the survival period averages almost 4 years in patients given postoperative radiation therapy. *Reticulum cell sarcoma* is by far the most common form and originates from perivascular or leptomeningeal histiocytes. Abundant reticulin fibers are present in these neoplasms. The presence of Reed-Sternberg cells is characteristic of the *Hodgkin's* variant of reticulum cell *sarcoma. Microglioblastoma* arises from microglial cells and is very rare. Mixed forms of reticuloendothelial sarcoma also occur. Influenza-like symptoms are present in a significant number of patients with reticuloendothelial neoplasms of the brain, suggesting the possibility that they may be caused by a filtrable virus.

Reticulum cell sarcoma

Microglioblastoma

6. Developmental Neoplasms

Developmental neoplasms associated with the central nervous system include *epidermal cyst* (cholesteatoma, pearly tumor), which arises from aberrant intracranial or intraspinal epithelium and grows slowly as nests of squamous cells, keratohyalin, and cholesterol crystals; *dermoid cyst,* which is similar but contains sebaceous glands and hairs; rare *teratomas; chordoma;* and *craniopharyngioma.*

CRANIOPHARYNGIOMA:

Craniopharyngioma constitutes about 5 percent of intracranial neoplasms. It derives from squamous epithelial nests from the craniopharyngeal canal within the pituitary gland [74] and occurs in children and young adults. The neoplasm is intrasellar and may be histologically benign or carcinomatous, the latter form tending to occur in younger individuals. *Rathke pouch (suprasellar) cyst* is a variant of craniopharyngioma and is derived from squamous cell nests in the capsule of the anterior pituitary. Occasionally such neoplasms are solid.

Pathologic changes

The *craniopharyngioma* is usually partly solid and partly cystic. It consists of interlacing strands of squamous epithelium in a fibrous stroma. Keratinized areas and foci of necrosis are common. Cholesterol crystals and calcification are present.

7. Metastatic Neoplasms

METASTATIC NEOPLASMS [75]:

Metastases to the brain are fairly common, occurring in about 20 percent of all fatal malignant neoplasms, but they are uncommon to the spinal cord. About 10 percent of intracranial neoplasms are metastatic. Malignant cells reach the brain by hematogenous routes, especially via cerebral arteries but also through the veins of Batson which drain into the vertebral veins; by direct invasion; and by meningeal spread.

Sources

The most common source of brain metastases is bronchogenic carcinoma. Other frequent primary sites are the mammary glands, kidneys, skin *(melanocarcinoma),* and gastrointestinal tract. Associated primary or metastatic neoplasm is found in the lungs in almost all patients with brain metastases.

Pathologic changes

Within the brain, *metastatic tumor* is found in the cerebrum in about 75 percent of cases, in the cerebellum in 30 percent, and in the brain stem in 10 percent. Focal or diffuse leptomeningeal involvement is found in about 60 percent. The metastatic lesions are very *often multiple.* They are usually well defined and unencapsulated. *Microscopically* they resemble the primary neoplasm.

REFERENCES

1. Kernohan, J. W., and Fletcher-Kernohan, E. M. The ependymomas. *Proc. Ass. Res. Nerv. Ment. Dis., 1935.* 16:182, 1937.
2. Jacobs, E. B., Landing, B. H., and Thomas, W., Jr. Vernicomyelia: Its bearing on theories of genesis of the Arnold-Chiari complex. *Amer. J. Path.* 39:345, 1961.
3. Vogel, F. S. The anatomic character of the vascular anomalies associated with anencephaly. *Amer. J. Path.* 39:163, 1961.
4. Nichols, J. Observations on the adrenal of the premature anencephalic fetus. *A.M.A. Arch. Path.* 62:312, 1956.
5. Miller, J. Q., Picard, E. H., Alkan, M. K., Warner, S., and Gerald, P. S. A specific congenital brain defect (arhinencephaly) in 13-15 trisomy. *New Eng. J. Med.* 268:120, 1963.
6. Love, J. G., Daly, D. D., and Harris, L. E. Tight filum terminale. *J.A.M.A.* 176:31, 1961.
7. Warkany, J. Etiology of mongolism. *J. Pediat.* 56:412, 1960.
8. Breg, W. R., Miller, O. J., and Schmickel, R. D. Chromosomal translocations in patients with mongolism and in their normal relatives. *New Eng. J. Med.* 266:845, 1962.
9. Murphy, E. S., Fujii, Y., Yasuda, A., and Sasabe, S. The tuberous sclerosis complex. *A.M.A. Arch. Path.* 65:166, 1958.
10. Perlstein, M. A., and Hood, P. N. Etiology of postneonatally acquired cerebral palsy. *J.A.M.A.* 188:850, 1964.
11. Towbin, A. Pathology of cerebral palsy. *A.M.A. Arch. Path.* 59:397, 529, 1955.
12. Spjut, H. J., and Luse, S. A. Chordoma: An electron microscopic study. *Cancer* 17:643, 1964.
13. Delta, B. G., Scott, R. B., and Booker, C. R. *Listeria* meningitis in the newborn. *Med. Ann. D.C.* 30:329, 1961.
14. Groover, R. V., Sutherland, J. M., and Landing, B. H. Purulent meningitis of newborn infants. *New Eng. J. Med.* 264:1115, 1961.
15. Shinner, J. J. St. Louis virus encephalomyelitis. *Arch. Path.* (Chicago) 75:309, 1963.
16. Kent, J. R., and Finegold, S. M. Human rabies transmitted by the bite of a bat, with comments on the duck-embryo vaccine. *New Eng. J. Med.* 263:1058, 1960.
17. Williams, H. W., and Chafee, F. H. Demyelinating encephalomyelitis in a case of tetanus treated with antitoxin. *New Eng. J. Med.* 264:489, 1961.
18. Sabin, A. B. Pathogenesis of poliomyelitis. *Science* 123:1151, 1956.
19. Baker, A. B., and Cornwell, S. Poliomyelitis XV. The spinal cord. *A.M.A. Arch. Path.* 61:185, 1956.
20. Magoffin, R. L., Lennette, E. H., Hollister, A. C., Jr., and Schmidt, N. J. An etiologic study of clinical paralytic poliomyelitis. *J.A.M.A.* 175:269, 1961.
21. Jarcho, L. W., Fred, H. L., and Castle, C. H. Encephalitis and poliomyelitis in the adult due to Coxsackie virus group B, type 5. *New Eng. J. Med.* 268:235, 1963.
22. Rab, S. M., and Choudhury, G. M. Landry-Guillain-Barré syndrome after chicken pox. *New Eng. J. Med.* 268:200, 1963.
23. Buff, B. H. Rabies: A summary of recent contributions to the literature (July 1958–June 1963). *Med. Ann. D.C.* 33:149, 1964.
24. Ross, E., and Armentrout, S. A. Myocarditis associated with rabies. *New Eng. J. Med.* 266:1087, 1962.

25. Newman, W., and Jacobson, A. S. Paraplegia and secondary amyloidosis. *Amer. J. Med.* 15:216, 1953.
26. Bardenwerper, H. W. Serum neuritis from tetanus antitoxin. *J.A.M.A.* 179:763, 1962.
27. Schumacher, G. A. Demyelinating diseases: Multiple sclerosis. *New Eng. J. Med.* 262:1119, 1960. (The last of an excellent four-part review on the demyelinating diseases; the others are 262:969, 1019, 1069.)
28. Ivers, R. R., McKenzie, B. F., McGuckin, W. F., and Goldstein, N. P. Spinal-fluid gamma globulin in multiple sclerosis and other neurologic diseases. *J.A.M.A.* 176:515, 1961.
29. Wolfe, H. J., and Pietra, G. G. The visceral lesions of metachromatic leukodystrophy. *Amer. J. Path.* 44:921, 1964.
30. Dawson, C. W., and Roberts, J. B. Charcot-Marie-Tooth disease. *J.A.M.A.* 188:659, 1964.
31. Teller, W. M., and Millichap, J. G. Ataxia-telangiectasis (Louis-Bar syndrome) with prominent sinopulmonary disease. *J.A.M.A.* 175:779, 1961.
32. Ayd, F. J., Jr. A survey of drug-induced extrapyramidal reactions. *J.A.M.A.* 175:1054, 1961.
33. England, A. C., Jr., and Schwab, R. S. Parkinson's syndrome. *New Eng. J. Med.* 265:785, 1961.
34. Doshay, L. J. Parkinson's disease. *J.A.M.A.* 174:1962, 1960.
35. Adner, M. M., Sherman, J. D., Ise, C., Schwab, R. S., and Dameshek, W. An immunologic survey of forty-eight patients with myasthenia gravis. *New Eng. J. Med.* 271:1327, 1964.
36. Becker, K. L., Titus, J. L., McConahey, W. M., and Woolner, L. B. Morphologic evidence of thyroiditis in myasthenia gravis. *J.A.M.A.* 187:994, 1964.
37. Drachman, D. B. Myasthenia gravis and the thyroid gland. *New Eng. J. Med.* 266:330, 1962.
38. Luse, S. A., and Smith, K. R., Jr. The ultrastructure of senile plaques. *Amer. J. Path.* 44:553, 1964.
39. Stehbens, W. E. Aneurysms and anatomical variation of cerebral arteries. *Arch. Path.* (Chicago) 75:45, 1963.
40. McDonald, C. A., and Korb, M. Intracranial aneurysms. *Arch. Neurol. Psychiat.* 42:298, 1939.
41. Patterson, J. C., and Cornish, B. R. Calcium concentrations in sclerotic cerebral arteries. *A.M.A. Arch. Path.* 62:177, 1956.
42. Gurdjian, E. S., Hardy, W. G., Lindner, D. W., and Thomas, L. M. Analysis of occlusive disease of the carotid artery and the stroke syndrome. *J.A.M.A.* 176:194, 1961.
43. Mannick, J. A., Suter, C. G., and Hume, D. M. The "subclavian-steal" syndrome: A further documentation. *J.A.M.A.* 182:254, 1962.
44. Sturgill, B. C., and Netsky, M. G. Cerebral infarction by atheromatous emboli. *Arch. Path.* (Chicago) 76:189, 1963.
45. Sherrick, J. C., and Amador, L. V. Cerebral infarction after carotid angiography. *Arch. Path.* (Chicago) 76:133, 1963.
46. Winter, W. J., and Gyori, E. Pathogenesis of small cerebral infarcts. *A.M.A. Arch. Path.* 69:224, 1960.
47. Walker, A. E., and Adamkiewicz, J. J. Pseudotumor cerebri associated with prolonged corticosteroid therapy. *J.A.M.A.* 188:779, 1964.
48. Frankel, S. A., and German, W. J. Glioblastoma multiforme. *J. Neurosurg.* 15:489, 1958.
49. Dunn, J., Jr., and Kernohan, J. W. Gliomatosis cerebri. *A.M.A. Arch. Path.* 64:82, 1957.

50. Feigin, I., Allen, L. B., Lipkin, L., and Gross, S. W. The endothelial hyperplasia of the cerebral blood vessels with brain tumors, and its sarcomatous transformation. *Cancer* 11:264, 1958.
51. Labitzke, H. G. Glioblastoma multiforme with remote extracranial metastases. *Arch. Path.* (Chicago) 73:223, 1962.
52. Oberman, H. A., Hewitt, W. C., Jr., and Kalivoda, A. J. Medulloblastomas with distant metastases. *Amer. J. Clin. Path.* 39:148, 1963.
53. Oberman, H. A., and Abell, M. R. Neurogenous neoplasms of the mediastinum. *Cancer* 13:882, 1960.
54. Bednar, B. Storiform neurofibromas of the skin, pigmented and nonpigmented. *Cancer* 10:368, 1957.
55. D'Agostino, A. N., Soule, E. H., and Miller, R. H. Sarcomas of the peripheral nerves and somatic soft tissues associated with multiple neurofibromatosis (von Recklinghausen's disease). *Cancer* 16:1015, 1963.
56. Carpenter, R. B., and Kernohan, J. W. Retroperitoneal ganglioneuromas and neurofibromas. *Cancer* 16:788, 1963.
57. Silver, L., Dahlin, D. C., Tyce, G. M., and Stickler, G. B. Ganglioneuroblastoma: Studies of pathologic changes and content of catecholamine. *Amer. J. Clin. Path.* 42:145, 1964.
58. Stowens, D. Neuroblastoma and related tumors. *A.M.A. Arch. Path.* 63:451, 1957.
59. Haber, S. L., and Bennington, J. L. Maturation of congenital extra-adrenal neuroblastoma. *Arch. Path.* (Chicago) 76:121, 1963.
60. Le Compte, P. M. Tumors of the carotid body and related structures. Section IV, Fascicle 16, in *Atlas of Tumor Pathology*. Washington: Armed Forces Institute of Pathology, 1951.
61. Barroso-Moguel, R., and Costero, I. Argentaffin cells of the carotid body tumor. *Amer. J. Path.* 41:389, 1962.
62. Glenner, G. G., Crout, J. R., and Roberts, W. C. A functional carotid-body-like tumor secreting levarterenol. *Arch. Path.* (Chicago) 73:230, 1962.
63. Perez, P. E., Harrison, E. G., Jr., and Re Mine, W. H. Vagal-body tumor (chemodectoma of the glomus intravagale). *New Eng. J. Med.* 263:1116, 1960.
64. Mendelow, H., and Slobodkin, M. Aortic-body tumor (chemodectoma) of the mediastinum. *Cancer* 10:1008, 1957.
65. Korn, D., Bensch, K., Liebow, A. A., and Castleman, B. Multiple minute pulmonary tumors resembling chemodectomas. *Amer. J. Path.* 37:641, 1960.
66. Napolitano, L., Kyle, R., and Fisher, E. R. Ultrastructure of meningiomas and their derivations and nature of their cellular components. *Cancer* 17:233, 1964.
67. Kepes, J., and Kernohan, J. W. Meningiomas: Problems of histological differential diagnosis. *Cancer* 12:364, 1959.
68. Noto, T. A., and Gyori, E. Malignant metastasizing meningioma. *Arch. Path.* (Chicago) 72:73, 1961.
69. Schechterman, L. Lindau's disease. *Med. Ann. D.C.* 30:64, 1961.
70. Lichtenstein, B. W. Sturge-Weber-Dimitri syndrome. *A.M.A. Arch. Neurol. Psychiat.* 71:291, 1954.
71. Noetzli, M., and Malamud, N. Postirradiation fibrosarcoma of the brain. *Cancer* 15:617, 1962.
72. Hitselberger, W. E., Kernohan, J. W., and Uihlein, A. Giant cell fibrosarcoma of the brain. *Cancer* 14:841, 1961.
73. Burstein, S. D., Kernohan, J. W., and Uihlein, A. Neoplasms of the reticuloendothelial system of the brain. *Cancer* 16:289, 1963.

74. Goldberg, G. M., and Eshbaugh, D. E. Squamous cell nests of the pituitary gland as related to the origin of craniopharyngiomas. *Arch. Path.* (Chicago) 70:293, 1960.
75. Chason, J. L., Walker, F. B., and Landers, J. W. Metastatic carcinoma in the central nervous system and dorsal root ganglia. *Cancer* 16:781, 1963.

GENERAL REFERENCES

Blackwood, W., McMenemey, W. H., Meyer, A., Norman, R. M., and Russell, D. S. *Neuropathology* (2d ed.). Baltimore: Williams & Wilkins, 1963.

Kernohan, J. W., and Sayre, G. P. Tumors of the central nervous system. Section X, Fascicles 35 and 37, in *Atlas of Tumor Pathology.* Washington: Armed Forces Institute of Pathology, 1952. (A masterly, well-organized, and splendidly illustrated review of a complex group of neoplasms.)

Russell, D. S., and Rubinstein, L. J. *Pathology of Tumours of the Nervous System* (2d ed.). Baltimore: Williams & Wilkins, 1963.

Stout, A. P. Tumors of the peripheral nervous system. Section II, Fascicle 6, in *Atlas of Tumor Pathology.* Washington: Armed Forces Institute of Pathology, 1949. (An authoritative and well-pictured presentation of peripheral neural neoplasms.)

27 THE ENDOCRINE SYSTEM; METABOLIC DISEASES

INTRODUCTION

The endocrine (ductless) glands make up a physiologic system of profound importance to the body as a whole. Each gland is concerned with the manufacture of one or more chemical substances (hormones) which are then secreted directly into the bloodstream, often for an ultimate effect on a distant organ or tissue. These internal secretions serve to *regulate various physiologic processes.* Hormones secreted by the endocrine glands determine *body size, vigor,* and *capacity for reproduction* through a complicated interlocking control of the metabolism of foods, minerals, and other substances essential for well-being.

Continuing checks and balances

Each endocrine gland has its own individual part to play in this process, but all are related to each other through a complicated system of checks and balances. The *anterior lobe of the pituitary is generally considered to be the "master gland,"* but it in turn is regulated, at least in part, by the central nervous system through the *hypothalamus.* The anterior lobe of the pituitary secretes a series of *tropic hormones* (gonadotropic, thyrotropic, adrenocorticotropic, to list only a few), each directed at a target endocrine gland, and thereby regulates the output of the target gland's hormone. The hormones secreted by each target gland serve in turn to determine the amount of each tropic hormone secreted by the pituitary.

Stress and adaptation: the alarm reaction

In addition to this system of regulation and counter-regulation that serves to meet the day-to-day metabolic needs of the body, the endocrines also provide a standby apparatus for use in physiologic emergencies. When this apparatus comes into full play, the combination of responses is known as the *adaptation syndrome.* It appears that *any damaging or even threatening event* can elicit this response: injury, infection, pain, fear – any situation producing *stress* – will cause the hypothalamus to direct the anterior lobe of the pituitary to release an excess of adrenocorticotropic hormone, thereby increasing the output of hormones by the adrenal cortex. The *adrenal cortical hormones* provide the necessary components for eliciting the adaptation syndrome. The acute form of this syndrome is the *alarm reaction,* best illustrated by a mental picture of a cornered cat, with back arched by tense muscles, fur on end, teeth and claws bared, and palpebral fissures widened. This reaction is marked physiologically by hyperglycemia, hypertension, tachycardia, and quickening of blood coagulation. The total effect of these responses is to bolster the defenses for the time of the emergency, to minimize blood loss, and to accelerate wound healing if injury should occur. This acute physiologic state must necessarily be short-lasting; if continued too long it may lead to exhaustion and even death. The milder, longer-lasting form of the adaptation syndrome is marked by the *formation of antibodies* in lymphatic tissue and their release into the bloodstream, and by the stimulation of tissue repair by an *acceleration of protein anabolism,* the *maintenance of blood pressure* under adverse circumstances, *regulation of nutrition,* etc.

Endocrine function in disease

It can readily be seen that the *endocrine glands play a part in many diseases,* and that endocrine function influences the outcome of many disorders in which the endocrine glands are not primarily affected. Thus an inadequate endocrine response might result in insufficient antibodies for defense against an infection, in a delay in wound healing, in a hypersensitive state, or in vascular collapse.

This chapter is limited largely to examination of those disease states in which actual anatomic abnormalities of the glands can be demonstrated. Usually these abnormalities are *neoplasms or hyperplasias resulting in hyperfunction of the glands,* or *destructive processes or atrophy resulting in hypofunction.* Theoretically *dysfunction of the endocrine glands* is also possible, resulting in the formation of a hormone which is chemically and physiologically different from the normal, but we have at present no adequate means for the recognition of these conditions, if they occur.

PITUITARY GLAND

1. General Considerations

Anatomy

The hypophysis or pituitary gland is located in the sella turcica of the sphenoid bone, and is connected with the hypothalamus by a thin neural stalk, the infundibulum. Functionally as well as anatomically the hypothalamus and the pituitary gland are closely related. The pituitary gland has two parts: the anterior lobe (adenohypophysis), in which most of the endocrine functions are localized, and the posterior lobe (neurohypophysis).

Anterior lobe hormones [1]

The anterior lobe ("master gland" of the endocrine system) is usually described as containing three types of cells, based on their histochemical reaction with the trichrome stain: the acidophil, basophil, and chromophobe (neutral) cells. The acidophil (eosinophilic) cells produce growth hormone, thyrotropin, and prolactin, and the basophil cells the gonadotropic hormones, male and female, and the adrenotropic hormone. No specific function has been ascribed to the chromophobe cells.

Posterior lobe hormones

The posterior lobe of the pituitary gland produces two hormones: *oxytocin* and *vasopressin.* Oxytocin produces powerful contractions of the uterus at term; synthetic oxytocin is widely used in obstetric practice. Vasopressin is predominantly a vasoconstrictor, tending to raise the blood pressure; it also has an antidiuretic action.

2. Pituitary Syndromes

Significant disturbances of pituitary function are rare. Theoretically these can be either an increase or a decrease in the production of each separate hormone, but this extreme variety is not recognized clinically. Thus an *overactivity* of the acidophilic cells is manifest by changes resulting from increased production of the growth hormone and not, as a rule, by changes resulting from increased production of the tropic hormones. Increased activity of the basophilic cells theoretically would be manifest by increased gonadotropic hormones and hence sexual precocity; however, sexual precocity is very rarely a result of pituitary lesions. Increased production of posterior pituitary hormones might theoretically be expected to cause hypertension as well as oliguria, but neither is recognized. *Decreased production* of pituitary hormones is usually manifest by multiple endocrine effects due to suppression of the various tropic hormones.

GIANTISM AND ACROMEGALY

Hyperfunction of the acidophil (eosinophil) cells is usually a result of an *eosinophilic adenoma;* the hyperfunction is usually manifest by *increased bone growth.* When the condition arises before epiphyseal closure has occurred, it results in abnormal tallness or *giantism;* this is arbitrarily set at above 6 feet 2 inches in females and 6 feet 6 inches in males [2]; heights of 7 to 8 feet are usual. When the hyperfunction has its onset after age 20, there is little opportunity for increase in height since the epiphyses of the long bones are already closed; instead the bone growth is manifest by a general increase in bone mass, the condition being known as *acromegaly.* This is especially evident in the lower jaw (prognathism), causing dental malocclusion; in the facial bones it causes a coarsening of the features; in the cranial bones, an increase in hat size; in the hands and feet, an increase in glove and shoe size. Other manifestations, such as headache and visual disturbances, are a result of the presence of a space-occupying mass in the region of the sella turcica (see section on Pituitary Neoplasms).

HYPOPHYSEAL CACHEXIA

Simmonds' disease (hypophyseal cachexia) is due to *extreme hypofunction* of the anterior lobe of the pituitary gland. It is usually a result of a destructive process, either *vascular* or *neoplastic.* Vascular processes include infarction and necrosis of the pituitary gland, usually ascribed to prolonged circulatory failure following *severe intrapartum or postpartum hemorrhage (Sheehan's syndrome)* [3]. Neoplasms causing Simmond's disease may be primary, either in the pituitary gland or in adjacent structures, or they may be metastatic, as from breast cancer. In Simmonds' disease there is *marked weight loss, weakness,* and a *very low basal metabolic rate. Subtypes* of Simmonds' disease are described [2] in which the chief manifestation is related to the target organ; thus there may be *myxedema* secondary to hypopituitarism and *adrenal cortical insufficiency* secondary to hypopituitarism. These manifestations may result from the same type of vascular or neoplastic lesions which cause in other cases the more profound hypophyseal cachexia.

DIABETES INSIPIDUS

Hypofunction of the posterior lobe of the pituitary gland usually results in *diabetes insipidus,* manifest by greatly increased thirst (polydipsia) and polyuria. There is no glycosuria or hyperglycemia. Deficiency of the antidiuretic hormone causes the convoluted tubules to lose their capacity for concentrating the urine. The basic lesion may be in the posterior lobe of the pituitary gland, in the bony sella turcica, or in the hypothalamus. Primary or secondary neoplasms, trauma, sarcoid, infection, or that rare disorder of the reticuloendothelial system, Hand-Schüller-Christian disease, may be causative. In the authors' experience, metastatic neoplasm is by far the most common cause of the syndrome.

FROEHLICH'S SYNDROME

Excessive obesity in childhood, in association with *sexual retardation,* is known as *Froehlich's syndrome.* The term is sometimes used erroneously for all cases of childhood obesity with delayed puberty, most of which are probably due to gluttony. The obesity portion of the picture in Froehlich's syndrome is probably due to injury of the appetite center in the hypothalamus, while the sex retardation is probably due to loss of gonadotropic hormone of the anterior lobe of the pituitary gland. A *craniopharyngioma* involving the sella turcica and hypothalamus is the usual cause for true Froehlich's syndrome.

3. Pituitary Neoplasms [4]

Clinical features

In most instances primary pituitary neoplasms are first noticed because of symptoms or signs suggestive of brain tumor – *headache, limitation of the visual fields, diplopia,* and the like (see Chapter 26). Some patients show endocrine disturbances resulting from pituitary hypofunction, these often being reflected in the target endocrine organs (gonadal deficiency, thyroid deficiency, diabetes mellitus). Rarely they are revealed as pituitary hyperfunction, chiefly somatic overgrowth. The occasional association of pituitary neoplasms with neoplasms of other endocrine glands has been noted [5].

Pathologic changes

Pituitary adenomas vary in size from microscopic to masses several centimeters in diameter. They may greatly enlarge the sella turcica as seen on lateral radiographs of the skull, and may compress nearby brain structures. After a certain size is reached, the neoplasm breaks through the diaphragm of the sella turcica and may erode the clinoid processes, as seen on skull radiographs. The extrasellar portion may be much larger than the intrasellar part. Many structures may be compressed by the growing neoplasm, particularly the optic chiasm, nerves, and tracts, and the non-neoplastic cells of the gland. With a large adenoma a thin shell of atrophic cells attached to the capsule may be all that remains of the gland. In most instances pituitary neoplasms are encapsulated, and are benign in the sense of not invading or metastasizing; however, because of their location and the difficulty experienced in their removal, many cause the death of the patient.

ADRENAL GLANDS

1. General Considerations

Anatomy

The adrenal (suprarenal) glands, right and left, lie in close relation to the upper pole of each kidney in the retroperitoneal space. Each adrenal gland consists of two parts: the cortex and the medulla; each part has its own specific hormones.

Adrenal cortex hormones

The *adrenal cortex* manufactures a number of *hormones,* including the following: (1) the *mineralocorticoids* (exemplified by *aldosterone*), which act upon the tubules of the kidney to conserve salt and water and to aid in the elimination of potassium, secreted by cells of the zona glomerulosa; (2) the *glucocorticoids* (such as *cortisone* and chemically related substances), which have a number of functions, including gluconeogenesis, antibody production, and excitation of the inflammatory response of the various tissues, secreted by zona fasciculata cells; and (3) *androgens,* which cause the rapid development of the genitals and secondary sex characteristics in both male and female, secreted by zona reticularis cells.

Adrenal medulla hormones

A hormone of the *adrenal medulla,* epinephrine, was the first *hormone* to be isolated and identified chemically. Both epinephrine and the chemically related substance from the adrenal medulla, norepinephrine, act upon the sympathetic nervous system, but their effects are different. Epinephrine causes vasodilatation and increased cardiac output; norepinephrine causes vasoconstriction and elevation of the systolic and diastolic blood pressure.

Methods of study

Clinical evaluation of adrenal disease has been much improved in recent years as the various hormones have been identified and as quantitative chemical methods for their estimation have been developed. Formerly adrenal function could be evaluated only indirectly, by studying water and electrolyte balance, observing the patient's response to the *glucose tolerance* test, or noting the effect of epinephrine upon the *circulating eosinophils* (Thorn test).

2. *Adrenal Syndromes*

A variety of clinical syndromes are described which result from abnormal function of the adrenal glands. *Overactivity of the cells of the adrenal cortex* may be characterized by either overproduction of the glucocorticoids or overproduction of the mineralocorticoids, chiefly aldosterone. *Destruction or exhaustion of the adrenal cortex* is characterized by acute or chronic insufficiency of the corticoids. *Overactivity of the adrenal medulla* is characterized by overproduction of epinephrine and related compounds. *Underactivity of the adrenal medulla* is apparently not recognized clinically.

Cushing's disease or syndrome: clinical features

When there is overproduction of the steroids of the adrenal cortex secondary to the overproduction of adrenocorticotropic hormone by basophils of the pituitary gland, it is usually spoken of as *Cushing's disease;* when unrelated to excess pituitary hormone, it is spoken of as *Cushing's syndrome.* In either case there is an *overproduction of the adrenal glucocorticoids.* The syndrome is more common in females than in males. The usual manifestations are: (1) *obesity,* chiefly of the trunk and face ("moonface" and "buffalo hump") rather than of the extremities; (2) *skin disorders,* such as acne and purplish striae of the thighs and abdomen; (3) *diminished sexual function* (amenorrhea in females; impotency in males); (4) *hypertension;* (5) *hirsutism* in females; (6) *diabetes mellitus,* or more often a diabetic type of glucose tolerance curve; and (7) *osteoporosis.*

Laboratory findings

Confirmation of the diagnosis of Cushing's syndrome is obtained by the demonstration of increased levels of 17-hydroxycorticosteroids in the plasma and urine. Glycosuria, a diabetic type of glucose tolerance curve, reduction of circulating eosinophils, and a tendency toward polycythemia are frequently noted.

Pathologic physiology

The excessive secretion of cortisol (hydrocortisone) and cortisone brings about increased gluconeogenesis by the diversion of certain amino and fatty acids for glucose production. The effects of the resultant decrease in protein synthesis include muscle wasting, osteoporosis, skin atrophy, cessation of growth in children, and perhaps amenorrhea. The *osteoporosis* involves flat bones and is due to decreased protein matrix formation and osteoblastic activity. Much of the excess glucose is reconverted to fat, which is deposited in the cheeks, shoulders, back, and abdominal wall, producing the peculiarly distributed *obesity.* Almost all patients develop a disturbance in carbohydrate metabolism. A decreased glucose tolerance test is most common. Diabetes mellitus occurs in about 15 percent of cases. The cause of the *hypertension* is obscure but may be related to the slight sodium retention effect of the glucocorticoids. Increased aldosterone secretion may also occur. The *acne and hirsutism* in female patients are due to an increase in androgenic hormone secretion by the adrenal cortical cells.

Pathologic changes: adrenal glands

In the *adrenals,* bilateral cortical *hyperplasia* is found in about 60 percent of the cases (in another 10 percent there is functional hyperplasia without apparent cellular changes), a cortical *adenoma* in 17 percent, and a cortical *adenocarcinoma* in 13 percent. Electron microscopic studies have demonstrated that the hyperplastic cells are zona fasciculata in type [6]. In cases with an adenoma or carcinoma the opposite adrenal is usually atrophic.

anterior pituitary

The most characteristic alteration in the *anterior pituitary gland* is *Crooke's hyaline change* in the basophilic cells. A dense hyaline mass is found in the cytoplasm of each affected basophil. Crooke's change is most likely retrogressive in nature due to the feedback effect of an elevated circulating glucocorticoid level. *Basophilic adenoma* or hyperplasia is found in less than 10 percent of cases. When either is present, excessive ACTH is secreted, with resultant adrenal hyperplasia. A chromophobe adenoma is found in the pituitary occasionally. A number of cases of Cushing's syndrome with adrenal hyperplasia have been associated with oat cell bronchogenic carcinoma, epithelial thymoma, islet cell carcinoma and carcinoid of the pancreas, ovarian adenocarcinoma, medullary thyroid carcinoma, and pheochromocytoma [7]. In most cases the neoplastic cells in these neoplasms produce ACTH or a similar compound. The *prolonged administration of cortisone or ACTH* produces Cushing's syndrome in some patients.

other changes

Other changes in Cushing's syndrome include myocardial hypertrophy due to hypertension; atrophy of skeletal muscles with extensive fatty infiltration; atrophy of skin in striae with dilatation of capillaries and venules, and hemorrhages to produce the purplish color; atrophy of the lymph nodes, thymus, and splenic white pulp due to the lympholytic effect of glucocorticoids; and steroid-induced peptic ulcer in occasional cases.

Outcome

Patients with Cushing's syndrome secondary to long-continued cortisone therapy (and the same is probably true of the cases due to primary adrenal cortical hyperplasia) often show a remarkable *susceptibility to bacterial infections.* Under these circumstances fulminant staphylococcal and tuberculous infections develop and cause death in short order, the symptoms of these infections meanwhile being largely masked by the well-being induced by the therapy. Presumably as a result of the same mechanism (suppression of antibody formation), *allergic manifestations tend to disappear* under cortisone therapy, and *wound healing is delayed* appreciably. When Cushing's syndrome is due to neoplasm or hyperplasia of the cells of the adrenal cortex, it is theoretically susceptible to cure by surgery, and some patients have been cured by this means. Commonly the complications of hypertension and diabetes determine the outcome.

HYPERALDOSTERONISM

Primary hyperaldosteronism [8] consists of hypertension, polyuria, hypokalemia, and severe muscle weakness, simulating paralysis. The syndrome can be identified by demonstrating abnormal amounts of aldosterone in the urine. In most instances it is associated with an adrenal cortical adenoma, occasionally with an adrenal carcinoma or adrenal hyperplasia. The adenomas consist almost entirely of zona glomerulosa cells or of a mixture of glomerulosa- and fasciculata-type cells [9]. Secondary aldosteronism may develop in cases of congestive heart failure, hepatic cirrhosis, or toxemia of pregnancy.

ADRENOGENITAL SYNDROME

The inherited types of *adrenogenital syndrome* are discussed on page 323. Noninherited cases in children and adults may result from adrenal cortical hyperplasia, adenoma, or carcinoma. Zona reticularis cells predominate in these lesions. In females excessive androgen secretion produces facial hirsutism and other masculinizing effects. In males estrogen secretion causes breast enlargement and other feminizing effects.

ACUTE ADRENAL CORTICAL INSUFFICIENCY: Manifestations

Certain systemic infections are sometimes marked by cyanosis, hypotension, purpura, and vascular collapse. The picture is most characteristically seen with *fulminant meningococcus bacteremia* (Waterhouse-Friderichsen syndrome), but may occur with other infections. Autopsy in such cases usually shows *bilateral adrenal cortical necrosis and hemorrhage,* suggesting hemorrhagic infarction. A similar clinical picture is sometimes seen as an acute crisis precipitated by stress of some sort in a patient with an essentially chronic, destructive lesion of the adrenal glands. Acute adrenal insufficiency occurs following unusual stress in patients receiving prolonged ACTH or cortisone therapy.

Outcome

In most cases the crisis of acute adrenal insufficiency proves fatal because of the profound circulatory collapse. Some patients have been saved by vigorous therapy with adrenal cortical steroids.

CHRONIC ADRENAL CORTICAL INSUFFICIENCY: Manifestations

Chronic adrenal cortical insufficiency, generally known as *Addison's disease,* is probably the best known and most common of the syndromes of adrenal disease. Addison, who described the syndrome in 1855, correctly related it to the destructive lesions observed in the adrenal glands. Clinically the disease occurs chiefly in middle life, and is manifest by weakness, hypotension, brownish black pigmentation of the skin (especially over exposed surfaces, scars, and creases), and varied gastrointestinal symptoms (vomiting, diarrhea, abdominal pain). If seen for the first time in crisis, circulatory collapse may be an additional finding.

Laboratory findings

Confirmation of the diagnosis is easily obtained if the condition is suspected. Urinary 17-ketosteroid levels are greatly reduced; serum sodium and chloride levels are low. The eosinophil count is generally slightly increased, and, more significantly, remains elevated following injection of ACTH.

Pathologic changes

In Addison's time, *tuberculosis of the adrenal glands* was the common cause of the syndrome; in such cases both glands are almost totally destroyed, being represented by caseous necrotic tissue. Calcium may be noted in the glands; occasionally calcium can be demonstrated on x-ray, and this may sometimes be of diagnostic value during life. Similar lesions may develop in disseminated *histoplasmosis.* In recent years the overall frequency of the disease seems to have declined, and *cortical atrophy* of the glands has become relatively more important. The cause for this atrophy is unknown, but commonly it is so extreme that the adrenal glands are easily missed at autopsy. They may be represented only by a small brownish area, corresponding to the adrenal medulla, found in an insignificant-looking pad of fat lying above each kidney. (When such cases are encountered at autopsy, it is well to save all the retroperitoneal fat so that it can be reexamined and blocked in its entirety if necessary.) Occasionally Addison's disease is a result of *bilateral adrenal metastases,* especially from bronchogenic carcinoma, or of *amyloid disease* of the adrenal glands. Other findings at necropsy in Addison's disease include enlargement of the thymus and lymphoid tissues, and a reduction in the size of the heart.

Outcome

Replacement therapy is required for the remainder of life. If this is carefully controlled, with special attention to the extra needs at the time of infections, surgery, pregnancy, and other periods of stress, the condition is compatible with near-normal existence.

HYPER-FUNCTION OF ADRENAL MEDULLA: Manifestations

Increased production of the two hormones – epinephrine and norepinephrine – of the adrenal medulla is usually due to tumor of the chromaffin cells of the medulla *(pheochromocytoma),* but may be due to tumor of the related chromaffin bodies of the sympathetic nervous system which are found in different parts of the retroperitoneal tissues. Both tumors are rare. The characteristic manifestations are a result of *paroxysmal hypertension,* often precipitated by exercise or change in position. The symptoms consist of throbbing headache, nausea, anxiety, palpitation, and often sweating. During such episodes the blood pressure may rise to very high levels, even to 300 mm. systolic and 170 mm. diastolic.

Laboratory findings

The most important confirmatory test for pheochromocytoma is the demonstration of increased quantities of catecholamines, such as epinephrine and norepinephrine, and vanillyl mandelic acid in the urine or blood. Less conclusive is the occurrence of a sudden paroxysm of hypertension following intravenous injection of histamine, or of a fall in blood pressure following intravenous injection of phentolamine.

Outcome

If a diagnosis of pheochromocytoma is made and the neoplasm successfully removed, the chance of cure is excellent. Surgery has its hazards, however, in that sudden paroxysms of hypertension may occur during the operation, or vascular collapse may follow the removal of the tumor because of sudden withdrawal of the accustomed hormone. If the cause of the paroxysmal hypertension is not recognized and treated, changes in the small blood vessels eventually occur, resulting in permanent hypertension. The outlook is then the same as in essential hypertension; cerebral hemorrhage is a common mode of exitus.

3. Adrenal Neoplasms [10]

CORTICAL ADENOMA

The most common neoplasm of the adrenal cortex is the *cortical adenoma.* It is an encapsulated nodule, bulging within the confines of the affected gland. On section it is soft and bright yellow, somewhat resembling the appearance of butter. In the majority of instances such neoplasms are *incidental findings at autopsy,* having caused no symptoms to signify their presence. Rarely they may be associated with Cushing's syndrome or one of its variants, or with hyperaldosteronism; the gross and microscopic findings in the neoplasms producing these various manifestations are not distinctive, insofar as is known. The constituent cells are usually arranged in cords closely related to vascular sinuses, and the cells themselves are rich in lipid. Usually the cells are regular in size and staining qualities, the nuclei being relatively small in proportion to the mass of cytoplasm.

CORTICAL CARCINOMA

Carcinoma of the adrenal cortex is rare; usually there is no evidence of endocrine hyperfunction. The component cells show marked pleomorphism, often with multinucleated giant cells. Venous and lymphatic invasion is commonly noted, and metastases occur in the regional lymph nodes, mediastinum, and lungs. Grossly and microscopically this neoplasm resembles the hypernephroma of the kidney.

PHEOCHROMOCYTOMA

The *pheochromocytoma* is usually classified as a tumor of the *adrenal medulla,* but it may also occur in other parts of the chromaffin system [11], usually located in the retroperitoneal tissues adjacent to the visceral sympathetic ganglia. In any of these sites it may cause the clinical syndrome described in the preceding section as *hyperfunction of the adrenal medulla.* Small tumors of this type, in the adrenal glands or elsewhere, apparently may cause no symptoms. These neoplasms are variable in size, most are encapsulated, and on section they are pink and soft. Microscopically they are composed of nests of polyhedral cells, usually constant in size and morphology. When the tissues are properly treated, these cells usually show characteristic cytoplasmic granules, i.e., the chromaffin reaction. A fine network of fibers usually separates the cell nests.

OTHER PRIMARY NEOPLASMS

Most other neoplasms arising in the adrenal medulla are derived from the cells of the sympathetic nervous system and have no endocrine effect. The *neuroblastoma* is an important malignant tumor of early childhood (see Chapters 16 and 26). The *sympathicoblastoma* and the *ganglioneuroma* are related tumors.

METASTATIC NEOPLASMS

Metastatic tumors of the adrenal glands are much more common than are primary tumors. In the authors' experience, breast cancer is the most common neoplasm in the female metastasizing to the adrenal glands and lung cancer the most common in the male. In most instances there is no recognizable clinical manifestation of the adrenal metastases. Perhaps the cachexia and hypotension of advanced neoplastic disease are due in part to adrenal metastases, but we have not been able to note any such correlation in the majority of cases. Rarely the clinical picture of chronic adrenal cortical insufficiency (Addison's disease) is seen with metastatic neoplasm of the adrenal glands.

THYROID GLAND

1. *General Considerations*

Anatomy

The thyroid gland arises as a ventral outpouching of the pharynx and migrates downward into the neck. Remnants of thyroid tissue are sometimes found in the base of the tongue or along the course of the thyroglossal duct, structures corresponding to the origin and migration of the gland in the embryo. In the adult the gland normally hugs the larynx and trachea, one lobe lying on either side and the two connected by the isthmus. The normal adult thyroid gland weighs 15 to 20 gm., but in some sections of the world the average is 30 gm.

Endocrine interrelationships

The thyroid gland is under the control of the anterior lobe of the pituitary gland, whose thyrotropic or thyroid-stimulating hormone (TSH) incites it to physiologic activity. The thyroid gland is also influenced by the adrenal cortex and influences in turn the function of the gonads and pancreatic islets. These interrelationships are complex and poorly understood.

Thyroxine

The chief active principle of the thyroid gland is an iodine-containing organic substance, *thyroxine;* several other chemically related iodine-containing compounds have also been isolated from the gland. According to Hamolsky and Freedberg [12], the thyroid gland traps iodine (derived from dietary sources) circulating in the blood and unites it with tyrosine to form thyroxine, which, bound to globulin, is then stored in the colloid of the thyroid follicles. The hormone is liberated as needed into the bloodstream, where it is bound to plasma protein. This protein-bound hormone then acts upon the peripheral tissues to produce the characteristic effects. These effects are extremely important and varied, and are presumably accomplished by *inhibition* or *enhancement* of the action of *various enzymes,* especially those concerned with energy production through oxidation. There are broad effects upon protein, carbohydrate, lipid, electrolyte, water, and vitamin metabolism. While the details of these actions of the thyroid gland are still quite clouded, it is known that growth may be impaired, glucose tolerance altered, blood cholesterol levels increased or decreased, and water retained or excreted, in instances of thyroid dysfunction.

Iodine and the thyroid gland

Iodine is not only an *essential component of the thyroid hormone,* but it is also apparently *essential for the maintenance of the structural integrity of the gland.* It has long been known that there is a greater frequency of diseases of the thyroid gland in geographic areas in which the iodine content of food and water is deficient. Experimental studies by Axelrad and Leblond [13] suggest that the first change induced by iodine deficiency is a reduction of circulating thyroid hormone. This, they believe, stimulates the hypophysis to increase its production of thyrotropic hormone, which in turn induces hyperplastic or neoplastic changes in the cells of the thyroid follicle, in proportion to the duration of the iodine deficiency state. In areas where there is no general deficiency of iodine in the diet, the sporadic occurrence of thyroid diseases may be related to individual factors affecting iodine absorption and usage, or to excess demand for the hormone, or perhaps to some inherent inability to manufacture the hormone.

Tests of thyroid function

The time-honored but now somewhat discredited *basal metabolism test* measures the total metabolic effect of thyroid function. The *serum cholesterol* level has long been known to provide an index of thyroid function; hyperthyroidism is generally characterized by a decrease in the blood cholesterol level, and hypothyroidism by an increase. The determination of *protein-bound iodine* (PBI), while generally valuable, suffers from defects that are unavoidable in any test based upon such small quantities as micrograms: the results are too easily thrown off by environmental factors. The test for butanol-extractable iodine (BEI) minimizes the potential errors in the chemical methods, but it does not abolish them entirely. The *uptake of radioactive iodine* (^{131}I) has added a new dimension to the physiologic evaluation of thyroid function.

2. *Thyroid Syndromes*

Basically there are only two thyroid syndromes, one of hyperfunction, the other of hypofunction. However, because of the interrelationships of the thyroid gland with other organ systems, and because of the differing manifestations at different ages, the direct syndromes may sometimes be overshadowed by their indirect effects, thereby multiplying the number.

HYPERTHYROIDISM:

Hyperthyroidism is variously known as *toxic goiter, Graves' disease,* or *exophthalmic goiter,* to mention only three of its synonyms.

Cause

The *cause* is uncertain. Since thyrotropin levels are normal or low in Graves' disease and the disorder is not relieved by hypophysectomy, the anterior pituitary does not appear to play an important role in its causation. A γ globulin known as *long-acting thyroid stimulator,* which produces thyroid hyperplasia, has been implicated in the etiology [1]. The origin of this thyroid stimulator is unknown. There is some evidence that iodine deficiency is involved in the causation of hyperthyroidism. The pathologic changes in the thyroid are quite comparable to those that have been produced experimentally by Axelrad and Leblond [13] in rats on a low iodine diet. Furthermore, the pathologic changes in the gland and the basal metabolic rate tend to return to normal, and symptoms of hyperthyroidism tend to improve, when iodine is administered.

Clinical features

The disease affects females more frequently than males (4:1), and is most common between 20 and 40 years of age. The usual clinical manifestations of the disease – tachycardia, excitability, tremors, weight loss, intolerance of heat, increased basal metabolic rate, and enlargement of the thyroid gland – are usually ascribed to increased output of thyroxine or related substances by the thyroid gland.

Pathologic changes

The *thyroid gland* is enlarged, vascular, and beefy. *Microscopically* the amount of colloid in the follicles is somewhat reduced and the cells lining the follicles are enlarged. Papillary projections into the follicles are frequent. Collections of lymphocytes, some having germinal centers, are commonly noted.

Related conditions:

thyroid heart disease

Usually hyperthyroidism responds to therapy, either medical or surgical or in combination, and the metabolic activity returns to normal or nearly so. Often, however, there are relapses over a period of many years. Usually the thyroid gland becomes permanently enlarged and often nodular. A significant number of such patients, perhaps 5 to 10 percent, will show cardiac symptoms. Usually these patients with thyrocardiac symptoms are aged 55 to 60, have a rapid pulse, often slight hypertension, and evidence of increased cardiac output. Atrial fibrillation and congestive heart failure are common. These patients do not have organic changes in their hearts; their heart "disease" can usually be cured if the thyroid hyperfunction can be brought under control.

exophthalmos

Protrusion of the eyes is related in some poorly understood way to hyperthyroidism. Sometimes the eye symptoms precede other evidences of thyroid hyperfunction, sometimes they accompany the clinical phase of hyperthyroidism, and in other instances exophthalmos first appears after thyroid function has returned to normal. The exophthalmos is probably due to an effect of long-acting thyroid stimulator on the mucopolysaccharides of the orbital mesenchymal tissue, which leads to the excessive binding of water. The resultant orbital edema, plus the infiltration of lymphocytes and fat in the extraocular muscles, pushes the eyes forward.

HYPOTHYROIDISM:

Hypothyroidism is a clinical syndrome due to a *deficiency of thyroid hormone.* It is characterized by a slowing of all body functions, a low basal metabolic rate, low PBI, and elevated serum cholesterol level. It may occur as a result of congenital absence of the thyroid gland, or it may be due to destructive diseases or total surgical removal of the gland, or to unexplained atrophy and fibrosis. The *clinical manifestations depend largely on the age at which the dysfunction appears.*

Cretinism

In the infant with *congenital hypothyroidism,* i.e., *cretinism,* both *physical and mental development are grossly retarded.* Physical changes are often present at birth but may not be recognized until months or years later. The facial features are coarse, the tongue is large and protuberant, and the skin is dry and somewhat thickened. Dentition, walking, and talking are all delayed. In such children the thyroid gland may be totally absent, or it may be enlarged and show colloid retention. Cretinism is much more common in those parts of the world where colloid goiter is endemic.

Myxedema

Myxedema is *acquired hypothyroidism.* It may occur in children (juvenile myxedema) or in adults. Females are much more frequently affected than males

(4:1). The *etiologic factors and pathologic changes vary.* In some cases the thyroid gland is small and fibrous without any cause being evident; in other cases the gland is enlarged and largely destroyed as a result of an inflammatory process (thyroiditis); in other cases the syndrome is a sequel of thyroidectomy or of therapy with radioactive iodine; rarely hypofunction is associated with an enlarged colloid gland. *Clinically* the skin is rough, dry, and thickened, but does not pit on pressure. The hair becomes thinner; this is especially notable in the eyebrows. Often there are anemia, lethargy, dullness, amenorrhea, and infertility. The basal metabolic rate and protein-bound iodine are low; the serum cholesterol level is elevated. When the nature of the illness is recognized promptly and replacement therapy adequate, all manifestations of the disease may clear up and the patient may live out a normally active life. In fatal cases the heart may show deposits of mucoid material between the muscle fibers (myxedema heart), pericardial effusion, and heart failure. The incidence of atherosclerosis is somewhat increased in patients with hypothyroidism.

3. Enlargement of the Thyroid Gland: Goiter

The term *goiter* means simply an *enlargement of the thyroid gland; struma* is sometimes used with the same meaning. Such enlargement may be a result of *hyperplasia* or *neoplasia* of the cells of the thyroid gland, of *inflammatory processes* affecting the gland, or of *distention of the follicles with colloid.* Goiter may be associated with a state of normal thyroid function (euthyroidism), with hyperthyroidism, or with hypothyroidism.

CONGENITAL GOITER

Rarely enlargement of the thyroid may be noted at birth. Congenital goiter is much more common in regions of endemic goiter, but it also occurs sporadically, sometimes in association with thyroid disease in the mother. The pathologic changes accounting for the enlargement are varied: simple hyperplasia of the cells lining the follicles is sometimes noted, but in other cases there is colloid retention. The functional status of the gland is also varied.

COLLOID GOITER: Relation to iodine deficiency

Diffuse enlargement of the thyroid gland without evidence of functional disturbance is common and is called *colloid goiter, simple goiter,* or *nontoxic goiter. Endemic goiter* describes the same pathologic state as the other terms given above, but its use is generally limited to the disorder occurring in a population group rather than in an individual. While there is some difference of opinion, the *chief etiologic factor of colloid goiter is probably iodine deficiency.* In those areas where the disease is endemic, as in mountainous areas generally and in the Great Lakes region of the United States, the soil and water are notably lacking in iodine content, and vegetables and dairy products are similarly deficient. The use of iodized salt has greatly reduced the frequency of the disease in these areas. Occasionally a goitrogenic substance seems to interfere with iodine uptake and to produce endemic goiter in an area where iodine intake is adequate [14]. Sporadic cases of colloid goiter may be due to such goitrogenic substances, or to individual differences in dietary habits or metabolic needs. Metabolic need for thyroid hormone is apparently greater in the female than in the male, and in the female the need is increased at puberty and at other times of stress. If the diet is deficient in iodine at the time of the increased demand for hormone, the thyroid gland is unable to manufacture the hormone to meet the need. This results in an increased output of thyrotropic hormone by the pituitary gland, and incites hyperplasia of the thyroid gland. When the demand for increased thyroid hormone subsides, the gland increases its stores of iodine in the colloid of the follicle. (This is the theoretical explanation for the fact that colloid goiter is more common in the female than in the male, and that it tends to appear first at a time of physiologic stress.) Hence *colloid goiter is the sequel of thyroid hyperplasia induced by iodine deficiency.*

Pathologic changes

The thyroid gland is often several times its normal size, and is firm and semitranslucent due to distention of the follicles by colloid. The cells lining the follicles are flattened against the fibrous septa.

NODULAR GOITER: Toxic and nontoxic

If subsequent demands are placed upon the thyroid gland, as with recurring physiologic stress, it presumably undergoes repeated *cycles of hyperplasia, involution,* and *colloid storage.* Over a period of years, the gland in such a case tends to become *progressively larger and somewhat nodular.* During the long history of thyroid disease in such a patient there are often periods during which signs of hyperthyroidism are manifest. Sometimes cardiac symptoms develop, as has been noted; such symptoms usually yield to therapy with iodine or antithyroid drugs. Nodular goiter is the most common type of thyroid disease for which thyroidectomy is done. Cysts, areas of old hemorrhage, fibrous and calcified areas, all are commonly noted.

Substernal thyroid gland

When the gland is greatly enlarged, it is common for its lower pole to lie in the upper portion of the thorax behind the sternum. Here it may *compress the trachea or superior vena cava,* producing distention of the veins of the head and upper chest, dyspnea, and other symptoms. Rarely a substernal portion of the thyroid gland may exist and cause symptoms without any evident enlargement of the cervical portion.

THYROID "ADENOMAS": Significance

Occasionally a single nodule stands out conspicuously from the rest of the gland and is easily palpable in the neck. Some students of thyroid disease believe that such nodules are fundamentally the same as the nodules commonly observed in enlarged thyroid glands (i.e., nodular goiter), while others believe that they are benign neoplasms. Axelrad and Leblond [13], from their studies in rats, believe that these nodules correspond to clones consisting of the whole progeny of single cells stimulated to neoplasia by iodine deficiency. The fact that these nodules, and, for that matter, thyroid carcinoma as well, occur predominantly in females with pathologic evidence of other thyroid disease suggests that they are a part of the general pattern of hyperplasia and involution of the cells of the follicle.

Pathologic types

A number of microscopic types of "adenomas" are described. The most common is the *follicular adenoma,* composed of glandlike spaces of varying size *(microfollicular* or *macrofollicular).* Some follicular adenomas contain very little colloid and the stroma has a loose structure suggesting the fetal thyroid gland; these have been called *fetal adenomas.* Some adenomas show only one or two follicles in a microscopic field and the cells are generally arranged in ribbonlike sheets; these have been designated *trabecular (embryonal) adenomas.* Others are composed of large pale cells and have been called *Hürthle cell adenomas.* The splitting of follicular adenomas into all these subvarieties serves no useful purpose and is only confusing. Separation of the follicular adenomas from the *papillary adenomas* does, however, seem useful, since *most papillary nodules are at least potentially malignant.* Microscopically the papillary adenomas show a branching epithelial growth projecting into a cystlike space containing stringy colloid. Small calcium masses, *psammoma bodies,* are commonly noted at the tips of the epithelial projections. In most instances there are no signs of thyroid dysfunction with either the follicular or the papillary adenomas.

THYROID CARCINOMA:

Carcinomas of the thyroid gland [15, 16] make up an important group of malignant neoplasms. They, like all thyroid diseases, are more frequent in females than in males. As a class they are slowly growing neoplasms, often being successfully controlled by surgery; never are they as frequent in statistics based on autopsies as they are in statistics based on surgical material. Usually they show no endocrine effect.

Pathologic criteria

The criteria for the pathologic diagnosis of thyroid cancer are generally the same as for the diagnosis of cancer in other organs. Unencapsulated fleshy nodules in the thyroid gland are particularly suspicious, as are fibrous foci in a nodular gland. Areas of hemorrhage and necrosis are also somewhat suspicious. Microscopically *cell anaplasia* and evidence of *capsular invasion* are important signs of thyroid cancer. *Venous invasion* is a particularly important sign and in some instances may be the only evidence that a neoplasm is malignant.

Papillary carcinoma

About half of all thyroid carcinomas have a *papillary structure,* either pure or mixed. If there is no gross evidence of invasion of normal tissues, the outlook is good and the cure rate is very high. Even when invasion and metastasis are evident, the 5-year survival rate may be 60 percent or better, since the tumor tends to grow very slowly. Metastases to the lungs may sometimes be evident on radiographs for 10 to 20 years before death. Metastasis to the regional lymph nodes is the usual method of spread. Uptake of ^{131}I by this form of thyroid cancer is generally minimal and hence surgery is the mode of therapy usually employed.

Follicular carcinoma

Follicular carcinoma makes up about 30 percent of all thyroid cancers and is slightly more aggressive in its growth pattern than is papillary carcinoma. If there is no gross evidence of tissue invasion, the 5-year survival rate is about 90 percent after simple excision; if tissue invasion is evident at the time of surgery, the 5-year survival rate is about 30 percent. Venous invasion and hematogenous metastasis are common in follicular carcinoma. In most patients with follicular carcinoma, the neoplastic tissue takes up radioactive iodine well and this form of therapy is often used effectively.

Undifferentiated carcinoma

In about 20 percent of the cases of thyroid cancer the tumor infiltrates in solid cell masses rather than forming papillae or follicles. The prognosis is much worse with these *undifferentiated carcinomas* than with papillary or follicular carcinomas. In some cases of undifferentiated carcinoma the characteristic cell is small, resembling the lymphocyte; in others there are numerous giant cells. This latter group *(giant cell carcinoma)* is very highly malignant, there being almost no 5-year survivors, even with radical surgery. Regional spread to the trachea and mediastinum is often the cause of death. Lymph node and hematogenous metastases are both common. Uptake of ^{131}I is generally poor. *Medullary carcinoma* [17] may show a spindle-cell or round-cell pattern, with small amyloid deposits. Electron microscopy indicates that the neoplasm arises from parafollicular cells. The medullary carcinoma may be a form of carcinoid tumor. It also may elaborate an ACTH-like compound which produces Cushing's syndrome.

Occult sclerosing carcinoma

Less common than any of these forms is the *occult sclerosing carcinoma* [18]. Usually these lesions have been discovered in scarred areas of thyroid glands removed because of hyperthyroidism or nodular goiter. The neoplasm is composed of atypical epithelium forming follicles and papillae and infiltrating surrounding structures. Metastasis is slow, and is chiefly to the cervical lymph nodes; none of the patients reported by Klinck and Winship died of their disease.

Thyroid cancer in children

Winship [19] has emphasized the importance of cancer of the thyroid gland in children. In some cases the neoplasm has followed irradiation of the thymus in infancy. Nodular enlargement of the thyroid gland in children is more commonly due to cancer than is the case in adults. The pathologic changes and natural history of thyroid cancer in children are the same as in adults.

OTHER THYROID NEOPLASMS

Carcinoma of the thyroid gland is the only malignant neoplasm of this organ that occurs with any frequency. *Lymphosarcoma* occasionally appears to arise within the thyroid gland, although more commonly it is secondarily involved from adjacent lymph nodes. *Teratomas* of the thyroid gland are usually congenital and may cause death from compression of the trachea. *Metastatic neoplasms* of the thyroid gland are found quite commonly if the thyroid tissue is carefully examined at autopsy, but such cases have little clinical significance.

"LATERAL ABERRANT THYROID"

There has been much discussion about the significance of the finding of thyroid tissue, usually quite well differentiated, in the soft tissues of the neck lateral to the thyroid gland. Certainly the last word on the subject has not been written, but at present it is the general opinion among pathologists that *nodules of thyroid tissue found in cervical lymph nodes represent metastases from thyroid cancer* rather than ectopic thyroid tissue.

4. Thyroiditis

THYROIDITIS [20]:

About 5 percent of thyroid glands removed surgically show on pathologic examination an inflammatory reaction of some degree of severity, often with extensive fibrous tissue proliferation. This is the group the pathologist designates as thyroiditis, and the group is of some clinical importance. Occasionally the disease is acute and of pyogenic origin; such patients experience pain over the gland and fever as conspicuous symptoms. More commonly the disease is chronic and the presenting complaint is a *tender swelling of the thyroid gland, with pain on swallowing.* Usually there is no real evidence of thyroid dysfunction; if any is noted, it is more apt to be hypofunction than hyperfunction. The surgeon often notes that the thyroid gland in these patients is unusually adherent to the strap muscles of the neck or to the trachea.

Causes

In most cases the etiologic agent of chronic thyroiditis is not known, although occasionally syphilis or radiation injury may be causal. Many patients with lymphatic thyroiditis have antibodies in their serum against human thyroid extract. Witebsky et al. developed artificial antibodies against thyroid substance in several species, and produced chronic thyroiditis in animals by injecting them with these antibodies [21]. The evidence suggests that *lymphocytic thyroiditis is due to an antigen-antibody process in which the patient's own thyroid provides the antigen.* Therefore, lymphocytic thyroiditis is considered to be an *auto-immune disorder.*

Pathologic types

Chronic thyroiditis has been separated into three types, based chiefly on their histologic features; whether they are fundamentally different diseases or stages of a single disease is unknown at present. The most common form is probably *lymphocytic thyroiditis (struma lymphomatosa, Hashimoto's disease),* in which the gland is diffusely enlarged and the acini are almost replaced by great numbers of lymphocytes, often gathered together to form lymph follicles. The acinar epithelium usually is pale and eosinophilic and appears moderately hyperplastic. One of our patients with Hashimoto's disease had also Mikulicz's disease of the submaxillary gland. *Granulomatous thyroiditis (de Quervain's thyroiditis, subacute thyroiditis)* is the second most frequent form. Giant cells are numerous; they are gathered about disrupted follicles, forming small focal lesions resembling tubercles. Their appearance suggests a foreign body reaction to the colloid material of the acini. Much rarer is *ligneous thyroiditis (Riedel's struma)* in which the gland is of woody consistency, densely adherent to surrounding structures, and often causes real difficulty in swallowing and breathing. The gland is white, sometimes gritty, and bears little gross resemblance to the normal thyroid gland; microscopically the lobular and acinar pattern is destroyed, being replaced by fibrous, often hyaline connective tissue containing lymphocytes and mononuclear cells.

ISLETS OF LANGERHANS: CARBOHYDRATE METABOLISM

1. General Considerations

Carbohydrate digestion and utilization [22]

Dietary carbohydrate, chiefly starch, is split by salivary and pancreatic enzymes into simple monosaccharides which are readily absorbed from the intestine. Proteins and fats may also yield monosaccharides by chemical conversion (gluconeogenesis). These monosaccharides, in the presence of insulin, are converted (in the liver) to glycogen, which is then stored in the cytoplasm of parenchymal cells of the liver and in the skeletal muscles. Glycogen in the muscles and liver is converted to glucose as needed, under the influence of insulin. Glucose circulates in the blood to all tissues of the body and is used for cell energy. Final products of its metabolism are usually carbon dioxide and water.

Action of insulin

Insulin, the chief hormone of the islets of Langerhans of the pancreas, increases carbohydrate combustion, decreases gluconeogenesis, and accelerates the formation of glycogen. In the normal individual responding to his own insulin, these actions result in the maintenance of the blood sugar and of glycogen stores, and in the ready release of glucose for energy. In the diabetic patient responding to the therapeutic administration of insulin, these actions cause a reduction of the hyperglycemia and lessen the catabolism of fat, thereby lessening ketosis. Oral hypoglycemic agents apparently act both by increasing insulin production in the pancreas and by inhibiting the action of insulin-destroying enzymes, thus permitting natural endogenous insulin to be more effective.

Blood sugar and glucose tolerance

The blood glucose value at any moment is determined by a number of processes including the *absorption* of carbohydrate in the diet, the *conversion* of monosaccharides to glycogen and of glycogen to glucose, and the *utilization* of glucose by tissue cells. The blood glucose level fluctuates, therefore, in relation to dietary intake and cell activity. After fasting (as before breakfast) the normal blood glucose is at its lowest level, approximately 80 mg. per 100 ml. of blood. About 30 minutes after ingestion of 100 gm. of glucose, as in the *glucose tolerance test,* the blood glucose normally rises to a level of about 150 mg. per 100 ml., returning to the fasting level about 1½ hours later. In patients with abnormalities of carbohydrate metabolism, this response to glucose loading may be abnormal. Thus a *failure of absorption* of carbohydrate (as in sprue) is manifest by a flat curve, in which the glucose level does not rise above 100 mg. per 100 ml. An *inability to use glucose* (as in diabetes mellitus) results in a high fasting level and a rise in the curve to 200 to 300 mg., followed by a sustained high level for several hours. For the diagnosis of incipient diabetes, cortisone is sometimes used in conjunction with glucose in the tolerance test. The glucose tolerance test is also commonly used in the study of patients suspected of having diseases of the other endocrine organs; characteristic patterns of response occur in a number of different disorders.

Glycosuria

In normal persons, glucose is filtered through the renal glomerulus but reabsorbed in the tubules; it appears in the urine only if the quantity of glucose in the filtrate exceeds that which the tubules can reabsorb. Normally there is no glycosuria unless the blood glucose level is above 150 mg. per 100 ml., this figure being the normal *renal threshold* for glucose. Occasionally a person in apparently good health will show glycosuria with a blood glucose level of 100 mg.; these individuals are said to have *renal glycosuria,* a metabolic fault which is apparently inherited. Occasionally sugars other than glucose (pentose, lactose, fructose, galactose) appear in the urine and give a positive test for sugar, i.e., for reducing substances; these sugars sometimes account for erroneous diagnoses of diabetes mellitus. Glycosuria may occasionally occur as a consequence of renal disease, due to a failure of tubular reabsorption of glucose; of course, true diabetes may also occur in such patients.

2. *Diabetes Mellitus*

Nature of the disease

Diabetes mellitus [23] is a fundamental disorder of carbohydrate metabolism; the essential feature is an *insufficient insulin effect.* This may be due to: (1) failure of the islets to produce or release sufficient insulin, (2) inefficient utilization of insulin, (3) insulin interference from other hormones (thyroid, adrenal, anterior pituitary) or an inhibitor, or (4) increased insulin destruction by tissue enzymes. This insulin defect interferes with storage of glycogen and with cell utilization of glucose, and leads to *hyperglycemia and glycosuria, the chief measurable aspects of the dysfunction.* The inability to use glucose results in dysfunction at the cell level, due to deficient energy production and accumulation of the breakdown products of fat.

Confusing terms

Diabetes insipidus has no relationship to diabetes mellitus; the former is a polyuria *(diabetes – a passing through)* associated with pituitary disease (page 715). *Bronze diabetes* (see Chapter 11) is a term describing two aspects of hemochromatosis, a many-faceted disorder of pigment metabolism; in this disease the pancreas is affected, resulting in a disturbance of carbohydrate metabolism resembling mild diabetes mellitus. When the term *diabetes* is used without qualification, diabetes mellitus is meant.

Etiologic factors

Diabetes mellitus is usually first manifest at *about age 50,* although it may occur much earlier, even in children. Several cases often appear in a family; diabetes seems to be inherited, although inconstantly and somewhat unpredictably. Sometimes it is transmitted as a mendelian recessive. Diabetes may also appear in families having no other known cases of the disease. *Females* are especially susceptible. *Obesity* is a common feature in adults with diabetes; by contrast, children with diabetes are often undernourished. *Diet* is of little etiologic importance in diabetes, except in relation to obesity. *Jews* have a particularly high incidence of diabetes, probably due both to inheritance and to a tendency toward obesity.

Exercise seems to lessen insulin requirements in patients with diabetes, but there is no evidence that lack of exercise causes the disease. *Infections* may precipitate recognition of the disease and certainly worsen it, but are probably not causal; brucellosis may apparently cause mild and transient diabetes in some instances. *Pancreatic diseases* (carcinoma, cysts, acute or chronic pancreatitis, hemochromatosis) or *pancreatectomy* may eliminate functioning islets and cause hyperglycemia and glycosuria. Insulin requirements in these conditions are usually less than those in spontaneous diabetes. *Disorders of the pituitary or adrenal gland* may sometimes cause hyperglycemia and glycosuria, and mild diabetes may be precipitated by the *therapeutic use of extracts of these glands. Thiazide derivatives,* commonly used in the treatment of hypertension and edema, *may cause hyperglycemia and glycosuria* [24]. The authors have seen two such cases; in one the blood sugar was 2700 mg. per 100 ml. just prior to death in "diabetic" coma; 3 months before, when thiazide therapy for hypertension was begun, this patient had had a blood glucose of 97 mg. per 100 ml.

Pathologic findings:

Demonstrable tissue changes due to diabetes are remarkably few. The earliest and most constant change is probably *disappearance of the granules in the beta cells of the islets* [25]. These granules are believed to be a stored precursor of insulin. This finding is not very dependable, however, because it is inconstant in elderly diabetics, and because postmortem autolytic changes may influence the interpretation. *Hyalinization or fibrosis of the islets* is encountered in about half the diabetics over age 50. Similar hyalin changes may be found in about 10 percent of nondiabetics. Young diabetics rarely show hyalinization or fibrosis and may, in fact, show islet hyperplasia. If death is a result of diabetic acidosis, there may be hydropic degeneration of islet cells and slight leukocytic infiltration between these cells. In some cases there may be a reduction of the number of islets.

autopsy findings

In addition to the more or less specific changes in the islets referred to above, certain pathologic findings are almost diagnostic when they occur; however, their absence does not justify the exclusion of diabetes. Sometimes the renal lesions, especially *necrotizing papillitis* and *intercapillary glomerulosclerosis,* are sufficiently distinctive to permit a strong suspicion of the presence of diabetes. If the diagnosis is suspected at the time of autopsy, perhaps because of the findings just given, or because of the *odor of acetone from the body cavities,* confirmation may be obtained by *chemical examination of bladder urine or of blood.* If lipemia has been present, as is often the case, there may be lipoid deposits in the subcutaneous tissues about the joints *(xanthoma diabeticorum),* in the Kupffer cells, or in the reticuloendothelial system generally. Glycogen deposits may occur in the nuclei of hepatic cells, or in the cytoplasm of renal tubule cells. Rarely in diabetics glycogen deposits may be sufficient to cause hepatomegaly.

Diabetes and other diseases:

Certain diseases, in addition to those mentioned above, are *commonly associated with diabetes mellitus* and are generally considered to be *complications* of diabetes. Most of these diseases also occur in nondiabetics, and are considered in more detail elsewhere.

vascular sclerosis

Atherosclerosis of medium-sized and large arteries is more common in diabetics than in nondiabetics, and occurs at an earlier age. The disturbance of lipoid metabolism that is a regular feature of diabetes is probably responsible; serum lipoprotein and cholesterol levels are often elevated, especially in patients whose diabetes is poorly controlled [26]. Coronary and extremity arteries are chiefly affected. Thrombosis of these vessels is common. *Coronary thrombosis* is especially important; when it occurs in a female before the menopause, either diabetes mellitus or familial hypercholesterolemia is usually present. *Gangrene of the feet* in both males and females is commonly of diabetic origin. Capillary basement membrane thickening is found in the skin of the toes of diabetics, as well as in the glomerular and retinal capillaries and elsewhere *(diabetic microangiopathy)* [27].

renal disease

Renal lesions are common in diabetic patients (see Chapter 22), but *glycosuria is not due to a demonstrable renal lesion.* A rather specific diabetic glomerular lesion is known as *intercapillary glomerulosclerosis (Kimmelstiel-Wilson disease);* it should be suspected when a diabetic patient shows proteinuria, changes in the eye grounds, edema, or hypertension. *Renal infections* are common and important in diabetics. Glycogen and lipid deposits may be found in the renal tubular epithelium. The nephrosclerosis of hypertensive disease is common but has no special features in the diabetic.

infections

Perhaps because of greater glucose concentration in the tissues, *diabetics have a general susceptibility to acute infections.* In most instances these infections are due to *pyogenic cocci,* but there is also a striking increase in *fungus* infections: mucormycosis seems to have a particular affinity for the diabetic. Boils, carbuncles, cellulitis, and renal infections are common. Any type of renal infection may occur in the diabetic, but *acute pyelonephritis* is especially common; a particularly characteristic form is associated with necrosis of the renal papillae. *Gangrene of the toes and feet* is due to a combination of vascular sclerosis, trauma, and infection. With any infection there is an increased tendency toward *acidosis.*

gallstones

Gallstones are common in diabetics, possibly due to abnormalities of lipid metabolism, or possibly because of obesity, age, and sex.

skin

Xanthoma diabeticorum has already been noted. These lesions may occasionally become necrotic and ulcerate (diabetic lipoid necrobiosis). Itching of the genitals (pruritis vulvae) is common, sometimes due to *Candida* infection, to which the diabetic appears to be especially susceptible.

eyes

Extensive *retinal changes* (hemorrhages, exudates) occur in diabetics and may cause blindness. These changes are due, at least in part, to minute *aneurysms of the retinal capillaries,* and occur in the same patients who show intercapillary glomerular lesions of the kidneys. *Cataracts* are frequent in diabetics.

nerves

Disorders of motor, sensory, and autonomic nerves (diabetic neuropathy) are occasionally noted in diabetics, especially when the diabetes is uncontrolled.

summary

In 120 known diabetics among 2500 patients autopsied at the George Washington University Hospital in a 10-year period the following complications were noted: myocardial infarction in 37; intercapillary glomerulosclerosis, 23; acute pyelonephritis, 10; acidosis, 10; other complications of diabetes, chiefly vascular, 11; in 43 the death was thought to be unrelated to diabetes or its complications.

Clinical features

Symptoms and signs in uncomplicated diabetes mellitus are usually vague; rarely can the diagnosis be more than suspected on clinical grounds alone. *Weakness* and *weight loss* are common and are presumably due to loss of caloric values because of glycosuria, plus impaired utilization of all nutrients at the cell level.

These symptoms in a child or young adult are particularly suggestive of diabetes. *Increased appetite and thirst* and *polyuria* result from the glycosuria which causes water diuresis, thus increasing water requirements. It is often the complications of diabetes which cause the patient to seek medical advice: *rapidly failing vision* due to diabetic retinopathy, *recurring boils or carbuncles,* or *pain or tingling in the feet* due to the vascular or neural changes of diabetes. In mild, asymptomatic cases of diabetes, the diagnosis is often due to chance: test for urinary sugar is usually part of the periodic health examination, and of the routine evaluation of a patient for elective surgery. When diabetes is carefully regulated by diet and by hypoglycemic agents as needed, the disease is quite compatible with a vigorous effective life, although the average life expectancy is somewhat shortened.

Diabetic coma

Diabetic coma is one of the most important complications of diabetes mellitus. It is a very complex metabolic disturbance, often precipitated by infection, trauma (including surgical trauma), or the omission of insulin therapy. The *blood sugar mounts, ketonemia and ketonuria appear, plasma potassium and carbon dioxide combining power fall,* and the patient becomes comatose. This is a true medical emergency, requiring prompt recognition and vigorous, carefully controlled management.

Childhood diabetes

Diabetes in children presents special problems in addition to those encountered in adult diabetics. There is often some *disturbance of growth,* reflecting pituitary and adrenal dysfunction. *Personality problems* often develop. Regulation is generally more difficult, especially during adolescence. This may be partly due to general endocrine lability at this period, but it also results from refusal of the child to follow the restrictive regime that is usually necessary to control the disease. Diabetic coma and hypoglycemia are both common.

Diabetes and pregnancy

Pregnancy and diabetes present problems to both the mother and the fetus. Acidosis is apt to occur during the last trimester, increasing fetal mortality. Polyhydramnios is very common. The infants of diabetic mothers are often abnormally large. Even with ideal diabetic and obstetric care, fetal mortality is 10 to 14 percent. Renal glycosuria commonly occurs during pregnancy, and lactosuria is often noted during the period of lactation. Because of all these facts, the diagnosis and management of diabetes during pregnancy and the puerperium require special skill.

3. Islet Cell Neoplasms of the Pancreas

Clinical features: hypoglycemia

Tumors of the islet cells of the pancreas are of special interest and importance because of their functional effects. Most cases that have been diagnosed clinically have produced a group of symptoms attributable to *excess insulin production and hypoglycemia.* Usually the symptoms come on some time after a meal; they can be prevented or relieved by taking sugar or orange juice. The symptoms of islet cell tumor, usually noted in the morning on arising, are weakness, drowsiness, faintness, sweating, mental confusion, coma, and convulsions. Some patients with this disease have been considered to have epilepsy or neurologic disorders. Usually these manifestations can be cured by surgery. A much more common cause of hypoglycemia is, of course, an overdosage of insulin in a diabetic patient. Hypoglycemia may also occur with hepatocarcinoma, adrenal cortical carcinoma, or peritoneal and retroperitoneal fibrous or mesothelial neoplasms, due to excessive glucose consumption or to secretion of an insulin-like substance by the tumor cells [28].

Zollinger and Ellison [29] have described several cases of islet cell tumors of the pancreas which were manifest by *gastric hyperacidity* and *hypersecretion,* and *recurrent intractable ulceration of the jejunum,* often with perforation. Such adenomas secrete a gastrin-like hormone. These patients usually do not show evidence of hypoglycemia. A relationship of the syndrome of Zollinger and Ellison to that of the malignant carcinoid has been suggested [30]. Theoretically removal of the tumor should correct the hyperacidity and cure the ulceration, but in most cases the underlying tumor has been recognized too late for this to be possible. Of islet cell tumors, benign and malignant, found at autopsy, about a third cause no clinical symptoms.

peptic ulceration

Most islet cell tumors are *adenomas,* but a small proportion are *carcinomas.* Adenomas may be small, often less than 1 cm. in diameter, and are difficult to identify. They are *multiple* in over 10 percent of the cases. Microscopically they consist of cords of small homogeneous cells, closely related to capillaries. Hyalinization and calcification in the tumors are common. Electron microscopy indicates that the ulcerogenic adenomas arise from alpha cells [32]. In the hypoglycemia-producing tumors the number and appearance of cytoplasmic granules are variable. These adenomas are presumed to arise from beta cells. Islet cell tumors metastasize slowly if at all, even when histologically malignant.

Pathologic changes [31]

PARATHYROID GLANDS: CALCIUM METABOLISM

1. General Considerations

Most diets, even when severely restricted, contain calcium in excess of body needs. Increased bodily requirements during pregnancy and lactation may cause a negative calcium balance, but rarely any manifest effect. The amount of calcium absorbed from the intestine is determined by the needs of the tissues, provided that vitamin D is available in normal quantity. *Vitamin D is apparently necessary for calcium absorption.*

Calcium intake

In health the adult human body contains about 2½ pounds of calcium, of which nearly 99 percent is found in the skeleton, about 1 percent in the soft tissues, and about 0.1 percent in blood and extracellular fluids. Of this last amount about 30 to 50 percent is bound to protein [33]; the remainder (less than 0.7 gm. in a normal 70-kg. male) is in ionic form and makes possible the *maintenance of the heartbeat, coagulation of blood, excitability of nerves and muscles,* and *permeability of cell membranes.* The blood calcium is maintained within narrow limits (9 to 11 mg. per 100 ml. of serum) in health by a feedback mechanism monitored by the *parathyroid glands* [34]: when the plasma calcium level falls, the parathyroid glands are stimulated to increased activity and cause the release of calcium from the bones into the plasma by osteoclastic resorption; when the plasma calcium level rises, parathyroid activity decreases. The hairline fineness of this regulation is evident when one notes that from a level of serum calcium signifying marked hypocalcemia (6 mg. per 100 ml.) to one of marked hypercalcemia (15 mg.), the total amount of calcium in question is only about 0.54 gm. – roughly the equivalent of the salt used on your breakfast eggs!

Calcium storage and utilization

Dietary calcium in excess of needs is largely excreted in the feces. A serum calcium level of about 7 to 8 mg. per 100 ml. is considered to be the renal

Calcium elimination

threshold; thus a small amount of calcium is normally present in the urine. Calcium is filtered through the glomerulus and reabsorbed in the tubule.

Parathyroid glands

The parathyroid glands are tiny tannish brown structures, in health rarely larger than 4 mm. in diameter. Usually there are four of them, two on each side, embedded in the loose connective tissue on the posterior and medial aspect of the thyroid gland, between it and the trachea. Grossly they are often confused with lymph nodes or with fat. Microscopically they consist of cords of cells somewhat resembling the islets of Langerhans. Physiologically these glands have a remarkable influence on calcium metabolism, and indirectly on many other physiologic processes.

Hypercalcemia: causes

Hyperparathyroidism is an important cause of hypercalcemia, but there may be other causes [35], including the following: *sarcoidosis; multiple myeloma; malignant neoplasms* of the lungs, kidneys, ovaries, stomach, and other sites, with or without metastases to bones; *massive doses of vitamin D,* as was formerly used therapeutically in rheumatoid arthritis; *high milk-alkali intake,* as for peptic ulcer; *continued immobilization,* as with body casts; *idiopathic infantile hypercalcemia;* certain cases of *dysfunction of the thyroid and adrenal glands;* and *prolonged androgen therapy.* The actual mechanism bringing about hypercalcemia is unknown in many of these conditions.

physiologic effects

Persistently high levels of blood calcium cause hypercalcinuria and frequently result in *renal damage,* often with *urinary calculi; metastatic calcification* (kidneys, lungs, stomach, and corneas) is another important sequel. Very high blood levels may cause *vomiting, coma,* and *death.* Lesser degrees of hypercalcemia may cause muscle hypotonicity and weakness, constipation, and shortening of the Q-T interval in the electrocardiogram.

Hypocalcemia: causes

Hypocalcemia is somewhat less common than hypercalcemia. It is an almost constant finding and is usually quite severe in *strumiprivous hypoparathyroidism,* i.e., when the parathyroid glands are removed or injured during surgical removal of the thyroid gland. Hypocalcemia may also occur in any condition causing severe alkalosis *(excess vomiting, hyperventilation, long-continued intake of sodium bicarbonate),* since hypocalcemia is part of the total ionic disturbance. Hypocalcemia may also occur in the following conditions: (1) *acute pancreatic necrosis,* presumably by the binding of calcium in the areas of fat necrosis [36]; (2) *rickets and osteomalacia,* due to inadequate vitamin D intake; (3) cases in which fat absorption (and therefore vitamin D absorption) is impaired, as in *sprue, celiac disease, cystic fibrosis of the pancreas, chronic pancreatitis, prolonged obstructive jaundice, external biliary fistula,* and *after gastrectomy* [37]; (4) *hypoproteinemia,* in which the low values are due to reduction of the nondiffusible calcium fraction, and hence are without physiologic effect; (5) *during lactation,* apparently from loss of calcium in the milk; (6) *chronic renal disease of childhood* (renal rickets) and occasionally of adults, related presumably to phosphate retention; and (7) occasionally in *osteoporosis* following the menopause or steroid therapy.

physiologic effects

Hypocalcemia results in *increased neuromuscular excitability,* leading to muscle cramps, carpopedal spasm, laryngeal stridor, convulsions, i.e., *tetany.*

Phosphorus metabolism

Some 90 percent of body phosphorus is in the skeleton, chiefly as crystalline calcium phosphate of the apatite series. The remainder is largely intracellular and plays an *important role in energy transfer.* The parathyroid glands control the plasma level of phosphorus (normal for adults: 3 to 4 mg. per 100 ml. of serum), apparently by regulating renal excretion: *overactivity of the parathyroid glands results in increased renal excretion of phosphorus.*

Calcium, phosphorus, and the parathyroid glands

Thus the *parathyroid glands act in two ways:* one results in *demineralization of bone,* producing hypercalcemia and hypercalcinuria, the other causes a *decrease in phosphorus reabsorption in the renal tubules,* resulting in hyperphosphaturia and hypophosphatemia. This two-way action of the parathyroid hormone results in a teeter-totter effect on blood levels of calcium and phosphorus: when one goes up, the other goes down. The product of the values for serum calcium and serum phosphorus, expressed in milligrams per 100 ml., remains relatively constant at 35 to 40, even in disease states. (The exception is that when renal insufficiency develops, phosphorus is retained more or less independently of calcium.) Thus the plasma levels of calcium and phosphorus are influenced by a complex "system" including the *parathyroid glands, kidneys, and bones.* Serious disturbances of any one of these organs may alter the plasma calcium and phosphorus levels and affect the function of the other two.

Normal bone formation

Normal bone formation occurs in two stages: (1) formation of the protein matrix of bone, known as osteoid, and (2) deposition of bone salts in the osteoid, apparently mediated by tissue concentration of alkaline phosphatase. Osteoid is formed by osteoblasts, and their activity can be estimated from the level of serum alkaline phosphatase, provided that the results of the test are not modified by liver dysfunction or jaundice. The normal deposits of mineral salts in osteoid is known as *ossification,* in contrast with *calcification,* which is often defined as abnormal deposition of calcium.

2. *Parathyroid Syndromes*

Only one hormone has been identified in the parathyroid glands, hence only two forms of abnormal function are recognized: *hyperfunction* and *hypofunction.* In both instances the effects are intimately related to calcium metabolism.

HYPERPARATHYROIDISM:

Hyperparathyroidism [38] is a disease affecting many organ systems, any of which may serve to cause symptoms. Truly it is like the elephant to the blind men in the story: the orthopedic surgeon gets one impression, the gastroenterologist another, the urologist a third; only one who understands the many aspects of disturbed calcium function can hope to comprehend the whole creature.

Bone manifestations

The best known manifestations of hyperparathyroidism relate to bone. *Long bones* in particular are affected, but characteristic x-ray changes also occur in vertebrae, skull, and jaws. Bone changes may be manifest clinically by bone pain, pathologic fractures, shortening of stature, or other skeletal deformity.

Digestive manifestations

Much less widely known are the *digestive tract* manifestations. It is important that these signs and symptoms be recognized since they may permit the early diagnosis of hyperparathyroidism before irreparable damage has been done to the kidneys and skeleton. Unexplained episodes of vomiting, often with severe abdominal pain and constipation, are usual symptoms, presumably due in some way to crises of hypercalcemia. *Peptic ulcers* may occur in patients with hypercalcemia. (Note that these manifestations are apparently due to the hypercalcemia rather than to the hyperparathyroidism per se; they may occur when hypercalcemia is a result of hypervitaminosis D or Boeck's sarcoid.) The reverse is also true: hypercalcemia may occur in patients with peptic ulcer, due to milk and alkali commonly used in the treatment of peptic ulcer. Such cases may give real difficulty in diagnosis, as noted by Kyle [39]. Acute pancreatic necrosis may also occur in patients with hyperparathyroidism, presumably because of hypercalcemia [40].

Urinary tract manifestations

Hypercalcemia, even of brief duration, is damaging to the kidneys [41], producing *injury to the tubular epithelium* and *interfering with tubular reabsorption. Polyuria* and *polydipsia* are commonly noted. Continued hypercalcemia and hypercalcinuria may lead to extensive deposits of calcium in the kidneys, eventually causing *renal insufficiency,* even without skeletal lesions being demonstrable. In some cases urinary calculi are formed, resulting in hematuria, pyuria, and pain. Hyperparathyroidism causes less than 5 percent of all kidney stones, and should be particularly suspected when *stones are multiple* or *bilateral* or *re-form after removal.* Stones lead to special complications in the urinary tract (see Chapter 22).

Primary and secondary hyperparathyroidism

Hyperparathyroidism may be *primary,* i.e., due to a benign tumor (adenoma) of one or more parathyroid glands, a primary hyperplasia, or rarely a primary carcinoma of the glands; or it may be *secondary.* The latter is usually associated with chronic renal disease with renal insufficiency, causing phosphate retention and stimulation of the parathyroid glands. These glands then become hyperplastic, causing demineralization of bones and elevation of the serum calcium to hypercalcemic levels. Any of the complications of hypercalcemia may then occur. In such cases of secondary hyperparathyroidism all the parathyroid glands are enlarged but no neoplasm is found. When primary hyperparathyroidism leads to nephrolithiasis or nephrocalcinosis and renal insufficiency, this too will result in phosphate retention and often a depression of the serum calcium to normal or low levels: *once renal failure has developed, the chemical studies prove much less diagnostic.* The distinction between the primary and secondary forms of the disease is important, since in primary hyperparathyroidism the renal and skeletal complications can be prevented or cured if the parathyroid adenoma can be found and removed. No such effect occurs with surgery in secondary hyperparathyroidism.

Pathologic changes:

The pathology of hyperparathyroidism is largely a study of *bone changes* and of the *effects of hypercalcemia.* The changes in the parathyroid glands may be either *hyperplasia,* in which the glands are enlarged due to an increase in the number of component cells, or *neoplasia* (see section following).

bone changes

The bones show widespread *focal decalcification,* followed in some instances by *cyst formation,* in others, possibly as a result of hemorrhage and minute fractures, by small *giant cell tumors* composed of osteoclasts, and in still others by *fibrosis* which obliterates the bony architecture. *Osteoid formation is active,* being manifest by high values of serum alkaline phosphatase; fractures heal readily but with excess callus formation. The skeletal disease, described before the relationship to the parathyroid glands was known, is called *osteitis fibrosa cystica (von Recklinghausen's disease of bone).*

metastatic calcification

Hypercalcemia results in deposition of calcium in certain tissues, apparently as a *consequence of a local ionic state resulting from the elimination of acid ions.*

This deposition of calcium in the tissues, known as *metastatic calcification,* occurs characteristically in three locations:

1. In the *kidneys,* calcium is seen first as small hematoxylin-staining masses in the lumen of the collecting tubules in the medulla; later the deposits may also be found in the interstitial tissue. Encrustations of calcium may occur in the mucosa of the pelvis and calyces. These may increase in size by further accretion until multiple large calculi fill the renal pelvis; separate calculi may be evident in the ureters and bladder. When the calcium deposits are confined to the renal parenchyma, the process is spoken of as *nephrocalcinosis;* when calculi are present in the renal pelvis or lower urinary tract, it is spoken of as *nephrolithiasis* or *urolithiasis.* kidneys

2. In the *lungs,* calcium is seen as splinters of hematoxylin-staining material in the alveolar walls; in one patient seen by the authors the deposits were so widespread as to give a sandy feel to the lungs at necropsy. Usually there are no clinical symptoms related to the alveolar deposits, although changes may be evident on radiographs of the thorax as a diffuse homogeneous increase in density. lungs

3. In the *stomach,* microscopic deposits of calcium occur in the interstitial tissue about the mouths of the glands of the fundus. Whether these deposits are in some way responsible for the gastrointestinal symptoms is unclear; peptic ulcers occurring with hyperparathyroidism may be either gastric or duodenal in location, while the calcium deposits are apparently confined to the fundus portion of the stomach. stomach

Occasionally calcium is deposited in other tissues than the three mentioned above, but in these sites no ionic explanation is offered. The deposits in the *corneas* of the eyes are of particular importance, since they may be visible on physical examination, thus giving a clue to the diagnosis of hypercalcemia; sometimes the corneal deposits result in impaired vision. Calcium may also be deposited in the thyroid gland and in the walls of arteries in any part of the body during the course of hypercalcemia; these deposits have no known special significance.

HYPOPARATHYROIDISM: Cause:

Hypoparathyroidism is a functional state in which demonstrable organ changes are minimal. The most common *cause* is accidental removal of the parathyroid glands during neck surgery, particularly thyroidectomy; occasionally hypoparathyroidism may be a result of destruction of the parathyroid glands, as by a neoplasm of the thyroid gland or larynx. With hyposecretion of parathyroid hormone there is *diminished excretion of phosphorus in the urine* and the *serum phosphorus level rises.* Because of the teeter-totter relationship of phosphorus and calcium, the *serum calcium level falls* as the serum phosphorus level rises. The serum calcium rarely falls below 5 to 7 mg. per 100 ml., apparently being maintained at this level by a passive chemical interchange with bone calcium.

Clinical features

The clinical manifestations of hypoparathyroidism are a *result of hypocalcemia.* When the serum calcium approaches the critical level, increased neuromuscular excitability develops, leading to muscle twitching and occasionally to a convulsive disorder resembling epilepsy, although there is usually no loss of consciousness. This excitable state, known as *tetany,* can be relieved by the intravenous administration of calcium. In its acute form, tetany usually occurs 1 or 2 days after total thyroidectomy or after removal of a parathyroid adenoma, and may cause death from laryngeal spasm or cardiac arrest unless recognized and treated promptly. Bone changes are usually not seen in acute tetany. Chronic forms of tetany may be due either to hypoparathyroidism or to other causes of hypocalcemia (see page 734). These patients may develop cataracts, trophic changes in the skin, teeth, and nails, mental retardation, and eventually extensive demineralization and softening of bones leading to multiple fractures.

3. Parathyroid Neoplasms

ADENOMA

Neoplasms of the parathyroid glands [42] are rare. In most instances they are benign *(adenomas)*. Usually the diagnosis of parathyroid adenoma is made on the basis of abnormal blood calcium, phosphorus, and alkaline phosphatase levels found during the study of a patient presenting bone, gastrointestinal, or renal symptoms. Often there is no mass palpable in the neck in such patients. Parathyroid adenomas are usually round or ovoid and rarely more than 3 cm. in diameter, often being much smaller. Since they may be indistinguishable grossly from lymph nodes, the surgeon usually has the pathologist do a frozen section on any suspicious nodule encountered during exploration of the neck or mediastinum: neoplasms of the parathyroid glands are often found at some distance from the normal location of these glands.

CARCINOMA

Carcinoma of the parathyroid glands is an extremely rare disease. Castleman [42] found parathyroid carcinoma in 3 percent of his cases of primary hyperparathyroidism, itself a rare disorder. Histologically the tumor consists of vacuolated cells arranged in cords and sheets, like those in the adenoma, but showing in addition evidence of capsular invasion, and sometimes invasion of veins and lymphatics.

4. Dystrophic Calcification

Nature of process

Calcium is often deposited in dead or dying tissues. This process, known as *dystrophic calcification* [43], has no known relation to the parathyroid glands or to hypercalcemia. Several theories have been advanced to explain the deposition of calcium in these tissues.

Calcification: in fatty tissues

Klotz proposed in 1905 a *chemical basis* to account for the deposition of calcium in damaged adipose tissue, or in tissues undergoing pathologic fatty changes (pancreatic fat necrosis, caseous tuberculous lesions, atheroma of vessels). Klotz showed that enzymes cause hydrolysis of fat, splitting it to fatty acid and diffusible glycerol. Calcium from blood was shown to unite chemically with the fatty acid residue in the tissues to form soap, which in turn was substituted to produce calcium phosphate and calcium carbonate.

in scar tissue

In the case of fibrous, hyaline, and scar tissues, it seems possible that there may be a *physical basis* for the deposition of calcium, based upon the relative alkalinity of the inert tissues. This might account for calcium deposition in the media of arteries in Mönckeberg's arteriosclerosis, in heart valves and serous membranes after inflammation, in hyaline scars, leiomyomas, or thrombi, or in the dead fetus in the abdominal cavity (lithopedion).

Relation to normal ossification

Both these old theories have been repeatedly questioned. There is a *high local concentration of alkaline phosphatase* in those tissues in which calcium is deposited. This fact brings the process of dystrophic calcification into line with the deposition of calcium in the osteoid matrix as a part of normal bone formation. Also, the calcium deposits in dead and dying tissue are chemically indistinguishable from those in normal bone and in metastatic calcification; they are composed of about nine parts calcium phosphate to one part calcium carbonate.

Calcinosis

Apparently not related to the deposition of calcium in fatty tissue or scar tissue is the deposition of calcium in the skin and subcutaneous tissues in the rare disease known as *calcinosis circumscripta,* and the additional deposits in muscles and tendons in *calcinosis universalis.* Clinically these cases may *resemble scleroderma* in the stiffness that is produced, particularly in the hands and about the joints, but it seems unlikely that the two diseases are related. The cause of calcinosis, as of scleroderma, is unknown; the parathyroid glands, kidneys, and serum calcium level are all normal.

THYMUS

1. General Considerations

The *thymus* is a lymphoepithelial structure whose function is poorly understood. The fact that it is relatively large at birth and during childhood and becomes atrophic after puberty indicates that it has some endocrine significance and suggests that the gland may *in some way be related to growth,* but no real evidence of such a function has ever been shown. Autopsies on infants and children who have died suddenly have often revealed large thymus glands, and many authors have speculated that there may be a relationship between *thymic enlargement and sudden death in childhood* (status thymicolymphaticus). Some deaths under these circumstances have been shown to be associated with a low level of gamma globulin in the serum [44]. Some cases of *acquired agammaglobulinemia* have also been noted on chest x-ray to have mediastinal, presumably thymic, masses. *Severe anemias* characterized specifically by erythroblastic hypoplasia of the bone marrow have also been described [45], and have responded to thymectomy by reticulocyte crisis and return of the blood picture to normal.

2. Thymic Neoplasms

MEDIASTINAL MASS

Neoplasms of the thymus gland [46] are rare, but they constitute an important segment of the *mediastinal tumors.* They occur in the upper mediastinum, anterior to the great vessels and the upper portion of the heart shadow, and may be confused with aortic aneurysms on chest radiographs. Sometimes they are manifest clinically by pressure symptoms, such as difficulty in breathing or edema of the face, at other times by myasthenia gravis.

THYMOMA

The *thymoma* [47], sometimes known as thymic lymphoepithelioma, is the most common thymic neoplasm. Although the term is used differently by some, the tendency is to restrict it to *benign neoplasms* of thymic origin characterized grossly by *encapsulation* and microscopically by a *mixed cellular pattern of lymphocytes and pale epithelial cells,* this pattern being divided into an irregular *lobulated structure* by bands of fibrous tissue. Clinically the thymoma rarely recurs after surgical excision, and distant metastases do not occur. Epithelial thymomas have secreted ACTH to produce adrenal hyperplasia and *Cushing's syndrome* in a number of patients. Electron microscopy has demonstrated neurosecretory granules in the neoplastic cells [48]. In about 25 percent of cases of *myasthenia gravis* a thymoma is present. The neoplasm is also present in about half the cases of selective erythroid aplastic anemia [49].

CARCI-NOMA

Thymic *carcinoma* is also described; this tumor has nests of *epithelial cells* separated by a *stroma containing many lymphocytes.* Some pathologists believe this tumor is a mediastinal teratoma or a metastatic growth from a seminoma of the testis.

LYMPHO-MAS

Lymphomas (Hodgkin's disease, lymphosarcoma) may also occur in the thymus. A peculiar hyperplastic lesion of the mediastinal nodes occurring in the region of the thymus and sometimes confused with thymoma has also been described [50].

GONADS

The ovaries and testes are, of course, part of the endocrine system and syndromes of hyperfunction and hypofunction are recognized. For convenience these have been considered under the genital system (Chapters 23 and 24) rather than in this chapter.

REFERENCES

1. Friesen, H., and Astwood, E. B. Hormones of the anterior pituitary body. *New Eng. J. Med.* 272:1216, 1272, 1328, 1965.
2. Lisser, H., and Escamilla, R. F. *Atlas of Clinical Endocrinology.* St. Louis: Mosby, 1957. (This very interesting book illustrates, with case histories, photographs, and radiographs, each of the common endocrine syndromes.)
3. Schneeberg, N. G., Perloff, W. H., and Israel, S. L. Incidence of unsuspected "Sheehan's syndrome." *J.A.M.A.* 172:20, 1960.
4. Kernohan, J. W., and Sayre, G. P. Tumors of the pituitary gland and infundibulum. Section X, Fascicle 36, in *Atlas of Tumor Pathology.* Washington: Armed Forces Institute of Pathology, 1956.
5. Zubrod, C. G., Pieper, W., Hilbish, T. F., Smith, R., Dutcher, T., and Wermer, P. Acromegaly, jejunal ulcers, and hypersecretion of gastric juice. *Ann. Intern. Med.* 49:1389, 1958.
6. Reidbord, H., and Fisher, E. R. Electron microscopic study of adrenal cortical hyperplasia in Cushing's syndrome. *Arch. Path.* (Chicago) 86:419, 1968.
7. Azzopardi, J. G., and Williams, E. D. Pathology of "nonendocrine" tumors associated with Cushing's syndrome. *Cancer* 22:274, 1968.
8. Conn, J. W. Primary aldosteronism, a new clinical syndrome. *J. Lab. Clin. Med.* 45:3, 1955. (The original description of the syndrome sometimes called Conn's disease.)
9. Neville, A. M., and Symington, T. Pathology of primary aldosteronism. *Cancer* 19:1854, 1966.
10. Karsner, H. Tumors of the adrenal. Section VIII, Fascicle, 29 in *Atlas of Tumor Pathology.* Washington: Armed Forces Institute of Pathology, 1950.
11. Lattes, R. Non-chromaffin paraganglioma of ganglion nodosum, carotid body, and aortic arch bodies. *Cancer* 3:667, 1950. (This paper includes a discussion of the differential points, clinical and pathologic, that permit a separation of the chromaffin and nonchromaffin paraganglia.)
12. Hamolsky, M. W., and Freedberg, A. S. The thyroid gland. *New Eng. J. Med.* 262:23, 70, 129, 1960. (These authors review the physiology and biochemistry

of the thyroid gland, and relate their studies to the laboratory tests available for the evaluation of function in the individual patient.)

13. Axelrad, A. A., and Leblond, C. P. Induction of thyroid tumors in rats by a low iodine diet. *Cancer* 8:339, 1955. (A review of the progressive pathologic alterations in the thyroid of animals deprived of iodine.)
14. Clements, F. W., and Wishart, J. W. Thyroid-blocking agent in etiology of endemic goiter. *Metabolism* 5:623, 1956. (Endemic goiter in a community in Australia is here ascribed to drinking milk from cows fed on a certain type of forage.)
15. Warren, S., and Meissner, W. A. Tumors of the thyroid gland. Section IV, Fascicle 14, in *Atlas of Tumor Pathology*. Washington: Armed Forces Institute of Pathology, 1953.
16. Russell, W. O., Ibanez, M. L., Clark, R. L., and White, E. C. Thyroid carcinoma. *Cancer* 16:1425, 1963.
17. Gonzalez-Licea, A., Hartmann, W. H., and Yardley, J. H. Medullary carcinoma of the thyroid. *Amer. J. Clin. Path.* 49:512, 1968.
18. Klinck, G. H., and Winship, T. Occult sclerosing carcinoma of the thyroid. *Cancer* 8:701, 1955.
19. Winship, T. Carcinoma of the thyroid in children. *Trans. Amer. Goiter Ass.* 364, 1951. (A comprehensive study of the problem, based on a review of published cases plus wide personal experience.)
20. Hazard, J. B. Thyroiditis: A review. *Amer. J. Clin. Path.* 25:289, 399, 1955.
21. Witebsky, E., Rose, N. R., Terplan, K., Paine, J. R., and Egan, R. W. Chronic thyroiditis and autoimmunization. *J.A.M.A.* 164:1439, 1957.
22. Lavine, R., and Haft, D. E. Carbohydrate homeostasis. *New Eng. J. Med.* 283:175, 237, 1970.
23. Beaser, S. B. Diabetes mellitus. *New Eng. J. Med.* 259:525, 573, 1958. (An excellent review of the fundamental aspects of diabetes, including biochemical theory, pathology, endocrine interrelationships, and ketosis.)
24. Goldner, M. G., Zarowitz, H., and Akgun, S. Hyperglycemia and glycosuria due to thiazide derivatives administered in diabetes mellitus. *New Eng. J. Med.* 262:403, 1960.
25. Bell, E. T. The pathologic diagnosis of diabetes mellitus (Editorial). *Amer. J. Clin. Path.* 25:299, 1955. (A very brief, concise review by a pathologist with very long experience.)
26. Lowry, A. D., Jr., and Barach, J. H. Study of serum lipoprotein and cholesterol determinations in 901 diabetics. *Diabetes* 6:342, 1957.
27. Banson, B. B., and Lacy, P. E. Diabetic microangiopathy in human toes. *Amer. J. Path.* 45:41, 1964.
28. Lowbeer, L. Hypoglycemia-producing extrapancreatic neoplasms. *Amer. J. Clin. Path.* 35:233, 1961.
29. Zollinger, R. M., and Ellison, E. H. Primary peptic ulceration of the jejunum associated with islet cell tumors of the pancreas. *Ann. Surg.* 142:709, 1955.
30. Thistlethwaite, J. R., and Horwitz, A. Ulcerogenic islet cell tumors of the pancreas. *Postgrad. Med.* 24:599, 1958.
31. Duff, G. L., and Murray, E. G. D. The pathology of islet cell tumors of the pancreas. *Amer. J. Med. Sci.* 203:437, 1942.
32. Greider, M. H., and Elliott, D. W. Electron microscopy of human pancreatic tumors of islet cell origin. *Amer. J. Path.* 44:663, 1964.
33. Copp, D. H. Calcium and phosphorus metabolism. *Amer. J. Med.* 22:275, 1957. (An excellent reference article on biochemistry and physiology.)
34. McLean, F. C. The ultrastructure and function of bone. *Science* 127:451, 1958. (A presentation of the chemistry of bone and an excellent discussion

concerning the feedback mechanism for the control of body calcium.)
35. Thomas, W. C., Jr., Connor, T. B., and Morgan, H. G. Diagnostic considerations in hypercalcemia, with a discussion of the various means by which such a state may develop. *New Eng. J. Med.* 260:591, 1959.
36. Edmondson, H. A., Berne, C. J., Homann, R. E., Jr., and Wertman, D. Calcium, potassium, magnesium, and amylase disturbances in acute pancreatitis. *Amer. J. Med.* 12:34, 1952.
37. Melick, R. A., and Benson, J. A., Jr. Osteomalacia following partial gastrectomy. *New Eng. J. Med.* 260:976, 1959.
38. Goldsmith, R. S. Hyperparathyroidism. *New Eng. J. Med.* 281:367, 1969.
39. Kyle, L. H. Differentiation of hyperparathyroidism and milk-alkali (Burnett) syndrome. *New Eng. J. Med.* 26:1035, 1954.
40. Lacher, M. J., Goldberg, J. A., Thomas, D. F., and Calvy, G. L. Hyperparathyroidism and pancreatitis. *New Eng. J. Med.* 261:239, 1959.
41. Carone, F. A., Epstein, F. H., Beck, D., and Levitin, H. The effects upon the kidney of transient hypercalcemia induced by parathyroid extract. *Amer. J. Path.* 36:77, 1960.
42. Castleman, B. Tumors of the parathyroid glands. Section IV, Fascicle 15, in *Atlas of Tumor Pathology*. Washington: Armed Forces Institute of Pathology, 1952.
43. Abraham, E. P. Necrosis, calcification, and autolysis. In Florey, H. (Ed.), *General Pathology* (4th ed.). Philadelphia: Saunders, 1970, pp. 431–450. (A good, concise presentation of the facts and theories of calcium deposition in tissues, particularly worthwhile in connection with dystrophic calcification.)
44. Spain, D. M., Bradess, V. A., and Greenblatt, I. J. Possible factor in sudden and unexpected death during infancy (low serum gamma globulin). *J.A.M.A.* 156:246, 1954.
45. Weinbaum, J. G., and Thompson, R. F. Erythroblastic hypoplasia associated with thymic tumor and myasthenia gravis. *Amer. J. Clin. Path.* 25:761, 1955.
46. Castleman, B. Tumors of the thymus gland. Section V, Fascicle 19, in *Atlas of Tumor Pathology*. Washington: Armed Forces Institute of Pathology, 1955.
47. Legg, M. A., and Brady, W. J. Pathology and clinical behavior of thymomas. *Cancer* 18:1131, 1965.
48. Kay, S., and Willson, M. A. Ultrastructural studies of an ACTH-secreting thymic tumor. *Cancer* 26:445, 1970.
49. Jacobs, E. M., Hutter, R. V. P., Pool, J. L., and Ley, A. B. Benign thymoma and selective erythroid aplasia of the bone marrow. *Cancer* 12:47, 1959.
50. Castleman, B., Iverson, L., and Menendez, V. P. Localized mediastinal lymph node hyperplasia resembling thymoma. *Cancer* 9:822, 1956.

GENERAL REFERENCES

Reifenstein, E. C., Jr. Endocrine glands. In Sodeman, W. A., and Sodeman, W. A., Jr. (Eds.), *Pathologic Physiology* (4th ed.). Philadelphia: Saunders, 1967. (A well-written section in a valuable book.)

Warren, S., LeCompte, P. M., and Legg, M. A. *The Pathology of Diabetes Mellitus* (4th ed.). Philadelphia: Lea & Febiger, 1966. (A comprehensive monograph stressing the complications of diabetes.)

28 THE MUSCULOSKELETAL SYSTEM

INTRODUCTION

Functions

The musculoskeletal system has many important functions. It is an *organ for locomotion and other mechanical work;* it is a rigid frame *providing support and protection of the viscera;* it *houses a factory for the manufacture of blood cells;* and *it is a reservoir for vital minerals* (calcium and phosphorus in bone) *and for energy-giving fuel* (glycogen in muscle). Its metabolic and hemopoietic functions have been considered in other chapters; here we are concerned chiefly with the musculoskeletal system as an organ for locomotion and support.

A machine

In these capacities, the muscles, bones, and joints act together as *a machine* – countering the force of gravity when standing erect, moving the weight of the body when walking, running, or climbing, and moving the weight of the body plus additional mass when lifting or carrying some object. The structure of bone combines *great strength* with *lightness,* at the same time providing space for the bone marrow; the tubular form of the long bones is particularly noteworthy in this regard. The skeletal machine is essentially *a series of levers of the third class,* i.e., the force acts between the fulcrum and the weight to be moved. The advantage of this type of lever in the case of the extremities is that the muscular force, acting through a short distance, can move the weight a much longer distance. The *muscles* provide the force to move the *bone* (lever) through an arc which turns around a *joint* (fulcrum). The muscles are arranged in functional groups about each joint: the *prime movers* contract to cause the intended movement, while the *antagonists* relax to permit the motion to remain under control; other muscle groups about related joints provide *fixation* of the part proximally so that the distal action can be effective.

Types of diseases

Because of their active motion and relatively exposed position, the *bones* are particularly subject to *trauma.* The *joints,* corresponding to the frictional surfaces, are subject to *wear* as the "machine" ages. The muscles may become ineffective as a result of disease of the nervous system, or may atrophy with disuse or cachexia, but *rarely are the muscles primarily affected by disease* in a way to cause a patient to seek medical attention.

BONES

1. Congenital Defects

OSTEOGENESIS IMPERFECTA

Osteogenesis imperfecta, also known as *osteopsathyrosis,* is a congenital disorder in which the *bones are imperfectly ossified. Fractures,* chiefly of the long bones, occur in utero or during birth. Fetal death is often due to *thoracic deformity* or *intracranial hemorrhage.* Affected bones have a cortex as thin and fragile as an eggshell. The skull may be only a fibrous membrane containing a few small plaques of bone. In those children who survive the neonatal period, a more widespread defect of mesenchymal tissues is sometimes seen: the teeth are soft, and the sclerae thin and translucent, giving a bluish appearance to the eyeballs; middle ear deafness is common. The disease is sometimes inherited, but with great variation in severity.

MARFAN'S SYNDROME

Marfan's syndrome is a rare congenital defect of connective tissues, involving the *cardiovascular system as well as the skeleton.* The defect – the exact biochemical nature is not known – occurs in families, being transmitted as a dominant trait. Affected individuals are usually tall and thin and have long slender fingers and hands *(arachnodactyly).* Curiously, there is a tendency to *subluxation of the lenses of the eyes.* An affected individual who dies in childhood or early youth often shows a *defect of the interatrial septum of the heart.* Those who survive to adult life are prone to develop *dissecting aneurysms* of the aorta or other vessels, or aortic insufficiency. The aneurysms apparently result from a deficiency of elastic tissue and an increase of mucopolysaccharide in the aortic wall. There is ordinarily no hypertension.

ACHONDROPLASIA

Achondroplasia is a *disorder of bone formation* resulting from defective cartilage. Some cases are apparently due to a hereditary fault but most affected children have normal parents, even if several siblings are affected. Cases of the latter type, thought due to mutation, are apparently more severe than cases in which one or both parents are affected [1]. Growth of the bones that develop from cartilage is greatly restricted, resulting in *short arms and legs* and a *depressed nasal bone,* while the head and torso appear more nearly of normal size. Although affected individuals are usually about half normal stature, they have well-developed muscles, and often find employment as circus acrobats because of their size and athletic prowess. It is said that the peculiar skeletal configuration in dogs of dachshund breed is due to a comparable defect.

OTHER FORMS

A number of other types of diffuse hereditary defects of bone formation are described, but they are rare. *Localized defects of bone formation,* as of the skull or vertebrae or extremities, may be found in those grossly deformed fetuses which are classed as *monsters* (see Chapter 12).

2. Mechanical Injury

The most common conditions affecting the bones are those due to *mechanical injury.* Highway, home, and industrial accidents cause the greatest number of cases. The injury may result in contusion or fracture of one or more bones, or in tearing of structures intimately related to bone, such as joints, tendons, or bursae. Mechanical injuries are considered in Chapter 9.

3. *Inflammatory Diseases*

ACUTE OSTEOMYELITIS:

Acute osteomyelitis is a *pyogenic inflammation* of bone and bone marrow. It may be a result of *direct implantation* of bacteria via a puncture wound (as in nail wounds of the feet), *extension* from an adjacent soft tissue infection (as a bone felon of a finger), or *hematogenous dissemination* (as from a skin or throat infection). In the last, the staphylococcus is the usual organism recovered in the blood culture; sometimes streptococci or other bacteria are the causative agent. Often there is a history of injury at the site of localization of the infection.

Clinical features

While osteomyelitis may occur at any age, the fulminating hematogenous form is more commonly observed in *children and adolescents, especially males.* In such cases, the onset may be sudden, often with *high fever* and *severe pain.* The patient tends to favor the affected part: if one of the lower extremities is affected, there is usually a tendency for the patient to limp; if an upper extremity is involved, the patient tends to hold it immobile against his side. Sometimes the affected extremity is held so still that paralysis is suspected. On examination there is usually marked tenderness, and some swelling and redness of the overlying skin. The child is often prostrated and acutely ill. Leukocytosis is usually marked.

Pathologic changes

The long bones of the extremities, especially the *tibiae, femora,* and *humeri,* are the ones usually affected in the hematogenous form. Bacteria spread along the small channels within the bone and a purulent exudate forms in these same areas, burrowing in all directions, elevating the overlying periosteum. Pressure builds up in the tissue spaces as the *pus collects; arteries and veins become compressed and thrombosed,* bone cells die and disappear from the bone lacunae, and eventually the fine osteoid of the bone becomes eroded and liquefied. In bones with rich arterial anastomoses the avascular necrosis may produce minimal structural damage; but in the metaphyses of the growing bones of children, the epiphyseal plate apparently is supplied by end arteries, and thrombosis of several of these vessels may cause serious damage, as was emphasized by Morse and Pryles [2]. It may take some time – on the average, about 17 days after the onset of symptoms – for characteristic radiographic evidence of bone destruction to be noted.

Outcome

In fulminant cases the *septic thrombi* in the venous channels of bone become softened by the action of bacterial and leukocytic enzymes, and embolism to the lungs occurs. The resulting infarcts of the lungs are septic, leading to the formation of multiple abscesses. It used to be common for death from sepsis to occur within a few days of the onset of symptoms, but this outcome is distinctly unusual at present when *antibiotics* are employed. The danger is that the *true nature of the condition may be overlooked,* perhaps being mistakenly diagnosed as acute rheumatic fever or a sprain, and antibiotics may be withheld. The usual course is for the infection to spread locally in the bone, causing the death of small bone fragments from ischemia. In about half the cases, some form of surgical procedure, usually *incision and drainage* of a soft tissue abscess, is necessary to evacuate pus and permit healing. If the periosteum remains viable, new bone will then be formed, repairing the defect. If the periosteum has been destroyed, or if the necrosis extends up to the articular cartilage, large *fragments of dead bone (sequestra)* may remain in the area, preventing normal healing of the part and acting as foreign bodies in the wound. In such cases it is usually necessary to remove each sequestrum, so that the *chronic suppurative process with draining sinuses* can resolve. Infection often spreads to the adjacent joint; this may lead to ankylosis. If the epiphysis is destroyed, the affected bone will not grow normally thereafter; the affected limb is thus shorter than its mate, resulting in asymmetry. These features are especially noteworthy when the lower limbs are affected, since limp results. In the upper extremities there is less apt to be a residual functional impairment.

CHRONIC OSTEOMYELITIS

Prior to the "antibiotic era" a series of recurrences *(chronic osteomyelitis)* would often follow an attack of acute osteomyelitis, each associated with a febrile episode and a *soft tissue abscess* requiring drainage. These recurrences sometimes repeated themselves at intervals over a period of several years, either attacking the same bone repeatedly or affecting widely scattered bones. Multiple *deep scars* marked the sites of the abscesses, and when a lower limb was affected, the gait was distorted by limb shortening and joint ankyloses. Sometimes *secondary amyloidosis* of the spleen, liver, and kidneys developed, resulting in death. Fortunately chronic osteomyelitis is today rare, presumably because of better control of the initial infection. There is still some tendency to recurrence, but it is not nearly what it used to be. If there is recurrence in the same bone, it usually means that a sequestrum is present and needs to be removed. *Brodie's abscess* is a circumscribed form of chronic osteomyelitis in a single bone, subject to periodic exacerbation. *Garre's sclerosing osteomyelitis* is a combination of periosteal and cortical bone infection associated with irregular growth of cortical bone.

TUBERCULOSIS OF BONE: Pathologic changes

Tuberculous osteomyelitis is sometimes due to infection by the bovine strain of *Mycobacterium tuberculosis;* more often the human strain is responsible. It is usually associated with a primary focus of tuberculosis in the respiratory or intestinal tract, but this focus is sometimes without symptoms. In recent years most of our cases of bone tuberculosis have been found in patients receiving long-term steroid therapy, as for rheumatoid arthritis; presumably this means that a previously dormant tuberculous infection has become activated. Chiefly affected are the small bones of the hands and feet *(tuberculous dactylitis)* or the vertebrae *(tuberculous spondylitis* or *Pott's disease);* sometimes the *ends of the long bones* are involved, chiefly the femora and tibiae. Bone destruction is much more extensive when weight-bearing bones are affected. The adjacent joints are usually involved; in most instances it appears that joint tuberculosis is secondary to involvement of the bone metaphyses. An area of bone necrosis develops and extends to involve the epiphysis and synovia. The affected joint becomes enlarged, tender, and fluctuant, but redness and heat are usually lacking (cold abscess). *Radiographic changes* are usually characteristic: bone destruction and regeneration, often in both bones adjacent to the affected joint. When the lumbar vertebrae are involved, the pus may burrow along a fascial plane, commonly within the sheath of one or both psoas muscles *(psoas abscess)* and form a soft fluctuant swelling below the inguinal ligament on the inner aspect of the thigh. The fluctuant mass tends to break down spontaneously, evacuating its liquid contents through one or more sinus tracts. *Multiple sinuses of the skin,* draining pus from an *abscess* located in an area which includes a joint, usually mean tuberculosis of one or both bones adjacent to that joint. Sometimes secondary pyogenic invaders may overshadow the picture, making the acid-fast organisms difficult to identify in smears. Occasionally fungus infections of the bones and joints, especially actinomycosis or blastomycosis, produce a similar pattern of bone destruction and skin sinuses.

Clinical features

Bone tuberculosis affects *children* more commonly than adults. It is essentially a *chronic disease,* lasting many months. *Limp* due to *pain* is the usual presenting symptom in tuberculosis of the long weight-bearing bones. Voluntary splinting may lessen motion at the affected joint, minimizing pain; when this splinting is relaxed during sleep, motion may occur, causing pain and the so-called *night cries. Swelling* of one or more of the proximal phalanges of the fingers is usually the first manifestation in tuberculous dactylitis. *Pain in the back* is usually evident with tuberculous spondylitis, but the cause may go unrecognized for some time. The pain is due to involvement of the vertebral bodies; not infrequently collapse of the affected vertebral body occurs, leading to compression of the spinal cord and *paraplegia.*

Outcome

Tuberculous dactylitis usually heals with only slight deformity. Tuberculosis of the long bones of the extremities is a more serious disease, but it, too, usually responds to *antituberculosis therapy,* supplemented in some instances with surgical immobilization. Tuberculosis of the vertebrae may heal, usually leaving an *angular kyphosis* of the spine (hunchback) when it does. *Miliary tuberculosis* sometimes occurs during the course of tuberculous osteomyelitis, and may cause death. *Tuberculous meningitis* may develop as a complication of tuberculous spondylitis; it results from spread of the bacilli from the vertebral bodies to the meninges of the spinal cord. *Secondary amyloid disease* is an important late sequel of tuberculosis of bones and joints.

SYPHILIS OF BONE

Bone syphilis is rarely seen today. The most common clinical form is probably the *epiphysitis* of congenital syphilis, in which an irregular zone of granulation tissue teeming with treponemas replaces the regular epiphyseal line, and causes chronic swelling adjacent to a joint. Sometimes bone enlargement and radiographic changes at the epiphyseal line aid in the diagnosis of congenital syphilis when other signs are inconclusive. Bone involvement may also occur in acquired syphilis; *periostitis,* causing pain and tenderness over the diaphysis of a long bone, is probably the most common form. *Gumma* of bone is very rare.

4. *Aseptic Necrosis of Bone*

General features

Aseptic necrosis is an uncommon disorder; it is a result of sudden occlusion of the blood supply. It is, in effect, *infarction of bone.* In children it sometimes occurs *without apparent cause,* or may be a result of *sudden trauma,* causing a *separation of the epiphysis* from the end of the bone, so-called epiphysitis, or slipped epiphysis. In the adult it is most commonly seen following *fracture of the head or neck of the femur,* obliterating the nutrient blood supply to the femoral head, which therefore becomes necrotic. Rarely aseptic necrosis may be a result of *embolism.* A particularly interesting form is that seen in *caisson workers* [3]; it is due to air embolism and affects chiefly the long bones at the knee and hip. Renewed interest in aseptic necrosis of bone has been aroused by the observations of Innes [4] and others that a similar condition occurs spontaneously in the hips of young rabbits and dogs. In these animals it seems to represent an inherited, or at least congenital, defect (dysplasia) in the structure of the femoral head and acetabulum, leading to a series of events which may include dislocation and aseptic necrosis of the femoral head.

Clinical types

Many clinical forms of this basic disease process have been described, particularly in children, depending upon the particular part affected and the radiographic findings. Most have been identified with the names of the surgeons or radiologists who described them. Thus we have *Osgood-Schlatter's disease* (osteochondrosis of the tibial tubercle), *Legg-Calvé-Perthes disease* (osteochondritis deformans juvenilis or coxa plana or osteochondrosis of the capitular epiphysis of the femur), *Köhler's disease* (osteochondritis of the tarsal navicular bone), and others. In each of these conditions, symptoms usually appear during childhood or adolescence, sometimes associated with direct trauma, more often not. There is *pain over the affected area;* usually a *limp* develops. Since the lesion usually affects a joint surface, *restriction of motion* is common. Radiographs may show no alterations in bone structure at first, although an abnormal relationship of the diaphysis and epiphysis is usually noted. In adults the condition is usually recognized some time after an injury, as when a fracture of the neck of the femur fails to heal because of ischemic necrosis of the femoral head.

Outcome

In children the necrotic bone may become organized by fibrous tissue and eventually new bone and cartilage may restore near-normal function. In other instances deformity of the joint persists, leading to some degree of permanent disability, such as limp, pain on motion, or restricted use of the part. Undoubtedly some cases of osteoarthritis in later life, particularly the monarticular forms, are a sequel of aseptic necrosis.

5. Metabolic Bone Disease

Definition

The term *metabolic bone disease* [5] is used for a group of diseases usually manifest by a *tendency to easy fracture (pathologic fracture),* by *skeletal deformity,* or by *x-ray changes,* rather than by pain, swelling, or fever. The term *excludes* primary and metastatic bone tumors, osteomyelitis, tuberculosis, and ordinary fractures. It *includes* those diseases of bone which are associated with disturbances of calcium metabolism (osteitis fibrosa cystica, rickets, osteomalacia) and also certain hereditary and acquired diseases associated with abnormalities of the organic matrix of bone. The hereditary diseases of this group are considered in an earlier section of this chapter. Rickets is discussed in Chapter 12, abnormalities of calcium metabolism in Chapter 27. Certain other important forms of metabolic bone diseases are now considered.

RENAL RICKETS

Any chronic renal disease with *renal insufficiency occurring in childhood* may cause a bone abnormality resembling rickets, hence known as *renal rickets.* It is due to the *low serum calcium level* which develops as a result of the retention of phosphates. The changes in the bone epiphyses closesly resemble those in true rickets. There is interference with body growth (renal dwarfism). The parathyroid glands usually show secondary hyperplasia. (See also Chapter 22.)

DE TONI-FANCONI SYNDROME

DeToni-Fanconi syndrome is a rare familial disease seen in children in which there is an excess loss of fixed base, including calcium, in the urine. Presumably it is due to a *defect of tubular reabsorption.* It results in a picture of disturbed calcium and electrolyte metabolism known as *renal tubular acidosis.* The bone lesions closely resemble those seen in rickets. (See also Chapter 22.)

OSTEOMALACIA

Osteomalacia, the *adult equivalent of rickets,* is rarely seen in the United States. It is a result of inadequate intake of calcium or vitamin D, and occurs in the female during pregnancy and lactation. Bone calcium is gradually depleted, since it is not replaced; the bones become soft and spongy. Bowing of the extremities, shortening of stature, and pathologic fractures may appear.

OSTEOPOROSIS:

Osteoporosis is the name given to a group of metabolic diseases of bone in which the *osteoid of bone is defective;* it is contrasted with rickets and osteomalacia, in which the osteoid is normal but mineralization is deficient. (The distinction between osteomalacia and osteoporosis is somewhat academic. When osteoid is defective, mineralization is usually defective also. In both cases the *bones appear rarefied on radiographs,* and are so soft at necropsy that they are easily cut with a knife.) While the precise cause of defective osteoid formation is not known, it is generally thought to be a result of failure of anabolic steroid hormone production [6]. Blood proteins, calcium, and phosphorus are usually normal, but *hypercalcemia* and *hypercalcinuria* may sometimes occur when osteoporosis is developing rapidly. The calcium content of bone is significantly reduced. In most cases, the *vertebrae* are the bones first and most severely affected, next the pelvic bones, and then the tubular bones of the extremities. Radiographs show a washed-out appearance of bone. The following are the most important types of osteoporosis.

Senile osteoporosis

The most common form of osteoporosis is that encountered in older people. This form *occurs earlier (age 40 to 50) in women* than in men and in them is commonly called postmenopausal osteoporosis. After age 50 it occurs at about the same frequency (23 percent) in both sexes, according to Caldwell's postmortem studies [6]. Later studies [7] suggest that osteoporosis in postmenopausal women can be postponed and lessened in severity by long-term estrogen therapy. Pain in the ribs or back following coughing or straining is the usual symptom; this may be due to pathologic fracture of vertebrae with compression of nerve roots. Fracture of the femur following a fall is an especially common manifestation. Shortening of stature and limitation of movement due to kyphosis may develop later.

Osteoporosis with endocrine disorders

Osteoporosis is an important manifestation of *hyperthyroidism* and also of *Cushing's syndrome:* in either instance it may mimic the osteoporosis of postmenopausal women. It may be due to overactivity of the adrenal cortex, to basophilic adenoma of the pituitary gland, or to *prolonged therapy with corticosteroids.*

Scorbutic osteoporosis

Vitamin C is an essential substance for the formation of the organic matrix of bone, and a lack of vitamin C is manifest by bone softening. In *children* hemorrhages in the periosteum and epiphysis cause pain and pseudoparalysis. In *adults* alterations in the gums may overshadow the pain in the extremities due to subperiosteal hemorrhages.

Disuse

Prolonged immobilization (as with chronic arthritis, or fractures treated with splints or casts) may cause marked osteoporosis.

Lathyrism

Very rarely osteoporosis may be seen in poisoning with the seeds of a flowering sweet pea, *Lathyrus odoratus* (hence *lathyrism* or *odoratism).* A nitrile damaging to connective tissues in general has been isolated from the seed and will produce the disease in experimental animals [8]. It is of interest that Hippocrates is said to have recognized this condition and to have associated it with peas in the diet [8].

Neoplastic osteoporosis

A generalized demineralization of bone indistinguishable clinically from the metabolic forms of osteoporosis is sometimes due to multiple myeloma or to metastatic carcinoma, particularly from the breast.

LOCALIZED BONE RESORPTION: In addition to these more or less *generalized forms* of bone softening, known as osteoporosis, *localized forms* of bone resorption may be seen.

Polyostotic fibrous dysplasia

Osteitis fibrosa disseminata (Albright's disease) is a rare disorder of children and young adults, associated with widespread but often *unilateral lytic lesions* in bone, sometimes resulting in pathologic fracture and deformity. The lesions resemble cysts on x-ray, but are actually focal nests of fibrous tissue (hence the synonym, *polyostotic fibrous dysplasia*) and cartilage. Premature sexual development and abnormalities of skin pigmentation complete the clinical picture known as Albright's syndrome. There are no known alterations in blood chemistry or endocrine function, although the disorder is generally believed to have an endocrine basis.

Monostotic fibrous dysplasia

Monostotic fibrous dysplasia is a condition similar histologically to polyostotic fibrous dysplasia but affecting single bones. Many so-called bone cysts are examples of this condition. In weight-bearing bones these lesions may cause pathologic fractures; in other bones (as the ribs), they usually go unnoticed until seen by chance on a radiograph.

Osteitis fibrosa cystica

The bone lesions of *hyperparathyroidism,* primary or secondary, are characterized by local fibrous and cystic changes and are often confused with other diseases in this category (see Chapter 27).

Lipoidoses

The lipoid storage diseases, particularly *Gaucher's disease* and *Hand-Schüller-Christian* disease (see Chapter 17), may show areas of bone resorption, especially in the bones of the face. *Eosinophilic granuloma* produces a more localized bone lesion but is generally believed related to the lipoidoses.

Hemolytic anemias

Congenital hemolytic anemias often show bone resorption, apparently due to erythroid hyperplasia of the bone marrow displacing normal bone structure (see Chapter 11). Resorptive *skull changes* are particularly characteristic.

Metastatic neoplasm

Metastatic neoplasm is probably the most common cause of local resorptive lesions of bone, but neoplasms of bone are not ordinarily considered under metabolic bone disease. Neoplasms having a tendency to metastasize to bone include: carcinoma of breast, lung, prostate, kidney, and thyroid, and lymphomas and leukemias. Multiple myeloma, a primary tumor of the bone marrow, also causes local lytic areas in bone. Tuberculosis of bone may produce local bone resorption in radiographs.

Osteitis deformans

Osteitis deformans (*Paget's disease* of bone) is an uncommon, sometimes familial, metabolic disease of bone; it is rarely seen before age 40. The pelvis, spine, skull, and tibiae are commonly involved; usually several bones are already affected when the disease is first recognized. The *bones are softened,* and *increased in diameter,* the normal architecture being distorted by *bone destruction plus active new bone formation.* Microscopically there is an irregular mosaic pattern of fibrous tissue and poorly calcified new bone. As the bones thicken, the skull becomes enlarged, the spine shortened, and the legs bowed, the latter causing an awkward gait. Blood calcium and phosphorus levels are usually normal, but the level of the blood *alkaline phosphatase* – the enzyme of new bone formation – is greatly elevated. The soft new bone provides a great increase in the number of vascular channels; sometimes this has a circulatory effect comparable to that of an arteriovenous shunt, returning an excess of blood to the right ventricle during effort; right heart failure is often the terminal phase [5]. Occasionally sarcoma develops in bones affected by Paget's disease.

6. Neoplasms of Bone and Cartilage

Neoplasms of bone and cartilage are considered together, since they usually arise within bone. X-rays of bone, consisting essentially of shadows of the gross tissue changes, often reveal to the experienced radiologist the exact nature of the various lesions, most of which are manifest by *pain* or *swelling* in the affected area. Mild trauma sometimes causes a fracture through an area of bone disease *(pathologic fracture)*, and the x-ray may reveal the reason for the unexpected break.

BENIGN NEOPLASMS: Osteoma:

Osteoma, the *benign tumor of osteoid tissue*, is a rare neoplasm in pure form. It may arise directly in the *bones of the skull* or *face*, or it may develop as the end result of ossification in a chondroma of the epiphyseal plate. *Grossly* the osteoma is a dense bony mass; *microscopically* the tumor cells resemble normal bone, but lack the regular organizational pattern of bone. Osteomas rarely become the site of malignant neoplastic growths.

variants

Variants of the osteoma include tumors having an admixture of bone and cartilage, known as the *osteochondromas*, and instances of local bone overgrowth due to trauma or infection. The localized overgrowth of new bone *(callus)* remaining after bone injury or fracture is not a neoplasm. The so-called *osteoid osteoma* is probably a chronic inflammatory lesion rather than a true neoplasm. Bone spurs or *exostoses* are common, probably being a result of trauma in most instances; they are not neoplasms. Bone formed in muscle *(myositis ossificans)*, often as a result of injury and hemorrhage, is not considered to be neoplastic, although in some instances the histologic pattern is so bizarre that the question is raised.

Chondroma:

The *chondroma*, or *benign tumor of cartilage*, is a common neoplasm of the small *bones of the hands and feet;* it may also be encountered at the *ends of the long bones*, or occasionally in flat bones, as in those of the pelvis. Rarely chondromas may arise in extraosseous cartilage, as in the tracheal rings. *Grossly* the chondroma is a firm, encapsulated nodule; on section it has a glairy translucent appearance to the cut surface, and a slick soapy feel. *Microscopically* the characteristic cell resembles the normal cell of adult hyaline cartilage, occurring haphazardly in a hyaline matrix. Chondromas, especially those appearing after puberty, seem to have a *potential for malignant change.* In long bones, cartilage tumors are always viewed with suspicion, even when the cartilage cells resemble those of normal cartilage. Chondromas of the small bones of hands or feet, or of the respiratory tract, rarely become malignant.

variants

Several variants of the chondroma are recognized. Cartilage-covered masses sometimes arise from the surface of bone or cartilage and protrude into the soft tissues; these are known as *ecchondroses.* A cartilaginous mass formed within the substance of bone is an *enchondrosis* or *enchondroma;* sometimes such a mass is part of a congenital disorder of bone formation. The *osteochondroma* is a benign tumor containing both bone and cartilage; sometimes multiple masses of this sort occur in the synovial lining of joints, a condition known as *osteochondromatosis.* The *epiphyseal chondroblastoma* (Codman's tumor) is a rare tumor which occurs chiefly in the male at the end of a long bone, usually first noted before puberty. Later, as the epiphyseal lines close, this tumor tends to be converted into bone and to fuse with normal bone. The *chondromyxoid fibroma* is a related tumor of bone, sometimes overdiagnosed as sarcoma.

(An unrelated tumor, the *chordoma*, may be confused with chondroma because of the similarity in spelling. The chordoma is a myxoid tumor arising from the notochord and occurring in relation to the vertebrae.)

Giant cell tumor: benign

The *benign giant cell tumor of bone* (osteoclastoma, giant cell sarcoma, benign synovioma) occurs chiefly in young adults. Its common sites are the *ends of the long bones*, especially at the knee, the *tendon sheaths* and *synovial membranes* near the large or small joints, and the *gingival ridge* of the mandible or maxilla. In the gingival ridge it constitutes an important segment of the neoplasms of the jaw known as *epulis*. Rarely the vertebrae are affected. *Grossly* the normal bone is replaced by soft, yellowish red, granular tissue; hemorrhages in the tumor are common, but fractures are rare. *Microscopically* the distinctive cell is the osteoclastic giant cell, which is smaller than the Langhans cell, and has centrally placed nuclei in most instances; spindle-shaped and round cells provide a background tissue which must be carefully studied for evidences of malignancy.

malignant

Although usually benign, *some tumors containing osteoclastic giant cells are frankly malignant* [9]. In addition, there is a tendency for benign giant cell tumor to become more aggressive if surgery has been incomplete or x-ray therapy unsuccessful. *Local recurrences* may then develop, and in rare cases there may be metastasis to the lungs. This change to a malignant tumor can usually be recognized microscopically on the basis of alterations in the spindle-shaped connective tissue cells; the osteoclasts usually show no sign of the change.

variants

Variants of the giant cell tumor sometimes occur during the course of osteitis fibrosa cystica, the non-neoplastic disease of bone resulting from *hyperparathyroidism;* in this condition multiple small, tumor-like masses showing osteoclastic giant cells may be noted. *Xanthomas* of bone, and the bulky inflammatory overgrowth of the synovial membrane known as *villonodular synovitis,* may closely simulate giant cell tumor of bone.

(Inflammatory and metabolic diseases of bone are often confused clinically with benign neoplasms. Among these diseases are bone cysts, fibrous dysplasia, eosinophilic granuloma, and the lipoid storage diseases.)

MALIGNANT NEOPLASMS: Osteogenic sarcoma:

Of the various forms of malignant tumors primary in bone, the most important is the *osteogenic sarcoma,* and even this is an *uncommon neoplasm.* It has one peak of incidence in the second and third decades, and another in later life, the latter apparently being secondary to chronic bone disease, particularly Paget's disease of bone and radiation osteitis. Important sites of occurrence of osteogenic sarcoma are the *ends of the long bones,* particularly of the lower extremities. *Grossly* the appearance is extremely variable: in some cases there is a soft bloody lesion destroying bone (osteolytic) and invading the soft tissues, whereas in other cases the periosteum is elevated as a result of the formation of sclerotic new bone (osteoblastic). *Microscopically* the pattern is also extremely variable both from case to case and also from area to area in the same case; this *pleomorphism is one of the most distinctive microscopic features* of the neoplasm. Multinucleated *tumor giant cells are numerous,* each one different from the others. Spindle-shaped connective tissue cells are also common. In the more sclerotic types, imperfect new bone trabeculae may be recognizable, the new bone tissue sometimes passing through a stage of cartilage formation. Large, thin-walled vascular channels, often lined by tumor cells, are a conspicuous feature of the softer, more hemorrhagic tumors.

variants

Of the several variants of osteogenic sarcoma, the so-called *bone aneurysm* is probably the most confusing, at least in name. This term is sometimes used for the soft pulsatile masses corresponding to the most malignant form of bone sarcoma, in which there are large vascular channels. The *parosteal (periosteal) sarcoma* is probably better considered as a fibrosarcoma of the periosteum, since it usually forms fibrous tissue rather than bone. It has a much better prognosis than do the true osteogenic sarcomas.

natural history

The *course of true osteogenic sarcoma is usually brief,* although with adequate treatment it is not quite as bad now as was once the case; the overall 5-year survival rate is about 22 percent and the 10-year survival rate about 19 percent [10]. In children the 5-year survival rate is considerably lower when the neoplasm is primary in the femur (16 percent) than when the tibia is the bone primarily affected (40 percent). Presumably surgical treatment is more effective in the latter. *Bone tissue is rapidly destroyed* (pathologic fracture may occur), *soft tissues are invaded,* and there is extensive hemorrhage. The affected extremity rapidly becomes an intolerably heavy and extremely painful burden. *Venous invasion* occurs early, often leading to widespread pulmonary metastases.

Chondrosarcoma:

Chondrosarcoma is a less common malignant neoplasm arising in bone, occurring usually about age 45. Its usual site is at the *end of a long bone,* often near the marrow cavity, but it may also arise in the *flat bones* of the pelvis or in the ribs. *Grossly* it is a lobulated tumor which often extends along the marrow cavity for some distance, eroding bone cortex and bulging into the soft tissues. On section it shows translucent areas having a slick soapy feel like that of mature hyaline cartilage. *Microscopically* the resemblance to the cells and matrix of hyaline cartilage is usually clear, even in those cases in which calcification and ossification have occurred.

natural history

The natural history of chondrosarcoma is usually longer than that of osteogenic sarcoma. In some cases, especially those in which the cartilage is growing in the marrow of long bones, it is possible to show that the malignant tumor has developed in a benign neoplasm of cartilage. The chondrosarcoma often follows a *protracted course* of many years' duration, finally causing death by pulmonary metastases. We have had one case in which, over a total period of about 20 years, chondrosarcoma appeared in three different bones – vertebra, calvaria, and tibia – apparently as separate primaries. Gottschalk and Allen [11] have shown that immature cartilage attracts sulfur and they have treated several chondrosarcoma patients with radioactive sulfur; there was some temporary improvement but all patients succumbed to their disease.

Ewing's tumor:

The *endothelial myeloma* of bone, more commonly known as Ewing's tumor, is a rare neoplasm, occurring chiefly at about age 10 to 25. Its sites of predilection are the *shafts of the long tubular bones;* it occurs less commonly in the flat bones such as the ribs and sternum. *Grossly* it is a soft gray tumor which arises in marrow, erodes the bone cortex from within, and often causes new bone formation beneath the periosteum. *Microscopically* the tumor is composed of uniform small cells resembling lymphocytes, having little cytoplasm. When new bone formation occurs in this tumor, it is secondary to recurring hemorrhage in bone and is not a result of bone formation by the neoplastic cells directly.

natural history

The natural history of this neoplasm is often confused by an early period in which the symptoms (pain, tender swelling, fever, and leukocytosis) lead to a diagnosis of osteomyelitis rather than neoplasm. *Metastases often appear in other bones,* a feature rarely noted in other neoplasms primary in bone. Metastases also occur in the lungs. Death usually occurs 2 to 3 years after onset. *X-ray therapy* often causes temporary improvement, but the outlook is even more *hopeless* than with osteogenic sarcoma.

Synovial sarcoma

Synovial sarcoma, a rare tumor also known as *synovioma,* arises from the synovial membrane of the joints and is therefore somewhat out of place under neoplasms of bone. It is included here because it is frequently confused with bone neoplasms and behaves essentially like a bone neoplasm. Grossly it is a soft, hemorrhagic tumor affecting the membranes of the joints and the ends of contiguous bones. *Microscopically* most synoviomas contain two types of cells: spindle-shaped *connective tissue cells* suggesting fibrosarcoma, and *cuboidal cells* resembling columnar epithelium. The latter, called synovioblasts, line microscopic *cleftlike spaces in the tumor.* The *natural history* of this tumor is one of slow local progression, often over a period of 3 or 4 years, followed later by metastases to the lungs. Sometimes synovial sarcoma extends to the regional lymph nodes, quite at variance with the usual course in other neoplasms of bone.

Miscellaneous forms

Certain systemic neoplasms, affecting primarily the reticuloendothelial system and therefore the bone marrow, may manifest themselves by bone pain or by pathologic fractures and be confused with true primary neoplasms of bone. The most important of these is *multiple myeloma,* but *reticulum cell sarcoma* and *Hodgkin's disease* may also present similar symptoms. These diseases are considered in Chapter 17.

METASTATIC TUMORS

Metastatic tumors of bone are much *more common than primary tumors,* especially after middle age. Carcinomas of the *prostate* almost regularly metastasize to bone, particularly the bones of the pelvis and lower spine. Carcinomas of the *lungs, breasts, thyroid gland,* and *kidneys* also metastasize to bone frequently, sometimes causing bone symptoms before there are symptoms related to the primary tumor. Any malignant tumor may on occasion metastasize to bone.

JOINTS

1. General Considerations

Types of joints

The joints form the connecting links between the rigid members of the skeleton, providing stability while permitting motion. *Three types of joints* are described: (1) *fibrous* joints, which unite bones at suture lines and permit little or no motion; (2) *cartilaginous* joints, such as occur between the bodies of two adjacent vertebrae, where no true joint space exists, but the intervertebral disk serves as a cushion to permit limited motion; and (3) *synovial* joints, in which a space filled with fluid (synovia) is interposed between two bones whose articular surfaces are covered with cartilage; these permit a wide range of motion. The last two types of joints, at which motion (and therefore friction) occurs, are of great clinical importance because of their proneness to disease.

Structure of joints

Gardner [12] has studied the structure of the moving joints with relation to the mechanical factors acting upon them. In the *vertebral column,* the nucleus pulposus of the intervertebral disk is a plastic mass which is held in shape by the cartilage plates covering the vertebral bodies above and below, and by the annulus fibrosus which surrounds the disk and contains it. The disk acts much as a pledget of soft rubber between two rigid blocks might act, permitting limited motion in all directions and serving as a shock-absorbing mechanism. In the *synovial joints,* where a much wider range of motion occurs, provision is made to minimize wear. The opposing bone surfaces are covered with *hyaline cartilage,* an avascular, relatively inert material, which yields to normal pressure without crushing or tearing and is self-polishing from the nature of its motion. The synovial joints are lined by *synovium,* a thin vascular connective tissue membrane having irregular folds and villi. Small fat pads are present in these folds, and these fat pads may serve a purpose by wiping the articular surfaces [12]. The *synovial fluid* is the most important substance for the lubrication of the synovial joints. It is a slippery, slightly viscid, clear fluid, apparently formed largely by dialysis through the synovial membrane from the blood plasma, although at least one component of synovial fluid appears to be derived from the articular cartilage itself [13]. Only minute quantities of the fluid are present in healthy joints – about 1 ml. in a knee joint, on an average [14]; the fluid is almost acellular and consists largely of water plus the mucopolysaccharide *hyaluronic acid,* which accounts for the viscidity. Hyaluronic acid is bound to protein in the synovial fluid, and this complex is capable of forming gels under pressure. These gels are believed to occupy the pits which form in the articular cartilage as a result of wear and tear, and to give up liquid synovia at times of heavy joint load, thus enhancing the lubricant action when needed [15].

Rheumatism and arthritis

The layman may use the term *rheumatism* to designate any painful disorder in which the principal symptoms are related to the joints or their anatomic supporting structures. The patient may include under this overall term such totally unrelated conditions as bone tumors and fractures involving joints, hemophilia, scurvy, and scleroderma, as well as diseases primary in the joints. *Arthritis* is a more restrictive term meaning *inflammation of a joint;* it is broad enough to cover all the bacterial and nonbacterial processes which may incite an inflammatory reaction in the joint tissues. Since most organic diseases of the joints do show features of inflammation, the term *arthritis* is generally used to cover *all joint diseases.* Obviously there are a number of subtitles.

Incidence and importance of arthritis

Evidence of arthritis has been revealed in the skeletal remains of the dinosaur and early man, and throughout the entire modern animal kingdom. Arthritis in man is said to cause total disability in 200,000 people in the United States, and 800,000 are partially disabled [16]. Lost wages due to arthritis amount to 7 million dollars in the United States each year [16]. It is also a problem of considerable importance to the farmer, whose annual losses from bovine arthritis run into millions of dollars [17].

Classification of arthritis

All attempts at the classification of arthritis are necessarily unsatisfactory, since the *causes of most cases of joint disease are largely unknown.* The best that can be done is to separate those diseases in which the cause is known from the much larger group in which it is unknown, and then to divide the unknown group along clinical lines.

2. *Acute Bacterial Arthritis*

Pathologic changes

Acute bacterial arthritis is usually due to a *pyogenic coccus* (staphylococcus, streptococcus, pneumococcus, gonococcus). The presence of these organisms in synovial fluid is usually the result of a septic state with hematogenous dissemination from some primary focus, such as the skin or urinary tract; occasionally the organisms reach the joint as a result of a penetrating wound or compound fracture involving the joint. Hyperemia and edema of the synovial membrane result, and there is an outpouring of polymorphonuclear neutrophils into the joint space. The result is usually a *suppurative arthritis,* the causative organisms being demonstrable on smear or culture of the synovial fluid, which has all the characteristics of an exudate. Fibrin is sometimes found in fluid of this type, but the viscosity of the fluid is less than normal [14]. Occasionally the infection spreads to the periarticular tissues.

Clinical features

Since acute bacterial arthritis is usually part of a general picture of sepsis, the patient is usually already acutely ill, with high fever and chills. With gonococcal arthritis the joint manifestations usually dominate the picture, although evidence of the venereal infection can often be obtained. The affected joint is swollen, reddened, and painful on motion. Sometimes several joints, chiefly the large ones, are involved.

Outcome

If the patient recovers from the general condition of sepsis, the likelihood of recovery from the arthritis is good. Often there is some restriction of motion due to a degree of fibrous ankylosis, but if effective therapy has been given promptly, there may be complete recovery of the joint.

3. *Chronic Bacterial Arthritis*

Certain bacterial infections of the joints tend to incite a chronic inflammatory reaction in the synovial tissues and adjacent bone, and may be confused clinically with rheumatoid arthritis or degenerative joint disease. The most important of these is tuberculosis.

TUBERCULOSIS

Joint tuberculosis is generally *secondary to bone tuberculosis* and the two are discussed together in an earlier section of this chapter.

SYPHILIS

Arthritis occurs with *syphilis* but the spirochete does not affect the joints directly; thus the arthritis occurring under these circumstances is not, strictly speaking, bacterial. The *joint changes are secondary to neurologic disturbances due to syphilis,* and are considered under degenerative joint disease.

BRUCELLOSIS

Brucellosis is another cause of chronic bacterial arthritis. Lowbeer [18] has described the arthritis and spondylitis that occur with human brucellar infection, and has studied the spontaneous and experimental lesions caused by brucellosis of bones and joints in animals. In most instances it appears that the intervertebral disks and vertebral bodies are directly affected, a *combined arthritis and osteomyelitis.* Abscesses and caseous foci occur, and in some instances extend to cause paravertebral abscesses. Lesions in other bones and joints also occur. Sometimes the arthritis is monarticular and destructive, leading to ankylosis of the joint. In other cases a polyarticular migratory arthritis, clinically resembling acute rheumatic fever, occurs and dominates the clinical picture [19]. As with rheumatic fever, this form is usually followed by complete recovery.

4. *Arthritis of Rheumatic Fever*

Pathologic changes

Rheumatic fever characteristically affects *preadolescent children,* and the arthritis is *acute, polyarticular,* and *migratory.* The cause is unknown, but a relationship to group A streptococcal infection is widely assumed. At the beginning the synovium shows an *acute inflammatory reaction,* with hyperemia, edema, and leukocytic infiltration; the synovial fluid is slightly turbid due to the presence of large numbers of polymorphonuclear cells [14], but is *sterile* on culture. Later mononuclear cells and lymphocytes predominate in both the synovium and the synovia. At no time are lesions seen in the synovium that are comparable to the Aschoff bodies of the myocardium (see Chapter 18).

Clinical features

As a rule the arthritis appears suddenly *several weeks after* an episode of *group A streptococcus infection* of the upper respiratory tract. First one large joint and then another is affected, becoming swollen, hot, and extremely painful on motion. As the condition spreads to a new joint, the inflammation in the old one tends to subside. Evidence of carditis or pleuritis often accompanies the arthritis.

Outcome

The *joints usually recover completely* following inflammation due to rheumatic fever. There is no tendency to ankylosis. The arthritis may recur with subsequent attacks of rheumatic fever, but the *prognosis is dependent upon the course of the cardiac disease,* not upon the joint lesions.

5. *Rheumatoid Arthritis*

Rheumatoid arthritis is a chronic inflammatory disease of the joints; it affects women chiefly (3 females:1 male) and has its onset characteristically in middle life.

Causes

Its cause or *causes remain obscure* after years of intensive study by a number of different groups of workers. Bacterial, mycoplasmal, and viral *infections, hypersensitivity states, endocrine imbalances,* and *other possibilities* have been investigated but *none has been proved to be the specific cause of rheumatoid arthritis.* Perhaps there is no single cause. Investigation of a comparable disease in swine [20] has thrown no light on the cause of the disease in man.

Pathologic changes: joints

The changes in the joints vary with the stage of the disease as well as from case to case. Studying *punch biopsies of the synovium* of the knee, Zevely and his co-workers [21] noted varying degrees of proliferation of synovial cells and fibroblasts, disarrangement of collagen fibers, edema, increased vascularity, and minimal cell infiltration, consisting chiefly of lymphocytes and plasma cells; however, the microscopic picture was not sufficiently distinctive to permit a differentiation to be made from lupus erythematosus, dermatomyositis, or Reiter's syndrome. In more advanced cases the synovium appears greatly thickened, the articular cartilage becomes eroded, exposing the bone irregularly in the joint, and granulation tissue comes to line the cavity. The *synovial fluid* in different cases of rheumatoid arthritis [14] varies in appearance from clear to frankly turbid, its cell count being between 450 and 66,000 cells per cubic millimeter. Viscosity of the fluid is generally much less than normal, and *cultures are sterile.*

other tissues

Changes in tissues other than those of the joints are also inconstant. *Subcutaneous nodules* occur in 15 to 20 percent of the cases, and their microscopic pattern is rather predictable: the center of the nodule is generally necrotic, eosinophilic, and somewhat granular; this area is surrounded by a zone of radially arranged elongated cells resembling the epithelioid cells of a tubercle, with lymphocytes and plasma cells interspersed. The *heart* shows endocardial or pericardial lesions in some cases, but in the authors' experience the frequency of valvular lesions nowhere approaches the figure of 65 percent that is sometimes quoted [16]. Lesions in small arteries, lymph nodes, and uveal tracts of the eyes have been described in occasional cases, but are neither frequent nor distinctive. With prolonged invalidism the bones develop *osteoporosis of disuse.*

Clinical features

Clinical manifestations are as variable as the pathologic findings. In some cases the onset is relatively acute, with fever, and with *pain, swelling, and stiffness in one or more joints.* In most cases the onset is more *insidious.* Any of the synovial joints may be affected, including the small joints of the fingers. *Multiple joints* are usually involved, often in more or less symmetric fashion, but the process is *not usually migratory;* instead of clearing up, the joint alterations lead to *deformity* with restriction of the range of motion. A particularly characteristic deformity is that of the hands, consisting of flexion and ulnar deviation of the fingers at the metacarpophalangeal joints. *Constitutional symptoms are inconstant;* weakness, anemia, leukopenia, splenic enlargement, and lymphadenopathy are occasionally noted. Cardiac symptoms are seldom evident. Subcutaneous nodules, when present, are usually found over bony prominences (as over the ulnas and clavicles). They must be searched for carefully, since the patient usually does not note their presence (they are usually painless); most are 0.5 to 2 cm. in diameter.

Laboratory findings

The sedimentation rate is usually increased, C-reactive protein is elevated, and agglutination of suspensions of sheep red cells, latex, or bentonite particles may be positive. These *tests for the "rheumatoid factor,"* while of some value, are certainly *nonspecific.* Positive tests may occur in a number of conditions in which the joints are not affected. These tests are dependent upon the presence of *abnormal globulins* in the serum. Electrophoretic studies often show an *elevation of the gamma globulin fraction* of the serum proteins. The thymol turbidity and zinc sulfate turbidity tests, also reflecting the presence of abnormal proteins, are often significantly elevated. Probably none of these empiric tests should be given any greater weight in the diagnosis of rheumatoid arthritis than is accorded the history, temperature, pulse rate, or degree of swelling of a joint.

Outcome

In a small percentage of cases the inflammatory process subsides, joint motility returns, and all symptoms and signs are resolved. Much more commonly the disease goes through a *series of remissions and exacerbations,* the net effect of which is *slow progression over a period of many years.* In the most severe cases there is *fibrous ankylosis of many joints,* usually a flexion deformity, with bedridden invalidism, muscle atrophy, and osteoporosis. Patients with advanced stages of this disease occupy a large fraction of the hospital beds used by the chronically ill. Nevertheless the disease is quite compatible with long life. Usually the patient finally succumbs to an infection, as of the respiratory tract; occasionally secondary amyloidosis supervenes; in some patients death results from iatrogenic factors, especially in relation to steroid therapy.

Special forms:

Since no specific cause of rheumatoid arthritis can be demonstrated in the tissues or body fluids, and since the tissue changes and clinical course are so variable, it is impossible to be certain that all cases classified as rheumatoid arthritis are in fact instances of the same disease. *It may well be that a number of different diseases producing similar effects are grouped together under the one diagnosis.* Several characteristic clinical patterns of progressive, inflammatory joint disease are recognized at present, and are generally considered as special forms of rheumatoid arthritis.

spondylitis

Rheumatoid spondylitis (Marie-Strümpell disease) is a particularly striking (and distressing) example. This disease is characterized by *inflammation of the cartilaginous joints between the vertebral bodies* and of the *gliding joints between the vertebral arches of the spine.* It usually begins in the lumbar area and extends upward. It leads to progressive *fibrous ankylosis* of the cartilaginous joints, often with *kyphosis* of such severity that the patient cannot raise his head to see in front at eye level. Kyphosis also leads to restriction of motion of the ribs and eventually to impaired pulmonary ventilation. This in turn may lead to cor pulmonale and heart failure. This disease differs from the usual type of rheumatoid arthritis in that *males are almost exclusively affected,* the onset is usually at an *earlier age* (about age 30), *iritis* is a common associated lesion (and sometimes leads to blindness), and *aortic insufficiency or stenosis* is sometimes noted. Perhaps some of these cases are due to brucellosis, a disease which also commonly causes spondylitis, affects males chiefly, has its onset in early adult life, and may cause iritis and aortic valve disease [22].

collagen diseases

Recurrent joint inflammation closely resembling rheumatoid arthritis is often noted as a feature of the collagen diseases, particularly *disseminated lupus erythematosus* and *polyarteritis.* These diseases, generally believed to be due to hypersensitivity, serve to emphasize that *hypersensitivity is the most widely held explanation for rheumatoid arthritis itself,* although the nature of the allergen(s) is unknown: certainly the joints frequently participate in allergic responses, as in serum sickness. A syndrome resembling rheumatoid arthritis in some cases, and disseminated lupus erythematosus in others, has been observed following the use of hydralazine (Apresoline) in the treatment of hypertension [23]. (For a fuller consideration of the hypersensitivity states and the collagen diseases, see Chapter 4.)

other forms

Still's disease is a form of chronic polyarthritis in children, often accompanied by splenomegaly. *Felty's syndrome* is a form of chronic polyarthritis in adults and is associated with splenomegaly and leukopenia. *Reiter's syndrome* is chronic polyarthritis, chiefly of males, with associated nonspecific urethritis and conjunctivitis; a recent outbreak of this syndrome followed an epidemic of bacillary dysentery (shigellosis) on an American naval vessel [24]. *Palindromic rheumatism* is a rare form of recurrent polyarthritis; it is characterized by many years of brief but severe episodes of joint swelling, usually with little residual joint disease. *Psoriatic arthritis* is a term that simply recognizes the occasional association of the chronic skin disease, *psoriasis,* with a polyarthritis which is otherwise typical of rheumatoid arthritis. An association of polyarthritis with *ulcerative colitis* is also noted in some patients, and with *intestinal lipodystrophy* in others, but it is difficult to make anything of the relationship.

6. *Acute Traumatic Arthritis*

Pathologic changes

Recurring *trauma* is undoubtedly of great importance in all types of arthritis, but under this heading we shall consider only those instances resulting from a single, well-recognized physical injury. The injury may be a direct one, causing *fracture of an articular surface* or *penetration of the joint by a foreign body,* or it may be an indirect one due to a twisting or wrenching motion or loss of balance, causing *rupture of ligaments or tendons* within the joint or external to it, *tears of the semilunar cartilage, disruption of the joint capsule* with *dislocation* or *subluxation,* and the like. Many such injuries occur as a result of *sporting accidents,* as in football or skiing; often the milder forms are termed sprains or strains. Recovery is usually complete if the injured structures lie outside the joint proper; only a slight serous effusion occurs in the joint and there is little inflammation of the synovium. If there is significant hemorrhage into the joint *(hemarthrosis),* as is often the case when structures within the joint are injured, recovery is delayed and often incomplete. *Blood incites an inflammatory reaction in the synovium* (as it does in other serous membranes), leading to the formation of fibrous and scar tissue and eventually to erosion of the articular surface, with limitation of motion. A similar clinical picture is sometimes seen in *hemophilia,* even without significant trauma. The end result of significant *joint hemorrhage* is often *degenerative joint disease.*

Clinical features

Usually symptoms follow directly upon the injury and are extreme: excruciating *pain on motion, swelling, and discoloration of periarticular tissues.* Radiographs often reveal small fractures, even when the clinical evaluation does not suggest such an injury. Occasionally joint injury is masked by other injuries, especially if the part is splinted while the patient is unconscious. In such a case the joint injury may not be evident until weight-bearing is resumed some time after the accident.

Outcome

If there has been real injury to the tissues within the joint or to the articular surfaces, *some disability is likely to persist, especially in the case of weight-bearing joints.* Loose bodies, derived from fractures of the articular surface or from fragments of meniscus, may remain in the joint cavity, causing either locking of the joint or some degree of restriction of motion. Injuries of the phalanges of the hands, such as follow baseball accidents, particularly in catchers, are often followed by stiff, painful fingers. A torn joint capsule may remain weak, permitting recurrent dislocation. A limp, favoring a joint that is only slightly painful, may result in unusual stresses in other joints, causing in time post-traumatic degenerative joint disease (see section following).

7. *Degenerative Joint Disease: Osteoarthritis*

Nature and cause

Degenerative joint disease is the most common of all the types of joint disease; some degree of degeneration and wear of the joints is almost inevitable with aging, and this is essentially the change that is implied by the term *osteoarthritis. Aging brings loss of elasticity of the joint capsules, articular cartilages,* and *ligaments,* as it does of other elastic tissues. This leads to a *lessening of joint stability,* and to a *greater tendency to joint wear.* One must add to this the *cumulative effect of multiple injuries,* large and small, direct and indirect, of *diminished vascular supply,* due to developing vascular sclerosis, of *obesity,* and of *occupation.* It is a great wonder that these moving parts stand up as well as they do to all this abuse: no manmade machine is so efficient!

Weight bearing and trauma

Naturally it is the *weight-bearing joints* that are first affected in most instances. As every athlete knows, "It's the legs that go first." An obese policeman, walking on hard pavements for many years, will almost certainly develop changes in the joints of his feet. Males are more often affected by osteoarthritis of the large joints than females, presumably because of greater exposure to injury. Degenerative changes in the small joints of the hands are about equally distributed between the sexes. If there is some form of static deformity of the spine, as from childhood poliomyelitis, or some congenital or acquired disease of bones or joints, this may result in compensatory adjustment of posture and gait so that unusual forces act upon certain joints, increasing the tendency to osteoarthritis. Loss of sense of pain and position, usually due to *neurosyphilis* (tabes dorsalis) or *syringomyelia,* leads to recurrent joint injury and an especially severe form of degenerative arthritis in which swelling is great and dissolution of all joint structures occurs *(Charcot's joint* or *neurotropic arthropathy).* Caisson workers, with their proneness to aseptic necrosis of bone from air embolism, commonly develop severe osteoarthritis of the large joints [3]. Other occupations cause recurrent injuries of specific joints, with residual degenerative joint disease: the knees in football players, shoulders and elbows in baseball pitchers, fingers of the unprotected hand in baseball catchers, ankles in ballet dancers, wrists and elbows in pneumatic drill workers (and carpal and tarsal joints in racehorses!).

Systemic factors

There is some evidence that *hereditary* and *systemic* factors may also contribute to the pathogenesis of osteoarthritis, at least in some instances [25]. The condition is common in that rare hereditary disorder known as *ochronosis,* presumably due to deposits of homogentisic acid in the articular cartilage. *Acromegaly* is frequently accompanied by osteoarthritis. Small laboratory animals are subject to osteoarthritis, presumably on a genetic basis.

Pathologic changes

Ackerman [26], studying early lesions of degenerative joint disease in legs amputated for other reasons, came to the conclusion that the *joint cartilage is the key to the tissue changes in osteoarthritis.* Due to the friction of weight bearing and motion and to the *loss of elasticity* in the cartilage, there is *thinning* of the articular cartilage, leading to *narrowing of the joint space* and to *loss of stability.* These changes in turn lead to fraying and *irregular erosion* of the cartilage, the latter change being evident as shallow pits on the articular surface. Cartilage, being an inert tissue, does not regenerate following injury; bone, as it becomes exposed on the joint surface, tends to react to recurrent injury by cellular overgrowth. This overgrowth leads to *gross irregularity of the joint surfaces* and to further fragmentation, so that *particles of bone and cartilage break loose into the joint cavity.* Bone overgrowth at the edges of the articular surface causes spurlike masses to project into the joint capsule, a condition easily noted on radiographs of the joint, and referred to as *lipping.*

Clinical features

The onset of osteoarthritis is so gradual as to go almost unnoticed in the majority of cases. With advancing years the transient aches and pains in the joints following exertion, probably due to beginning joint changes, are usually attributed to being "out of condition," as noted by Schubert [27]. There is often *some restriction of motion* (as inability to squat) and *some discomfort in an unaccustomed position* (as on one's knees to tack down a carpet). Even when symptoms are no more pronounced than this, *radiographs may show extensive changes.* If symptoms are present and are related to a specific joint, they are generally a result of *recent trauma* or a sequel of *unusual trauma in early life.* (This situation often leads to court disagreements between members of the medical profession. A workman will claim disability as a result of recent joint injury, but the radiographs may show only chronic proliferative changes and lipping that must from their very nature antedate the injury. The plaintiff's physician will emphasize the lack of symptoms prior to the injury, while the defendant's expert will claim that symptoms represent only the natural progression of preexisting disease [27].) There are *no constitutional symptoms* related to osteoarthritis although there may, of course, be symptoms due to aging generally. Physical examination usually shows limitation of motion and pain on motion in the chiefly affected joint with lesser changes in the other joints. *Heberden's nodes,* bony nodules on the lateral and medial aspects of the distal interphalangeal joints of the fingers, are often evident and are generally considered to support a diagnosis of degenerative arthritis. *Radiographs usually show characteristic changes,* but *laboratory tests,* including the sedimentation rate and C-reactive protein, usually give *normal results* in osteoarthritis. The exception to this statement is the occasional patient in whom rheumatoid arthritis and osteoarthritis coexist, in the same or in different joints.

Outcome

Usually *life is not shortened as a result of osteoarthritis.* In most instances there is *slow progression of the disease* without striking new developments. Sometimes an obese person with degenerative arthritis of hip or knee following an old injury will have a great deal of pain and discomfort, and be confined to a wheelchair. More often the patient learns to accept his joint disease as a part of growing old, and regulates his activities accordingly.

8. Degeneration and Herniation of the Nucleus Pulposus

Pathologic changes

Alteration of the nucleus pulposus of the vertebral column, while unrelated to osteoarthritis, is also a result of degenerative changes. According to Putschar, in his discussion of Hansen's paper [28], the intervertebral disks begin to show retrogressive changes at about age 20. These consist of *loss of vascularity, dehydration,* and *chemical alterations,* which tend to modify disk response to motion and weight bearing, making the disk more prone to protrusion through weak spots in the annulus fibrosus. Herniation of the nucleus pulposus occurs chiefly in the *lumbar or cervical portions of the vertebral column,* presumably because there is a greater range of motion of the spine at these levels. Cervical lesions are sometimes the result of whiplash injuries. Herniation may occur at any point on the circumference of the disk, but it produces symptoms only when the projection occurs posteriorly or posterolaterally, *compressing the spinal cord or the nerve roots.* (It is of interest that disk herniation and its clinical effects were recognized by a veterinarian in dogs some 30 years before the lesions were identified in man. The disorder is apparently common in dachshunds of any age, and occurs in older dogs of many breeds. Comparable lesions of the intervertebral disks have been observed in cats, horses, cattle, pigs, and camels [28].)

Clinical features

In the lumbar area the protrusions usually occur below the level of the spinal cord proper, resulting in compression of the cauda equina or nerve roots, thus producing *pain along the course of the sciatic nerves* (sciatica), and sometimes motor changes as well. In the cervical region the herniated mass is usually smaller, presumably because the weight compressing the affected disk is less; nerve roots are chiefly affected, producing *pain in the arms* and occasionally paralysis or muscle atrophy. Since herniation often occurs suddenly with lifting or twisting motions, pain may come on with lightning-like suddenness, causing the victim to fall to the floor. With prolonged rest there is usually gradual lessening of pain, but individuals once affected are prone to recurrences of herniation, either at the same or at different levels.

9. Gout

Nature of the disease

Gout is a constitutional disorder occurring chiefly in males; it is manifest by joint disease and is associated with an inherited *defect of uric acid metabolism* which is transmitted as a dominant gene. The disease occurs in two forms: *acute gouty arthritis,* in which there is sudden severe inflammation, usually of a single joint, and *chronic tophaceous gout,* in which there are multiple joint deformities and extensive deposits of urates in the tissues.

Uric acid metabolism

Normally in man, uric acid is formed from purines derived from the breakdown of cell nuclei and from dietary sources; all other nitrogenous substances are split to urea and excreted as such. In patients with *"primary" gout,* or with familial hyperuricemia without gout, *uric acid may be formed in excess* as the result of blockage of alternate pathways for the elimination of precursor substances [29]; the total yield of uric acid may then be greater than the kidneys can excrete. With an excess of urates in the blood, these relatively insoluble substances tend to be deposited in the tissues *(tophaceous gout). Hyperuricemia* (usually given as above 7.5 mg. uric acid per 100 ml. of serum in the male and above 6.5 mg. in the female) may also occur under some circumstances when the normal metabolic pathways of uric acid are not at fault. Thus hyperuricemia and acute gout may occur in *leukemia* or *polycythemia* when there is excessive destruction of cell nuclei, or *following the use of chlorothiazide* for the treatment of hypertension; these cases are sometimes referred to as *"secondary" gout.*

The enigma of gout

Hyperuricemia is not always associated with joint disease; apparently some additional factor, as yet unknown, is necessary to produce the clinical picture of gout. Seegmiller and his associates [30] suggest that an inflammatory reaction must develop to the crystals of monosodium urate which are deposited in the synovium, and that this depends upon a number of systemic and local factors. It is acute gout that presents the enigma: the crises which occur in this form are not related to sudden rises in the level of uric acid in the blood. Chronic tophaceous gout seems more clearly related to persistent hyperuricemia than does acute gout. In this connection the metabolism of uric acid in reptiles and birds is of interest. In these "uricotelic" animals, uric acid (rather than urea) is the natural end product of nitrogenous metabolism, and the avian kidney can eliminate uric acid in large quantities. Schlumberger [31] reports that with renal disease parakeets and other birds develop synovial and other lesions closely simulating human tophaceous gout.

Pathologic changes

There have been few studies of the synovial membrane during an attack of *acute gouty arthritis.* Chemical determination of uric acid in synovial fluid of patients with gout yields values that equal those in the serum; a similar balance is noted in normal persons [14]. The lesions of *chronic tophaceous gout* are better known. Firm nodular masses *(tophi)* occur beneath the skin of the ears, in the periarticular tissues of the fingers, toes, and elbows, and in the synovial membranes and articular cartilages of the large joints. When incised, these masses are chalky white and somewhat pasty, often with gritty calcium masses interspersed. Microscopically *sheaves of needle-like crystals* can be demonstrated in tissues treated with xanthydrol, and polarized light reveals that these crystals are doubly refractile. A characteristic tissue reaction consisting of foreign-body giant cells, lymphocytes, and monocytes occurs at the periphery of the tophi. Similar, although smaller, deposits of urates are frequently noted in the renal medulla, chiefly in the interstitial tissues but also in the tubules, and in about 10 percent of fatal cases uric acid calculi will be found in the urinary tract. Vascular disease related to hypertension is commonly noted in patients with chronic gout, but the lesions are in no way specific for gout.

Clinical features

The acute attack of gout often follows a period of intemperate eating or drinking; it begins frequently with an *abrupt onset, often at night, of acute inflammation of the metatarsophalangeal joint of one of the great toes,* the classic *podagra.* Spontaneous and complete recovery usually occurs in a few days, without other joints being affected. Subsequent attacks occur at intervals of a year or so, gradually becoming more frequent and perhaps affecting larger joints, although *usually monarticular* in form in the single attack. Serum uric acid levels are only slightly elevated during the acute attacks. *Colchicine* therapy is effective in preventing and relieving attacks of acute gout, but it has no effect upon the uric acid level in the blood [30]. After 10 years or so, about half the patients who have recurrent attacks of gouty arthritis develop chronic tophaceous gout. The urate deposits occur in the hands and feet, and the skin over the large nodular lesions sometimes ulcerates. The deposits in the synovial membranes and articular cartilages cause a *progressive deforming arthritis.* Prophylactic treatment with uricosuric agents plus a restrictive diet sometimes forestalls the development of tophaceous gout; however, there is some danger of the development of uric acid calculi during the period of therapy with these drugs, because of the large amounts of uric acid eliminated in the urine. The renal complications of gout are usually manifest by mounting azotemia and evidence of impaired renal function, but when proteinuria and hypertension develop, they are usually a result of complicating nephrosclerosis.

Outcome

Most patients with gout live out their usual life span, although handicapped by progressive disease of the joints. Gout seems to predispose its victims to *vascular disease;* hypertension commonly occurs, and often causes death from coronary or cerebral thrombosis in the sixth or seventh decade. Gouty nephritis, with or without calculi, may cause death in azotemia at about the same age.

10. Hypertrophic Pulmonary Osteoarthropathy

Nature of the process

Hypertrophic pulmonary osteoarthropathy, a peculiar thickening and widening of the bones and periarticular tissues of the *distal phalanges of the fingers and toes,* has long been known, and its *association with chronic pulmonary disease* has also long been recognized. It is not so generally known that an active inflammatory process in the joints of the hands, wrists, feet, and ankles sometimes occurs in these patients, and may be confused with rheumatoid arthritis.

Pathologic changes

The pain, swelling, and tenderness of the large joints, and the clubbing of fingers and toes, are due to the *deposition of calcium in the subperiosteal tissues about the joints.* These proliferative bone changes may come on with amazing rapidity, especially in children. The authors have seen a striking degree of clubbed fingers, plus acute arthritis of the ankles, develop within a period of 4 months in a 70-year-old man with a myxoma of the left atrium.

Causes

When the condition was first described, its relationship to chronic pulmonary disease was reported. Since then, clubbed fingers have been noted in association with an ever-widening range of diseases, including the following: (1) *respiratory* – tuberculosis, lung abscess, bronchiectasis, empyema, bronchiogenic carcinoma, mediastinal diseases; (2) *circulatory* – many types of congenital heart disease, especially those associated with chronic cyanosis, and arteriovenous communications in the peripheral vessels; (3) *digestive* – biliary cirrhosis and liver abscess, steatorrhea due to various causes, and ulcerative colitis. (It should be emphasized that clubbed fingers occur only *occasionally* in the disorders mentioned, and that the factor or factors specifically responsible for the development of the bone changes is not known, in spite of centuries of familiarity with the process.) It is said that clubbing of the fingers may occur in the absence of any of the diseases mentioned, but the authors have never observed significant clubbing at autopsy without finding one of the diseases listed above. Obviously periosteal ossification may occur from other causes, and may be confused with periarticular calcification (as in Heberden's nodes of osteoarthritis), but this is another question.

11. Neoplasms of Joints

Since neoplasms of joints usually affect the bones as well as the joints, and since they are usually *considered clinically as bone tumors,* they are discussed in the earlier section of this chapter along with neoplasms of bones. *Synovioma* is the important – though rare – *malignant* neoplasm of the joints. *Giant cell tumor* is the important – and fairly common – *benign* neoplasm of joints, also affecting bones and tendons. A related and somewhat rarer condition is known as *pigmented villonodular synovitis.* It represents a bulky overgrowth of the synovium of a large joint; there are extensive hemosiderin deposits, which are sometimes present in sufficient quantity to outline the neoplasm within the joint cavity on radiographs. The knee is usually affected and there is often a history of prior trauma. There is some question whether the process is a true benign neoplasm, or a non-neoplastic overgrowth of connective tissue in response to injury and hemorrhage. The lesion sometimes seems invasive and in some cases there are microscopic areas very reminiscent of giant cell tumor; hence most pathologists consider it as a benign neoplasm.

BURSAE

The bursae are flat, thin-walled, poorly defined spaces containing synovial fluid and lying adjacent to bones and joints. They apparently serve to facilitate joint motion by permitting the soft tissues to slip easily over the joints.

BURSAL CYSTS

The bursal sacs are not particularly subject to disease. The most common abnormality of a bursa is *ganglion,* a cystic lesion which occurs usually at the *wrist* and occasionally on the dorsum of the foot. Apparently it occurs as a result of an effusion into a bursa, or perhaps of a herniation of the synovial sac of one of the small joints. It shows as a soft, rounded, fluctuant, usually painless swelling beneath the skin. Cystic bursal lesions occasionally develop in connection with other joints: *Baker's cyst* occurs *in the popliteal space* and occasionally extends upward or downward in the soft tissues of the leg for some distance; it usually communicates with the knee joint. Bursal cysts have a *dense fibrous wall* divided by fibrous septa. The cyst fluid is watery or mucinous and may contain small, flat, seedlike particles.

BURSITIS

Inflammation of the bursae may occur. Often this is a result of *mild recurrent injury,* as is the case in "housemaid's knee," affecting the prepatellar bursae. Bursitis may also follow local or systemic *bacterial infections.* More commonly no actual cause is found. The bursae about the shoulders are among those most frequently affected, and may cause considerable discomfort. In most instances the process is chronic. The tissue changes consist of fibrosis and lymphocytic infiltration of the bursal wall, often with calcium deposits, and an increase of mucoid synovia in the bursal space.

MUSCLES

Chemistry and physiology

The shortening of voluntary muscle fibers is said to result from *two kinds of filaments* within the myofibril sliding past each other. These filaments, one composed of the protein *myosin* and the other of the protein *actin,* have been identified clearly in electron micrographs [32]. Energy for the action is derived from enzymatic splitting of a phosphate group from *adenosine triphosphate.* Normal muscles contain two forms of *myoglobin,* which can be separated chromatographically [33]. Attempts have been made to identify chemical and physiologic differences between normal and diseased muscle, but to date these have been inconclusive [34].

Nature of muscle diseases

Diseases of the muscles, except for those due to trauma or direct infection, are *rare.* Veterinarians tell us that *selenium,* and certain plants eaten by grazing animals, will cause generalized *muscle diseases in sheep and goats* [35]. An acute, reversible muscle syndrome has been described in some individuals consuming large amounts of *alcoholic beverages* [36]; phosphorylase activity seemed to be at fault in these cases. Some muscle diseases are *hereditary,* often sex-linked. These genetically determined diseases of muscle are of several types. *McArdle's disease* is the only one in which the nature of the metabolic defect is known – a *hereditary lack of skeletal muscle phosphorylase* [37] resulting in an inability to use muscle glycogen. As a result, muscle cramps are noted after moderate exercise, such as stair climbing or lifting. If exercise is continued, myoglobinuria may follow.

Laboratory findings

Certain enzyme tests of the blood, especially *creatine phosphokinase (CPK)* and *aldolase,* will reveal evidence of active muscle disease. Elevations of lactic dehydrogenase (LDH) and glutamic oxalic transaminase (GOT) levels also may be noted, but these enzymes are less specific for muscle than are the first two mentioned. Both skeletal and cardiac muscle show high CPK activity. Values for this enzyme may be increased 100-fold in certain types of muscle disease: childhood forms of muscular dystrophy, polymyositis, and acute myocardial infarction. Direct injury of muscles and even strenuous exercise such as the squat-jump may cause transient elevations. In severe cases of muscle injury, such as crushing of an extremity or acute destructive disease, myoglobin may appear in the urine. *Myoglobinuria* may be associated with renal failure, similar in many ways to that seen with hemoglobinuria.

Classification of muscle disease

Adams [35] has suggested that the muscle diseases can be better understood if we divide them into three categories, as follows:

I. *Diseases which cause disorder of motility*
   A. Neural and spinal atrophy
   B. Progressive muscular dystrophy
   C. Polymyositis
II. *Diffuse muscle diseases without much disturbance of motility,* usually metabolic or inflammatory in nature and part of a systemic disease (as Zenker's degeneration, trichinosis, sarcoidosis)
III. *Diseases localized to a single muscle,* as may be due to trauma, infection, neoplasm, or the like

ATROPHY

Neural and spinal atrophy is the muscle change resulting from interruption of the motor nerve supply, whether in the motor cortex, the lateral columns, the anterior horn cells of the spinal cord, or the peripheral nerves. In this group the *diseases of the nervous system are primary* and the muscular weakness is secondary. There is an *infantile form* (infantile muscular atrophy, Werdnig-Hoffman disease) in which some unknown destructive process affects scattered motor neurons, finally ending in most instances with *death from bulbar paralysis.* The affected muscles are wasted in appearance; microscopically atrophic muscle fibers are scattered among fibers having a normal appearance. In the more massive forms of spinal atrophy, including *amyotrophic lateral sclerosis, poliomyelitis, Guillian-Barré syndrome,* and *Jamaica ginger paralysis,* the entire mass of muscle fibers may show atrophy, and may eventually almost disappear. Kohn [38] suggests that the muscle changes in denervation atrophy are a result of activation of an autolytic system affecting the proteins in nonfunctioning muscle.

DYSTROPHY: Clinical types

Much more complex is the *genetically determined, sex-linked* condition known as *progressive muscular dystrophy.* A number of different forms have been described, affecting different muscle groups and having onset at different ages. The *pseudohypertrophic form* of Duchenne is the most common. It affects chiefly the pelvifemoral muscles, with onset at about age 3 to 6 years and death before age 20. Other forms affect the *facial and shoulder muscle groups* (Landouzy-Dejerine), the *shoulder and pelvic muscles* (Erb), or may be limited to the *eye muscles* (progressive ophthalmoplegia). One form, *Steinart's myotonic dystrophy,* is characterized by myotonia (i.e., sustained muscular contraction after stimulation) and, in addition, cataracts, testicular atrophy, and baldness. There is some question whether these several forms are fundamentally different or whether they represent varying penetrance or expression of a single basic defect. It appears that, in a given kindred, each case is strikingly like the others [39], and that there may be gradations between the different "types." *Cardiac involvement,* manifest generally by electrocardiographic changes, is commonly noted; in some instances cardiac failure occurs. Inheritance is believed to be typically *X-linked,* transmitted by females and appearing only in males. Serum levels for the enzymes, *creatine phosphokinase* and *aldolase,* are greatly elevated, especially in the younger patients, and it appears likely that enzyme level elevations can be detected even before the onset of muscle weakness [39]. Transaminase levels are also elevated but not as strikingly.

Microscopic changes

Microscopically there is a broad range of changes in muscle, from almost no abnormality in the youngest individuals affected to almost complete replacement of muscle bundles by adipose and fibrous tissue in the oldest patients. The essential change is *degeneration of the muscle fiber,* and there is no significant difference in the histologic manifestations of the different clinical types. Extremely large muscle fibers are mingled with narrow atrophic fibers; the nuclei of the muscle cells tend to migrate toward the center of the fibers from the normal sarcolemmal position; a floccular degeneration, with disorientation of the sarcolemmal fibers, is frequently seen; *ringed fibers* are the most striking change noted, consisting of a beltlike ring of striated fibers encircling more or less normal muscle fibers. There is almost no evidence of phagocytosis or of muscle fiber regeneration.

POLYMYOSITIS

Polymyositis is a somewhat controversial disease in that *skin lesions* and *connective tissue diseases* (lupus erythematosus, scleroderma, rheumatoid arthritis) are sometimes but not always associated. These combined cases, often called *dermatomyositis,* show exactly the same muscle lesions as do the cases in which the muscles only are affected [35]. The condition may occur at any age, including later life. The onset is usually rapid, the patient becoming bedfast because of muscle weakness within a few weeks. The proximal limb and the trunk muscles are the groups usually affected, but the muscles of the larynx and pharynx may also be involved. The muscles are not tender and there is usually no fever. *Creatine excretion is increased* and creatinine excretion decreased. Blood levels of *creatine phosphokinase and aldolase are greatly increased,* and occasionally myoglobin is excreted in the urine, due to the rapidity of *rhabdomyolysis.* Some patients die in the acute phase of the illness, either as a result of *pharyngeal paralysis* or from *lower nephron nephrosis,* but the great majority survive. Some recover almost completely but others have persistent muscle disability. *Microscopically* there is evidence of *active destruction of the muscle fibers,* with infiltration by lymphocytes, macrophages, and plasma cells, and with active phagocytosis of sarcolemmal fragments. Older, burnt-out cases may resemble progressive muscular dystrophy, although persistent inflammatory changes and evidence of regeneration usually serve to identify the case of polymyositis.

SYSTEMIC DISEASES AFFECTING MUSCLE

The muscles may be affected during the course of a number of systemic diseases. Perhaps the first to be described was *Zenker's hyaline degeneration* of voluntary muscle, seen especially in protracted febrile illnesses such as typhoid fever, in which marked dehydration occurs. The muscle fibers become coagulated and homogeneous, losing their cross striations. The rectus abdominis muscles are most commonly affected. *Trichinosis,* due to invasion of the muscles by *Trichinella spiralis,* is contracted by eating infested pork that has not been well cooked. Due to improved conditions on the farms and thanks to meat inspection, the frequency of trichinosis has decreased sharply in the United States in the last 20 years [40]. (For a further discussion of trichinosis, see Chapter 8.) The skeletal muscles are frequently affected in *polyarteritis* and other *collagen-vascular diseases,* even without the fullblown picture of polymyositis. *Boeck's sarcoid* sometimes involves the muscles generally, and random muscle biopsy has occasionally proved of value in the diagnosis of sarcoid. The microscopic changes are those characteristic of the disease – noncaseating granulomas with foreign-body giant cells and occasionally refractile inclusion bodies.

LOCALIZED MUSCLE DISEASES

The muscles are often affected by trauma and bacterial invasion. *Clostridial myositis* is an essential feature of gas gangrene: the organisms, and the gas formed by them, spread within as well as between the muscle fibers, producing coagulation necrosis and an inflammatory reaction. *Chronic myositis* due to tuberculosis, syphilis, or fungus infection is sometimes seen, but this is usually a consequence of similar involvement of adjacent bones and joints. Boeck's sarcoid may sometimes cause a palpable, localized, nodular form of myositis rather than systemic muscle disease. *Neoplasms of muscle,* both primary and secondary, are relatively rare; they are considered in Chapter 14.

IDIOPATHIC RHABDOMYOLYSIS

It has already been noted that *myolysis and myoglobinuria* may be important features in some cases of polymyositis. In addition, there is another condition, apparently rare, in which paroxysmal myolysis occurs, as a result of *unusual exercise* rather than as a result of muscle disease per se. This disorder, *idiopathic rhabdomyolysis,* seems to be *familial* and to occur chiefly in *males.* There may be no evidence of muscle disease on biopsy in spite of the fact that muscle enzymes may be strikingly elevated during an attack [41]. The *renal manifestations* of this form of myoglobinuria are identical to those seen following crushing muscle injury, and similar to those seen with the hemoglobinopathies.

MYOSITIS OSSIFICANS

Myositis ossificans is a peculiar disorder in which *bone is formed within one or more muscles.* The localized form is usually a result of trauma to the muscle with hemorrhage into its substance. The generalized form is of unknown cause, is sometimes familial, occurs chiefly in children, and may be associated with congenital anomalies, especially of the thumbs or big toes, resulting in shortening of those digits. In its fully developed stage the afflicted individual becomes virtually a *"stone man."* In both the localized and generalized forms, osteoid seems to arise from *alteration of fibrous connective tissue,* sometimes through an intermediate step in which cartilage is evident. The osteoid in such cases may be very cellular and may suggest the *microscopic* picture of osteogenic sarcoma. Occasionally a true osteogenic sarcoma arises in the muscle tissue of an extremity (extra-osseous osteogenic sarcoma).

TENDONS AND TENDON SHEATHS

TENO-SYNO-VITIS

Tenosynovitis is inflammation of a tendon sheath; it occurs chiefly in the hands and wrists or feet and ankles. The inflammation may be related to *recurrent mild injury* (as in pianists and typists), it may be a sequence of *acute trauma and infection* (usually streptococcal) occurring in the hand, or it may be *tuberculous,* associated with tuberculous dactylitis. There is an inflammatory exudate of the lining of the tendon sheaths; this is often associated with the formation of fibrin, followed by the development of adhesions between the tendon and the lining of its sheath. With time such adhesions result in contractures and distortions of the affected tissues. The most common form is *Dupuytren's contracture,* occurring chiefly in males and causing a thickening and shortening of the palmar fascia and related tendons, with flexion deformity of the third, fourth, and fifth fingers.

REFERENCES

1. Potter, E. L. *Seminar on Diseases of the Perinatal Period.* Chicago: American Society of Clinical Pathologists, 1965.
2. Morse, T. S., and Pryles, C. V. Infections of the bones and joints in children. *New Eng. J. Med.* 262:846, 1960. (A summary of clinical experience with skeletal infections in which antibiotics have been used.)
3. Coley, B. L., and Moore, M., Jr. Caisson disease with special reference to the bones and joints. *Ann. Surg.* 3:399, 1940.
4. Innes, J. R. M. "Inherited dysplasia" of the hip joint in dogs and rabbits. *Lab. Invest.* 8:1170, 1959. (This paper, and the discussion by C. N. Barron, shine interesting sidelights on Legg-Calvé-Perthes disease in children.)
5. Snapper, I. *Bone Diseases in Medical Practice.* New York: Grune & Stratton, 1957. (This clinical presentation of metabolic bone diseases is abundantly illustrated with excellent radiographs.)
6. Caldwell, R. A. Observations on the incidence, aetiology and pathology of senile osteoporosis. *J. Clin. Path.* 15:421, 1962. (A postmortem study of bone changes with aging.)
7. Davis, M. E., Strandjord, N. M., and Lanzl, L. H. Estrogens and the aging process. *J.A.M.A.* 196:129, 1966. (This controlled, prospective study of osteoporosis in menopausal women shows the beneficial effects of long-term estrogen therapy.)
8. Dasler, W. Experimental lathyrism. *Chicago Med. Sch. Quart.* 18:1, 1957.
9. Hutter, R. V. P., Worcester, J. N., Jr., Francis, K. C., Foote, F. W., Jr., and Stewart, F. W. Benign and malignant giant cell tumors of bone: A clinicopathological analysis of the natural history of the disease. *Cancer* 15:653, 1962.
10. Hayles, A. B., Dahlin, D. C., and Coventry, M. B. Osteogenic sarcoma in children. *J.A.M.A.* 174:1174, 1960.
11. Gottschalk, R. G., and Allen, H. C., Jr. Selective uptake of radioactive sulfur by human chondrosarcomas. *Cancer Res.* 12:266, 1952.

12. Gardner, E. Comparative arthrology. *Lab. Invest.* 8:1160, 1959. (An interesting description of the structure and mechanical aspects of joints.)
13. Sandson, J. Human synovial fluid: Detection of a new component. *Science* 155:839, 1967.
14. Ropes, M. W., and Bauer, W. *Synovial Fluid Changes in Joint Disease.* Cambridge, Mass.: Harvard University Press, 1953.
15. Lubrication of joints (Editorial). *Lancet* 1:609, 1969.
16. Primer on the rheumatic diseases, prepared by a committee of the American Rheumatism Association. *J.A.M.A.* 171:1205, 1345, 1680, 1959.
17. Shupe, J. L. Degenerative arthritis in the bovine. *Lab. Invest.* 8:1190, 1959.
18. Lowbeer, L. Skeletal and articular involvement in brucellosis of animals. *Lab. Invest.* 8:1448, 1959.
19. Johnson, L. C. Discussion of Lowbeer's paper [18].
20. Sikes, D. A rheumatoidlike arthritis in swine. *Lab. Invest.* 8:1406, 1959.
21. Zevely, H. A., French, A. J. Mikkelsen, W. M., and Duff, I. F. Synovial specimens obtained by knee joint punch biopsy. *Amer. J. Med.* 20:510, 1956.
22. Peery, T. M. Brucellosis and heart disease. I. The shaky foundations of rheumatic heart disease. *Postgrad. Med.* 19:323, 1956.
23. Perry, H. M., and Schroeder, H. A. Syndrome simulating collagen disease caused by hydralazine (Apresoline). *J.A.M.A.* 154:670, 1954.
24. Noer, H. R. An "experimental" epidemic of Reiter's syndrome. *J.A.M.A.* 197:693, 1966.
25. Sokoloff, L. The biology of degenerative joint disease. *Perspect. Biol. Med.* 7:94, 1963. (An erudite essay on the subject of osteoarthritis and its varied causes.)
26. Ackerman, L. V., and Butcher, H. R. *Surgical Pathology* (4th ed.). St. Louis: Mosby, 1968.
27. Schubert, R. R. The arthritides in industry. In Moritz, A. R., and Helberg, D. S. (Eds.), *Trauma and Disease.* Brooklyn, N. Y.: Central, 1959.
28. Hansen, H.-J. Comparative views on the pathology of disc degeneration in animals. *Lab. Invest.* 8:1242, 1959.
29. Gutman, A. B., and Yü, T.-F. Uric acid metabolism in normal man and in primary gout. *New Eng. J. Med.* 273:252, 313, 1965. (A well-written study of the chemical pathways for elimination of uric acid.)
30. Seegmiller, J. E., Laster, L. and Howell, R. R. Biochemistry of uric acid and its relation to gout. *New Eng. J. Med.* 268:712, 764, 821, 1963.
31. Schlumberger, H. G. Synovial gout in the parakeet. *Lab. Invest.* 8:1304, 1959. (A fascinating report.)
32. Huxley, H. E. The mechanism of muscular contraction. *Sci. Amer.* 213:18, 1965.
33. Perkoff, G. T. Studies of human myoglobin in several diseases of muscle. *New Eng. J. Med.* 270:263, 1964.
34. Genetics and biochemistry of muscular dystrophy (Editorial). *New Eng. J. Med.* 270:1107, 1965.
35. Zimmerman, H. M., and Adams, R. D. *Seminar on Diseases of Nervous Tissue and Muscle.* Chicago: American Society of Clinical Pathologists, 1959. (Cases of different types of muscle diseases are discussed and their histologic features illustrated.)
36. Perkoff, G. T., Hardy, P., and Velez-Garcia, E. Reversible acute muscular syndrome in chronic alcoholism. *New Eng. J. Med.* 274:1277, 1966.
37. Rowland, L. P., Fahn, S., and Schotland, D. L. McArdle's disease: Hereditary myopathy due to absence of muscle phosphorylase. *Arch. Neurol.* (Chicago) 9:325, 1963.

38. Kohn, R. R. Denervation muscle atrophy: An autolytic system in vitro. *Amer. J. Path.* 47:315, 1965.
39. Mabry, C. C., Roeckel, I. E., Munich, R. L., and Robertson, D. X-linked pseudohypertrophic muscular dystrophy with a late onset and slow progression. *New Eng. J. Med.* 273:1062, 1965. (A report of a carefully studied kindred; enzyme and histologic studies are especially valuable.)
40. Zimmermann, W. J. The present status of trichinosis in the United States. *Bull. Path.* 7:30, 1966.
41. Tavill, A. S., Evanson, J. M., Baker, S. B. de C., and Hewitt, V. Idiopathic paroxysmal myoglobinuria with acute renal failure and hypercalcemia. *New Eng. J. Med.* 271:282, 1964.

29 THE SKIN

The skin, interposed between the individual and his environment, may be affected as a result of changes either in the environment or in the body. Lesions resulting from external causes are brought about largely by physical and chemical agents such as mechanical trauma, ultraviolet light, x-radiation, heat, and corrosives.

DEFINITIONS RELATED TO DERMATOLOGIC PATHOLOGY

GROSS SKIN CHANGES

Some terms relating to gross skin changes are defined below.

Bulla. A large blister, such as that seen in pemphigus and second-degree burns.

Comedo. An inspissated secretion in a sebaceous gland duct; blackhead.

Erythema. A more or less diffuse redness due to hyperemia, as in first-degree burns.

Keratosis. A localized, usually scaly skin thickening.

Lichenification. An irregular skin thickening with cracks and hyperpigmentation.

Macule. A flat, usually red or brown skin lesion.

Papule. A raised, pointed or rounded, usually red lesion.

Pustule. A raised, pus-containing, yellowish lesion with a red border.

Verruca. An elevated, rough, warty lesion.

Vesicle. A small blister, often occurring in clusters, as in poison ivy.

Wheal. A firm, sharply circumscribed, plateau-like lesion which occurs in allergic or inflammatory skin reactions.

MICROSCOPIC SKIN CHANGES

Some terms relating to microscopic skin changes are defined below.

Acantholysis. A loss of epidermal cellular cohesion due to degeneration of intercellular bridges.

Acanthosis. A thickening of the malpighian (prickle cell) layer of the epidermis.

Dyskeratosis. A disarrangement of the normal polarity of the epidermal cells with the focal presence of atypical cells, which occurs in premalignant lesions.

Hyperkeratosis. A piling up of surface keratin in the stratum corneum.

Parakeratosis. The persistence of nuclei in the stratum corneum due to imperfect keratin formation.

Spongiosis. A loose sponginess of the epidermis due to intercellular edema.

EPIDERMAL HYPERPLASIAS

CALLUS

CLAVUS

CUTANEOUS HORN

Callus is a marked hyperkeratosis due to surface friction. On a toe it is painful and is called a *clavus (corn),* being caused by an ill-fitting shoe. *Cutaneous horn* (cornu cutaneum) is a keratinous excrescence on the skin. Huge masses of keratin accumulate in a tremendously thickened stratum corneum to produce a papillomatoid "horn" somewhat in the manner in which the horn of the rhinoceros normally develops. A cutaneous horn may occur on a senile keratosis or an epidermoid carcinoma of the skin. Other than being a cosmetic blemish, the horn itself has no clinical manifestations. A cutaneous horn measures from a few millimeters to several centimeters in length. *Grossly* it is a hard, curved, rough-surfaced, reddish brown, hornlike mass projecting from the skin surface. *Microscopically* it consists of sheets of eosinophilic keratin with occasional foci of parakeratosis.

VIRAL HYPERPLASIAS

Molluscum contagiosum and *verruca vulgaris* are epidermal hyperplasias produced by viruses; they are discussed in Chapter 7.

ACANTHOSIS NIGRICANS

Acanthosis nigricans occurs in three forms: (1) The childhood type *(benign or juvenile acanthosis nigricans)* is a genodermatosis (a skin disorder due to an inborn developmental defect). It may be present at birth or begin in childhood or puberty. Endocrine disturbances, such as gigantism or acromegaly, Cushing's syndrome, Stein-Leventhal syndrome, and diabetes mellitus, are significantly associated with it [1]. (2) *Malignant acanthosis nigricans* almost always occurs in adults and is inexplicably associated with malignant neoplasms [2]. In about 75 percent of the cases the tumor is an adenocarcinoma, and about half the neoplasms arise in the stomach. (3) *Pseudoacanthosis nigricans* occurs in the body creases of obese, light-skinned individuals. In all three forms there are *brown or black warty patches,* especially in the axillae and submammary folds and on the neck and genital regions. *Microscopically* there is a marked papillary hyperkeratosis with slight acanthosis and basal melanin pigmentation. Thick keratin plugs are present between the finger-like epidermal projections.

SEBORRHEIC KERATOSIS

Seborrheic keratosis (verruca pigmentosum, senile wart) is common on older persons, especially on the trunk. *Grossly* the lesion is elevated, brown, greasy, and friable. Attachment to the underlying dermis is loose. *Microscopically* there are hyperkeratosis and basal cell papillomatosis (a papillary upward proliferation of basal cells), with fine, brown, granular *melanin pigmentation.* Keratin nests or plugs and islands of dermis appear in the acanthotic epidermis.

ICHTHYOSIS

Ichthyosis may be congenital (congenita) or may develop later (vulgaris), the early form being much more severe. *Ichthyosis vulgaris* is inherited as an autosomal dominant trait. The congenital form may be inherited as a recessive or an X-linked trait. In ichthyosis, dry, rough "fish scales" appear, being most pronounced on the extensor surfaces of the extremities. *Microscopically* in ichthyosis vulgaris there is moderate hyperkeratosis with a decrease in or obliteration of the stratum granulosum. Parakeratosis is absent, and the stratum spinosum is thin. Keratotic plugs are frequent in the hair follicles. Ichthyosis congenita is similar except that hyperkeratosis is marked.

INFLAMMATIONS

1. Specific Inflammations

Skin inflammations occur in numerous specific infections such as scarlet fever, erysipelas, impetigo contagiosa, tuberculosis (lupus vulgaris), leprosy, syphilis (secondary and tertiary syphilides), numerous viral diseases (the exanthemata of smallpox, chickenpox, measles, German measles, herpes zoster), fungus infections (blastomycosis, coccidioidomycosis, dermatomycosis), parasitic infestations (ground itch of hookworm disease), and arthropodal infestations such as scabies. Ionizing radiation may produce atrophic changes in the dermis (radiation dermatitis). In sarcoidosis, rheumatoid arthritis, and various metabolic disorders such as gout, diabetes mellitus, and lipid storage diseases, specific cutaneous or subcutaneous changes occur. All these have been discussed under the specific disease state.

2. Nonspecific Inflammations

The *nonspecific skin inflammations* constitute a miscellaneous group of disorders which are by and large idiopathic. Although in some cases the precipitating cause is known, the disease is modified by other factors such as individual hypersensitivity. Secondary factors such as scratching, bacterial infection, and topical agents often modify the basic disease process. Some of these disorders are probably not truly inflammatory in nature.

ACUTE DERMATITIS

Acute dermatitis occurs in the contact reaction due to poison ivy *(Rhus toxicodendron)* and in skin hypersensitivity to other agents. Subjectively there is intense itching and even burning. *Grossly* the affected skin areas are swollen, reddened, and vesiculated. *Microscopically* the vesicles are intra-epidermal, with cellular necrosis. There is also spongiosis. In the superficial dermis there are edema, capillary dilatation, and a mainly perivascular infiltration with neutrophils, eosinophils, and lymphocytes.

SUBACUTE DERMATITIS

Subacute dermatitis is exemplified by the idiopathic nummular eczema, in which there is itching. The involved skin areas show pinpoint-sized vesicles. The *microscopic findings* are parakeratosis, acanthosis, spongiosis, and small vesicles in the epidermis. The underlying dermis is infiltrated with lymphocytes and with smaller numbers of neutrophils, eosinophils, and macrophages.

CHRONIC DERMATITIS

Chronic dermatitis is typified by atopic dermatitis (neurodermatitis disseminata) and lichen simplex chronicus (neurodermatitis circumscripta). There are patchy lichenification, fissuring, and scarring. *Microscopically* there are hyperkeratosis with focal parakeratosis, marked acanthosis, slight spongiosis, and rete peg elongation. In the superficial dermis the perivascular infiltrate consists chiefly of lymphocytes, with fewer eosinophils and macrophages.

ACNE VULGARIS

Acne vulgaris is a persistently chronic disorder which usually appears during adolescence, involving the face and upper chest and back. Sebaceous gland ducts become blocked, and sebum accumulates. When sebaceous follicles rupture, keratin in the comedos stimulates foreign body reactions. Lipolytic enzymes elaborated by bacteria act on lipids in sebum to release free fatty acids which mediate papule and pustule *(pimple)* formation [3]. *Microscopically* the papules show a lymphocytic and plasmocytic infiltrate, with occasional foreign-body giant cells about pilosebaceous glands which contain inspissated sebum. The sebaceous glands are atrophic and fragmented. Bacterial infection, almost always by *Corynebacterium acnes* and *Staphylococcus albus* or *epidermidis,* causes pustulation and subcutaneous abscesses. Foreign-body giant cells are common about ruptured follicles. In the later stages dermal fibrous scarring develops in some of the lesions.

PITYRIASIS ROSEA

Pityriasis rosea is of unknown cause and usually lasts 4 to 6 weeks. The disease occurs most often in the spring and summer in children and young adults. It begins with a *herald patch* on the trunk, followed by the appearance of numerous similar round or oval, pinkish buff (salmon-colored) patches on the trunk. Thin scales, which have been likened to cigarette paper, overlie the lesions. Localized lesions on the lower abdomen or axilla occasionally occur. *Microscopically* there is a nonspecific chronic dermatitis with moderate parakeratosis and acanthosis, spongiosis, and intracellular edema. There are occasional small vesicles in the epidermis. A lymphocytic infiltrate with some neutrophils is found in the underlying dermis.

URTICARIA PIGMENTOSA

Urticaria pigmentosa is a rare, idiopathic, chronic, usually generalized, pruritic condition which most commonly becomes manifest in the first year of life. It typically occurs in light-skinned boys. A diffuse, yellowish to reddish brown maculopapular rash covers the skin of the back, head, palms, and soles. The lesions are oval and measure up to 2.5 cm. in diameter. They become wheals when irritated. *Microscopically* there is a dense infiltrate of the edematous outer dermis consisting mainly of *mast cells* (tissue basophils). These cells contain basophilic cytoplasmic granules which can be demonstrated with the Giemsa stain. Eosinophils are scattered through the infiltrate. In some cases numbers of mast cells are found in the bone marrow, and small foci of cystic osteoporosis contain spindle-shaped mast cells *(mast cell granuloma of bone)* [4]. In about 20 percent of cases of urticaria pigmentosa developing in later childhood or early adulthood, *systemic mastocytosis* occurs [5]. Infiltrates of tissue mast cells are found in the liver, spleen, lymph nodes, gastrointestinal tract, and kidneys.

LICHEN PLANUS

Lichen planus is a subacute or chronic dermatitis of unknown cause. It persists for months or years and usually causes severe pruritis. The flexor surfaces of the wrists, forearms, and legs are most often involved, but the disease may be generalized. The buccal mucosa is not infrequently affected. *Grossly* there are small, angulated, plateau-like, violaceous papules. *Microscopically* the epidermis shows moderate hyperkeratosis, no parakeratosis, hyperplasia of the stratum granulosum, and uneven acanthosis with irregular elongations of the rete pegs (which are often pointed and so have a *"sawtooth" appearance*), and degeneration of the stratum basale. A heavy lymphocytic infiltrate is present in the upper dermis and crowds up against the epidermis, so that the epidermodermal junction is obscured. Oral lesions are similar to the cutaneous ones. In *lichen planus follicularis* the lesions are centered about hair follicles, the hairs being absent and the follicles containing keratin plugs. The rare *bullous lichen planus* is characterized by extensive separation at the epidermodermal junction so that bullae are formed.

PSORIASIS

Psoriasis is a fairly common chronic, recurrent skin disease which is sometimes associated with rheumatoid arthritis. The extensor surfaces of the elbows and knees are most commonly affected, but the entire skin may be involved (exfoliative psoriasis). The lesions *grossly* are sharply outlined, dry, dun red to brown papules and plaques covered with layered fine silvery scales. Scraping of these scales produces multiple bleeding points. *Microscopically* in the epidermis there are marked laminated parakeratosis, in which the layers are separated by slitlike spaces; *Munro microabscesses* filled with neutrophils in the stratum corneum; absence of the stratum granulosum; thinning of the stratum malpighii over the edematous and club-shaped dermal papillae; and elongation and terminal broadening of the rete pegs. In the dermal papillae the capillaries are dilated. A moderate infiltration of lymphocytes and macrophages, with some neutrophils in the early lesions, is found in the upper dermis. Quiescent psoriatic lesions show hyperkeratosis rather than parakeratosis.

KERATOSIS FOLLICULARIS

Keratosis follicularis (Darier's disease) is characterized by a fairly extensive papular or papulovesicular eruption; it occurs chiefly on the face, neck, and extremities in adolescents. The lesions may coalesce to form crusty, warty foci. Lesions develop often on the buccal mucosa and, less commonly, on the laryngeal, pharyngeal, and vulvar mucosa. *Microscopically* there are hyperkeratosis; keratotic plugs in the hair follicles and elsewhere (the name *keratosis follicularis* is not strictly correct); dyskeratotic *corps ronds* (these are cells with large, round, strongly basophilic nuclei and a homogeneous, deeply eosinophilic cytoplasm surrounded by a halo; they are found in the stratum malpighii and granulosum and represent premature keratinization); *grains,* which are much smaller than corps ronds, in the stratum corneum; acanthosis; *epidermal lacunae,* which are due to small cleavages just above the stratum basale and which contain grains and corps ronds; and elongated and tortuous projections of the dermal papillae, lined by a single basal cell layer, into the lacunae as villi. Mucosal lesions are similar to the cutaneous ones except that hyperkeratosis is slight or absent.

CHRONIC DISCOID LUPUS ERYTHEMATOSUS

Chronic discoid lupus erythematosus is a form of this collagen vascular disease which is limited to the skin. Sometimes the localized skin disease eventuates in disseminated lupus erythematosus. Like the latter, discoid lupus appears most commonly in young women. There is a sharply delimited, swollen, erythematous rash with a "butterfly" distribution over the cheeks (less often other areas exposed to sunlight are affected). *Microscopically* there are hyperkeratosis with keratotic plugging of hair follicles; thinning of the stratum malpighii alternating with foci of acanthosis; *liquefactive degeneration of the stratum basale,* the sine qua non of the diagnosis of cutaneous lupus; edema of the dermis with vascular dilatation; degeneration of the dermal collagen, which becomes basophilic, in exposed skin areas; fragmentation of elastic fibrils; and a mainly perifollicular lymphocytic infiltrate, with a few plasmocytes and macrophages.

DERMATITIS HERPETIFORMIS

Dermatitis herpetiformis (Duhring's disease) is chronic, recurrent, and characterized by itching. It may occur during pregnancy *(herpes gestationis).* There is a symmetric distribution of groups of papules, vesicles, and, rarely, bullae surrounded by zones of erythema. The lesions occur most commonly on the shoulders, extensor surfaces of the extremities, and buttocks. *Microscopically* the epidermis is only slightly affected, but there is subepidermal vesicle or bulla formation with a usually marked, predominantly eosinophilic infiltrate of these lesions as well as of the surrounding edematous dermis.

ACUTE PEMPHIGUS

Acute pemphigus is a fulminating, usually fatal *bullous dermatitis* which develops in association with smallpox vaccination, bites, skin infections, and debilitating diseases, or spontaneously. It occurs most commonly in Jews and Italians. *Clinically* there are high fever, dehydration, and collapse. When a nonvesiculated skin area is pressed or rubbed, the epidermis is denuded *(Nikolsky's sign). Vesicles and bullae,* the latter measuring up to 10 cm. in diameter, appear suddenly in the mouth and extensively over the skin. They contain straw-colored fluid early, but this may become hemorrhagic or purulent. Rupture of bullae frequently occurs. *Microscopically* the vesicles and bullae result from cleavage at the epidermodermal junction or within the stratum spinosum. The underlying dermis is edematous. In secondarily infected cases neutrophils and sometimes eosinophils are present within vesicles.

PEMPHIGUS VULGARIS

Pemphigus vulgaris is a severe *bullous dermatitis* characterized by itching and burning. It occurs most often in the fifth through the seventh decade of life, and its incidence is about the same in men and women. Before adrenal steroid therapy the disease was often fatal. The skin of the axillae and groin is particularly affected; however, any part of the cutaneous surface may be involved, and oral lesions are almost always present and may be the first to appear. The bullae are soft and break easily, releasing fluid with an offensive odor. Early *microscopic changes* are spongiosis and acantholysis in the lower stratum malpighii. Clefts and later bullae develop suprabasally. Degenerated squamous cells *(Tzanck cells)* are found singly and in clusters within the bullae. Young bullae have a floor consisting of a single layer of basal cells, but in older ones there are several cell layers. Early the dermal infiltrate consists of a few eosinophils, but with time a considerable number of eosinophils and plasmocytes are found.

PEMPHIGUS ERYTHEMATODES

In *pemphigus erythematodes* (Senear-Usher syndrome) an eruption consisting of vesicles, bullae, and reddened, scaly patches appears on the face, trunk, extremities, and, in severe cases, buccal mucosa. *Microscopically* the bullae are formed by cleavage, usually at the epidermodermal junction. The *erythematous foci* show parakeratosis and moderate acanthosis and spongiosis; liquefactive degeneration at the epidermodermal junction; and a heavy infiltration of lymphocytes, macrophages, and neutrophils in the superficial dermis. After a series of remissions and exacerbations, during which the patient has few systemic manifestations, the disease evolves into *pemphigus vulgaris or pemphigus foliaceus.*

PEMPHIGUS FOLIACEUS

In *pemphigus foliaceus,* soft, oozing bullae gradually involve almost the entire body. Then most of the bullae disappear and thick, scaly lesions develop. *Microscopically* the bullae show a separation of the stratum corneum from the spinous layer. The underlying dermis is often infiltrated with eosinophils. Later the lesions consist of marked hyperkeratosis with keratotic plugging of hair shafts; parakeratosis; acantholysis and cleavage in the stratum granulosum with shrinkage and hyperchromatism of its cells; and acanthosis. Fogo selvagem is an endemic form of pemphigus foliaceus in parts of Brazil.

PEMPHIGUS VEGETANS

Pemphigus vegetans begins as bullae which later heal as warty masses. *Microscopically* the bullous lesions are the same as those of pemphigus vulgaris, except that there is an extensive downward growth of epidermal strands. In the verrucous lesion there are intra-epidermal abscesses filled with eosinophils early, papillomatosis, acanthosis, an irregular downward projection of broad squamous strands, and villus formation by upward growth of edematous dermal papillae.

EPIDERMOLYSIS BULLOSA

Epidermolysis bullosa appears shortly after birth as a genodermatosis or between the ages of 10 and 30 as an acquired disease. In the *simple form* of epidermolysis, vesicles and bullae typically develop by cleavage between the stratum corneum and stratum granulosum. They may appear following slight injury to the skin over any part of the body and heal without permanent damage. In the *dystrophic form* the extremities are frequently involved, and lesions sometimes appear on the buccal mucosa. Vesicles and bullae are usually produced by separation at the epidermodermal junction. Regression of these lesions leads to hyperpigmentation and slight scarring of the skin, the formation of small epidermal inclusion cysts (milia), and atrophy or destruction of the nails. Severe cases of dystrophic epidermolysis bullosa may be fatal in infants.

ERYTHEMA MULTIFORME

Erythema multiforme is an acute dermatosis which is part of a self-limited systemic disease with fever and sore throat. The skin lesions are pleomorphic with macules, papules (the most common manifestations), vesicles, and bullae. The papules often enlarge peripherally and clear centrally to form the typical *iris lesions. Microscopically* the macules and papules show spongiosis and intracellular edema in the epidermis, with edema and a perivascular, mainly lymphocytic infiltrate in the dermis. The vesicles and bullae form by complete separation of the epidermis from the dermis. In the detached epidermis, necrotic squamous cells are often seen. The lesions may be hemorrhagic.

GRANULOMA ANNULARE

Granuloma annulare is a chronic, asymptomatic dermatosis of young adults characterized by ring-shaped clusters of small, firm, light red nodules; these appear most commonly on the fingers, dorsum of the hands, elbows, and feet. *Microscopically* the dermal nodules show central fibrinoid necrosis of collagen with epithelioid cells and occasional multinucleated giant cells at the periphery. The lesions may be indistinguishable from subcutaneous rheumatic nodules.

NECROBIOSIS LIPOIDICA DIABETICORUM

Diabetic lipid necrobiosis is a skin manifestation of hyperlipemia, lipid material being deposited in the dermis and initiating a granulomatous foreign body reaction. About 90 percent of the cases of lipid necrobiosis are associated with diabetes mellitus; the lesions sometimes precede the onset of clinical diabetes. Occasionally trauma initiates the skin changes. *Grossly* lipid necrobiosis is an oval or round, sharply outlined, firm plaque with a violaceous border and yellow, frequently ulcerated center. The lesions are often multiple and are most common on the lower extremities, but also occur on the forearms, neck, and face. *Microscopically* in the outer and mid-dermis there are tuberculoid granulomata. In the center of the lesions the dermal collagen is swollen, granular, and afibrillar. Peripherally there are small epithelioid cell collections with occasional multinucleated giant cells. Occasional lipid vacuoles may be found intracytoplasmally in these cells.

EXFOLIATIVE DERMATITIS

Generalized exfoliative dermatitis is often a manifestation of a drug reaction, especially to arsenicals and occasionally to penicillin. About 25 percent of the cases are associated with a lymphoma. There is an extensive epidermal peeling which may lead to a severe loss of serous fluid. The condition is occasionally fatal. *Microscopically* in the epidermis there are parakeratosis; severe intercellular and intracellular edema, especially in the outer malpighian layer; acanthosis; elongation of the rete pegs; and a migration of inflammatory cells. When the edema in the outer stratum malpighii is marked, cells in this zone may exfoliate with the parakeratotic cells of the stratum corneum. In the dermis there are edema and a rather pronounced inflammatory infiltrate. *Exfoliative dermatitis of the newborn* (Ritter's disease) is caused by *Staphylococcus aureus.*

3. Panniculitides

The *panniculitides* are inflammations of the subcutaneous fat.

ERYTHEMA NODOSUM

Erythema nodosum is a panniculitis that is often associated with systemic diseases such as tuberculosis and rheumatic fever. Tender, bright red, slightly elevated nodules 1 to 5 cm. in diameter develop along the shins typically. *Microscopically* the lesions are mainly in the superficial subcutaneous tissue. Early there is a nonspecific patchy infiltration of the subcutaneous fat with neutrophils and lymphocytes. A *vasculitis* is present, particularly in the veins, with infiltration of the walls, marked endothelial proliferation, and, rarely, thrombosis. Later tuberculoid granulomata, which are sometimes infiltrated with neutrophils, are found in the adipose tissue.

ERYTHEMA INDURATUM

Erythema induratiŏn occurs in hematogenous tuberculosis in women with a fairly strong immunity to *Mycobacterium tuberculosis.* Chronic, recurrent nodules develop on the calves and slowly progress to bluish red plaques which usually ulcerate. Tubercles with caseation necrosis are found in the subcutaneous fat, and there is also a nonspecific infiltration of lymphocytes and plasmocytes. *M. tuberculosis* may be identified in the tubercles. The inflammatory lesions produce atrophy of the adipose tissue. The blood vessels show endothelial and fibrous proliferation, lymphocytic infiltration, and thrombosis, which results in further necrosis.

WEBER-CHRISTIAN DISEASE

Nodular, nonsuppurative, relapsing, febrile panniculitis (Weber-Christian disease) is characterized by crops of hard, tender subcutaneous nodules, most often on the extremities. There is slight erythema of the overlying skin, which becomes depressed in the last phase of the nodule. Occasionally the skin ulcerates and discharges an oily fluid. *Microscopically* in early lesions there is an extensive, predominantly neutrophilic infiltrate between the cells of the subcutaneous fat. In the second phase there is fat necrosis with numerous lipid-laden macrophages with a foamy cytoplasm and some foreign-body giant cells containing lipid material. Fibrous scarring in the adipose tissue occurs in the third phase, fibroblastic proliferation being followed by the laying down of collagen. Occasionally internal adipose tissues (omentum and mesentery) are involved in the disease. Rare cases of *systemic nodular panniculitis* with fever, anemia, leukopenia, and thrombocytopenia occur [6]. Lesions are found in the bone marrow fat, lymph nodes, spleen, and liver.

DEGENERATIONS

SENILE ELASTOSIS

Degenerative changes are common in the skin, especially in elderly persons. *Senile elastosis* is the cause of the loss of skin elasticity in old people. It is most marked on exposed area of the skin, such as the face and backs of the hands.

Microscopically the dermal elastic fibers are swollen and stain basophilically. The overlying epidermis and the nearby sweat and sebaceous glands are often atrophic. Other lesions, such as epidermoid carcinoma, are frequent in skin showing senile elastosis.

Elastosis perforans serpiginosa [7] is a rare degeneration of dermal elastic tissue which typically involves the skin of the back or sides of the neck. It occurs about five times as frequently in men as in women. The lesions may represent an auto-immune reaction to altered elastic fibers. *Grossly* firm, red papules, each measuring up to 4 mm. and covered by a thin scale, are arranged in a snakelike or circular pattern over an area up to 4 cm. in diameter. *Microscopically* the superficial dermal elastic fibers are thickened and tangled. Portions of the abnormal elastic tissue are extruded into or through the epidermis via tortuous microsinuses. The elastic fibers in these channels bear a striking resemblance to fungal hyphae. In the dermis there is an infiltration of lymphocytes and macrophages, with a few foreign-body giant cells.

ELASTOSIS PERFORANS SERPIGINOSA

In the hereditary *pseudoxanthoma elasticum* the skin is excessively lax, especially over the neck, axillae, groin, elbows, and popliteal regions. Soft yellow papules and plaques appear symmetrically in the involved areas. *Microscopically* the dermal elastic tissue is seen as focally calcified, basophilic masses of fragmented curved or spiral fibers. In about half the cases, angioid streaks are seen in the fundus of the eye due to degenerative changes in the choroidal arteries and the elastic fibers of the lamina vitrea. Changes also occur in the walls of muscular arteries due to degeneration of elastic or collagen fibers, and hemorrhages may result.

PSEUDOXANTHOMA ELASTICUM

In *colloid milium,* discrete, round, yellow nodules measuring about 2 mm. in diameter appear in skin areas exposed to sunlight, especially the forehead and backs of the hands. On cut surface the nodules are gelatinous. *Microscopically* small pools of acidophilic, homogeneous colloid-like material are found in the outer dermis. Intact fibroblast nuclei and small blood vessels are present within these pools. The gelatinous substance is believed to represent degenerated elastic tissue or collagen or to be a derivative of blood plasma.

COLLOID MILIUM

Lipid proteinosis (lipoglycoproteinosis, Urbach-Wiethe's disease) [8] is rare and chronic. It is characterized by the deposition of lipid, protein, and carbohydrate material in the dermis and submucosa of the lips, mouth, tongue, pharynx, and larynx. Skin lesions are common on the eyelids, face, hands, elbows, knees, axillary regions, and scrotum. *Grossly* there are numerous papules, nodules, and firm plaques, some of which are ulcerated, on the skin and mucous membranes. *Microscopically* hyalin deposits thicken capillary walls and, in the skin, surround sweat glands. Later, hyalin replaces the collagenous and elastic fibers, and stainable lipid and carbohydrate material is present. These changes are probably due to degeneration of the collagen and elastic tissue.

LIPID PROTEINOSIS

NEOPLASMS [9]

1. *Benign Epidermal Neoplasms*

Squamous papilloma may occur as a true neoplasm on the skin, but many papillomatous lesions are verrucae (warts) caused by a virus, with marked proliferation of the epidermis.

PAPILLOMA

KERATOACANTHOMA: *Keratoacanthoma* (verrugoma, molluscum sebaceum, self-healing epithelioma of the skin) [10] may easily be confused with epidermoid carcinoma. However, it is benign and disappears spontaneously in a few months if untreated. The lesion is probably hyperplastic rather than neoplastic. Keratoacanthoma occurs about twice as often in men as in women and is most frequent in persons between 50 and 70 years of age. It appears most commonly on the face (especially about the mouth) and lower extremities. Often the lesions are multiple. *Causative factors* appear to include: occupational exposure to carcinogens, trauma, cigarette smoking, exposure to sunlight, and possibly a virus [11].

Pathologic changes: *Grossly* the lesion is a well-defined flat, papillary, or depressed keratotic focus 0.5 to 2 cm. in diameter. The flat lesions may show a central ulcerated crater. *Microscopically* differentiation from epidermoid carcinoma can be difficult. The keratoacanthoma consists of masses of active squamous cells with central keratotic foci. At the base there may be apparent invasion, but the "invading" foci of squamous cells are usually fairly well differentiated and relatively inactive, and they stain more acidophilically than the actively infiltrating foci in epidermoid carcinoma.

2. Precancerous Epidermal Lesions

SENILE KERATOSIS: *Senile keratosis (solar keratosis)* is frequent in the aged and in those exposed to arsenic or radiation. It occurs especially on the face and dorsum of the hands, but may appear anywhere on the skin. Similar lesions appear on the mucous membranes of the lips, mouth, tongue, vulva, and cervix in *leukoplakia.* Pathologic changes: *Grossly* irregular brown scaly patches appear on the skin. *Microscopically* there are hyperkeratosis, parakeratosis, and dyskeratosis (hyperchromatism, mitoses, irregularity in nuclear size and shape, and loss of polarity) in the basal and malpighian layers. Infiltration of lymphocytes in the superficial dermis and degeneration of dermal collagen and elastic tissue occur.

BOWEN'S DISEASE: *Bowen's disease* is a subject of dispute. Some pathologists use the term to indicate an intra-epidermal (preinvasive or in situ) carcinoma; others, a premalignant dyskeratosis. About 20 percent of these lesions become invasive carcinoma. Similar histologic changes occur on the glans penis and vulva in *Queyrat's erythroplasia.* Pathologic changes: *Grossly* in Bowen's disease there are irregular, scaly, slowly growing brownish patches on the trunk, buttocks, and extremities. *Microscopically* numerous *dyskeratotic cells* with one or two hyperchromatic nuclei surrounded by a cytoplasmic halo are found throughout the epidermis. *Hyperkeratosis or parakeratosis* may be marked.

XERODERMA PIGMENTOSUM: *Xeroderma pigmentosum* is inherited as an autosomal recessive and becomes manifest in childhood. There is marked hypersensitivity to ultraviolet light, and the tendency to develop epidermoid or basal cell carcinoma is pronounced. Dermal fibroblasts in patients with xeroderma pigmentosum lack the ability of normal fibroblasts to repair ultraviolet radiation damage to deoxyribonucleic acid [12]. Pathologic changes: *Grossly* there are patches of scaling and mottled pigmentation of the skin. *Microscopically* hyperkeratosis, atrophy of the malpighian layer, and increased melanin in the basal layer are found. Some patients with xeroderma pigmentosum have neurologic manifestations such as mental deficiency, ataxia, choreoathetosis, and deafness (DeSanctis-Cacchione syndrome).

3. Malignant Epidermal Neoplasms

EPIDERMOID CARCINOMA:

Epidermoid carcinoma of the skin constitutes about 15 percent of all cancer in males and 10 percent in females, and causes about 2 percent of cancer deaths. The fundamental cause is unknown, but certain factors appear to be causally related:

1. *Ultraviolet rays* [13]. The lesions are more common on exposed than on unexposed parts of the body and occur frequently in persons heavily exposed to sunlight, such as farmers. The frequency is higher in tropical and subtropical zones than in temperate regions.

2. *Chronic irritation.* Epidermoid carcinoma is common in old scars from burns or osteomyelitis.

3. *Ionizing radiation.* The lesion may occur in areas subjected to prolonged or severe radiation.

4. *Carcinogenic hydrocarbons.* Lesions were formerly common on the scrotum in chimney sweeps and on the skin of mule spinners.

5. *Infrared rays or heat.* Kangri burn cancer occurs on the abdominal wall of natives of Kashmir who wear a charcoal heater beneath their clothing.

6. *Arsenic.* Lesions are common in industrial workers.

Pathologic changes

Epidermoid carcinoma occurs most commonly on the *exposed surfaces* (such as the face or hands), especially over bony prominences. Early there is slight thickening of the skin or mucosa. Later an *ulcer* with thick, indurated edges appears and will not heal. *Microscopically* columns, sheets, and clusters of atypical squamous cells invade the dermis. Well-differentiated (grade I) squamous carcinoma shows amorphous keratin masses *(epithelial pearls)* within sheets of cells. Anaplastic (grade IV) neoplasms show little or no differentiation and no pearl formation. Dermal lymphocytic infiltration is common in the lower-grade squamous carcinomas.

Metastases

Metastases are mainly to *regional lymph nodes,* but late in the course metastases may be widespread.

BASAL CELL CARCINOMA:

Basal cell carcinoma (rodent ulcer) is relatively benign and metastasizes extremely infrequently [14]. It occurs predominantly in fair-skinned persons on the region of the *face* bounded by the hairline, ears, and upper lip. Exposure to bright sunlight appears to be a causative factor. Its *origin* is from the cells of the basal layer of the epidermis or the hair follicles.

Pathologic changes

Grossly it is a slowly growing lesion, beginning as a *papule* which soon ulcerates centrally. The *ulcer* border is waxy and rolled. The neoplasm, if neglected, may eventually erode deeply and invade the underlying bone. The lesions may be multiple. *Microscopically* solid sheets of small, hyperchromatic, basophilic cells extend in columns from the epidermis into the dermis. The columns often have club-shaped endings. Cyst formation may occur within large sheets of basal cells. Heavy pigmentation with melanin is sometimes present. *Multicentric basal cell carcinoma* (superficial epitheliomatosis) occurs as scaly plaques. Several separate foci of atypical basal cells are found. *Intra-epidermal* (Jadassohn) *basal cell carcinoma* grows outward to involve all layers of the epidermis, but does not extend into the dermis.

BASOSQUAMOUS CARCINOMA

Basosquamous carcinoma shows both squamous and basal cell elements. The prognosis is worse than in pure basal cell carcinoma because of the squamous character of the neoplasm. This squamous component may metastasize, as in pure epidermoid carcinoma.

4. Neoplasms Arising From Dermal Vessels

LYMPHANGIOMA

Lymphangioma is a benign neoplasm derived from lymph vessels. It is often congenital. Such tumors also occur in the tongue *(macroglossia)* or lips *(macrocheilia)*. *Grossly* the neoplasm may be local or diffuse. Often it is a soft pink nodule. *Microscopically* there is a proliferation of lymph vessels which may be small (capillary) or large (cavernous). *Cystic hygroma* (lymphangioma cysticum colli) is a congenital cavernous lymphangioma of the neck and submaxillary regions.

LYMPHANGIOSARCOMA

Lymphangiosarcoma occurs, especially in the lymphedematous arm, following extirpation of the axillary lymph nodes during radical mastectomy *(Stewart-Treves syndrome)* [15]. The neoplasm is bulky and red. *Microscopically* atypical endothelial cells are seen in sheets and sometimes lining lymphatic spaces.

HEMANGIOMA:

Hemangioma is a benign neoplasm derived from small blood vessels. About 50 percent of these neoplasms appear on the head. It is often congenital, and many regress spontaneously after birth.

Capillary hemangioma

Capillary hemangioma (port-wine stain, vascular nevus, birthmark) shows a network of small capillaries often filled with blood. The capillaries are often lined with a single layer of endothelium. When endothelial proliferation is marked, forming several layers about each vessel, the neoplasm is called a *hemangioendothelioma,* although some reserve this term for a malignant tumor. *Grossly* the hemangioma is bright red. The *skin of the head and face* is the most common site of occurrence; mucous membranes of the lips, tongue (macroglossia), gingiva, nose, and rectum, and the brain are other frequent sites.

Cavernous hemangioma

Cavernous hemangioma is less common than the capillary type. The red neoplasm consists of large sinusoids lined by endothelium. No definite capsule is formed. The neoplasm is usually small and may be multiple. It occurs most commonly in the *liver;* other sites of occurrence are the skin, lips, and skeletal muscles. A cavernous hemangioma arising high in the papillae and so closely associated with the epidermis as to appear within it in places is known as an *angiokeratoma* (telangiectatic wart).

Hemangiopericytoma

Hemangiopericytoma is usually benign and derives from the pericytes of Zimmerman which are found outside the capillary basement membrane. *Grossly* a painless skin nodule is found. *Microscopically* blood-filled capillaries ringed by proliferated pericytes are present. The latter are round or elongated and lie outside the vascular reticulin sheath. Each pericyte is surrounded by reticulin fibers, as is demonstrated by silver stains. An example of a comparable retroperitoneal neoplasm arising from pericytes around lymph vessels *(lymphangiopericytoma)* has been reported [16].

Sclerosing hemangioma (dermatofibroma) is considered by some pathologists to be due to obliteration of a hemangioma; others interpret it as a fibrous neoplasm. It is usually found on an extremity and may be multiple. *Grossly* sclerosing hemangioma is an elevated, yellow or orange, cutaneous nodule. *Microscopically* there are tightly wound spirals of spindle cells; numerous small, endothelially lined spaces; and lipid-laden macrophages with intracytoplasmic vacuoles. Hemosiderin granules are found within the phagocytic cells. Foreign-body giant cells may be present.

Sclerosing hemangioma

Primary solitary angiosarcoma, a malignant tumor derived from endothelium, is rare. Less anaplastic examples are sometimes called hemangioendothelioma. Widespread visceral metastases may occur.

ANGIOSARCOMA:

Kaposi's sarcoma [17] is a more frequently occurring type of angiosarcoma, but it is also an uncommon disease. It occurs chiefly in Italians and Ashkenazi Jews, but the disease is also common among Bantus in southern Africa. *Over 90 percent of the cases are in men.* Kaposi's sarcoma appears simultaneously with a lymphoma in a significant number of cases.

Kaposi's sarcoma:

Early reddish purple, discrete or grouped, tender nodules appear on the skin, especially of the hands and feet. Later large areas of skin may be involved, and lesions occur in the gastrointestinal tract submucosally, liver, lungs, and, less often, the brain and bones. It is not certain whether these represent multicentric primaries or metastases. *Microscopically* early Kaposi's sarcoma is like a hemangioma, with hemosiderin in phagocytic cells in the stroma. Later there are abortive capillaries lined by large, atypical, spindle-shaped endothelial cells. The stroma is infiltrated by macrophages and lymphocytes. Death is usually due to hemorrhage.

pathologic changes

Glomangioma (glomus tumor) is a benign neoplasm derived from the neuromyoarterial glomus apparatus, an arteriovenous shunt found in the skin of the fingertips, in the scapular and coccygeal regions, and about joints. The *glomus* consists of an afferent artery (Sucquet-Hoyer canal or shunt) surrounded by glomus cells, which are thought to control the flow of blood by their contractility, and an efferent vein. Associated with the shunt are numerous nonmedullated nerves and smooth muscle bundles. The neoplasm usually produces a *burning pain.* It appears in nailbeds most commonly, but also occurs elsewhere on the extremities. Subungual tumors are more common in women than in men; others are more common in men than in women.

GLOMANGIOMA:

Grossly the glomangioma is an unencapsulated, purplish red nodule several millimeters in diameter. *Microscopically* it varies from sheets of glomus cells with few vascular spaces to many large sinusoids with a few peritheliomatously arranged glomus cells. Each cell is surrounded by a thin reticulin fiber, with silver stains. Electron microscopy demonstrates that glomus cells have large numbers of cytoplasmic myofibrils and a thick enveloping sheath [18]. They are almost identical to arterial smooth muscle cells.

Pathologic changes

5. Dermal Appendage Neoplasms

Sweat gland adenoma (syringadenoma) may be solid or cystic. The histologic appearance is bewilderingly varied, a typical feature being clusters of small dark cells separated by thin lines of stroma. Islands of hyaline cartilage may be included *(mixed tumor of the skin)* [19]. *Dermal eccrine cylindroma* [20] is a

SWEAT GLAND NEOPLASMS

syringadenoma appearing on the neck, head, and scalp *(turban tumor).* Multiple lesions are common and may form clusters. *Grossly* the cylindroma is a firm, pink or red nodule measuring up to 6 cm. in diameter. Hyalinized collagenous bands separate cords and nests of basophilic epithelial cells which sometimes line cysts or ductlike spaces. The *eccrine acrospiroma* [21] is grossly grayish tan and unencapsulated. *Microscopically* it consists of nests or sheets of cells, some of which have an eosinophilic and some a clear cytoplasm. Sometimes there may be a trabecular or sievelike pattern.

Sweat gland adenocarcinoma (syringocarcinoma) [22] is rare and of low-grade malignancy. However, widespread metastases can occur. Sweat gland carcinoma appears most often in the axillae, vulva, and scrotum, where apocrine sweat glands are normally present. *Grossly* it is a firm, red or purple, raised nodule. *Microscopically* varisized and disorganized glandular structures are lined or filled by atypical epithelial cells.

SEBACEOUS GLAND NEOPLASMS

Sebaceous gland adenoma occurs as a yellow papule in the skin of the nose, cheeks, or forehead. *Microscopically* an overgrowth of sebaceous glands, sometimes with basal cell proliferation, is found. *Associated lesions* may include nevi, verrucae, or tuberous sclerosis in many cases.

Sebaceous gland carcinoma is rare and of low-grade malignancy.

HAIR FOLLICLE NEOPLASMS

Trichoepithelioma (epithelioma adenoides cysticum, Brooke tumor) arises from hair follicles, is benign and familial, and appears as multiple nodules on the face and chest. *Microscopically* the overlying epidermis is intact. Numerous cystic spaces are found, containing keratinized debris and lined by stratified squamous epithelium, from which nests of basal cells proliferate.

Trichochlamydoacanthoma [23] is rare and arises from the lower hair sheath on the scalp. It has a central keratin-filled crater surrounded above by squamous epithelium and below by outer hair sheath epithelium.

In *trichochlamydocarcinoma* there are clusters and sheets of atypical outer hair sheath epithelium. Metastases are rare.

6. Dermal Cysts

EPIDERMAL INCLUSION CYST

Epidermal inclusion cyst (wen, sebaceous cyst) is common and arises from included epidermal elements within the dermis. It is lined by stratified squamous epithelium and contains laminated keratinized debris. There is a fibrous wall. Rupture leads to a dermal foreign body reaction to the keratohyalin in the lining. An inclusion cyst may attain enormous size.

Trichlamydocyst (hair sheath cyst) [23] almost always occurs on the scalp and in women. It is filled with keratin and is lined with several layers of epithelial cells, some of which have a clear cytoplasm. These cells contain glycogen and lipid.

Calcifying epithelioma (pilomatrixoma) [24] is a dermal cyst in which plaques of calcification and cholesterol deposits with a foreign body reaction are found. Electron microscopy indicates that the cyst arises by proliferation and keratinization of hair matrix cells.

Dermoid cyst is a congenital inclusion in the skin. Its wall contains a variety of skin elements.

7. *Pigment Cell Neoplasms*

NEVUS:

A *nevus (mole)* is any benign neoplasm arising from melanocytes, which are discussed in relation to melanin pigment metabolism on page 279. It may occur anywhere on the skin, being most common on the face, neck, and back, and occasionally in the eye. The average number is 20 per person.

Junctional nevus

Junctional nevus is common on the palms, soles, and genitalia, but may appear anywhere on the skin. Some probably arise in a preexisting lentigo. Thc junctional nevus is considered *potentially premalignant,* because in occasional cases it progresses to a melanocarcinoma. *Grossly* the junctional nevus is typically flat, hairless, small, and brown. *Microscopically* small clusters of melanocytes are found in the basal and lower malpighian layers. Some cells contain brown pigment; others are clear. "Skip" lesions with multiple foci of involvement and intervening normal epidermis are common. The dermis is not involved.

Intradermal nevus

Intradermal nevus is the most common type of mole. The pigment cells are thought to reach the dermis by the process of *Abtropfung* (dropping) from the epidermis. *Grossly* the lesion is typically elevated, brown, and often hairy. It is usually small, but may become enormous. *Microscopically* cords and clusters of *nevus cells* (large, pale, often pigmented, polyhedral cells) lie in the superficial and deep dermis. These are both melanocytes and melanophores. The amount of fine, brown, granular melanin varies greatly; it lies both within the cytoplasm and extracellularly. The disks of eosinophilic collagenous tissue within such a nevus are *lâmes foliacées.*

Compound nevus

Compound nevus shows a combination of junctional and intradermal elements. It is the *common type of mole in children* and is unusual in adults. The compound nevus is considered potentially premalignant in adults because of the junctional element.

Blue nevus

Blue nevus (Jadassohn-Tièche nevus) is common on the face, dorsum of the hands and feet, and soles. *Grossly* it is small, flat or slightly elevated, and bluish black. *Microscopically* interlacing bundles of spindle cells associated with a large amount of brown granular melanin are found deep in the dermis. These cells are melanocytes and melanophores. Electron microscopy indicates that the melanocytes originate from Schwann cells [25]. *Mongolian spot* (dermal melanocytosis) is histologically the same as the blue nevus. The spot is congenital in the skin of the sacrococcygeal region and disappears by the fourth year. The differentiation between a cellular blue nevus and melanocarcinoma can be difficult. In the former, junctional activity is absent, the margins push aside rather than invade the surrounding dermis, mitoses are rare, the cytoplasm is scanty and fibrillar, and associated neuroid structures are frequent [26]. Rarely *malignant blue nevus* may occur. Metastases are to regional lymph nodes and distant organs.

JUVENILE MELANOMA

Juvenile melanoma [27] occurs in white children and occasionally in young or even older adults. Even though it is histologically very similar to melanocarcinoma, this neoplasm remains localized and is clinically benign. The face is the most common site. *Grossly* the neoplasm is heavily pigmented, being tan, dark brown, blue, or bluish black. It is usually elevated and well demarcated and measures up to 2 cm. in diameter. *Microscopically* [28] most are *spindle cell nevi,* which consist of sheets of long, spindly or fusiform cells with large nuclei and abundant cytoplasm associated with varying amounts of melanin pigment. *Epithelioid cell nevi* are made up of large cells with very abundant acidophilic or amphophilic cytoplasm, and 1 to 6 nuclei. Some of the giant cells are of the Touton type with centrally clustered nuclei. Some juvenile melanomas contain a mixture of the two cell types.

MELANOCARCINOMA:

Melanocarcinoma (malignant melanoma) [29] is an extremely malignant neoplasm arising from melanocytes in the skin or uveal tract, and rarely from the conjunctiva and other mucous membranes. It is rare before puberty. Most cases develop in the 25 to 50 age group, and the incidence in males and females is about equal. In whites it is four times as common as in Negroes, the highest incidence being in fair-skinned blondes. Chronic irritation of and the use of electrocoagulation on apparent nevi are sometimes implicated in the onset of melanoma.

Clinical features

Clinically it is usually preceded by a flat, brown junctional nevus, although it may appear to arise de novo on the palms, soles, and genitalia. The lesion becomes progressively darker and darker.

Pathologic changes

Grossly melanocarcinoma is elevated or flat and is usually darkly pigmented, although an amelanotic type occurs. *Microscopically* sheets and clusters of atypical polyhedral or spindle cells arise from the lower epidermal layers and deeply invade the dermis. The cell type varies tremendously from tumor to tumor, ranging in appearance from that of squamous carcinoma to fibrosarcoma (formerly called melanosarcoma). Variable amounts of brown pigment are present, the cells commonly being loaded with melanin. Some melanocarcinomas are excised before dermal invasion has occurred or extended beyond the upper layers *(superficial melanoma).* In these cases there is marked junctional activity with many atypical melanocytes containing melanin granules in an otherwise clear cytoplasm. *In the underlying dermis there is a marked infiltration of lymphocytes and plasmocytes,* and numerous pigment-laden macrophages are seen.

Metastases [30]

Spread is via lymphatics early, with later extensive hematogenous spread. Regional lymph nodes are involved frequently. *Hematogenous metastases* are common in the skin, lungs, liver, pancreas, intestines, heart, adrenals, kidneys, and brain. Transplacental metastasis from mother to fetus has occurred in a few cases [31].

Prognosis

The *prognosis* is always serious. It is somewhat better in women than in men. Melanocarcinoma may spread rampantly during pregnancy, but in large series the prognosis is not appreciably different in pregnant and nonpregnant women [32]. The overall 5-year survival rate is about 35 percent. With superficial melanocarcinoma it is about 75 percent.

8. Lymphomas

SKIN IN LYMPHOMAS

Infiltration of the dermis by malignant cells to form papules, plaques, or nodules occurs occasionally in the *leukemias and lymphomas,* such as lymphosarcoma, Hodgkin's granuloma, and reticulum cell sarcoma. Rarely a lymphoma will become manifest by an apparently primary lesion in the skin. *Exfoliative dermatitis and generalized herpes zoster* may also develop in cases of lymphoma.

Mycosis fungoides is a rare and peculiar entity which sometimes results from involvement of the skin by cells arising in an underlying malignant lymphoma, such as reticulum cell sarcoma, Hodgkin's granuloma, or lymphosarcoma. However, in numerous cases no lymph node or visceral involvement has been found. In the early *erythematous (premycotic) stage* a pruritic, eczematoid or psoriasiform, red to brown, scaly eruption appears. The *microscopic picture* is often not diagnostic, since it may reveal only a nonspecific dermal chronic inflammatory reaction and psoriasis-like epidermal changes. Sometimes large, even binucleated, atypical reticulum cells are spotted in the superficial dermis. In the *plaque stage,* sharply defined, bluish red, raised plaques appear. *Microscopically* these show *Darier-Pautrier microabscesses* containing atypical reticulum cells or lymphocytes in the stratum spinosum; and a diffuse pleomorphic outer dermal infiltrate consisting of atypical reticulum cells, Reed-Sternberg cells, eosinophils, macrophages, lymphocytes, and many plasmocytes. Some of the latter are binucleated *(Marschalko cells).* In the *tumor stage,* frequently ulcerated, fungoid masses develop in the skin due to the extensive proliferation of the neoplastic and inflammatory cells.

MYCOSIS FUNGOIDES

9. Metastatic Neoplasms

Metastatic neoplasms reach the skin by direct extension or via lymph or blood vessels. Common metastases are from breast, kidney, lung, gastrointestinal tract, pancreas, thyroid gland, and prostate gland carcinomas, malignant melanomas, lymphomas, and sarcomas. The *metastatic tumor lies in the dermis,* and the overlying dermis is usually intact.

METASTASES TO SKIN

REFERENCES

1. Winkelmann, R. K., Scheen, S. R., Jr., and Underdahl, L. O. Acanthosis nigricans and endocrine disease. *J.A.M.A.* 174:1145, 1960.
2. Curth, H. O., Hilberg, A. W., and Machacek, G. F. The site and histology of the cancer associated with malignant acanthosis nigricans. *Cancer* 15:364, 1962.
3. Freinkel, R. K. Pathogenesis of acne vulgaris. *New Eng. J. Med.* 280:1161, 1969.
4. Stark, E., Van Buskirk, F. W., and Daly, J. F. Radiologic and pathologic bone changes associated with urticaria pigmentosa. *A.M.A. Arch. Path.* 62:143, 1956.
5. Caplan, R. M. Urticaria pigmentosa and systemic mastocytosis. *J.A.M.A.* 194:1077, 1965.
6. Steinberg, B. Systemic nodular panniculitis. *Amer. J. Path.* 29:1059, 1953.
7. Greenblatt, M. Elastosis perforans serpiginosa. *Arch. Path.* (Chicago) 75:177, 1963.
8. McCusker, J. J., and Caplan, R. M. Lipoid proteinosis (lipoglycoproteinosis). *Amer. J. Path.* 40:599, 1962.
9. Lund, H. Z. Tumors of the skin. Section 1, Fascicle 2, in *Atlas of Tumor Pathology*. Washington: Armed Forces Institute of Pathology, 1957.
10. Grinspan, D., and Abulafia, J. Idiopathic cutaneous pseudoepitheliomatous hyperplasia. *Cancer* 8:1047, 1955.
11. Ghadially, F. N., Barton, B. W., and Kerridge, D. F. The etiology of keratoacanthoma. *Cancer* 16:603, 1963.

12. Reed, W. B., Landing, B., Sugarman, G., Cleaver, J. E., and Melnyk, J. Xeroderma pigmentosum. *J.A.M.A.* 207:2073, 1969.
13. Blum, H. F. Sunlight as an environmental factor in cancer of the skin. *Milit. Med.* 117:202, 1955.
14. Baxter, H. A., and Pirozynski, W. J. Metastasizing basal cell carcinoma. *Amer. J. Clin. Path.* 48:53, 1967.
15. Nelson, W. R., and Morfit, H. M. Lymphangiosarcoma in the lymphedematous arm after radical mastectomy. *Cancer* 9:1189, 1956.
16. Enterline, H. T., and Roberts, B. Lymphangiopericytoma. *Cancer* 8:582, 1955.
17. Cox, F. H., and Helwig, E. B. Kaposi's sarcoma. *Cancer* 12:289, 1959.
18. Venkatachalam, M. A., and Greally, J. G. Fine structure of glomus tumor: Similarity of glomus cells to smooth muscle. *Cancer* 23:1176, 1969.
19. Stout, A. P., and Gorman, J. C. Mixed tumors of the skin of the salivary gland type. *Cancer* 12:537, 1959.
20. Crain, R. C., and Helwig, E. B. Dermal cylindroma (dermal eccrine cylindroma). *Amer. J. Clin. Path.* 35:504, 1961.
21. Johnson, B. L., Jr., and Helwig, E. B. Eccrine acrospiroma. *Cancer* 23:641, 1969.
22. Miller, W. L. Sweat gland carcinoma. *Amer. J. Clin. Path* 47:767, 1967.
23. Holmes, E. J. Tumors of lower hair sheath. *Cancer* 21:234, 1968.
24. McGavran, M. H. Ultrastructure of pilomatrixoma (calcifying epithelioma). *Cancer* 18:1445, 1965.
25. Merkow, L. P., Burt, R. C., Hayeslip, D. W., Newton, F. J., Slifkin, M., and Pardo, M. A cellular and malignant blue nevus: A light and electron microscopic study. *Cancer* 24:888, 1969.
26. Rodriguez, H. A., and Ackerman, L. V. Cellular blue nevus. *Cancer* 21:393, 1968.
27. Hendrix, R. C. Juvenile melanomas, benign and malignant. *A.M.A. Arch. Path.* 58:636, 1954.
28. Kernen, J. A., and Ackerman, L. V. Spindle cell nevi and epithelioid cell nevi (so-called juvenile melanomas) in children and adults. *Cancer* 13:612, 1960.
29. Allen, A. C., and Spitz, S. Malignant melanoma, clinicopathological analysis of criteria for diagnosis and prognosis. *Cancer* 6:1, 1953.
30. Das Gupta, T., and Brasfield, R. Metastatic melanoma. *Cancer* 17:1323, 1964.
31. Brodsky, I., Baren, M., Kahn, S. B., Lewis, G., Jr., and Tellem, M. Metastatic malignant melanoma from mother to fetus. *Cancer* 18:1048, 1965.
32. George, P. A., Fortner, J. G., and Pack, G. T. Melanoma with pregnancy. *Cancer* 13:854, 1960.

GENERAL REFERENCES

Allen, A. C. *The Skin: A Clinicopathologic Treatise* (2d ed.). New York: Grune & Stratton, 1967. (An enormous, thorough, and copiously illustrated documentary on skin diseases.)

Lever, W. F. *Histopathology of the Skin* (4th ed.). Philadelphia: Lippincott, 1967. (A concise discussion of dermatologic disorders with a strong emphasis on the microscopic changes.)

30 ORGANS OF THE SPECIAL SENSES

DISEASES OF THE EYES

DEFINITIONS

Because the language of clinical ophthalmology and ophthalmic pathology contains numerous terms not generally used elsewhere, the definitions of such words may be helpful in the study of the diseases of the "precious jewels" man wears in his head.

Blindness. Central visual acuity less than 20/200, accompanied by limitation of the field of vision to an angle of 20°. About 350,000 persons in the United States are blind in both eyes and 1.5 million are blind in one eye.

Coloboma. Absence of a segment of an eye structure due to developmental defect, disease, or surgery.

Cyclitic membrane. An inflammatory fibrovascular band between the ciliary body and anterior vitreous surface.

Drusen. Small hyaline excrescences on the lamina vitrea or optic disk.

Emmetropia. Condition of normal refraction in the eye in which parallel light rays are focused on the retina.

Epiphora. Excessive lacrimation or tearing.

Hyperopia. Condition in which vision for distant objects is superior to that for near objects; farsightedness. It is due to a developmental flatness of the globe or a refractive error, so that parallel light rays are focused behind the retina.

Hyphema. Hemorrhage into the anterior chamber of the eye.

Hypopyon. Presence of pus in the anterior chamber.

Hypotony. Decreased intraocular pressure.

Iris bombé. A forward bulging of the iris peripherally due to increased posterior chamber pressure caused by annular synechiae between the iris and lens about the pupil.

Keratic precipitates (K.P.). Aggregates of lymphocytes, plasmocytes, and macrophages adherent to the deep corneal surface; large masses are called *"mutton fat" deposits.*

Leukoma. A dense, large, opaque, white corneal scar.

Macula. A fairly large and dense corneal scar.

Nebula. A small, thin corneal scar.

Phlyctenule. A small, red, superficially ulcerated conjunctival nodule consisting of lymphocytes.

Photophobia. Abnormal sensitivity of the eyes to light.

Phthisis bulbi. A disorganized shrinkage of the eyeball following extensive infection, injury, or necrosis, due to cicatricial contraction. The globe is small and firm with a wrinkled surface.

Scotoma. A blind or dark spot in the visual field.

Staphyloma. A bulging of the sclera or cornea due to thinning resulting from defective development or disease.

Synechia. An adhesion between the iris and cornea (anterior synechia) or iris and lens (posterior synechia).

1. Developmental Defects

EYES AS A WHOLE

Malformations involving the eyes as a whole include: the extremely rare *anophthalmos,* a complete absence of the eyes in which the lids may or may not be developed; *cyclops,* in which there is a single central eye due to fusion of the two optic vesicles; *supernumerary eyes* (when there are three eyes, the nose and mouth are duplicated; when there are four eyes, the entire face is duplicated, as in Janus monsters); *abnormalities of position,* such as the widely set eyes in hypertelorism and the forwardly displaced eyes (exophthalmos) of oxycephaly and platybasia; unilateral or bilateral *microphthalmia,* in which the eyes are abnormally small; and *macrophthalmia* (*buphthalmos,* megalophthalmos), in which the eyes are abnormally large, the cornea being enlarged, the anterior chamber deepened, the optic nerve cupped, and the sclera thinned so that it appears bluish. Arachnodactyly is sometimes associated with macrophthalmia.

MYOPIA

Myopia (nearsightedness) is frequently familial, and hereditary factors are important. It is due to *enlargement and lengthening of the posterior segment* of the eyes, much of which occurs during the growth period. As a result, parallel light rays are focused in front of the retina. *Stationary (simple) myopia* is mild, develops in childhood, and does not progress after the cessation of body growth. Simple myopic eyes are little different from emmetropic ones.

Progressive myopia begins in childhood and worsens throughout life, becoming very severe. The *optic disk* is somewhat flattened temporally, and a white area *(scleral crescent)* is seen lateral to the disk. Beyond this there is a pigmented and vascular *choroidal crescent.* These crescents are due to scleral thinning and the drawing away of the choroid and retinal pigment epithelium from the disk margin as the posterior segment enlarges. Temporally the pigment epithelium and lamina vitrea end at a distance from the disk margin, leaving uncovered choroid. The latter does not reach to the disk border, leaving exposed sclera. Thus the two crescents are formed. Nasally, choroid, lamina vitrea, and pigment epithelium may overlap up to half the width of the nerve head. In the *retina* the rods and cones and pigment epithelium degenerate slowly and progressively, especially over scleral staphylomata. The *choroid* atrophies, and branching clefts develop in the lamina vitrea *(lacquer cracks).* The *sclera* becomes thin, especially at the posterior pole and sides of the optic nerve. An equatorial staphyloma may result from the thinning.

EYELIDS

Anomalies of the eyelids include: *ablepharon,* in which the eyelids are absent, the eyes being exposed; *ankyloblepharon,* in which the lids are fused; *cryptophthalmos,* in which the eyes are hidden by the overlying skin, no evidence of lid formation being present; *coloboma* (a vertical fissure) of one or both upper lids; and, rarely, *ectropion* (eversion) and *entropion* (inversion). An *epicanthus* (a fold of skin covering the inner or, extremely rarely, the outer canthus) which in the Mongolian race is normal at the inner canthus, occurs abnormally in mongolism (Down's syndrome) and bilateral renal agenesis. *Distichiasis* is the presence of an accessory row of eyelashes.

LACRIMAL APPARATUS

Anomalies of the lacrimal secretory apparatus include: *agenesis; facial fissure,* in which a lacrimal duct opens onto the cheek; and *duct atresia* or *stenosis. Anomalies of the excretory portion* are: *atresia* of the punctum lacrimale and/or lacrimal canaliculi, *cyst* of a canalicus or lacrimal sac, and a *fistula* from the sac to the subcutaneous tissue of the lower lid.

CONJUNCTIVA

Congenital defects of the conjunctiva include: *hereditary intra-epithelial dyskeratosis,* characterized by focal, gelatinous plaques in which acanthosis, prickle cell vacuolation, and dyskeratosis are found microscopically in the conjunctival and buccal mucosa [1]; junctional or compound *nevus,* which appears as a flat brown spot measuring 1 to 3 mm. in diameter on the bulbar conjunctiva and may undergo malignant change later in life; and *dermoid tumor,* which occurs most commonly astride the limbus above or below the cornea and is frequently associated with coloboma of the eyelid. It is a solid choristoma, measuring up to 1.5 cm. in diameter, covered by squamous epithelium, and containing hair follicles, sebaceous glands, collagenous bundles, and adipose tissue. *Dermolipoma* is a variant in which fat is predominant.

CORNEA

Corneal anomalies are rare and include: *megalocornea,* in which the cornea is abnormally large, reaching 2 cm. in diameter, and which is associated with myopia and subluxation or dislocation of the lens; *microcornea,* in which the cornea is smaller than normal and which is usually accompanied by microphthalmia, marked hyperopia, and a predisposition to glaucoma; and *dermoid tumor. Congenital corneal opacity* may be due to focal absence of Descemet's membrane; collagenous thickening and central displacement of Schwalbe's ring with veil-like lateral projections *(posterior embryotoxon, Axenfeld's syndrome);* and intra-uterine keratitis. The latter may be related to *congenital anterior staphyloma,* in which the thin, diffusely opaque cornea bulges forward and is lined by adherent iris.

IRIS, CILIARY BODY, AND CHOROID

Malformations of the iris include: the very rare *aniridia* (complete absence); *coloboma; albinism* (absence of pigment, which is usually inherited as a recessive and in which vision is typically very poor); *nevi,* which rarely undergo malignant change; *heterochromia iridis,* in which the two eyes are different in color; *corectopia* (eccentric pupil); *polycoria,* in which there are two or more pupillary openings; *persistence of the pupillary membrane,* which is usually partial and too delicate to interfere with vision; *congenital anterior synechiae,* which may occur alone or as thick cords in posterior embryotoxon; and *incomplete separation of the iris root* from the trabecular meshwork. The last two defects are causes of congenital glaucoma. *Aniridia* is significantly associated with nephroblastoma (Wilms' tumor) [2]. *Coloboma of the ciliary body* is usually associated with a similar defect in the iris and absence of the ciliary muscle. Anterior or posterior *displacement of the ciliary processes* occurs, and *long* but otherwise normal *ciliary processes* are commonly seen. *Malformations of the choroid* are: the usually unilateral *coloboma,* which is typically due to incomplete closure of the fetal fissure and is often associated with coloboma of the iris; and absence of choroidal pigment in *albinism.*

LENS

Lenticular defects include: the rare *aphakia* (absence); *microphakia* (abnormally small lens); *spherophakia* (rounded lens); *coloboma* (a notched defect at the equator); *ectopia lentis* (abnormal position); *lenticonus,* in which the cortex bulges through a thin segment of the anterior or posterior lens capsule; and *congenital cataract.* The last is often due to intra-uterine infection of the embryonic lens epithelium by rubella virus. Such cataracts may be unilateral or bilateral. They are nuclear, dense, and pearly white. A chronic nongranulomatous iridocyclitis with focal necrosis of pigment epithelium in the ciliary body often accompanies rubella cataracts [3]. *Dislocation or subluxation of the lens* occurs in childhood in Marfan's syndrome, due to a developmental weakness of the zonular ligament.

VITREOUS BODY

Developmental anomalies of the vitreous (hyaloid) body are: *persistence of the primary vitreous,* in which all or part of the hyaloid vascular system present during early development fails to regress; and the usually unilateral *persistent hyperplastic primary vitreous,* in which the fibrovascular tunic of the lens and the hyaloid vessels fail to disappear. Blood vessels and fibrous tissue grow into the lens through a defect in its posterior capsule, and a dense fibrovascular membrane containing hyaloid artery remnants forms behind the lens. This gives a white pupillary reflex like that seen with a retinoblastoma. The membrane often is attached to the retina peripherally. Hemorrhage into the membrane and vitreous sometimes occurs postnatally, and its organization may cause retinal detachment. After birth the lens becomes cataractous, and glaucoma commonly follows due to a pupillary block by the swollen lens or the formation of synechiae.

RETINA

Retinal defects are uncommon and include: *coloboma,* which typically is in the lower nasal region; the presence of *medullated nerve fibers,* usually near the optic disk; *grouped pigmentation,* in which proliferation of the cells of the retinal pigment epithelium produces dark plaques over which rods and cones are absent; and the usually familial and bilateral *retinal dysplasia,* which sometimes occurs in conjunction with persistent hyperplastic primary vitreous. Proliferation and infolding of the outer retinal layers produces a fibrous retrolental mass containing disorganized retinal elements. Tubular structures with a rosette-like appearance on cross section are present. Contraction of this mass may detach relatively normal portions of the retina. *Retinal dysplasia* occurs in infants with trisomy 13-15 in association with arhinencephaly, harelip, cleft palate, and cardiac defects [4]. The eyes are small (microphthalmos), and an island of cartilage is sometimes found within fibrous tissue which traverses a coloboma in the ciliary body or iris.

SCLERA

In *blue sclera* the outer coat of both eyes is abnormally and uniformly thin and transparent, uveal pigment being visible through it. The condition is usually hereditary and associated with osteogenesis imperfecta.

2. Inflammations

EYELIDS: Dermatitis

Dermatitis of the eyelids is common because of the delicacy of these structures. It is usually allergic in origin and may be caused by atropine used to dilate the pupils, local anesthetic agents, chemicals present in eyelash dyes and other cosmetics, and poison ivy. The lids are red and edematous, and there is a lymphocytic dermal infiltration.

Blepharitis

Blepharitis is an inflammation of a lid margin due to infection of sebaceous glands. The inflammation is usually chronic with acute exacerbations. There are photophobia, excessive lacrimation, itching, and loss of eyelashes. The lid margin is red and covered with scales, which are greasy in the *seborrheic form,* and dried secretions. Edema, congestion, perifollicular abscesses, and lymphocytic infiltration are found. Hordeola, corneal ulcers, and chronic conjunctivitis are commonly associated with blepharitis.

Hordeolum

Hordeolum (sty) is an acute, circumscribed, suppurative inflammation of a gland of Zeis or Moll (external hordeolum) or a meibomian gland (acute chalazion, internal hordeolum). It is usually caused by *Staphylococcus aureus* or *epidermidis. Clinically* there are a feeling that a foreign body is in the eye, pain, photophobia, and epiphora. A reddish swelling appears near the eyelash roots and develops into an abscess filled with yellow pus and measuring 3 to 10 mm. in diameter. The abscess not uncommonly ruptures spontaneously.

Chalazion

Chalazion is a chronic granuloma of the eyelid due to infection and obstruction of a meibomian gland or its duct. The inspissated sebaceous material incites a foreign-body giant cell reaction in the surrounding tissue. A round or oval mass a few millimeters in diameter develops in the lid. It causes no symptom except an occasional feeling of pressure.

Other lid infections

The eyelids may be involved in a number of infectious diseases which affect the skin, such as erysipelas, syphilis (as a chancre or diffuse tarsitis), herpes zoster, molluscum contagiosum, vaccinia, blastomycosis, sporotrichosis, and trichophytosis.

LACRIMAL APPARATUS: Dacryoadenitis

Dacryoadenitis is an inflammation of a lacrimal gland. It may occur in mumps and in some cases of conjunctivitis. Chronic, often bilateral enlargement, with or without concomitant salivary gland involvement, occurs in Sjögren's syndrome in which there are keratoconjunctivitis sicca (dry eyes), xerostomia (dry mouth), and polyarthritis [5]. The lacrimal glands show moderate to extensive lymphocytic infiltration.

Dacryocystitis

Dacryocystitis connotes an inflammation of a lacrimal sac resulting from obstruction of the corresponding nasolacrimal duct. The inflammation is typically chronic with acute exacerbations. Streptococci and pneumococci are common causative organisms. Swelling of the sac is noted, and mucopurulent material can be expressed from a tear point on pressure. A mucocele may form within the sac. In *chronic dacryocystitis* the sac wall is densely infiltrated with lymphocytes and plasmocytes. *Acute dacryocystitis* is almost always secondary to a chronic inflammation, organisms escaping into the tissues about the sac (peridacryocystitis). An abscess may form and perforate spontaneously, producing a *lacrimal fistula.*

ORBIT: Cellulitis

Acute inflammation of the orbit occurs as a cellulitis usually, a soft tissue or subperiosteal abscess forming less commonly. *Cellulitis of the orbit* is usually secondary to inflammation of surrounding structures (acute panophthalmitis; ethmoid, frontal, sphenoid, or maxillary sinusitis; osteomyelitis of the frontal or a maxillary bone; dental infections; or infections of the region drained by the facial vein). The orbital tissues are edematous, hyperemic, and infiltrated with neutrophils. Thrombosis of the regional veins may progress to cavernous sinus thrombophlebitis.

Acute tenonitis

Acute tenonitis is an inflammation of Tenon's capsule. *Clinically* there are chemosis (a pink bulbar conjunctival swelling over the sclera and as a ring about the corneal limbus), lid swelling, exophthalmos, and pain on rotation of the eye.

Chronic inflammation

Chronic orbital inflammation is typically granulomatous and often nonspecific. Tuberculosis, syphilis, and fungus infections such as mucormycosis and sporotrichosis may involve the orbit.

CONJUNCTIVA: Acute conjunctivitis

Acute conjunctivitis (pinkeye) is an inflammation of the bulbar and palpebral conjunctiva, and is caused by several organisms (*Moraxella lacunata, Hemophilus aegyptius* [Koch-Weeks bacillus], *Corynebacterium xerose,* streptococci, staphylococci, pneumococci, and gonococci). The viral conjunctivitides are discussed in Chapter 7. *Purulent conjunctivitis* is usually due to gonococci; it is discussed as ophthalmia neonatorum on page 608. Most cases of bacterial conjunctivitis are catarrhal. Children are affected more often than adults, and transmission is by personal contact or by fomites. *Clinically* after a short incubation period the conjunctiva becomes intensely injected, and there are a scratching sensation and mild photophobia. The discharge is serous or mucinous, and it may dry overnight to fuse the lids together. *Pathologically* the conjunctiva is edematous and infiltrated with neutrophils, and its blood vessels are dilated and congested.

Chronic conjunctivitis

Chronic conjunctivitis may be caused by bacteria, such as pneumococci, streptococci, or staphylococci; irritating fumes, such as tobacco smoke; or allergies, such as to dust or pollens. *Clinically* there are moderate conjunctival thickening and reddening, with itching in the allergic cases.

Parinaud's conjunctivitis

Parinaud's conjunctivitis is rare and is almost always unilateral; it is characterized by focal ulcerations over submucosal nodules, eyelid swelling, enlargement of the preauricular lymph nodes, fever, and eosinophilia. A gram-positive, alga-like bacterium, probably a strain of *Leptotrichia buccalis,* appears to be the usual cause, but a similar picture occurs in oculoglandular tularemia and in cases of cat-scratch fever and lymphogranuloma venereum with ocular involvement. The nodules consist of macrophages and necrotic cellular debris, with a surrounding lymphocytic and plasmocytic infiltrate.

Other conjunctival inflammations

Conjunctivitis occurs as part of *Reiter's syndrome* together with urethritis and arthritis (see page 105), and in *mucosal respiratory (Stevens-Johnson) syndrome* (see page 461). *Conjunctival infection* is caused rarely by *Mycobacterium tuberculosis* and certain fungi such as *Pityrosporum ovale, Streptothrix foersteri, Candida albicans, Sporotrichum schenkii, Rhinosporidium seeberi,* and *Blastomyces dermatiditis.* In many of these infections the lesions are granulomatous. *Helminths* which infest the conjunctiva include *Loa loa, Onchocerca volvulus,* and *Trichinella spiralis.* The last-named produces chemosis and also involves the extraocular muscles.

Vernal conjunctivitis

Vernal conjunctivitis, so named because it is typified by flare-ups during several successive springs, is allergic in causation and usually occurs in young individuals. Epiphora and conjunctival redness and itching are common. Large, plateau-like papules occur in the palpebral or perilimbar conjunctiva. The mucosa is thickened, and tonguelike processes lick into the submucosa, which is heavily infiltrated with eosinophils.

CORNEA:

Keratitis is an inflammation of the cornea and may be ulcerative, in which the irritant comes from outside the body, or deep, in which corneal infection is hematogenous or by extension from the iris or sclera. Many ulcerative cases are associated with conjunctival involvement *(keratoconjunctivitis).* In some cases organisms are introduced directly into the cornea by foreign bodies. Viral and gonococcal infections are discussed on pages 153 and 608, respectively.

Acute purulent keratitis:

Acute purulent keratitis (serpiginous ulcer) is a severe pyogenic infection produced by bacteria such as pneumococci, streptococci, staphylococci, gonococci, and *Pseudomonas aeruginosa,* the latter infections being especially serious; and by fungi such as *Aspergillus* species, *Candida albicans, Cephalosporium serrae,* and *Nocardia* species. *Corneal injury due to an abrasion or foreign body* is usually necessary for invasion to occur, although the gonococcus can penetrate the intact cornea. *Mycotic keratitis* [6] is increasing in frequency, especially in patients using eye drops containing an antibiotic or corticosteroid. *Clinically* a rapidly enlarging yellow focus appears in the cornea, and later the anterior chamber becomes cloudy. Pain, excessive tearing, and photophobia are severe, and involvement of the iris leads to a small, fixed pupil.

pathologic changes

The *pathologic changes* include mucosal ulceration with an undermined border, a stromal neutrophilic infiltrate, a sterile hypopyon and acute inflammation of the iris, and sometimes corneal perforation. The inflammatory reaction is most striking at the progressing edge of the ulcer. *Healing* is by fibrous corneal scarring, with formation of a nebula, macula, or leukoma. When corneal perforation has occurred, a dense cicatrix containing prolapsed uveal tissue (adherent leukoma) may develop; or there may be a bulging cicatrix of the cornea with prolapse of the iris into it *(anterior staphyloma).* Simple bulging of the cornea without iris involvement is called *keratectasia.* In many cases *peripheral anterior synechiae* (PAS) form between the cornea and iris, and these commonly produce secondary glaucoma. The synechiae may be appositional, due to gluing of the iris root to the trabecular meshwork, or nonappositional, due to organization of an exudate.

Marginal keratitis

Marginal (catarrhal) ulcer of the cornea usually is a complication of acute or chronic conjunctivitis due to *Moraxella lacunata, Hemophilus aegyptius,* streptococci, or staphylococci. *Clinically* there is moderate pain; a marginal gray ulcer with adjacent conjunctival injection is noted. *Pathologically* there is a small, superficial ulcer with a neutrophilic stromal infiltrate. Bacteria are rarely found in these lesions.

Ring abscess

Ring abscess of the cornea is caused by pyogenic infection following a perforating injury or intraocular surgery. Extensive central corneal necrosis, especially in the deeper layers, results. An intense neutrophilic infiltration is found. The process usually progresses to massive destruction of the eye.

Chronic serpiginous ulcer

Chronic serpiginous (Mooren's) ulcer of the cornea is a rare, idiopathic keratitis. The condition is bilateral in up to 50 percent of the cases. An ulcer begins at the corneal margin, and, over a period of months and often accompanied by intense pain, it enlarges to involve the entire cornea. The ulcer edges are undermined, and the limbus and adjacent sclera may be affected. There is a stromal chronic inflammatory reaction. Healing is by a thin corneal scar that allows some vision.

Ring ulcer

Ring ulcer is similar to the chronic serpiginous type, but its progress is more rapid, the limbus and sclera are not involved, and the inflammatory reaction is more marked. Systemic disease, such as periarteritis nodosa, lupus erythematosus, or bacillary dysentery, is often associated with ring ulcers.

Phlyctenular keratoconjunctivitis

Phlyctenular keratoconjunctivitis is an allergic reaction to bacterial products, especially to tuberculoprotein. In the perilimbar conjunctiva and cornea, papules infiltrated with lymphocytes develop. Superficial ulceration occurs over the papules. In the conjunctiva, healing usually leaves the structure intact, but in the cornea, vascularization and scarring may seriously impair vision.

Herpetic keratitis

Herpetic keratitis (dendritic ulcer) is caused by the virus of herpes simplex (see page 151). *Clinically* the lesions are quite painful. At first a row of tiny vesicles appears in the central cornea. These soon ulcerate, and the process extends rapidly in a dendrite-like pattern. This progresses to the formation of a leaf-shaped ulcer. The epithelial cells adjacent to the ulcer contain intranuclear acidophilic inclusions (Lipschütz bodies). The ulcers may heal with slight scarring, which may interfere with vision; or the lesions may develop into a recurrent metaherpetic keratitis, the ulcers being round or oval with scalloped borders in which the epithelium is adherent to Bowman's membrane. Herpes virus bodies cannot be found in the metaherpetic lesions, which are thought to be neurotrophic in origin. *Disciform keratitis* is another sequela, although it may also be caused by other viruses and trauma. There is a disklike edema of the corneal stroma, and the underlying Descemet's membrane is thrown into folds (striate keratopathy). Most cases clear with a slight posterior corneal opacity. However, if the lesion becomes chronic, deep vessels proliferate into it and an opaque scar results.

Interstitial keratitis

Interstitial (deep stromal) *keratitis* may develop by extension of inflammatory processes in the conjunctiva and outer cornea, sclera, or uvea. It occasionally occurs in *tuberculosis,* typical epithelioid (but rarely caseating) tubercles being found in the deep layers of the cornea. *Mycobacterium tuberculosis* is not found in the lesions. In *congenital syphilis,* bilateral interstitial keratitis usually occurs between the ages of 5 and 15 and is probably due to hypersensitivity, since treponemas are not found in the lesions. The corneal stromal fibers degenerate, and the stroma is very heavily infiltrated with lymphocytes. Later fibrosis and vascularization develop, with severe impairment of vision. *Cogan's syndrome* [7] is a nonspecific interstitial keratitis associated with vestibulo-auditory dysfunction due to cochlear inflammation and sometimes with systemic vascular lesions. It is probably a hypersensitivity reaction.

SCLERA

Scleritis is an inflammation of the sclera; *episcleritis* is an inflammation of the episcleral tissue. Such inflammations may be caused by penetrating wounds or by extension of an infection, such as syphilis or tuberculosis, within the eye. The zone about the limbus is the most common site for scleritis, so the deep cornea is often involved *(sclerokeratitis).* Scleral inflammation is characterized by severe pain and photophobia, frequently with signs of an underlying uveitis. The sclera becomes purplish due to congestion. The inflammation sometimes persists for months, and healing may result in a focal thinning and transparency. A staphyloma may develop. Episcleritis is similar except that the congested tissues appear red, and thinning does not accompany healing. In patients with *rheumatoid arthritis,* nodules similar to those in subcutaneous tissues occur in the sclera, usually between the limbus and equator. Diffuse involvement causes extensive scleral thickening *(brawny scleritis).*

INTRINSIC STRUCTURES OF THE EYE:

Most *acute suppurative inflammations of the inner eye* are due to organisms introduced during or following trauma. However, any of the ocular structures may become infected in septicemia or pyemia. *Abscess of the vitreous* is a rare complication of meningococcemia. Depending on the structure(s) involved, the process is known as *acute iridocyclitis* (inflammation of the iris and ciliary body) *uveitis* (inflammation of the entire uveal tract, i.e., the iris, ciliary body, and choroid), *choroiditis,* or *chorioretinitis* (inflammation of the choroid and retina).

Panophthalmitis

Endophthalmitis is an inflammation of the vitreous, retina, and uveal tract. *Panophthalmitis* is an inflammation of the entire eye and is usually secondary to a penetrating wound. The tissues are edematous and infiltrated by polymorphonuclear leukocytes, and the chambers are filled with pus. *Phthisis bulbi* is the end result of the subsidence of the inflammatory reaction.

Acute iridocyclitis

Acute iridocyclitis manifests itself *clinically* by severe pain, epiphora, iridal congestion, decreased intraocular pressure, and a miotic pupil which is dilated with difficulty. Mild cases clear in a few days, while in severe cases complications may result in diminution of vision. *Acute plastic iritis* occurs in patients with *rheumatoid arthritis.* The eyes are fiery red and a proteinaceous exudate fills the anterior chamber. It usually clears in about 6 weeks. *Pathologically* in iridocyclitis the iris and ciliary body are edematous, hyperemic, and infiltrated with neutrophils. A fibrinous exudate forms on the posterior surface of the iris and may become adherent to the lens capsule. *Hypotony* is due to inability of the ciliary epithelium to produce aqueous humor. *Complications* are usually the result of repeated attacks and include organization of the fibrinous exudate to form fibrous synechiae between the iris and the cornea and/or lens. Formation of a *ring (annular) synechia* about the pupil *(seclusion of the pupil)* obstructs the flow of fluid from the posterior to the anterior chamber so that the trapped posterior chamber fluid pushes the iris forward peripherally *(iris bombé).* The protruded iris may become adherent to the cornea. In some cases a pupillary membrane dense enough to interfere with vision forms *(occlusion of the pupil).* Occasionally ciliary exudates organize to produce fibrous adhesions to the anterior vitreous surface *(cyclitic membrane),* sometimes causing a retrolental opacity. Contraction of these adhesions may detach the retina near the ora serrata.

Chronic iridocyclitis

Chronic nongranulomatous iridocyclitis follows the acute form directly or after a subacute phase. *Clinically* chronic inflammation of the anterior uvea is characterized by slight pain and congestion, keratic precipitates, secondary glaucoma due to anterior or posterior synechiae, and seclusion of the pupil. The affected tissues show focal aggregates of lymphocytes and a diffuse infiltration with plasmocytes associated with numerous Russell bodies.

Chronic cyclitis

Chronic cyclitis [8] is an uncommon entity which probably represents a hypersensitivity reaction. It is usually bilateral and is characterized by the insidious development of visual blurring in young individuals. Dustlike particles are seen in the *anterior vitreous* due to a lymphocytic infiltrate. The *ciliary body* is thickened due to stromal fibrosis and moderate lymphocytic and plasmocytic infiltrate. Its epithelium is atrophic. A cyclitic membrane is formed, and the *lens* becomes cataractous. Macular edema and cystoid degeneration also occur.

Granulomatous endophthalmitis:

Granulomatous endophthalmitis occurs in tuberculosis, leprosy, sarcoidosis, syphilis, brucellosis, fungus infections, toxoplasmosis, helminthic infestations, sympathetic ophthalmia, and phacoanaphylaxis (discussed as a complication of cataract on page 811). In the infectious forms the organisms usually reach the inner eye hematogenously. *Hypersensitivity* plays a role in causing tissue damage in many forms of uveitis. The finding of a significant incidence of positive complement fixation tests against lens and uveal antigens in patients with uveitis indicates that *auto-immune mechanisms* are factors in continuing the tissue reaction, regardless of the original inciting cause [9].

tuberculosis

Tuberculosis may localize anteriorly as an iridocyclitis, tiny yellow tubercles appearing on the iris. Large *"mutton fat" precipitates* consisting of neutrophils, lymphocytes, and macrophages are seen on the corneal endothelium, and lymphocytic nodules are found at the pupillary border. If the process extends into the cornea or sclera, staphylomata may develop, and spontaneous rupture of the globe sometimes occurs. Posterior localization produces a *chorioretinitis.* Severe infections may progress to involve all the ocular structures *(tuberculous panophthalmitis).* In *tuberculous endophthalmitis* the granulomatous intraocular lesions consist of tubercles with caseation necrosis, but *M. tuberculosis* is rarely identified in the lesions.

leprosy

Lepromatous leprosy involves the anterior uvea, sclera, and cornea, the tissues being infiltrated with foamy macrophages filled with *M. leprae.* There is surprisingly little inflammatory response.

syphilis

Syphilis is an unusual cause of endophthalmitis today. In late *secondary syphilis,* orange-red "papules" 2 to 3 mm. in diameter may appear at the pupillary border, producing the clinical picture of acute iritis. These nodules microscopically are miliary gummata. In *tertiary syphilis,* gummata occur rarely in the iris, ciliary body (where they may reach a large size), and choroid. In *syphilitic choroiditis,* multiple granulomatous foci, 1 to 2 mm. in size, with infiltration of the adjacent retina and sclera are found. Many of these lesions appear in congenital syphilis, and their healing gives the equatorial zone of the fundus a "salt and pepper" appearance due to the presence of tiny foci of hyperpigmentation and depigmentation. In *optic neuritis,* which usually occurs in the secondary stage, a destructive granuloma occurs typically at or near the optic disk, with a lymphocytic and plasmocytic infiltrate into the retina. *Treponema pallidum* is rarely demonstrated in any of the ocular syphilitic lesions.

sarcoidosis

Sarcoidosis is now recognized as an important cause of endophthalmitis, especially in Negroes. Ocular manifestations appear in about half of sarcoid cases, sometimes in association with parotid gland lesions in uveoparotid fever. The *iris and ciliary body* are most commonly involved, noncaseating tuberculoid granulomata forming nodular masses within and upon the surfaces of these structures. Greasy *keratic precipitates* form on the corneal endothelium. Small sarcoid granulomata may occur in the *choroid, retina, or optic nerve.* Calcific deposits may appear in the cornea *(band keratopathy)* as a result of hypercalcemia in sarcoidosis.

brucellosis

In *acute brucellosis,* iritis is a rare manifestation. Somewhat more commonly uveitis occurs in *chronic brucellosis.* Granulomatous foci consisting of masses of epithelioid cells – sometimes with necrotic centers filled with neutrophils – surrounded by lymphocytes occur in the uveal tract, retina, and optic nerve. Brucella are very difficult to isolate, and the diagnosis of ocular involvement is usually presumptive.

mycotic endophthalmitis

Intraocular fungus infections [10] may result from perforation of a mycotic corneal ulcer; direct penetration of a corneal ulcer by *Mucor* species; introduction during a penetrating wound or surgery; or hematogenous spread, as in *Candida albicans* mycotemia, aspergillosis, blastomycosis, coccidioidomycosis, cryptococcosis, and histoplasmosis. *Postoperative infections* following intracapsular cataract extraction are characterized by numerous tiny abscesses in the ciliary body and anterior vitreous. The *vitreous, choroid, and retina* are commonly involved in mycotic endophthalmitis and show focally suppurative granulomata which usually reveal the causative organism. Although *Histoplasma capsulatum* has never been demonstrated in the eye, it is considered to be an *important cause of chorioretinitis.* The most characteristic lesions attributed to histoplasmosis are tiny, disseminated, round, yellowish white, *lymphocytic choroidal nodules* [11]. A hypothetical histoplasmosis lesion, based on a significant incidence of positive histoplasmin and histoplasmosis complement fixation tests, calcified lung lesions, and residence in an endemic area, is *disciform detachment of the macula* [12]. In this lesion blood or serum is present between the lamina vitrea and pigment epithelium, pushing the retina forward.

histoplasmosis

toxoplasmosis

In both the congenital and acquired forms of *toxoplasmosis, chorioretinitis* is a frequent manifestation, occurring in over 90 percent of congenital infections. The *choroid* and often the *adjacent sclera* are focally thickened near the equator or the posterior pole of the orbit by a granulomatous infiltrate of epithelioid and giant cells, lymphocytes, and plasmocytes. The segment of *retina* overlying the granuloma is necrotic, and *Toxoplasma gondii* can be identified in this necrotic focus either lying free or encysted within retinal cells. The remaining retina is swollen and diffusely infiltrated by mononuclear cells, as is the *choroid.* Healed lesions form a *chorioretinal scar,* loss of pigment producing a white spot.

helminthic endophthalmitis

Nematodal infestation of the inner eye occurs in *visceral larva migrans* due to *Toxocara canis* or *T. cati.* It most often develops before the age of 10. One eye becomes blind without associated symptoms. A completely detached retina is found attached to a fibrous retrolental mass. Within this granulomatous focus, nematode larval fragments can be identified in about 50 percent of the cases. The membrane is infiltrated with numerous eosinophils. *Ocular cysticerciasis* is most commonly subretinal or subhyaloidal but occurs behind the choroid and in the vitreous or anterior chamber. There is little inflammatory reaction while the *Taenia solium* larva is alive or well preserved. When it degenerates, a giant cell layer abuts the cyst wall. A marked lymphocytic and plasmocytic infiltration with numerous Russell bodies surrounds the giant cells, and there is peripheral fibrosis.

sympathetic ophthalmia

Sympathetic ophthalmia (sympathetic uveitis) is the development of a bilateral granulomatous inflammation of the uveal tract following a perforating wound of the anterior segment of one eye. If the wounded eye is not promptly enucleated, sympathetic uveitis follows about 5 percent of such injuries, and blindness may result. The lesion apparently is an *auto-immune reaction to released uveal pigment. Microscopically* the uveal tissues are densely infiltrated by lymphocytes with islands of epithelioid cells. Eosinophils are occasionally numerous, and *Dalen-Fuchs' nodules* composed of clusters of epithelioid cells may be found between the lamina vitrea and pigment epithelium of the retina.

3. Mechanical Injuries

Mechanical injury is the most common form of eye disease. It may be produced by a contusion, concussion, penetrating wound, or perforating wound of the eye.

CONTUSION

Ocular contusion may result from a direct blow, as of a fist or boxing glove, or indirectly from blast injury, an automobile or plane crash, a fall, or a bullet wound of the head. Intraocular hemorrhage and displacement or rupture of eye structures commonly follow contusion. Subcutaneous *hemorrhage into the eyelids* (black eye, shiner) with marked edema is caused by blunt force injury such as a fist blow. The hemorrhage is slowly resorbed. Severe contusion injury of the *cornea* is rare, but Bowman's and/or Descemet's membrane may be torn, with resultant keratitis and edema. *Hyphema* frequently occurs. Small hemorrhages do not clot, and the blood may leave the anterior chamber through the trabecular meshwork. Larger hemorrhages fill the chamber and often clot. Secondary glaucoma may develop due to blockage of the anterior chamber angle or pupil by organization of such a clot. In rare cases the anterior and posterior chambers are filled by fibrous tissue.

The *iris* may suffer sphincter muscle injury *(iridoplegia),* with resultant dilatation of the pupil, stromal atrophy, recession (wedging of a fold of iris into the space about the lens), or rupture. Rupture occurs as a radial tear beginning at the pupillary margin or as a separation of the iris root from the ciliary body *(iridodialysis).* Rupture is accompanied by hemorrhage, and a long-lasting or recurring hemorrhage may result in the formation of synechiae between the iris, cornea, and lens.

Contusion injury of the ciliary body may consist of ciliary muscle tears with resultant cycloplegia, avulsion of the ciliary muscle from the scleral spur *(cyclodialysis),* or rupture and necrosis of the ciliary processes. Ciliary body tears are accompanied by hemorrhage into the posterior chamber and vitreous, or directly into the anterior chamber due to rupture of anterior ciliary vessels. Either open- or closed-angle *glaucoma or hypotony,* due to failure of aqueous humor secretion, may follow contusion of the ciliary body. *Open-angle glaucoma* results from damage to the trabecular meshwork associated with a tear which produces a wide, deep chamber angle [13]. The increased pressure may develop long after the injury. *Closed-angle glaucoma* is caused by organization of a blood clot or synechia formation in the chamber angle.

Contusion damage to the choroid may be in the form of hemorrhage into the stroma or subretinal space, detachment from the ciliary body, a usually crescentic tear lying between the optic disk and macula or temporal to the macula, and traumatic choroiditis secondary to hemorrhage and necrosis.

In the *retina,* contusion may express itself as edema, which is typically most marked around the macula and may lead to cystoid degeneration there; hemorrhage, which may be resorbed innocuously or eventuate in cystoid degeneration or extensive gliosis of the retina; a tear at the ora serrata *(retinal dialysis or disinsertion);* detachment due to subretinal hemorrhage or serous fluid accumulation or to organization of a vitreous hemorrhage; or *concussion of the retina (commotio retinae),* the mechanism of which is poorly understood but is probably related to injury of the retinal capillaries and arterioles. Extensive edema and small hemorrhages appear in the retina, giving it a snowy appearance on funduscopic examination. The edema and hemorrhages usually clear with slight residual damage.

Rupture of the zonular fibers by a contusing force leads to subluxation or to complete dislocation of the *lens.* Dislocation into the anterior chamber causes pupillary and filtration angle block and results in glaucoma. A powerful contusing force may rupture the lens capsule, usually at the equator. Most cases of *contusion cataract* develop without capsular rupture, a rosette-like opacity appearing in the posterior cortex. *Vossius' ring* of pigment (melanin or hemosiderin) frequently appears on the anterior lens capsule surface. Extremely forceful blunt trauma may cause rupture of the globe, usually at the equator where the sclera is thin or at the limbus. Explosive loss of ocular structures and massive hemorrhage often occur, and if the eye is not enucleated, phthisis bulbi results.

PENETRATING AND PERFORATING WOUNDS:

Penetrating or perforating wounds of the eye occur as a laceration, puncture wound, surgical incision, or rupture resulting from contusion. They may be inflicted by a knife, ice pick or other pointed weapon, missile or other flying object, and stationary structures hit during automobile accidents or falls. Such wounds of the anterior segment, involving the conjunctiva, cornea, iris, and lens, are common. When they are small and uncomplicated by infection or a residual foreign body, healing is often accomplished with only slight scarring and visual loss. An *abrasion of the cornea* usually involves only the epithelium and heals by migratory re-epithelialization within a week. *Penetrating corneal wounds* reaching the stroma heal by fibroblastic proliferation with scar formation and without replacement of the defect in Bowman's membrane. Following a small perforation of the cornea, the broken segment of Descemet's membrane is reformed by the adjacent endothelial cells.

Complications

Complications of penetrating or perforating wounds occur when they are large, deep, infected, and/or associated with a residual foreign body. *Early complications* include *expulsive hemorrhage* from the choroid which may propel ocular structures such as the retina, vitreous, lens, and iris out through the wound; angle closure *glaucoma* due to organization of a hyphema or formation of synechiae; *cataract* secondary to injury to the lens capsule; *phacoanaphylactic endophthalmitis,* which is due to hypersensitivity to released lens protein and occasionally also involves the uninjured eye; *endophthalmitis or panophthalmitis* resulting from infection and necrosis; *sympathetic ophthalmia* in both the injured and opposite eye due to hypersensitivity to released uveal pigment; and *retinal detachment* due to hemorrhage. *Late complications* include *glaucoma* due to synechia formation, pupillary block by occlusion or seclusion, fibrosis of the trabecular meshwork, or the ingrowth of surface corneal epithelium into the anterior chamber angle; and *retinal detachment* due to organization of a vitreous hemorrhage or inflammatory reaction.

INTRAOCULAR FOREIGN BODIES: *Foreign bodies* propelled into the eye during penetrating or perforating injury include pieces of metal, wood, or stone, animal or vegetable matter, eyelashes, and bone fragments. Their presence enhances the deleterious effects of the associated trauma by the reaction of ocular tissues to them and/or the introduction of bacteria or fungi. The degree and type of reaction vary. Animal and vegetable materials evoke a marked foreign-body giant cell reaction and are often contaminated with infectious organisms. Many types of clean metallic foreign bodies stimulate a very slight inflammatory reaction; however, those containing iron and copper may provoke widespread changes in the eye.

Siderosis: *Ferrous* foreign bodies cause *siderosis.* The extent of the damage is dependent on the size, degree of hardness (soft iron products are especially dangerous), location in the eye, and encapsulation of the iron-containing body. If it is quickly and completely walled off, the reaction to it is localized. Otherwise, iron becomes oxidized, and absorption may lead to its distribution throughout the eye with the formation of insoluble iron-protein complexes within cells, particularly those of the cornea, iris, ciliary, and lens epithelium and the retina. *Siderosis bulbi* is characterized by a rusty brown pigmentation of involved tissues; a brown anterior subcapsular cataract; retinal degeneration; and glaucoma, probably due to iron pigment absorption by the trabecular meshwork fibers.

Chalcosis: *Chalcosis* is the term used for similar changes due to intraocular foreign bodies containing copper alloys. These may produce a pigmented corneal ring, cataract formation, and retinal atrophy.

Argyrosis: *Argyrosis* is a grayish black pigmentation of the cornea and choroid occurring in silversmiths and individuals following prolonged local or systemic use of medicinal silver compounds. The metal is deposited in Bowman's membrane and the lamina vitrea.

4. Glaucoma

DEFINITION: *Glaucoma* is a complex of diseases *characterized by an elevated intraocular pressure.* This is almost always due to tissue changes which decrease the outflow of aqueous humor from the eyes. A *glaucomatous pressure* is one which is incompatible with the continued health and function of the eye. *Pressures above 23 mm. of mercury can damage the eye by capillary compression.* Patients with an intraocular pressure less than 30 mm. are usually not treated until Bjerrum's scotoma, a sickle-shaped enlargement of the physiologic blind spot, or a visual field loss is present. It is estimated that 2 percent of persons in the United States over 40 have some degree of glaucoma. It is the cause of about 15 percent of blindness; about 45,000 persons are blind and another 150,000 have decreased vision due to glaucoma.

NORMAL AQUEOUS HUMOR: An understanding of the *physiology of aqueous humor flow and the fine anatomy of the anterior chamber of the eye* is essential in regard to glaucoma. *Aqueous humor* is formed by the epithelium of the ciliary body at the rate of about 2 cubic millimeters per minute. *Hyposecretion* occurs: in acute iridocyclitis, with retinal detachment, after certain surgical procedures, and following administration of carbonic anhydrase inhibitors. *Hypersecretion* causes less than 1 percent of open-angle glaucoma. The fluid flows from the posterior chamber through the pupil into the anterior chamber where it is filtered through the trabecular meshwork into the canal of Schlemm, from which it returns to the venous system. The *trabecular meshwork* lies in the corneoscleral groove. About 75 percent of aqueous humor outflow resistance is in the meshwork, which consists of interconnecting, endothelially covered bands. The aqueous humor flows through oval perforations in the meshwork which connect by tortuous pathways. *Schlemm's canal* is an "outpost of the venous system." The canal runs a tortuous course in the posterior part of the internal scleral sulcus. Numerous collector channels drain Schlemm's canal and anastomose with the deep intrascleral venous plexus.

Glaucoma may be *classified* as congenital (developmental) glaucoma; primary angle closure glaucoma; primary open-angle glaucoma; secondary glaucoma; and absolute glaucoma.

CONGENITAL GLAUCOMA

Congenital glaucoma is recognized at birth in about 50 percent of the cases and by the age of 1 year in almost 90 percent. Involvement is bilateral in about 65 percent. The defect is probably transmitted as a simple recessive trait. The infant has constant light sensitivity, blepharospasm, and excessive tearing. The cornea becomes hazy or cloudy due to edema, and it may appear like white porcelain. *Pathologically the most consistent finding is an anterior insertion of the iris on the trabecular meshwork.* The longitudinal fibers of the ciliary muscle insert more anteriorly than normally, many inserting directly into the trabecular bands instead of the scleral spur. When the muscle contracts, the meshwork collapses and Schlemm's canal is flattened. The ciliary body and processes are often pulled centrally by the zonular fibers of an abnormally small lens, so that *microphakia* may be a factor in the development of congenital glaucoma [14]. *Defective formation of the anterior chamber angle* is due to failure of the normal cleavage between the trabecular fibers and the iris root by which the anterior chamber angle opens late in gestation. In occasional cases Schlemm's canal is not formed or there is a prominent Schwalbe's ring. Late in the course of congenital glaucoma the eye becomes very large in all directions *(buphthalmos)* since all coats stretch readily in infancy. *The anterior chamber is deep, and the angle is wide.* The iris root and trabecular meshwork degenerate, and Schlemm's canal often disappears. The *retina* shows severe degenerative changes, but the *nerve head* may show only a moderate cupping, probably because of scleral stretching.

PRIMARY ANGLE CLOSURE GLAUCOMA

Primary angle closure glaucoma is paroxysmal and is related to the development of an abnormally narrow anterior chamber angle. The anterior chamber loses depth with age, possibly due to enlargement of the lens. *Highly hyperopic eyes* are especially prone to acute angle closure glaucoma due to an associated narrow angle. *Acute attacks* may be precipitated by mydriatics, dark adaptation, and emotional shock (possibly by swelling of the ciliary body which pushes the iris forward). In acute glaucoma the eye is stony hard and markedly congested with a dilated pupil and edematous cornea. There are eye pain, headache, nausea, vomiting, and some loss of vision. Milder attacks are characterized by halos about lights, due to corneal edema. In the early stages of primary angle closure glaucoma the intraocular pressure fluctuates markedly, and the glaucoma is reversible. Between attacks the tension may be normal and only a shallow anterior chamber and narrow angle are found. With repeated attacks anterior synechiae form, angle closure becomes permanent, and the glaucoma is irreversible. *Pathologically the essential feature is contact between the iris and trabecular meshwork.* Early there are no actual adhesions, but with long contact *peripheral anterior synechiae develop. The meshwork undergoes fibrosis and degenerative changes, and Schlemm's canal is compressed* and later obliterated. The outflow of aqueous is decreased to zero, so that changes in the eye develop more rapidly and are more severe than in other types of glaucoma.

PRIMARY OPEN-ANGLE GLAUCOMA

Primary open-angle glaucoma (chronic simple glaucoma) is a slowly progressive disease in which the anterior chamber angle may vary from excessively wide to somewhat narrow. It is more common in men than women up to the age of 50, and then occurs about equally in both sexes in older persons. This suggests a hormonal factor, probably relaxin, which facilitates aqueous outflow in premenopausal women [15]. The *disease is bilateral* and increases in severity and frequency with age. The rise in intraocular pressure may be intermittent early. A decrease in aqueous outflow is present very early and may be greater than would be expected from the degree of pressure rise. The *principal pathologic changes* are probably in the trabecular meshwork due to degeneration and sclerosis of its collagen fibers, especially those adjacent to Schlemm's canal. The intertrabecular spaces adjacent to the canal are narrowed and even closed. However, these changes could be an effect rather than the cause of the increased pressure. *Narrowing of the collector channels and/or episcleral veins* may also produce outflow resistance in primary open-angle glaucoma.

SECONDARY ANGLE-CLOSURE GLAUCOMA

Secondary glaucoma is usually unilateral. Except for the pupillary block type, it is almost always due to changes in the anterior chamber. *Secondary angle-closure glaucoma may result from pupillary block* in iritis and partial lens dislocation, or following cataract extraction (due to forward protrusion of the vitreous face). *Iris bombé* develops because of the increased posterior chamber pressure and closes the anterior chamber angle. *Angle closure is most often due to the formation of peripheral anterior synechiae, as in acute and chronic iridocyclitis; penetrating wounds; contusion; vascular disease of the posterior segment of the eye* (diabetes; central retinal vein or artery occlusion; Eales' disease – retinal hemorrhages in young males often associated with tuberculosis; and retinal vasculitis); *intraocular neoplasms* (by pushing the iris forward, an associated iridocyclitis, or invasion of the angle); and *essential atrophy of the iris,* in which iris displacement and hole formation results in peripheral anterior synechiae. Synechia formation in vascular diseases is poorly understood but may be due to the development of new vessels in the anterior ciliary body, trabecular area, and anterior iris surface with extension into the angle.

SECONDARY OPEN-ANGLE GLAUCOMA

Secondary open-angle glaucoma is due to particulate matter in the trabecular meshwork. In *acute iridocyclitis,* inflammatory cells may block the meshwork, but glaucoma is not common because aqueous production is decreased. Glaucoma is more common in *chronic anterior uveitis.* The trabeculae become scarred, thickened, and matted together, obliterating the trabecular spaces in prolonged cases. Sometimes the meshwork is directly involved in the inflammatory process *(trabeculitis).* In *phacolytic glaucoma* associated with hypermature cataract, macrophages containing phagocytized lens material plug the meshwork spaces. The pressure may become very high in severe cases. Pseudoexfoliation of the lens capsule produces *glaucoma capsulare* due to meshwork blocking by the sloughing of periodic acid-Schiff- and colloidal iron-positive material which has been deposited on the anterior lens capsule in anterior chamber disease. The material is gray, fluffy, and dandruff-like, and it is found on the zonule of the lens, iris, and cornea as well as in the trabecular meshwork. Granules are present within macrophages and endothelial cells in the meshwork. *Pigmentary glaucoma* is rare and idiopathic, occurring bilaterally in myopic young individuals. Melanin granules block the meshwork and float in the anterior chamber. The iris epithelium is depigmented. In *diffuse iris melanoma,* loosely adherent neoplastic cells may shed and enter the meshwork, as may cells from lymphomas and juvenile xanthogranuloma. *Choroidal neoplasms,* even small ones, may cause glaucoma in an obscure manner. *Increased venous pressure* (as in a carotid arterial-cavernous sinus communication) or *obstruction of venous outflow* (due to orbital neoplasm or thrombophlebitis) may cause secondary open-angle glaucoma. *Trauma is an important cause;* glaucoma may result from erythrocytes in the meshwork or clotted blood in the angle resulting from anterior chamber hemorrhage in ocular contusion. *Penetrating injuries* may lead to epithelial or endothelial proliferation over the meshwork, although peripheral anterior synechia formation and angle closure is a more common cause following such injuries.

EFFECTS OF GLAUCOMA

The effects of glaucoma on ocular tissues are widespread and may be severe. The *corneal epithelium* becomes edematous in acute or chronic glaucoma, and bullae may form in long-standing cases *(bullous keratopathy).* A degenerative pannus may form between the epithelium and Bowman's membrane, and the endothelium may become atrophic. The *sclera* may bulge under a prolonged increased pressure, especially in children, producing a *scleral staphyloma.* These are most common along the equator at the perforations of vortex veins. They may also occur at the limbus *(intercalary staphyloma)* and adjacent to the ciliary body *(ciliary staphyloma)* in association with inflammation and scleral softening in these areas. The *lens* is not directly affected by the increased pressure, but *cataracts* are almost always present in prolonged glaucoma, possibly due to alterations in aqueous humor composition. The *iris* shows ischemic necrosis in acute glaucoma due to interference with its nerve and blood supply. The stroma and sphincter almost completely disappear, producing a fixed dilated and oval pupil. The entire *uveal tract* becomes atrophic in long-standing glaucoma, the *choroid* being least affected. *Ciliary epithelial atrophy* reduces aqueous production. Peripapillary choroidal atrophy with hyperplasia of the overlying pigment epithelium produces the *peripapillary glaucomatous halo.* The *retina* shows degenerative changes in the nerve fiber and ganglion cell layers with gliosis. *Optic disk* changes cause most of the visual impairment. The disk becomes *cupped,* and there is atrophy of nerve fibers and supporting cells. The *cribriform plate* is bowed backward. Usually the *nerve* shows a columnar gliosis, but in some cases this is absent and large cystoid cavernous spaces filled with mucoid material are found. *Nerve fiber damage* is probably due to their stretching, compression, and angulation as they cross the disk and enter the cribriform plate. *Visual loss* is partly due to interference with the blood supply to the retinal ganglion cells.

ABSOLUTE GLAUCOMA

Absolute glaucoma is the end stage of chronic simple glaucoma. The eyes are blind, painful, and chronically inflamed. The cornea is usually cloudy, the lens may contain a cataract, and the optic nerve is deeply cupped and atrophic.

5. *Degenerations*

EYELIDS: Blepharochalasis

Blepharochalasis is a peculiar atrophy and slackening of the skin of the eyelid; it is associated with repeated episodes of edema. The skin becomes finely wrinkled, and enlarged blood vessels are visible beneath it. Eventually the upper lid comes to hang down over the lash border. *Senile atrophy* occurs in an older age group than blepharochalasis and is due to elastic degeneration in the dermis.

Ectropion

Senile ectropion is an eversion of the lower lid usually and is common in persons exposed to sunlight and wind occupationally and in fair-skinned individuals. Ectropion may also result from scarring of either lid by inflammation or a burn. In ectropion the palpebral conjunctiva is exposed and covered with dried secretions.

Entropion

Entropion is an inversion of a lid and may be due to scar contraction, as following trachoma or a burn, or to spasm of the orbicularis muscle (spastic entropion). The inverted eyelashes cause the sensation of a foreign body and may produce corneal abrasion.

Xanthelasma

Xanthelasma palpebrarum is the presence of soft, yellow to brown, oval papules on the eyelids of middle-aged persons as part of a xanthomatosis, or sometimes without apparent cause. The dermis is heavily infiltrated with foamy, lipid-laden macrophages and occasional Touton giant cells.

CONJUNCTIVA: Pinguecula; Pterygium

Pinguecula is a focal degeneration of the bulbar conjunctiva near the limbus. It is closely related to the *pterygium,* a winglike plaque usually lying across the nasal half of the conjunctiva and cornea. Occasionally the process affects the temporal side of the eye. It is due to repeated exposure to wind and dust in hot, dry climates. Pupillary involvement by the membrane diminishes vision. *Grossly* both the pinguecula and pterygium are raised and pearly gray or yellow. *Microscopically* the epithelium shows alternating foci of atrophy and acanthosis with hyperkeratosis and dyskeratosis. In the submucosa there are elastic degeneration and hyalinization of collagen, together with chronic inflammation and telangiectasia.

CORNEA:

The *cornea* is subject to multifold *degenerations* due to keratitis, systemic disease, or aging; and *dystrophies* related to developmental and frequently hereditary factors. The *degenerations* typically begin peripherally in the elderly and cause no visual loss in the early stages. The *dystrophies* usually start centrally in younger persons and are responsible for definite sight impairment. They are basically nutritional or metabolic disturbances in the cornea.

Degenerations: pannus; band keratopathy; lipid keratopathy

A *pterygium* may extend over the cornea from the conjunctiva and is covered by conjunctival epithelium. *Degenerative pannus* is associated with corneal edema and is formed by hyalin deposition between the epithelium and Bowman's membrane. *Band keratopathy* is the deposition of calcium in Bowman's membrane in old blind eyes, as in absolute glaucoma; chronic iridocyclitis; and the hypercalcemia of sarcoidosis, hyperparathyroidism, and hypervitaminosis D. *Lipid keratopathy* is the formation of a cholesterol-containing plaque in or next to a vascularized segment of corneal stroma, usually in patients with hypercholesterolemia.

arcus senilis; bloodstaining

Arcus senilis is the formation of a gray or white ring near the corneal periphery. It is common in elderly persons and is due to the accumulation of lipid material in the corneal stroma. *Hassall-Henle bodies* (warts) are senile, focal hyaline thickenings at the periphery of Descemet's membrane. Corneal clouding at birth or during infancy occurs in *gargoylism* (Hurler's disease) because of the storage of glycoprotein and acid mucopolysaccharide there. In *cystinosis* fine, bright cystine crystals are deposited in the anterior corneal stroma. In *ochronosis* melanin pigment appears in the stroma peripherally. The *Kayser-Fleischer ring* in hepatolenticular degeneration results from the laying down of greenish black copper sulfide in Descemet's membrane peripherally. *Bloodstaining of the cornea* follows hyphema associated with glaucoma, hemoglobin pigments appearing throughout the stroma and clearing slowly.

Dystrophies: keratoconjunctivitis sicca

Keratoconjunctivitis sicca is due to a degeneration of the lacrimal glands as part of *Sjögren's syndrome* and occurs preponderantly in women recently past the menopause. It is usually bilateral, one eye being affected before the other, and is characterized by *inadequate lacrimation and conjunctival and corneal dryness* with punctate erosions and stromal opacities. The lacrimal gland changes are due to an *auto-immune reaction* and consist of secretory epithelial atrophy and a marked lymphocytic infiltration. Sjögren's syndrome also consists of salivary gland degeneration with decreased salivation, atrophic rhinitis, and a chronic polyarthritis. Lymphocytosis and sometimes eosinophilia are found in the peripheral blood. *Decreased lacrimation* also results from congenital defects or surgical excision of a lacrimal gland or its duct.

keratoconus

Keratoconus is an idiopathic, usually bilateral dystrophic degeneration of the corneal stroma which begins at about the age of 10, progresses for about 5 years, and then stops. There is thinning of the stromal lamellar fibers of the central cornea so that it gives under the intraocular pressure and assumes a conical shape. Bowman's membrane becomes fibrillar, then wavy, and numerous breaks occur in it. A narrow zone of pigment (Fleischer ring) surrounds the cone. Perforation of Descemet's membrane leads to corneal opacities.

granular dystrophy

macular dystrophy

lattice dystrophy

The *heredofamilial stromal dystrophies* are: *granular dystrophy,* transmitted as a dominant, in which discrete, gray, granular or ringlike opacities develop in the center of the cornea; *macular dystrophy,* inherited as a recessive, in which poorly demarcated gray opacities appear with a diffuse cloudiness of the cornea between them; and *lattice dystrophy,* transmitted as a dominant and characterized by branching linear opacities in the central cornea. *Microscopically* [16] in the *granular form* the opacities are foci of finely granulated stromal hyalin degeneration; in the *macular type* the opacities show the accumulation of acid mucopolysaccharide within and between corneal fibroblasts [17]; and in *lattice dystrophy* amyloid accumulates between the epithelium and Bowman's membrane, and there is a focal amyloid deposition in the outer layers of the stroma [18].

endothelial dystrophy

Fuchs' dystrophy

Endothelial dystrophy (cornea guttata) is bilateral and is typified by a marked laminar thickening of Descemet's membrane and the presence of subendothelial wartlike excrescences centrally on the membrane. The endothelial cells show degenerative changes. As a result excessive amounts of water are absorbed into the cornea, and *Fuchs' epithelial dystrophy* ensues. The cornea becomes cloudy, especially centrally, due to edema of the epithelium and stroma. In severe cases bullae form and a degenerative pannus develops.

IRIS

In *diabetes mellitus* a pathognomonic lacy vacuolization of the pigment epithelium of the iris may occur. The lesion is due to extensive glycogen storage.

LENS: Cataract:

A *cataract* is an opacity of the lens. The opacification is often due to the accumulation of interfibrillar fluid and the precipitation of proteins within the lens. Cataract may be congenital or it may be due to trauma; intraocular inflammation; physical agents such as ionizing and microwave radiation, infrared radiation (as in glassblowers and others exposed occupationally to high temperatures), and electric or lightning shock; intraocular foreign bodies containing toxic metals (iron, copper); drugs such as adrenocorticosteroids, triparanol, busulfan, 2,3-dinitrophenol, and ergot; diabetes mellitus; tetany; and, most commonly of all, senile degeneration.

congenital cataract

Congenital cataract is often associated with other ocular malformations. It is sometimes due to persistence of the embryonic perilenticular vascular network over the anterior or posterior pole. *Zonular (lamellar) cataract* is almost always bilateral and is probably due to injury to one or more groups of newly formed lenticular fibers in the embryo. In some cases the rubella virus is the injurious agent. Congenital cataracts are often familial or hereditary. This is true of the *nuclear cataract,* a small opacity in the center of the embryonal nucleus which interferes only slightly with vision; the rare *coralliform cataract,* which is a branching lustrous opacity; and the *coronary* (cerulean) *cataract,* which appears at the time of puberty and consists of flaky or punctate opacities in the shape of a wreath.

traumatic cataract

Traumatic cataract may be caused by a penetrating wound or contusion of the eye. When the lens capsule is penetrated, it often retracts elastically away from the perforation site. Portions of the exposed lenticular cortex and nucleus degenerate and are removed by phagocytic cells. Optically dense new fibers fill the defect. A similar opacity may follow the surgical removal of a cataract from within the capsule. Lens epithelium may regenerate to form a new dense, ring-shaped lens about the equatorial zone *(Sommering's ring).* In *postcontusion cataracts* a ring-shaped opacity conforming to the pupillary outline *(Vossius' ring)* may form due to blood or iris pigment adherent to the lens; or a star-shaped or leaf-shaped opacity (posterior rosette-shaped cataract) may occur due to suture line separation by the force of the blow. The former type clears rapidly; the latter improves within weeks, but leaves a residual opacity.

cataract due to foreign body

Cataract due to an intraocular metallic foreign body is known as siderosis of the lens when the offending metal is iron and chalcosis when it is copper. In *siderosis* iron is taken up by the subcapsular epithelium and later by the lens fibers. Their degeneration leads to cataract formation. In *chalcosis* copper is deposited in the lens capsule and just beneath it. The resulting cataract has a radiating pattern which gives it a sunflower appearance.

cataract due to therapeutic agents

Discrete small *posterior subcapsular cataracts* have developed in a number of patients receiving moderate or high doses of *adrenocorticosteroids over prolonged periods* [19]. Severe visual impairment does not occur with steroid-induced cataracts. *Bilateral involvement* occurs in almost all the cases. A number of cases of cataract associated with *triparanol* [20] occurred before the drug was withdrawn. Linear white, branching opacities which sometimes coalesced to a honeycomb pattern appeared beneath the anterior and posterior lens capsules.

irradiation cataract

In cataract due to ionizing radiation the opacity begins in the posterior cortex and may extend over a period of years to involve the entire lens. *Cataract due to infrared radiation* is characterized by splitting and sloughing of the outer layer of the lens capsule. This process is most marked in the peripupillary zone.

electric or lightning cataract

Cataract due to electric or lightning shock usually occurs in the eye nearer the point of contact and appears a few months after the shock. It begins as flakelike subcapsular opacities which progress within months or a year to clouding of a quadrant or the entire lens. Cataract does not occur with psychiatric electroshock therapy.

cataract in tetany or diabetes

Cataracts in cases of tetany and in diabetes mellitus in young persons are bilateral and characterized by flaky opacities in the subcapsular cortex of the lens. In older diabetics cataracts are of the senile type.

cataracta complicata

Cataracta complicata is the term applied to a lenticular opacity complicating intraocular disease. It occurs in cases of chronic uveitis, retinitis pigmentosa, and retinal detachment due to an interference with lens nutrition. The opacity begins in the cortex near the posterior pole, becomes progressively larger and thicker as dense new fibers are laid down, and gradually involves the entire lens. In *severely myopic eyes* cataracts occur more often and at an earlier age than in hyperopic or normal eyes. Such cataracts are typically due to nuclear sclerosis.

senile cataract

Senile cataract is the category into which spontaneous lenticular opacities in persons beyond middle age are placed. The *cause* is most likely senescent degenerative changes in the lens. The condition becomes progressively more frequent with increasing age, and by the age of 80 over 85 percent of persons have some degree of lenticular opacity. *Pathologically* two forms occur: the nuclear (sclerotic) and the cortical (liquefactive). In *nuclear sclerosis* there are gradual enlargement, increased yellowness and density, and loss of transparency of the nucleus. Occasionally the nucleus or even the entire lens becomes dark brown or black. In the *cortical type,* fluid accumulates in and between lenticular fibers early. With time the fibers become edematous and fragmented. In the optically opaque *mature cataract* the degenerated fibers commonly become a mass of strongly acidophilic morgagnian globules. Still later the cortex develops into a homogeneous, poorly staining fluid structure. In the *hypermature cataract* this lens fluid has been lost through the intact capsule, and the lens is collapsed and wrinkled. In the *morgagnian cataract* the entire cortex is liquefied and milky, and the nucleus sinks downward into it. *Clinically* nuclear sclerosis produces myopia by increasing the refractive index of the lens, so that farsighted persons find that they can read better without glasses ("second sight"). Their distance vision is affected, and over a period of years there is a gradual diminution of sight. Cortical opacities are somewhat more rapidly progressive and interfere considerably with vision.

complications of cataract

The *complications of cataract* are *phacogenic glaucoma and endophthalmitis. Glaucoma* may be due to interference with intraocular fluid flow by pupillary block due to an intumescent (markedly swollen) mature cataract, or by escaped liquefied lens protein from hypermature cataracts. This fluid is phagocytized by macrophages which plug the anterior chamber angle *(phacolytic glaucoma).* Rarely hyaline flakes exfoliated from the lens capsule may block the chamber angle. *Phacoanaphylactic endophthalmitis* is due to a hypersensitivity reaction to released lens protein. A tuberculoid granulomatous reaction occurs on the surface of the lens and about separated lenticular fragments in the vitreous or aqueous humor. Synechiae plaster the lens to the iris. Sympathetic uveitis occasionally develops, and phacoanaphylaxis may be bilateral. In *phacotoxic uveitis,* which is probably a variant of the previous lesion, macrophages and a few neutrophils accumulate on the lens surface, and there is a heavy lymphocytic and plasmocytic infiltration of the anterior uvea. Both types of endophthalmitis are uncommon among cases of cataract.

VITREOUS LAMINA AND BODY: Drusen

Drusen (verrucae) are nodular thickenings on the lamina vitrea (Bruch's membrane) which develop after middle age usually. The excrescences are hyaline material secreted by retinal pigment epithelial cells and may become calcified. Excessive deposits centrally may produce retinal degeneration.

Synchysis scintillans is the presence of white, bright cholesterol and fatty acid bodies in the vitreous gel in persons beyond middle age. In *asteroid hyalosis* (nivea), crystalline calcium soap particles are innocuously present in the vitreous of older persons. In *muscae volitantes* ("spots before the eyes"), no morphologic cause is found in the vitreous. *Opacities of the vitreous* are common in older persons and following chorioretinal hemorrhage or inflammation. They range from dustlike particles to membranes or threads. *Liquefaction of the vitreous* is common in patients with severe myopia and in elderly individuals.

RETINA: Retrolental fibroplasia

Retrolental fibroplasia is an oxygen-induced degeneration in the premature infant in whom the *peripheral retina* is not completely vascularized. In such an infant an *increased oxygen tension* causes an immediate but transient closing down of terminal arterioles and the arterial side of the capillary bed [21]. With continued increased oxygen levels an irreversible vaso-obliteration occurs. The involved vessels degenerate, and vasoproliferation from adjacent vessels begins. *Newly formed capillaries* invade the retina, penetrate the internal limiting membrane, and grow into the vitreous. *Endothelial proliferation* produces glomeruloid capillary tufts, and reactive gliosis may occur in the retina. *Retinal detachment* may be caused by organization of vitreous hemorrhages and exudates and the formation of a preretinal membrane. In severe cases a completely detached retina and organized vitreous form an *opaque retrolental mass* giving a white cat's-eye reflex *(leukocoria)* which is difficult to distinguish from that of a retinoblastoma. In fibroplasia there may be a temporary secondary glaucoma without buphthalmos, but in advanced cases the eye becomes phthisical *(enophthalmos)*. In less severe cases the retina may be only partially involved, mainly on the temporal side in 90 percent of such cases. In some cases *only the temporal side* is involved, that half being fully vascularized later than the nasal side. *Unilateral cases and ones in full-term babies occur,* probably due to variations in retinal vascularization. *Myopia* is fairly frequently associated with mild retrolental fibroplasia.

Retinitis pigmentosa

Retinitis pigmentosa is a recessively inherited premature degeneration of the neuroepithelium which begins early in life and slowly progresses to blindness at the age of 50 to 60. The process begins peripherally and gradually extends centrally, sparing the macula until the very late stages. The rod and cone layer almost entirely disappears, and the ganglion cells are reduced in number. The fundus becomes slate gray in color due to excessive pigment deposits in the foci of degeneration by the pigment epithelium. Retinitis pigmentosa is sometimes associated with congenital deaf-mutism and the Laurence-Moon-Biedl syndrome.

Peripheral cystoid degeneration

Peripheral cystoid degeneration (Blessig's or Iwanoff's cysts) is so common as to be considered physiologic in older persons. The cysts usually appear after age 20 and increase in number and size with age. They begin at the ora serrata and extend backward, and arise first in the outer plexiform layer. Their enlargement and coalescence may lead to splitting of the retina into two layers *(retinoschisis)*.

Senile retinoschisis

Senile retinoschisis occurs with severe cystoid degeneration, especially on the temporal side. It is often bilaterally symmetric. The process is frequently slowly progressive, extending circumferentially more than posteriorly. *Microscopically* the inner wall of the cyst usually consists of a glial membrane with sclerotic vessels coursing through it. The outer wall maintains its structure, and the rods and cones are well preserved. Holes are frequent in the inner membrane and may also occur in the outer layers, leading to retinal detachment. Even without detachment an absolute scotoma is produced by the destruction of neural pathways.

Peripheral chorioretinal degeneration

Peripheral chorioretinal degeneration typically appears after age 40, progresses with age, and is bilateral. The process is most common inferiorly near the ora serrata, but in the elderly may occur patchily around the entire peripheral retina. *Grossly* the lesions vary from a tiny round or oval depigmented spot to large patches with scalloped edges, usually with some pigment remaining centrally or heaped up at the periphery. *Microscopically, all retinal layers* are often involved. Pigment epithelium, sensory cells, and the outer nuclear layers are completely absent. In the *choroid* the vessels are obliterated and replaced by fibrosis with marked stromal hyalinization, and the *choriocapillaris* is usually absent. When the retinal vessels are similarly affected, the degeneration is profound and hole formation is common. The *vitreous* becomes adherent over the degenerated foci, and tension on *vitreoretinal adhesions* during eye movements may produce retinal hole formation. If a blood vessel is included in the tear, vitreous hemorrhage follows. *Retinochoroidal adhesions* may be firm enough peripherally to prevent detachment so that the tears in the regions of degeneration are arrowhead- or horseshoe-shaped with the convexity toward the optic disk. Most of these tears occur superiorly and temporally. Occasionally stellate and, rarely, round holes develop. *Horseshoe tears are a frequent cause of retinal detachment,* and peripheral chorioretinal degeneration probably underlies the majority of retinal separations.

Lattice degeneration

Lattice degeneration of the retina is seen as patches of intersecting thin gray lines in the peripheral retina. Broad bands concentric with the ora serrata may develop. *Microscopically* there is degeneration of the retina and vitreous, and the blood vessels show hyaline thickening and luminal obliteration in the atrophic foci.

Retinal disinsertion

Disinsertion (dialysis) of the retina from its attachment to the ora serrata occurs spontaneously or as a result of peripheral retinal atrophy and cystoid degeneration or trauma, such as contusion. The dialysis most often is in the inferior temporal portion of the insertion. In adults disinsertion stops at the ora; in children ciliary epithelium may be separated.

Retinal detachment:

Detachment of the retina is a separation of the neuroepithelial layers from the pigment epithelium layer, thus depriving the former of an adequate blood supply. Such a detachment is due to the accumulation of fluid in the potential space between these two portions of the retina, a vestige of the central cavity of the embryonic optic vesicle. *Fluid accumulations may come about by extravasation from the choroid or retina* in chorioretinitis, choroidal or retinal neoplasms, hypertensive retinopathy, or retinal venous occlusion; *by the contraction of vitreous fibrous bands* which have been formed following intraocular trauma, inflammation, neovascularization, or hemorrhage and are attached to the inner retina, the contraction pulling apart the layers of the retina; *or by the pouring of fluid from the vitreous into the space through a retinal hole or tear (rhegmatogenous retinal detachment)* [22]. The last is present in about 7 percent of persons over the age of 40. However, the incidence of actual retinal detachment in such persons is about 0.14 percent. Such retinal openings may occur following ocular contusion (as in boxers) or mild trauma, especially in myopic eyes, or they may develop spontaneously. Peripheral cystoid degeneration and retinal atrophy predispose to hole or tear formation. The openings are horseshoe- or hairpin-shaped, crescentic or round. Once vitreous fluid seeps through a retinal defect, it tends to dissect through the subretinal space, peeling off more and more of the sensory retina.

clinical features

Clinically there is typically a sudden loss of a field of vision. With time the field loss extends, and central vision fails. In untreated cases almost total blindness usually results from progression of the detachment to involve most of the retina. On funduscopic examination the detached retina is elevated above the intact portions, and its vessels appear almost black. One or more tears are usually found through which the dark red choroid can be seen.

pathologic changes

In the detached portions of the retina the *rods and cones,* especially of the macula, degenerate after 4 to 6 weeks, with later *microcystoid degeneration* of the other layers. The cysts coalesce and form bullae. The underlying *pigment epithelium* proliferates, and drusen form on Bruch's membrane. Glial and fibrous proliferation may close retinal holes or tears, and trap the subretinal fluid. Adhesions may develop at the margins of the detachment, preventing its extension. Cellular, pigment, and cholesterol debris in the fluid act as irritants to produce a uveitis. This in turn may lead to synechia formation and *secondary glaucoma. Laser* (light amplification by the stimulated emission of *radiation*) used in the treatment of retinal detachment produces a small chorioretinal burn where the beam is focused. With a *ruby laser beam* (wave length 6940 angstroms), vesiculation occurs in the pigment epithelium, which absorbs about 70 percent of the light at this wave length [23]. Degenerative changes occur in the adjacent choroid layer. *A neodymium laser beam* (wave length 10,600 angstroms) produces degeneration mainly in the neural layers of the retina.

6. *Retinopathies Associated With Vascular Disturbances*

CENTRAL RETINAL ARTERY OR VEIN OCCLUSION

Atherosclerosis may develop in the central retinal artery, and thrombosis or other types of occlusion may occur on the plaques. *Central retinal arterial occlusion* within the optic nerve produces infarction of the entire inner half of the retina. Occlusion of veins is frequent where they are crossed and compressed by arterial branches with which they share a common adventitia. *Central retinal vein thrombosis* occurs in the segment within the lamina cribrosa of the sclera. A massive hemorrhagic infarct commonly develops in the retina. The streaklike hemorrhages may rupture into the vitreous and subretinal space. Later vascular proliferation occurs on the nerve head and anterior iridal surface *(rubeosis iridis),* and fibrovascular anterior synechiae develop. These occlude the anterior chamber angle and lead to glaucoma.

RETINAL ARTERIOLOSCLEROSIS:

Clinicopathologically changes in *retinal arteriolosclerosis* are classified in five groups. *Group I* includes the cases in which there is *retinal arteriolosclerosis* without loss of vision or evidence of retinal damage. On examination the vessels are seen as tortuous silver or copper wires, and the veins are compressed where the arterioles cross them, producing *arteriovenous nicking. Pathologically* there is a luminal narrowing due to a patchy hyaline intimal thickening of the arterioles. These changes are most constant and marked in individuals with *benign essential hypertension,* but they also occur in diabetics and elderly persons without hypertension. *Group II (retinal arteriolosclerosis with retinopathy)* includes more advanced cases in which small, round, well-defined white plaques *(retinal infarcts),* due to arteriolar occlusions, are found. The infarcts involve the superficial layers (inner nuclear and plexiform layers, ganglion cells, and nerve fibers). There also may be round or flame-shaped retinal hemorrhages. The infarcts and hemorrhages are common about the nerve head and macula. Visual loss is usually noted only when the macular area is involved.

Group III includes early cases of malignant hypertension and eclampsia in which there is *diffuse retinal arteriolar constriction.* All the arterioles are narrowed due to severe, irregular, and at times transient arteriolar spasm. No retinal change nor visual loss is found at this stage.

Hypertensive retinopathy

Group IV is *diffuse retinal arteriolar constriction with retinopathy (angiospastic hypertensive retinopathy)* and may develop rapidly in malignant hypertension and eclampsia. Central vision is commonly severely reduced due to macular involvement. In *toxemia of pregnancy* the retinal changes and visual loss often clear completely following return of the blood pressure to normal. The retinal arterioles show severe angiospasm in eclampsia, and in *malignant hypertension* there is also a smudgelike necrosis of the wall of terminal arterioles and capillaries. The retina is edematous and shows *exudates* (pools of edema fluid containing lipid, protein, and fibrin), hemorrhages, and whitish or grayish spots with fluffy borders. In the macular region the spots may form a stellate figure *(macular star)*. Arteriovenous nicking is usually quite marked. *Cotton-wool spots* are tiny, white, superficial retinal infarcts. Microscopically they are disk-shaped foci of nerve fiber layer thickening and necrosis. They contain several *cytoid* (cell-like) *bodies* which derive from degenerating axis cylinders. These bodies are globular and strongly acidophilic, have an even more deeply acidophilic or sometimes basophilic nucleoid mass, and measure 10 to 20μ in diameter.

Hypertensive neuroretinopathy

Group V is *diffuse retinal arteriolar constriction with neuroretinopathy (hypertensive neuroretinopathy)*. The changes are those described in Group IV, plus edema of the optic disk. *Retinal detachment* not uncommonly occurs in cases of groups IV and V due to the severe retinal edema with subretinal fluid accumulation.

DIABETIC RETINOPATHY: Clinical features

Diabetic retinopathy is commonly seen in patients who have had diabetes for over 15 years. While it is most frequent in patients past middle age, severe retinopathy may occur in young persons. Only about 50 percent of the cases of diabetic retinopathy also have retinal arteriolosclerosis. *Clinically* small round or oval, white or yellow (fatty) retinal deposits, petechiae, and other small hemorrhages are seen ophthalmoscopically. In severe cases the macular region may have a fluffy snowbank-like appearance, large hemorrhages are common, and vision is impaired to 20/200 or less.

Pathologic changes

Microscopically saccular *capillary microaneurysms* filled with a globoid mass of hyalin rich in mucopolysaccharides and similar to the glomerular capillary lesions of diabetic glomerulosclerosis are found. Microaneurysms occur in both arteriolar and venular capillaries. They are associated with a decreased ratio of pericytes to endothelial cells [24]. The loss of pericytes may produce a weakness of the vessel wall which results in microaneurysm formation. Petechiae result from aneurysmal ruptures and occur deep within the retina. The white deposits *(hard exudates)* consist of puddles of inspissated proteinaceous material in the outer plexiform layer. Yellowish deposits are made up of collections of lipid-laden macrophages *(circinate retinitis)*. Retinal hemorrhages may occur superficially and become organized, new capillaries forming on the surface *(retinitis proliferans)*. Vitreous contraction may produce retinal detachment.

SEPTIC EMBOLISM

In *septicemia,* especially in subacute bacterial endocarditis, petechiae and white spots with hemorrhagic halos *(Roth spots)* commonly appear (septic retinitis). The spots are microinfarcts caused by arteriolar occlusion by minute septic emboli.

PURTSCHER'S TRAUMATIC RETINOPATHY

Purtscher's traumatic retinopathy results from *fat embolism in the retinal and choroidal capillaries* following fractures due to crushing injuries of the chest or an extremity. Varisized distinct grayish white exudates, sometimes surrounded by hemorrhage, are found in the inner layers of the retina, especially near the disk and macula. Severe visual loss results.

7. Neoplasms

EYELIDS:

The *skin of the eyelids* is a common site for epithelial neoplasms. *Squamous papilloma* develops at the lid margin and on the palpebral conjunctiva and is often multiple. *Seborrheic keratosis,* which is not a true neoplasm, appears fairly frequently on the lid skin. *Senile keratosis* is found somewhat less often. *Basal cell carcinoma* is distinctly the most common malignant neoplasm of the eyelids. About 80 percent of these tumors develop at the inner canthus or on a lower lid, especially at the lid margin. *Epidermoid carcinoma* is seen much less frequently than the basal cell type. Both may be related to occupational exposure to sunlight and wind and to ill-fitted spectacle guards.

Basal cell carcinoma

Adnexal neoplasms

Neoplasms arising in the lid adnexa are uncommon and include sweat and sebaceous gland adenoma and carcinoma. Extramammary Paget's disease of the eyelid occurs with *adenocarcinoma of Moll's glands,* which are apocrine in type [25]. The *lacrimal glands* may be the site of mixed tumor, adenoid cystic and mucoepidermoid carcinoma, and adenocarcinoma similar to those seen in the salivary glands.

Pigment cell neoplasms

Junctional, compound, and intradermal *nevi* are common on the eyelids. A *premalignant melanosis,* in which there are the microscopic changes of a junctional nevus with excessive pigment formation involving the lid skin, palpebral and bulbar conjunctiva, and limbus, may occur. *Melanocarcinoma* infrequently develops on an eyelid.

CONJUNCTIVA

Epithelial neoplasms arising from the bulbar conjunctival mucosa are uncommon. Squamous papilloma, leukoplakia, carcinoma in situ, and invasive epidermoid carcinoma occur, especially about the limbus and other exposed conjunctival areas. The latter are typically superficially infiltrating and slowly growing. Occasionally metastases to the preauricular and upper cervical lymph nodes develop. *Nevi* are fairly common on the bulbar conjunctiva and at the limbus. At the latter site *malignant melanoma* is especially likely to occur, but its prognosis is much less serious than in cutaneous melanocarcinoma.

CORNEA

Occasionally *epidermoid carcinoma* arises on the *corneal mucosa,* particularly at the site of a pterygium. It grows slowly and invades the eye late in its course.

UVEA: Ciliary adenoma

Adenoma of the ciliary epithelium is an uncommon, usually asymptomatic, round or oval mass measuring up to 1 mm. in diameter. It arises by the invagination of nonpigment and pigment epithelial cells into the ciliary body and the proliferation of the nonpigmented epithelium in the form of rosettes. The tumor is surrounded by pigment epithelium. Rarely an adenoma arises from the iris epithelium.

Ciliary carcinoma

Adenocarcinoma of the ciliary epithelium is rare and appears to develop in a benign ciliary tumor, especially following inflammation of the anterior uvea. *Microscopically* the neoplasm consists of sheets of undifferentiated cuboidal epithelial cells with varying numbers of tubular structures lined by single layers of atypical epithelium. It may invade the iris root or press against the lens, producing a cataract. Metastases do not occur.

Diktyoma

Diktyoma (embryonal medullo-epithelioma) *of the ciliary epithelium* is an unusual, often congenital neoplasm which arises from the nonpigmented epithelium. It is the ciliary counterpart of the retinoblastoma. A white flat tumor slowly extends from the ciliary body over the iris, posterior corneal surface, and anterior lens surface. These structures are later invaded and destroyed. *Microscopically* the neoplasm is almost stromaless, and there are membrane-like foci resembling embryonic retinal tissue, nonpigmented ciliary epithelium, and retinoblastoma; in some cases there are foci of pigment epithelium, cartilage, and/or neuroglial tissue. The membranes often surround a cavity, as in the primary optic vesicle. A differentiated tumor of this group is called a *teratoneuroma.* Metastases do not occur.

Nevi

Nevi (benign melanomas) commonly appear in the uveal tract as small brown plaques, and on the iris are called freckles. *Microscopically* they consist of clusters of small, spindle-shaped melanocytes which are typically loaded with melanin pigment.

Malignant melanoma:

Malignant melanoma of the uveal tract is the most important of all intraocular neoplasms. Uveal malignant melanomas arise from branching stromal melanocytes, possibly from Schwann sheath cells of ciliary nerves, and rarely from the pigment epithelium. They arise in the choroid much more often than in either the iris or the ciliary body. Choroidal melanomas originating near the macula are typically smaller at the time of discovery than those developing peripherally, because the former interfere with vision early. Visual disturbances are produced by interfering with the blood supply of the rods and cones of the overlying retina and by retinal detachment resulting from a collection of serous fluid in the subretinal space.

clinical features

Uveal melanoma usually becomes manifest in persons past middle age, but there is evidence that its growth not uncommonly begins in the early adult years. The neoplasm is rare in Negroes, and its frequency is about the same in the two sexes. Bilateral uveal melanomas are rare.

pathologic changes

Grossly choroidal melanoma early is a disk-shaped, pinkish to dark brown mass located most commonly in the posterior segment. Eventually it breaks through the lamina vitrea and invades the retina, forming a mushroom or collar button-shaped mass in which the head of the neoplasm is much larger than the tumor base. In the *ciliary body* the neoplasm may grow circularly within the body *(ring melanoma)* or it may implant on the iris and extend through that structure to involve the anterior chamber angle and produce glaucoma. Increased intraocular pressure is commonly caused by *melanoma of the iris* (glaucoma occurs in about one-third of all cases of uveal melanoma, sometimes without apparent cause). Iris melanoma [26] may grow as a localized or diffuse mass or as a ring melanoma.

Microscopically, according to Callender's classification, *uveal melanomas* show six different growth patterns with varying prognoses. Least malignant, with a 5-year survival rate of 95 percent, is the *spindle A type* in which the melanoma consists of sheets of nevus-like cells with an elongated nucleus containing a longitudinal chromatin bar. The *spindle B type* is the most common cell form; its 5-year survival rate is about 85 percent. This neoplasm is made up of plump spindle-shaped cells with a large, prominently nucleolated nucleus. The *fascicular type* is the least common form of melanoma; it has a survival rate of about 80 percent. It contains both spindle A and B cells, and their nuclei are frequently palisaded, in some cases around blood vessels and in others as in neurilemmomas. The uncommon *epithelioid type* has the poorest prognosis, with a 5-year survival figure of about 30 percent. It consists of pleomorphic sheets and clusters of varisized epithelium-like cells which are sometimes arranged alveolarly. The *mixed type* has a survival rate of roughly 50 percent. The *necrotic type,* in which there is such extensive loss of structure that classification is impossible, has a 55 percent survival for 5 years. The amount of melanin pigment in all types of uveal melanoma varies from none occasionally (amelanotic melanoma) to an enormous deposition of pigment which is often especially dense about foci of necrosis.

Metastases

Extraocular extension has been reported in from 10 to 40 percent of the cases of choroidal melanoma. Metastases are even less frequent with ciliary or iris melanomas. The periorbital tissues may be invaded through the sclera or by means of emissary veins. Melanomas occasionally invade the optic nerve. *Distant metastases are hematogenous and are most common in the liver.* Not infrequently, widespread and fatal metastases appear more than 5 years after enucleation of the affected eye.

Other neoplasms

Leiomyoma occasionally arises in the iris from the sphincter or dilator pupillae, those derived from the latter often being pigmented. Rarely a benign smooth muscle neoplasm develops from the ciliary muscle. *Neurilemmoma* arises rarely from the sheath of a ciliary nerve.

RETINA: Retinoblastoma

Retinoblastoma [27] is the most common malignant intraocular neoplasm of infancy and childhood. It *arises from retinal neuroblasts* and probably has its inception during intra-uterine life, although it is usually not apparent at birth. About 75 percent of these tumors are diagnosed by the age of 3 years. Retinoblastoma occurs with equal frequency in boys and girls, and occasionally several children in a family are affected. *In about 20 percent of the cases the neoplasm is bilateral,* and in about 85 percent of unilateral cases it is multicentric. The mortality rate is about 20 percent, most deaths occurring within a year after discovery. Among cases in which there is no invasion of the optic nerve in the enucleated eye, the survival rate is over 90 percent. Rarely a retinoblastoma becomes completely necrotic, and phthisis bulbi results.

clinical features

Clinically the pupil of the involved eye becomes white or gray, and a yellow reflex is seen behind the pupil when light is shone into it (amaurotic cat's-eye reflex). Ophthalmic examination reveals a white or gray mass projecting from the retina. The neoplasm is radiosensitive. However, in some cases in which a cure has been achieved a radiation-induced osteogenic sarcoma or fibrosarcoma has developed in the orbital region after 5 to 10 years.

pathologic changes

The neoplasm usually arises in the posterior retinal hemisphere. It may grow mainly *endophytically* into the vitreous humor with seeding onto the lens, ciliary body, and iris, or *exophytically* with invasion of the subretinal space and choroid. In either form secondary foci of tumor tissue are common on the retina and the optic disk. *Extension is common along the optic nerve,* intracranial invasion being the cause of death in about 50 percent of fatal cases. *Microscopically* the retinoblastoma consists of small cells with prominent, hyperchromatic nuclei. In well-differentiated examples there are numerous *Flexner-Wintersteiner rosettes* in which the cells are arranged circularly with their cytoplasmic processes extending centrally. Electron microscopy demonstrates that the rosette cells possess many features in common with photoreceptor cells of the retina [28]. Undifferentiated neoplasms contain few or no rosettes and show numerous mitoses. *Foci of necrosis with calcification* are common in retinoblastomas.

metastases

Besides the common extension along the optic nerve and into the subarachnoid space and brain, hematogenous spread to distant sites such as the lungs and long bones may occur.

Angiomatosis

Angiomatosis of the retina (von Hippel's disease) has been mentioned on page 706. On the inner retinal surface a mass consisting of many tiny vascular spaces interspersed with proliferated glial tissue is formed. A large artery supplies the tumor with blood, and a dilated vein, often containing oxygenated blood because of arteriovenous fistula formation, drains it. Eventually the enlarging mass causes retinal detachment and blindness. The angiomatosis may involve both eyes.

METASTATIC NEOPLASMS

Metastatic neoplasms are rare in the eye and occur more often in the left than in the right eye. *Ocular metastases are usually hematogenous* through the ciliary artery. The uveal tract, especially the choroid, is the usual site of implantation. *Mammary carcinoma* is the most common source of metastases; bronchogenic carcinoma is also an important source. Infiltration of the inner eye may occur in the leukemias and lymphomas. Metastatic neoplasm often diffusely invades and thickens the choroid and produces retinal detachment.

8. Diseases of the Optic Disk and Nerve

CONGENITAL MALFORMATIONS

Coloboma of the optic nerve is a rare defect in which a portion of the nerve is absent, usually in the lower half. The corresponding visual field is lost. *Congenital optic atrophy* is sometimes familial and is characterized by a white disk and intra-uterine atrophy of the distal portion of the optic nerves. The affected infants are born blind.

OPTIC NEURITIS:

Anterior optic neuritis is an inflammation of the optic nerve which is visible on ophthalmoscopic examination. It may be caused by extension of an infection in an adjacent or nearby structure, such as meningitis, encephalitis, sinusitis, or orbital cellulitis; hematogenous infections, such as syphilis, certain fungus diseases, septicemia, or mumps; systemic poisoning by methyl alcohol, lead, or thallium; or multiple sclerosis.

Clinical features

Clinically there is a sudden marked, almost always unilateral loss of vision. The disk is hyperemic and elevated 1 to 3 diopters; its edges are blurred *(papillitis).* A large central scotoma is present.

Pathologic changes

The general changes include severe congestion of the vessels of the disk and surrounding retina, frequently with hemorrhages. The nerve head and retina are edematous. Specific changes vary according to the cause of the neuritis.

RETROBULBAR NEURITIS

Retrobulbar (posterior optic) *neuritis* is an inflammation of the second cranial nerve; there is no ophthalmoscopic evidence. About two-thirds of these cases occur in patients with multiple sclerosis. Other causes are extension of a sinusitis or meningitis to involve the nerve, hematogenous infection, or poisoning by methyl alcohol or thallium. *Clinically* there is a sudden central visual loss with a large scotoma. On examination the fundus is normal. Spontaneous recovery is common, especially in patients with multiple sclerosis. The *pathologic changes* vary with the cause. Those due to multiple sclerosis include focal demyelinization, chronic inflammation, and gliosis.

PAPILLEDEMA:

Papilledema (choked disk) is a swelling of the optic nerve head usually produced by stasis in the central retinal vein caused by increased intracranial pressure. Another factor is the transmission of the elevated intracranial pressure along the meningeal sheaths of the optic nerves. *Increased pressure within the cranial cavity* may be produced by a brain tumor or abscess, meningitis, cerebral hemorrhage, or cavernous sinus thrombosis. Posterior fossa neoplasms cause papilledema when they are relatively small, whereas frontal or temporal lobe tumors reach a large size before papilledema becomes apparent. Occasionally sudden *hypotony* resulting from intraocular surgery or from a penetrating eye wound results in papilledema. Less often a sharp rise in intraocular pressure causes it by interfering with venous outflow at the lamina cribrosa.

Clinical features

Clinically, the optic disks are elevated, often to 6 to 8 diopters, the condition almost always being bilateral. The retinal veins are tortuous and engorged, while the arterioles are normal; hemorrhages are common. Loss of vision occurs late in the course; it begins as enlargements of the physiologic blind spots, followed by a concentric contraction of the visual fields as optic atrophy progresses. When the nerves become atrophic, the disks usually flatten. Symptoms of the increased intracranial pressure, such as headache and projectile vomiting, are also present.

Pathologic changes

As fluid collects, the *nerve fibers* become edematous. The *retina* is pushed away from the disk margins by the fluid accumulation, and becomes folded. Serous fluid forms in the subretinal space.

PSEUDO-PAPILLEDEMA

Pseudopapilledema is an anomalous elevation of the optic disk which is often confused with true papilledema. It is usually first detected in childhood and is bilateral in the great majority of cases. About half the patients complain of headaches, and a few note blurring of vision or diplopia. The disk elevation is due to the *presence of hyaline bodies (drusen) within the optic disk* [29].

OPTIC ATROPHY

Optic atrophy is a loss of substance in the optic nerve and may be due to optic or retrobulbar neuritis, glaucoma, increased intracranial pressure, thrombosis or embolism in the central artery, neoplasms, or trauma. In *ascending optic atrophy* the initiating lesion is intraocular, and the atrophy extends inward in the direction of the optic chiasm. In *descending optic atrophy* the cause is usually intracranial, and the degeneration proceeds outward along the nerve. *Simple optic atrophy* is not preceded by inflammation or edema and is characterized by decreased size of the nerve with a variable loss of neurofibrils. The nerve head is pale or ghostly white and sharply defined on ophthalmoscopic examination. In *postneuritic optic atrophy* there are foci of gliosis in the degenerated nerve because of the preceding inflammation. The nerve head is pale or white, with indistinct borders. In cases of *atrophy due to glaucoma* the optic disk is deeply cupped.

NEOPLASMS: Melanocytoma

Melanocytoma of the optic disk is histologically benign and appears to arise from melanocytes in the lamina cribrosa. It occurs more commonly in Negroes than in white persons. The neoplasm grows as a small, jet black, nodular mass in the nerve head and occasionally the surrounding retina. *Microscopically* it consists of closely packed polyhedral cells with abundant cytoplasm which is bursting with melanin granules.

Glioma

Since the optic nerve is a fiber tract of the central nervous system with neuroglial supporting tissue, *gliomas* may arise in the nerve. They usually develop in childhood, and there is a slowly progressive visual loss with exophthalmos. The gliomas occur in the orbital or intracranial segments of the nerve and vary from the most common grade I astrocytoma to the unusual glioblastoma multiforme (astrocytoma, grade III or IV). In about 15 percent of the cases there are stigmata of neurofibromatosis.

The optic nerve has a meningeal covering from which a *meningioma* occasionally arises, usually in the intracranial segment of the nerve. It is not unlike meningiomas developing elsewhere. The adjacent bone undergoes marked proliferation (hyperostosis). Optic meningioma occurs in adults and produces a gradually increasing exophthalmos, loss of ocular movements, and optic atrophy.

Meningioma

DISEASES OF THE EARS

1. Developmental Defects

Congenital absence of the entire external ear is very, very rare, failure of development of some portion being somewhat more common. Absence of considerable portions of the external ear is usually associated with defective formation of the middle ear, and hearing is severely impaired or absent. *Microtia* is the presence of an abnormally small, normally shaped pinna; in *macrotia* this part is abnormally large. In cases of bilateral renal agenesis the external ears are flat and large, being set lower and more horizontally than usual. *Satyr ear* is a usually hereditary abnormality in shape, the external ear being pointed. In an extreme form, more common in females than males and often associated with deafness due to maldevelopment of the auditory nerve nuclei, the ear is triangular in shape. *Darwinian tubercle* is a nodular thickening of the helix. *Fibroepithelial polypoid masses* resulting from faulty growth of the aural part of the first branchial arch may appear just anterior to the tragus or on the cheek. A congenital *aural fistula (ear pit)* is a small, blind, epithelially lined invagination usually opening anterior to the tragus. *Synotia* results from developmental arrest, the ears lying horizontally beneath the mandible and meeting in the midline; it is always accompanied by mandibular hypoplasia. *Congenital middle ear deafness* (which often cannot be detected for several months) is usually associated with maternal rubella in early pregnancy.

2. Nondevelopmental Diseases of the External Ear and Tympanic Membrane

OTITIS EXTERNA

Otitis externa is an infection of the external ear and may be in the form of herpes zoster (due to a specific virus) with vesicles on the auricle and external auditory canal; leprosy; otomycosis of the auditory canal (usually due to *Aspergillus* and *Mucor* species), which is common in swimmers; or bacterial infection of the canal.

NONINFECTIOUS LESIONS:

Noninfectious lesions of the external ear include frostbite; *cauliflower ear* in boxers and wrestlers due to trauma with an overgrowth of cartilage caused by increased perichondrial activity; *chondrodermatitis nodularis chronica helicis* in which a painful nodule occurs in the helix in men (due to focal proliferation of the epidermis with central ulceration, necrosis of dermal collagen, a chronic inflammatory infiltrate into the dermis and perichondrium [perichondritis],and cystic degeneration of the cartilage), the cause of which is possibly trauma; *calcification of the cartilage* in hypercalcemia, Addison's disease, and systemic chondromalacia; and *tophi of gout.*

Neoplasms

Basal cell and epidermoid carcinomas are common in the skin of the ear. Neoplasms of the ceruminous glands [30] are very rare. These modified sweat glands lie deep in the dermis of the external auditory canal. Most of the ceruminous tumors are *adenomas or mixed tumors* with glandular and cartilaginoid components. These histologically benign neoplasms have a tendency to recur after surgical removal. Extremely rarely cylindromatous *ceruminous gland carcinoma* occurs.

MYRINGITIS

Myringitis is an infection of the tympanic membrane; it is caused by extension to the eardrum of an inflammatory process in the external auditory canal or middle ear, and by herpes zoster *(bullous myringitis)*. The membrane is usually most affected in its upper half, especially along the line of the handle of the malleus. This part is usually bulging in acute bacterial infections, and may rupture. Pain, loss of hearing, and tinnitus on the affected side are common. *Acute traumatic rupture* of the eardrum sometimes occurs in the left ears of women due to slaps ("lover's-tap ear").

3. Diseases of the Middle Ear and Air Cells

OTITIS MEDIA: Causes

Otitis media is an inflammation of the middle ear and may be acute or chronic. Common causes are beta-hemolytic streptococci, pneumococci, and staphylococci. Pneumococci are especially likely to lead to intracranial complications such as epidural abscess and leptomeningitis. Otitis media is most frequently due to *ascending infections along the eustachian tube* and is common, especially in children, as a complication in cases of scarlet fever, pharyngitis, tonsillitis, diphtheria, measles, influenza, and colds.

Clinical features

Clinically there are earache, fever, angry redness, and outward bulging of the tympanic membrane, sometimes perforation of the drum with drainage of pus from the middle ear, tinnitus, and impairment of hearing on the affected side. Signs of the underlying disease are also found.

Pathologic changes:

In *acute otitis media* the middle ear is filled with a purulent exudate (mucoserous in infections with organisms of low virulence). The mucosa of the middle ear and eustachian tube is edematous and is desquamated in places. Usually the process clears without residual damage, but occasionally fibrous adhesions form and interfere with the movements of the ossicles. Impairment of hearing or complete deafness results in such cases. *Chronic otitis media* may result in the formation of a *secondary cholesteatoma* (pearly tumor) by the ingrowth of squamous epithelium from Shrapnell's membrane. It is a pearly gray mass which most commonly develops in the upper portion of the middle ear in young adults who have had suppurative otitis media in childhood. Microscopically there are concentric rings of keratinized squamous cells with cholesterol deposits between them. The lining consists of squamous cells with a definite basal layer. *Aural polyp* is a soft, reddish mass of granulation tissue up to 1 cm. in diameter which grows into and may fill the external auditory canal in some cases of chronic suppurative otitis media. The vascular granulation tissue is infiltrated with mononuclear cells principally and is covered by cuboidal or squamous epithelium.

(Margin notes: cholesteatoma; aural polyp)

Complications

Complications of acute otitis media include mastoiditis, petrositis, labyrinthitis, thrombophlebitis, epidural abscess, meningitis, brain abscess, and hydrocephalus. *Thrombophlebitis* commonly occurs in the numerous small veins draining the petrous bone area, especially from the region of the mastoid air cells. These veins drain into the superior and inferior petrosal sinuses, thence into the sigmoidal sinus and the jugular bulb and vein. Septic thrombi may be carried to the lungs, setting up multiple abscesses.

SECRETORY OTITIS MEDIA

Secretory otitis media is caused by a block in the eustachian tube, usually produced by adenoids. A negative pressure develops in the middle ear, so that there is a transudation of fluid from the vessels, and the drums are retracted. The serous fluid is loculated and may persist for years. A 30 to 40 percent hearing loss is commonly found.

AEROTITIS MEDIA:

Aerotitis media (otic barotrauma) occurs in persons flying in nonpressurized aircraft. As the air pressure falls during ascent, air trapped in the middle ear under ground level pressure pushes the tympanic membrane outward. During descent the outside air pressure becomes greater than the middle ear pressure, so that a partial vacuum develops there and the membrane is pushed inward. Inflammation of the eustachian tube underlies the pressure differential. The resulting ear pain may be excruciating.

Pathologic changes

In the *acute form* of aerotitis media [31] the mucosa becomes edematous and its blood vessels are engorged. Submucosal hemorrhages are found, and there may be bleeding into the middle ear cavity. Straw-colored, clear fluid of low viscosity resembling serum collects in the cavity, probably due to the negative pressure there when a partial vacuum develops. The eustachian tube contains blood and mucus but may not be obstructed. In the *recurrent form,* granulation tissue is present in the middle ear and mastoid air cells; in the *chronic form,* fibrosis of the middle ear is found.

TUBERCULOUS OTITIS MEDIA

Tuberculosis may extend to the middle ear via the eustachian tube or hematogenously. There is extensive damage due to caseation necrosis within the middle ear and tuberculous osteomyelitis of the surrounding bone.

RADIATION OTITIS MEDIA

Radiation otitis media [32] occurs in some patients receiving x-ray or other types of ionizing radiation therapy to the auricular region. The mucosa of the middle ear becomes edematous, and the lining cells slough. Sterile fluid accumulates in the cavity. Hearing loss occurs in many cases receiving 4000 to 6000 R.

MASTOIDITIS

Mastoiditis is an inflammation of the mastoid air cells which communicate with the middle ear. *Acute mastoiditis* is due to an extension of an otitis media into the air cells. Their mucosa is edematous, and they are filled with an acute inflammatory exudate. An *acute osteomyelitis of the mastoid bone* may result. Erosion of the tip of this bone leads to the development of a deep cervical abscess or a cellulitis. An *epidural abscess* is produced by destruction of the inner table of the mastoid bone.

PETROSITIS

Petrositis [33] is an inflammation of the apical air cells which are sometimes present in the petrous portion of the temporal bone. As with mastoiditis, its incidence has been greatly reduced by the antibiotic therapy of otitis media. *Pathways* by which purulent exudate may reach the petrous pyramid are: (1) from the tympanic space above and behind the superior semicircular canal, (2) from the peritubal cells into the pyramids, and (3) from the peritubal cells by way of the carotid canal into the tip. The thin mucoperiosteum of the infected petrous air cells is eroded, and *osteomyelitis of the surrounding bone* develops. *Septic thrombophlebitis* is common, and the process may extend into the sigmoid and other large venous sinuses. A *cholesteatoma* may develop in the petrous air cells in chronic cases. *Clinically* in petrositis, pain in, around, or behind the ipsilateral eye or in the temporoparietal region is the most typical symptom. Early the pain is due to irritation of the great superficial petrosal nerve; later the ophthalmic nerve is involved. The appearance of *Gradenigo's syndrome* indicates an extension of the infection beyond the petrous bone to involve the abducens and trigeminal nerves. The patient develops pain in the ipsilateral temporal region and paralysis of the ipsilateral lateral rectus extraocular muscle.

NEOPLASMS

Neoplasms of the middle ear are rare. The most common type is *epidermoid carcinoma* [34]. Most cases occur in persons over 50. About 70 percent of the patients have had chronic otitis media for years. Occasionally adenocarcinoma and rhabdomyosarcoma develop in the middle ear.

4. Diseases of the Inner Ear

LABYRINTHITIS

Labyrinthitis is an inflammation of the inner ear, which may involve either the cochlear or vestibular part or both. Middle ear infections reach the inner ear through the fenestra cochleae (round window), fenestra ovale (oval window), or the fissula ante fenestram. Labyrinthitis may also be secondary to a meningitis. If cells of the organ of Corti or the hair cells of the semicircular canals are destroyed, there will be permanent loss in the functions of hearing or equilibration.

OTOSCLEROSIS:

Otosclerosis (otospongiosis) is an osteodystrophy of the bony capsule of the inner ear which may produce progressive, although usually not total, bilateral deafness. The *cause* is uncertain, but otosclerosis appears to be inherited as an autosomal dominant with limited penetrance. There is a familial history in 40 percent of the cases. The incidence of Rh negative blood is somewhat higher among otosclerotics than in the general population [35]. The disease is as common in women as in men, and some cases have their onset or become worse during the menarche or pregnancy. Otosclerosis develops in about half of all patients with osteogenesis imperfecta.

Clinical features

Clinically in about 50 percent of the patients the onset of deafness occurs between 16 to 30 years. In most cases there is tinnitus, and vertigo occurs in some. Deafness usually begins in one ear (in 10 percent of patients it remains unilateral for years) and becomes bilateral and more and more severe over a period of months or even years. The low tones by air are lost first, the high tone perception disappearing later in the course. The patient speaks softly because of increased bone conduction. In about 20 percent of the cases there is redness of the promontory of the eardrum due to increased vascularity (Schwartze's sign).

Pathologic changes

The *bony lesions resemble those of osteitis deformans.* There is a lacunar absorption of the bone of the otic capsule, with replacement by immature, vascular, spongy new bone which contains basophilic cementum *("blue" bone).* This is resorbed and replaced by more mature, weblike, lamellar bone. These gradual resorptions and replacements produce a *mosaic pattern.* Later the involved bone becomes dense, avascular, and eosinophilic *("red" bone),* the sclerotic phase of the disease. The process usually begins in the bone between the fenestra ovale and cochlea. *Deafness* begins when the process involves the foot plate of the stapes in the fenestra ovale and produces bony *stapes ankylosis* [36], which interferes with the transmission of sound waves to the perilymph of the cochlea.

HYDROPS OF THE LABYRINTH:

Hydrops of the labyrinth (endolymphatic hypertension, *Ménière's disease*) [37] is characterized *clinically* by tinnitus, sound perception distortion, and progressive hearing impairment, followed after several years by attacks of vertigo lasting minutes or hours and sometimes associated with nausea and vomiting. The disorder usually begins in middle age, and men are affected more frequently than women. In about 80 percent of the cases the involvement is *unilateral.* In attacks there is a *sudden increase in endolymphatic fluid* due to *capillary dilatation and increased permeability in the stria vascularis* of the cochlear portion of the labyrinth where the endolymphatic fluid originates. The vascular reaction is variously explained as being allergic or psychogenic. Intermittent rupture and repair of Reissner's membrane, with contamination of potassium-rich endolymph with sodium-rich perilymph, may explain the periodicity of attacks.

Pathologic changes

The increased endolymphatic fluid tension produces *severe dilatation of the cochlear duct and saccule. Reissner's vestibular membrane,* which forms the roof of the cochlear duct, is *ballooned out* by the excessive pressure. The *hair cells of the organ of Corti,* which rests on the basilar membrane of the cochlear duct, show degenerative changes.

DIABETES MELLITUS

Diabetes mellitus may cause *inner ear lesions* [38] characterized *clinically* by a slowly progressive perceptive hearing loss or by Ménière-like episodes with sudden hearing loss and vestibular signs and symptoms. The *Ménière-like attacks* may be due to hemorrhage from fragile capillaries in the stria vascularis of the cochlear duct or to an increased sensitivity of the strial epithelium to the vasomotor crises which are common in diabetics. The inner ear lesions are in the form of a *diabetic angiopathy.* The *capillaries of the stria vascularis* show thickening of their walls due to the presence of partly homogeneous and partly netlike or lamellated, periodic acid-Schiff (PAS) stain positive precipitates.

5. Diseases of the Structures Related to the Ears

OSTEOMA

Osteoma of the temporal bone arises fairly commonly from the osteocartilaginous junction of the external auditory canal, usually in males in the 15 to 25 age group. Trauma or inflammation precedes the bony proliferation in a number of cases, and these tumors may represent exostoses rather than true neoplasms. *Osteoma of the mastoid portion of the temporal bone* [39] is rare. Most cases appear after puberty, being more common in girls than boys. The neoplasm may grow forward and close off the external auditory canal, causing a hearing loss. Mastoid osteoma usually arises from the cortex of the mastoid body. Microscopically it consists of compact lamellated bone with well-developed haversian canals.

GLOMUS JUGULARE TUMOR

Glomus jugulare tumor [40] is a rare nonchromaffin paraganglioma arising in the jugular body of Guild which lies in the adventitia of the jugular bulb just below the bony floor of the middle ear. A similar neoplasm develops very rarely in the glomus (paraganglion) tympanicum which is situated submucosally in the promontory of the middle ear in close association with the tympanic branch of the glossopharyngeal nerve. These neoplasms are more common in women than men. *Clinically* there are progressive deafness and tinnitus in and a discharge from the ear on the affected side. A red or gray polypoid mass bulges under the tympanic membrane or into the external auditory canal. The mass bleeds profusely when manipulated. *Grossly* these neoplasms are polypoid, soft, dark red or reddish brown, and hemorrhagic. *Microscopically* they resemble the carotid body tumor closely, showing nests of chief paraganglion cells which average 15μ in diameter and have a finely granular eosinophilic cytoplasm. Each cell nest is surrounded by a thin but extremely vascular stromal wall. The neoplasms are *histologically benign,* but they are *aggressive,* invading the petrous portion of the temporal bone over a long period of time and even extending into the brain. Isolated cases with distant metastases have occurred.

Diseases of the nose are discussed with the respiratory system in Chapter 19, and diseases of the tongue are treated with the digestive system in Chapter 20.

REFERENCES

1. Von Sallmann, L., and Paton, D. Hereditary benign intraepithelial dyskeratosis. I. Ocular manifestations. *A.M.A. Arch. Ophthal.* 63:421, 1960.
2. Fraumeni, J. F., Jr., and Glass, A. G. Wilms' tumor and congenital aniridia. *J.A.M.A.* 206:825, 1968.
3. Zimmerman, L. E. Recent developments concerning the pathology and pathogenesis of ocular malformations in rubella. *Med. Ann. D.C.* 36:723, 1967.
4. Zimmerman, L. E., and Font, R. L. Congenital malformations of the eye. *J.A.M.A.* 196:684, 1966.
5. Font, R. L., Yanoff, M., and Zimmerman, L. E. Benign lymphoepithelial lesion of the lacrimal gland and its relationship to Sjögren's syndrome. *Amer. J. Clin. Path.* 48:365, 1967.
6. Zimmerman, L. E. Mycotic keratitis. *Lab. Invest.* 11:1151, 1962.
7. Fisher, E. R., and Hellstrom, H. R. Cogan's syndrome and systemic vascular disease. *Arch. Path.* (Chicago) 72:96, 1961.
8. Kimura, S. J., and Hogan, M. J. Chronic cyclitis. *Arch. Ophthal.* (Chicago) 71:101, 1964.
9. Perkins, E. S., and Wood, R. M. Auto-immunity in uveitis. *Brit. J. Ophthal.* 48:61, 1964.
10. Fine, B. S. Intraocular mycotic infections. *Lab. Invest.* 11:1161, 1962.
11. Walma, D., Jr., and Schlaegel, T. F., Jr. Presumed histoplasmic choroiditis. *Amer. J. Ophthal.* 57:107, 1964.
12. Van Metre, T. E., Jr., and Maumanee, A. E. Specific ocular uveal lesions in patients with evidence of histoplasmosis. *Arch. Ophthal.* (Chicago) 71:314, 1964.
13. Wolff, S. M., and Zimmerman, L. E. Chronic secondary glaucoma associated with retrodisplacement of iris root and deepening of the anterior chamber angle secondary to contusion. *Amer. J. Ophthal.* 54:547, 1962.
14. Maumanee, A. E. Further observations on the pathogenesis of congenital glaucoma. *Amer. J. Ophthal.* 55:1163, 1963.
15. Paterson, G. D., and Miller, S. J. H. Hormonal influence in simple glaucoma. *Brit. J. Ophthal.* 47:129, 1963.
16. Jones, S. E., and Zimmerman, L. E. Histopathologic differentiation of granular, macular, and lattice dystrophies of the cornea. *Amer. J. Ophthal.* 51:394, 1961.
17. Klintworth, G. K., and Vogel, F. S. Macular corneal dystrophy. *Amer. J. Path.* 45:565, 1964.
18. Klintworth, G. K. Lattice corneal dystrophy. An inherited variety of amyloidosis restricted to the cornea. *Amer. J. Path.* 50:371, 1967.

19. Giles, C. L., Mason, G. L., Duff, I. F., and McLean, J. A. The association of cataract formation and systemic corticosteroid therapy. *J.A.M.A.* 182:719, 1962.
20. Bellows, J. G. Lens opacities produced by cataractogenic agents with special reference to triparanol cataract. *Amer. J. Ophthal.* 55:537, 1963.
21. Patz, A. The role of oxygen in retrolental fibroplasia. *Pediatrics* 19:504, 1957.
22. Pilkerton, R., and O'Rourke, J. Rhegmatogenous retinal detachment. *Med. Ann. D.C.* 35:481, 1966.
23. Wolbarsht, M. L., Fligsten, K. E., and Hayes, J. R. Retina: Pathology of neodymium and ruby laser burns. *Science* 150:1453, 1965.
24. Yanoff, M. Diabetic retinopathy. *New Eng. J. Med.* 274:1344, 1966.
25. Whorton, C. M., and Patterson, J. B. Carcinoma of Moll's glands with extramammary Paget's disease of the eyelid. *Cancer* 8:1009, 1955.
26. Zimmerman, L. E. Clinical pathology of iris tumors. *Amer. J. Clin. Path.* 39:214, 1963.
27. Zimmerman, L. E. Retinoblastoma. *Med. Ann. D.C.* 38:366, 1969.
28. Ts'O, M. O., Fine, B. S., and Zimmerman, L. E. The Flexner-Wintersteiner rosettes in retinoblastoma. *Arch. Path.* (Chicago) 88:664, 1969.
29. Hoyt, W. F., and Pont, M. E. Pseudopapilledema: Anomalous elevation of optic disk. *J.A.M.A.* 181:191, 1962.
30. Cankar, V., and Crowley, H. Tumors of ceruminous glands. *Cancer* 17:67, 1964.
31. Senturia, B. H., Gessert, C. F., Carr, C. D., and Baumann, E. S. Aerotitis media. *Arch. Otolaryng.* (Chicago) 74:141, 1961.
32. Borsanyi, S., Blanchard, C. L., and Thorne, B. The effects of ionizing radiation on the ear. *Ann. Otol.* 70:255, 1961.
33. Hambley, W. M. Petrositis. *Laryngoscope* 71:800, 1961.
34. Tucker, W. N. Cancer of the middle ear. *Cancer* 18:642, 1965.
35. Proctor, B. Chronic progressive deafness. *Arch. Otolaryng.* (Chicago) 74:446, 1961.
36. Henner. R., Guilford, F. R., Shea, J. J., Jr., and Jeantet, C. Histopathology of the otosclerotic footplate. *Laryngoscope* 70:506, 1960.
37. Altmann, F. Ménière's disease. *J.A.M.A.* 176:215, 1961.
38. Jorgensen, M. B. The inner ear in diabetes mellitus. *Arch. Otolaryng.* (Chicago) 74:373, 1961.
39. Schwartz, L. J. Osteoma of the mastoid. *Arch. Otolaryng.* (Chicago) 74:350, 1961.
40. Foote, E. L. Tumors of the glomus jugulare. *Amer. J. Clin. Path.* 41:72, 1964.

GENERAL REFERENCES

Ash, J. E., Beck, M. R., and Wilkes, J. D. Tumors of the upper respiratory tract and ear. Section IV, Fascicles 12 and 13, in *Atlas of Tumor Pathology*. Washington: Armed Forces Institute of Pathology, 1964, pp. 215–262.

Barsky, D. *Color Atlas of Pathology of the Eye*. New York: McGraw-Hill, 1966.

Hogan, M. J., and Zimmerman, L. E. (Eds.). *Ophthalmic Pathology* (2d ed.). Philadelphia: Saunders, 1962.

Reese, A. B. Tumors of the eye and adnexa. Section X, Fascicle 38, in *Atlas of Tumor Pathology*. Washington: Armed Forces Institute of Pathology, 1956.

INDEX